UNIPA Springer Series

M000011934

Editors-in-Chief

Eleonora Riva Sanseverino, Department of Engineering, University of Palermo, Palermo, Italy

Series Editors

Carlo Amenta, Department of Economics, Management and Statistics, University of Palermo, Palermo, Italy

Marco Carapezza, Department of Human Sciences, University of Palermo, Palermo, Italy

Marcello Chiodi, Department of Economics, Management and Statistics, University of Palermo, Palermo, Italy

Andrea Laghi, Department of Surgical and Medical Sciences and Translational Medicine, Sapienza University of Rome, Rome, Italy

Bruno Maresca, Department of Pharmaceutical Sciences, University of Salerno, Fisciano, Italy

Giorgio Domenico Maria Micale, Department of Industrial and Digital Innovation, University of Palermo, Palermo, Italy

Arabella Mocciaro Li Destri, Department of Economics, Management and Statistics, University of Palermo, Palermo, Italy

Andreas Öchsner, Department of Engineering and Information Technology, Griffith University, Southport, QLD, Australia

Mariacristina Piva, Department of Economic and Social Sciences, Catholic University of the Sacred Heart, Piacenza, Italy

Antonio Russo, Department of Surgical, Oncological and Oral Sciences, University of Palermo, Palermo, Italy

Norbert M. Seel, Department of Education, University of Freiburg Freiburg im Breisgau, Germany

Antonio Russo • Marc Peeters
Lorena Incorvaia • Christian Rolfo
Editors

Practical Medical Oncology Textbook

Volume II

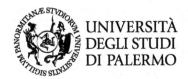

UNIVERSITÀ
DEGLI STUDI
DI PALERMO

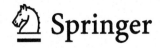

Springer

Editors
Antonio Russo
Department of Surgical
Oncological and Oral Sciences
University of Palermo
Palermo, Italy

Lorena Incorvaia
Department of Biomedicine
Neuroscience and Advanced Diagnostics
University of Palermo
Palermo, Italy

Marc Peeters
Oncology Department
University of Antwerp
Edegem, Belgium

Christian Rolfo
Center for Thoracic Oncology
Tisch Cancer Institute
Mount Sinai System &
Icahn School of Medicine
Mount Sinai, New York, USA

ISSN 2366-7516   ISSN 2366-7524   (electronic)
UNIPA Springer Series
ISBN 978-3-030-56053-9   ISBN 978-3-030-56051-5   (eBook)
https://doi.org/10.1007/978-3-030-56051-5

This Springer imprint is published by the registered company Springer Nature Switzerland AG
The registered company address is: Gewerbestrasse 11, 6330 Cham, Switzerland

Preface

Clinical oncology is a rapidly evolving field. Within just a few years, increase in understanding of the molecular and immunological basis of cancer provided a strong base to clinical development of novel treatment options for patients across many cancer types. Several targeted therapies and immunotherapy are changing the clinical landscape and the natural history of many tumors, with an impact on patients survival. To maximize the patient benefit, prognostic and predictive biomarkers are under investigation to identify patients who will likely benefit from therapy, and multimodal diagnostic tools, such as liquid biopsy, are opening new frontiers to cancer diagnosis, screenings and therapeutic decisions.

In this textbook, many specialists in the field have covered many aspects of medical oncology. The first general section provides a comprehensive overview and background information on tumor biology and genetics, innovative technologies for clinical and translational research, and covers introductory topics on the main treatment modalities in the care of cancer patients. The following chapters are included in the clinical section on tumor presentations, diagnosis, prognosis, until the current state-of-the-art of medical treatment. It provides a systematic overview of all types of solid tumors, including epidemiology and cancer prevention, genetic aspects of hereditary cancers, differential diagnosis, typical signs and symptoms, diagnostic strategies and staging, and treatment modalities. Special attention is given to new and innovative treatments for cancer patients, such as targeted therapy and immunotherapy.

This textbook combines, therefore, essential information on clinical cancer medicine with a guide to the latest advances in molecular oncology and tumor biology. Expert commentaries at the end of each chapter highlight key points, offer hints for deeper insights, suggest further reading and discuss clinical application through the description of cases.

This textbook offers an invaluable, practice-oriented tool for medical students just beginning their clinical oncology studies, as well as medical oncology residents and young professionals.

Antonio Russo
Palermo, Italy

Marc Peeters
Edegem, Belgium

Lorena Incorvaia
Palermo, Italy

Christian Rolfo
New York, NY, USA

Contents

Volume II

IV Clinical Oncology: Diagnosis and Treatment of Solid Tumors

Contributors

Alberto Abrate Department of Surgical, Oncological and Oral Sciences, University of Palermo, Palermo, Italy
alberto.abrate@gmail.com

Vincenzo Adamo Department of Human Pathology, University of Messina & Medical Oncology Unit, A.O. Papardo, Messina, Italy
vadamo@unime.it

Marco Maria Aiello Oncology Unit, Policlinico - Vittorio Emanuele Hospital, Catania, Italy
marcomaria.aiello@gmail.com

Laura Ajello Cardiology Unit, Department for the Treatment and Study of Cardiothoracic Diseases and Cardiothoracic Transplantation, IRCCS-ISMETT, Palermo, Italy
lajello1305@libero.it

Filippo Alongi Department of Radiation Oncology, Ospedale Sacro Cuore-Don Calabria, Verona, Italy
filippo.alongi@sacrocuore.it

Valentina Ambrosini Nuclear Medicine Service - PET Unit, Policlinico S. Orsola-Malpighi, Bologna University, Bologna, Italy
valentina.ambrosini@aosp.bo.it

Grazia Arpino Medical Oncology Unit, Department of Clinical Medicine and Surgery, University of Naples "Federico II", Naples, Italy
grazia.arpino@unina.it

Paolo A. Ascierto Department of Melanoma and Cancer Immunotherapy, Istituto Nazionale Tumori IRCCS Fondazione Pascale, Napoli, Italy
p.ascierto@istitutotumori.na.it

Giuseppe Badalamenti Department of Surgical, Oncological and Oral Science, University of Palermo, Palermo, Italy
giuseppe.badalamenti@unipa.it

Miguel Barbosa Centro Hospitalar de Trás-os-Montes e Alto Douro, Vila Real, Portugal
miguelbarbosa75@gmail.com

Nadia Barraco Department of Surgical, Oncological and Oral Sciences, University of Palermo, Palermo, Italy
barraconadia@gmail.com

Viviana Bazan Department of Biomedicine, Neuroscience and Advanced Diagnostics (Bi.N.D.), University of Palermo, Palermo, Italy
viviana.bazan@unipa.it

Alfredo Berruti Clinical Oncology, Department of Medical and Surgical Specialties, Radiological Sciences and public Health, University of Brescia at ASST Spedali Civili di Brescia, Brescia, Italy
alfredo.berruti@gmail.com

Alessandro Bertani Department for the Treatment and Study of Cardiothoracic Diseases and Thoracic Transplantation, IRCCS–ISMETT (Istituto Mediterraneo per i Trapianti e Terapie ad alta specializzazione)/University of Pittsburgh Medical Center Italy, Palermo, Italy
abertani@ismett.edu

Davide Bimbatti Medical Oncology 1 Unit, Department of Oncology, Istituto Oncologico Veneto IOV IRCCS, Padova, Italy
Davide.Bimbatti@gmail.com

Andrea Botticelli   Sant'Andrea Hospital, University "La Sapienza", Rome, Italy
andrea.botticelli@uniroma1.it

Andrea Boutros   Department of Internal Medicine and Medical Specialties (DiMI), School of Medicine, University of Genova, Genova, Italy
boutros.andrea@gmail.com

Davide Brocco   Department of Medical, Oral and Biotechnological Sciences, Section of Medical Oncology, Centro Scienze dell'Invecchiamento e Medicina Traslazionale – CeSI-MeT, University G. D'Annunzio, Chieti, Italy
davideabilly@gmail.com

Enrico Bronte   Department of Surgical, Oncological and Oral Sciences, University of Palermo, Palermo, Italy
enrico.bronte@gmail.com

Oronzo Brunetti   Medical Oncology Unit, Istituto Tumori "Giovanni Paolo II", Bari, Italy
dr.oronzo.brunetti@tiscali.it

Giuseppe Buono   Medical Oncology Unit, Department of Clinical Medicine and Surgery, University of Naples "Federico II", Naples, Italy
giuseppe.buono@unina.it

Silvio Buscemi   Department of Surgical, Oncological and Oral Sciences, University of Palermo, Palermo, Italy
silvio.buscemi@unipa.it

Valentina Calò   Department of Surgical, Oncological and Oral Sciences, University of Palermo, Palermo, Italy
valentinacalo74@gmail.com

Giuseppina Calareso   Department of Radiology, Fondazione IRCCS Istituto Nazionale dei Tumori, Milan, Italy
giuseppina.calareso@istitutotumori.mi.it

Massimiliano Cani   Department of Surgical, Oncological, and Oral Sciences, University of Palermo, Palermo, Italy
massi.cani@gmail.com

Enrica Capelletto   Department of Oncology, University of Turin, Orbassano, Italy
enrica.capelletto@gmail.com

Ettore Domenico Capoluongo   Department of Molecular Medicine and Medical Biotechnology, Federico II University-CEINGE, Advanced Biotechnology, Naples, Italy
capoluongo@ceinge.unina.it

Claudia Cardone   Department of Precision Medicine, Medical Oncology, Università degli Studi della Campania Luigi Vanvitelli, Naples, Campania, Italy
cardone.cla@gmail.com

Paolo G. Casali   University of Milan and Fondazione IRCCS Istituto Nazionale Tumori, Milan, Italy
paolo.casali@istitutotumori.mi.it

Francesca Caspani   Medical Oncology Unit, ASST Sette Laghi, Circolo Hospital, Varese, Italy

Giuseppe Castaldo   CEINGE Advanced Biotechnologies, University Federico II, Naples, Italy
giuseppe.castaldo@unina.it

Luisa Castellana   Department of Surgical, Oncological and Oral Sciences, University of Palermo, Palermo, Italy
luisa.castellana@you.unipa.it

Marta Castiglia   Department of Surgical, Oncological and Oral Sciences, University of Palermo, Palermo, Italy
martacastiglia@gmail.com

Carlos Centeno   Department of Palliative Medicine and Symptom Control, Clínica Universidad de Navarra, Pamplona, Spain

IdiSNA, Instituto de Investigación Sanitaria de Navarra, Pamplona, España

ATLANTES Research Program, Institute for Culture and Society (ICS), University of Navarra, Pamplona, Spain
ccenteno@unav.es

Maria Angela Cerruto   Urology Unit, University of Verona, Verona, Italy
mariaangela.cerruto@univr.it

Marcello Ciaccio   Department of Laboratory Medicine, University-Hospital, Palermo, Italy

Department of Biomedicine, Neurosciences and Advanced Diagnostics, Institute of Clinical Biochemistry, Clinical Molecular Medicine and Laboratory Medicine, University of Palermo, Palermo, Italy
marcello.ciaccio@unipa.it

Chiara Ciccarese   University of Verona, Medical Oncology Unit, Verona, Italy
ciccarese.c@gmail.com

Mauro Cives   Department of Biomedical Sciences and Human Oncology, University of Bari "Aldo Moro", Bari, Italy
mauro.civ@tiscali.it

Mélanie Claps   Medical Oncology, ASST Spedali Civili di Brescia - Università degli Studi di Brescia, Brescia, Italy
melanieclaps@gmail.com

Andreia Coelho   Hospital de Santo Espirito da Ilha Terceira, Medical Oncology, Angra do Heroismo, Portugal
andreiamachadocoelho@gmail.com

Pier Franco Conte   Division of Oncology 2, Istituto Oncologico Veneto IRCCS, Padova, Italy
pierfranco.conte@unipd.it

Lidia Rita Corsini   Department of Surgical, Oncological and Oral Sciences, University of Palermo, Palermo, Italy
lidiarita.corsini@you.unipa.it

Deborah Cosentini   Medical Oncology, ASST Spedali Civili di Brescia - Università degli Studi di Brescia, Brescia, Italy
daborah.cosentini@gmail.com

Sofia Cutaia   Department of Surgical, Oncological and Oral Sciences, University of Palermo, Palermo, Italy
sofia.cutaia@you.unipa.it

Romano Danesi   Unit of Clinical Pharmacology and Pharmacogenetics, Department of Clinical and Experimental Medicine, University of Pisa, Pisa, Italy
romano.danesi@unipi.it

Maria Vittoria Dieci   Division of Oncology 2, Istituto Oncologico Veneto IRCCS, Padova, Italy

Department of Surgery, Oncology and Gastroenterology, University of Padova, Padova, Italy
mariavittoria.dieci@unipd.it

Maurizio D'Incalci   Department of Oncology, Istituto di Ricerche Farmacologiche "Mario Negri", Milan, Italy
maurizio.dincalci@marionegri.it

Sinziana Dumitra   Department of Surgery, Fondazione IRCCS Istituto Nazionale dei Tumori, Milan, Italy
sinziana.dumitra@gmail.com

Iñaki Eguren-Santamaría   Department of Oncology, Clínica Universidad de Navarra, Pamplona, Spain
ieguren@unav.es

Daniele Fanale   Department of Surgical, Oncological and Oral Sciences, University of Palermo, Palermo, Italy
fandan@libero.it

Emanuela Fantinel   University of Verona, Medical Oncology Unit, Verona, Italy
manuf86@hotmail.it

Ivan Fazio   Radiotherapy Unit, Casa di Cura Macchiarella, Palermo, Italy
ivanfazio@alice.it

Nicola Fazio   Division of Gastrointestinal Medical Oncology and Neuroendocrine Tumors, European Institute of Oncology, IEO, IRCCS, Milan, Italy
nicola.fazio@ieo.it

Manuela Federico   Radiotherapy Unit, Casa di Cura Macchiarella, Palermo, Italy
manuela.fed@gmail.com

Eugenio Fiorentino   Department of Surgical, Oncological and Oral Sciences, University of Palermo, Palermo, Italy
eugenio.fiorentino@unipa.it

Tindara Franchina   Department of Human Pathology, University of Messina, Messina, Italy
tindifra@yahoo.it

Fabio Fulfaro   Department of Surgical, Oncological and Oral Sciences, University of Palermo, Palermo, Italy
fabio.fulfaro@unipa.it

Patricia Gago   Centro Hospitalar de Trás-os-Montes e Alto Douro, Vila Real, Portugal
patriciafgago@gmail.com

Donata Galbiati   Head and Neck Medical Oncology Unit, Fondazione IRCCS Istituto Nazionale dei Tumori, Milan, Italy
donata.galbiati@istitutotumori.mi.it

Massimo Galia   Department of Biomedicine, Neurosciences and Advanced Diagnostics (BiND), University of Palermo, Palermo, Italy
massimo.galia@unipa.it

Antonio Galvano   Department of Surgical, Oncological and Oral Sciences, University of Palermo, Palermo, Italy
antonio.galvano@unipa.it

Andrea Casadei Gardini   Department of Medical Oncology, UNIMORE, Modena, Italy
casadeigardini@gmail.com

Cristina Scalici Gesolfo   Section of Urology, Department of Surgical, Oncological and Oral Sciences, University of Palermo, Palermo, Italy
cristinasc1986@gmail.com

Ignacio Gil-Bazo   Department of Oncology, Clínica Universidad de Navarra, Pamplona, Spain

Program of Solid Tumors, Center for Applied Medical Research, Pamplona, Spain

Navarra Health Research Institute (IDISNA), Pamplona, Spain

Centro de Investigación Biomédica en Red de Cáncer (CIBERONC), Madrid, Spain
igbazo@unav.es

Antonio Giordano   Sbarro Institute for Cancer Research and Molecular Medicine, Center for Biotechnology, College of Science and Technology, Temple University, Philadelphia, PA, USA
president@shro.org

Mario Giuliano   Medical Oncology Unit, Department of Clinical Medicine and Surgery, University of Naples "Federico II", Naples, Italy

Lester and Sue Smith Breast Center at Baylor College of Medicine, Houston, TX, USA
m.giuliano@unina.it

Stefania Gori   Department of Oncology, IRCCS Ospedale Sacro Cuore Don Calabria, Negrar di Valpolicella, Verona, Italy
stefania.gori@sacrocuore.it

Antonino Grassadonia   Department of Medical, Oral and Biotechnological Sciences, Section of Medical Oncology, Centro Scienze dell'Invecchiamento e Medicina Traslazionale – CeSI-MeT, University G. D'Annunzio, Chieti, Italy
grassadonia@unich.it

Gaia Griguolo   Division of Oncology 2, Istituto Oncologico Veneto IRCCS, Padova, Italy

Department of Surgery, Oncology and Gastroenterology, University of Padova, Padova, Italy
gaia.griguolo@iov.veneto.it

Valerio Gristina   Department of Surgical, Oncological and Oral Sciences, University of Palermo, Palermo, Italy
valerio.gristina@you.unipa.it

Alessandro Gronchi   Department of Surgery, Fondazione IRCCS Istituto Nazionale dei Tumori, Milan, Italy
alessandro.gronchi@istitutotumori.mi.it

Salvatore Gruttadauria   Department for the Treatment and Study of Abdominal Diseases and Abdominal Transplantation, IRCCS–ISMETT (Istituto Mediterraneo per i Trapianti e Terapie ad alta specializzazione)/University of Pittsburgh Medical Center Italy, Palermo, Italy
sgruttadauria@ismett.edu

Fiorella Guadagni   Department of Human Sciences and Quality of Life Promotion, San Raffaele Roma Open University, Rome, Italy
fiorella.guadagni@sanraffaele.it

Aurelia Ada Guarini   Department of Surgical, Oncological and Oral Sciences, University of Palermo, Palermo, Italy
aurelia.guarini@gmail.com

Valentina Guarneri   Division of Oncology 2, Istituto Oncologico Veneto IRCCS, Padova, Italy

Department of Surgery, Oncology and Gastroenterology, University of Padova, Padova, Italy
valentina.guarneri@unipd.it

Roberto Iacovelli   Oncologia Medica, Fondazione Policlinico Universitario Agostino Gemelli IRCCS, Rome, Italy
roberto.iacovelli@alice.it

Lorena Incorvaia   Department of Biomedicine, Neuroscience and Advanced Diagnostics, University of Palermo, Palermo, Italy
lorena.incorvaia@unipa.it

Alessandro Inno   Department of Oncology, IRCCS Ospedale Sacro Cuore Don Calabria, Negrar di Valpolicella, Verona, Italy
alessandro.inno@sacrocuore.it

Lavinia Insalaco   Department of Surgical, Oncological and Oral Sciences, University of Palermo, Palermo, Italy
lavinia.insalaco@you.unipa.it

Juan Lucio Iovanna   Centre de Recherche en Cancérologie de Marseille (CRCM), INSERM U1068, CNRS UMR 7258, Aix-Marseille Université et Institut Paoli-Calmettes, Parc Scientifique et Technologique de Luminy, Marseille, France
juan.iovanna@inserm.fr

Michele Iuliani   Medical Oncology Department, University Campus Bio-Medico, Rome, Italy
m.iuliani@unicampus.it

Nicola Alessandro Iacovelli   Radiation Oncology Department, University of Milan, Milan, Italy
nicolaalessandro.iacovelli@istitutotumori.mi.it

Giuseppe La Tona   Department of Biomedicine, Neuroscience and Advanced Diagnostic (BiND), University of Palermo, Palermo, Italy
giuseppe.la_tona@unipa.it

Nicla La Verde   Oncology Unit, ASST Fatebenefratelli Sacco Presidio Ospedaliero Fatebene-fratelli, Milan, Italy
nicla.laverde@fbf.milano.it

Fiorenza Latteri   Medical Oncology Department, Azienda Ospedaliera Garibaldi, Catania, Italy
sotolatteri@hotmail.com

Stefano Lepori   IRCCS National Cancer Institute, Department of Gynecologic Oncology, Milan, Italy
ste.lepori@tiscali.it

Laura Deborah Locati   Head and Neck Medical Oncology Unit, Fondazione IRCCS Istituto Nazionale dei Tumori, Milan, Italy
laura.locati@istitutotumori.mi.it

Claudio Longhitano   Center of Experimental Oncology and Hematology, A.O.U. Policlinico "G. Rodolico - S. Marco", Catania, Italy
longhitanoclaudio@hotmail.it

Valter D. Longo   Department of Surgical, Oncological and Oral Sciences, Surgical Oncology Unit, University of Palermo, Palermo, Italy

IFOM FIRC Institute of Molecular Oncology, Milan, Italy

Eli and Edythe Broad Center for Regenerative Medicine and Stem Cell Research at USC, Keck School of Medicine, University of Southern California, Los Angeles, CA, USA
vlongo@usc.edu

Domenica Lorusso   Fondazione Policlinico Universitario A Gemelli IRCCS, Rome, Italy
Università Cattolica del Sacro Cuore, Rome, Italy
domenica.lorusso@policlinicogemelli.it

Ina Macaione   University of Palermo, Palermo, Italy
inamacaione@gmail.com

Giorgio Madonia   Department of Surgical, Oncological and Oral Sciences, University of Palermo, Palermo, Italy
giorgio.madonia@you.unipa.it

Massimo Di Maio   Division of Medical Oncology, "Ordine Mauriziano" Hospital, Department of Oncology, University of Turin, Torino, Italy
massimo.dimaio@unito.it

Umberto Malapelle   Department of Public Health, University of Naples Federico II, Naples, Italy
umberto.malapelle@unina.it

Giuseppa Maltese   Fondazione IRCCS Istituto Nazionale dei Tumori, Milan, Italy
Giusi.maltese@hotmail.it

Lucia Mangone   AUSL Reggio Emilia, Reggio Emilia, Italy
mangone.lucia@ausl.re.it

Maria La Mantia Department of Surgical, Oncological and Oral Sciences, University of Palermo, Palermo, Italy
maria.lamantia@unipa.it

Paolo Marchetti Oncology Unit, "Sapienza" University of Rome, Rome, Italy
paolo.marchetti@uniroma1.it

Antonio Marchetti Center of Predictive Molecular Medicine, University-Foundation, Chieti, Italy
antonio.marchetti@unich.it

Erika Martinelli Medical Oncology, Università degli Studi della Campania "Luigi Vanvitelli", Napoli, Italy
erika.martinelli@unicampania.it

Giulia Martini Medical Oncology, Università degli Studi della Campania "Luigi Vanvitelli", Napoli, Italy
giulia.mart14@gmail.com

Federica Martorana Center of Experimental Oncology and Hematology, A.O.U. Policlinico "G. Rodolico - S. Marco", Catania, Italy
fede.marto.fm@gmail.com

Renzo Mazzarotto Radiotherapy Unit, University of Verona, Verona, Italy
renzo.mazzarotto@aovr.veneto.it

Antonella Mazzonello Radiotherapy Unit, Casa di Cura Macchiarella, Palermo, Italy
antonellamazzonello@alice.it

Puja Mehta Division of Cardiology, Department of Medicine, Emory University, Atlanta, GA, USA
Puja.Mehta@cshs.org

Riccardo Memeo U.O.D. Chirurgia Epatobiliopancreatica, Ospedale "F. Miulli", Acquaviva delle Fonti, Bari, Italy
drmemeo@yahoo.it

Massimo Midiri Department of Biomedicine, Neurosciences and Advanced Diagnostics (BiND), University of Palermo, Palermo, Italy
massimo.midiri@unipa.it

Mario G. Mirisola Department of Surgical, Oncological and Oral Sciences, Section of Medical Oncology, University of Palermo, Palermo, Italy
mario.mirisola@unipa.it

Elena Monti Department of Biotechnology and Life Sciences (DBSV), University of Insubria, Varese, VA, Italy
elena.monti@uninsubria.it

Claudia Mosillo Medical Oncology Unit, "Sapienza" University of Rome, Rome, Italy
claudiamosillo@hotmail.it

Clara Natoli Department of Medical, Oral and Biotechnological Sciences, Section of Medical Oncology, Centro Scienze dell'Invecchiamento e Medicina Traslazionale – CeSI-MeT, University G. D'Annunzio, Chieti, Italy
clara.natoli@unich.it

Laura Noto UOC Oncologia Medica, Azienda Ospedaliera Universitaria Policlinico San Marco, Catania, Italy
lauranoto1983@hotmail.it

Silvia Novello Department of Oncology, University of Turin, Orbassano, Italy
silvia.novello@unito.it

Giuseppina Novo   Department of Internal Medicine and Specialities (DIBIMIS), Cardiology Unit, University of Palermo, Palermo, Italy
giuseppina.novo@unipa.it

Salvatore Novo   Department of Internal Medicine and Specialities (DIBIMIS), Cardiology Unit, University of Palermo, Palermo, Italy
salvatore.novo@unipa.it

Laura Ottini   Department of Molecular Medicine, Sapienza University of Rome, Rome, Italy
laura.ottini@uniroma1.it

Alberto Paderno   Department of Otorhinolaryngology, Head and Neck Surgery University of Brescia, Brescia, Italy
alberto.paderno@unibs.it

Duilio Pagano   Department for the Treatment and Study of Abdominal Diseases and Abdominal Transplantation, IRCCS–ISMETT (Istituto Mediterraneo per i Trapianti e Terapie ad alta specializzazione)/University of Pittsburgh Medical Center Italy, Palermo, Italy
d.pagano@ismett.edu

Francesco Pantano   Medical Oncology Department, University Campus Bio-Medico, Rome, Italy
f.pantano@unicampus.it

Susmita Parashar   Division of Cardiology, Department of Medicine, Emory University, Atlanta, GA, USA
smallik@emory.edu

Hector Josè Soto Parra   Medical Oncology Department, Azienda Ospedaliera Garibaldi, Catania, Italy
hsotoparra@yahoo.it

Francesco Passiglia   Department of Oncology, University of Torino, AOU S. Luigi Gonzaga, Orbassano, Italy
francesco.passiglia@unito.it

Marc Peeters   Oncology Department, University of Antwerp, Edegem, Belgium

Center for Oncological Research, Antwerp University Hospital, Edegem, Belgium
marc.peeters@uza.be

Francesco Pepe   University of Naples Federico II, Department of Public Health, Naples, Italy
francesco.pepe4@unina.it

Alessandro Perez   Department of Surgical, Oncological and Oral Sciences, University of Palermo, Palermo, Italy
ale-like@libero.it

Francesco Perrone   Clinical Trials Unit, Istituto Nazionale per lo Studio e la Cura dei Tumori "Fondazione Giovanni Pascale"-IRCCS, Naples, Italy
f.perrone@istitutotumori.na.it

Patrick Pessaux   Institut Hospitalo-Universitaire (IHU), Institute for Minimally Invasive Hybrid Image-Guided Surgery, Université de Strasbourg, Strasbourg, France
patrick.pessaux@ihu-strasbourg.eu

Angelica Petrillo   University of study of Campania "L. Vanvitelli"- Medical Oncology, Naples, Italy
angelic.petrillo@gmail.com

Cesare Piazza   Department of Otorhinolaryngology, Maxillofacial and Thyroid Surgery, Fondazione IRCCS, National Cancer Institute of Milan University of Milan, Milan, Italy
cesare.piazza@istitutotumori.mi.it

Sabino De Placido　Medical Oncology Unit, Department of Clinical Medicine and Surgery, University of Naples "Federico II", Naples, Italy
sabino.deplacido@unina.it

Luca Pompella　University of Study of Campania "L. Vanvitelli", Caserta, Italy
luca.pompella@icloud.com

Camillo Porta　Division of Medical Oncology, IRCCS San Matteo University Hospital Foundation, Pavia, Italy
c.porta@smatteo.pv.it

Giuseppe Procopio　Fondazione Istituto Nazionale Tumori, Milano, Italia
giuseppe.procopio@istitutotumori.mi.it

Paola Queirolo　IRCCS Ospedale Policlinico San Martino, Genoa, Italy
paola.queirolo@hsanmartino.it

Sara Ramella　Radiation Oncology, Campus Bio-Medico University, Rome, Italy
s.ramella@unicampus.it

Raffaele Ratta　Fondazione IRCCS Istituto Nazionale Tumori, Medical Oncology, Milan, Italy
Raffaele.Ratta@istitutotumori.mi.it

Elisabetta Razzaboni　Servizio di Psicologia Ospedaliera A.O.U. Policlinico di Modena, Modena, Italy
elisabetta.razzaboni@gmail.com

Giuseppe Lo Re　Department of Biomedicine, Neurosciences and Advanced Diagnostics (BiND), University of Palermo, Palermo, Italy
giuseppe.lore01@unipa.it

Marzia Del Re　Clinical Pharmacology and Pharmacogenetics Unit, Department of Clinical and Experimental Medicine, University of Pisa, Pisa, Italy
marzia.delre@ao-pisa.toscana.it

Carlo Resteghini　Head and Neck Medical Oncology Unit, Fondazione IRCCS Istituto Nazionale dei Tumori, Milan, Italy
carlo.resteghini@istitutotumori.mi.it

Giulia Ribelli　Medical Oncology Department, University Campus Bio-Medico, Rome, Italy
g.ribelli@unicampus.it

Enrico Ricevuto　Department of Biotechnological and Applied Clinical Sciences, University of L'Aquila, L'Aquila, Italy

Oncology Territorial Care, S. Salvatore Hospital, Oncology Network ASL1 Abruzzo, University of L'Aquila, L'Aquila, Italy
enrico.ricevuto@univaq.it

Giuseppina Rosaria Rita Ricciardi　Department of Human Pathology, University of Messina & Medical Oncology Unit, A.O. Papardo, Messina, Italy
giusyricciardi81@hotmail.it

Carla Germana Rinaldi　Radiation Oncology, Campus Bio-Medico University, Rome, Italy
c.rinaldi@unicampus.it

Sergio Rizzo　Department of Oncological, Surgical and Oral Science, University of Palermo, Palermo, Italy
sergiorizzo77@gmail.com

Elisa Roca　ASST Spedali Civili di Brescia - Università degli Studi di Brescia, Brescia, Italy
elisaroca@gmail.com

Christian Rolfo   Center for Thoracic Oncology, Tisch Cancer Institute, Mount Sinai System & Icahn School of Medicine, Mount Sinai, New York, USA
christian.rolfo@uza.be

Roberta Elisa Rossi   Gastrointestinal and Hepato-Pancreatic Surgery and Liver Transplantation Unit, Fondazione IRCCS Istituto Nazionale Tumori (INT, National Cancer Institute) and Università degli Studi di Milano, Milan, Italy
Robertaelisa.rossi@gmail.com

Antonio Russo   Department of Surgical, Oncological and Oral Sciences, University of Palermo, Palermo, Italy
antonio.russo@unipa.it

Alessandro Russo   Department of Human Pathology, University of Messina & Medical Oncology Unit, A.O. Papardo, Messina, Italy
alessandro-russo@alice.it

Ilaria Sabatucci   Department of Gynecologic Oncology, IRCCS National Cancer Institute, Milan, Italy
Fondazione IRCCS Istituto 21Nazionale dei Tumori, Milan, Italy
Sabatucci.ilaria@gmail.com

Daniele Santini   Medical Oncology Department, University Campus Bio-Medico, Rome, Italy
d.santini@unicampus.it

Francesco Schettini   Medical Oncology Unit, Department of Clinical Medicine and Surgery, University of Naples "Federico II", Naples, Italy
francescoschettini1987@gmail.com

Silvana Sdao   Department of Radiology, Ospedale Alessandro Manzoni, Lecco, Italy
silvana.sdao@istitutotumori.mi.it

Nicola Silvestris   Medical Oncology Unit, Istituto Tumori "Giovanni Paolo II", Bari, Italy

Department of Internal Medicine and Oncology, University of Bari, Bari, Italy
nicola.silvestris@uniba.it

Franco Silvestris   Department of Biomedical Sciences and Human Oncology, University of Bari "Aldo Moro", Bari, Italy
francesco.silvestris@uniba.it

Alchiede Simonato   Section of Urology, Department of Surgical, Oncological and Oral Sciences, University of Palermo, Palermo, Italy
alchiede.simonato@unipa.it

Sonia Simonetti   Medical Oncology Department, University Campus Bio-Medico, Rome, Italy
s.simonetti@unicampus.it

Antonio Giovanni Solimando   Department of Internal Medicine and Oncology, University of Bari, Bari, Italy
antonio.solimando@uniba.it

Francesca Spada   Division of Gastrointestinal Medical Oncology and Neuroendocrine Tumors, European Institute of Oncology, IEO, IRCCS, Milan, Italy
francesca.spada@ieo.it

Simona De Summa   Molecular Diagnostics and Pharmacogenetics Unit – IRCCS Istituto Tumori "Giovanni Paolo II", Bari, Italy
s.desumma@oncologico.bari.it

Antonella Surbone   New York University Medical School, New York, NY, USA
antonella.surbone@gmail.com

Pierosandro Tagliaferri   Medical Oncology Unit, Department of Experimental and Clinical Medicine, Magna Græcia University and Cancer Center, Catanzaro, Italy
tagliaferri@unicz.it

Enrica Teresa Tanda   IRCCS Ospedale Policlinico San Martino, Genoa, Italy
enrica.tanda@gmail.com

Pierfrancesco Tassone   Medical Oncology Unit, Department of Experimental and Clinical Medicine, Magna Græcia University and Cancer Center, Catanzaro, Italy
tassone@unicz.it

Antonio Teira   Centro Hospitalar de Trás-os-Montes e Alto Douro, Vila Real, Portugal
antonioteira@gmail.com

Albert J. ten Tije   Medical-oncologist, University Hospital Antwerp, Edegem, Belgium
BertJan.tenTije@uza.be

Nicola Tinari   Department of Medical, Oral and Biotechnological Sciences, Section of Medical Oncology, Centro Scienze dell'Invecchiamento e Medicina Traslazionale – CeSI-MeT, University G. D'Annunzio, Chieti, Italy
nicola.tinari@unich.it

Giuseppe Tirino   University of study of Campania "L. Vanvitelli"- Medical Oncology, Naples, Italy
giuseppe.tirino@unicampania.it

Patrizia Toia   Department of Biomedicine, Neurosciences and Advanced Diagnostics (BiND), University of Palermo, Palermo, Italy
toiapatrizia@gmail.com

Stefania Tommasi   Molecular Diagnostics and Pharmacogenetics Unit – IRCCS Istituto Tumori "Giovanni Paolo II", Bari, Italy
s.tommasi@oncologico.bari.it

Giuseppe Tonini   Medical Oncology Department, University Campus Bio-Medico, Rome, Italy
g.tonini@unicampus.it

Paolo Tralongo   Medical Oncology Unit, Umberto I Hospital, Siracusa, Italy
tralongo@raosr.it

Antonino Carmelo Tralongo   Medical Oncology Unit, ASST Sette Laghi, Circolo Hospital, Varese, Italy
antonino.tralongo@guest.marionegri.it

Elisa Tripodi   Department of Gynecologic Oncology, IRCCS National Cancer Institute, Milan, Italy
elisa.tripodi@istitutotumori.mi.it

Claudia Trojaniello   IRCCS Istituto Nazionale Tumori Fondazione G Pascale, Napoli, Italy
c.trojanello@istitutotumori.na.it

Giancarlo Troncone   Department of Public Health, University of Naples "Federico II", Naples, Italy
giancarlo.troncone@unina.it

Mauro Truini   Società Italiana di Anatomia Patologica e Citologia Diagnostica, Milano, Italy
mauroa.truini@gmail.com

Marco Tucci   Department of Biomedical Sciences and Human Oncology, University of Bari "Aldo Moro", Bari, Italy
marco.tucci@uniba.it

Jhony Alberto De La Cruz Vargas   Universidad Ricardo Palma Instituto de Investigación en Ciencias Biomedicas, Lima, Peru
jhony.delacruz@urp.edu.pe

Elena Verzoni   Fondazione IRCCS Istituto Nazionale Tumori, Milan, Italy
Elena.Verzoni@istitutotumori.mi.it

Elena Vigliar   Department of Public Health, University of Naples "Federico II", Naples, Italy
elena@vigliar.it

Paolo Vigneri   Center of Experimental Oncology and Hematology, A.O.U. Policlinico "G. Rodolico - S. Marco", Catania, Italy
vigneripaolo@gmail.com

Bruno Vincenzi   Department of Medical Oncology, Università Campus Bio-Medico di Roma, Rome, Italy
b.vincenzi@unicampus.it

Ferdinando De Vita   University of study of Campania "L. Vanvitelli"- Medical Oncology, Naples, Italy
ferdinando.devita@unicampania.it

Francesco Vitale   Department of Science for Health Promotion, Mother to Child Care, Internal Medicine and Excellence Specialties "G. D'Alessandro", University of Palermo, Palermo, Italy
francesco.vitale@unipa.it

Clinical Oncology: Diagnosis and Treatment of Solid Tumors

Contents

Locoregional and Locally Advanced Breast Cancer

Gaia Griguolo, Maria Vittoria Dieci, Valentina Guarneri, and Pier Franco Conte

Breast Cancer

Contents

© Springer Nature Switzerland AG 2021
A. Russo et al. (eds.), *Practical Medical Oncology Textbook*, UNIPA Springer Series,
https://doi.org/10.1007/978-3-030-56051-5_30

Learning Objectives

By the end of this chapter, the reader will:

— Have learned the basic concepts of breast cancer epidemiology
— Understand relevant prognostic and predictive factors in breast cancer
— Be aware of clinical presentation and diagnostic strategies in breast cancer
— Have learned the basic principles of breast cancer management and treatment

30.1 Epidemiology

Breast cancer (BC) is a major public health problem throughout the world. It represents the second most frequently diagnosed cancer worldwide and the most frequently diagnosed cancer among women, accounting for nearly 1.7 million cancer cases diagnosed worldwide per year. It is also the second leading cause of cancer deaths in women worldwide [1].

However, there is a significant heterogeneity in incidence rates between high incidence areas (developed Western countries, such as the United States and Western Europe) and low incidence areas (such as Africa and Asia).

In the United States, the incidence of BC has shown a consistent increase up to the first years of the twenty-first century, probably due to the increasing implementation of mammography screening programs and to the extensive use of hormonal replacement therapy in menopausal women. On the contrary, BC mortality has consistently decreased in several Western countries during the last decades, thanks to the extensive use of screening and advances in adjuvant systemic treatments [2]. Nevertheless, BC is still the leading cause of cancer-related deaths in European women. Moreover, incidence in low-income nations is increasing [3]. BC in males is rare, contributing to approximately 1% of cases.

30.2 Risk Factors for Breast Cancer

Multiple factors are associated with an increased risk of developing BC, such as age, gender, family history, genetic alterations, diet, and life style. However, most of these factors carry a small/moderate increase in risk for any individual woman. In fact, BC pathogenesis is often linked to a complex interaction among multiple factors, and it has been estimated that approximately half of BC cases do not have any identifiable risk factor beyond increasing age and female sex. Age is indeed the most relevant risk factor for BC in women with the incidence

Table 30.1 WHO classification of breast tumors. (Adapted from Lakhani et al. 2012)

Epithelial tumors
Microinvasive carcinoma
Invasive breast carcinoma
Invasive carcinoma of no special type (NST)
Invasive lobular carcinoma
Tubular carcinoma
Cribiform carcinoma
Mucinous carcinoma
Carcinoma with medullary features
Carcinoma with apocrine differentiation
Carcinoma with signet ring differentiation
Invasive micropapillary carcinoma
Metaplastic carcinoma
Rare types
Carcinoma with neuroendocrine features
Secretory carcinoma
Invasive papillary carcinoma
Acinic cell carcinoma
Mucoepidermoid carcinoma
Polymorphous carcinoma
Oncocytic carcinoma
Lipid rich carcinoma
Glycogen rich clear cell carcinoma
Sebaceous carcinoma
Salivary gland/skin adnexal type tumors
Precursor lesions
Ductal carcinoma in situ
Lobular neoplasia
Lobular carcinoma in situ
Classic lobular carcinoma in situ
Pleomorphic lobular carcinoma in situ
Atypical lobular hyperplasia
Intraductal proliferative lesions
Epithelial-myoepithelial tumors
Papillary lesions
Mesenchymal tumors
Fibroepithelial tumors
Fibroadenoma

(continued)

◼ Table 30.1 (continued)

Phyllodes tumor
Hamartoma
Tumors of the nipple
Nipple adenoma
Syringomatous adenoma
Paget disease of the nipple
Malignant Lymphoma
Metastatic tumors
Tumors of the male breast
Gynaecomastia
Invasive carcinoma
In situ carcinoma
Clinical patterns
Inflammatory carcinoma
Bilateral breast carcinoma

of BC doubling on average every 10 years until menopause [4].

For men, major risk factors include hormonal imbalances (especially gynecomastia and cirrhosis), radiation exposure, and positive family history and genetic predisposition.

30.2.1 Hormonal and Reproductive Factors

The increase in the incidence of BC with age is at least partly explained by the role played by sex hormones in the etiology of the human BC. In fact, several evidences point out the pro-tumor role played by exposure to hormones in human BC.

BC incidence increases steeply with age until menopause and then plateaus, highlighting the role of ovarian function. Moreover, estrogen deprivation via iatrogenic premature menopause can reduce BC risk: premenopausal women undergoing oophorectomy without subsequent hormone replacement therapy have reduced risk of BC later in life, with magnitude of risk reduction increasing as the age at oophorectomy decreases [5]. The total duration of ovarian function (and thus of exposure to endogenous estrogens) seems relevant. There appears to be a relative 20% increase in BC risk for women with early menarche (<11 years of age) as compared to women with first menarche at 13 years of age [6].

The relationship with pregnancy is more complicated. Nulliparous women are at greater risk of BC than parous women (relative risk ≈ 1.4) and women whose first pregnancy occurs after age 30 have a higher BC risk as compared with women who had a pregnancy before that age [5–7]. However, BC risk increases transiently for the 10 years after a pregnancy and then declines. This appears to be related to the differentiating effect exerted by hormones on the mammary gland during pregnancy [7]. Abortion, either spontaneous or induced, does not increase the risk of BC [8].

Breastfeeding has a protective effect in lowering the risk of BC, particularly for longer durations. This effect might be linked to the inhibition of ovarian function and to structural modifications of the glandular tissue during breastfeeding.

Reproductive history and breastfeeding may at least partly part account for differences in BC risk between developed and developing nations.

Exposure to exogenous hormones also contributes to BC risk. In the Women's Health Initiative, use of combined estrogen and progestin hormone replacement therapy increased the risk of BC diagnosis (relative risk ≈ 1.5), while use of estrogen only formulations did not [9, 10]. The incidence was noted after 2 years of hormone replacement therapy and decreased after 5 years from therapy termination.

30.2.2 Dietary and Lifestyle Factors

Several studies have tried to investigate the impact of diet on BC risk. However, the results of cohort studies and meta-analyses are not always consistent, probably due to the intrinsic difficulties in accurately assessing the composition of diet over long periods of time and the effect of single components on cancer risk. The most consistent results point out that alcohol consumption is a risk factor for BC and that BC risk increases linearly with the amount of alcohol consumed (10% relative risk increase for every 10 g/day of alcohol) [11]. Risk might be enhanced by decreased intake of vitamin C, folate, and β-carotene.

In addition, existing evidence, even if not totally consistent, suggests that a diet rich in fruit, vegetables, whole grain cereals, and fiber and low in fats and refined carbohydrates might reduce BC risk.

Even if data regarding the accordant of diet composition of BC risk is not completely consistent, consistent evidence is available associating obesity with both increased risk of BC development (in postmenopausal women) and increased BC mortality. In fact, during early adult life, obesity is associated with a lower incidence of BC before menopause, but no reduction in breast mortality. After menopause, overweight women have a 1.5-fold greater risk of developing BC than normal weight women, which increases to twofold in case of obesity [12]. In particular, weight gain after age 18 is associated with a substantial increase in postmenopausal BC [13].

On the contrary, physical exercise has been pointed out as a protective factor, and several studies have estimated that a regular physical activity reduces the relative risk of developing BC by 10–20%.

Smoking is also associated with an increase in BC risk, in addition to an increased risk of other cancers.

30.2.3 Environmental Factors

Among environmental factor, exposure to ionizing radiation is the best-known risk factor for BC risk. This has been observed in atomic bombing survivors and in patients receiving diagnostic or therapeutic irradiation. A marked increase in BC risk is observed in women who received mantle irradiation for the treatment of Hodgkin lymphoma before 15 years of age [14].

30.2.4 Family History and Inherited Predisposition to Breast Cancer

A family history of BC is a well-recognized risk factor: overall, the risk of developing BC of a woman with a first-degree relative with BC is increased 1.5–3-fold as compared to a woman with negative family history. However, the risk carried by family history depends on number of relatives affected, the exact relationship, age at diagnosis, and the number of unaffected relatives.

Only 5–10% of women diagnosed with BC have a clearly identifiable hereditary predisposition.

The most frequent and best-known genetic alterations are germline mutations in the BC susceptibility genes *BRCA1* and *BRCA2*. These mutations are inherited in an autosomal dominant manner with varying penetrance. These genes encode proteins involved in homologous recombination repair and contribute to maintain the genomic integrity of the cell. Pathogenic mutations in these genes frequently result in a loss of the functional protein produced by that allele. When the second allele of the gene is altered by a somatic event (double hit), there is a complete absence of functional protein in the cell, which leads to genomic instability. BRCA1 and BRCA2 germline mutations are relatively rare, being present in less than 1% of the general population (2% in individuals of Ashkenazi Jewish ancestry).

BRCA pathogenic mutation carriers have an estimated lifetime risk of BC ranging between 26% and 85%. *BRCA1* mutations are associated with a higher incidence of triple-negative BCs, while the phenotype of *BRCA2* associated cancers does not significantly differ from that seen in sporadic tumors [15, 16].

BRCA mutations also carry a significant lifetime risk of ovarian cancer, which ranges from 16% to 63% and 10% to 27%, respectively, for *BRCA1* and *BRCA2* [17]. *BRCA1* or *BRCA2* mutations have also been associated with male BC, fallopian tube cancer, pancreatic cancer, and prostate cancer.

However, not every BRCA1 or BRCA2 mutation is pathogenic and different mutations have been shown to carry different risk of developing cancer.

The presence of a *BRCA1* or *BRCA2* mutation may be suggested by family history, personal history of cancer, and cancer phenotype. Models are available to estimate the likelihood of mutation and evaluate referral to a genetic counselor. The implications of genetic testing are considerable for both patients and their family members and should be discussed prior to undertaking genetic testing.

If a *BRCA1/2* mutation carrier is identified, management strategies available for risk reduction include intensive surveillance, chemoprevention with selective estrogen receptor modulators (SERMs), and risk-reducing surgery (breast and salpingo-ovarian). Prospective studies demonstrated an 80–100% reduction in BC mortality in *BRCA* mutation carriers undergoing prophylactic mastectomy [18, 19]. Prophylactic bilateral salpingo-oophorectomy has the added benefit of reducing the risk of ovarian carcinoma (HR = 0.21), for which effective screening is not available, and concomitantly reduces BC risk (HR = 0.49) [20].

In families where a *BRCA* mutation is known to be present, women who test negative for the mutation are not at increased risk for BC development and do not require special surveillance.

Other genetic mutations are associated with increased BC risk: germinal mutations of *TP53* (Li-Fraumeni syndrome), *PTEN* (Cowden syndrome), and of both alleles of *ATM* (ataxia-telangiectasia syndrome) each account for <1% of cases. Mutations in CDH1 are associated with a predisposition to diffuse gastric cancer and lobular BC. Moreover, mutations in low-penetrance genes account for a significant number of non-*BRCA1* or -*BRCA2* BCs: *PALB2*, *CHEK2,* and *ATM* in heterozygosity are among these [21, 22].

Even in the absence of a known inherited predisposition, women with a family history of BC face some level of increased risk, likely from some combination of shared environmental exposures, unexplained genetic factors, or both.

30.2.5 Personal History of Breast Cancer and Benign Breast Disease

Women with a previous diagnosis of breast carcinoma have an increased risk (two- to sixfold relative risk increase) of developing a contralateral BC; however, the absolute annual risk usually remains below 1%.

Benign breast lesions are classified as proliferative or non-proliferative. Non-proliferative lesions do not increase BC risk, while proliferative lesions are a risk factor for BC. Proliferative disease without atypia usually results in a small increase in risk (relative risk ≈ 1.5–2.0), while proliferative disease with atypical hyperplasia carries a greater risk of cancer development (relative risk ≈ 4.0–5.0) [23]. A previous diagnosis of breast carcinoma in situ carries an even greater risk of developing BC (relative risk ≈ 10).

30.2.6 Mammary Density

Mammographic breast density is an index of the ratio between glandular-stromal tissue and adipose tissue in the breast. High breast density not only makes detection of BC more difficult but is also an important predictor of BC risk. Women with >75% breast density have 4.7-fold increase in BC risk than those with <10% breast density, even after adjustment for other risk factors [24].

Breast density is mainly genetically determined, although it has been shown to vary due to postmenopausal hormone replacement therapy.

30.3 Breast Cancer Prevention

30.3.1 Breast Cancer Screening for the General Population

If diagnosed based on clinical signs and symptoms, most BCs present as large nodules or with axillary node involvement. Mammography can detect smaller, clinically asymptomatic tumors or noninvasive lesions.

As disease extension is one of the principle factors determining BC prognosis, this has led to the implementation of mammographic screening programs aiming to early detection and treatment of BC, thus reducing its mortality.

Estimates of the effect of mammography screening on BC mortality vary from trial to trial: a UK review of randomized, controlled mammography trials estimated a 20% relative BC mortality reduction in women aged between 50 and 70 years old [25], while more modern case-control and cohort studies conducted in Europe and Canada have reported up to a 40% relative reduction in BC mortality for women more than 50 years of age. However, screening programs carry the risk of false-positive results, with consequent over-diagnosis and overtreatment, and risk of false-negative results, that might instill a false feeling of security among patients and doctors and delay diagnosis.

In women aged between 50 and 69 years benefits appear to outweigh risks and mammography screening, repeated every 2 years, is recommended by most countries [26].

For the age group 40–49 years, evidence of effectiveness of mammography screening is limited. Meta-analyses stratified by age have shown that reduction in BC mortality is smaller (15%) in women <50 years of age and the risk of false-positives is higher, due to lower incidence of BC in this population. Therefore, no consensus exists regarding extension of population screening to women aged between 45 and 49 years and in the age group 70–74 [9]. Moreover, no consensus exists regarding the use of ultrasound for BC screening, due to the possible increase in false-positive results [27].

Regular auto palpation of the breasts is also recommended by several countries.

30.3.2 Management of High-Risk Patients

There is no formal and unambiguous definition of which patients should be considered at *high risk* for BC. Without question, BRCA mutation carriers and women with a similar risk based on family history are considered at high risk. Other high-risk groups can include women who received mantle irradiation and those diagnosed with lobular carcinoma in situ (LCIS) or atypical hyperplasia.

The Gail model [28], which calculates a woman's risk of developing BC based on age at menarche, age at first live birth, number of previous breast biopsies, presence or absence of atypical hyperplasia, and number of first-degree female relatives with BC, has been used in several cancer prevention trials to define high-risk population. However, no clear consensus exists regarding which model should be used.

Management strategies for high-risk women include intensive surveillance, chemoprevention with endocrine agents, and, for extremely selected patients, prophylactic surgery.

30.3.2.1 BC Screening for High-Risk Patients

Annual MRI concomitantly or alternating (every 6 months) with mammography, starting 10 years younger than the youngest case in the family, is recommended for patients at high risk of BC (proven BRCA mutations or similar risk due to genetic factors or history of prior thoracic irradiation) [27] as it can detect BC at a more favorable stage than mammography screening alone. However, MRI screening is not recommended for women with atypical hyperplasia as no benefit was observed [27, 29].

30.3.2.2 Chemoprevention

Chemoprevention is an option, in addition to surveillance strategies, for patients at high risk of BC. Endocrine treatments, such as SERMs (selective estrogen receptor modulators) and aromatase inhibitors (AIs) have been evaluated in clinical trials to prevent BC occurrence.

Tamoxifen reduces the incidence of HR+ BC (a 48% reduction in a meta-analysis of 4 randomized trials), while no effect is seen in HR− cancers [30, 31]. In the largest of these studies, the NSABP P1 trial, a 49% risk reduction was seen with tamoxifen, with a reduction in both invasive and noninvasive carcinoma, and for women of all ages. A particular benefit was seen in women with atypical hyperplasia, with an 84% reduction in cancer incidence in this group. However, treatment with tamoxifen carries some well-known side effects: in these trials, tamoxifen users had an increase in thromboembolic events (RR 1.9) and endometrial cancer (RR 2.4). Therefore, despite the proven efficacy, use of tamoxifen as chemoprevention has been limited by concerns about side effects and the small absolute differences in outcomes.

Raloxifene, another SERM used for the treatment and prevention of osteoporosis, was compared to tamoxifen as chemopreventive agent in the NSABP-P2 STAR trial [32]. No difference in the incidence of invasive cancer was observed between tamoxifen and raloxifene, while more cases of noninvasive cancer were noted in the raloxifene group. Raloxifene has a more favorable side-effect profile, with less hysterectomies and endometrial cancers and significantly fewer thromboembolic events and cataracts. However, history of deep vein thrombosis, stroke, pulmonary embolism, or transient ischemic attacks is considered a contraindication to the use of both tamoxifen and raloxifene.

AIs have also been tested for BC prevention, with a reduction in invasive BC, limited to HR+ cancers. However, the side-effect profile of these drugs (arthralgia, osteoporosis) represents a limit for their use in a preventive setting [33].

30.4 Pathological Classification of Breast Cancer

Historically, classification of invasive BCs has been based on its morphologic appearance in light microscopy. The WHO (World Health Organization) classification system (□ Table 30.1), based on the growth pattern and cytologic features of the invasive tumor cells, recognizes invasive "ductal" and "lobular" carcinoma [34]; however, this does not imply that the former originates in the ducts and the latter in the lobules of the breast. In fact, regardless of histologic type, most invasive BCs arise from epithelial cells of the terminal duct lobular unit.

30.4.1 Invasive Ductal Carcinoma

The most common histologic type of BC is invasive ductal carcinoma, representing 65–80% of BC cases. Most classification systems use the terms *infiltrating ductal carcinoma, not otherwise specified* (NOS) or *infiltrating carcinoma of no special type* interchangeably, to emphasize that diagnosis of invasive ductal carcinoma is made by exclusion (when tumors do not present characteristics classifying them into other special categories of invasive mammary carcinoma) [34].

30.4.2 Invasive Lobular Carcinoma

Invasive lobular carcinoma is the second most common histologic type, comprising 10–15% of BC cases. It is often multifocal or multicentric, and not rarely bilateral. It is characterized by neoplastic epithelial glandular cells, which infiltrate the surrounding stroma by circling the mammary ducts. This often leads to an underestimation of tumor size by radiological techniques. It characteristically lacks expression of E-cadherin (an epithelial cell membrane molecule involved in cell-cell adhesion), a feature that distinguishes lobular from ductal disease, both in situ and invasive.

30.4.3 Special Types of Breast Carcinoma

Rarer special types comprise approximately 10% of invasive BCs and often carry a distinct prognosis as compared to ductal invasive carcinoma. BCs with pure tubular, mucinous, papillary, or cribriform features are recognized to have a more favorable outcome than ductal BC, while micropapillary tumors have a high incidence of systemic recurrence [35]. Other cancers, not considered to be typical BCs, can occur in the breast, such as cystosarcoma phyllodes, angiosarcoma, and primary lymphoma.

30.4.4 Carcinoma In Situ

Carcinoma in situ is defined as the proliferation of malignant-appearing mammary epithelial cells that remain confined within the basement membrane without evidence of invasion in the stroma.

Ductal carcinoma in situ (DCIS) comprises 80–85% of in situ carcinomas and involves ductal epithelial cells. The number of ductal carcinomas in situ diagnosed has dramatically increased with the diffusion of screening mammography (15–30% of cancers detected in mammography screening programs are DCIS, especially in women aged 49–69 years), raising the problem of its management. In fact, concordance between risk factors and shared genetic alterations suggests that DCIS and invasive carcinoma might be part of the same pathologic process, and DCIS is generally considered a precursor of invasive BC. This has led to an aggressive treatment of all DCIS (see ▶ Sect. 30.11).

Lobular neoplasia is instead defined from a morphological point of view as "a proliferation of generally small and often loosely cohesive cells originating in the terminal duct lobular unit, with or without pagetoid involvement of terminal ducts" [34], a definition generally used to cover both LCIS and ALH.

Patients with LCIS treated by biopsy alone have a substantially increased risk of BC compared with women without LCIS (30–40% lifetime risk) and, although the risk for development of BC is bilateral, subsequent ipsilateral carcinoma is more likely than contralateral. This supports the view that ALH and LCIS act both as precursor lesions and as risk indicators. However, the relative risk for subsequent BC is lower in women diagnosed with ALH than in those with LCIS.

The management of lobular neoplasia must address the bilateral risk, and options include surveillance, chemoprevention, and prophylactic bilateral mastectomy. Surveillance is most commonly used, and mammography is the standard imaging technique for these patients. Prophylactic mastectomy reduces BC risk among high-risk women by approximately 90%, but there is no data indicating that the incidence of subsequent cancer is reduced by other surgical approaches, such as excision to negative margins or subsequent irradiation.

30.5 Prognostic and Predictive Pathological Factors in Breast Cancer

30.5.1 Grading

The most commonly evaluated microscopic feature is grading, which describes the grade of differentiation of a BC. Grading can be based solely on nuclear characteristics (nuclear grading) or, more commonly, on a combination of architectural and nuclear characteristics (histologic grading). In the Elston-Ellis modification of the original Scarff-Bloom-Richardson grading system, tubule formation, nuclear pleomorphism, and mitotic activity are each scored on a scale of 1–3 [36] and added. Tumors with scores of 3–5 are designated as grade 1 (well differentiated), those with sums of 6–7 as grade 2 (moderately differentiated), and those with sums of 8–9 as grade 3 (poorly differentiated). Histologic grading has prognostic significance. However, the clinical use of grade to coadjuvate clinical decision has not been implemented worldwide due to persistent challenges in standardization and inter-operator discrepancies.

30.5.2 Hormone Receptors (HR)

Estrogen (ER) and progesterone receptor (PgR) expression is evaluated using immunohistochemistry and the percentage of positive BC cells is reported (a cutoff of 1% or more positive tumor cells is generally used to define a tumor as positive). Around 80% of BCs are classified as hormone-receptor-positive.

Estrogen and progesterone receptor expression are extremely useful prognostic and predictive factors (e.g., only patients with hormone receptor-positive BC benefit from hormonal treatment) [37].

30.5.3 HER2

HER2 (human epidermal growth factor receptor 2), a transmembrane receptor of the epidermal growth factor receptor (EGFR) family with tyrosine kinase activity, is overexpressed in 15–20% of BCs. It activates pro-survival intracellular signaling pathways and is associated with clinically aggressive disease and a propensity for visceral relapses. Overexpression is generally linked to *HER2/neu* gene amplification.

In clinical practice, *HER2* status is evaluated by either immunohistochemistry or in situ hybridization. Immunohistochemical scores of 0 or 1+ are considered negative, while tumors with HER2 expression 3+ are considered positive. Cases classified as 2+ by immuno-histochemistry are evaluated using in situ hybridization: if *HER2* gene amplification is identified, the tumor is considered HER2-positive and can be treated with anti-*HER2* therapies. *HER2* status is the major predictor for benefit from *HER2*-targeted therapies [38].

30.5.4 Proliferation

Proliferation of tumor cells is usually evaluated by immunohistochemistry. Antibodies directed toward cell cycle proteins, such as Ki-67 or MIB-1, are used, thus measuring the percentage of cells in the G1 phase. Proliferation is a significant adverse prognostic factor in BC. However, due to persistent inter-operator discrepancies, this evaluation has not been implemented in clinical practice worldwide.

30.6 Molecular Classification of Breast Cancer

BC is a biologically heterogeneous disease, and it has long been appreciated that tumors with different biologic features have different clinical outcomes and responses to therapy. Clinically, BC is divided into three subgroups based on immunochemistry and in situ hybridization: HR-positive, HER2-positive, and triple-negative BC. Each of these subtypes presents specific clinical characteristics and therapeutic possibilities.

During the last 15 years, advances in molecular biology and gene expression profiling have led to the classification of BC into four intrinsic molecular subtypes (Luminal A, Luminal B, HER-2 enriched, Basal-like) and a normal breast-like group, which have been extensively characterized [39, 40].

These entities have shown significant differences in terms of incidence, risk factors, prognosis, and treatment sensitivity, giving additional information from that provided by evaluation of ER, PgR, and HER2. Moreover, intrinsic molecular subtypes only partially overlap with tumor phenotype as defined using ER, PgR, and HER2, with a discordance rate of around 30% [41].

30.6.1 Luminal A

Luminal A is the most common subtype and represents 50–60% of all BCs. It is characterized by expression of ER-activated genes, which are typically expressed in the luminal epithelium lining of mammary ducts [42]. As compared to Luminal B tumors, Luminal A tumors have lower expression of proliferation/cell cycle-related

genes (e.g., MKI67 and AURKA) and higher expression of luminal-related proteins such as PgR [41]. Immunohistochemical profile is usually characterized by the expression of ER, PgR, and absence of HER2 expression. Luminal A tumors are also frequently characterized by low proliferation rate as measured by Ki67, a low degree of nuclear polymorphism and a low histological grade.

Patients with luminal A BCs have a good prognosis, the relapse rate of this subtype being significantly lower than in the other subtypes [39]. Recurrence is common in bone, whereas liver, lung, and central nervous system metastases occur less frequently than in other subtypes [42].

30.6.2 Luminal B

Luminal B represents 10–20% of all BCs. Compared to luminal A tumors, it presents a more aggressive phenotype, higher histological grade, higher proliferation rate and a worse prognosis [39]. Luminal B tumors more frequently (16.4–20.8%) present HER2-overexpression [41].

The pattern of distant relapse also differs, and although the bone is still the most common site of recurrence, this subtype more frequently presents visceral metastatic sites such as the liver. Luminal B tumors are more chemosensitive and usually benefit more from adjuvant chemotherapy [42].

30.6.3 HER2-Enriched

HER2-enriched BC is characterized at RNA and protein level by high expression of HER2, of HER2-related genes (such as other genes in the HER2 amplicon) and proliferation-related genes, intermediate expression of luminal-related genes (e.g., ESR1 and PgR), and low expression of basal-related genes. HER2-enriched BC is biologically aggressive and intrinsically carries a poor prognosis [39]. However, introduction of HER2-targeted treatment has substantially improved outcomes, both in the early and advanced settings [43].

30.6.4 Basal-Like

Approximately 15% of BCs are classified as basal-like [41]. This subtype is characterized by high expression of proliferation-related genes and keratins typically expressed by the basal layer of the skin (e.g., keratins 5, 14, and 17), and very low expression of luminal-related genes [41]. Basal-like tumors generally present high grade, high mitotic indices and are characterized by the lack of expression of ER, PgR, and HER2. Patients with basal-like BC have poor prognosis, with higher relapse rates and short overall survival [39, 40].

30.6.5 Normal-Like Subtype

This subtype is poorly characterized, and its clinical significance remains undetermined. There are even doubts about its actual existence. In fact, some researchers believe the normal-like subtype might be a technical artifact due to contamination with normal tissue. Indeed, in a large series of samples where neoplastic cells were isolated by microdissection, no cases of normal breast-like subtype were found, supporting this hypothesis [42].

30.6.6 Gene Expression Prognostic Signatures

As previously discussed, gene expression profiles can be used to gain additional prognostic and/or predictive information to complement pathology assessment and to predict the benefit of adjuvant chemotherapy. Several of these gene signatures are commercially available, such as MammaPrint, Oncotype DX Recurrence Score, Prosigna, and Endopredict. The more clinically mature are MammaPrint and Oncotype DX.

In fact, the MammaPrint assay has been cleared by the US Food and Drug Administration for use in women younger than 61 years old with stage I or II, node-negative BC, to assess patient's risk for distant metastases. This 70-gene assay has been evaluated in the prospective MINDACT study [44], which enrolled women independently from BC grade, receptor status, and lymph node involvement. In this study, women with a low risk according to the 70-gene prognostic assay and high clinical risk (as calculated by the online tool Adjuvant! Online) were randomized to receive chemotherapy or not. Distant disease-free survival at 5 years was similar for these patients with or without chemotherapy, pointing out that MammaPrint can be used to avoid chemotherapy in a subgroup of clinically high-risk patients.

Similar evidence exists to support the use of the Oncotype DX test in node-negative HR+ BC. The OncotypeDX Recurrence Score (RS) is based on the quantitative assessment of 21 genes relevant to BC biology and is a continuous, numeric result that correlates with distant metastatic recurrence in node-negative BC

patients treated with tamoxifen and with prognosis of postmenopausal women with node-positive tumors receiving endocrine treatment [45, 46]. In the prospective TAILORx (Trial Assigning Individualized Options for Treatment Rx) trial patients with HR-positive, HER2-negative, lymph node-negative BC were tested using Oncotype DX. Patients with RS <11 received endocrine therapy alone and had a 5-year distant recurrence-free survival of 99.3% without chemotherapy [47]. Patients in the intermediate-risk group (RS 11-25) were randomized to receive chemotherapy or not and the study showed non-inferiority of endocrine treatment alone in terms of disease-free survival in this group. However, subgroup analysis showed that significant benefit from adding chemotherapy exists in some subgroups of patients with intermediate risk according to OncotypeDX (such as young patients ≤50 years of age) [48]. The WSG PLAN B trial, another large randomized trial, tested the use of Oncotype DX in clinically high-risk pN0-N1 HR-positive BC patients. In this trial, patients with RS < 11 received endocrine therapy alone and had a 5-year disease-free survival of 94% without chemotherapy [49]. The RxPONDER trial is also currently testing the role of OncotypeDX in patients with HR+ HER2− BC with lymph node involvement.

For Prosigna, a 50-gene intrinsic subtype classifier that categorizes cancers into luminal A, luminal B, HER2, or basal-like subtypes [50], retrospective analyses of data from prospective trials show independent prognostic information beyond traditional pathologic markers. However, we are still waiting for data from its validation prospective randomized clinical trial, the OPTIMA trial.

For the EPclin Risk Score, a BC recurrence test integrating both gene expression data (EndoPredict) and clinicopathological features designed to accurately predict 10-year risk of distant recurrence in ER+ HER2- BC with node-negative (N0) or node-positive (N1), only retrospective analyses of data from several large prospective trials are currently available.

30.7 Clinical Presentation and Diagnosis

Most BCs are diagnosed by mammography screening in the absence of any sign or symptom.

When this is not the case, the most frequent sign of BC is the presence of a palpable, non-tender, hard breast nodule with unclear margins. Sometimes a retraction of the nipple or the skin of the breast can be present. Less frequently, BC presents with discharge of secretion or bleeding from the nipple, usually in relation with Paget disease or ductal papillomas.

In more advanced cases, the first sign of BC can be the presence of hard, fixed, non-tender lymph nodes in the axilla (or more rarely supra or infraclavicular region), eventually accompanied by lymphedema of the arm. More rarely, BC might present with mastitis or as an inflammatory carcinoma, with the diffuse involvement of the entire breast, which shows signs of inflammation (edematous, erythematous, warm, tender, enlarged breast).

30.7.1 Clinical Examination of the Breast

Breast examination includes the neck, chest wall, both breasts, and axillae and is part of a complete physical examination.

Inspection: Visual inspection of the breasts is an important component of clinical examination. The patient should be examined in both upright (arms relaxed, arms raised over the head, hands pressing on the hips) and supine positions. Asymmetry, bulging areas, skin changes (retraction, edema, dermatological lesions), and position of the nipple (inversion or retraction) should be evaluated. Spontaneous discharge should also be investigated, without squeezing the nipple.

Palpation: A first bimanual examination of the breasts should be performed with the patient in sitting position, supporting the breast with one hand and examining the breast with the other. Bimanual examination is then completed with arms raised above her head. Palpation should extend from the midaxillary line to the lateral edge of the sternum and from the clavicle to infra-mammary ridge to cover all the perimeter of the breast. Using three levels of pressure will help detect asymmetric thickenings or masses that can occur at different depths in the breast tissue. Palpation should include the careful application of pressure to the retroareolar region to check for abnormal discharge.

Regional Lymph node Examination: Clavicular and axillary lymph nodes should be examined in sitting position to allow best access to the deepest nodes. Patient should relax her shoulders and allow the examiner to support her arm while the axilla is palpated. Attention should be given to cervical, supraclavicular, infraclavicular, and axillary nodal basins. The presence of any palpable nodes and their characteristics, whether they are soft and mobile or firm, hard, tender, fixed, or matted, should be noted.

Assessment for distant metastases (bones, liver, and lungs, or neurological examination if symptoms are present) should also be conducted.

30.7.2 Imaging Techniques for Breast Cancer Diagnosis and Local Staging

The most commonly used imaging technique for BC is mammography. Mammography is used for BC screening in asymptomatic women and for differential diagnostic in patients presenting with clinical suspect of BC. Breast neoplasia usually appears at mammography as radio opaque nodule with spiculated margins. In some cases, microcalcifications are present.

Ultrasonography is often used to complement mammography and clinical examination. It is particularly useful in young women in which higher breast density might affect the sensitivity of mammography. With this exception, the sensitivity of ultrasonography is generally lower than that of mammography, even if it has a higher specificity to distinguish benign and malignant lesions. For this reason, it should be used after mammography to better characterize lesions. Ultrasonography also allows to explore regional lymph nodes and can be used to guide biopsy of suspicious lesions.

Bilateral mammography and ultrasound of the breast and regional lymph nodes are therefore usually considered standard imaging evaluation at BC diagnosis [27].

Contrast-enhanced MRI is not routinely recommended and is generally used as second-level imaging technique. It has higher sensitivity than mammography, but less specificity and its use might lead to an increase in false-positive rate. MRI is used for surveillance in women at high risk of BC or BRCA1/BRCA2 mutation carriers, in patients with breast implants, in equivocal cases at first-level imaging techniques, for staging of multifocal or bifocal lesions (particularly in lobular BC), and for evaluation of pectoral muscle infiltration. MRI may also be recommended before neoadjuvant chemotherapy, for evaluating the response to primary systemic therapy or when conventional imaging findings are inconclusive (such as a positive axillary lymph node status with an occult primary tumor in the breast) [27]. Outside these indications, MRI is generally not recommended routinely as it has a substantial false-positive rate and several studies have shown an association between MRI use and greater unwarranted use of mastectomy [51].

30.7.3 Biopsy and Diagnosis

The presence of carcinoma can only be determined by tissue biopsy. Several biopsy techniques are available: fine-needle aspiration (FNA), core needle biopsy, and excisional biopsy.

Needle biopsy techniques are usually preferred to avoid surgical scars. FNA is easily performed. However, it requires a trained cytopathologist, does not reliably distinguish invasive cancer from DCIS and often does not permit a reliable immunohistochemical characterization. For this reason, FNA use is currently only recommended to confirm involvement of axillary lymph nodes but not to evaluate primary breast lesions. Core needle biopsy, instead, provides histologic specimen suitable for interpretation by any pathologist and for ER, PR, and *HER2* testing. If preoperative systemic therapy is planned, a core needle biopsy is mandatory to ensure a complete diagnosis and assessment of biomarkers. A marker, such as a surgical clip, should be left in place into the tumor at biopsy, to ensure surgical resection of the correct site. Both core needle biopsies of breast lesions and FNA of axillary lymph nodes are usually performed using ultrasonography guiding to reduce the risk of false-negative results due to inappropriate sampling. When lesions are difficult to identify at ultrasonography (e.g., microcalcifications), mammographic guidance and vacuum-assisted biopsy can be used. False-negative rates of core biopsy are now reliably <1%.

For this reason, excisional biopsy is now a diagnostic technique reserved to patients with imaging abnormalities that cannot be targeted for core biopsy. In addition, surgical biopsy can also be indicated following core biopsy in specific cases:

- Failure to sample calcifications
- Diagnosis of atypical ductal hyperplasia
- Diagnosis of atypical lobular hyperplasia or lobular carcinoma in situ (controversial)
- Lack of concordance between imaging findings and histologic diagnosis
- Radial scar (differential diagnosis with tubular carcinoma)
- Papillary lesions (differential diagnosis with papillary carcinoma in situ)

30.7.4 Breast Cancer Staging

Once BC has been diagnosed, its extension and its prognosis should be accurately evaluated in order to define the most appropriate treatment.

Extension of the disease is usually assessed using the classical TNM staging system in which "T" refers to tumor, "N" to nodes, and "M" to metastasis. Definitions for classifying the primary tumor are the same for clinical and pathologic classification, while the clinical and pathologic classification for N staging are different (◨ Table 30.2).

◨ **Table 30.2**	AJCC Clinical and Pathological TNM staging
T category	*T criteria*
TX	Primary tumor cannot be assessed
T0	No evidence of primary tumor
Tis(DCIS)[a]	Ductal carcinoma in situ
Tis(Paget)	Paget disease of the nipple NOT associated with invasive carcinoma and/or carcinoma in situ (DCIS) in the underlying breast parenchyma. Carcinomas in the breast parenchyma associated with Paget disease are categorized based on the size and characteristics of the parenchymal disease, although the presence of Paget disease should still be noted
T1	Tumor ≤20 mm in greatest dimension
T1mi	Tumor ≤1 mm in greatest dimension
T1a	Tumor >1 mm but ≤5 mm in greatest dimension (round any measurement >1.0–1.9 mm to 2 mm).
T1b	Tumor >5 mm but ≤10 mm in greatest dimension
T1c	Tumor >10 mm but ≤20 mm in greatest dimension
T2	Tumor >20 mm but ≤50 mm in greatest dimension
T3	Tumor >50 mm in greatest dimension
T4	Tumor of any size with direct extension to the chest wall and/or to the skin (ulceration or macroscopic nodules); invasion of the dermis alone does not qualify as T4
T4a	Extension to the chest wall; invasion or adherence to pectoralis muscle in the absence of invasion of chest wall structures does not qualify as T4

◻ Table 30.2 (continued)

T4b	Ulceration and/or ipsilateral macroscopic satellite nodules and/or edema (including peau d'orange) of the skin that does not meet the criteria for inflammatory carcinoma
T4c	Both T4a and T4b are present
T4d	Inflammatory carcinoma (see "Rules for Classification")
T suffix	Definition
(m)	Select if synchronous primary tumors are found in single organ.
N category	*N criteria*
cNX[a]	Regional lymph nodes cannot be assessed (e.g., previously removed)
cN0	No regional lymph node metastases (by imaging or clinical examination)
cN1	Metastases to movable ipsilateral Level I, II axillary lymph node(s)
cN1mi[b]	Micrometastases (approximately 200 cells, larger than 0.2 mm, but none larger than 2.0 mm)
cN2	Metastases in ipsilateral Level I, II axillary lymph nodes that are clinically fixed or matted; *or* in ipsilateral internal mammary nodes in the absence of axillary lymph node metastases
cN2a	Metastases in ipsilateral Level I, II axillary lymph nodes fixed to one another (matted) or to other structures
cN2b	Metastases only in ipsilateral internal mammary nodes in the absence of axillary lymph node metastases
cN3	Metastases in ipsilateral infraclavicular (Level III axillary) lymph node(s) with or without Level I, II axillary lymph node involvement; *or* in ipsilateral internal mammary lymph node(s) with Level I, II axillary lymph node metastases; *or* metastases in ipsilateral supraclavicular lymph node(s) with or without axillary or internal mammary lymph node involvement
cN3a	Metastases in ipsilateral infraclavicular lymph node(s)
cN3b	Metastases in ipsilateral internal mammary lymph node(s) and axillary lymph node(s)
cN3c	Metastases in ipsilateral supraclavicular lymph node(s)

[a]The cNX category is used sparingly in cases where regional lymph nodes have previously been surgically removed or where there is no documentation of physical examination of the axilla.

[b]cN1mi is rarely used but may be appropriate in cases where sentinel node biopsy is performed before tumor resection, most likely to occur in cases treated with neoadjuvant therapy.

N category	*N criteria*
pNX	Regional lymph nodes cannot be assessed (e.g., not removed for pathological study or previously removed)
pN0	No regional lymph node metastasis identified or ITCs only
pN0(i+)	ITCs only (malignant cell clusters no larger than 0.2 mm) in regional lymph node(s)
pN0(mol+)	Positive molecular findings by reverse transcriptase polymerase chain reaction (RT-PCR); no ITCs detected
pN1	Micrometastases; or metastases in 1–3 axillary lymph nodes; and/or clinically negative internal mammary nodes with micrometastases or macrometastases by sentinel lymph node biopsy
pN1mi	Micrometastases (approximately 200 cells, larger than 0.2 mm, but none larger than 2.0 mm)
pN1a	Metastases in 1–3 axillary lymph nodes, at least one metastasis larger than 2.0 mm
pN1b	Metastases in ipsilateral internal mammary sentinel nodes, excluding ITCs
pN1c	pN1a and pN1b combined
pN2	Metastases in 4–9 axillary lymph nodes; or positive ipsilateral internal mammary lymph nodes by imaging in the absence of axillary lymph node metastases
pN2a	Metastases in 4–9 axillary lymph nodes (at least one tumor deposit larger than 2.0 mm)
pN2b	Metastases in clinically detected internal mammary lymph nodes with or without microscopic confirmation; with pathologically negative axillary nodes

(continued)

▣ Table 30.2 (continued)

pN3	Metastases in 10 or more axillary lymph nodes *or* in infraclavicular (Level III axillary) lymph nodes *or* positive ipsilateral internal mammary lymph nodes by imaging in the presence of one or more positive Level I, II axillary lymph nodes *or* in more than three axillary lymph nodes and micrometastases or macrometastases by sentinel lymph node biopsy in clinically negative ipsilateral internal mammary lymph nodes *or* in ipsilateral supraclavicular lymph nodes
pN3a	Metastases in 10 or more axillary lymph nodes (at least one tumor deposit larger than 2.0 mm) *or* metastases to the infraclavicular (Level III axillary lymph) nodes
pN3b	pN1a or pN2a in the presence of cN2b (positive internal mammary nodes by imaging) *or* pN2a in the presence of pN1b
pN3c	Metastases in ipsilateral supraclavicular lymph nodes
M category	*M criteria*
cM0	No clinical or radiographic evidence of distant metastases[a]
cM0(i+)	No clinical or radiographic evidence of distant metastases in the presence of tumor cells or deposits no larger than 0.2 mm detected microscopically or by molecular techniques in circulating blood, bone marrow, or other nonregional nodal tissue in a patient without symptoms or signs of metastases
cM1	Distant metastases detected by clinical and radiographic means
pM1	Any histologically proven metastases in distant organs; or if in nonregional nodes, metastases greater than 0.2 mm

Pathologic stage after neoadjuvant therapy is designated with the prefix "yp." Complete response is defined as the absence of invasive carcinoma in the breast and axillary nodes and has been clearly associated with significant improvement in disease-free survival and overall survival for the individual patient [52].

However, the principal aim of a staging system is to group patients with respect to prognosis. Despite its importance, the TNM staging has been progressively superseded by the biological characterization of the disease, which defines subgroups with different outcomes and different response to specific treatments.

This has led to a recent radical change in the staging of BC. In 2018, the Eighth edition of the American Joint Committee on Cancer (AJCC) included, in addition to the classic anatomic parameters (T, N, and M), prognostic biological parameters (grade, ER, PgR, and HER2). Moreover, the new AJCC classification also takes into account results of prognostic multigene signatures, which can be used to more accurately stratify individual patient prognosis (▣ Table 30.3).

30.7.5 Imaging for Breast Cancer Staging and Other Pre-treatment Evaluations

In stage I–II BC without clinical suspicious of metastasis, asymptomatic distant metastases are very rare, and patients do not appear to benefit from comprehensive laboratory (including tumor markers) or radiological staging. For this reason, international guidelines do not recommend the use of imaging techniques (such as total body TC scan or bone scan) for the preoperative staging of these patients [27].

More comprehensive staging including a chest radiography or CT scan, an abdominal ultrasound or CT scan, and a bone scan can be considered for patients with clinically positive axillary nodes, large tumors (e.g., ≥5 cm), aggressive biology or clinical signs or symptoms suspicious for metastases.

Bone scan is a very sensitive technique for identifying bone metastases. However, its specificity is very low and the number of false-positives is high. Therefore, any suspicious alteration identified by bone scan should be confirmed by another imaging technique (X-ray/segmental CT scan/segmental MRI).

Functional/anatomical imaging, such as fluorodeoxyglucose positron emission tomography (FDG-PET)/CT, can be useful when conventional methods are inconclusive. It can also replace traditional imaging for staging in high-risk patient candidates to neoadjuvant chemotherapy, as well as those with locally advanced/inflammatory BC, in consideration of their high risk of metastatic disease.

Other pre-treatment assessments include: complete personal medical history, family history relating to breast/ovarian and other cancers, physical examination, a full blood count, liver and renal function tests, and alkaline phosphatase and calcium levels. Accurately assessing the menopausal status of the patient is also

Table 30.3 AJCC Pathological Prognostic Staging system. (Adapted from 8th ed). Pathological prognostic stage does not apply to patients treated with systemic or radiation prior to surgical resection

TNM	Grade	HER2 status	ER status	PR status	Pathological prognostic stage
Tis N0 M0	Any	Any	Any	Any	0
T1^a N0 M0 T0 N1mi M0 T1^a N1mi M0	G1	Positive	Positive	Positive	IA
				Negative	IA
			Negative	Positive	IA
				Negative	IA
		Negative	Positive	Positive	IA
				Negative	IA
			Negative	Positive	IA
				Negative	IA
	G2	Positive	Positive	Positive	IA
				Negative	IA
			Negative	Positive	IA
				Negative	IA
		Negative	Positive	Positive	IA
				Negative	IA
			Negative	Positive	IA
				Negative	IB
	G3	Positive	Positive	Positive	IA
				Negative	IA
			Negative	Positive	IA
				Negative	IA
		Negative	Positive	Positive	IA
				Negative	IA
			Negative	Positive	IA
				Negative	IB
T0 N1^b M0 T1^a N1^b M0 T2 N0 M0	G1	Positive	Positive	Positive	IA
				Negative	IB
			Negative	Positive	IB
				Negative	IIA
		Negative	Positive	Positive	IA
				Negative	IB
			Negative	Positive	IB
				Negative	IIA

(continued)

◻ Table 30.3 (continued)

TNM	Grade	HER2 status	ER status	PR status	Pathological prognostic stage
	G2	Positive	Positive	Positive	IA
				Negative	IB
			Negative	Positive	IB
				Negative	IIA
		Negative	Positive	Positive	IA
				Negative	IIA
			Negative	Positive	IIA
				Negative	IIA
	G3	Positive	Positive	Positive	IA
				Negative	IIA
			Negative	Positive	IIA
				Negative	IIA
		Negative	Positive	Positive	IB
				Negative	IIA
			Negative	Positive	IIA
				Negative	IIA
T2 N1[c] M0 T3 N0 M0	G1	Positive	Positive	Positive	IA
				Negative	IIB
			Negative	Positive	IIB
				Negative	IIB
		Negative	Positive	Positive	IA
				Negative	IIB
			Negative	Positive	IIB
				Negative	IIB
	G2	Positive	Positive	Positive	IB
				Negative	IIB
			Negative	Positive	IIB
				Negative	IIB
		Negative	Positive	Positive	IB
				Negative	IIB
			Negative	Positive	IIB
				Negative	IIB

Table 30.3 (continued)

TNM	Grade	HER2 status	ER status	PR status	Pathological prognostic stage
	G3	Positive	Positive	Positive	IB
				Negative	IIB
			Negative	Positive	IIB
				Negative	IIB
		Negative	Positive	Positive	IIA
				Negative	IIB
			Negative	Positive	IIB
				Negative	IIIA
T0 N2 M0 T1ª N2 M0 T2 N2 M0 T3 N1ᶜ M0 T3 N2 M0	G1	Positive	Positive	Positive	IB
				Negative	IIIA
			Negative	Positive	IIIA
				Negative	IIIA
		Negative	Positive	Positive	IB
				Negative	IIIA
			Negative	Positive	IIIA
				Negative	IIIA
	G2	Positive	Positive	Positive	IB
				Negative	IIIA
			Negative	Positive	IIIA
				Negative	IIIA
		Negative	Positive	Positive	IB
				Negative	IIIA
			Negative	Positive	IIIA
				Negative	IIIB
	G3	Positive	Positive	Positive	IIA
				Negative	IIIA
			Negative	Positive	IIIA
				Negative	IIIA
		Negative	Positive	Positive	IIB
				Negative	IIIA
			Negative	Positive	IIIA
				Negative	IIIC

(continued)

Table 30.3 (continued)

TNM	Grade	HER2 status	ER status	PR status	Pathological prognostic stage
T4 N0 M0 T4 N1c M0 T4 N2 M0 Any T N3 M0	G1	Positive	Positive	Positive	IIIA
				Negative	IIIB
			Negative	Positive	IIIB
				Negative	IIIB
		Negative	Positive	Positive	IIIA
				Negative	IIIB
			Negative	Positive	IIIB
				Negative	IIIB
	G2	Positive	Positive	Positive	IIIA
				Negative	IIIB
			Negative	Positive	IIIB
				Negative	IIIB
		Negative	Positive	Positive	IIIA
				Negative	IIIB
			Negative	Positive	IIIB
				Negative	IIIC
	G3	Positive	Positive	Positive	IIIB
				Negative	IIIB
			Negative	Positive	IIIB
				Negative	IIIB
		Negative	Positive	Positive	IIIB
				Negative	IIIC
			Negative	Positive	IIIC
				Negative	IIIC
Any T Any N M1	Any	Any	Any	Any	IV

If T1N0M0 or T2 N0 M0 with ER-positive, HER2 negative and Oncotype Dx score is less than 11, then the pathological prognostic stage group is IA

[a]T1 includes T1mi

[b]N1 does not include N1mi. T1 N1mi M0 and T0 N1mi M0 cancers are included for prognostic staging with T1 N0 M0 cancers of the same prognostic factor status

[c]N1 includes N1mi. T2, T3, and T4 cancers and N1mi are included for prognostic staging with T2 N1, T3 N1, and T4 N1, respectively

imperative, and pre-treatment serum estradiol and follicle-stimulating hormone levels should be measured in case of doubt. In patients planned for (neo)adjuvant treatment, with anthracyclines and/or trastuzumab, evaluation of cardiac function with measurement of ejection fraction should also be performed [27].

30.8 Management of Nonmetastatic Breast Cancer

Treatment of BC patients should be carried out in "breast units" defined as specialized departments that treat a high volume of BC patients. Treatment should be provided by a multidisciplinary team, which includes at least one surgeon, radiation oncologist, medical oncologist, radiologist, and pathologist, who are specialized in BC. The breast team may include plastic/reconstructive surgeons, psychologists, physiotherapists, and geneticists [53]. The choice of treatment strategy, based on tumor burden, location and biological characteristics as well as on age and patient's comorbidities, should be extensively discussed with the patient and take into account her/his preferences.

Apart from metastatic disease, treatment of BC patients should take into account two components:
- Locoregional treatment (surgery and radiotherapy) aiming to the radical excision of macroscopic disease, local staging of the disease and treatment of residual tumor cells in the breast and nodes in order to limit the risk of locoregional recurrence
- Systemic treatment aiming to eradicate systemic micrometastases, which might have originated even from early-stage BC, reducing the risk of distant and locoregional recurrence at the same time

Locoregional treatment of BC is mainly guided by the evaluation of disease operability. Metastatic disease is generally considered a contraindication to surgical and local treatment, even if in some selected cases of oligometastatic disease locoregional treatments might be proposed with a potentially curative intent. Patients with T4 tumors or N2/N3 nodal disease are not candidates for surgery upfront and should be treated with neoadjuvant systemic therapy in order to shrink the tumor, allowing radical operability. However, in the N3 category, patients with N3a-b disease are considered operable and are managed as locally advanced operable BC, while patients with N3c disease (involvement of ipsilateral supraclavicular nodes) are considered inoperable and are managed as such.

Patients with lesser extent of disease are usually managed with surgery upfront. However, neoadjuvant systemic therapy can be used in these patients to allow breast conservation in a woman who would otherwise require mastectomy or to test chemosensitivity in patients with sure indication to chemotherapy (e.g., TN/HER2+ BC) (◘ Fig. 30.1).

The possibility of hereditary cancer should also be explored, allowing for appropriate genetic counseling and testing of the patient and, if needed, prophylactic procedures. In younger premenopausal patients, fertility issues should also be discussed [27].

30.8.1 Local Management of Breast Cancer: Surgery

Breast surgery represents a cornerstone in the treatment of BC. In fact, surgery is capable of eradicating macroscopic disease in breast. However, increasing knowledge of BC biology has led to the understanding that most BCs are capable of micro-metastasizing even in early stage. Over the last century, this has led to a progressive decrease in surgical aggressiveness (both on the breast and on the axilla) and a parallel increase in the use of adjuvant system treatments.

For almost one century, from its first use in 1882 to the mid-twentieth century, *Halsted's radical mastectomy* has been the classical surgical procedure for BC. This intervention involved the removal of mammary gland, nipple, skin, underlying chest muscle (including pectoralis major and pectoralis minor), and axillary lymph nodes. It was an extremely disfiguring and invalidating surgery and is nowadays used only in extremely selected cases (e.g., infiltration of the pectoralis major).

Less invasive mastectomies have been subsequently employed:
- *Patey's conservative radical mastectomy*: which preserves the pectoralis major while removing the pectoralis minor.
- *Madden's modified radical mastectomy*: which preserves both the pectoralis major and the pectoralis minor.
- *Simple mastectomy, a* term used to define a procedure in which the entire mammary gland is removed, but both pectoral muscles and axillary lymph nodes are undisturbed.

Today, mastectomy generally includes removal of the breast tissue from the clavicle to the rectus abdominous and between the sternal edge and the latissimus dorsi muscles. It also removes the nipple-areolar complex (NAC), the excess skin of the breast, and the fascia of the pectoralis major muscle. When mastectomy is

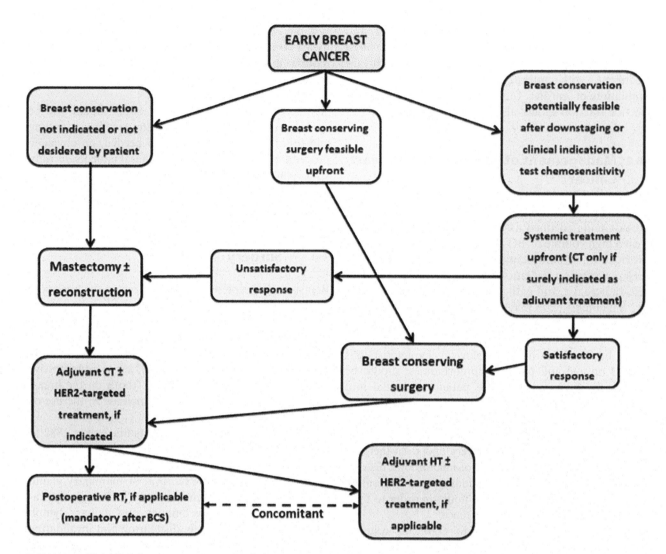

● **Fig. 30.1** Multidisciplinary management of early breast cancer

accompanied by axillary dissection, it is also termed modified radical mastectomy.

To ameliorate esthetic results, skin-sparing or nipple sparing mastectomy can be used. In skin-sparing mastectomy, skin excision is limited to the NAC and excisional biopsy scar, preserving the skin envelope of the breast and facilitating reconstruction. Traditionally, skin-sparing mastectomy included resection of the NAC to avoid the risk of leaving behind malignancy within the ducts of the nipple. Nipple-sparing mastectomy preserves the NAC (after residual cancer beneath the nipple is excluded by intraoperative frozen assessment) and generally guaranties excellent cosmetic results.

Over the last 50 years, the major change in the surgical treatment of primary BC has been a shift toward *breast-conserving treatment* (BCT). The goal of BCT is to use the combination of conservative surgery and radiotherapy to provide survival equivalent to mastectomy with preservation of the cosmetic appearance and a low rate of recurrence in the treated breast. Medical contraindications to the use of BCT are generally infrequent and currently, in Western Europe, 60%–80% of newly diagnosed cancers are amenable to breast conservation. Despite improvements in esthetic results, there is concern regarding the increase in rates of voluntary mastectomy (due to patient choice and not to medical reasons) in the last years. Moreover, many patients also ask for voluntary contralateral (prophylactic) breast amputation. Although patient's choice should be taken into account, physicians have a clear ethical responsibility to completely inform patients about the options and consequences.

30.8.1.1 Breast Conservation Treatment: Modalities and Risk of Local Relapse

BCT involves the combination of conservative surgery and radiotherapy for the local treatment of BC.

Conservative surgery is usually achieved through on of two main surgical procedures:

- Quadrantectomy, which implies the surgical removal of the tumor plus a large portion of surrounding healthy mammary gland, overlying skin and the pectoral fascia section beneath it.
- Lumpectomy (also known as wide local excision) only involves surgical removal of the tumor and a small portion of surrounding breast tissue.

A large number of randomized clinical trials have been conducted comparing mastectomy and BCT, and have demonstrated equivalent survival, even at long follow-up (20-year follow-up reports of the two largest studies, the NSABP B-06 and Milan I trials are available) [54, 55]. Moreover, the incidence of local relapse (LR) after BCT has declined over time, from 8–19% at 10-years in initial randomized trials to 2–7% in more recent studies. This decrease results from improved mammographic and pathologic evaluation and more frequent use of adjuvant systemic therapy.

Risk factors for locoregional recurrence after BCT can be divided into patient, tumor, and treatment factors:

- Young age (<35 or 40) is associated with increased risk of LR after BCT (even when correction is for pathologic features is applied) and is also a risk factor for LR after mastectomy
- Inherited susceptibility: BRCA1 and BRCA2 mutation carriers have a substantial risk of contralateral and late ipsilateral BC (most are second primary cancers). In these patients, the option of bilateral mastectomy should be considered (especially in young and early-stage patients) to avoid the long-term risk of a second BC in either breast.
- Margin of resection: patients with negative margins have lower rates of LR after BCT. However, there is no standard definition of a close margin and the impact of close margins on local relapse is controversial. To date, "no ink on tumor" (the absence of cancer cells at inked surfaces) remains the standard for an adequate margin in invasive cancer [56].
- Tumor biology is the most significant determinant of likelihood of LR after BCT (and mastectomy): patients with triple-negative BC are at higher risk, regardless of surgical technique.

- Supplementary irradiation to primary tumor area (boost) reduces (by 40%) the risk of ipsilateral LR, but does not impact survival [57].
- The use of adjuvant systemic therapy after BCT also significantly reduces the risk of LR

BCT requires careful patient selection and a multidisciplinary approach. A recent preoperative mammographic evaluation is necessary to determine patient eligibility (evaluate extent of the disease, presence or absence of multicentricity or microcalcifications) and should include evaluation of the contralateral breast to exclude synchronous lesions.

Some patients still undergone mastectomy due to the following:

- Tumor size (relative to breast size)
- Tumor multicentricity
- Inability to achieve negative surgical margins after multiple resections
- Patient choice
- Absolute or relative contraindications to RT, such as:
  - Ongoing pregnancy (absolute)
  - Diffuse suspicious microcalcifications (absolute)
  - Active connective tissue disease involving the skin (e.g., scleroderma and lupus) (relative)
  - Tumors >5 cm (relative)
  - Focally positive margin (relative)
  - Prophylactic bilateral mastectomy for risk reduction is under consideration (relative)

Whole-breast irradiation (WBI) is effective at eradicating subclinical multicentric foci of breast carcinoma present at the time of diagnosis but does not prevent subsequent development of new cancers in the treated breast. Therefore, patients who elect BCT require life-long follow-up for the development of new cancers in the treated and contralateral breast.

30.8.1.2 Breast Reconstruction After Breast Surgery

For women undergoing mastectomy and wishing for breast reconstruction, a wide range of surgical options are available. The best technique should be discussed individually taking into account anatomic, treatment and patient preference.

The two major reconstructive techniques involve the following:

- Use of implants and/or tissue expanders (best suited for small/medium sized breasts with minimal ptosis)
- Use of myocutaneous tissue flaps (more flexible in the size and shape of the reconstructed breast)

For autologous tissue flaps, tissue can be taken from the latissimus dorsi muscle, from the transverse rectus abdominis muscle, from the free deep inferior epigastric perforator flap, from the superior gluteal artery-based perforator flap, or from the free gracilis-based flap. It generally tolerates postoperative RT better than implant-based reconstruction with more favorable esthetic outcomes. If postmastectomy radiotherapy is indicated, a temporary implant is usually positioned before RT.

Reconstruction may be immediate or delayed. Immediate reconstruction has the advantages of avoiding a second operative procedure and the psychological impact of breast loss. However, some patients might be advised against immediate reconstruction for oncological reasons (e.g., inflammatory BC).

30.8.1.3 Advances in Axillary Management

For many years, complete axillary dissection with removal of axillary lymph nodes has been considered standard surgical management of the axilla for patients with invasive BC and a critical component of the cure of BC. This idea was undermined by the NSABP B-04 trial, in which clinically node-negative patients were randomized to radical mastectomy (including axillary dissection), total mastectomy with RT to regional lymphatics, or total mastectomy and observation, in which delayed axillary dissection was only performed if axillary lymph nodes metastases developed. In this trial, patients treated with axillary surgery did not show a survival benefit [54].

Nevertheless, as lymph node status is one of the strongest predictors of long-term prognosis in primary BC, axillary dissection continued to be used primarily as staging procedure, while maintaining local disease control in the axilla and some therapeutic value for some patients with axillary nodal metastases.

However, axillary dissection is associated with high incidence (up to 25%) of upper limb lymphedema, which increases significantly (up to 40%) when axillary dissection is combined with RT to the axilla and that can become an invalidating sequela. On this basis, lymphatic mapping and sentinel node biopsy progressively replaced axillary dissection as staging procedure of choice in clinically node-negative patients. In the American College of Surgeons Oncology Group (ACOSOG) Z10 trial, a sentinel node could be identified in >95% of cases with the use of blue dye alone, radiocolloid alone, or the combination of the two. Complications were rare and lymphedema only occurred in 5% of patients [58]. Moreover, despite a 10% false-negative rate, patients treated by sentinel node biopsy alone showed an extremely low rate of LR in the axilla if the sentinel node did not contain metastases. Contraindications to the procedure included pregnancy and lactation (rela-

tive), and locally advanced BC (LABC). The presence of isolated tumor cells (<0.2 mm deposits) and micrometastases (>0.2 mm, <2.0 mm) in axillary nodes does not associate with any significant overall survival difference, and no difference in LR rate was observed if axillary dissection was omitted in these patients [59, 60]. Therefore, the routine use of serial sections and IHC to detect micrometastases is not warranted.

Traditionally, the presence of macrometastases in the sentinel node mandated axillary lymph node clearance. The ACOSOG Z0011 prospective randomized study tested the need for axillary dissection in clinically node-negative women with macrometastases to less than three sentinel nodes. Almost 900 patients were randomized. Five-year nodal recurrence rate was very low in both arms (0.5% in the dissection arm and 0.9% in the sentinel node biopsy alone arm) and no trend toward a survival benefit for dissection was observed. As expected, morbidity was significantly lower in the sentinel node group. However, all patients in this study underwent BCT (consequently receiving irradiation of the low axilla by breast radiotherapy tangents) and 97% of patients received systemic therapy. Therefore, these findings do not apply to women with clinically positive nodes, extensive nodal involvement, those undergoing partial breast irradiation or treatment with mastectomy [59].

Another option for the management of axilla in patients with clinically negative nodes and sentinel lymph node metastases is axillary irradiation. In fact, the AMAROS trial randomized these patients to receive irradiation of axillary and supraclavicular fields or axillary dissection and did not show a significant difference in 5-year disease-free survival (1.0% vs 0.5%) with lower incidence of lymphedema in patients treated with radiotherapy as compared to those who received surgery (14% vs 28%) [61].

At present, it is clear that axillary dissection is no longer the standard approach for all patients with positive sentinel nodes treated with BCT including whole-breast RT. However, which is the optimal approach for these patients remains a matter of debate.

Another matter of debate is axillary approach in patients receiving neoadjuvant treatment. If preoperative systemic treatment is planned, ultrasound-guided fine-needle aspiration or core biopsy of suspicious lymph nodes before treatment should be carried out as a minimum. In patients with clinically and imaging negative axilla, the best timing to carry out sentinel lymph node biopsy (if before or after preoperative therapy) remains controversial. If fact, the SENTINA and ACOSOG Z1071 trials reported lower detection rates and higher rates of false-negatives when SLNB is carried out after systemic therapy, compared with SNLB that is carried out before neoadjuvant chemotherapy [62, 63]. However, if the axilla is negative at imaging evaluation before treatment and three or more lymph nodes are excised, a post-systemic therapy SNLB can be considered [27].

30.8.2 Local Management of Breast Cancer: Radiotherapy

30.8.2.1 Radiotherapy after Breast-Conserving Treatment

Whole-breast RT is strongly recommended after breast-conserving surgery [72], as it reduces the risk of LR and long-term BC-related mortality (3.8% reduction in BC mortality at 15 years). In elderly (>70 years old), selected patients with low risk of recurrence (small, biologically indolent tumors) receiving endocrine treatment omission of RT after breast-conserving surgery can be discussed in case of comorbidities.

Boost irradiation further reduces the risk of LR and is indicated for patients with unfavorable risk factors such as age <50 years, grade 3 tumors, extensive DCIS, vascular invasion, or focally positive margin [73, 74].

Traditionally, doses used for local and/or regional adjuvant irradiation are 45–50 Gy in 25–28 fractions followed by a 10–16 Gy boost in 2 Gy doses. Shorter fractionation schemes (e.g., 15–16 fractions with 2.5 Gy doses) have been tested showing similar efficacy without increases in side effects and are now considered a standard for whole-breast RT after breast-conserving surgery in most low-risk patients. However, young patients, patients with node-positive or high-grade tumors, and patients undergoing mastectomy and/or additional regional irradiation were under-represented in these trials and use of shorter fractionation schemes should be carefully evaluated case by case.

Another alternative schedule is accelerated partial breast irradiation (APBI), which is based on the rationale that most LR occur in the proximity of the primary tumor site. APBI can be performed using a number of different techniques, including interstitial brachytherapy, three-dimensional conformal external beam irradiation, intracavitary brachytherapy, and intraoperative radiotherapy. APBI by intraoperative radiotherapy was tested in two randomized trials, the ELIOT (single dose of electrons) and TARGIT (single intraoperative dose 50 kV X-rays) trials, which reported a significantly higher ipsilateral breast recurrence with APBI as compared to whole-breast radiotherapy [75, 76]. Despite this, APBI might be considered for the treatment of patients with an extremely low risk of LR (>60 years old, not BRCA mutated patients with unicentric, unifocal, node-negative, non-lobular BC, <2 cm, without

extensive intraductal components or vascular invasion, with negative margins, which will receive adjuvant hormonal treatment) [77].

30.8.2.2 Radiotherapy After Mastectomy

The use of postmastectomy RT has been evolving over the last decade. In fact, postmastectomy RT has been always recommended for high-risk patients, including positive resection margins, cutaneous involvement or ulceration, four or more involved axillary lymph nodes, and large tumors (>5 cm). However, it has been recently shown that, in node-positive BC patients, postmastectomy RT reduces by 10% the 10-year risk of any recurrence (locoregional and distant) and by 8% the 20-year risk of BC-related mortality, independently from the number of involved axillary lymph nodes and the administration of adjuvant systemic treatment [78]. Based on these data, postmastectomy RT should also be considered for patients with 1–3 positive lymph nodes carefully evaluating on an individual patient basis (taking into account patient age and biological characteristics) [78, 79].

Older trials usually used large RT fields encompassing the chest wall and all regional lymph nodes. The European Society for Radiotherapy and Oncology guidelines advise to include only the most caudal lymph nodes surrounding the sub-clavicular arch and the base of the jugular vein, while the resected part of the axilla (after axillary lymph node dissection) should not be irradiated, except in cases of residual disease after surgery. The Danish population-based study, in which left-sided BC patients received medial supraclavicular RT, while right-sided patients also received RT to the internal mammary nodes, seems to point out the importance of including internal mammary lymph nodes in the regional target volume.

30.8.2.3 Regional Irradiation After Breast-Conserving Surgery

Whole-breast RT is considered the standard after breast-conserving surgery [72]. However, a number of findings also support the use of regional RT in intermediate/high-risk patients treated with BCT. The MA.20 trial randomized high-risk node-negative or node-positive patients treated with breast-conserving surgery to breast irradiation alone or breast irradiation plus regional RT (including internal mammary and medial supraclavicular fields). Most patients included had 1–3 involved lymph nodes. The addition of regional RT prolonged isolated locoregional disease-free survival, distant disease-free survival and disease-free survival (82% vs 77% at 10-year follow-up), but did not have a significant impact on overall survival (82.8% vs 81.8% at 10-year follow-up) [64]. However, benefits and risks should be carefully evaluated on an individual patient basis taking into account also patient age and biological characteristics.

30.8.2.4 Radiotherapy for Unresectable Disease

Patients who present with unresectable non-metastatic disease are usually treated with primary systemic therapy. If disease is rendered resectable, it is then usually treated with surgery, followed by RT, in analogy with LABC. If the disease remains unresectable, however, RT can be considered to treat all sites of the original tumor extension with a boost to residual disease.

30.8.2.5 Toxicities of Breast Radiotherapy

Breast RT is generally well tolerated with few long-term toxicities. However, irradiation of the heart or of coronary arteries can result in premature ischemic heart disease [65]. A proportional relationship between RT dose to the heart and subsequent heart disease has been reported. Nevertheless, the absolute increase in lifetime risk is small and the risk of cardiac mortality is generally small as compared to the survival benefit from RT (both in BCT and postmastectomy). Moreover, current RT techniques spare most of the heart, reducing cardiac risk.

30.8.3 Adjuvant Systemic Treatment

The goal of adjuvant systemic therapy is to prevent BC recurrence by eradicating occult micrometastases already present at time of diagnosis. In fact, the hypothesis that, even in early stages of BC development, tumor cells are disseminated throughout the body has been validated through decades of clinical investigation. Approximately half of the decline in BC mortality observed in Westerns countries has been attributed to the use of adjuvant therapy [2].

Up to date, three systemic treatment modalities are available as adjuvant therapy for early-stage BC: endocrine treatment; chemotherapy and anti-*HER2* targeted treatment.

Selection of adjuvant treatment is based on predicted sensitivity to the specific treatment modality and on individual's risk of relapse (◘ Table 30.4). Chemotherapy is used for HR− tumors and alongside with HER2 targeted treatment in *HER2*+ tumors. Patients with HR+ tumors are candidates for adjuvant endocrine therapy and, for high-risk patients with chemosensitive tumors, chemotherapy is added.

The estimation of recurrence risk is obtained taking into account several *prognostic factors*:

- Nodal status: Nodal status is the most important prognostic factor (risk increases progressively with number of positive lymph nodes.

- Tumor size: Risk of recurrence increases with tumor size.
- Patient age: Very young patients ($\leq$35 years) have a poorer prognosis than older patients. Usually, BCs in these patients tend to be more often of higher grade and HR negative than in older patients. These differences probably explain in part the worse outcomes observed in very young patients [66].
- Grade: A high tumor grade (G3) is a negative prognostic factor.
- Proliferation (Ki67): High tumor proliferation is a negative prognostic factor. No clear cut-off exists, but 20% positivity for Ki67 is usually considered high proliferation.
- Histotype: Some rare special BC histotypes (e.g., tubular, mucinous, cribriform, and medullary) carry a better prognosis and a lower metastatic potential, while other rare histotypes, such as metaplastic BC have a worse prognosis.
- HR status: BCs are considered positive for HR if at least 1% of tumor cells express ER or PgR. However, tumors with an expression between 1% and 10% often present a clinical history similar to that of HR− tumors. Higher expression of HRs is associated with better prognosis.
- HER2 status: HER2 positivity is associated with more aggressive tumor biology in the absence of HER2-targeted treatment.
- Gene expression profiles: As previously discussed, several multigene tests have been recently introduced in clinical practice to select early BC patients with good prognosis which might be spared chemotherapy.

The choice of adjuvant treatment also takes into account the predicted sensitivity to the specific treatment, which is based on some *predictive factors*:

- HR status: Sensitivity to endocrine treatment is generally higher for tumors with higher levels of expression of HR as compared to tumors with lower levels. In fact, even if BCs are considered eligible for endocrine treatment if at least 1% of tumor cells express ER or PgR, it is well known that tumors with an expression between 1% and 10% are less sensitive to endocrine treatment.
- HER2 status: HER2 positivity is associated with sensitivity to HER2-targeted treatment and is used to select patients eligible for anti-HER2 treatment in clinical practice. HER2 is also a marker of benefit from adjuvant chemotherapy (HER2 overexpression being associated with a higher benefit from anthracycline-based chemotherapy) [67].
- Proliferation (Ki67): Tumors with high proliferation rates are more sensitive to chemotherapy and usually have a reduced sensitivity to endocrine treatment. In

Table 30.4 Surrogate intrinsic subtypes and recommended adjuvant therapy (Modified from Senkus et al. 2015)

Surrogate intrinsic subtype	IHC definition	Recommended adjuvant therapy
Luminal A-like	ER-positive HER2-negative Ki67 low[a] PgR high[b] low-risk molecular signature (if available)	ET alone in the majority of cases Consider CT if: high tumor burden (four or more positive LN, T3 or higher) or grade 3
Luminal B-like (HER2-negative)	ER-positive HER2-negative *and either* Ki67 high[a] *or* PgR low[b] high-risk molecular signature (if available)	ET + CT for majority of cases
Luminal B-like (HER2-positive)	ER-positive HER2-positive	CT + anti-HER2 + ET for all patients If contraindications for the use of CT, one may consider ET + anti-HER2
HER2-positive (non-luminal)	ER and PgR negative HER2-positive	CT + anti-HER2
Triple-negative (ductal)	ER and PgR negative HER2-negative	CT

ET endocrine therapy, *CT* chemotherapy, *LN* lymph node
[a]Ki-67 scores should be interpreted in the light of local laboratory values: as an example, if a laboratory has a median Ki-67 score in receptor-positive disease of 20%, values of 30% or above could be considered clearly high; those of 10% or less clearly low
[b]Suggested cut-off value is 20%

fact, Ki67 and PgR can be used as an IHC surrogate to distinguish Luminal A tumors from Luminal B tumors, which are more likely to be chemosensitive, for which chemotherapy is generally recommended in addition to endocrine treatment. However, IHC assessment of Ki67 is subjective and the St Gallen Consensus Guidelines recommend using the criteria of "clearly high" (>30%) and "clearly low" (<10%). Unclearly defined tumors according to IHC surrogates might benefit from gene expression profiling to more accurately estimate the potential benefit of adding chemotherapy (Table 30.4).

The final decision should also incorporate the predicted treatment sequelae, the patient's biological age, general health status, comorbidities, and preferences.

30.8.3.1 Endocrine Treatment

Adjuvant endocrine treatment is indicated for all patients with detectable HR expression (defined as ≥1% of invasive cancer cells) irrespective of the use of chemotherapy and/or targeted therapy. The choice of agent and its duration is primarily determined by the patient's menopausal status and risk of relapse. Differences in side-effect profiles are also present and may be taken into consideration in the decision. Tamoxifen and AIs are associated with different safety profiles. Tamoxifen is associated with an increased risk of thromboembolic complications and endometrial hyperplasia (including endometrial cancer) and should not be administered in patients using strong and moderate CYP2D6 inhibitors due to drug interaction. Patients treated with AIs are at increased risk of arthralgias and bone loss: adequate calcium and vitamin D3 intake should be administered, and they should undergo periodic assessment of their bone mineral density. All endocrine treatments can cause or worsen menopausal symptoms.

Standard duration of adjuvant endocrine treatment is at least 5 years, as shorter durations have been shown to result in inferior outcomes.

For postmenopausal women, endocrine treatment options include AIs and tamoxifen. Tamoxifen might still be a valid option for selected patients. Five years of adjuvant tamoxifen result in a 41% reduction in BC recurrence rate (HR = 0.59) and a 34% reduction in death rate (HR = 0.66) for women with HR+ BC [68]. The ATLAS trial, comparing 10 years to 5 years of adjuvant tamoxifen, have shown an improvement in overall survival and disease-free survival with the longer duration [69]. This finding is of particular relevance for women who lack the option of receiving extended adjuvant endocrine therapy with an AI, as for example premenopausal women (see the following) [27]. AIs are not appropriate for premenopausal patients not receiving ovarian suppression, as residual ovarian function can increase aromatase production overcoming the effects of AIs.

AIs can be used upfront (non-steroidal AI and exemestane), after 2–3 years of tamoxifen (non-steroidal AI and exemestane) or as extended adjuvant therapy, after 5 years of tamoxifen (letrozole and anastrozole) [27]. In the upfront setting, 5 years of AIs significantly reduce BC mortality as compared with 5 years of tamoxifen (15% more) and should be used upfront as treatment of choice in postmenopausal patients at high risk for relapse or with lobular histology [27]. For lower risk patients, the sequence can be decided on an individual basis, taking into account the

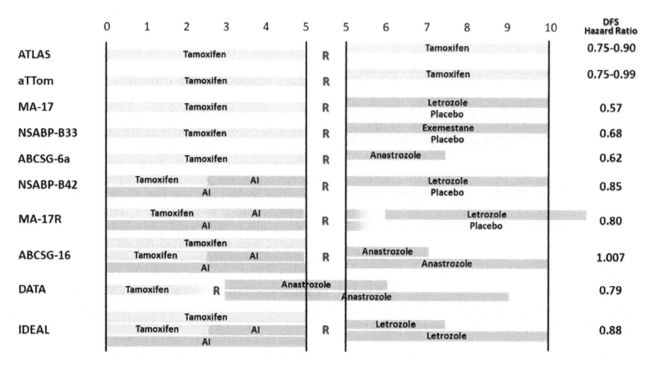

Fig. 30.2 Extended adjuvant endocrine treatment trials

different side-effect patterns. However, AIs should be considered at some point in the treatment program of postmenopausal women either as initial therapy or as sequential therapy after 2–3 years of tamoxifen [70]. The optimal duration and regimen of adjuvant ET is currently unknown. The extension of endocrine therapy beyond 5 years, underscoring the long natural history of HR+ BC, might be of benefit after initial tamoxifen, with improved outcomes seen in the ATLAS, aTTom, MA.17, and NSABP-B33 trials, but is of lesser benefit after initial AIs (IDEAL, NSABP-B42, MA-17R) (■ Fig. 30.2). Due to associated adverse effects, and limited absolute benefit in low-risk disease, it is more appropriate to reserve extended ET for high-risk disease.

Premenopausal women may be treated with tamoxifen alone, tamoxifen + ovarian function suppression (OFS), or an AI + OFS, according to estimated risk of relapse and patient's preference.

The combination of an AI + OFS has been shown to reduce recurrence as compared with tamoxifen + OFS, and the addition of OFS to tamoxifen has been shown to reduce recurrence as compared to tamoxifen alone. However, the addition of OFS to endocrine treatment also significantly increases adverse effects, in particular menopausal and sexual symptoms. For this reason, AI + OFS can be considered for higher risk cases (e.g., those treated with adjuvant chemotherapy), for which the absolute benefit over tamoxifen +/– OFS is greater [71].

Monitoring the bone health of these young women, especially those taking AIs or OFS, is crucial.

Tamoxifen alone can be enough for very-low-risk premenopausal patients, where outcomes are good and, in rare cases where both tamoxifen and AIs are not tolerated, a GnRH agonist alone may be considered. For premenopausal women not receiving OFS, prolongation of tamoxifen duration to 10 years, according to the ATLAS trial, might be of benefit as an improvement in overall survival and disease-free survival has been reported with the longer duration [69]. In patients becoming postmenopausal during the first 5 years of tamoxifen, switch to AIs should be considered [27].

30.8.3.2 Chemotherapy

Adjuvant chemotherapy, consisting of multiple cycles of polychemotherapy, is a well-established strategy for lowering the risk of BC recurrence and improving survival. Chemotherapy is recommended in the vast majority of triple-negative (with the possible exception of low-risk rare histological subtypes), HER2+ BCs (apart from selected cases with very low risk, such as T1aN0) and in high-risk HR+ HER2- tumors.

Over time, several chemotherapy regimens have been tested for the adjuvant treatment of BC:

- *First-generation regimens*: the combination of cyclophosphamide, methotrexate and 5-fluorouracil (CMF) was the first widely used regimen. Today it may still be used in selected patients.

- *Second-generation regimens*: anthracycline containing regimens (such as EC: epirubicin-cyclophosphamide or AC: adriamycin-cyclophosphamide) were proven to be more efficient in terms of relapse reduction (11%) and mortality reduction (16%) as compared to the same duration of first generation CMF. However, anthracyclines are associated with cardiotoxicity and might be contraindicated in case of concomitant cardiomyopathy or important cardiovascular risk factors.
- *Third-generation regimens:* The addition of taxanes to anthracyclines (in combination or sequentially) improves the efficacy of chemotherapy, at the cost of increased non-cardiac toxicity (peripheral neuropathy) [27]. Anthracyclines-taxanes based regimens reduce BC mortality by about one-third [72]. On this basis, for women who warrant chemotherapy, sequential regimens (AC/EC for 3–4 cycles followed by paclitaxel or docetaxel) are today considered the "gold standard." After four cycles of anthracyclines, weekly paclitaxel or three-weekly docetaxel (more myelotoxic) are the preferred regimens. Sequential regimens present the best efficacy combined with less toxicity as compared to combination regimens (such as TAC: docetaxel-adriamycin-cyclophosphamide) or TEC (docetaxel-epirubicin-cyclophosphamide).

The addition of 5-fluorouracil to EC (epirubicin and cyclophosphamide)-paclitaxel sequence does not improve efficacy [73]. Similarly, the addition of other drugs such as capecitabine or gemcitabine to an anthracycline-taxane regimen was not successful in phase 3 trials.

Chemotherapy is usually administered for four to eight cycles (12–24 weeks), depending on individual risk of recurrence and selected regimen. For high-risk tumors, the use of dose-dense schedules (biweekly instead of three-weekly administration with granulocyte colony-stimulating factor support) should be considered [27]. High-dose chemotherapy with stem cell support should not be used.

As an alternative to four cycles of anthracycline-based chemotherapy, taxane-based regimens, such as four cycles of docetaxel and cyclophosphamide (TC), have been developed, showing superior disease-free survival and overall survival [74]. However, these regimens are less efficacious than sequential regimens (a small 2.5% difference in invasive disease-free survival was reported when 6 cycles of TC were compared with the sequential regimen). Therefore, these regimens are not a standard for all patients, but can be used as an effective anthracycline-free option for selected patients (i.e., those with cardiac risk factors or at intermediate risk of relapse).

For patients with triple-negative BC, several neoadjuvant trials have tested the addition of platinum to a neoadjuvant anthracycline-taxane combination or sequence, improving pathological complete response. However, only some of these studies reported a consensual improvement in disease-free survival [75]. Since platinum adds toxicity and no robust, prospective randomized data exists on its use in the adjuvant setting, its addition is not routinely recommended. However, its use can be discussed with triple-negative BC patients.

In young BC patients receiving chemotherapy, the impact on subsequent fertility should be discussed. Fertility preservation techniques, such as oocyte cryopreservation or embryo cryopreservation, are available. Moreover, GnRH agonists can be used during chemotherapy to prevent chemotherapy-related ovarian failure, resulting in less premature ovarian failures and more pregnancies [76]. A decision should be taken in a case-by-case manner, after discussion with the patient regarding benefits and risks.

In general, chemotherapy should not be used concomitantly with endocrine treatment, which is usually started after chemotherapy completion, and radiotherapy, if planned, usually follows chemotherapy. Radiotherapy can be safely delivered concomitantly with trastuzumab, endocrine treatment and non-anthracycline–non-taxane-based chemotherapy [27].

30.8.3.3 Bone-Stabilizing Agents

In early BC, bisphosphonates were initially used to prevent side effects of adjuvant endocrine treatments on bone. However, several large clinical trials have shown outcome benefits for oral and intravenous adjuvant bisphosphonates. The large EBCTCG meta-analysis showed that adjuvant bisphosphonates reduced BC recurrence in bone, and improved BC survival [77]. However, the benefit appears to higher in postmenopausal patients, or in premenopausal patients receiving adjuvant ovarian suppression. Prophylactic use of bisphosphonates is not formally approved in most countries.

30.8.3.4 HER2-Targeted Treament

For HER2+ BC, the addition of trastuzumab (anti-HER2 monoclonal antibody) to adjuvant chemotherapy nearly halves recurrence risk translating into a 10% absolute improvement in long-term disease-free survival and 9% increase in 10-year overall survival. Subset analyses demonstrated comparable relative risk reduction regardless of tumor size, nodal status, or hormone receptor status.

Due to its cardiotoxicity risk, trastuzumab should not be routinely administered concomitantly with anthracyclines. However, combination with non-anthracycline-based chemotherapy, endocrine treatment and radiotherapy is safe. Moreover, concurrent administration of trastuzumab and chemotherapy is more active than sequential therapy, and for most patients, sequential anthracycline-based followed by taxane–trastuzumab-based regimen is the preferred choice.

Trastuzumab cardiotoxicity is typically characterized by a decrease in left ventricular ejection fraction (LVEF), which is usually asymptomatic, and often resolves with drug withdrawal. In these cases, rechallenge with trastuzumab is usually feasible. Rarely, trastuzumab cardiotoxicity may evolve in symptomatic cardiac failure. Risk factors for cardiac dysfunction with adjuvant trastuzumab include anthracycline administration, preexisting cardiac disease (e.g., borderline normal LVEF or hypertension), and age >65 years. All patients being considered for adjuvant trastuzumab require baseline determination and subsequent 3-monthly monitoring of LVEF. Cardiologist input is recommended in case of cardiotoxicity.

Standard trastuzumab duration is 12 months, as in most studies trastuzumab was administered for 12 months. Several trials tested different trastuzumab durations. The HERA trial failed to demonstrate an additional benefit for 2 years vs 1 year of trastuzumab administration [78], while the PHARE and HORG trials failed to demonstrate the non-inferiority of 6 months of trastuzumab [79, 80]. The SOLD and ShortHER trial, which tested 9 weeks of trastuzumab, also failed to demonstrate non-inferiority of the shorter regimen. However, subgroup analysis suggests that in patients with stage I-II HER2+ BC the shorter regimen might have similar efficacy, with less cardiotoxicity [81, 82]. Moreover, results from the large randomized Persephone trial, enrolling more than 4000 women, have recently shown in patients treated with 6 months of trastuzumab a similar rate of disease-free survival as those treated for 12 months (4-years disease-free survival rate was 89.4% in the 6-month group and 89.8% in the 12-month group) with less cardiotoxicity (4% of patients had to stop the drug early due to cardiac toxicity vs 8%). On this basis, a shorter duration of trastuzumab might be considered in selected patients with low risk of recurrence or cardiac risk factors.

To reduce cardiac toxicity, anthracycline-free regimens such as TCH (docetaxel-carboplatin-trastuzumab) have also been proposed. However, efficacy also appeared to be lower than with the anthracycline-taxane sequence plus trastuzumab (5-year disease-free survival of 81% for TCH vs 84% for anthracycline-taxane sequence plus trastuzumab, the study was not powered for this comparison).

Moreover, in node-negative patients with tumor diameters up to 3 cm, a small prospective non-randomized trial of 12 weeks of paclitaxel plus trastuzumab, followed by 1 year of adjuvant trastuzumab, yielded a remarkably low risk of recurrence (3-year invasive disease-free survival of 98·7%) and can be considered an option for these low-risk HER2+ BCs. This regimen might also represent an option for patients with HER2+ N0 tumors 5–10 mm, which were not included in the seminal trials but that have a relatively high failure risk, particularly in HR− disease.

HR+/HER2+ early BCs are usually treated with chemotherapy followed by endocrine treatment, in combination with trastuzumab. No randomized data exist to support an endocrine therapy-trastuzumab combination without chemotherapy in this group.

Treatment escalation using a second HER2-targeting agent has been tested.

In the neoadjuvant setting, dual HER2 blockade (trastuzumab + lapatinib, trastuzumab + pertuzumab) associated with chemotherapy has led to improvements in pathological complete response (pCR) rate as compared with chemotherapy plus trastuzumab and is currently approved in several countries. However, for the combination of trastuzumab and lapatinib, the significant pathological complete response advantage observed in NeoALTTO did not translate into a significant survival advantage 29. Similarly, no significant survival advantage was observed from the addition of lapatinib in the adjuvant setting. Therefore, the combination of trastuzumab and lapatinib cannot be recommended [27]. By contrast, the combination of trastuzumab and pertuzumab combination received approval by both the US FDA and EMA for the neoadjuvant setting. In the adjuvant setting, the large randomized APHINITY trial, testing the addition of pertuzumab to standard chemotherapy plus trastuzumab, showed a small but statistically significant decrease in the risk of invasive recurrence (3-year rates of invasive-disease-free survival were 94.1% vs 93.2%). The difference was more relevant in patients with node-positive disease (3-year invasive-disease-free survival rate 92.0% vs 90.2%) and in HR− tumors. Based on these data, the combination of pertuzumab and trastuzumab has been approved in several countries. However, in consideration of its limited impact, risks and benefits for the specific patient should be carefully assessed.

The administration of neratinib for one additional year after completion of adjuvant trastuzumab has been tested in the large randomized ExteNET trial. A 5-year invasive disease-free survival benefit was reported for patients receiving neratinib (90.2% vs 87.7%), and the benefit was more evident in the HR+ subgroup (5-year invasive disease-free survival 91.2% vs 86.8%, HR 0.60), while the HR− cohort did not show a significant benefit (88.9% vs 88.8%, HR 0.95). Based on these data, the adjuvant use of neratinib for high-risk HER2+ BC has been approved in the United States and in Europe (only in the HR+ subgroup) (◘ Fig. 30.3).

30.8.4 Preoperative Systemic Therapy

In early BC, preoperative chemotherapy is equally effective as postoperative chemotherapy in terms of disease-free survival and overall survival. Therefore, in addition to patients with inoperable BC, neoadjuvant systemic therapy has also emerged as an option for patients in which BCT is not feasible upfront, due to tumor size, provided that the patient has a clear indication for adjuvant chemotherapy. Overtreatment for simple local tumor reduction should indeed be avoided and neoadjuvant systemic therapy should only be given if the same therapy is indicated in the adjuvant setting.

Nevertheless, neoadjuvant treatment represents an opportunity for several BC patients. Prospective, randomized trials of patients with operable BC have shown high rates of clinical response to neoadjuvant chemotherapy (50–85%, higher in HER+ and triple-negative BC), and 25–30% of patients who were not candidates for BCT upfront were able to undergo the procedure after preoperative treatment. Moreover, pCR, defined as the absence of residual invasive cancer in the breast and axilla following preoperative therapy, can be achieved in a significant number of patients (15–40%). A meta-analysis including over 13.000 BC patients has shown that patients achieving pCR have better long-term outcomes, with lower risk of cancer recurrence, as compared to women with residual cancer [52]. Since pCR is strongly correlated with patient outcome in triple-negative and HER2+ BC, neoadjuvant therapy has become a preferred option for these patients. In fact, response allows refined counseling about the expected individual prognosis.

In the neoadjuvant setting, it is generally recommended to deliver all planned chemotherapy before surgery without unnecessary breaks to maintain dose intensity and increase the probability of pCR. After delivery of 6–8 cycles of sequential anthracyclines-taxanes, additional chemotherapy in the adjuvant setting has no proven benefit, even in the absence of pCR. However, several clinical trials are now specifically available for patients with HER2+ and triple-negative BC with residual disease. Indeed, the KATHERINE trial, which randomized HER2+ BC patients with resid-

ual disease after standard neoadjuvant treatment to receive trastuzumab emtansine (TDM-1) vs trastuzumab to complete one-year of anti-HER2 therapy, reported a significant improvement in invasive disease-free survival with TDM-1. In a similar context, the CreateX trial recently reported the potential efficacy of 6 months of adjuvant capecitabine in patient with HER2- residual disease after neoadjuvant treatment.

Neoadjuvant endocrine therapy can also be used to increase BCT rates. In postmenopausal women with HR+ tumors, the preoperative use of an AI or tamoxifen significantly increases the likelihood of breast conservation (30–40% after 4 months of treatment). In clinical practice, neoadjuvant endocrine therapy (4–8 months) is typically reserved for women not considered candidates for neoadjuvant chemotherapy (i.e., comorbidities or tumor subtypes less responsive to chemotherapy such as the lobular subtype). Due to limited data, preoperative endocrine treatment is not routinely recommended in premenopausal patients outside clinical trials.

Surgery after neoadjuvant chemotherapy has dramatically changed. Initially, the rule was to excise the original tumor bed; however, currently "no ink on tumor" is considered a standard even in the post-neoadjuvant setting. Percutaneous placement of marker clips within the primary tumor prior to the initiation of neoadjuvant treatment provides a landmark for excision in case of complete response.

Radiotherapy is generally planned based on pre-treatment disease extension.

In some rare cases, a disease progression might be observed during neoadjuvant treatment. These cases usually receive non-cross resistant chemotherapy or salvage radiotherapy to achieve radical surgery.

30.9 Follow-Up for Breast Cancer Survivors

Following initial treatment for BC, patients require surveillance for LR, contralateral BC, and distant metastatic disease. Moreover, monitoring of late treatment side effects and management of endocrine treatment is needed. Even if the maximum risk of recurrence is in the first 5 years after surgery, women with HR+ BC remain at risk for many years after treatment.

The principal aim of follow-up in BC survivors is identifying potentially curable disease, in order to improve patient outcome. Locoregional recurrences and new contralateral cancers are potentially curable, so there is a clear indication for women to undergo an annual mammography and breast examination. By contrast, it is not clear if early detection of distant meta-

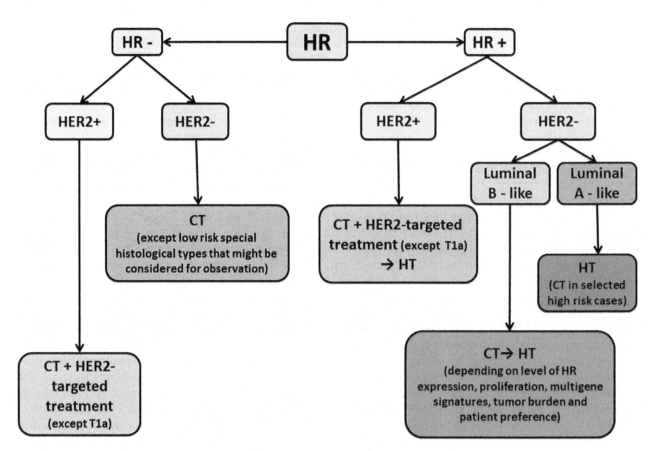

Fig. 30.3 Flowchart of adjuvant systemic treatment decision according to tumor biology

static disease can improve patient outcome. Randomized trials have compared intensive surveillance with imaging (chest X-ray, bone scan, and liver ultrasound) and blood exams (blood counts, liver function tests, and serum tumor markers) against regular physical examination and annual mammography, with additional testing performed only if clinically indicated. Intensive surveillance only achieved a modest increase in early detection of metastases in asymptomatic patients, but no impact on overall survival was observed. Based on these data, surveillance guidelines for women with early-stage BC emphasize the importance of careful history and examination to elicit symptoms or signs of recurrence and minimize the role of routine imaging and laboratory testing [27]. However, these guidelines might change in the future as efficacy of treatment in the metastatic setting increases.

30.10 Inflammatory Breast Cancer

Inflammatory BC accounts for 1–5% of all cases of BC and is characterized by diffuse erythema and edema of breast skin (peau d'orange) usually associated with a diffuse thickening of the breast. The clinical presentation results from tumor emboli in the dermal lymphat-

ics. Inflammatory BC typically has a rapid onset and is often initially mistaken as infection. Once diagnosis is achieved, inflammatory BC is treated with neoadjuvant chemotherapy followed if possible by mastectomy. BCT is contraindicated in patients with inflammatory BC, even if a complete response is achieve, due to its diffuse nature.

30.11 Management of In Situ Malignancy

30.11.1 Surgery for In Situ Malignancy

DCIS can be treated with total mastectomy or BCT provided that adequate resection margins can be achieved. No DCIS on inked margins is considered a minimal requirement. However, no clear consensus exists regarding what should be considered an adequate margin and circumferential margins <2 mm are generally considered less than adequate. Axillary lymph node evaluation is not generally required for DCIS. Nevertheless, sentinel lymph node biopsy can be used for large and/or high-grade tumors, especially if treated with mastectomy, in case an invasive cancer is subsequently accidentally identified in the surgical specimen. Lobular neoplasia (formerly called LCIS) is only regarded as a risk factor for future development of invasive cancer and does not require active treatment. However, its pleomorphic variant may behave similarly to DCIS and is usually treated accordingly (multidisciplinary evaluation needed).

30.11.2 Radiotherapy for In Situ Malignancy

WBRT after breast-conserving surgery for DCIS decreases the risk of LR. The decrease is evident in all subgroups; however, in some patients with low-risk DCIS (<10 mm, G1/G2 nuclear grade, adequate surgical margins), the risk of local recurrence is so low that omitting RT can be an option. After total mastectomy with clear margins for DCIS, postmastectomy RT is not recommended.

30.11.3 Systemic Adjuvant Therapy for In Situ Malignancy

In patients undergoing BCT for HR+ DCIS, tamoxifen decreases the risk of both invasive and noninvasive recurrences and reduces the incidence of second primary (contralateral) BC, without effects on overall survival. Following mastectomy, tamoxifen can decrease the risk of contralateral BC. However, the use of endocrine treatment is sometimes limited by concerns about side effects and by the absence of survival benefit.

30.12 Management of Locoregional Recurrence

Locoregional recurrence (LRR) after BC includes breast recurrences after BCT, chest wall recurrence after mastectomy, and regional nodal recurrences. It accounts for about 15% of all BC recurrences and is associated with higher stage, young age, positive margins, and intrinsic subtype (lower risk in Luminal A). Locoregional recurrence is an important predictor of metastatic disease: more than 60% of patients with LRR will eventually develop metastases (patients with short disease-free intervals, lymph node recurrence, skin lesions, and HR− tumors being at higher risk).

For this reason, patients with LRR should be accurately restaged to exclude concurrent metastatic disease.

Once metastatic disease has been ruled out, patients with LRR are treated with curative intent. Treatment is multidisciplinary and individualized based on site, prior local and systemic therapy. Usually, the first step is surgical resection. Women previously treated with BCT are treated with salvage mastectomy, patients with localized chest wall recurrences undergo surgical excision and axillary dissection is indicated for axillary nodal recurrences. Radiotherapy can also be used based on site of recurrence and previous irradiation fields.

Systemic therapy following local management is also recommended. For HR+ BC, LRR warrants the introduction or switching of endocrine therapy (e.g., for recurrences on tamoxifen, AIs should be considered). For HER2+ LRR, initiation or re-institution of anti-*HER2* therapy in an adjuvant fashion should be considered. The role of chemotherapy in this setting is more controversial, especially for patients previously treated with adjuvant chemotherapy. The CALOR trial randomized patients to "adjuvant" chemotherapy following optimal resection of LRR and a reduction in subsequent cancer recurrence, and an improvement in overall survival was observed. However, benefit was more evident in HR− tumors and no significant benefit was observed in the HR+ cohort. For patients previously treated with adjuvant chemotherapy, a non-overlapping regimen may be considered based on disease-free interval.

Case Study: Locally Advanced HER2-Positive Breast Cancer

Women, 60 years old
- *Family history* negative for malignancy
- *APR:* hypertension, hypercholesterolemia, emphysema
- *APP:* autopalpation of a mammary mass and axillary mass
- *Objective examination*: Palpable mass in the left breast (2 cm); palpable lymph nodes in the left axilla *cT1c cN2*
- *Bilateral Mammography and Ultrasonography*: in the superior external quadrant of the left breast radio opaque speculated nodule of about 1.9 cm of diameter; in the left axilla suspicious enlarged lymph nodes of 2.5 cm of maximum diameter

Question

What action should be taken?
(1) Surgery (2) Fine-needle cytology of breast mass (3) Fine-needle biopsy of the breast mass

Answer

Fine-needle biopsy of the breast mass
   Histological examination:
   Infiltrating ductal carcinoma, grade 3
   Er 0; PgR 0, Ki-67 40%, HER2 Score 3+

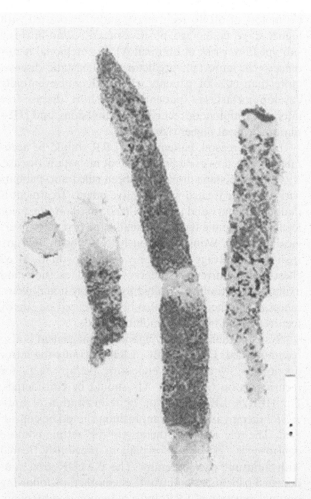

+ *Fine-needle biopsy of the axillary lymph node*
Histological examination:
Metastasis of infiltrating ductal carcinoma

Question

What action should be taken?
(1) Surgery (2) Start systemic treatment (3) Complete staging

Answer

Complete staging
CT scan *(thorax-abdomen):* 2 cm mass in the left breast, enlarged left axillary lymph nodes. No other lesions suspicious for metastases.

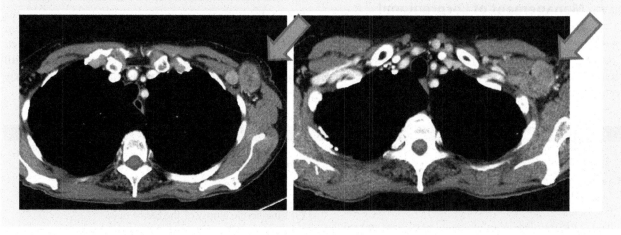

Bone scan: Negative

Blood tests: Normal results, CA15.3, and CEA within normality limits

Question

What action should be taken?

(1) Surgery (2) Start systemic therapy (3) Other
Answer

Start systemic therapy

Taxane + Trastuzumab (+ Pertuzumab, if available) for 3 months

⇩

Epirubicin-Cyclophosphamide for 4 cycles (3 months)

Response evaluation after neoadjuvant therapy: Complete clinical response; complete radiological response

Question

What action should be taken?

(1) Surgery (2) Continue systemic therapy (3) Start radiotherapy

Answer

Surgery: Quadrantectomy (superior external) of the left breast + axillary dissection

Histological examination:
Pathological complete response

Question

What action should be taken?

(1) Stop all treatment (2) Continue HER2-targeted treatment and start RT (3) Others

Answer

Continue HER2-targeted treatment and start RT

Trastuzumab 8 mg/kg q3w was continued for 9 months (1 year of treatment in total)

Radiation therapy delivered to the remaining breast (50 Gy + 16 Gy boost) + Regional RT

Key Points

– The importance of a correct diagnosis: histopathological diagnosis should be obtained by biopsy
– Importance of a correct staging before treatment in locally advanced breast cancer
– Use of neoadjuvant treatment in locally advanced breast cancer
– Importance of biological characteristics in treatment choice

Case Study: A Case of Triple-Negative Breast Cancer

Woman, 65 years old
– *Family history* negative for malignancy
– *APR:* negative
– *APP:* enlarged red breast since one month
– *Objective examination:* Skin edema and palpable supero-medial nodule in the right breast (4 cm)
– *Bilateral mammography and ultrasonography:* a 35 × 30 mm lesion in the upper medial quadrant of the right breast with multiple homolateral axillary lymph nodes
– *cT4b cN1*

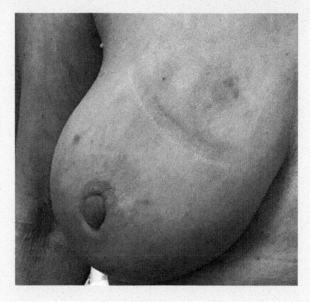

Question

What action should be taken?
   (1) Surgery (2) Biopsy (3) Other

Answer

Fine-needle biopsy of the breast mass
   Histological examination:
   Infiltrating ductal carcinoma, grade 3
   ER 0% PgR 0% Ki-67 80% HER2 0
   CT scan (thorax-abdomen): negative for metastasis
   Bone scan: negative for metastasis

Question

What action should be taken?
   (1) Surgery (2) Start systemic therapy (3) Start Radiotherapy

Answer

Start systemic therapy
   Weekly paclitaxel 80 mg/kg for 10 doses
   After 10 doses, *worsening of pain, edema, and erythema in the right breast -> Clinical progression of disease*

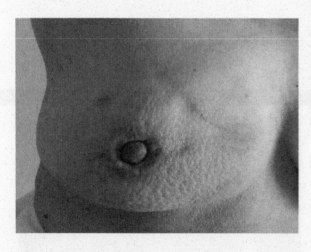

Restaging: Chest-abdomen CT scan (negative)
   Breast ultrasound: a 40 × 35 mm lesion in the upper medial quadrant of the right breast with multiple homolateral axillary lymph nodes

Question

What action should be taken?
   (1) Surgery (2) Switch to non-cross resistant systemic therapy (3) Best Supportive Care

Answer

Switch to non-cross resistant systemic therapy
   Epirubicin-Cyclophosphamide for 3 cycles (patient refuses to continue) with marginal clinical tumor response
   Surgery: Right mastectomy and homolateral axillary dissection
   Histological examination:
   Infiltrating ductal carcinoma ypT3 (6.5 cm) ypN3 (12 affected lymph nodes/13 resected lymph nodes)
   ER 0%, PR 0%, Ki67 50%, HER2 0
   At clinical examination: edema and erythema around the surgical scar

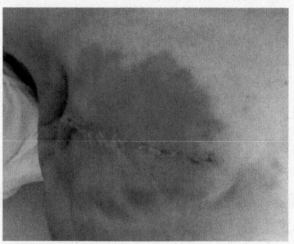

Skin biopsy: infiltrating ductal carcinoma G3 (triple-negative IHC) -> *locoregional recurrence*
   Patient starts salvage radiotherapy + Carboplatin

Key Points

- Importance of clinical examination in breast cancer staging and re-evaluation of response to treatment
- Importance of readapting treatment based on response
- Importance of biological characteristics in treatment choice

Expert Opinion
Antonio Russo

Key Points

Breast cancer is a major public health problem throughout the world.

- Multiple factors are associated with an increased risk of developing BC, such as age, gender, family history, genetic alterations, diet, and life style.
- In women, aged between 50 and 69 years, benefits of population mammography screening appear to outwait risks, and mammography screening, repeated every 2 years, is recommended by most countries.
- Management strategies for high-risk women include intensive surveillance, chemoprevention with endocrine agents, and, for extremely selected patients, prophylactic surgery.
- Breast cancer is a biologically heterogeneous disease. Biological characteristics of the disease play a fundamental role in treatment choice.
- Histopathological diagnosis of breast cancer should be obtained by biopsy.
- Treatment of breast cancer patients should be provided by a multidisciplinary team and should be carried out in "breast units" defined as specialized departments that treat a high volume of BC patients.
- Locoregional treatment (surgery and radiotherapy) aims to the radical excision of macroscopic disease, local staging of the disease, and treatment of residual tumor cells in the breast and nodes in order to limit the risk of locoregional recurrence.
- Systemic treatment aims to eradicate systemic micrometastases which might have originated even from early stage BC, reducing the risk of distant and locoregional recurrence at the same time.

1. Breast cancer (BC) is the most frequent cancer in women (1.7 million cancer diagnosed per year), and today regarded as a major public health issue. In the last decades, there has been an increase in incidence and a reduction of mortality, probably due to the diffusion of screening campaigns.
2. BC is linked to several risk factors such as age, family history, or genetic predisposition (i.e., mutation in BRCA1, BRCA2 genes), parity, BMI, combined hormone replacement therapy (estrogen and progesterone), cigarette smoke, previous radiotherapy in thoracic region, and prior diagnosis of BC. It is almost likely that these factors interact in a multimodal manner; it is although possible to identify high-risk women who can be submitted previously to screening programs or preventive treatments (i.e., intense surveillance, chemoprevention with endocrine agents or prophylactic mastectomy).
3. Screening programs have changed the history of this neoplasm: mammography can detect small, non-palpable lesions. In women between 50 to 69 years of age, benefits of mammography appear higher than its risks; otherwise, limited evidence of effectiveness regard 40–49 year-old women.
4. According to the latest WHO classification, it is possible to recognize different types: invasive ductal carcinoma (the most frequent form), invasive lobular carcinoma (the second most frequent one), special types (i.e., pure tubular, mucinous, papillary etc.), and carcinoma in situ. It is possible to use also a molecular classification for BC that recognize five types: Luminal A, B, HER-2 enriched, basal-like, and normal-like, considering the expression of different genes. The most important prognostic and predictive factors are grading (1–3), estrogen and progesterone receptors, HER2 expression, and cellular proliferation.
5. Clinical presentation usually consists in the evidence of a palpable, non-tender, hard nodule; sometimes, the involvement of the nipple or the evidence of a cutaneous inflammation (inflammatory carcinoma), with edema, tenderness, and erythema is possible. Otherwise, it is possible to detect a nodule during the mammographic screening. Clinical examination is the first step, quite useful to understand the involvement of axillary supraclavicular, infraclavicular lymph nodes. Then a mammography is mandatory often accompanied by US, which allows to study regional lymph nodes. Biopsy ensures the presence of a BC, and it is essential to classify it; two methods can be used: FNA (usually used to assess axillary lymphnodes) or core needle biopsy; excisional biopsy nowadays is used just in particular features.
6. Treatments differ depending on stage and biology. Locoregional approaches consist in surgery (quadrantectomy, lumpectomy, or mastectomy with different techniques) and radiotherapy. Systemic therapies can be used in the neoadjuvant setting in order to shrink the tumor burden and allowing radical operability. After mastectomy, reconstructive techniques are usually implied using myocutaneous tissue flaps or implants and/or tissue expanders.

    Radiotherapy is strongly recommended after breast-conserving surgery reducing the risk of local recurrence of BC and post-mastectomy radiation and regional radiation can be used in higher-risk patients. Adjuvant therapy has the role to prevent BC recurrence, and it can consist in endocrine treatment, chemotherapy, and anti-HER2-targeted treatment (trastuzumab) considering the characteristics of the BC.
7. Follow-up is essential to early diagnose local and locoregional recurrences, contralateral BC, distant metastases and to monitor long-term treatment toxicities.

Recommendations

- Cardoso F, Kyriakides S, Ohno S, Penault-Llorca F, Poortmans P, Rubio IT, Zackrisson S, Senkus E. ESMO early breast cancer: ESMO clinical practice guidelines published in 2019. Ann Oncol. 2019;30:1194–220.
- Paluch-Shimon S, Cardoso F, Sessa C, Balmana J, Cardoso MJ, Gilbert F, Senkus E. Prevention and screening in BRCA mutation carriers and other breast/ovarian hereditary cancer syndromes: ESMO clinical practice guidelines published in 2016. Ann Oncol. 2016;27(suppl 5):v103–v110.
- NCCN guidelines for breast cancer.
- ESMO ▶ www.esmo.org/Guidelines/Breast-Cancer/Early-Breast-Cancer
- NCCN ▶ www.nccn.org/professionals/physician_gls/default.aspx#breast

Hints for a Deeper Insight

- Harbeck N, Penault-Llorca F, Cortes J, et al. Breast cancer. Nat Rev Dis Prim. 2019;5. ▶ https://doi.org/10.1038/s41572-019-0111-2.
- Burstein HJ, Curigliano G, Loibl S, et al. Estimating the benefits of therapy for early-stage breast cancer: the St. Gallen International Consensus Guidelines for the primary therapy of early breast cancer 2019. Ann Oncol. 2019;30:1541–57.
- Tung NM, Boughey JC, Pierce LJ, et al. Management of hereditary breast cancer: American Society of Clinical Oncology, American Society for Radiation Oncology, and Society of Surgical Oncology Guideline. J Clin Oncol. 2020:JCO2000299.
- Burstein HJ, Lacchetti C, Griggs JJ. Adjuvant endocrine therapy for women with hormone receptor-positive breast cancer: ASCO clinical practice guideline focused update. J Oncol Pract. 2019;15:106–7.
- EUSOMA. The requirements of a specialist breast unit. Eur J Cancer. 2000;36:2288–93.
- Breast Cancer Screening, Mammography, and Other Modalities: ▶ https://www.ncbi.nlm.nih.gov/pubmed/27741212.
- Global, Regional, and National Cancer Incidence, Mortality, Years of Life Lost, Years Lived With Disability, and Disability-Adjusted Life-Years for 29 Cancer Groups, 1990–2017: A Systematic Analysis for the Global Burden of Disease Study: ▶ https://www.ncbi.nlm.nih.gov/pubmed/31560378.
- Cardiotoxicity in breast cancer treatment: What about left ventricular diastolic function and left atrial function? ▶ https://www.ncbi.nlm.nih.gov/pubmed/31573712.
- 11 years' follow-up of trastuzumab after adjuvant chemotherapy in HER2-positive early breast cancer: final analysis of the HERceptin Adjuvant (HERA) trial: ▶ https://www.ncbi.nlm.nih.gov/pubmed/28215665.
- Imaging in the evaluation and follow-up of early and advanced breast cancer: When, why, and how often? ▶ https://www.ncbi.nlm.nih.gov/pubmed/27422453.

References

1. Torre LA, Siegel RL, Ward EM, Jemal A. Global cancer incidence and mortality rates and trends–an update. Cancer Epidemiol Biomark Prev. 2016;25:16–27.
2. Berry DA, Cronin KA, Plevritis SK, et al. Effect of screening and adjuvant therapy on mortality from breast cancer. N Engl J Med. 2005;353:1784–92.
3. Jemal A, Bray F, Center MM, Ferlay J, Ward E, Forman D. Global cancer statistics. CA Cancer J Clin. 2011;61:69–90.
4. McPherson K, Steel CM, Dixon JM. ABC of breast diseases. Breast cancer-epidemiology, risk factors, and genetics. BMJ. 2000;321:624–8.
5. Trichopoulos D, MacMahon B, Cole P. Menopause and breast cancer risk. J Natl Cancer Inst. 1972;48:605–13.
6. Bernstein L, Ross RK. Endogenous hormones and breast cancer risk. Epidemiol Rev. 1993;15:48–65.
7. Rosner B, Colditz GA, Willett WC. Reproductive risk factors in a prospective study of breast cancer: the Nurses' Health Study. Am J Epidemiol. 1994;139:819–35.
8. Melbye M, Wohlfahrt J, Olsen JH, Frisch M, Westergaard T, Helweg-Larsen K, Andersen PK. Induced abortion and the risk of breast cancer. N Engl J Med. 1997;336:81–5.
9. Chlebowski RT, Hendrix SL, Langer RD, et al. Influence of estrogen plus progestin on breast cancer and mammography in healthy postmenopausal women: the Women's Health Initiative Randomized Trial. JAMA. 2003;289:3243–53.
10. Beral V, Collaborators MWS. Breast cancer and hormone-replacement therapy in the Million Women Study. Lancet. 2003;362:419–27.
11. Chen WY, Rosner B, Hankinson SE, Colditz GA, Willett WC. Moderate alcohol consumption during adult life, drinking patterns, and breast cancer risk. JAMA. 2011;306:1884.
12. Neuhouser ML, Aragaki AK, Prentice RL, et al. Overweight, obesity, and postmenopausal invasive breast cancer risk. JAMA Oncol. 2015;1:611.
13. Keum N, Greenwood DC, Lee DH, Kim R, Aune D, Ju W, Hu FB, Giovannucci EL. Adult weight gain and adiposity-related cancers: a dose-response meta-analysis of prospective observational studies. JNCI J Natl Cancer Inst. 2015;107(2):djv088. https://doi.org/10.1093/jnci/djv088.
14. Elkin EB, Klem ML, Gonzales AM, et al. Characteristics and outcomes of breast cancer in women with and without a history of radiation for Hodgkin's lymphoma: a multi-institutional, matched cohort study. J Clin Oncol. 2011;29:2466–73.
15. Lakhani SR, Van De Vijver MJ, Jacquemier J, Anderson TJ, Osin PP, McGuffog L, Easton DF. The pathology of familial breast cancer: predictive value of immunohistochemical markers estrogen receptor, progesterone receptor, HER-2, and p53 in patients with mutations in BRCA1 and BRCA2. J Clin Oncol. 2002;20:2310–8.
16. Incorvaia L, Fanale D, Bono M, et al. BRCA1/2 pathogenic variants in triple-negative versus luminal-like breast cancers: genotype-phenotype correlation in a cohort of 531 patients. Ther Adv

30

Med Oncol. 2020;12:1758835920975326. Published 2020 Dec 16. https://doi.org/10.1177/1758835920975326.

17. Narod SA. Modifiers of risk of hereditary breast cancer. Oncogene. 2006;25:5832–6.

18. Hartmann LC, Schaid DJ, Woods JE, et al. Efficacy of bilateral prophylactic mastectomy in women with a family history of breast cancer. N Engl J Med. 1999;340:77–84.

19. Meijers-Heijboer H, van Geel B, van Putten WLJ, et al. Breast cancer after prophylactic bilateral mastectomy in women with a *BRCA1* or *BRCA2* mutation. N Engl J Med. 2001;345:159–64.

20. Rebbeck TR, Kauff ND, Domchek SM. Meta-analysis of risk reduction estimates associated with risk-reducing salpingo-oophorectomy in BRCA1 or BRCA2 mutation carriers. J Natl Cancer Inst. 2009;101:80–7.

21. Bono M, Fanale D, Incorvaia L, et al. Impact of deleterious variants in other genes beyond BRCA1/2 detected in breast/ovarian and pancreatic cancer patients by NGS-based multi-gene panel testing: looking over the hedge [published online ahead of print, 2021 Aug 6]. ESMO Open. 2021;6(4):100235. https://doi.org/10.1016/j.esmoop.2021.100235.

22. Fanale D, Incorvaia L, Filorizzo C, et al. Detection of germline mutations in a cohort of 139 patients with bilateral breast cancer by multi-gene panel testing: impact of pathogenic variants in other genes beyond BRCA1/2. Cancers (Basel). 2020;12(9):2415. Published 2020 Aug 25. https://doi.org/10.3390/cancers12092415.

23. Dupont WD, Page DL. Risk factors for breast cancer in women with proliferative breast disease. N Engl J Med. 1985;312:146–51.

24. Boyd NF, Guo H, Martin LJ, et al. Mammographic density and the risk and detection of breast cancer. N Engl J Med. 2007;356:227–36.

25. Independent UK Panel on Breast Cancer Screening. The benefits and harms of breast cancer screening: an independent review. Lancet. 2012;380:1778–86.

26. Lauby-Secretan B, Scoccianti C, Loomis D, Benbrahim-Tallaa L, Bouvard V, Bianchini F, Straif K, International Agency for Research on Cancer Handbook Working Group. Breast-cancer screening — viewpoint of the IARC Working Group. N Engl J Med. 2015;372:2353–8.

27. Senkus E, Kyriakides S, Ohno S, Penault-Llorca F, Poortmans P, Rutgers E, Zackrisson S, Cardoso F, ESMO Guidelines Committee. Primary breast cancer: ESMO Clinical Practice Guidelines for diagnosis, treatment and follow-up. Ann Oncol. 2015;26:v8–v30.

28. Gail MH, Brinton LA, Byar DP, Corle DK, Green SB, Schairer C, Mulvihill JJ. Projecting individualized probabilities of developing breast cancer for white females who are being examined annually. J Natl Cancer Inst. 1989;81:1879–86.

29. Mainiero MB, Lourenco A, Mahoney MC, et al. ACR appropriateness criteria breast cancer screening. J Am Coll Radiol. 2016;13:R45–9.

30. Fisher B, Costantino JP, Wickerham DL, et al. Tamoxifen for prevention of breast cancer: report of the National Surgical Adjuvant Breast and Bowel Project P-1 Study. J Natl Cancer Inst. 1998;90:1371–88.

31. Cuzick J, Powles T, Veronesi U, Forbes J, Edwards R, Ashley S, Boyle P. Overview of the main outcomes in breast-cancer prevention trials. Lancet. 2003;361:296–300.

32. Vogel VG, Costantino JP, Wickerham DL, et al. Effects of tamoxifen vs raloxifene on the risk of developing invasive breast cancer and other disease outcomes: the NSABP Study of Tamoxifen and Raloxifene (STAR) P-2 trial. JAMA. 2006;295:2727.

33. Visvanathan K, Hurley P, Bantug E, et al. Use of pharmacologic interventions for breast cancer risk reduction: American Society of Clinical Oncology Clinical Practice Guideline. J Clin Oncol. 2013;31:2942–62.

34. Lakhani S, Ellis IO, Schnitt SJ, Tan PH, van de Vijver MJ. WHO classification of tumours of the breast. 4th ed. Lyon: WHO – OMS – AIRC; 2012.

35. Dieci MV, Orvieto E, Dominici M, Conte P, Guarneri V. Rare breast cancer subtypes: histological, molecular, and clinical peculiarities. Oncologist. 2014;19:805–13.

36. Elston CW, I.O E (1998) Assessment of histologic grade. The Breast.

37. Hammond MEH, Hayes DF, Dowsett M, et al. American Society of Clinical Oncology/College Of American Pathologists guideline recommendations for immunohistochemical testing of estrogen and progesterone receptors in breast cancer. J Clin Oncol. 2010;28:2784–95.

38. Wolff AC, Hammond MEH, Hicks DG, et al. Recommendations for human epidermal growth factor receptor 2 testing in breast cancer: American Society of Clinical Oncology/College of American Pathologists clinical practice guideline update. J Clin Oncol. 2013;31:3997–4013.

39. Parker JS, Mullins M, Cheang MCU, et al. Supervised risk predictor of breast cancer based on intrinsic subtypes. J Clin Oncol. 2009;27:1160–7.

40. Perou CM, Sørlie T, Eisen MB, et al. Molecular portraits of human breast tumours. Nature. 2000;406:747–52.

41. Prat A, Pineda E, Adamo B, Galván P, Fernández A, Gaba L, Díez M, Viladot M, Arance A, Muñoz M. Clinical implications of the intrinsic molecular subtypes of breast cancer. Breast. 2015;24:S26–35.

42. Yersal O, Barutca S. Biological subtypes of breast cancer: prognostic and therapeutic implications. World J Clin Oncol. 2014;5:412.

43. Slamon DJ, Leyland-Jones B, Shak S, et al. Use of chemotherapy plus a monoclonal antibody against HER2 for metastatic breast cancer that overexpresses HER2. N Engl J Med. 2001;344:783–92.

44. Cardoso F, van't Veer LJ, Bogaerts J, et al. 70-gene signature as an aid to treatment decisions in early-stage breast cancer. N Engl J Med. 2016;375:717–29.

45. Paik S, Shak S, Tang G, et al. A multigene assay to predict recurrence of tamoxifen-treated, node-negative breast cancer. N Engl J Med. 2004;351:2817–26.

46. Dowsett M, Cuzick J, Wale C, et al. Prediction of risk of distant recurrence using the 21-gene recurrence score in node-negative and node-positive postmenopausal patients with breast cancer treated with anastrozole or tamoxifen: a TransATAC study. J Clin Oncol. 2010;28:1829–34.

47. Sparano JA, Gray RJ, Makower DF, et al. Prospective validation of a 21-gene expression assay in breast cancer. N Engl J Med. 2015;373:2005–14.

48. Sparano JA, Gray RJ, Makower DF, et al. Adjuvant chemotherapy guided by a 21-gene expression assay in breast cancer. N Engl J Med. 2018;379:111–21.

49. Nitz U, Gluz O, Christgen M, et al. Reducing chemotherapy use in clinically high-risk, genomically low-risk pN0 and pN1 early breast cancer patients: five-year data from the prospective, randomised phase 3 West German Study Group (WSG) PlanB trial. Breast Cancer Res Treat. 2017;165:573–83.

50. Chia SK, Bramwell VH, Tu D, et al. A 50-gene intrinsic subtype classifier for prognosis and prediction of benefit from adjuvant tamoxifen. Clin Cancer Res. 2012;18:4465–72.

51. Katipamula R, Degnim AC, Hoskin T, et al. Trends in mastectomy rates at the Mayo Clinic Rochester: effect of surgical year and preoperative magnetic resonance imaging. J Clin Oncol. 2009;27:4082–8.

52. Cortazar P, Zhang L, Untch M, et al. Pathological complete response and long-term clinical benefit in breast cancer: the CTNeoBC pooled analysis. Lancet. 2014;384:164–72.

53. Cardoso F, Loibl S, Pagani O, et al. The European Society of Breast Cancer Specialists recommendations for the management of young women with breast cancer. Eur J Cancer. 2012;48:3355–77.

54. Fisher B, Anderson S, Bryant J, Margolese RG, Deutsch M, Fisher ER, Jeong J-H, Wolmark N. Twenty-year follow-up of a randomized trial comparing total mastectomy, lumpectomy, and lumpectomy plus irradiation for the treatment of invasive breast cancer. N Engl J Med. 2002;347:1233–41.

55. Veronesi U, Cascinelli N, Mariani L, Greco M, Saccozzi R, Luini A, Aguilar M, Marubini E. Twenty-year follow-up of a randomized study comparing breast-conserving surgery with radical mastectomy for early breast cancer. N Engl J Med. 2002;347:1227–32.

56. Moran MS, Schnitt SJ, Giuliano AE, et al. Society of Surgical Oncology–American Society for Radiation Oncology consensus guideline on margins for breast-conserving surgery with whole-breast irradiation in stages I and II invasive breast cancer. J Clin Oncol. 2014;32:1507–15.

57. Bartelink H, Maingon P, Poortmans P, et al. Whole-breast irradiation with or without a boost for patients treated with breast-conserving surgery for early breast cancer: 20-year follow-up of a randomised phase 3 trial. Lancet Oncol. 2015;16:47–56.

58. Posther KE, McCall LM, Blumencranz PW, et al. Sentinel node skills verification and surgeon performance: data from a multicenter clinical trial for early-stage breast cancer. Ann Surg. 2005;242:593–9; discussion 599–602

59. Giuliano AE, Ballman KV, McCall L, et al. Effect of axillary dissection vs no axillary dissection on 10-year overall survival among women with invasive breast cancer and sentinel node metastasis. JAMA. 2017;318:918.

60. Galimberti V, Cole BF, Viale G, et al. Axillary dissection versus no axillary dissection in patients with breast cancer and sentinel-node micrometastases (IBCSG 23-01): 10-year follow-up of a randomised, controlled phase 3 trial. Lancet Oncol. 2018;19:1385–93.

61. Donker M, van Tienhoven G, Straver ME, et al. Radiotherapy or surgery of the axilla after a positive sentinel node in breast cancer (EORTC 10981-22023 AMAROS): a randomised, multicentre, open-label, phase 3 non-inferiority trial. Lancet Oncol. 2014;15:1303–10.

62. Kuehn T, Bauerfeind I, Fehm T, et al. Sentinel-lymph-node biopsy in patients with breast cancer before and after neoadjuvant chemotherapy (SENTINA): a prospective, multicentre cohort study. Lancet Oncol. 2013;14:609–18.

63. Boughey JC, Suman VJ, Mittendorf EA, et al. Sentinel lymph node surgery after neoadjuvant chemotherapy in patients with node-positive breast cancer. JAMA. 2013;310:1455.

64. Whelan TJ, Olivotto IA, Parulekar WR, et al. Regional nodal irradiation in early-stage breast cancer. N Engl J Med. 2015;373:307–16.

65. Darby SC, Ewertz M, McGale P, et al. Risk of ischemic heart disease in women after radiotherapy for breast cancer. N Engl J Med. 2013;368:987–98.

66. Nixon AJ, Neuberg D, Hayes DF, Gelman R, Connolly JL, Schnitt S, Abner A, Recht A, Vicini F, Harris JR. Relationship of patient age to pathologic features of the tumor and prognosis for patients with stage I or II breast cancer. J Clin Oncol. 1994;12:888–94.

67. Wolff AC, Hammond MEH, Hicks DG, et al. Recommendations for human epidermal growth factor receptor 2 testing in breast Cancer: American Society of Clinical Oncology/College of American Pathologists Clinical Practice Guideline Update. J Clin Oncol. 2013;31:3997–4013.

68. Early Breast Cancer Trialists' Collaborative Group (EBCTCG). Effects of chemotherapy and hormonal therapy for early breast cancer on recurrence and 15-year survival: an overview of the randomised trials. Lancet. 2005;365:1687–717.

69. Davies C, Pan H, Godwin J, et al. Long-term effects of continuing adjuvant tamoxifen to 10 years versus stopping at 5 years after diagnosis of oestrogen receptor-positive breast cancer: ATLAS, a randomised trial. Lancet. 2013;381:805–16.

70. Burstein HJ, Prestrud AA, Seidenfeld J, et al. American Society of Clinical Oncology Clinical Practice Guideline: update on adjuvant endocrine therapy for women with hormone receptor–positive breast cancer. J Clin Oncol. 2010;28:3784–96.

71. Burstein HJ, Lacchetti C, Anderson H, et al. Adjuvant endocrine therapy for women with hormone receptor–positive breast cancer: American Society of Clinical oncology clinical practice guideline update on ovarian suppression. J Clin Oncol. 2016;34:1689–701.

72. Early Breast Cancer Trialists' Collaborative Group (EBCTCG), Peto R, Davies C, et al. Comparisons between different polychemotherapy regimens for early breast cancer: meta-analyses of long-term outcome among 100 000 women in 123 randomised trials. Lancet. 2012;379:432–44.

73. Del Mastro L, De Placido S, Bruzzi P, et al. Fluorouracil and dose-dense chemotherapy in adjuvant treatment of patients with early-stage breast cancer: an open-label, 2 × 2 factorial, randomised phase 3 trial. Lancet. 2015;385:1863–72.

74. Jones S, Holmes FA, O'Shaughnessy J, et al. Docetaxel with cyclophosphamide is associated with an overall survival benefit compared with doxorubicin and cyclophosphamide: 7-year follow-up of US Oncology Research Trial 9735. J Clin Oncol. 2009;27:1177–83.

75. Poggio F, Bruzzone M, Ceppi M, Pondé NF, La Valle G, Del Mastro L, de Azambuja E, Lambertini M. Platinum-based neoadjuvant chemotherapy in triple-negative breast cancer: a systematic review and meta-analysis. Ann Oncol. 2018;29:1497–508.

76. Lambertini M, Moore HCF, Leonard RCF, et al. Gonadotropin-releasing hormone agonists during chemotherapy for preservation of ovarian function and fertility in premenopausal patients with early breast cancer: a systematic review and meta-analysis of individual patient–level data. J Clin Oncol. 2018;36:1981–90.

77. Early Breast Cancer Trialists' Collaborative Group (EBCTCG). Adjuvant bisphosphonate treatment in early breast cancer: meta-analyses of individual patient data from randomised trials. Lancet. 2015;386:1353–61.

78. Cameron D, Piccart-Gebhart MJ, Gelber RD, et al. 11 years' follow-up of trastuzumab after adjuvant chemotherapy in HER2-positive early breast cancer: final analysis of the HERceptin Adjuvant (HERA) trial. Lancet. 2017;389:1195–205.

79. Mavroudis D, Saloustros E, Malamos N, Kakolyris S, Boukovinas I, Papakotoulas P, Kentepozidis N, Ziras N, Georgoulias V, Breast Cancer Investigators of Hellenic Oncology Research Group (HORG), Athens, Greece. Six versus 12 months of adjuvant trastuzumab in combination with dose-dense chemotherapy for women with HER2-positive breast cancer: a multicenter randomized study by the Hellenic Oncology Research Group (HORG). Ann Oncol. 2015;26:1333–40.

80. Pivot X, Romieu G, Debled M, et al. 6 months versus 12 months of adjuvant trastuzumab for patients with HER2-positive early breast cancer (PHARE): a randomised phase 3 trial. Lancet Oncol. 2013;14:741–8.

81. Conte P, Frassoldati A, Bisagni G, et al. Nine weeks versus 1 year adjuvant trastuzumab in combination with chemotherapy: final results of the phase III randomized Short-HER study. Ann Oncol. 2018;29(12):2328–33. https://doi.org/10.1093/annonc/mdy414.

82. Joensuu H, Fraser J, Wildiers H, et al. Effect of adjuvant trastuzumab for a duration of 9 weeks vs 1 year with concomitant chemotherapy for early human epidermal growth factor receptor 2–positive breast cancer. JAMA Oncol. 2018;4:1199.

Metastatic Breast Cancer

Giuseppe Buono, Francesco Schettini, Grazia Arpino, Mario Giuliano, and Sabino De Placido

Breast Cancer

Contents

© Springer Nature Switzerland AG 2021
A. Russo et al. (eds.), *Practical Medical Oncology Textbook*, UNIPA Springer Series,
https://doi.org/10.1007/978-3-030-56051-5_31

31.1 Introduction

Breast cancer (BC) represents the most common malignancy among women worldwide. It has been estimated that 1.67 million of new cancer cases were diagnosed in 2012, with incidence rates ranging from 27 per 100,000 in Middle Africa and Eastern Asia to 92 per 100,000 in Northern America. Despite the overall increased incidence of BC occurred worldwide in the past decades, since the late 1990s, there was a constant reduction of mortality, especially in western countries, probably due to improvement of treatment strategies, as well as early diagnosis [1]. As matter of fact, only about 6% of BC cases present at diagnosis as metastatic "de novo" disease [2]. Additionally, 20–30% of patients diagnosed at early stages are expected to develop metastatic disease [3].

Traditionally, BCs are divided into different subtypes defined by immunohistochemistry (IHC), according to the expression of estrogen receptor (ER), progesterone receptor (PgR), grading, proliferative index ki67, and overexpression/amplification of human epithelial growth factor receptor 2 (HER2).

According to the 15th St. Gallen International Breast Cancer Conference Expert Panel [4], BC could be divided in four IHC subtypes: (1) luminal A-like tumors, which are typically low-grade, strongly ER/PgR-positive, and HER2-negative and have low proliferative fraction; (2) luminal B-like tumors, which are ER-positive but may have variable degrees of ER/PgR expression, are higher grade, have higher proliferative fraction, and can be also subdivided in luminal B HER2-positive and luminal B HER2-negative [5], according to the presence of HER2 amplification/overexpression; (3) HER2-positive tumors, which are ER/PgR-negative and HER2-positive; (4) triple-negative, which are ER/PgR-negative and HER2-negative, and corresponds to the most aggressive histological subtype.

This classification still represents the mainstay for treatment choice even if gene expression profiling demonstrated to give additional prognostic information and to be more accurate in the definition of tumor cell biology than IHC. Indeed, within the same BC intrinsic subtype, a variety of biological distinct entities can be identified; as an example, within the triple-negative BC (TNBC) subgroup, several molecular subtypes have been recognized, as shown by Lehmann and colleagues, who classified TNBC into six distinct subtypes, namely, basal-like 1 and 2, mesenchymal and mesenchymal-stem-like, immunomodulatory, and luminal androgen receptor, with potential clinical implications [6].

The risk and the pattern of BC recurrence is correlated to the initial tumor stage at presentation and to tumor biology. HER2-positive and TNBCs tend to relapse within the first 5 years after initial diagnosis of

early BC, whereas in hormone receptor (HR)-positive tumors, late relapses are more frequent. Tumor biology could also influence the specific sites of recurrence. In a study by Kennecke et al. [7] high rates of brain metastases were demonstrated among HER2-enriched (28.7%), basal-like (25.2%), and non-basal triple-negative (22%) tumors, whereas they were less frequent in the luminal/HER2 (15.4%) and other groups ($p = 0.001$). In contrast, bone was the predominant metastatic site for the luminal A (66.6%), luminal B (71.4%), and luminal/HER2 (65%) groups and the least a common site of metastases in the basal group (39%).

Breast cancer can metastasize anywhere in body, but the most common metastatic sites are bones, lungs, lymph nodes, liver, and brain, being the bone the most frequent initial metastatic site [8].

Metastatic BC is currently considered an incurable disease. Therefore, the main treatment objectives are improving quality of life and prolonging patient survival. In this scenario, systemic treatments represent the mainstay in the therapeutic management of metastatic BC, whereas local therapies, such as surgery and radiotherapy, are limited to peculiar situations (◘ Fig. 31.1).

Three major therapeutic subtypes are considered for the choice of systemic treatment of metastatic BC: HR+/HER2-negative, HER2+, and triple-negative disease. Systemic treatment options for each therapeutic subtype are described separately in the next paragraphs.

31.2 Systemic Treatment

31.2.1 HR+/HER2-Negative Disease

HR+/HER2-negative (HER2−) BCs accounts for about 65% of all breast cancers. Endocrine-based therapies represent the mainstay of treatment for this BC subtype, even in presence of visceral disease [9]. Chemotherapy, instead, is the required treatment in the presence of "visceral crisis," defined by the 3rd ESO-ESMO International Consensus Guidelines for Advanced Breast Cancer (ABC) as "severe organ dysfunction as assessed by signs and symptoms, laboratory studies and rapid progression of disease. Visceral crisis is not the mere presence of visceral metastases but implies important visceral compromise leading to a clinical indication for a more rapidly efficacious therapy, particularly since another treatment option at progression will probably not be possible" [10]. Fortunately, visceral crisis is not a common clinical presentation of HR+/HER2− metastatic BC.

Another important aspect which can guide treatment choice is the presence of endocrine resistance, which is empirically classified in primary and secondary resistance. Primary (de novo) endocrine resistance is defined by the presence of a BC relapse within the first 2 years

Fig. 31.1 Clinical management of metastatic breast cancer: general aspects. *Evaluation of Ki67 is relatively important to guide treatment decision in MBC. It can serve as an indicator of biologic aggressiveness and endocrine sensitivity (i.e., luminal A vs luminal B tumors). **Locoregional treatment to be performed with curative intent only in selected cases before or after systemic treatment (i.e., isolated local relapses, oligometastatic disease)

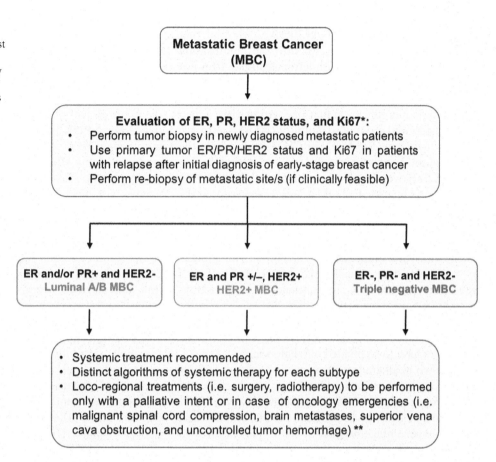

of adjuvant endocrine therapy (ET) or during the first 6 months of ET, when administered for metastatic disease. Secondary (acquired) endocrine resistance is typically defined by the presence of tumor relapse between 2 years after the beginning and 1 year after the end of adjuvant ET or by disease progression after 6 months of ET in the metastatic setting [10]. Importantly, in the presence of primary endocrine resistance, the probability of response to ET is very low; thus chemotherapy or molecularly targeted agents (see below) should be the preferred option. On the contrary, the probability of response to ET is substantially higher in the presence of acquired endocrine resistance and maximum in endocrine sensitive metastatic BC. Therefore, it is crucial to correctly predict the potential endocrine sensitivity, in order to define the best treatment option for each patient.

Our understanding about the molecular mechanisms of endocrine resistance has evolved over the past two decades. Among the different potential mechanisms identified as responsible for the development of endocrine resistance, two have been particularly studied in the last few years: genome aberrations affecting the gene encoding for ER (ESR1), considered as drivers of resistance to endocrine therapy in 15–40% of patients [11]; and activation of mammalian target of rapamycin (mTOR) signaling pathway mediated by various mechanisms,

including overexpression of human epidermal growth factor receptor family members, activating mutations in PIK3CA (gene encoding for phosphatidylinositol-4, 5-bisphosphate 3-kinase – PI3K catalytic subunit alpha), in AKT1 (encoding for serine-threonine kinase 1 – AKT), and HER2, found in 30%, 4%, and 2% of patients, respectively [11]. In addition, cyclin-dependent kinase 4 (CDK4) and CDK6 have been recently identified as key drivers of tumor cell proliferation in HR+/HER2− BC [11]. Furthermore, the amplification of FGFR1 (the gene encoding fibroblast growth factor receptor 1), found in 10% of patients, was also investigated for its role in BC oncogenesis and endocrine resistance [11].

Basing on these evidences, the treatment for HR+/HER2− metastatic BC has been radically changed over the past few years by the introduction of several targeted agents administered in combination with ET, such as the selective CDK4/6 inhibitors palbociclib, ribociclib, and abemaciclib. These drugs have been studied in various lines of therapy, but their clinical benefit was demonstrated primarily in the first- and second-line setting. In first line, the randomized phase III clinical trial PALOMA 2 clearly demonstrated the advantage of adding palbociclib to the aromatase inhibitor letrozole in women with endocrine sensitive metastatic BC: median progression-free survival (PFS) was 24.8 vs. 14.5 months in palbociclib vs. placebo group ($p < 0,0001$) [12]. A very similar trial, the MONALEESA 2, showed that the addition of ribociclib to letrozole significantly improved PFS compared with letrozole alone: PFS not reached vs. 14.7 months in ribociclib vs. placebo group ($p = 0,00000329$) [13]. More recently, also abemaciclib demonstrated its efficacy in first-line setting when added to a nonsteroidal aromatase inhibitor (NSAI – letrozole or anastrozole) in the MONARCH 3 study where the combination treatment showed similar advantages in terms of PFS over the placebo group ($p = 0.000021$) [14].

In second line, the PALOMA 3 study showed that the addition of palbociclib to the selective estrogen receptor downregulator (SERD) fulvestrant in patients with acquired endocrine resistance improved PFS when compared with fulvestrant alone: PFS 9.5 vs. 4.6 months ($p < 0.0001$) [15]. Finally, the MONARCH 2 trial assessed the benefit of adding abemaciclib to fulvestrant in endocrine-resistant patients: PFS 16.4 vs. 9.3 months ($p < 0.001$) [16]. Overall, the three CDK4/6 inhibitors showed a similar and good safety profile, although some differences have to be pointed out. Palbociclib and ribociclib resulted in all grade neutropenia in 66.5% and 59.3% respectively, while abemaciclib therapy was complicated by neutropenia only in 26.5% of patients. However, 13.4% of patients treated with abemaciclib experienced diarrhea, while this percentage was about 1% in patients treated with palbociclib and ribociclib.

Altogether these results suggest a remarkable benefit that can be obtained by adding CDK4/6 inhibitors to ET, and this leads to a substantial change in treatment algorithms for HR+/HER2− metastatic BC. Indeed, to date, CDK4/6 inhibitors are considered the standard for either first or second line of therapy (basing on previous treatment) associated with letrozole or fulvestrant, respectively (see ◘ Fig. 31.2).

As mentioned before, the activation of the mTOR signaling pathway is another important mechanism of treatment resistance in HR+/HER2− metastatic BC [11]. The clinical relevance of mTOR blockade has been assessed by the BOLERO 2 trial [17], in which patients, previously treated with an NSAI, were randomized to receive exemestane + everolimus vs. exemestane + placebo. The median PFS per central assessment was 11.0 vs. 4.1 months in the treatment vs. placebo group ($p < 0.001$). Currently, the mTOR inhibitor everolimus is indicated in the treatment of HR+/HER2− metastatic BC progressing after NSAI therapy, administered either in the adjuvant or metastatic setting (◘ Fig. 31.2).

Recently, other trials have investigated the effect of PI3K/AKT/mTOR pathway inhibition by the use of PI3K inhibitors. The PIK3CA gene is frequently mutated in breast cancer: it is estimated that 30% of luminal HR+/HER2− BCs harbor an activating PIK3CA mutation [11], which lead to overactive downstream signaling and mediate proliferation and survival,

as well as capability of migration and invasion of tumor cells [11]. Currently, there are several PI3K inhibitors in clinical development, and they could be classified in two major categories: pan-PI3K inhibitors and isoform specific inhibitors (designed to be selective to one or more of the four isoforms of the catalytic subunit of PI3K). The pan-isoform PI3K inhibitor buparlisib has been studied in the phase III randomized BELLE2 study [11], which investigated the efficacy of buparlisib plus fulvestrant versus placebo plus fulvestrant in 1147 postmenopausal women with metastatic BC progressed on an aromatase inhibitor. PFS was significantly improved from 5.0 to 6.9 months (HR 0.78, 95% CI 0·67–0·89; $p < 0·001$) by the addition of buparlisib. However, the treatment was complicated by several side effects: hyperglycemia, rash, fatigue, elevated transaminase, stomatitis, nausea, vomiting, and diarrhea. Mood disorders such as anxiety, irritability, and depression were also frequent, because the drug is able to cross the blood-brain barrier. BELLE2 study did not support the use of buparlisib, because of the small magnitude of benefit and induced toxicity [11].

Isoform-specific PI3K inhibitors aim to more selectively inhibit the driver oncogene and thus reduce toxicity and more potently inhibit the targeted oncogene. The ongoing phase III trial SANDPIPER and the recently published phase III trial SOLAR-1, enrolled patients with HR+/HER2-negative MBC to receive the alfa-selective PI3K inhibitors taselisib and alpelisib, respectively, in combination with fulvestrant. Alpelisib + fulvestrant showed a significant PFS improvement compared to fulvestrant alone in first-/second-line patients with tumors harboring a PIK3CA-mutation (HR: 0.65, 95% CI: 0.50–0.85, $p<0.001$). The study did not show any benefit for the PIK3CA-wild type cohort (HR: 0.85, 95% CI: 0.58–1.25). All patients had been pretreated with an aromatase inhibitor in the neo/adjuvant or metastatic setting. The combination was well tolerated, although G3-4 adverse events were more frequent with alpelisib and mainly represented by hyperglycemia (32.7%), diarrhea (6.7%), rash (9.9%) and fatigue (3.5%) [11, 18].

Despite the positive results achieved by ET combined with several target therapies, ET alone could still be considered a valid treatment option in the first-line setting, for some patients with endocrine sensitive disease. As support to this hypothesis, in the recent randomized phase III FALCON trial [19], fulvestrant confirmed to be a good treatment option in endocrine naïve patients, as it was superior to the aromatase inhibitor anastrozole (PFS was 16.6 vs. 13.8 months, $p = 0.0486$). Of note, the difference between the two endocrine agents was significant only in patients without visceral disease, where treatment with fulvestrant was associated with a particularly long median PFS (24 months).

In this complex therapeutic scenario, defining an optimal treatment algorithm is challenging, and several

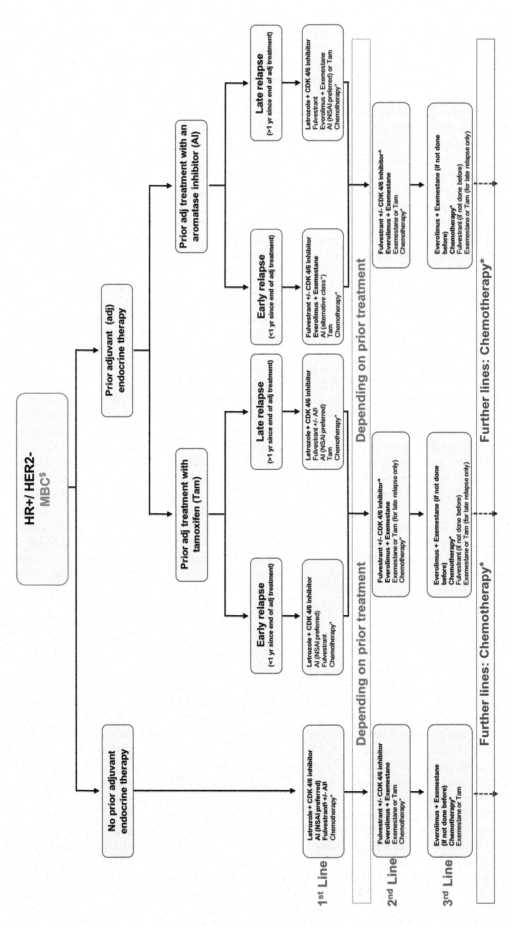

■ **Fig. 31.2** Systemic treatment algorithm for HR+/HER2– metastatic breast cancer. *Additional abbreviations:* NSAI: Nonsteroidal aromatase inhibitor. §The present treatment algorithm applies to postmenopausal patients. For premenopausal patients consider adding LH-RH therapy (to induce pharmacological menopause) to endocrine +/– targeted agents. *Chemotherapy always preferred in case of symptomatic visceral disease. For the choice of chemotherapy scheme, please refer to treatment algorithm of triple-negative MBC. In case of objective response/stable disease achieved by chemotherapy, consider to continue with maintenance endocrine therapy or metronomic chemotherapy (in the absence of a clear standard). §Not yet authorized by AIFA. °Steroidal inhibitor if previously it was administered a nonsteroidal inhibitor, and vice versa. ^CDK 4/6 inhibitors can be administered only one time

treatment options could be considered in each case (● Fig. 31.2). Therefore, the identification of predictive biomarkers of response, useful to guide treatment choice, is critical. Unfortunately, no predictive biomarkers for CDK4/6 inhibitors have been identified with certainty so far [11]. On the contrary, ESR1 mutations showed to be predictive of response in patients treated with everolimus and fulvestrant. Finally, the benefit associated with PI3K inhibitors seems to rely on the presence of PIK3CA mutations [18].

In patients with endocrine refractory disease and/or with visceral crisis, the standard indication is to perform chemotherapy with or without targeted agents. In this case the treatment algorithm is the same of that adopted in triple-negative metastatic BC with only few exceptions (see section entitled "Triple-Negative Disease" and ● Fig. 31.4).

31.2.2 HER2+ Disease

HER2-positive tumors accounts for about 15–20% of all BCs. Despite the aggressive biology of HER2+ BC, which is responsible for its relatively poor prognosis, the introduction of effective anti-HER2 therapies has dramatically changed the natural history of this disease. Importantly, HER2 signaling pathway represents the main driver of proliferation and survival in HER2+ cancer cell. Thus, complete inhibition of HER2 pathway represents the most effective treatment for this BC subtype [20].

HER2 status is assessed by immunohistochemistry and/or by fluorescence in situ hybridization (FISH) [21]. Considering the possibility of discordance in HER2 status between primary and metastatic tumor (discordance rate up 25%), and the critical importance of anti-HER2 therapies in this disease subtype, re-biopsy should be always taken into consideration if clinically possible, in case of relapse of HER-negative primary tumors [20].

The first anti-HER2 agent successfully introduced into clinical practice is trastuzumab, which is a monoclonal antibody directed against the extracellular domain of HER2 receptor. Trastuzumab inhibits the omo- and heterodimerization of HER2 receptors, impeding the activation of downstream signaling, determining increased endocytotic destruction of the receptor, and finally inducing immune-mediated cytotoxicity (ADCC – antibody-dependent cell-mediated cytotoxicity). For many years, the anti-HER2 monoclonal antibody trastuzumab in combination with a taxane (paclitaxel or docetaxel) has been the standard first-line treatment for HER2-positive metastatic BC basing on the pivotal trial carried out by Slamon and colleagues [20].

Recently, the phase III randomized trial CLEOPATRA [22, 23] showed that the addition of the humanized monoclonal antibody pertuzumab to the standard first-line therapy with trastuzumab and docetaxel was associated with a significant improvement of overall survival (OS) and PFS (OS 56.5 vs. 40 months for the standard and experimental treatment, respectively). Basing on these positive results, dual HER2 blockade with trastuzumab and pertuzumab in combination to a taxane has become the new standard first-line therapy for HER2-positive metastatic BC patients. The reason for the remarkable improvement of patient outcome achieved by the addition of pertuzumab to anti-HER2 therapy relies on the fact that this monoclonal antibody is designed to bind the extracellular dimerization domain of HER2 and inhibit the ability of this receptor to interact with other HER family members (HER1, HER2, HER3, and HER4), determining a complete and effective inhibition of HER signaling.

Another novel anti-HER2 drug, successfully tested in metastatic BC is the antibody-drug conjugate trastuzumab emtansine (TDM1). TDM1 is a complex molecule where the antibody trastuzumab is linked to the microtubule inhibitory agent emtansine (DM1). The molecular structure of TDM1 allows intracellular drug delivery of the potent cytotoxic drug emtansine to HER2-overexpressing cells, thereby improving the therapeutic index and minimizing exposure of normal tissue. The efficacy of TDM1 as second-line therapy for HER2+ metastatic BC was shown in the EMILIA trial, where this agent determined a significant improvement of both PFS and OS in comparison with the combination of the oral chemotherapy agent capecitabine together with the dual HER1/HER2 tyrosine kinase inhibitor lapatinib, which was the standard second-line therapy at the time of study beginning [24]. Additional trials evaluated TDM1 in subsequent lines of therapy [25, 26]. Finally, TDM1 alone or in association with pertuzumab did not demonstrate to be superior to docetaxel + trastuzumab in the first-line setting [27]. Therefore, TDM1 is currently recommended in second or subsequent line of therapy (● Fig. 31.3).

An additional treatment option for HER2+ metastatic BC to be administered as second or subsequent line of therapy is lapatinib in association with capecitabine. This option could be particularly useful in patients with brain metastases, since lapatinib has been shown to penetrate the blood-brain barrier [21]. Of note brain metastases represent a major clinical challenge in HER2-positive BC since they occur in up to 50% of patients with this disease subtype [21, 28]. T-DM1 also demonstrated to be effective in case of brain metastases, in a retrospective subgroup analysis of the EMILIA trial [29].

Heavily pre-treated patients could benefit from the re-challenge of trastuzumab combined with different chemotherapy agents [21] (● Fig. 31.3).

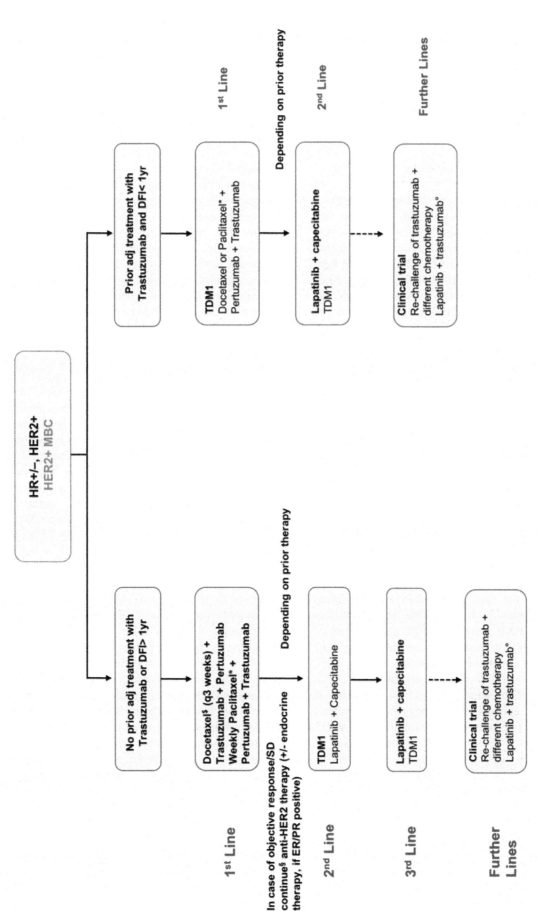

Fig. 31.3 Systemic treatment algorithm for HER2+ metastatic breast cancer. *Additional abbreviations:* DFI: Disease-free interval (from the end of adjuvant treatment). §At least 6 cycles should be administered. *Alternative to docetaxel in case of reported unacceptable toxicity or known intolerance.§Switch to maintenance therapy when maximum tolerability is reached. °Not reimbursed

Finally, for patients with HR+/HER2+ disease, anti-HER2 therapy combined with endocrine treatment is a valid option, either as maintenance therapy in case of objective response/stable disease achieved with chemotherapy + anti-HER2 therapy or as upfront treatment in patients who are not fit for chemotherapy.

31.2.3   Triple-Negative Disease

Triple-negative breast cancers (TNBC) subgroup accounts for about 15% of all BCs and is characterized by the absence of estrogen and progesterone receptor expression and the lack of overexpression/amplification of HER2 [30]. Patients affected by TNBC do not benefit from either endocrine or anti-HER2 therapies; thus standard treatment choice in this subgroup of patients is chemotherapy with or without targeted agents. The prognosis of TNBC patients remains poor (fewer than 30% of patients with metastatic TNBC survive 5 years after diagnosis) [31] due to the lack of specific "target" therapies and to the rapid onset of metastasis (probably due to the very high proliferative index), despite the high response of this BC subgroup to chemotherapeutic agents [30]. In general, international guidelines [10, 32] recommend the use of sequential single-agent chemotherapy, whereas the combination of chemotherapeutic agents (poly-chemotherapy) should be adopted for patients with symptomatic and rapidly progressive disease, which requires rapid tumor debulkying. However, only patients without impairment of multi-organ function are eligible for poly-chemotherapy, as it is associated with higher risk of toxicity. The most effective sequencing of chemotherapy agents in the treatment of metastatic TNBC has yet to be defined. In the following paragraphs, the most active chemotherapy-based therapeutic schemes for both TNBC and endocrine-refractory HR+/HER2− metastatic BC are reported.

- *Anthracyclines* [33]: these drugs are among the most active class of chemotherapy agents in breast cancer, achieving an overall response rate (ORR) in HER2-negative disease between 30% and 50%. It consists of doxorubicin, epirubicin and pegylated liposomal doxorubicin. The latter showed similar PFS and OS results comparing to the traditional form of anthracyclines, with lower rates of cardiotoxicity. Due to the frequent use of antracyclines in the neo-/adjuvant setting and considering the probability of cardiotoxicity due to the exceeding of cumulative dose levels (ranging from 450 mg/m² for doxorubicin to 900 mg/m² for epirubicin), their use in metastatic setting can be limited, although liposomal anthracyclines allow to expose the patients to much higher cumulative doses without a substantial increase of the risk of cardiotoxicity. A recent meta-analysis comparing anthracyclines and taxanes showed a modest superiority in ORR (38% vs. 33%) and PFS (7 vs. 5 months) in favor of anthracyclines group of patients. However, the strength and clinical applicability of these results were limited due to trial heterogeneity and by the cumulative toxicity in patients which were treated in adjuvant setting. As mentioned before, the combination of anthracyclines with other chemotherapy agents (i.e., taxanes, cyclophosphamide, etc.) is associated with superior ORR and PFS at the cost of higher toxicity rates.

- *Taxanes* [33]: are anti-mitotic agents widely and commonly used in BC. Taxane-based schemes are among the most effective systemic therapies in metastatic BC. This class of drugs includes docetaxel, paclitaxel, and nab-paclitaxel (paclitaxel bound to nanomolecules of albumin). The latter is a novel formulation, which requires a shorter infusion time and does not need steroid pre-medication, because of its albumin-bound formulation, and is associated with a lower risk of allergic reactions. Taxanes can be administered as single agents (for paclitaxel a weekly schedule is preferred) or in association with other chemotherapy drugs, including anthracyclines. Moreover, weekly paclitaxel associated with the antivascular endothelial growth factor (VEGF) monoclonal antibody bevacizumab is one of the standard options as first-line treatment for HER2− metastatic BC. However, the use of bevacizumab is still debated as the combination of bevacizumab + chemotherapy determined improvement of PFS but was not associated with improvement of overall survival (OS) in any of the prospective randomized trials that tested this treatment strategy.

- *Eribulin* [33]: this chemotherapeutic agent is currently approved for the treatment of HER2+ metastatic BC patients who progressed after receiving anthracyclines and taxanes. It blocks cell cycle in the M phase by inhibiting microtubule polymerization.

- *Capecitabine* [33]: is an oral chemotherapy agent, pro-drug of the anti-metabolite 5-fluorouracil (5-FU). It can used in the first-line metastatic setting (especially in patients pre-treated with anthracyclines and taxanes in neo-/adjuvant setting), because of its oral administration and relatively advantageous safety profile.

- *Vinorelbine* [33]: is a commonly used chemotherapy agent in TNBC and is a semi-synthetic vinca alkaloid, with activity in heavily pretreated patients (ORR: 25–45%). This agent can be administered alone or in combination with capecitabine.

- *Gemcitabine* [33]: this antimetabolite is typically administered in combination with other drugs, such as taxanes or platinum salts, since it showed low response rates when administered as single agent.

- *Platinum salts* [33]: these drugs (i.e., carboplatin and cisplatin) cause DNA crosslink strand breaks resulting in tumor cell apoptosis. The association of cisplatin and paclitaxel resulted in a better PFS when compared with gemcitabine and paclitaxel in unselected metastatic TNBC patients [30]. In the phase III Triple-Negative Breast Cancer Trial (TNT) [30], carboplatin monotherapy was directly compared with docetaxel in patients with metastatic TNBC. Overall, carboplatin was not superior to docetaxel. However, in patients carrying BRCA1/2 mutations carboplatin was significantly superior to docetaxel. Similar results were also found in the non-randomized TBCRC009 trial [30], where BRCA-mutated patients demonstrated increased response rates with platinum therapy. These studies are paving the way to an increasing use of platinum salts in metastatic TNBC patients, especially for those carrying mutations of BRCA genes.

To date the optimal treatment algorithm for metastatic TNBC and endocrine-refractory HER2− disease is still debated, and several options can be considered for each line of therapy (◘ Fig. 31.4), according to previous treatments, disease burden, comorbidity, expected toxicity, and patients' preferences.

Besides chemotherapy, other biologically targeted agents (in addition to bevacizumab) have been recently tested in HER2-negative metastatic BC. In particular, the poly (ADP-ribose) polymerase (PARP) inhibitors olaparib and talazoparib showed to improve PFS in *BRCA*-mutated patients with HER2− metastatic BC, comparing with physician's choice chemotherapy [34, 35]. PARP is a constitutively expressed nuclear enzyme that modulates DNA repair and cell survival. In response to DNA single-strand and double-strand breaks, it has been reported an immediate catalytic activation [31]. In normal cells with no mutations of BRCA1 and BRCA2 genes, double-strand breaks can be repaired by homologous recombination, but in BRCA1- or BRCA2-mutated cells, homologous recombination is not functioning, and thus DNA strand breaks rely on PARP action for repair [31]. Hence, inhibition of PARP leads to severe toxicity in BRCA1- and BRCA2-mutated cells, causing the so-called synthetic lethality [31]. Importantly, sensitivity to PARP inhibition depends also on homologous recombination deficiency (HRD) which can produce a similar phenotype termed "*BRCA*ness" [31]. These results are particularly important, as they represent the first evidence of efficacy for treatments developed to inhibit selective targets in TNBC. Moreover, approximately 10–20% of TNBC patients harbor germline *BRCA* mutations, and additional cases can show "*BRCA*ness" [36].

Recently, immunotherapy showed, for the first time, to be active and effective in TNBC, as the addition of the atezolizumab, a humanized programmed death-ligand 1 (PD-L1) antibody, to nab-paclitaxel prolonged PFS in both the intention-to-treat population and the PD-L1-positive patient subgroup and OS among sub-jects with PD-L1-positive tumors (25.0 vs. 15.5 months, HR: 0.62) [36].

Moreover, increasing evidence suggest a potential role of anti-androgen therapy in a subset of TNBC. The expression of the androgen receptor (AR) has been described in TNBC in a range from 12 to 60%, especially in LAR subtype by Lehman and colleagues [37]. In a meta-analysis of 13 studies including 2826 patients with metastatic TNBC, it was demonstrated a rate of AR positivity of 24.4% [30]. In this context two phase II studies [37] demonstrated promising response rates with anti-androgen therapy in patients with >10% of AR expression by IHC.

Finally, many other therapeutic strategies are currently being investigated in metastatic TNBC, including among others immune checkpoint inhibitors, PI3K/AKT pathway inhibitors, and MAPK pathway inhibitors.

31.3 Local Therapies for Metastatic BC

Although systemic treatments represent the mainstay of therapy for metastatic BC, locoregional treatments performed by surgery or radiotherapy and other techniques may be useful to prevent cancer-related complications and to palliate symptoms (◘ Fig. 31.1).

Radiation therapy has a central role in palliative care, especially in case of (1) brain metastases [radio-surgery (Gamma Knife or stereotaxic treatment) if there are few (<5 lesions) and small (<2–3 cm) metastases, or whole brain irradiation]; (2) symptomatic bone disease or risk of bone fracture; (3) medullar compression, due to vertebral fracture or endo-canalar disease; and (4) mediastinal syndrome (rare in BC), typically due to massive metastatic involvement of mediastinal nodes.

Breast surgery is indicated in case of a local relapse of BC, if there are no other metastatic sites. In metastatic de novo BCs, some evidences from retrospective and non-randomized studies seem to suggest a potential benefit deriving from the excision of primary BC in presence of metastatic disease [38]. Finally, several clinical reports suggest potential clinical benefit using locoregional treatment approaches in combination with systemic therapies for the management of oligometastatic BC, although data from prospective randomized trials are still lacking (see below) [39].

31.3.1 Management of Oligometastatic Disease

The state of "oligometastatic" breast cancer is defined by the presence of solitary or few evaluable lesions, usually in number ≤5 [40]. This particular kind of metastatic disease is estimate to represent up to 10% of patients with newly diagnosed metastatic BC [40]. Importantly

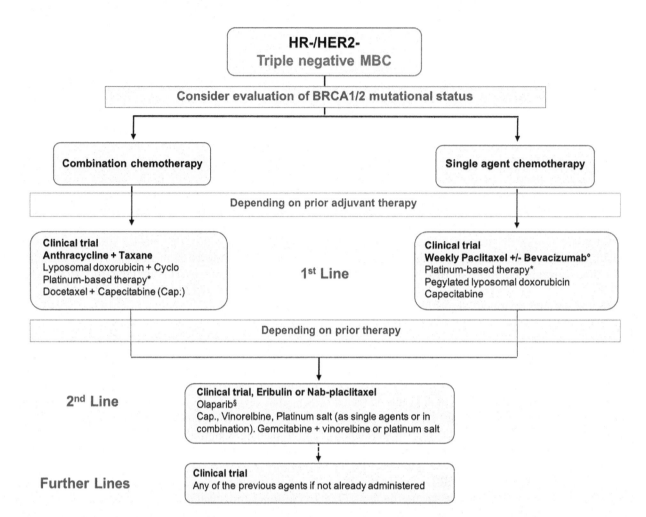

◻ Fig. 31.4 Systemic treatment algorithm for HR-/HER2-metastatic breast cancer. *Additional abbreviations*: Cyclo: Cyclophosphamide; Cap: Capecitabine. *Platinum salt: either carboplatin or cisplatin. Platinum salts are important treatment options either in first- or second line for patients pre-treated with anthracyclines and taxanes, and in presence of BRCA1/BRCA2 mutations. °Combination of paclitaxel + bevacizumab should be considered also for patients with symptomatic visceral disease. Switch to maintenance therapy (bevacizumab +/− capecitabine) when maximum tolerability is reached. §To be approved in patients with BRCA1 or BRCA2 mutations

some of these patients could benefit from more aggressive treatment approaches administered with curative intent. Multimodal treatments are typically represented by of systemic therapy together with surgery or radiotherapy [40].

A meta-analysis by Harris et al. [40] of 28.693 MBC patients demonstrated a better 3 years OS in patients undergoing surgery of primary breast cancer, particularly in patients with smaller tumors, lower burden of metastatic disease, and fewer comorbidities, while no differences were found regarding hormone receptor status, grading, and site of metastasis. However, two randomized trials [40] failed to demonstrate a survival benefit in patients receiving surgery after systemic therapy for metastatic disease.

As mentioned before, liver represents a common metastatic site in BC, but isolated liver metastases are presents only in 4–5% of patients. Locoregional treatment approaches for liver metastases are surgical excision, transcatheter arterial chemoembolization (TACE),

and radiofrequency ablation (RFA). Several lines of evidence support the use of these techniques in patients with isolated liver metastases [40].

The role of locoregional treatment of lung metastases is still unclear in BC. No studies directly compared systemic therapy alone vs. the combination with locoregional treatments.

Bone-only metastases occur in 17–37% of patients with distant relapses [40]. Radiotherapy remains the treatment approach for bone metastases, in particular to vertebral and extremities stabilization (to reduce the risk of bone fractures) and for pain relief. However, patients treated with stereotactic body radiation therapy (SBRT) demonstrated to achieve a potential survival benefit [40].

It is estimated that about 10–15% of all MBC patients develop symptomatic brain metastases and this risk is higher in triple-negative and HER2+ breast cancer. Survival of patients with central nervous system (CNS) metastases remains poor, ranging from 2 to 16 months [40, 41]. Locoregional treatment approaches are represented by surgery, stereotactic radiosurgery (SRS), and whole brain RT (WBRT). The first two treatments are adopted in patients with limited number (1–3) and small CNS metastases, whereas WBRT is used for the remaining cases.

Overall, despite the lack of randomized trials, multimodal treatment of oligometastatic BC could represent an important strategy to improve patient outcome. However, selecting the oligometastatic patients who can benefit the most from multimodal aggressive treatment approaches remains a major challenge.

Expert Opinion
Antonio Russo

Key Points
1. Breast cancer can diffuse to other organs, and the most frequent sites of metastases are the lymph nodes, bone, liver, lung, and brain. Metastatic disease is not a curable condition, and even if with new treatments in the last years, there has been an improved survival and a better quality of life for these patients.
2. In case of hormone receptors positive and HER-2-negative breast cancer, treatment is based on endocrine therapy (ET), after having evaluated the condition of endocrine resistance which can be primary or secondary. Together with ET in first and second line of therapy, it is possible to administer new drugs such as palbociclib, ribociclib, and ademaciclib, which are CDK4/6 (involved in the resistance mechanisms) inhibitors. Palbociclib can be also added to fulvestrant in second-line treatment; another treatment is represented by everolimus, an mTOR (a factor which cause resistance) inhibitor.
3. For HER-2-positive BC, therapy consists in the administration of trastuzumab with taxane (paclitaxel or docetaxel); recently pertuzumab has been studied in this setting of patients, observing a better OS and PFS; this is the reason why the new standard of care is based on the use of trastuzumab, pertuzumab, and taxane. Another innovation is the antibody-drug conjugate trastuzumab emtansine (TDM1) which is recommended in second or subsequent lines of therapy.
4. Triple-negative BCs are characterized by a poor prognosis. Different therapeutic strategies can be used and based on chemotherapy anthracyclines, taxanes, eribulin, capecitabine, vinorelbine, gemcitabine, and platinum salts are used. It is quite important to remind that chemotherapy should be used also in HR+/HER2− BCs in case of organ crisis, also during the treatment with ET. Interesting updates come from immunotherapy: atezolizumab a PD-L1 antibody, added to nab-paclitaxel, has prolonged PFS in both the intention-to-treat population and the PD-L1-positive patient subgroup, and OS among subjects with PD-L1-positive tumors.
5. Also in the metastatic setting, locoregional treatments can be used for palliative intent and to prevent cancer-related complications. Even the absence of strong evidences, in case of oligometastatic disease, it could be useful combination of locoregional and systemic treatments. Radiotherapy (RT) is suggested when there is a bone involvement and a whole brain RT should be chosen in case of encephalic metastases.

Recommendations
- ESMO
- ▶ www.esmo.org/Guidelines/Breast-Cancer/4th-ESO-ESMO-International-Consensus-Guidelines-for-Advanced-Breast-Cancer-ABC-4
- ASCO
- ▶ https://www.asco.org/practice-guidelines/quality-guidelines/guidelines/breast-cancer#/9786
- ▶ https://www.asco.org/practice-guidelines/quality-guidelines/guidelines/breast-cancer#/11751
- ▶ https://www.asco.org/practice-guidelines/quality-guidelines/guidelines/breast-cancer#/9781

Hints for a Deeper Insight
- Atezolizumab for the treatment of triple-negative breast cancer: ▶ https://www.ncbi.nlm.nih.gov/pubmed/30474425
- Current state of clinical trials in breast cancer brain metastases: ▶ https://www.ncbi.nlm.nih.gov/pubmed/31555454
- Everolimus-based combination therapies for HR+, HER2− metastatic breast cancer: ▶ https://www.ncbi.nlm.nih.gov/pubmed/30092555
- Fulvestrant and palbociclib combination in heavily pretreated hormone receptor-positive, HER2-negative metastatic breast cancer patients: ▶ https://www.ncbi.nlm.nih.gov/pubmed/31612291

References

1. http://globocan.iarc.fr/old/FactSheets/cancers/breast-new.asp.

2. https://seer.cancer.gov/statfacts/html/breast.html.

3. Early Breast Cancer Trialists' Collaborative Group (EBCTCG). Effects of chemotherapy and hormonal therapy for early breast cancer on recurrence and 15-year survival: an overview of the randomised trials. Lancet. 2005;365:1687–717.

4. Curigliano G, et al. De-escalating and escalating treatments for early-stage breast cancer: the St. Gallen International Expert Consensus Conference on the Primary Therapy of Early Breast Cancer 2017. Ann Oncol. 2017;28:1700–12.

5. Schettini F, et al. Hormone receptor/human epidermal growth factor receptor 2-positive breast cancer: where we are now and where we are going. Cancer Treat Rev. 2016;46:20–6.

6. Lehmann BD, et al. Identification of human triple-negative breast cancer subtypes and preclinical models for selection of targeted therapies. J Clin Invest. 2011;121(7):2750–67.

7. Kennecke H, et al. Metastatic behavior of breast cancer subtypes. J Clin Oncol. 2010;28:3271–7.

8. Lee YT, et al. Breast carcinoma: pattern of metastasis at autopsy. J Surg Oncol. 1983;23(3):175–80.

9. Cardoso F, et al. 1st International Consensus guidelines for advanced breast cancer (ABC1). Breast. 2012;21:242–52.

10. Cardoso F, et al. 3rd ESO-ESMO International Consensus guidelines for advanced breast cancer (ABC3). Ann Oncol. 2017;28:16–33.

11. Turner N, et al. Advances in the treatment of advanced oestrogen-receptor-positive breast cancer. Lancet Series. 2016; https://doi.org/10.1016/S0140-6736(16)32419-9.

12. Finn RS, et al. Palbociclib and letrozole in advanced breast cancer. N Engl J Med. 2016;375:1925–36.

13. Hortobagyi G, et al. Ribociclib as first-line therapy for HR-positive, advanced breast cancer. N Engl J Med. 2016;375: 1738–48.

14. Goetz MP, et al. MONARCH 3: abemaciclib as initial therapy for advanced breast cancer. J Clin Oncol. 2017 Nov 10;35(32):3638–46.

15. Cristofanilli M, et al. Fulvestrant plus palbociclib versus fulvestrant plus placebo for treatment of hormone-receptor-positive, HER2-negative metastatic breast cancer that progressed on previous endocrine therapy (PALOMA-3): final analysis of the multicentre, double-blind, phase 3 randomised controlled trial. Lancet Oncol. 2016;17(4):425–39.

16. Sledge GW Jr, et al. MONARCH 2: abemaciclib in combination with fulvestrant in women with HR+/HER2− advanced breast cancer who had progressed while receiving endocrine therapy. J Clin Oncol. 2017;35(25):2875–84.

17. Piccart M, et al. Everolimus plus exemestane for hormone-receptor-positive, human epidermal growth factor receptor-2-negative advanced breast cancer: overall survival results from BOLERO-2. Ann Oncol. 2014;25(12):2357–62.

18. André F, Ciruelos E, Rubovszky G, Campone M, Loibl S, et al. Alpelisib for PIK3CA-Mutated, Hormone Receptor–Positive Advanced Breast Cancer. New Engl J Med. 2019;380: 1929–40.

19. Robertson JFR, et al. Fulvestrant 500 mg versus anastrozole 1 mg for hormone receptor-positive advanced breast cancer (FALCON): an international, randomised, double-blind, phase 3 trial. Lancet. 2016;388(10063):2997–3005.

20. Loibl S, Gianni L. HER2-positive breast cancer. Lancet Series. 2016; https://doi.org/10.1016/S0140-6736(16)32417-5.

21. Wolf AC, et al. Recommendations for human epidermal growth factor receptor 2 testing in breast cancer: American Society of Clinical Oncology/College of American Pathologists clinical practice guideline update. J Clin Oncol. 2013;31:3997–4013.

22. Swain SM, et al. Pertuzumab, trastuzumab, and docetaxel in HER2-positive metastatic breast cancer. N Engl J Med. 2015;372: 724–34.

23. Baselga J, et al. CLEOPATRA: a phase III evaluation of pertuzumab and trastuzumab for HER2-positive metastatic breast cancer. Clin Breast Cancer. 2010;10:489–91.

24. Verma S, et al. Trastuzumab emtansine for HER2-positive advanced breast cancer. N Engl J Med. 2012;367:1783–91. Erratum in: N Engl J Med 2013; 368: 2442.

25. Krop IE, et al. Trastuzumab emtansine versus treatment of physician's choice for pretreated HER2-positive advanced breast cancer (TH3RESA): a randomised, open-label,phase 3 trial. Lancet Oncol. 2014;15:689–99.

26. Wildiers H, et al. Trastuzumab emtansine improves overall survival versus treatment of physician's choice in patients with previously treated HER2-positive metastatic breast cancer: fi nal overall survival results from the phase 3 TH3RESA study. Cancer Res. 2016;76:S5–05 (abstr.

27. Ellis PA, et al. Phase III, randomized study of trastuzumab emtansine (T-DM1) ± pertuzumab (P) vs trastuzumab + taxane (HT) for fi rst-line treatment of HER2-positive MBC: primary results from the MARIANNE study. J Clin Oncol. 2015; 33:507.

28. Pivot X, et al. CEREBEL (EGF111438): a phase III, randomized, open-label study of lapatinib plus capecitabine versus trastuzumab plus capecitabine in patients with human epidermal growth factor receptor 2-positive metastatic breast cancer. J Clin Oncol. 2015;33:1564–73.

29. Krop IE, et al. Trastuzumab emtansine (T-DM1) versus lapatinib plus capecitabine in patients with HER2-positive metastatic breast cancer and central nervous system metastases: a retrospective, exploratory analysis in EMILIA. Ann Oncol. 2015;26:113–9.

30. Denkert C, et al. Molecular alterations in triple-negative breast cancer - the road to new treatment strategies. Lancet Series. 2016; https://doi.org/10.1016/S0140-6736(16)32454-0.

31. Bianchini G, et al. Triple-negative breast cancer: challenges and opportunities of a heterogeneous disease. Nat Rev Clin Oncol. 2016;13(11):674–90.

32. Partridge AH, et al. Chemotherapy and targeted therapy for women with human epidermal growth factor receptor 2-negative (or unknown) advanced breast cancer: American Society of Clinical Oncology Clinical Practice Guideline. J Clin Oncol. 2014;32:3307–29.

33. Zeichner SB, et al. A review of systemic treatment in metastatic triple-negative breast cancer. Breast Cancer. 2016(10):25–36. https://doi.org/10.4137/BCBCR.S32783.

34. Robson M, et al. Olaparib for metastatic breast cancer in patients with a germline BRCA mutation. N Engl J Med. 2017;377(6):523–33.

35. Litton J, et al. EMBRACA: a phase 3 trial comparing talazoparib, an oral PARP inhibitor, to physician's choice of therapy in patients with advanced breast cancer and a germline BRCA mutation. Abstract GS6-07, Presented at San Antonio Breast Cancer Symposium, December 8, 2017.

36. Schmid P, et al. Atezolizumab and nab-paclitaxel in advanced triple-negative breast cancer. N Engl J Med. 2018;379(22): 2108–21.

37. Lee A, et al. Triple negative breast cancer: emerging therapeutic modalities and novel combination therapies. Cancer Treat Rev. 2018;62:110–22.

38. Criscitiello C, et al. Surgery of the primary tumor in de novo metastatic breast cancer: to do or not to do? EJSO. 2015;41:1288–92.

39. Pagani O, et al. International guidelines for management of metastatic breast cancer: can metastatic breast cancer be cured? J Natl Cancer Inst. 2010;102(7):456.

40. Di Lascio S, Pagani O. Oligometastatic breast cancer: a shift from palliative to potentially curative treatment? Breast Care. 2014;9:7–14.

41. Galanti D, Inno A, La Vecchia M, et al. Current treatment options for HER2-positive breast cancer patients with brain metastases. Crit Rev Oncol Hematol. 2021;161:103329. https://doi.org/10.1016/j.critrevonc.2021.103329.

Lung Cancer

*Francesco Passiglia, Valerio Gristina, Christian Rolfo,
Nadia Barraco, Viviana Bazan, and Antonio Russo*

Thoracic Cancers

Contents

Francesco Passiglia, Valerio Gristina, and Christian Rolfo should be considered equally co-first authors.

© Springer Nature Switzerland AG 2021
A. Russo et al. (eds.), *Practical Medical Oncology Textbook*, UNIPA Springer Series,
https://doi.org/10.1007/978-3-030-56051-5_32

Learning Objectives

By the end of the chapter, the reader will
- Be able to apply diagnostic, staging, and treatment procedures of lung cancer
- Learn the basic concepts of epidemiology, pathology, and molecular biology of lung cancer
- Reach in-depth knowledge of diagnosis and treatment of lung cancer
- Be able to put acquired knowledge into clinical practice management of lung cancer patients

32.1 Introduction

Lung cancer was the most important epidemic of the twentieth century, and it's likely to remain a major public health problem also in the twenty-first century. We can ascribe different "primates" to lung cancer among all other epithelial malignant neoplasms:
- Lung cancer is the most frequent malignant tumor after non-melanocytic skin cancer.
- Lung cancer is the leading cause of cancer-related mortality worldwide.

- Lung cancer is the first malignant epithelial tumor to be successfully treated with single-agent targeted therapy.
- Lung cancer is the first malignant epithelial tumor to be successfully treated with single-agent immunotherapy.
- Lung cancer is the first malignant epithelial tumor to include liquid biopsy in the clinical management of patients.

32.2 Epidemiology

Over the last century, lung cancer switched from a rare disease to the most common malignant neoplasm in most countries and the first cause of cancer death worldwide, with about 1 of 4 cancer deaths due to lung cancer and a 5-year survival estimated to be 18%, ranging from 55% for localized disease to 4.5% for advanced disease [1] (◘ Fig. 32.1).

The American Cancer Society's estimates for lung cancer in the United States for 2017 were [2]:
- About 222,500 new cases of lung cancer (116,990 in men and 105,510 in women).
- About 155,870 deaths from lung cancer (84,590 in men and 71,280 in women).

◘ **Fig. 32.1** Five-year relative survival by stage at diagnosis

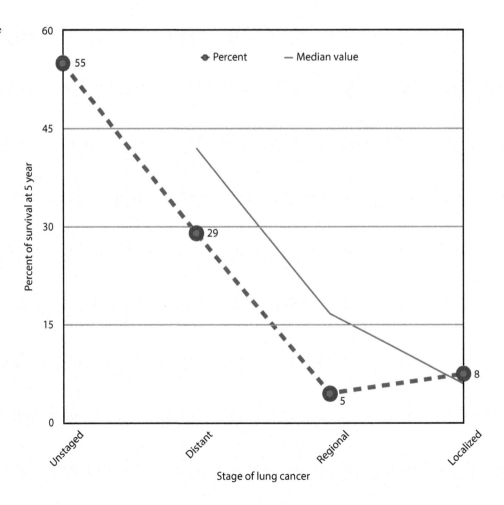

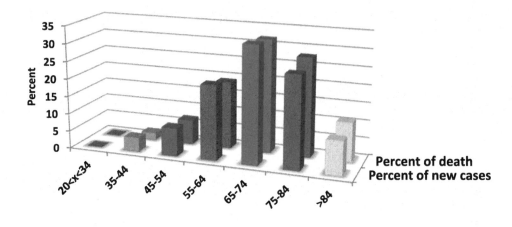

Fig. 32.2 Percent of new cases and death by age

The incidence of lung cancer increases in people who are 65 or older, and it is very rare under age 40, with an average age at the time of diagnosis of 70 years old [1, 2]. The percent of lung cancer deaths is highest among people aged 65–74 with a median age at death of 72 years old [1, 2] (Fig. 32.2).

Lung cancer has been historically most common in men; however, in the last few decades, the incidence of this disease increased among women. Since 1985 the estimated number of lung cancer cases worldwide increased by 51%, with a 44% increase in men and about 76% increase in women [2]. Interestingly women with lung cancer were usually younger at the time of diagnosis, never or former smokers, reporting adenocarcinoma as most common subtype and better survival at any stage as compared with man [3–5].

The patterns of lung cancer incidence are mainly dependent from the tobacco consumption, being tobacco smoking the main cause of lung cancer accounting for 87% of lung cancer deaths in men and for 70% in women [6], with other factors as genetic susceptibility, poor diet, asbestos, radon, and indoor air pollution less contributing to the descriptive epidemiology of this disease [7, 8] (Fig. 32.3).

A significant reduction in tobacco consumption would result in the prevention of a large fraction of lung cancers. In countries with effective tobacco control measures, the incidence of new lung cancer has begun to decline in men and is reaching a plateau for women, making lung cancer a paradigm of the superiority of prevention over treatment [9, 10].

Lung cancer in never smokers is not a rare disease especially in Asian countries and adenocarcinoma subtype, with 15% of cases in men and 53% in women, overall accounting for 25% worldwide [7]. Thus, it is emerging as a distinct disease entity with specific molecular and genetic features.

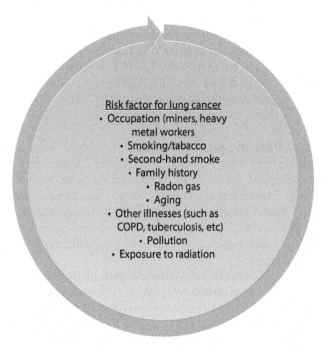

Fig. 32.3 Risk factors for lung cancer

32.3 Screening

Lung cancer diagnosis is usually performed at advanced stages with the majority of patients presenting with metastatic, not curable disease. Most early-stage lung cancers are asymptomatic, often detected by imaging procedures performed for other reasons [11–13]. Therefore, early detection by screening could be a valuable approach to detect the disease earlier, at asymptomatic and potentially curable stage [14].

Screening trials evaluating chest radiography and sputum cytology failed to demonstrate a significant decrease in lung cancer-related mortality [15, 16]. More recently the National Lung Screening Trial (NLST) demonstrated a 20% reduction in mortality with low-dose computed tomography (LDCT) screening as compared to chest radiography in over 53,000 current or former heavy smokers [17], leading several US organizations to recommend screening for high-risk individuals in specialized centers with multidisciplinary expertise [18, 19]. Likewise, the final results of the Dutch-Belgian Randomized Lung Cancer Screening (NELSON) trial have recently shown that LDCT screening in a high-risk population reduced mortality by about 33% in women and 24% in men among more than 15,000 individuals across a 10-year follow-up period [20]. It should be noted that the interval between screens in NELSON was 2 years after the first screen and 2.5 years after the second screen, while the interval in NLST was 1 year.

However, considering the high rate of over-diagnosis of indolent cancers (20–25% of surgery performed in LDCT screening trial have been performed for benign lesions) and the fear of radiation exposure, screening with LCDT has not been endorsed in Europe yet, while an annual screening with chest LDCT in high-risk individuals (30 pack-year smoking history) from age 55 to 80 years is currently recommended in the United States.

32.4   Pathological Features

Pathological diagnosis is recommended prior to any curative treatment and should be made according to the 2015 World Health Organization (WHO) classification. In ◘ Table 32.1, we summarized the current approach for the histologic classification of surgically resected lung cancers.

The recent WHO classification, with its further subclassification of (surgically resected) adenocarcinoma (◘ Table 32.2) by the International Association for the Study of Lung Cancer (IASLC), the American Thoracic Society (ATS), and the European Respiratory Society (ERS), showed differences in metastatic pattern, recurrence, and survival between different histological subtypes which could influence initial treatment decisions.

Non-small cell lung cancer (NSCLC) accounts for 85–90% of lung cancers including the three main histological subtypes: squamous cell carcinoma (30%), adenocarcinoma (40%), and large cell carcinoma (3–9%) [21, 22]. Immunohistochemistry (IHC), including p63, p40, and CK5/6 for squamous cell carcinoma and TTF1, napsin A, and CK7 for adenocarcinoma, is generally required to increase the specificity of diagnosis in the small sample setting and reduce the NSCLC-NOS (not otherwise specified) rate [23–25]. Large cell carcinoma is a tumor lacking morphologic or IHC evidence of clear lineage, with negative or uninformative stains for both squamous cell and adenocarcinoma (◘ Fig. 32.4).

◘ **Table 32.1** Current classification of lung cancer

Category	Description
Adenocarcinoma	Pre-invasive lesions Minimally invasive adenocarcinoma Invasive adenocarcinoma Variants of invasive adenocarcinoma
Squamous cell carcinoma	Pre-invasive lesions Keratinizing Nonkeratinizing Basaloid carcinoma
Large cell carcinoma	
Neuroendocrine tumors	Pre-invasive lesions Carcinoid tumors (typical and atypical carcinoid) Large cell neuroendocrine carcinoma Small cell carcinoma
Adenosquamous carcinoma	
Sarcomatoid carcinoma	Pleomorphic Spindle cell Giant cell carcinoma Carcinosarcoma Pulmonary blastoma
Other unclassified carcinoma	Lymphoepithelioma-like carcinoma NUT carcinoma
Salivary gland tumors	Mucoepidermoid carcinoma Adenoid cystic carcinoma Epithelial-myoepithelial carcinoma Pleomorphic adenoma
Papillomas	Squamous cell papilloma Glandular papilloma Mixed squamous cell and glandular papilloma
Adenomas	Sclerosing pneumocytoma Alveolar adenoma Papillary adenoma Mucinous cystadenoma Pneumocytic adenomyoepithelioma Mucous gland adenoma
Mesenchymal tumors	
Lymphohistiocytic tumors	
Tumors of ectopic origin	
Metastatic tumors	

■ Table 32.2 Classification of lung adenocarcinomas in resection specimens

Category	Description
Pre-invasive lesions	Atypical adenomatous hyperplasia Adenocarcinoma in situ (<3 cm, formerly solitary BAC): non-mucinous, mucinous, mixed
Minimally invasive adenocarcinoma (<3 cm lepidic predominant tumor with <5 mm invasion)	Non-mucinous Mucinous Mixed
Invasive adenocarcinoma	Lepidic predominant (formerly non-mucinous BAC pattern with >5 mm invasion) Acinar predominant Papillary predominant Micropapillary predominant Solid predominant
Variants of invasive adenocarcinoma	Mucinous adenocarcinoma (including formerly mucinous BAC) Colloid Fetal (low and high grade) Enteric

BAC bronchioloalveolar carcinoma

Neuroendocrine malignant tumors account for about 15% of lung cancers, including large cell neuroendocrine carcinoma (LCNEC) (2%) and small cell lung cancer (SCLC) (13%). Immunohistochemistry to confirm the diagnosis of SCLC (synaptophysin, chromogranin A, CD56, thyroid transcription factor 1, and MIB-1) is not mandatory, but should be used in case of any doubt [26] (■ Fig. 32.4). SCLC originates from neuroendocrine cell precursors and is characterized by rapid growth, high response to both chemotherapy and radiotherapy, and development of treatment resistance in all patients with advanced disease [27].

Changes in composition and patterns of tobacco consumption have also led to a significant change in the distribution of lung cancer histological subtypes. Squamous cell carcinoma which was historically considered as the most common subtype in males with smoking history is now decreasing, while adenocarcinoma is increasing in both genders [28]. Smoking cessation possibly has contributed also to the decline of SCLC diagnosis [29].

The last pathologic classification of 2011 highlighted the concept that personalized medicine for patients with advanced lung cancer is determined by histology and genetics and that tissue/cell management of small biopsy/cytology samples is critical for pathologic and molecular diagnosis in order to prevent the loss of tissue in less important analysis [21, 30].

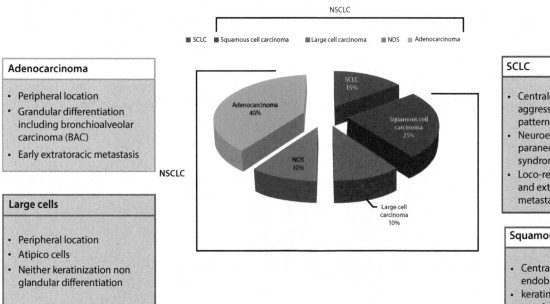

■ Fig. 32.4 Histological subtypes of lung cancer: Pathological features

32.5 Molecular Biology

The identification of genomic alterations as oncogene drivers in a subset of lung cancer led to a radical shift from pathological to molecular classification, establishing a new paradigm for the diagnosis and treatment of this disease known as "personalized medicine" (◘ Fig. 32.5).

Epidermal growth factor receptor (EGFR)-activating mutations have been identified in about 40–60% of Asian [31–33], 15–20% of Caucasian [34, 35], and 30% of Latin American [36] NSCLC patients. Exon 19 deletion (Del19) and point mutation in exon 21 (L858R) account for 90% of overall EGFR-activating mutations [37], but there are also uncommon mutations in exon 18 (E709 and G719X) and in exon 21 (T854 and L861X) resulting in a constitutively activated EGFR [38]. The interaction of EGFR extracellular domain with specific ligands induced homo-dimerization or hetero-dimerization with other HER family member receptors, resulting in the activation of TK domain and tyrosine autophosphorylation. Activating mutations significantly increased autophosphorylation of intracellular tyrosine residues with the subsequent constitutive activation of downstream RAS/RAF/ERK/MAPK and PI3K/AKT pathways, ultimately favoring tumor cell proliferation, angiogenesis, and metastatic potential [37, 39] (◘ Fig. 32.6). The EGFR mutation was the first molecular alteration in lung cancer that has been associated with clinical sensitivity to tyrosine kinase inhibitor (TKI) selectively targeting and inhibiting EGFR.

Based on currently available published data, EGFR mutations are more frequent in female, Asian, never-smoker patients with adenocarcinoma subtype. Thus, EGFR mutational testing is currently recommended in all patients with newly diagnosed advanced adenocarcinoma or large cell carcinoma and in squamous cell carcinoma patients who are never smoker and former light smokers (<15 pack-years). Based on expert consensus opinion, mutational analysis should be performed on tissue specimens, and the commonly used methods for EGFR mutation detection are reported in ◘ Table 32.3.

However, EGFR mutation analysis on circulating tumor DNA (ctDNA) demonstrated an adequate diagnostic accuracy [40, 41] as compared to tumor tissue analysis and is currently recommended as an alternative approach in a subgroup of patients with newly diagnosed metastatic disease who can't undergo biopsy or received uninformative results from tissue molecular analysis. In contrast to EGFR where strong data exists, the assessment of other genomic alterations using ctDNA in treatment-naive patients is more limited. However, as endorsed by most international scientific societies, the detection of an actionable alteration in ctDNA, if using a validated assay, would eventually represent sufficient evidence to initiate targeted treatment, albeit not without reimbursement variations among all the different countries. Nonetheless, a negative finding of either EGFR or other genomic alterations using ctDNA should be considered not conclusive, and, when feasible due to patients' performance status, a tissue re-biopsy should be performed (◘ Fig. 32.7).

The EML4-ALK rearrangements have been detected as potent oncogene drivers in about 3–8% of NSCLC patients [42], resulting in a constitutive activation of the intracellular domain of ALK receptor and downstream RAS/MAPK, PI3K/AKT, and JAK/STAT3 signaling pathways [43], thus emerging as a predictive biomarker of clinical response to ALK inhibitors. Similarly ROS proto-oncogene 1 (ROS1) rearrangements occur in about 1–2% of NSCLC patients and were associated with a great response rate to ALK inhibitors [44, 45]. Both ALK and ROS1 rearrangements are more frequent in never smokers and younger people with adenocarcinoma, while are not associated with gender or ethnicity.

◘ **Fig. 32.5** From histological to molecular subtypes of lung cancer

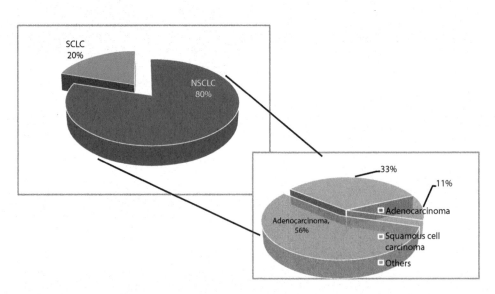

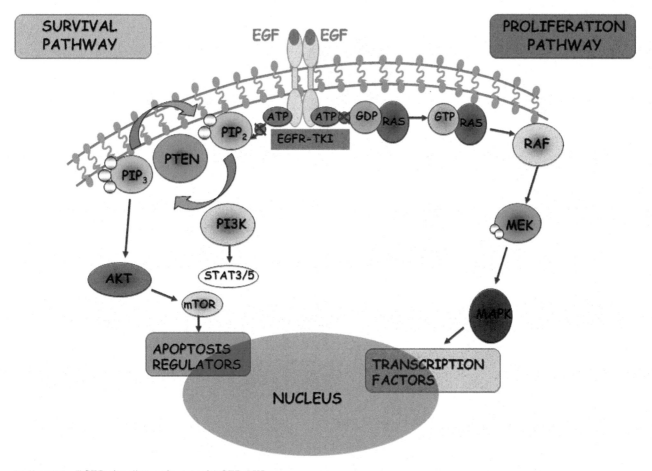

□ **Fig. 32.6** EGFR signaling pathway and EGFR TKI

□ **Table 32.3** Methods for EGFR mutation detection on tumor samples

Method	Tumor DNA required (%)	EGFR mutations detected	Deletions and insertions
Sanger direct sequencing	25	Known and new	Yes
Real-time/ TaqMan PCR	10	Known only	No
Cobas	5–10	Known only	Yes
Pyrosequencing	5–10	Known only	Yes
MALDI-TOF MS-based genotyping	5	Known only	No
Allelic-specific PCR/ARMS	1	Known only	No
PNA-LNA-PCR clamp	1	Known only	No
Massively parallel NGS	0.1	Known and new	Yes

The ALK/ROS1 analysis should be performed on the same patient population tested for EGFR. Fluorescence in situ hybridization (FISH) using break-apart probes on tissue specimens has been the standard Food and Drug Administration (FDA)-approved tool [46, 47] (□ Fig. 32.8). However, several studies showed a high concordance between FISH and immunohisto-chemistry (IHC) for ALK detection [48–54], suggesting IHC as a reliable screening assay for ALK rearrangements which has been adopted worldwide. Although FISH analysis on cytologic preparations is not recommended, however cell blocks may be acceptable.

Since both EGFR mutations and ALK rearrangements predicted therapeutic benefit with their respective targeted drugs in patients with adenocarcinoma, biomarker testing has been implemented and integrated into treatment decision process. The recent development of next-generation sequencing (NGS) accomplishes massive parallel gene mutation analysis and requires low amount of tissue, favoring the identification of several targetable molecular alterations, including BRAF, HER2, and MET mutations and RET and NTRK gene fusions, which may allow access to targeted treatments in the context of clinical trials (□ Fig. 32.8). Molecular

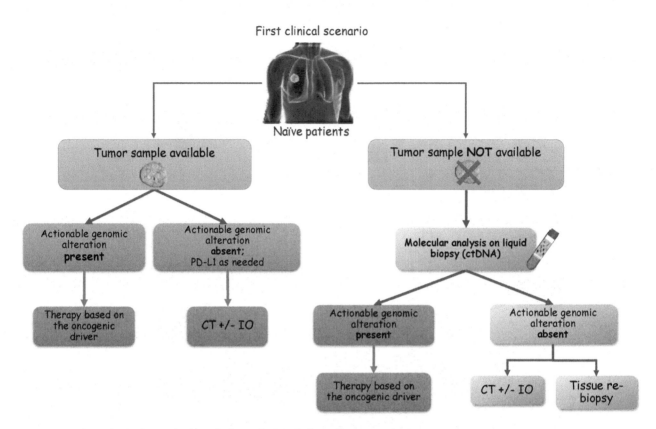

◻ Fig. 32.7 Mutation testing at the time of advanced NSCLC diagnosis

alterations in different signaling pathways have been recently identified also in squamous cell carcinoma, including PI3KCA, PTEN, AKT, FGFR, RAS, TP53, CDKN2A, and RB1, offering new avenues of investigation for targeted treatment [55]. Despite many efforts, very few data are currently available for SCLC, revealing FGFR1, JAK2, and SOX2 gene amplifications and TP53, RB, and PTEN gene mutations [56, 57] among the most common genetic alterations, but their predictive roles need to be investigated in clinical trials.

32.6 Clinical Features

The majority of patients with lung cancer are symptomatic at the time of initial presentation, with only 5–15% of asymptomatic people in whom lung cancer is detected incidentally on a chest x-ray for other indications or in the context of screening clinical trials [11, 12]. Most symptoms may be ascribed to the loco-regional intra-thoracic tumor invasive growth and/or to the development of extra-thoracic metastasis. In a small subgroup of patients, symptoms may be related to specific paraneoplastic syndromes which require differential diagnosis with other clinical conditions [58] (◻ Fig. 32.9).

Among the most common symptoms caused by local tumor growth, cough and dyspnea are reported in up to

60% of cases [59], and hemoptysis is reported in about one third of patients [60], while some people may refer persistent chest pain or discomfort, even if no invasion of the chest wall, mediastinum, or pleura occurred. Systemic and not specific symptoms such as fatigue and weight loss frequently occur in about 70% of patients at the time of lung cancer diagnosis. However, because these symptoms are reported also in other lung diseases associated with smoke exposure, such as COPD, special attention should be posed to any relevant symptom changing pattern in high-risk patients.

Dysphagia [61], dysphonia or hoarseness [62], and diaphragmatic paralysis may be related to the loco-regional intra-thoracic tumor growth, respectively, invading the esophagus, left recurrent laryngeal nerve, and phrenic nerve. Malignant pleural and pericardial effusions are caused by either direct tumor invasion or hematological/lymphatic spread of cancer cells, respectively, occurring in 10–20% and 5–10% of people with lung cancer [63, 64]. The "superior vena cava syndrome" occurs in less than 5% of patients with initial diagnosis of lung cancer. It is caused by obstruction or compression of vena cava by tumor and is characterized by head and neck swelling, dilatation of the veins on both neck and chest wall, cough, dizziness, headache, dyspnea, and chest pain [65, 66]. Lung cancer growing in the apex of the upper lobe, known as Pancoast tumor, may cause the

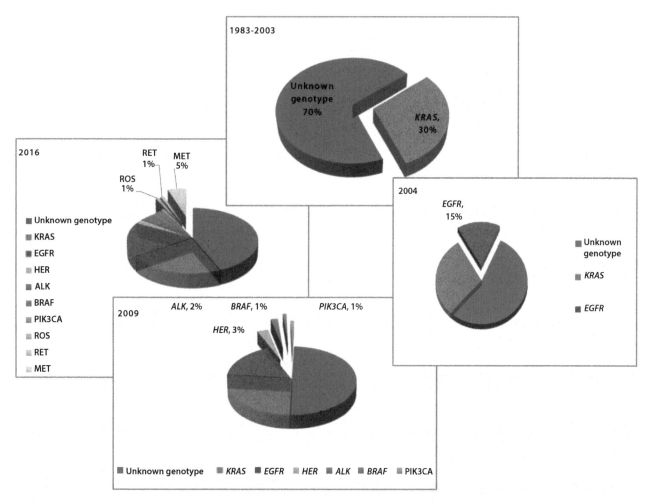

Fig. 32.8 Progress in identifying molecular alterations in lung adenocarcinoma

Fig. 32.9 Clinical presenting symptoms and signs in lung cancer

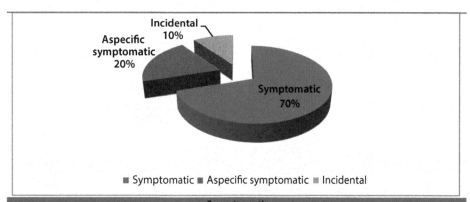

Symptomatic	
Local tumor growth	Cough, hemoptysis, dyspnea, chest pain
Loco-regional growth	Pleuro-pericardial effusion, hoarseness, superior vena cava syndrome, disphagia, Pancoast syndrome
Extra-thoracic metastasis	Bone, brain, liver, andrenal gland, others
Paraneoplastic syndromes	Muscoloskeletal, cutaneous, endocrinologic, hematologic, neurologic, miscellaneous

"Horner syndrome," overall occurring in about 4% of cases at initial presentation. It's characterized by enophthalmos, ptosis, miosis, and hemi-facial anhidrosis due to the invasion of the sympathetic chain and stellate ganglion by the tumor and is often associated with pain and muscle wasting in the arm and hand due to the invasion of the brachial plexus and chest wall pain due to the invasion of ribs and vertebrae by the tumor [67].

A significant subgroup of patients may present symptoms caused by distant tumor metastasis at the time of lung cancer diagnosis. Bone metastasis may cause pain, pathological fractures, hypercalcemia, and rarely spinal cord compression which is characterized by local pain, paralysis, sensory loss, and sphincter dysfunction and requires urgent intervention [68]. Brain metastasis is often symptomatic with variable clinical presentation including headache, focal or generalized seizures, nausea and vomiting, confusion, or visual alterations [69]. Lung cancer metastasis may occur also at other sites, including the liver, adrenal gland, and lymph nodes, with clinical presentation varying according to patient's symptoms (Fig. 32.10).

Paraneoplastic syndromes include a large spectrum of endocrine, neurologic, dermatologic, hematologic, and metabolic clinical manifestations due to the production of bioactive substances (e.g., hormone-like peptides, prostaglandins, cytokines, etc.) by tumor cells in the absence of a direct invasion/obstruction of vital organs by the tumor [70]. Paraneoplastic syndromes occur in about 10% of patients with lung cancer, mostly SCLC, and may be classified according to the clinical presentation (Table 32.4).

A careful evaluation of the aforementioned clinical manifestations and syndromes by physicians is crucial for the early detection of lung cancer, ultimately resulting in better patients' survival outcomes.

32.7 Diagnosis and Staging

The diagnostic evaluation should initially focus on careful physical examination and personal patient's history, to identify new symptoms or a significant change in the usual respiratory symptoms [58]. For all the patients with suspected lung cancer, an urgent referral for non-invasive chest imaging is recommended, including radiographs, computed tomography (CT), and positron emission tomography (PET) [71]. Chest radiography plays a crucial role in the diagnostic workup of lung cancer especially in the primary care setting [72]. However, even if it may lead to the identification of a suspected tumor, it has no sufficient diagnostic accuracy to differentiate benign from malignant lesions, often requiring additional imaging examinations, even in the case of negative result [73]. Conventional contrast-enhanced chest CT is considered the best exam to detect lung cancer, as it provides detailed information on anatomic location, margins, invasion of surrounding structures or chest wall, and mediastinal lymph node involvement [74]. PET with fluorodeoxyglucose (FDG) is very accurate for differentiating benign from malignant lesions, but plays a crucial role in the mediastinal staging, since it has shown to have both higher sensitivity and specificity than CT [75]. The overall diagnostic information which emerged from non-invasive imaging (CT, PET, or combined PET-CT), including size and location of the tumor, presence of mediastinal or distant metastasis, and the patient's clinical status, will guide the most appropriate strategy to achieve the final diagnosis and staging of lung cancer with the least risk to the patients (Fig. 32.11). Bronchoscopy with biopsy and transbronchial needle aspiration (TBNA) is the most common procedure used to obtain a pathological diagnosis

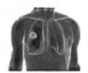

BRAIN	BONE	LIVER	BRAIN
• SCLC 50%	• SCLC 30-40%	• SCLC 25%	• SCLC 20-40%
• NSCLC 25-30%	• NSCLC 30-40%	• NSCLC 5%	• NSCLC 10%
Symptoms	Symptoms	Symptoms	Symptoms
• Headache;	• Pain and morbidity;	• Abdominal pain/	• Black pain;
• nausea/vomiting;	• pathologic fractures;	discomfort;	• abdominal pain;
• neurological/psychiatric	• spinal cord	• nausea;	• hemorrhage;
symptoms.	compression.	• weight loss;	

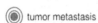 tumor metastasis

 Fig. 32.10 Symptoms caused by tumor metastasis at the time of lung cancer diagnosis

◻ **Table 32.4** Classification of paraneoplastic syndromes in lung cancer

Syndrome	Lung cancer subtype	Cause
Acromegaly	Carcinoid tumors Small cell lung cancer	Growth hormone
Carcinoid syndrome	Carcinoid tumors Large cell carcinoma Small cell lung cancer	Serotonin
Ectopic adrenocorticotropic hormone (ACTH) syndrome	Carcinoid tumors Small cell lung cancer	ACTH Corticotropin-releasing hormone
Encephalomyelitis/sensory neuropathy	Small cell lung cancer	Anti-HU antibody and Hu-D antigen
Hypertrophic pulmonary osteoarthropathy	Non-small cell lung cancer Small cell lung cancer	Prostaglandin-E Inflammatory cytokines
Granulocytosis	Non-small cell lung cancer	Colony-stimulating factor (CSF) Granulocyte-CSF Granulocyte macrophage CSF Interleukin (IL)-6
Hypercalcemia	Non-small cell lung cancer	Parathormone Parathyroid hormone-related peptide
Hyponatremia	Small cell lung cancer Non-small cell lung cancer	Arginine vasopressin Atrial natriuretic peptide
Lambert-Eaton syndrome	Small cell lung cancer	Anti-P/Q channel antibody and P/Q type calcium channel (antigen)
Retinopathy	Small cell lung cancer	Antirecoverin antibody and specific antigen to photoreceptor cells
Thrombocytosis	Non-small cell lung cancer Small cell lung cancer	IL-6
Thromboembolism	Non-small cell lung cancer Small cell lung cancer	Procoagulants Inflammatory cytokines Tumor interaction with host cells

of NSCLC, especially in presence of central lesions [76]. Additional tools for biopsy include both endobronchial ultrasound (EBUS) and endoscopic ultrasound (EUS)-guided biopsy [77–79]. For peripheral pulmonary nodules not detectable by bronchoscopy, CT-guided trans-thoracic biopsy (TTB) may be considered as an alternative approach [80, 81], while in patients with pleural effusion at initial presentation, thoracentesis with cytological examination of pleural fluid should be performed [82], and, if negative, image-guided pleural biopsy or video-assisted thoracoscopy surgery (VATS) is recommended [83]. For patients in whom SCLC is suspected on the basis of both clinical and imaging findings, the easiest method among sputum cytology, bronchoscopy, trans-thoracic biopsy, and thoracentesis should be used to obtain a pathological diagnosis [76]. The diagnostic strategy should be individualized for each patient and should be decided within a multidisciplinary team.

Mediastinum staging plays a crucial role in the diagnostic workup of intra-thoracic NSCLC and significantly influences patients' prognosis and treatment strategy with the final aim of identifying patients who may benefit from surgery from those who will receive other forms of therapy. Because of the high frequency of false positive imaging tests, all patients with mediastinal lymph node involvement on CT or PET should undergo invasive tissue sampling by EBUS or EUS to confirm node disease, and if results are negative, mediastinoscopy is recommended [76, 84, 85]. For tumors without mediastinal involvement on CT or PET, invasive mediastinal staging is advised only in case of central lesion and/or a tumor size >3 cm, while peripheral tumors <3 cm should not receive additional examinations [86]. Screening for brain metastases by MRI might be useful in patients considered for curative therapy, while it's recommended in all patients reporting CNS-related symptoms. Finally, abdomen CT scan and bone scan should be performed in all patients to exclude the presence of distant metastasis [87].

During the 16th World Congress of Lung Cancer, the Union for International Cancer Control (UICC) presented the revised tumor, node, and metastasis

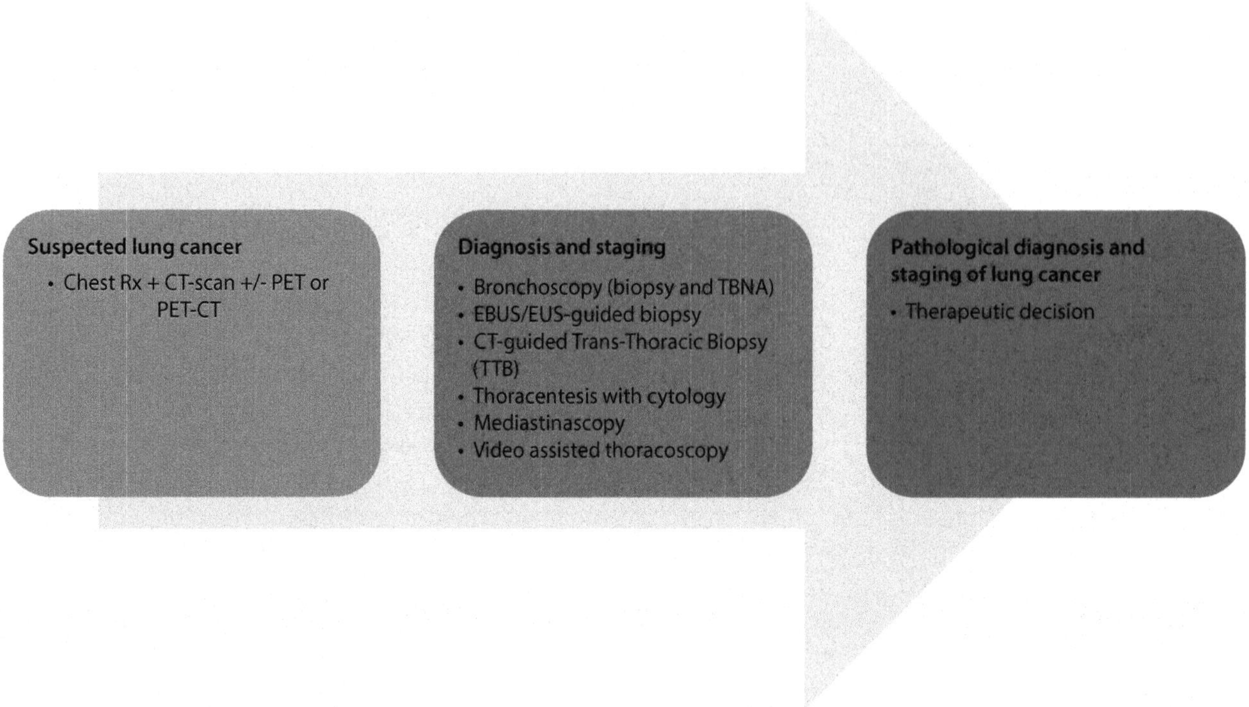

◘ Fig. 32.11 Diagnostic algorithm in patients with suspected lung cancer

(TNM) classification of lung cancer (UICC TNM 8) [88], as shown in ◘ Table 32.5, which should be used for both NSCLC and SCLC.

The practice of classifying cancer according to anatomical extent named "stage" derives from the observation that patients' survival rates correlated with their tumor extension at the time of diagnosis [88] (◘ Table 32.6). The TNM tumor staging remains the most important parameter informing clinicians about the prognosis for survival and guiding treatment planning and monitoring in lung cancer patient.

32.8   Treatment

32.8.1   Localized Disease

Despite recent advances in diagnostic procedures, only 20% of NSCLC patients have early-stage disease at the time of diagnosis, thus potentially operable [1] (◘ Fig. 32.12).

The recommended treatment of patients with stage I–II NSCLC is curative-intent surgical resection [89] for all patients who are considered clinically "operable," with a 5-year survival rate reported to be 40–60% for stage I and 20–35% for stage II [1]. The current gold standard is lobectomy [90] with hilar and mediastinal lymph node sampling or dissection [91]. Either open thoracotomy or VATS is recommended as an appropriate surgical approach to the expertise of the surgeon, even if VATS should be preferred in stage I tumors [92]

because it was associated with lower post-operative morbidity/mortality, resulting in improved quality of life [93]. Alternative approaches, including segmentectomy or wedge resection, could be reserved to patients with limited cardiopulmonary function [94–96]. Systematic nodal dissection of a minimum of six nodes/ stations, three of which should be mediastinal including the subcarinal station, should be guaranteed to ensure "R0 resection" [91]. Curative stereotactic body radiotherapy (SABR) should be offered to patients with a peripherally located stage I NSCLC who have clinical comorbidities or are at very high surgery-related risk and those who refuse to undergo surgical procedure [97–99]. For patients with multifocal NSCLC, radical surgical resection whenever possible or alternatively SABR [100] is recommended after discussion within a multidisciplinary tumor board [83].

Adjuvant platinum doublet chemotherapy is recommended for all patients with stage II and III surgically resected disease [83]. Two meta-analyses demonstrated that post-operative platinum-based chemotherapy led to more than 10% reduction in the risk of death resulting in 5% absolute 5-year survival rate improvement [101, 102]. On the basis of the results of the JBR.10 and ANITA trials, cisplatin-vinorelbine is currently considered as the best regimen for adjuvant setting [103, 104]. The role of adjuvant therapy in stage I is still controversial, with a small survival benefit limited to patients with stage IB disease with tumor >4 cm [104, 105]. In the decision process for adjuvant therapy, several factors, including time from surgery, age, and pre- and post-operative morbidi-

Table 32.5 The eight edition of the TNM clinical classification of lung cancer

TNM clinical classification	
T	*Primary tumor*
TX	Primary tumor cannot be assessed or tumor proven by the presence of malignant cells in sputum or bronchial washing but not visualized by imaging/bronchoscopy
T0	No evidence of primary tumor
Tis	Carcinoma in situ
T1	Tumor 3 cm or less in greatest dimension, surrounded by lung or visceral pleura, without bronchoscopic evidence of invasion more proximal than lobar bronchus (not in the main bronchus) T1a(mi): Minimally invasive adenocarcinoma T1a: Tumor <1 cm in greatest dimension T1b: Tumor >1 cm but <2 cm in greatest dimension T1c: Tumor >2 cm but <3 cm in greatest dimension
T2	Tumor >3 cm but <5 cm or tumor with any of the following features: involves the main bronchus regardless of distance from the carina but without involvement of the carina; invades the visceral pleura; and associated with atelectasis or obstructive pneumonitis that extends to the hilar region, involving part or all of the lung T2a: Tumor >3 cm but <4 cm in greatest dimension T2b: Tumor >4 cm but <5 cm in greatest dimension
T3	Tumor >5 cm but <7 cm in greatest dimension or associated with separate tumor nodules in the same lobe as the primary tumor or directly invades any of the following structures: chest wall (including the parietal pleura and superior sulcus tumors), phrenic nerve, and parietal pericardium
T4	Tumor >7 cm in greatest dimension or associated with separate tumor nodules in a different ipsilateral lobe than that of the primary tumor or invades any of the following structures: diaphragm, mediastinum, heart, great vessels, trachea, recurrent laryngeal nerve, esophagus, vertebral body, and carina
N	*Regional lymph nodes*
Nx	Regional lymph nodes cannot be assessed
N0	No regional lymph node metastasis
N1	Metastasis in ipsilateral peribronchial and/or ipsilateral hilar lymph nodes and intrapulmonary nodes, including involvement by direct extension
N2	Metastasis in ipsilateral mediastinal and/or subcarinal lymph nodes
N3	Metastasis in contralateral mediastinal, contralateral hilar, ipsilateral or contralateral scalene, or supraclavicular lymph nodes
M	*Distant metastasis*
M0	No distant metastasis
M1	Distant metastasis present M1a: Separate tumor nodules in a contralateral lobe; tumor with pleural or pericardial nodules or malignant pleural or pericardial effusion M1b: Single extra-thoracic metastasis M1c: Multiple extra-thoracic metastases in one or more organs

ties, should be taken into account and discussed within a multidisciplinary tumor board. Several studies and meta-analysis suggested that the estimated benefit from neoadjuvant chemotherapy is similar to that expected with adjuvant chemotherapy [106–108]; thus, it may be considered as a feasible and ethical approach for patients with stage II–IIIA NSCLC. However, adjuvant treatment is currently preferred because of major evidence base and clinical experience (Fig. 32.13).

Based on the efficacy interim analysis of the phase III ADAURA trial, adjuvant osimertinib has recently led to significantly improved disease-free survival (DFS) compared with placebo in NSCLC patients presenting with the complete resection of primary tumor with stage IB to IIIA and harboring EGFR common mutations. In patients with stage II to IIIA median DFS rate was not even yet reached, while the 2-year DFS was 90% with osimertinib for up to three years versus 44% with placebo with most of patients not experiencing central nervous disease relapse. No new safety signals have been observed. Even if final overall survival (OS) analyses are pending, in the EGFR-mutated radically resected NSCLC this trial might be already considered practice-changing as opposed to the current standard of care based on adjuvant cisplatin-based chemotherapy [109]. The ongoing ITACA trial aims to identify predictive tumor molecular biomarker, such as excision repair cross-complementation group 1 (ERCC1) and thymidylate synthase (TS), useful to select patients who may derive the most clinical benefit from adjuvant chemotherapy. Post-operative radiotherapy (PORT) should be considered only after R1 resection or N2 pathological disease discovered at sur-

gery [83]. Even if the updated results of the PORT meta-analysis showed a not clear benefit in patients with N2 pathological disease undergoing PORT after radical surgery [110], PORT is largely adopted in clinical practice. However, even if possibly retaining a role in the ablative treatment of low-volume recurrences in brain and other sites (so-called oligometastases) and as conventional chemoradiotherapy to the thorax in patients who develop isolated nodal recurrences, mediastinal post-operative radiotherapy should not be used routinely in completely resected pN2 patients with radical surgery remaining a single local modality to be followed by a watch-and-wait strategy, as recently confirmed by the LungART primary end-point analyses [111].

Only 5% of patients with SCLC have "very limited" stage I disease (T1-2, N0-1, M0) at the time of diagnosis, thus potentially benefiting from curative surgery with 5-year survival rate reported to be around 50% [112, 113]. Surgical resection with mediastinal lymph node dissection followed by four cycles of systemic platinum doublet chemotherapy is recommended as standard of care, while concurrent chemoradiotherapy may be considered as an alternative option in patients who have high perioperative risk after discussion within a multidisciplinary team [27] (◘ Fig. 32.14).

◘ **Table 32.6** Stage grouping and 5-year OS according to the 8th TNM Clinical classification

Stage	T	N	M	5-year OS
Occult carcinoma	Tx	N0	M0	
Stage 0	Tis	N0	M0	
Stage IA1	T1a, T1a(mi)	N0	M0	92%
Stage IA2	T1b	N0	M0	83%
Stage IA3	T1c	N0	M0	77%
Stage IB	T2a	N0	M0	68%
Stage IIA	T2b	N0	M0	60%
Stage IIB	T1a, T1b, T1c	N1	M0	53%
	T2a, T2b	N1	M0	
	T3	N0	M0	
Stage IIIA	T1a, T1b, T1c	N2	M0	36%
	T2a, T2b	N2	M0	
	T3	N1	M0	
	T4	N1	M0	
Stage IIIB	T1a, T1b, T1c	N3	M0	26%
	T2a, T2b	N3	M0	
	T3	N2	M0	
	T4	N2	M0	
Stage IIIC	T3	N3	M0	13%
	T4	N3	M0	
Stage IVA	Any T	Any N	M1a M1b	10%
Stage IVB	Any T	Any N	M1c	0%

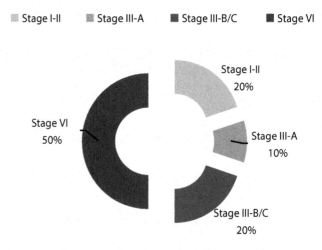

◘ **Fig. 32.12** Percentage of disease staging at the time of lung cancer diagnosis

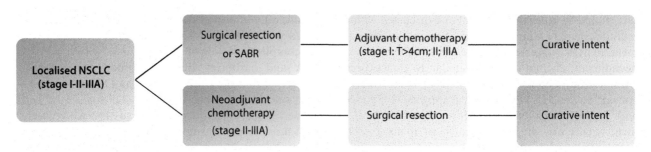

◘ **Fig. 32.13** Therapeutic algorithm for early-stage NSCLC

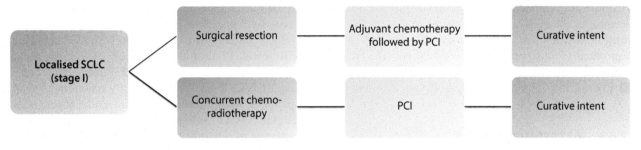

Fig. 32.14 Therapeutic algorithm for early-stage SCLC

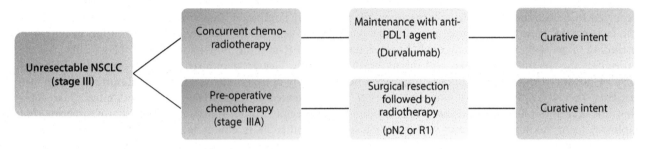

Fig. 32.15 Therapeutic algorithm for stage III NSCLC

Fig. 32.16 Therapeutic algorithm for locally advanced SCLC

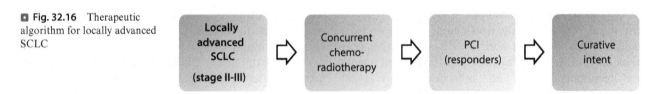

32.8.2 Locally Advanced Disease

Stage III account for 25–30% of NSCLC, including a heterogeneous group of tumors with a very controversial treatment. Patients with locally advanced stage IIIA NSCLC may be candidate to surgical therapy if they have T4, N0, or single-station N2 disease with nodal staging performed by invasive methods or if they obtained nodal downstaging after pre-operative induction chemotherapy. Several studies included in the LACE meta-analysis demonstrated a 4.2% absolute 5-year survival rate improvement for patients who received adjuvant therapy, including those with stage IIIA N0-1, suggesting platinum-vinorelbine as the best regimen [102]. Eligibility for pre-operative or post-operative platinum doublets with or without radiotherapy should be evaluated in the context of an experienced multidisciplinary team. For all other patients with unresectable stage IIIA or IIIB disease, concurrent chemoradiation is currently recommended as the treatment of choice with 5-year survival rate reported to be 10% [83]. A meta-analysis including seven randomized studies demonstrated a 5.7% absolute 3-year survival rate improvement with concurrent versus sequential treatment in patients with IIIB NSCLC, even if at the cost of increased toxicity [114]. However, sequential chemother-

apy followed by definitive radiotherapy is considered as an alternative valid option, especially for elderly or frail patients with clinical comorbidities. Different platinum-based combinations may be used on the clinical center experience [115–117]. Recently the randomized phase III PACIFIC study compared the anti-PDL1 monoclonal antibody durvalumab vs placebo as maintenance therapy in patients with stage III unresectable NSCLC after definitive concurrent chemoradiation, showing a significant PFS improvement in patients receiving durvalumab [118], which represents a new standard of care in this setting of patients (⦾ Fig. 32.15).

Patients with T1-4, N1-3, and M0 SCLC represent about one third of overall SCLC population. Several studies and meta-analysis demonstrated that concurrent radiochemotherapy is the best treatment option for such patients with "limited disease" and good performance status and platinum-etoposide is the most used chemo-regimen [119]. However, sequential chemotherapy followed by radiotherapy may be considered as an alternative valid option when concurrent treatment is not feasible [27]. A meta-analysis including about 1000 patients with limited disease who had complete response to chemoradiotherapy showed that prophylactic cranial irradiation (PCI) significantly improved patients' survival and reduced the risk of brain metastasis at 3 years, without any impact on extracranial disease [120]. Because of the high incidence of brain metastasis in the natural history of the disease, all patients who responded to initial therapy should be considered for PCI within 6 months from treatment beginning [27] (■ Fig. 32.16).

32.8.3 Metastatic Disease

The majority of patients have distant metastasis at the time of NSCLC diagnosis, with median survival reported to be 6 months without any treatment [1]. In the last two decades, the advent of new effective drugs including targeted therapies and immunotherapies revolutionized the treatment strategies and the natural history of advanced disease, significantly improving both patients' survival and quality of life. The decision of first-line therapy should be discussed within a multidisciplinary team, taking into account both tumor histology and molecular profile, along with age, PS, comorbidities, and preference of patients [121].

■ **Oncogene-Addicted NSCLC**

For about 20% of patients whose tumors harbor oncogenic drivers, including both EGFR-activating mutations and ALK/ROS1 rearrangements, targeted agents are recommended as an upfront therapy [121] (■ Fig. 32.17). The recent advent of next-generation sequencing (NGS) in many centers favored molecular testing for multiple gene alterations, including BRAF, HER2, and MET alterations, as well as ROS1, RET, and NTRK fusions which may currently allow access to targeted treatment only in late lines of therapy in the context of a clinical trial [121].

Eight randomized phase III trials [33, 122–128] demonstrated that EGFR TKIs gefitinib, erlotinib, and afatinib significantly improved response rate (RR), progression-free survival (PFS), tolerability, and QoL as compared to platinum-based chemotherapy in about 12–15% of patients with metastatic NSCLC harboring EGFR (exon 19 deletion and exon 21 L858R point mutation)-activating mutations (■ Table 32.7). Thus, molecular EGFR testing is currently recommended in all patients with newly diagnosed, advanced, non-squamous NSCLC and in never/former and light smokers with squamous subtype before starting the first-line therapy in order to select the best treatment for each patient [121].

Recently the randomized phase III FLAURA trial [129] compared third-generation TKI osimertinib to first-generation TKI gefitinib or erlotinib in untreated EGFR-mutant NSCLC patients. The results of this study clearly demonstrated that upfront osimertinib nearly doubled median PFS and duration of response, presented with less toxicities and with intracranial activity against brain metastasis (BM) that is superior than all other TKIs, emerging as the most effective and better tolerated drug currently available for first-line treatment of EGFR-positive NSCLC patients (■ Table 32.8). Accordingly, the final results of the study have recently proved that osimertinib achieved a clinically meaningful improvement in median OS of almost 7 months (38.6 versus 31.8 months) in the same setting of patients [130].

Noteworthy, these EGFR mutations proved to be strong predictors of response to TKIs with the most "common" type of activating or sensitizing EGFR mutation being the in-frame deletion of exon 19 (about 45% of EGFR mutations), followed by the L858R point mutation of exon 21 (about 40% of EGFR mutations). The remaining 10% of EGFR mutations appeared to harbor heterogeneous molecular alterations within exons 18–21 (so-called "uncommon" mutations) with clinically variable responses to targeted drugs and shorter survival rates when compared to classical mutations [131].

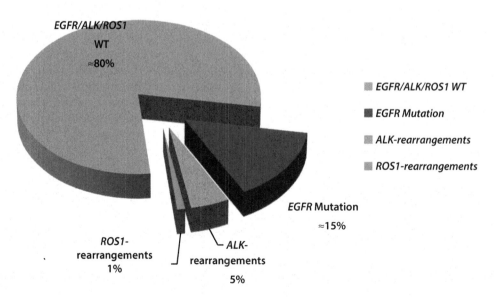

■ **Fig. 32.17** Targetable oncogenic drivers in patients with advanced NSCLC

Table 32.7 Randomized phase III trials of EGFR TKI vs chemo as the first-line treatment in EGFR+ NSCLC

Study	Treatment	N (EGFR mut+)	PFS months (EGFR mut+)	HR for PFS (EGFR mut +)	OS months (EGFR mut+)	HR for OS (EGFR mut+)
IPASS Mok 2009	Gefitinib Chemo	132 129	9.5 6.3	0.48 (0.36–0.66)	21.6 21.9	0.91 (0.76–1.10)
First-SIGNAL Han 2012	Gefitinib Chemo	26 16	8.0 6.3	0.54 (0.26–1.10)	27.2 25.6	1.043 (0.49–2.18)
NEJ002 Maemondo 2010	Gefitinib Chemo	114 110	10.8 5.4	0.30 (0.22–0.41)	30.5 23.6	0.887 (0.63–1.24)
WJTOG3405 Mitsudomi 2010	Gefitinib Chemo	86 86	9.2 6.3	0.49 (0.34–0.71)	35.5 38.8	1.185 (0.76–1.82)
OPTIMAL Zhou 2011	Erlotinib Chemo	82 72	13.7 4.6	0.16 (0.10–0.26)	22.6 28.8	1.04 (0.69–1.58)
EURTAC Rosell 2012	Erlotinib Chemo	86 87	9.7 5.2	0.37 (0.25–0.54)	25.8 20.8	0.86 (0.54–1.38)
LUX-Lung 3 Sequist 2013	Afatinib Chemo	230 115	11.1 6.9	0.58 (0.43–0.78)	28.2 28.2	0.88 (0.66–1.17)
LUX-Lung 6 Wu 2014	Afatinib Chemo	242 122	11.0 5.6	0.28 (0.20–0.39)	23.1 23.5	0.93 (0.72–1.22)

Table 32.8 Efficacy and tolerability of EGFR TKIs as the first-line treatment in EGFR+ NSCLC

	Gefitinib	Erlotinib	Afatinib	Dacomitinib	Osimertinib
ORR	71.2%	64%	69%	75%	80%
PFS	9.5 months	9.7 months	11.1 months	14.7 months	18.9 months
Severe AEs	28.7%	32%	49%	63%	34%

Similarly, the ALK TKI crizotinib has shown to improve RR, PFS, and QoL as compared to first-line platinum chemotherapy and has been recommended as an upfront treatment in 3–8% of NSCLC harboring ALK rearrangements [132]. Thus, routine screening testing for ALK by IHC should be performed simultaneously to EGFR mutations in the same patient population, followed by the break-apart fluorescence in situ hybridization (FISH) analysis to confirm definitive positivity [121].

Recently the phase III randomized J-ALEX [133] and ALEX [134] studies compared the new-generation ALK inhibitor alectinib vs crizotinib in untreated ALK-rearranged NSCLC patients. Treatment with alectinib was associated with longer PFS and better tolerability than crizotinib, and, most importantly, it prevented the occurrence of BMs, emerging as the new standard of

Table 32.9 Efficacy and tolerability of ALK inhibitors as the first-line treatment in ALK+ NSCLC

	ORR	CNS ORR	PFS (months)	Any grade AEs	Grade 3–5 AEs
Alectinib	82.9%	81%	N.R	97%	41%
Crizotinib	75.5%	50%	11.1	97%	50%

care worldwide (◘ Table 32.9). Likewise, according to the planned interim analysis of the CROWN trial, the third generation ALK TKI lorlatinib led to a 72% improvement in PFS along with numerical improvements in best overall response when compared with crizotinib as a first-line treatment approach, finally resulting in a higher incidence of grade 3/4 adverse events without an increased treatment discontinuation rate [135, 136].

As regards other second-generation ALK TKIs, brigatinib showed superiority to crizotinib in the phase III ALTA-1L trial as well as the third-generation ALK inhibitor lorlatinib, demonstrating a significant intracranial activity. Of significance, no randomized trials comparing alectinib with the other second-generation or third-generation ALK TKIs have been published.

Interestingly, the addition of immune checkpoint inhibitors to both first- and third-generation EGFR TKIs did not lead to any significant enhancement of clinical activity when compared to EGFR TKI alone in TKI-naïve and TKI-pre-treated NSCLC patients, however at the cost of unexpected toxicities, ultimately resulting in the limitation of further active investigation [135].

As far as other targetable alterations are concerned, BRAF mutations are identified in 2–4% of lung adenocarcinomas, half of whom presenting with a BRAF V600 mutation. Based on the results of the phase II BRF113928 trial, the combination of dabrafenib and trametinib is now approved in the first-line treatment of patients with BRAF V600 mutations, reporting excellent results that were similar in treated and untreated patients with an average ORR of 64% and a median PFS of 10 months along with a manageable safety profile, especially in the BRAF V600E population [137]. Furthermore, the discovery of new highly selective KRAS inhibitors such as AMG510 and MRTX849 eliciting partial responses in phase I trials has provided a renewed opportunity to better understand the role of KRAS mutation as an oncogenic driver, occurring in 20–30% of NSCLC patients [138]. Recently, the list of actionable targets in lung cancer has been expanded with the FDA approval of capmatinib for MET exon 14 skipping mutations, larotrectinib and entrectinib for NTRK-rearranged tumors [139, 140], and selpercatinib for RET fusion-positive NSCLCs. Other experimental molecular targets include HER-2 mutations, which recently have been shown to be therapeutically exploitable with novel potent anti-HER2 agents, such as T-DM1 and trastuzumab deruxtecan (DS-8201a) [141], and NRG1 gene fusions [142]. Moreover, the introduction of new targeted agents in clinical practice modified the lung cancer treatment strategy and was accompanied by the emergence of a new spectrum of toxicities. Skin rash, diarrhea, and asymptomatic hypertransaminasemia were the most common adverse events associated with EGFR TKIs, while visual disorders, gastrointestinal disturbances, and elevated liver enzymes were associated with ALK inhibitors [143], thus requiring an active involvement and

a close collaboration between oncologists and family physicians in all phases of patients' care.

■ **Acquired Resistance**

Even if oncogene-addicted NSCLC patients benefited from TKIs, the majority of them experienced disease progression within 10–12 months of therapy, due to the development of acquired resistance by cancer cells [144] (◘ Fig. 32.18).

The exon 20 T790M mutation is the most common finding detected in 50–60% of EGFR-mutated resistant tumors progressing to first-/second-generation EGFR TKIs. It involves the ATP-binding pocket of the receptor and results in an increased ATP affinity, causing resistance to competitive reversible EGFR TKIs [145].

The third-generation TKI osimertinib, targeting both EGFR-activating and EGFR-resistant T790M mutations, has shown to significantly improve RR, PFS, OS, and QoL as compared to standard platinum chemotherapy in patients with EGFR-mutated NSCLC who progressed to first-line EGFR TKI and were T790M-positive [146]. The results of the randomized phase III AURA trial [146] have led to the recent approval of osimertinib as new standard of care in this subset of patients emphasizing the importance of a genotype-guided approach to second-line therapy [121].

Thus, tumor re-biopsy at the time of disease progression should be considered in all patients who progressed to prior EGFR TKI [121]. Even if tissue biopsy remains the current gold standard, it is limited by several features, such as the difficult access to different tumor sites, the invasiveness of procedures, the tumor heterogeneity, and the low patients' compliance [147]. An increasing number of studies and meta-analysis [40, 41, 148, 149] evaluated the diagnostic accuracy of ctDNA for the detection of EGFR mutations in the plasma of patients with advanced NSCLC, overall suggesting a high concordance rate between these two testing methods and ultimately leading to the introduction of ctDNA in clinical practice. Molecular testing by ctDNA has been recommended as the first step of tumor genotyping for all patients who progressed to first- or second-generation EGFR TKI [121]. However, because of 30% potential false negative rate associated with this method [150], ctDNA analysis must be always followed by tissue biopsy in all cases who are T790M-negative on plasma [121]. Interestingly, the location of metastatic site appeared to significantly influence the ability to identify EGFR-activating and EGFR-resistant T790M mutations, leading to a higher diagnostic accuracy of ctDNA analysis in the event of extra-thoracic disease [151]. With the increasing upfront use of osimertinib considering the impressive results of the aforementioned FLAURA study, the detection of T790M mutation in this setting would become of secondary importance, since its loss has been usually associated with early resistance to osimertinib in the light of

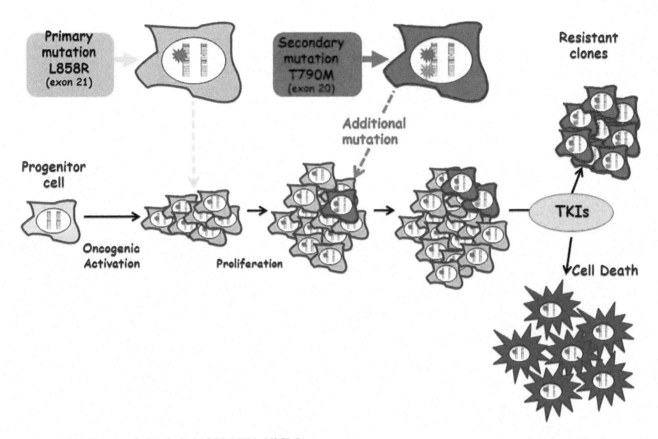

Fig. 32.18 Clonal evolution during EGFR TKI in NSCLC

the drug mechanism of action. Even if the mutational status of T790M could be readily monitored in plasma in order to precede a proven radiological progression of disease, other multiple resistance mechanisms need to be considered in this regard. Further implementation of liquid biopsy in monitoring the response to osimertinib and detecting the wide spectrum of molecular alterations responsible for treatment failure (either EGFR-dependent or EGFR-independent) is warranted and eagerly awaited in both ongoing and future clinical trials. In this context, liquid biopsy using ctDNA analysis has proved to be feasible and reliable for detecting most of genomic alterations [152] (■ Fig. 32.19).

Besides T790M mutation, other molecular alterations have been detected in EGFR-positive resistant tumors, including the amplification of the mesenchymal-epithelial transition (MET) factor receptor tyrosine kinase (20%), Her-2 amplification (12%), phenotypic change from NSCLC to SCLC (4%), and modifications in other parallel signaling pathways (■ Fig. 32.20), and new targeted agents are currently under investigation in clinical trials [144]. Waiting for the new tailored agents, platinum chemotherapy is currently recommended as the standard treatment for all patients who progressed to EGFR TKI and are T790M-negative on tumor tissue analysis.

Unfortunately, ALK-positive patients treated with crizotinib also relapse after a variable period of drug sensitivity because of the development of acquired resistance [153]. Different resistance mechanisms to crizotinib have been identified, including secondary mutations in the ATP-binding pocket of the receptor or the amplification of the ALK fusion gene or the activation of other oncogenic drivers such as increased EGFR phosphorylation and mutation, Kit amplification and mutation, and KRAS mutation, which may cause resistance independent of ALK [154, 155] (■ Fig. 32.21).

Second-generation ALK inhibitors ceritinib [156] and alectinib [157] have shown to significantly improve both RR, PFS, OS, and QoL as compared to platinum chemotherapy in ALK-rearranged patients who progressed to crizotinib, thanks to their ability to target the most frequent secondary mutations in the ALK domains and their higher activity against brain metastasis [158]. Although the new ALK inhibitors showed a selective spectrum of activity according to the different tumor-resistant mutations (ALK-dependent and ALK-independent), a genotype-guided approach is strongly encouraged within clinical trials but not currently recommended at the time of disease progression in clinical practice. Thus, both ceritinib and alectinib may be used in ALK-positive NSCLC patients who failed

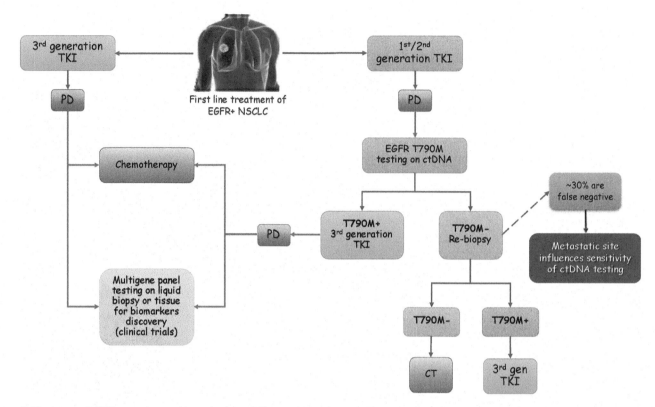

Fig. 32.19 EGFR mutation testing at the time of disease progression to EGFR TKI

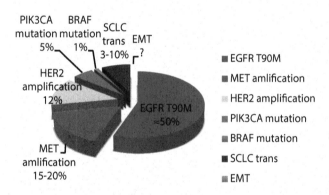

Fig. 32.20 Molecular mechanisms of acquired resistance to first-generation EGFR TKIs

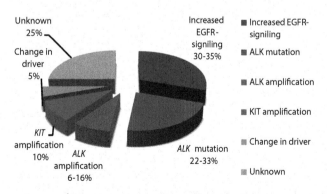

Fig. 32.21 Molecular mechanisms of acquired resistance to first-generation ALK inhibitors

crizotinib, reserving platinum combinations to further line of therapy [159]. As ctDNA and tissue NGS techniques continue to advance in this regard, a better understanding of the optimal treatment sequencing is warranted.

For all oncogene-addicted NSCLC patients who experienced limited and asymptomatic radiological progression at a single site, including the brain, bone, or adrenal gland, and were still dependent from the oncogenic signaling, continuing the TKI beyond PD in combination with local treatment, such as surgery or radiotherapy, may represent a reasonable option and could be considered on an individualized basis after discussion within a multidisciplinary team [121] (◘ Fig. 32.22).

■ Non-oncogene-Addicted NSCLC

The advent of immunotherapy has recently led to a paradigm shift of first-line treatment for about 30% of patients with advanced NSCLC whose tumors overexpressed PD-L1 >50% by IHC analysis on tumor tissue samples [121, 160]. The results of the phase III KEYNOTE-024 randomized trial [161] showed that the anti-PD1 checkpoint inhibitor pembrolizumab significantly improved RR, PFS, OS, and QoL as compared to platinum chemotherapy, becoming the new standard of care in this subset of patients. Adding immunotherapy to first-line platinum regimens [162] as well as combin-

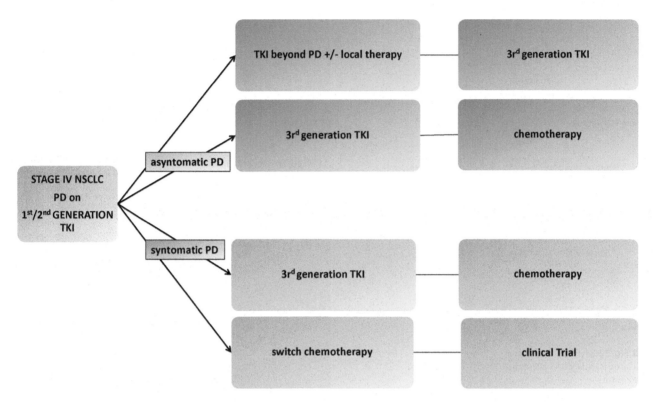

□ Fig. 32.22 Therapeutic options in oncogene-addicted NSCLC patients who failed first-line treatment based on TKIs

ing different anti-PD1/CTLA4 immunotherapeutic agents [163] emerged also as effective and tolerable first-line options in patients with advanced NSCLC, irrespective of PD-L1 expression. Despite some initial concerns of toxicity profiles, patients treated with the association of immune checkpoint inhibitors (pembrolizumab or atezolizumab) with platinum-based chemotherapy had improved OS, PFS, and ORR when compared to chemotherapy alone, making these regimens the current standard of care in the first-line treatment of non-oncogene-addicted NSCLC fit patients. In contrast, the results of those trials investigating the combination immunotherapy when compared to chemotherapy are difficult to interpret: the CheckMate 227 trial evaluating the association of the anti-PD1 nivolumab with the anti-CTLA4 ipilimumab showed initial improvement in PFS and later on in OS rates only in PD-L1-positive patients while being amended to use tumor mutation burden (TMB) or PD-L1 as a primary endpoint [164], whereas the MYSTIC trial evaluating the combination of the anti-PD-L1 durvalumab with the anti-CTLA4 tremelimumab did not significantly improve OS or PFS in PD-L1 selected patients [165].

For all other patients with EGFR-/ALK-/PD-L1-negative, advanced NSCLC, without major comorbidities, platinum combinations should be recommended as an upfront treatment, according to the tumor histological subtype [121]. Particularly up to six cycles of plati-

num combinations with a third-generation cytotoxic agent, including gemcitabine, vinorelbine, or taxanes, are recommended in patients with both squamous and non-squamous subtypes, while four cycles of platinum-pemetrexed followed by less toxic maintenance pemetrexed monotherapy until disease progression or unacceptable toxicities may be preferred in non-squamous NSCLC [166, 167]. Randomized trials and meta-analysis showed that the addition of bevacizumab to paclitaxel/carboplatin regimens improved OS in patients with non-squamous subtype and PS 0–1 and may be considered as an effective treatment option in these patients [168, 169] (□ Fig. 32.23). The randomized phase III SQUIRE trial [170] showed that the addition of the anti-EGFR monoclonal antibody necitumumab to platinum-gemcitabine led to a small benefit in patients with squamous EGFR-expressing tumors assessed by IHC [171], but this combination should be carefully evaluated due to the limited clinical improvement.

Different treatment options are currently available for patients with clinical or radiological progression to first-line treatment. Before the advent of chemo-immunotherapy, single-agent Immunotherapy, including the PD1 checkpoint inhibitors nivolumab and pembrolizumab and the PD-L1 inhibitor atezolizumab, represented the new standard of care in pre-treated NSCLC patients [121, 160]. Four phase III randomized studies demonstrated that PD1/PDL1 inhibitors are

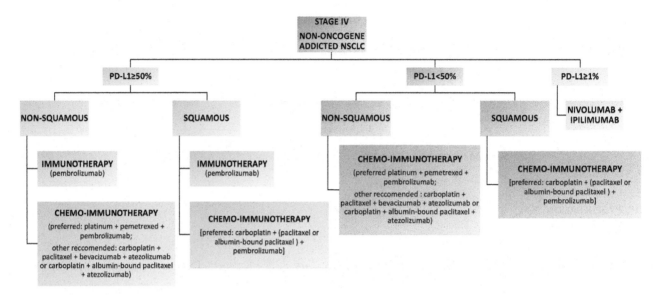

Fig. 32.23 Therapeutic upfront options in non-oncogene-addicted NSCLC patients

Fig. 32.24 Immune-related adverse events with checkpoint inhibitors

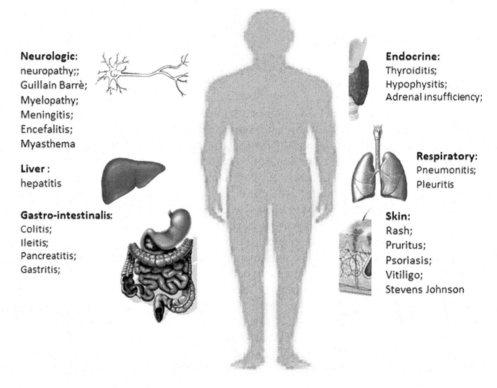

Neurologic:
neuropathy;;
Guillain Barrè;
Myelopathy;
Meningitis;
Encefalitis;
Myasthema

Liver :
hepatitis

Gastro-intestinalis:
Colitis;
Ileitis;
Pancreatitis;
Gastritis;

Endocrine:
Thyroiditis;
Hypophysitis;
Adrenal insufficiency;

Respiratory:
Pneumonitis;
Pleuritis

Skin:
Rash;
Pruritus;
Psoriasis;
Vitiligo;
Stevens Johnson

more effective and better tolerated than second-line single-agent docetaxel [172–175] and are currently recommended in NSCLC patients who experienced progression after platinum combinations regardless of tumor histological subtype and PD-L1 status, except for pembrolizumab, which was approved only for PD-L1-positive (IHC > 1%) tumors [121]. In this setting, an indirect comparison seemed to favor nivolumab and pembrolizumab in terms of response rates when compared to atezolizumab, whereas nivolumab appeared to be associated with a significant lower incidence of adverse events as compared to pembrolizumab and atezolizumab [176].

The use of immunotherapeutic agents in clinical practice was associated with the emergence of a new spectrum of toxicities (■ Fig. 32.24) derived from autoimmune response against normal tissues. Even if not frequently reported, immune-related toxicities

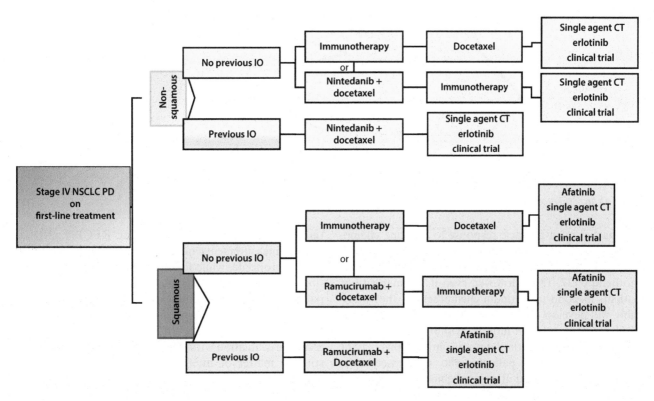

Fig. 32.25 Therapeutic options in non-oncogene-addicted NSCLC patients who failed first-line platinum chemotherapy

may be life-threatening, thus requiring an urgent and adequate pro-active management [177, 178].

Antiangiogenic agents such as the multi-kinase inhibitor nintedanib and the anti-VEGFR2 monoclonal antibody ramucirumab have been investigated in combination with docetaxel in two randomized phase III LUME-Lung1 [179] and REVEL [180] trials, showing to significantly improve OS of pre-treated NSCLC patients with adenocarcinoma and all histological subtypes, respectively. In the LUX-Lung 8 trial [181], the EGFR TKI afatinib showed significant improvements in PFS and OS as compared to erlotinib in pre-treated squamous EGFR wild-type NSCLC, emerging as an additional option in later lines of therapy. In the absence of direct comparisons among these new approved agents as well as of validated predictive biomarkers, the decision of second-line therapy should take into account several factors, including first-line treatment, tumor histology, best response and toxicities to prior treatment, and patients' comorbidities and preference in order to select the most effective and tolerable treatment for each patient (■ Fig. 32.25).

■ **Brain and Bone Metastasis**

The brain is the most common site of metastatic recurrence, followed by the bone, lung, liver, and adrenal glands. About 50% of patients with oncogene-addicted NSCLC will develop brain metastasis in the natural his-

tory of their disease [182]. Different from first-generation TKIs, the new EGFR TKI osimertinib [129, 183], as well as the new ALK inhibitor alectinib [134, 184], showed great activity against brain metastasis because of their ability to penetrate the blood-brain barrier (BBB) [185], emerging as new effective treatment options for patients with asymptomatic disease. For all other patients with symptomatic brain metastasis or EGFR-/ALK-negative tumors, the multimodality treatment, including surgical resection, stereotactic radiotherapy (SRS), whole brain radiotherapy, and systemic chemotherapy, should be offered or combined according to the patient's prognosis and number of metastatic sites [121].

All the patients with advanced NSCLC and bone metastasis should receive zoledronic acid or denosumab to prevent skeletal-related events (SRE), including pathological fracture, radiation or surgery to bone, or spinal cord compression. Palliative radiation should be offered to all patients with symptomatic bone lesions to achieve symptom control and is also effective in treating pain related to chest wall, soft tissue, or neural invasion [121].

■ **Extensive-Stage SCLC**

Chemotherapy with platinum-etoposide up to six cycles has been recommended as first-line treatment for all patients with metastatic SCLC and PS 0–1 for many years. Thoracic radiotherapy may be considered in patients who achieved complete extra-thoracic response

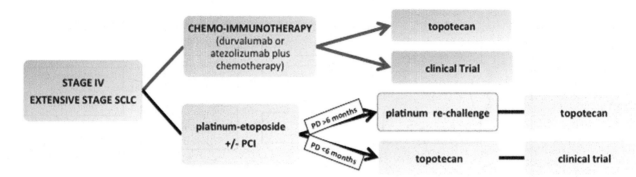

◻ Fig. 32.26   Therapeutic algorithm in patients with extensive-stage SCLC

and partial intra-thoracic response to first-line chemotherapy, while PCI should be offered to all patients with extensive-stage SCLC who responded to first-line chemotherapy [27, 186]. However, even if the majority of patients respond to platinum chemotherapy, they inevitably will develop disease progression with median survival reported to be 3 months without any treatment [187]. Re-challenge with platinum combinations may be considered in those patients who progressed after 6 months from the end of prior chemotherapy. Second-line therapy with topotecan is recommended as standard of care in all patients who failed prior platinum chemotherapy and have PS 0–1 [27, 186].

Additionally, the combination of the anti-PD-L1 atezolizumab with platinum doublet followed by maintenance atezolizumab has been already approved and used in clinical practice in the United States, demonstrated to significantly achieve longer median OS rates (12.3 vs 10.3 months) in the IMpower133 randomized trial [188]. Likewise, the FDA approved durvalumab in combination with etoposide and either carboplatin or cisplatin as first-line treatment of such patients, since median OS was 13.0 months in the durvalumab plus chemotherapy arm compared with 10.3 months in the chemotherapy alone arm [189].

After first-line failure in small cell lung cancer, clinical trials with novel immunotherapeutic agents including anti-PD1/PD-L1 inhibitors and the DLL3-targeted antibody-drug conjugate rovalpituzumab showed encouraging activity in patients with recurrent SCLC and are currently under investigation in randomized studies [190, 191] (◻ Fig. 32.26).

32.9   Response Evaluation

Response evaluation should be performed every 2 months for patients undergoing systemic therapy, preferably using the same radiological investigation of ini-

tial diagnosis/staging. CT scan using RECIST criteria v1.1 for measurements and response reporting is considered appropriate, while follow-up with PET is not routinely recommended. In oncogene-addicted NSCLC patients, treatment beyond RECIST disease progression is a common approach especially in patients with asymptomatic and limited PD [121]. The best criteria for response evaluation with immunomodulatory agents are still the matter of intense work and debate. Even if RECIST criteria have been adopted in the majority of clinical trials which have led to the approval of such agents, the "immune-RECIST" criteria have been recently developed by the RECIST working group to be adopted in the next cancer immunotherapy trials as well as in clinical practice [192].

32.10   Follow-Up

Due to the aggressive nature of this disease, generally close follow-up, including both clinical and radiological evaluation at least every 2–3 months after initial treatment, is advised but should also depend on individual basis [121].

Summary of Clinical Recommendations

— *AIOM*
   ▶ http://www.aiom.it/professionisti/documenti-scientifici/linee-guida/1,413,1,#TopList
— *ESMO*
   ▶ http://www.esmo.org/Guidelines/Lung-and-Chest-Tumours
— *NCCN*
   ▶ https://www.nccn.org/professionals/physician_gls/pdf/nscl.pdf
   ▶ https://www.nccn.org/professionals/physician_gls/pdf/sclc.pdf

Man: 55 years old
- *Family history*: negative for malignancy
- *APR*: hypertension
- *Smoke history*: former smoker (1 pack/day for 20 years)

- *APP*: cough
- *ECOG PS*: 0
- *CT scan total body*: multiple lung bilateral nodules, mediastinal lymph node metastasis

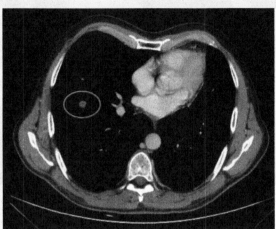
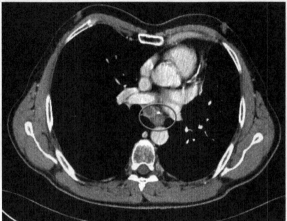

Bronchoscopy with biopsy: lung adenocarcinoma
Clinical stage (8th TNM staging system): stage IV (M1a)

Question

Which action should be taken?

(1) Surgery (2) Medical therapy (3) Mutational analysis

Answer

Mutational analysis: EGFR, EML/ALK, ROS1: wild-type

PD-L1 assessment: PD-L1 expression 5%

⇩

Medical therapy: cisplatin-pemetrexed × 4 cycles
- *Response evaluation after 3 months of chemotherapy*: Stable disease (SD)

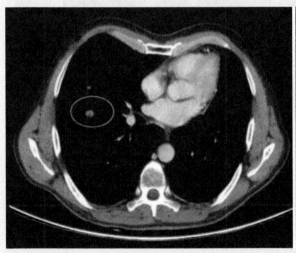
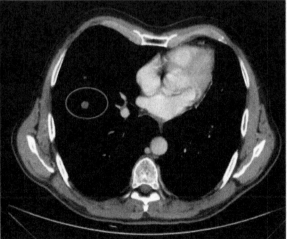

– *Response evaluation after 9 months of maintenance therapy with pemetrexed*: progression disease (PD)

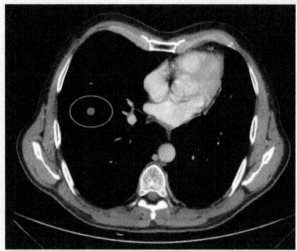 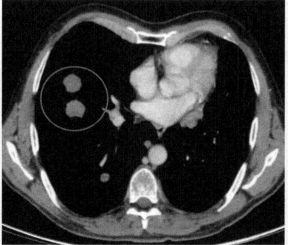

After 3 months

After 12 months

Question

Which action should be taken?

(1) Immunotherapy (2) Chemotherapy plus nintedanib (3) Chemotherapy

Answer

Begins nivolumab 3 mg/kg q 14

– *Response evaluation after 3 months of therapy with nivolumab*: partial response (PR)

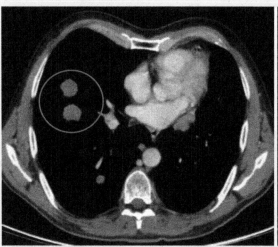 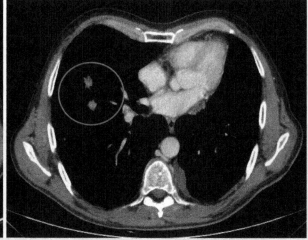

Before Nivolumab

After 3 months Nivolumab

Key Points

– Importance of a correct staging and histological diagnosis

– Importance of histology and mutational analysis for first-line therapeutic choice

– Importance of PD-L1 expression for first- and second-line therapeutic choice

Case Study: Oncogene-Addicted Advanced NSCLC

Woman: 45 years old
- *Family history*: negative for malignancy
- *APR*: negative
- *Smoking history*: never smoker
- *APP*: dyspnea, cough
- *ECOG PS*: 1
- *PET-CT total body*: left lobe nodule, bilateral mediastinal lymph node metastasis *(PET 11)*

Bronchoscopy with trans-bronchial needle aspiration (TBNA): lung adenocarcinoma
Clinical stage (8th TNM staging system): stage IIIB

Question

Which action should be taken?
(1) Surgery (2) Definitive chemoradiotherapy (3) Mutational analysis

Answer

Mutational analysis: exon 19 deletion of EGFR

⇩

Gefitinib 250 mg os/day
- *Response evaluation after 3 months of therapy*: partial response (PR) (PET 16)

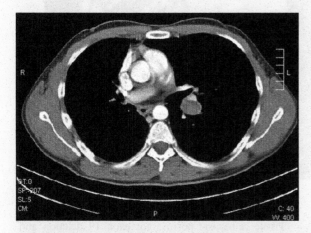

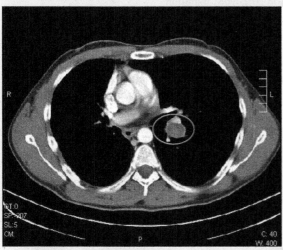

Before therapy

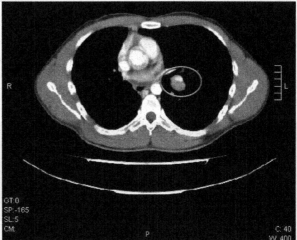

After 3 months therapy

■ *Response evaluation after 12 months of therapy*: progression disease (PD) (PET e RMN 17)

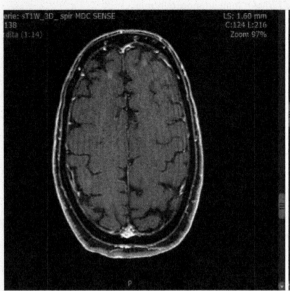

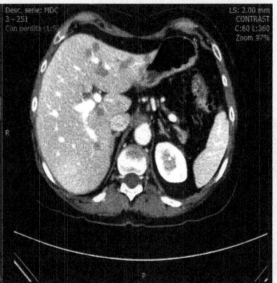

Multiple asymptomatic brain lesions   Multiple liver lesions

Question

Which action should be taken?

(1) Whole brain radiotherapy (2) Chemotherapy (3) Re-biopsy

Answer

Liquid biopsy: mutational analysis on ctDNA: no evidence of EGFR-T790M mutation

Tissue re-biopsy: positive for exon 19 deletion and exon 20 T790M mutation

Osimertinib 80 mg os/day

■ *Response evaluation after 3 months of therapy with osimertinib*: partial response (PR)

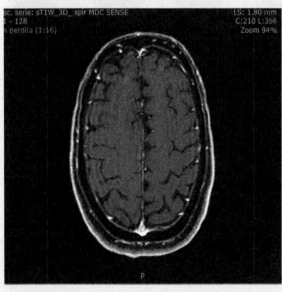

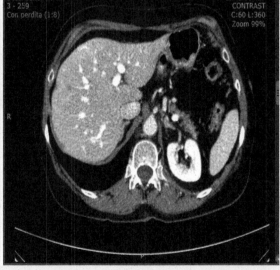

Key Points

■ Importance of histology and mutational analysis for first-line therapeutic choice

■ Importance of re-biopsy at the time of EGFR+ NSCLC radiological progression

■ Great intracranial activity of third-generation EGFR TKI

Expert Opinion
Giorgio Vittorio Scagliotti

Key Points

- Lung cancer remains the first cause of cancer death in both women and men, and, despite several therapeutic improvements over the last 15 years, 5-year survival rates remain disappointing.

- Further studies are clearly needed to implement lung cancer screening strategies to reduce significantly lung cancer mortality. Selection of high-risk participants for LDCT screening is improved by the use of multivariate risk prediction models. Additionally, a range of recruitment strategies will be required based on available health infrastructure and the distribution of the high-risk population. Simplified management algorithms for pulmonary nodules, incorporating risk prediction models and image analysis techniques, will likely lead to reduction in downstream investigations and surgery for benign disease.

- Smoking cessation is critical to the overall benefit and cost-effectiveness of a lung cancer screening program. The best strategy to optimize the intervention and integrate it into a program is not known.

- Morphological staging of lung cancer has almost reached the "efficacy" plateau, and future initiatives should integrate molecular data.

- Molecular, biological, and histological heterogeneities represent major challenges in the majority of lung cancers.

- With the completion of the human genome, we understand now that life is based on dynamic molecular networks rather than on a direct connection between genotype and phenotype.

Hints for Deeper Insight

The application of precision medicine is anticipated to improve all areas of medicine, including predicting an individual's risk of disease, disease prognosis, and risk of side effects versus positive response to disease treatment approaches.

Tissue remains the issue in the era of targeted therapies and immunotherapy because of the clear need to identify the subset of patients who benefit most from these tailored approaches. Histological and biological heterogeneities are well-known phenomena, which might significantly impact our capability to detect specific molecular targets as well as prediction of sensitivity to specific molecular targeted agents. The heterogeneity of response and outcome associated with specific molecular features is more likely a reflection of biological heterogeneity than technical issues, which might not be captured in small biopsies, fine needle aspirates, or tissue microar-rays consisting of small selected tissue cores. To address all these issues, potential exploration of genomic altera-tions in several biological fluids, such as blood, represents a reasonable alternative with huge potential applications in the near future when test sensitivity will be optimized. The unit in precision medicine is a "biomarker ensemble" that includes a predictive biomarker, hypothesized to play a crucial role in the disease pathway; a diagnostic assay, used to determine a patient's biomarker status; and final a therapeutic agent, intended to be more effective for patients who are "biomarker-positive." If one of the three basic elements is lacking, we are lying down outside of the framework of precision medicine.

With the current emphasis on biomarker-driven drug development and the increasing inclusion of integral and integrated biomarkers in our trials, it is necessary to ensure that fit-for-purpose assays of these biomarkers are incorporated in study protocols. Briefly, markers are inte-gral when they are essential for conducting the study as they define eligibility, stratification, and monitoring of the disease or study endpoints. Markers are considered integrated when they actually are testing a hypothesis based on preexisting data and not simply generating hypotheses.

The genomic revolution encompasses only a portion of the emerging hallmarks of cancer, which include enabling characteristics and a better understanding of the tumor microenvironment. In this context, an under-standing of the immune landscape of cancers, including immune evasion strategies, has led to breakthrough ther-apeutic advances for patients with non-small cell lung cancer and has created a platform for future therapeutic developments.

We are at the beginning of a creative period of bot-tom-up research activity, organized through pilot projects of increasing scope and scale, from which best practices will progressively emerge. In particular, given the size and diversity of the healthcare enterprise, a single approach to data gathering that will populate the space is probably not appropriate for all contributors. As in any initiative of this complexity, we will need the right level of coordination and encouragement of the many players who must coop-erate to create a higher level of biomedical knowledge.

In this patient-centered context, patients and their advocates are and will be more critical, each and every day, first to promote the right social pressure for the sys-tematic implementation of the results of preclinical and clinical research and, second, to develop a work in prog-ress and continuous discussion with the regulatory bodies and national healthcare systems in an attempt to guaran-tee drug accessibility to every patient, as well as help national authorities to maintain the long-term financial sustainability of the healthcare systems.

Suggested Reading

1. Pass H, Scagliotti GV, Ball D, editors. IASLC thoracic oncology textbook. Elsevier Publisher; 2016.
2. Curtius K, Nicholas A, Wright NA, Graham TA. An evolutionary perspective on field cancerization. Nat Rev Cancer. 2018;18:19–32.
3. Cohen JD, et al. Detection and localization of surgically resectable cancers with a multi-analyte blood test. Science. 2018;359(6378):926–30. ▶ https://doi.org/10.1126/science.aacr3247.
4. Schreiber RD, Old LJ, Smyth MJ. Cancer immuneediting: Integrating Immunity's roles in cancer suppression and promotion. Science. 2011;331:1565–70.
5. Abbosh C, et al. Phylogenetic ctDNA analysis depicts early-stage lung cancer evolution. Nature. 2017;545:446–51.
6. Houghton AM. Mechanistic links between COPD and lung cancer. Nat Rev Cancer. 2013;13:233–45.

References

1. Cancer CSFLaB. https://seer.cancer.gov/statfacts/html/lungb.html.
2. Siegel RL, Miller KD, Jemal A. Cancer statistics, 2018. CA Cancer J Clin. 2018;68(1):7–30.
3. Pesch B, Kendzia B, Gustavsson P, et al. Cigarette smoking and lung cancer--relative risk estimates for the major histological types from a pooled analysis of case-control studies. Int J Cancer. 2012;131(5):1210–9.
4. Radzikowska E, Głaz P, Roszkowski K. Lung cancer in women: age, smoking, histology, performance status, stage, initial treatment and survival. Population-based study of 20 561 cases. Ann Oncol. 2002;13(7):1087–93.
5. Jemal A, Ma J, Rosenberg PS, Siegel R, Anderson WF. Increasing lung cancer death rates among young women in southern and midwestern States. J Clin Oncol. 2012;30(22):2739–44.
6. Centers for Disease Control and Prevention (CDC). Smoking-attributable mortality, years of potential life lost, and productivity losses--United States, 2000–2004. MMWR Morb Mortal Wkly Rep. 2008;57(45):1226–8.
7. Sun S, Schiller JH, Gazdar AF. Lung cancer in never smokers--a different disease. Nat Rev Cancer. 2007;7(10):778–90.
8. Straif K, Benbrahim-Tallaa L, Baan R, et al. A review of human carcinogens--part C: metals, arsenic, dusts, and fibres. Lancet Oncol. 2009;10(5):453–4.
9. Warren GW, Marshall JR, Cummings KM, et al. Practice patterns and perceptions of thoracic oncology providers on tobacco use and cessation in cancer patients. J Thorac Oncol. 2013;8(5):543–8.
10. Moolgavkar SH, Holford TR, Levy DT, et al. Impact of reduced tobacco smoking on lung cancer mortality in the United States during 1975–2000. J Natl Cancer Inst. 2012;104(7):541–8.
11. Chute CG, Greenberg ER, Baron J, Korson R, Baker J, Yates J. Presenting conditions of 1539 population-based lung cancer patients by cell type and stage in New Hampshire and Vermont. Cancer. 1985;56(8):2107–11.
12. Filderman AE, Shaw C, Matthay RA. Lung cancer. Part I: Etiology, pathology, natural history, manifestations, and diagnostic techniques. Investig Radiol. 1986;21(1):80–90.
13. Raz DJ, Glidden DV, Odisho AY, Jablons DM. Clinical characteristics and survival of patients with surgically resected, incidentally detected lung cancer. J Thorac Oncol. 2007;2(2):125–30.
14. Field JK, Oudkerk M, Pedersen JH, Duffy SW. Prospects for population screening and diagnosis of lung cancer. Lancet. 2013;382(9893):732–41.
15. Melamed MR, Flehinger BJ, Zaman MB, Heelan RT, Perchick WA, Martini N. Screening for early lung cancer. Results of the Memorial Sloan-Kettering study in New York. Chest. 1984;86(1):44–53.
16. Fontana RS, Sanderson DR, Woolner LB, Taylor WF, Miller WE, Muhm JR. Lung cancer screening: the Mayo program. J Occup Med. 1986;28(8):746–50.
17. Aberle DR, Adams AM, Berg CD, et al. Reduced lung-cancer mortality with low-dose computed tomographic screening. N Engl J Med. 2011;365(5):395–409.
18. Bach PB, Mirkin JN, Oliver TK, et al. Benefits and harms of CT screening for lung cancer: a systematic review. JAMA. 2012;307(22):2418–29.
19. Wender R, Fontham ET, Barrera E, et al. American Cancer Society lung cancer screening guidelines. CA Cancer J Clin. 2013;63(2):107–17.
20. de Koning HJ, van der Aalst CM, de Jong PA, et al. Reduced lung-cancer mortality with volume CT screening in a randomized trial. N Engl J Med. 2020;382(6):503–13.
21. Travis WD, Brambilla E, Noguchi M, et al. International Association for the Study of Lung Cancer/American Thoracic Society/European Respiratory Society international multidisciplinary classification of lung adenocarcinoma. J Thorac Oncol. 2011;6(2):244–85.
22. Travis WD, Brambilla E, Riely GJ. New pathologic classification of lung cancer: relevance for clinical practice and clinical trials. J Clin Oncol. 2013;31(8):992–1001.
23. Ordóñez NG. Thyroid transcription factor-1 is a marker of lung and thyroid carcinomas. Adv Anat Pathol. 2000;7(2):123–7.
24. Kaufmann O, Fietze E, Mengs J, Dietel M. Value of p63 and cytokeratin 5/6 as immunohistochemical markers for the differential diagnosis of poorly differentiated and undifferentiated carcinomas. Am J Clin Pathol. 2001;116(6):823–30.
25. Pelosi G, Pasini F, Olsen Stenholm C, et al. p63 immunoreactivity in lung cancer: yet another player in the development of squamous cell carcinomas? J Pathol. 2002;198(1):100–9.
26. Flieder DB. Neuroendocrine tumors of the lung: recent developments in histopathology. Curr Opin Pulm Med. 2002;8(4):275–80.
27. Früh M, De Ruysscher D, Popat S, et al. Small-cell lung cancer (SCLC): ESMO Clinical Practice Guidelines for diagnosis, treatment and follow-up. Ann Oncol. 2013;24(Suppl 6):vi99–105.
28. Gabrielson E. Worldwide trends in lung cancer pathology. Respirology. 2006;11(5):533–8.
29. Parsons A, Daley A, Begh R, Aveyard P. Influence of smoking cessation after diagnosis of early stage lung cancer on prognosis: systematic review of observational studies with meta-analysis. BMJ. 2010;340:b5569.
30. Travis WD, Brambilla E, Noguchi M, et al. Diagnosis of lung cancer in small biopsies and cytology: implications of the 2011

International Association for the Study of Lung Cancer/ American Thoracic Society/European Respiratory Society classification. Arch Pathol Lab Med. 2013;137(5):668–84.

31. Mitsudomi T, Kosaka T, Endoh H, et al. Mutations of the epidermal growth factor receptor gene predict prolonged survival after gefitinib treatment in patients with non-small-cell lung cancer with postoperative recurrence. J Clin Oncol. 2005;23(11): 2513–20.

32. Takano T, Ohe Y, Sakamoto H, et al. Epidermal growth factor receptor gene mutations and increased copy numbers predict gefitinib sensitivity in patients with recurrent non-small-cell lung cancer. J Clin Oncol. 2005;23(28):6829–37.

33. Han JY, Park K, Kim SW, et al. First-SIGNAL: first-line single-agent iressa versus gemcitabine and cisplatin trial in never-smokers with adenocarcinoma of the lung. J Clin Oncol. 2012;30(10):1122–8.

34. Sharma SV, Bell DW, Settleman J, Haber DA. Epidermal growth factor receptor mutations in lung cancer. Nat Rev Cancer. 2007;7(3):169–81.

35. Rosell R, Moran T, Queralt C, et al. Screening for epidermal growth factor receptor mutations in lung cancer. N Engl J Med. 2009;361(10):958–67.

36. Arrieta O, Cardona AF, Federico Bramuglia G, et al. Genotyping non-small cell lung cancer (NSCLC) in Latin America. J Thorac Oncol. 2011;6(11):1955–9.

37. Bronte G, Rolfo C, Giovannetti E, et al. Are erlotinib and gefitinib interchangeable, opposite or complementary for non-small cell lung cancer treatment? Biological, pharmacological and clinical aspects. Crit Rev Oncol Hematol. 2014;89:300–13.

38. Passiglia F, Rizzo S, Rolfo C, et al. Metastatic site location influences the diagnostic accuracy of ctDNA EGFR- mutation testing in NSCLC patients: a pooled analysis. Curr Cancer Drug Targets. 2018;18(7):697–705. https://doi.org/10.2174/1568009618 666180308125110.

39. Arteaga CL. Overview of epidermal growth factor receptor biology and its role as a therapeutic target in human neoplasia. Semin Oncol. 2002;29(5 Suppl 14):3–9.

40. Qiu M, Wang J, Xu Y, et al. Circulating tumor DNA is effective for the detection of EGFR mutation in non-small cell lung cancer: a meta-analysis. Cancer Epidemiol Biomark Prev. 2015;24(1):206–12.

41. Luo J, Shen L, Zheng D. Diagnostic value of circulating free DNA for the detection of EGFR mutation status in NSCLC: a systematic review and meta-analysis. Sci Rep. 2014;4:6269.

42. Shaw AT, Yeap BY, Mino-Kenudson M, et al. Clinical features and outcome of patients with non-small-cell lung cancer who harbor EML4-ALK. J Clin Oncol. 2009;27(26):4247–53.

43. Chiarle R, Voena C, Ambrogio C, Piva R, Inghirami G. The anaplastic lymphoma kinase in the pathogenesis of cancer. Nat Rev Cancer. 2008;8(1):11–23.

44. Shaw AT, Ou SH, Bang YJ, et al. Crizotinib in ROS1-rearranged non-small-cell lung cancer. N Engl J Med. 2014;371(21): 1963–71.

45. Kazandjian D, Blumenthal GM, Luo L, et al. Benefit-risk summary of crizotinib for the treatment of patients with ROS1 alteration-positive, metastatic non-small cell lung cancer. Oncologist. 2016;21(8):974–80.

46. Camidge DR, Kono SA, Flacco A, et al. Optimizing the detection of lung cancer patients harboring anaplastic lymphoma kinase (ALK) gene rearrangements potentially suitable for ALK inhibitor treatment. Clin Cancer Res. 2010;16(22): 5581–90.

47. Bergethon K, Shaw AT, Ou SH, et al. ROS1 rearrangements define a unique molecular class of lung cancers. J Clin Oncol. 2012;30(8):863–70.

48. Yi ES, Boland JM, Maleszewski JJ, et al. Correlation of IHC and FISH for ALK gene rearrangement in non-small cell lung carcinoma: IHC score algorithm for FISH. J Thorac Oncol. 2011;6(3):459–65.

49. Selinger CI, Rogers TM, Russell PA, et al. Testing for ALK rearrangement in lung adenocarcinoma: a multicenter comparison of immunohistochemistry and fluorescent in situ hybridization. Mod Pathol. 2013;26(12):1545–53.

50. Sakai Y, Nakai T, Ohbayashi C, et al. Immunohistochemical profiling of ALK fusion gene-positive adenocarcinomas of the lung. Int J Surg Pathol. 2013;21(5):476–82.

51. Park HS, Lee JK, Kim DW, et al. Immunohistochemical screening for anaplastic lymphoma kinase (ALK) rearrangement in advanced non-small cell lung cancer patients. Lung Cancer. 2012;77(2):288–92.

52. Martinez P, Hernández-Losa J, Montero M, et al. Fluorescence in situ hybridization and immunohistochemistry as diagnostic methods for ALK positive non-small cell lung cancer patients. PLoS One. 2013;8(1):e52261.

53. Conklin CM, Craddock KJ, Have C, Laskin J, Couture C, Ionescu DN. Immunohistochemistry is a reliable screening tool for identification of ALK rearrangement in non-small-cell lung carcinoma and is antibody dependent. J Thorac Oncol. 2013;8(1):45–51.

54. Alì G, Proietti A, Pelliccioni S, et al. ALK rearrangement in a large series of consecutive non-small cell lung cancers: comparison between a new immunohistochemical approach and fluorescent in situ hybridization for the screening of patients eligible for crizotinib treatment. Arch Pathol Lab Med. 2014;138:1449–58.

55. Network CGAR. Comprehensive genomic characterization of squamous cell lung cancers. Nature. 2012;489(7417):519–25.

56. Peifer M, Fernández-Cuesta L, Sos ML, et al. Integrative genome analyses identify key somatic driver mutations of small-cell lung cancer. Nat Genet. 2012;44(10):1104–10.

57. Sos ML, Dietlein F, Peifer M, et al. A framework for identification of actionable cancer genome dependencies in small cell lung cancer. Proc Natl Acad Sci U S A. 2012;109(42):17034–9.

58. Spiro SG, Gould MK, Colice GL, American College of Chest Physicians. Initial evaluation of the patient with lung cancer: symptoms, signs, laboratory tests, and paraneoplastic syndromes: ACCP evidenced-based clinical practice guidelines (2nd edition). Chest. 2007;132(3 Suppl):149S–60S.

59. Pretreatment evaluation of non-small-cell lung cancer. The American Thoracic Society and the European Respiratory Society. Am J Respir Crit Care Med. 1997;156(1):320–32.

60. Hamilton W, Peters TJ, Round A, Sharp D. What are the clinical features of lung cancer before the diagnosis is made? A population based case-control study. Thorax. 2005;60(12):1059–65.

61. Stankey RM, Roshe J, Sogocio RM. Carcinoma of the lung and dysphagia. Dis Chest. 1969;55(1):13–7.

62. Kamel EM, Goerres GW, Burger C, von Schulthess GK, Steinert HC. Recurrent laryngeal nerve palsy in patients with lung cancer: detection with PET-CT image fusion -- report of six cases. Radiology. 2002;224(1):153–6.

63. Sahn SA. Pleural diseases related to metastatic malignancies. Eur Respir J. 1997;10(8):1907–13.

64. Kim SH, Kwak MH, Park S, et al. Clinical characteristics of malignant pericardial effusion associated with recurrence and survival. Cancer Res Treat. 2010;42(4):210–6.

65. Yellin A, Rosen A, Reichert N, Lieberman Y. Superior vena cava syndrome. The myth--the facts. Am Rev Respir Dis. 1990;141(5 Pt 1):1114–8.

66. Rice TW, Rodriguez RM, Light RW. The superior vena cava syndrome: clinical characteristics and evolving etiology. Medicine (Baltimore). 2006;85(1):37–42.

67. Arcasoy SM, Jett JR. Superior pulmonary sulcus tumors and Pancoast's syndrome. N Engl J Med. 1997;337(19):1370–6.

68. Coleman RE. Metastatic bone disease: clinical features, pathophysiology and treatment strategies. Cancer Treat Rev. 2001;27(3):165–76.

69. Cheng H, Perez-Soler R. Leptomeningeal metastases in non-small-cell lung cancer. Lancet Oncol. 2018;19(1):e43–55.

70. Pelosof LC, Gerber DE. Paraneoplastic syndromes: an approach to diagnosis and treatment. Mayo Clin Proc. 2010;85(9):838–54.

71. Ost DE, Jim Yeung SC, Tanoue LT, Gould MK. Clinical and organizational factors in the initial evaluation of patients with lung cancer: diagnosis and management of lung cancer, 3rd ed: American College of Chest Physicians evidence-based clinical practice guidelines. Chest. 2013;143(5 Suppl):e121S–41S.

72. Christensen JD, Patz EF. Future trends in lung cancer diagnosis. Radiol Clin N Am. 2012;50(5):1001–8.

73. Silvestri GA, Gonzalez AV, Jantz MA, et al. Methods for staging non-small cell lung cancer: diagnosis and management of lung cancer, 3rd ed: American College of Chest Physicians evidence-based clinical practice guidelines. Chest. 2013;143(5 Suppl):e211S–50S.

74. Patel VK, Naik SK, Naidich DP, et al. A practical algorithmic approach to the diagnosis and management of solitary pulmonary nodules: part 1: radiologic characteristics and imaging modalities. Chest. 2013;143(3):825–39.

75. Voigt W. Advanced PET imaging in oncology: status and developments with current and future relevance to lung cancer care. Curr Opin Oncol. 2018;30:77–83.

76. Rivera MP, Mehta AC, Wahidi MM. Establishing the diagnosis of lung cancer: diagnosis and management of lung cancer, 3rd ed: American College of Chest Physicians evidence-based clinical practice guidelines. Chest. 2013;143(5 Suppl):e142S–65S.

77. Adams K, Shah PL, Edmonds L, Lim E. Test performance of endobronchial ultrasound and transbronchial needle aspiration biopsy for mediastinal staging in patients with lung cancer: systematic review and meta-analysis. Thorax. 2009;64(9):757–62.

78. Gu P, Zhao YZ, Jiang LY, Zhang W, Xin Y, Han BH. Endobronchial ultrasound-guided transbronchial needle aspiration for staging of lung cancer: a systematic review and meta-analysis. Eur J Cancer. 2009;45(8):1389–96.

79. Um SW, Kim HK, Jung SH, et al. Endobronchial ultrasound versus mediastinoscopy for mediastinal nodal staging of non-small-cell lung cancer. J Thorac Oncol. 2015;10(2):331–7.

80. Capalbo E, Peli M, Lovisatti M, et al. Trans-thoracic biopsy of lung lesions: FNAB or CNB? Our experience and review of the literature. Radiol Med. 2014;119(8):572–94.

81. Beslic S, Zukic F, Milisic S. Percutaneous transthoracic CT guided biopsies of lung lesions; fine needle aspiration biopsy versus core biopsy. Radiol Oncol. 2012;46(1):19–22.

82. Vial MR, Eapen GA, Casal RF, et al. Combined pleuroscopy and endobronchial ultrasound for diagnosis and staging of suspected lung cancer. Respir Med Case Rep. 2018;23:49–51.

83. Postmus PE, Kerr KM, Oudkerk M, et al. Early and locally advanced non-small-cell lung cancer (NSCLC): ESMO Clinical Practice Guidelines for diagnosis, treatment and follow-up. Ann Oncol. 2017;28(suppl_4):iv1–iv21.

84. Czarnecka-Kujawa K, Yasufuku K. The role of endobronchial ultrasound versus mediastinoscopy for non-small cell lung cancer. J Thorac Dis. 2017;9(Suppl 2):S83–97.

85. Sehgal IS, Dhooria S, Aggarwal AN, Behera D, Agarwal R. Endosonography versus mediastinoscopy in mediastinal staging of lung cancer: systematic review and meta-analysis. Ann Thorac Surg. 2016;102(5):1747–55.

86. Vilmann P, Clementsen PF, Colella S, et al. Combined endobronchial and esophageal endosonography for the diagnosis and staging of lung cancer: European Society of Gastrointestinal Endoscopy (ESGE) guideline, in cooperation with the European Respiratory Society (ERS) and the European Society of Thoracic Surgeons (ESTS). Endoscopy. 2015;47(6):545–59.

87. Ettinger DS, Wood DE, Aisner DL, et al. Non-small cell lung cancer, version 5.2017, NCCN clinical practice guidelines in oncology. J Natl Compr Cancer Netw. 2017;15(4):504–35.

88. Goldstraw P, Chansky K, Crowley J, et al. The IASLC lung cancer staging project: proposals for revision of the TNM stage groupings in the forthcoming (eighth) edition of the TNM classification for lung cancer. J Thorac Oncol. 2016;11(1):39–51.

89. Rosen JE, Keshava HB, Yao X, Kim AW, Detterbeck FC, Boffa DJ. The natural history of operable non-small cell lung cancer in the national cancer database. Ann Thorac Surg. 2016;101(5):1850–5.

90. Ginsberg RJ, Rubinstein LV. Randomized trial of lobectomy versus limited resection for T1 N0 non-small cell lung cancer. Lung Cancer Study Group. Ann Thorac Surg. 1995;60(3):615–22; discussion 622–613.

91. Rami-Porta R, Wittekind C, Goldstraw P, International Association for the Study of Lung Cancer (IASLC) Staging Committee. Complete resection in lung cancer surgery: proposed definition. Lung Cancer. 2005;49(1):25–33.

92. Petrella F, Spaggiari L. The smaller the better: a new concept in thoracic surgery? Lancet Oncol. 2016;17(6):699–700.

93. Bendixen M, Jørgensen OD, Kronborg C, Andersen C, Licht PB. Postoperative pain and quality of life after lobectomy via video-assisted thoracoscopic surgery or anterolateral thoracotomy for early stage lung cancer: a randomised controlled trial. Lancet Oncol. 2016;17(6):836–44.

94. Veluswamy RR, Ezer N, Mhango G, et al. Limited resection versus lobectomy for older patients with early-stage lung cancer: impact of histology. J Clin Oncol. 2015;33(30):3447–53.

95. Koike T, Kitahara A, Sato S, et al. Lobectomy versus segmentectomy in radiologically pure solid small-sized non-small cell lung cancer. Ann Thorac Surg. 2016;101(4):1354–60.

96. Linden PA, Bueno R, Colson YL, et al. Lung resection in patients with preoperative FEV1 < 35% predicted. Chest. 2005;127(6):1984–90.

97. Baumann P, Nyman J, Hoyer M, et al. Outcome in a prospective phase II trial of medically inoperable stage I non-small-cell lung cancer patients treated with stereotactic body radiotherapy. J Clin Oncol. 2009;27(20):3290–6.

98. Ricardi U, Filippi AR, Guarneri A, et al. Stereotactic body radiation therapy for early stage non-small cell lung cancer: results of a prospective trial. Lung Cancer. 2010;68(1):72–7.

99. Timmerman R, Paulus R, Galvin J, et al. Stereotactic body radiation therapy for inoperable early stage lung cancer. JAMA. 2010;303(11):1070–6.

100. Chang JY, Liu YH, Zhu Z, et al. Stereotactic ablative radiotherapy: a potentially curable approach to early stage multiple primary lung cancer. Cancer. 2013;119(18):3402–10.

101. Chemotherapy in non-small cell lung cancer: a meta-analysis using updated data on individual patients from 52 randomised clinical trials. Non-small Cell Lung Cancer Collaborative Group. BMJ. 1995;311(7010):899–909.

102. Pignon JP, Tribodet H, Scagliotti GV, et al. Lung adjuvant cisplatin evaluation: a pooled analysis by the LACE Collaborative Group. J Clin Oncol. 2008;26(21):3552–9.

103. Douillard JY, Rosell R, De Lena M, et al. Adjuvant vinorelbine plus cisplatin versus observation in patients with completely resected stage IB-IIIA non-small-cell lung cancer (Adjuvant Navelbine International Trialist Association [ANITA]): a randomised controlled trial. Lancet Oncol. 2006;7(9):719–27.

104. Butts CA, Ding K, Seymour L, et al. Randomized phase III trial of vinorelbine plus cisplatin compared with observation in com-

pletely resected stage IB and II non-small-cell lung cancer: updated survival analysis of JBR-10. J Clin Oncol. 2010;28(1): 29–34.

105. Strauss GM, Herndon JE, Maddaus MA, et al. Adjuvant paclitaxel plus carboplatin compared with observation in stage IB non-small-cell lung cancer: CALGB 9633 with the Cancer and Leukemia Group B, Radiation Therapy Oncology Group, and North Central Cancer Treatment Group Study Groups. J Clin Oncol. 2008;26(31):5043–51.

106. Burdett S, Stewart LA, Rydzewska L. A systematic review and meta-analysis of the literature: chemotherapy and surgery versus surgery alone in non-small cell lung cancer. J Thorac Oncol. 2006;1(7):611–21.

107. Song WA, Zhou NK, Wang W, et al. Survival benefit of neoadjuvant chemotherapy in non-small cell lung cancer: an updated meta-analysis of 13 randomized control trials. J Thorac Oncol. 2010;5(4):510–6.

108. NSCLC Meta-analysis Collaborative Group. Preoperative chemotherapy for non-small-cell lung cancer: a systematic review and meta-analysis of individual participant data. Lancet. 2014;383(9928):1561–71.

109. Wu Y, Tsuboi M, M.D., He J et al. Osimertinib in Resected EGFR-Mutated Non–Small-Cell Lung Cancer. NEJM 2020, 10.1056/NEJMoa2027071.

110. PORT Meta-analysis Trialists Group. Postoperative radiotherapy for non-small cell lung cancer. Cochrane Database Syst Rev. 2000;(2):CD002142.

111. Yu JB, Decker RH, Detterbeck FC, Wilson LD. Surveillance epidemiology and end results evaluation of the role of surgery for stage I small cell lung cancer. J Thorac Oncol. 2010;5(2): 215–9.

112. Le Pechoux C, Pourel N, Barlesi F et al. An international randomized trial, comparing post-operative conformal radiotherapy (PORT) to no PORT, in patients with completely resected non-small cell lung cancer (NSCLC) and mediastinal N2 involvement: Primary end-point analysis of LungART. Annals of Oncology (2020) 31 (suppl_4): S1142-S1215. 10.1016/annonc/annonc325.

113. Schreiber D, Rineer J, Weedon J, et al. Survival outcomes with the use of surgery in limited-stage small cell lung cancer: should its role be re-evaluated? Cancer. 2010;116(5):1350–7.

114. Aupérin A, Le Péchoux C, Rolland E, et al. Meta-analysis of concomitant versus sequential radiochemotherapy in locally advanced non-small-cell lung cancer. J Clin Oncol. 2010;28(13):2181–90.

115. Yamamoto N, Nakagawa K, Nishimura Y, et al. Phase III study comparing second- and third-generation regimens with concurrent thoracic radiotherapy in patients with unresectable stage III non-small-cell lung cancer: West Japan Thoracic Oncology Group WJTOG0105. J Clin Oncol. 2010;28(23):3739–45.

116. Hanna N, Neubauer M, Yiannoutsos C, et al. Phase III study of cisplatin, etoposide, and concurrent chest radiation with or without consolidation docetaxel in patients with inoperable stage III non-small-cell lung cancer: the Hoosier Oncology Group and U.S. Oncology. J Clin Oncol. 2008;26(35):5755–60.

117. Albain KS, Crowley JJ, Turrisi AT, et al. Concurrent cisplatin, etoposide, and chest radiotherapy in pathologic stage IIIB non-small-cell lung cancer: a Southwest Oncology Group phase II study, SWOG 9019. J Clin Oncol. 2002;20(16):3454–60.

118. Antonia SJ, Villegas A, Daniel D, et al. Durvalumab after chemoradiotherapy in stage III non-small-cell lung cancer. N Engl J Med. 2017;377(20):1919–29.

119. Baas P, Belderbos JS, Senan S, et al. Concurrent chemotherapy (carboplatin, paclitaxel, etoposide) and involved-field radiotherapy in limited stage small cell lung cancer: a Dutch multicenter phase II study. Br J Cancer. 2006;94(5):625–30.

120. Aupérin A, Arriagada R, Pignon JP, et al. Prophylactic cranial irradiation for patients with small-cell lung cancer in complete remission. Prophylactic Cranial Irradiation Overview Collaborative Group. N Engl J Med. 1999;341(7):476–84.

121. Novello S, Barlesi F, Califano R, et al. Metastatic non-small-cell lung cancer: ESMO Clinical Practice Guidelines for diagnosis, treatment and follow-up. Ann Oncol. 2016;27(suppl 5):v1–v27.

122. Mok TS, Wu YL, Thongprasert S, et al. Gefitinib or carboplatin-paclitaxel in pulmonary adenocarcinoma. N Engl J Med. 2009;361(10):947–57.

123. Mitsudomi T, Morita S, Yatabe Y, et al. Gefitinib versus cisplatin plus docetaxel in patients with non-small-cell lung cancer harbouring mutations of the epidermal growth factor receptor (WJTOG3405): an open label, randomised phase 3 trial. Lancet Oncol. 2010;11(2):121–8.

124. Maemondo M, Inoue A, Kobayashi K, et al. Gefitinib or chemotherapy for non-small-cell lung cancer with mutated EGFR. N Engl J Med. 2010;362(25):2380–8.

125. Rosell R, Carcereny E, Gervais R, et al. Erlotinib versus standard chemotherapy as first-line treatment for European patients with advanced EGFR mutation-positive non-small-cell lung cancer (EURTAC): a multicentre, open-label, randomised phase 3 trial. Lancet Oncol. 2012;13(3):239–46.

126. Zhou C, Wu YL, Chen G, et al. Erlotinib versus chemotherapy as first-line treatment for patients with advanced EGFR mutation-positive non-small-cell lung cancer (OPTIMAL, CTONG-0802): a multicentre, open-label, randomised, phase 3 study. Lancet Oncol. 2011;12(8):735–42.

127. Sequist LV, Yang JC, Yamamoto N, et al. Phase III study of afatinib or cisplatin plus pemetrexed in patients with metastatic lung adenocarcinoma with EGFR mutations. J Clin Oncol. 2013;31(27):3327–34.

128. Wu YL, Zhou C, Hu CP, et al. Afatinib versus cisplatin plus gemcitabine for first-line treatment of Asian patients with advanced non-small-cell lung cancer harbouring EGFR mutations (LUX-Lung 6): an open-label, randomised phase 3 trial. Lancet Oncol. 2014;15(2):213–22.

129. Soria JC, Ohe Y, Vansteenkiste J, et al. Osimertinib in untreated EGFR-mutated advanced non-small-cell lung cancer. N Engl J Med. 2018;378(2):113–25.

130. Ramalingam SS, Vansteenkiste J, Planchard D, et al. Overall survival with osimertinib in untreated. N Engl J Med. 2020;382(1):41–50.

131. Gristina V, Malapelle U, Galvano A, et al. The significance of epidermal growth factor receptor uncommon mutations in non-small cell lung cancer: a systematic review and critical appraisal. Cancer Treat Rev. 2020;85:101994.

132. Mok T, Kim DW, Wu YL, et al. First-line crizotinib versus pemetrexed cisplatin or pemetrexed carboplatin in patients with advanced ALK-positive non-squamous non small-cell lung cancer: results of a phase III study (PROFILE 1014). In J Clin Oncol. 2014;32(5s):(suppl; abstr 8002).

133. Hida T, Nokihara H, Kondo M, et al. Alectinib versus crizotinib in patients with ALK-positive non-small-cell lung cancer (J-ALEX): an open-label, randomised phase 3 trial. Lancet. 2017;390(10089):29–39.

134. Peters S, Camidge DR, Shaw AT, et al. Alectinib versus crizotinib in untreated ALK-positive non-small-cell lung cancer. N Engl J Med. 2017;377(9):829–38.

135. List A, Barraco N, Bono M, Insalaco L, Castellana L, Cutaia S, Ricciardi MR, Gristina V, Bronte E, Pantuso G, Passiglia F. Immuno-targeted combinations in oncogene-addicted non-small cell lung cancer. Transl Cancer Res. 2018;8:S55–63.

136. Solomon B, Bauer TM, De Marinis F et al. Lorlatinib vs crizotinib in the first-line treatment of patients (pts) with advanced ALK-positive non-small cell lung cancer (NSCLC): Results of

137. the phase III CROWN study. Annals of Oncology (2020) 31 (suppl_4): S1142-S1215. 10.1016/annonc/annonc325.

137. Planchard D, Smit EF, Groen HJM, et al. Dabrafenib plus trametinib in patients with previously untreated BRAF. Lancet Oncol. 2017;18(10):1307–16.

138. Seton-Rogers S. KRAS-G12C in the crosshairs. Nat Rev Cancer. 2020;20(1):3.

139. Drilon A, Laetsch TW, Kummar S, et al. Efficacy of larotrectinib in TRK fusion-positive cancers in adults and children. N Engl J Med. 2018;378(8):731–9.

140. Doebele RC, Drilon A, Paz-Ares L, et al. Entrectinib in patients with advanced or metastatic NTRK fusion-positive solid tumours: integrated analysis of three phase 1-2 trials. Lancet Oncol. 2020;21(2):271–82.

141. Rolfo C, Russo A. Mutations in non-small cell lung cancer: a herculean effort to hit the target. Cancer Discov. 2020;10(5):643–5.

142. Russo A, Lopes AR, McCusker MG, et al. New targets in lung cancer (excluding EGFR, ALK, ROS1). Curr Oncol Rep. 2020;22(5):48.

143. Rolfo C, Passiglia F, Ostrowski M, et al. Improvement in lung cancer outcomes with targeted therapies: an update for family physicians. J Am Board Fam Med. 2015;28(1):124–33.

144. Rolfo C, Giovannetti E, Hong DS, et al. Novel therapeutic strategies for patients with NSCLC that do not respond to treatment with EGFR inhibitors. Cancer Treat Rev. 2014;40(8):990–1004.

145. Passiglia F, Bronte G, Castiglia M, et al. Prognostic and predictive biomarkers for targeted therapy in NSCLC: for whom the bell tolls? Expert Opin Biol Ther. 2015:1–14.

146. Mok TS, Wu YL, Ahn MJ, et al. Osimertinib or platinum-pemetrexed in EGFR T790M-positive lung cancer. N Engl J Med. 2017;376(7):629–40.

147. Chouaid C, Dujon C, Do P, et al. Feasibility and clinical impact of re-biopsy in advanced non small-cell lung cancer: a prospective multicenter study in a real-world setting (GFPC study 12-01). Lung Cancer. 2014;86(2):170–3.

148. Wu Y, Liu H, Shi X, Song Y. Can EGFR mutations in plasma or serum be predictive markers of non-small-cell lung cancer? A meta-analysis. Lung Cancer. 2015;88(3):246–53.

149. Qian X, Liu J, Sun Y, et al. Circulating cell-free DNA has a high degree of specificity to detect exon 19 deletions and the single-point substitution mutation L858R in non-small cell lung cancer. Oncotarget. 2016;7(20):29154–65.

150. Oxnard GR, Thress KS, Alden RS, et al. Association between plasma genotyping and outcomes of treatment with osimertinib (AZD9291) in advanced non-small-cell lung cancer. J Clin Oncol. 2016;34(28):3375–82.

151. Passiglia F, Rizzo S, Rolfo C, et al. Metastatic site location influences the diagnostic accuracy of ctDNA EGFR- mutation testing in NSCLC patients: a pooled analysis. Curr Cancer Drug Targets. 2018;18:697–705.

152. Russo A, Incorvaia L, Del Re M, et al. The molecular profiling of solid tumors by liquid biopsy: a position paper of the AIOM-SIAPEC-IAP-SIBioC-SIC-SIF Italian Scientific Societies [published online ahead of print, 2021 Jun 3]. ESMO Open. 2021;6(3):100164. https://doi.org/10.1016/j.esmoop.2021.100164.

153. Rolfo C, Passiglia F, Castiglia M, et al. ALK and crizotinib: after the honeymoon…what else? Resistance mechanisms and new therapies to overcome it. Transl Lung Cancer Res. 2014;3(4):250–61.

154. Camidge DR, Pao W, Sequist LV. Acquired resistance to TKIs in solid tumours: learning from lung cancer. Nat Rev Clin Oncol. 2014;11(8):473–81.

155. Costa DB. Resistance to ALK inhibitors: pharmacokinetics, mutations or bypass signaling? Cell Cycle. 2017;16(1):19–20.

156. Shaw AT, Kim TM, Crinò L, et al. Ceritinib versus chemotherapy in patients with ALK-rearranged non-small-cell lung cancer previously given chemotherapy and crizotinib (ASCEND-5): a randomised, controlled, open-label, phase 3 trial. Lancet Oncol. 2017;18(7):874–86.

157. Larkins E, Blumenthal GM, Chen H, et al. FDA approval: alectinib for the treatment of metastatic, ALK-positive non-small cell lung cancer following crizotinib. Clin Cancer Res. 2016;22(21):5171–6.

158. Gadgeel SM, Shaw AT, Govindan R, et al. Pooled analysis of CNS response to alectinib in two studies of pretreated patients with ALK-positive non-small-cell lung cancer. J Clin Oncol. 2016;34(34):4079–85.

159. Metro G, Tazza M, Matocci R, Chiari R, Crinò L. Optimal management of ALK-positive NSCLC progressing on crizotinib. Lung Cancer. 2017;106:58–66.

160. Incorvaia L, Fanale D, Badalamenti G, et al. Programmed death ligand 1 (PD-L1) as a predictive biomarker for pembrolizumab therapy in patients with advanced non-small-cell lung cancer (NSCLC). Adv Ther. 2019;36(10):2600–17.

161. Reck M, Rodríguez-Abreu D, Robinson AG, et al. Pembrolizumab versus chemotherapy for PD-L1-positive non-small-cell lung cancer. N Engl J Med. 2016;375(19):1823–33.

162. Langer CJ, Gadgeel SM, Borghaei H, et al. Carboplatin and pemetrexed with or without pembrolizumab for advanced, non-squamous non-small-cell lung cancer: a randomised, phase 2 cohort of the open-label KEYNOTE-021 study. Lancet Oncol. 2016;17(11):1497–508.

163. Hellmann MD, Rizvi NA, Goldman JW, et al. Nivolumab plus ipilimumab as first-line treatment for advanced non-small-cell lung cancer (CheckMate 012): results of an open-label, phase 1, multicohort study. Lancet Oncol. 2017;18(1):31–41.

164. Reck M, Borghaei H, O'Byrne KJ. Nivolumab plus ipilimumab in non-small-cell lung cancer. Future Oncol. 2019;15(19):2287–302.

165. Rizvi NA, Cho BC, Reinmuth N, et al. Durvalumab with or without tremelimumab vs standard chemotherapy in first-line treatment of metastatic non-small cell lung cancer: the MYSTIC phase 3 randomized clinical trial. JAMA Oncol. 2020;6:661–74.

166. Scagliotti GV, Parikh P, von Pawel J, et al. Phase III study comparing cisplatin plus gemcitabine with cisplatin plus pemetrexed in chemotherapy-naive patients with advanced-stage non-small-cell lung cancer. J Clin Oncol. 2008;26(21):3543–51.

167. Paz-Ares LG, de Marinis F, Dediu M, et al. PARAMOUNT: final overall survival results of the phase III study of maintenance pemetrexed versus placebo immediately after induction treatment with pemetrexed plus cisplatin for advanced nonsquamous non-small-cell lung cancer. J Clin Oncol. 2013;31(23):2895–902.

168. Sandler A, Yi J, Dahlberg S, et al. Treatment outcomes by tumor histology in Eastern Cooperative Group Study E4599 of bevacizumab with paclitaxel/carboplatin for advanced non-small cell lung cancer. J Thorac Oncol. 2010;5(9):1416–23.

169. Reck M, von Pawel J, Zatloukal P, et al. Overall survival with cisplatin-gemcitabine and bevacizumab or placebo as first-line therapy for nonsquamous non-small-cell lung cancer: results from a randomised phase III trial (AVAiL). Ann Oncol. 2010;21(9):1804–9.

170. Thatcher N, Hirsch FR, Luft AV, et al. Necitumumab plus gemcitabine and cisplatin versus gemcitabine and cisplatin alone as first-line therapy in patients with stage IV squamous non-small-cell lung cancer (SQUIRE): an open-label, randomised, controlled phase 3 trial. Lancet Oncol. 2015;16(7):763–74.

171. Genova C, Socinski MA, Hozak RR, et al. EGFR gene copy number by FISH may predict outcome of necitumumab in squa-

mous lung carcinomas: analysis from the SQUIRE study. J Thorac Oncol. 2018;13:228–36.

172. Brahmer J, Reckamp KL, Baas P, et al. Nivolumab versus docetaxel in advanced squamous-cell non-small-cell lung cancer. N Engl J Med. 2015;373(2):123–35.

173. Borghaei H, Paz-Ares L, Horn L, et al. Nivolumab versus docetaxel in advanced nonsquamous non-small-cell lung cancer. N Engl J Med. 2015;373:1627–39.

174. Herbst RS, Baas P, Kim DW, et al. Pembrolizumab versus docetaxel for previously treated, PD-L1-positive, advanced non-small-cell lung cancer (KEYNOTE-010): a randomised controlled trial. Lancet. 2016;387(10027):1540–50.

175. Rittmeyer A, Barlesi F, Waterkamp D, et al. Atezolizumab versus docetaxel in patients with previously treated non-small-cell lung cancer (OAK): a phase 3, open-label, multicentre randomised controlled trial. Lancet. 2017;389(10066):255–65.

176. Passiglia F, Galvano A, Rizzo S, et al. Looking for the best immune-checkpoint inhibitor in pre-treated NSCLC patients: an indirect comparison between nivolumab, pembrolizumab and atezolizumab. Int J Cancer. 2018;142(6):1277–84.

177. Champiat S, Lambotte O, Barreau E, et al. Management of immune checkpoint blockade dysimmune toxicities: a collaborative position paper. Ann Oncol. 2016;27(4):559–74.

178. Michot JM, Bigenwald C, Champiat S, et al. Immune-related adverse events with immune checkpoint blockade: a comprehensive review. Eur J Cancer. 2016;54:139–48.

179. Reck M, Kaiser R, Mellemgaard A, et al. Docetaxel plus nintedanib versus docetaxel plus placebo in patients with previously treated non-small-cell lung cancer (LUME-Lung 1): a phase 3, double-blind, randomised controlled trial. Lancet Oncol. 2014;15(2):143–55.

180. Garon EB, Ciuleanu TE, Arrieta O, et al. Ramucirumab plus docetaxel versus placebo plus docetaxel for second-line treatment of stage IV non-small-cell lung cancer after disease progression on platinum-based therapy (REVEL): a multicentre, double-blind, randomised phase 3 trial. Lancet. 2014;384(9944):665–73.

181. Soria JC, Felip E, Cobo M, et al. Afatinib versus erlotinib as second-line treatment of patients with advanced squamous cell carcinoma of the lung (LUX-Lung 8): an open-label randomised controlled phase 3 trial. Lancet Oncol. 2015;16(8):897–907.

182. Liao BC, Lee JH, Lin CC, et al. Epidermal growth factor receptor tyrosine kinase inhibitors for non-small-cell lung cancer patients with leptomeningeal carcinomatosis. J Thorac Oncol. 2015;10(12):1754–61.

183. Goss G, Tsai CM, Shepherd FA, et al. CNS response to osimertinib in patients with T790M-positive advanced NSCLC: pooled data from two phase II trials. Ann Oncol. 2017;29:687–93.

184. Gadgeel S, Shaw AT, Barlesi F, et al. Cumulative incidence rates for CNS and non-CNS progression in two phase II studies of alectinib in ALK-positive NSCLC. Br J Cancer. 2018;118(1):38–42.

185. Ballard P, Yates JW, Yang Z, et al. Preclinical comparison of osimertinib with other EGFR-TKIs in EGFR-mutant NSCLC brain metastases models, and early evidence of clinical brain metastases activity. Clin Cancer Res. 2016;22(20):5130–40.

186. Stinchcombe TE. Current treatments for surgically resectable, limited-stage, and extensive-stage small cell lung cancer. Oncologist. 2017;22(12):1510–7.

187. Cheng S, Evans WK, Stys-Norman D, Shepherd FA, Lung Cancer Disease Site Group of Cancer Care Ontario's Program in Evidence-based Care. Chemotherapy for relapsed small cell lung cancer: a systematic review and practice guideline. J Thorac Oncol. 2007;2(4):348–54.

188. Horn L, Mansfield AS, Szczęsna A, et al. First-line atezolizumab plus chemotherapy in extensive-stage small-cell lung cancer. N Engl J Med. 2018;379:2220–9.

189. Paz-Ares L, Dvorkin M, Chen Y, et al. Durvalumab plus platinum-etoposide versus platinum-etoposide in first-line treatment of extensive-stage small-cell lung cancer (CASPIAN): a randomised, controlled, open-label, phase 3 trial. Lancet. 2019;394(10212):1929–39.

190. Rudin CM, Pietanza MC, Bauer TM, et al. Rovalpituzumab tesirine, a DLL3-targeted antibody-drug conjugate, in recurrent small-cell lung cancer: a first-in-human, first-in-class, open-label, phase 1 study. Lancet Oncol. 2017;18(1):42–51.

191. Antonia SJ, López-Martin JA, Bendell J, et al. Nivolumab alone and nivolumab plus ipilimumab in recurrent small-cell lung cancer (CheckMate 032): a multicentre, open-label, phase 1/2 trial. Lancet Oncol. 2016;17(7):883–95.

192. Seymour L, Bogaerts J, Perrone A, et al. iRECIST: guidelines for response criteria for use in trials testing immunotherapeutics. Lancet Oncol. 2017;18(3):e143–52.

Malignant Pleural Mesothelioma

Enrica Capelletto and Silvia Novello

Thoracic Cancers

Contents

© Springer Nature Switzerland AG 2021
A. Russo et al. (eds.), *Practical Medical Oncology Textbook*, UNIPA Springer Series,
https://doi.org/10.1007/978-3-030-56051-5_33

By the end of the chapter the reader will:

- Be able to apply the right clinical and diagnostic procedures to easily recognize malignant pleural mesothelioma
- Have learned the basic concepts of epidemiology, risk factors and genetic predisposition
- Have reached in-depth knowledge of main treatment modalities
- Be able to put acquired knowledge into clinical practice

33.1 Introduction

Malignant pleural mesothelioma (MPM) is a rare and aggressive disease arising from the mesothelial cells of the pleural cavity, with a close relationship to the asbestos fibres exposure and an increasing incidence worldwide (■ Fig. 33.1).

Systemic chemotherapy with antifolate agents and platinum compounds still represents the standard of care for the vast majority of patients at the time of diagnosis.

The role of multimodal approaches, combining systemic treatment with radiotherapy and/or surgery, is still debated, because of the absence of adequate clinical trials designed to evaluate these strategies in patients with an early disease at diagnosis.

Despite some preliminary promising results of immunotherapy and the emerging role of biological agents for the treatment of MPM, a deeper knowledge of its pathogenesis is needed, in order to improve diagnostic tools and treatment outcomes.

33.2 Origin and Histologic Subtypes

The neoplastic transformation of the mesothelial layer leads to the onset of MPM. According to the World Health Organization (WHO) Classification of Tumours of the Pleura [1], the major MPM histologic types encounter:

- Epithelioid, with histological appearance resembling epithelial neoplasia (i.e. carcinomas)
- Sarcomatoid, with histological appearance resembling mesenchymal neoplasia (i.e. sarcomas)
- Biphasic, with the two previous variously combined together (■ Fig. 33.2)

Patients with sarcomatoid and biphasic tumours have significantly poorer survival compared to patients with epithelioid disease.

33.3 Epidemiology and Risk Factors

MPM is considered to be a relatively rare tumour with an estimated 2500 new cases in the United States every year and a poor survival rate (■ Fig. 33.3a). Incidence began to rise in 1975 and peaked around 1995, concur-

33

■ **Fig. 33.1** Schematic presentation of unilateral malignant pleural mesothelioma (MPM) and its strict correlation to the inhaled asbestos fibres. (Photo credit: Dreamstime)

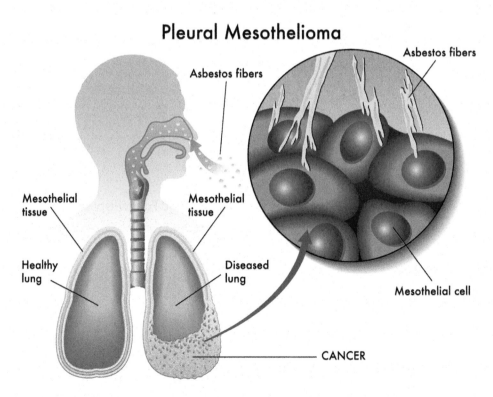

Pleural Mesothelioma

Asbestos fibers
Asbestos fibers
Mesothelial tissue
Mesothelial tissue
Healthy lung
Diseased lung
Mesothelial cell
CANCER

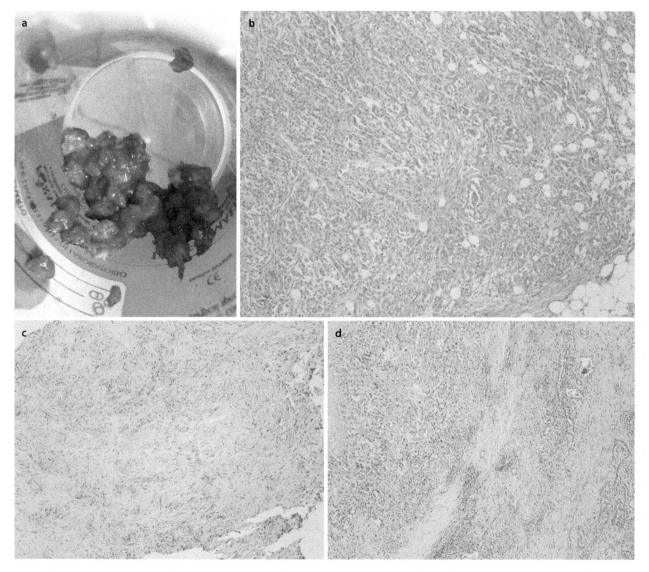

Fig. 33.2 Macroscopic aspect of a pleural tumour **a**. Microscopic aspect of epithelioid **b**, sarcomatoid **c** and biphasic **d** MPM stained with haematoxylin-eosin. (Courtesy of Dr. Luisella Righi)

rently with the diminishing of occupational and environmental exposure to asbestos (■ Fig. 33.3b) (SEER programme).

Professional exposure to asbestos and other mineral fibres accounts for more than 80% of the cases and makes the MPM a preventable disease. The latency time from exposure to the onset of the disease can range from 20 to 70 years and seems to be dose dependant, with a premature presentation in heavily exposed patients [3], even if there are also data suggesting a relationship between the disease and a minimal exposure [4].

In the past decades in Europe, Australia and Japan, the incidence of MPM has increased slowly, and the expected peak of incidence is between 2015 and 2025 [5]. The continued use of asbestos in the developing world and the scant regulation about the handling of many asbestos products even in some Western countries could

unfortunately lead to an imminent global epidemic of MPM.

Exposure to ionizing radiations, for occupational reasons or therapeutic use for other malignancies, has also been recently described as a risk factor for MPM [6, 7].

33.4 Genetic Predisposition

Up to 20% of MPM patients do not recognize a clear exposure to asbestos, suggesting that genetic predisposition may play a central role in the pathogenesis of the disease.

A germline mutation in the BRCA1-associated protein 1 (BAP1) tumour suppressor gene, coupled with the loss of the second BAP1 allele, has been recently

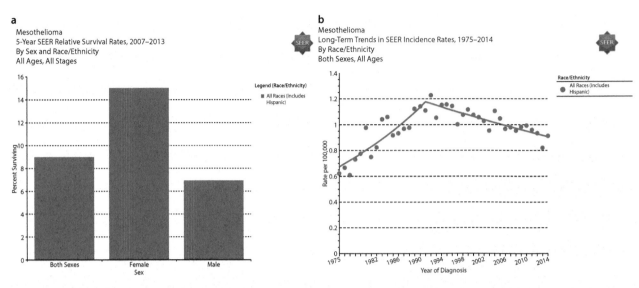

■ **Fig. 33.3** 5-year relative survival rate by sex **a** and age-adjusted incidence rates **b** for MPM. (Photo credit: SEER*Explorer: An interactive website for SEER cancer statistics [Internet]. Beta Version. Surveillance Research Program, National Cancer Institute. [Cited 2017 Apr 14]. Available from ▸ https://seer.cancer.gov/explorer/ [2])

described in up to 50% of familiar cases of MPM in the presence of a modest environmental or occupational exposure to asbestos [8, 9].

The prevalence of germline BAP1 mutations is described in 6% of cases in a large asbestos-exposed cohort of patients with both mesothelioma and a family history of cancer [10].

Somatic loss of the NF2 and CDKN2A/ARF tumour suppressor genes has also been related to a higher incidence of MPM, even if with a lower frequency than BAP1 mutations [8].

33.5 Clinical Features

Median age of onset of MPM is between 65 and 70 years old, with a higher prevalence in men (80% of cases). Female incidence rate is fourfold lower than male and has remained unchanged over the past four decades in Western countries [5].

Patients typically present with shortness of breath, chest wall pain and weight loss. At physical evaluation, unilateral pleural effusion can be often detected as the main cause of respiratory symptoms and pain (■ Fig. 33.4). Initial symptoms are insidious and not specific, leading often to a late diagnosis, and complications due to "local invasion" are extremely common. Local complications include superior vena cava obstruction, cardiac tamponade, spinal cord compression, phrenic nerve or recurrent laryngeal nerve paralysis, dysphagia, subcutaneous involvement and direct extension through the chest wall.

MPM's spreading to the controlateral pleural cavity or to the abdomen across the diaphragm is uncommon, observed in about 10–20% of cases. Peritoneal involvement may cause ascites or bowel obstruction with high morbidity for the rapid symptoms' deteriorations [11].

Haematogenous metastasis is rare, but could potentially arise in any extrathoracic organs, strongly affecting prognosis.

33.6 Diagnosis

In the suspect of MPM, standard work-up includes:
- Chest X-ray
- Computed tomography (CT) scan of the chest and upper abdomen
- Thoracentesis (when needed, with examination of the pleural effusion)
- General laboratory blood tests

A detailed occupational history, with emphasis on asbestos exposure, is mandatory, as well as the familiar anamnesis with particular attention to other malignancy.

Chest X-ray still represents the first radiological assessment performed in the vast majority of cases of MPM. Significant volumes of pleural effusions can mask pleural or pulmonary lesions, and, conversely, small malignant pleural effusions could not be detectable with this technique. When patient's symptoms and the documented exposure to asbestos are suggestive for MPM, computed tomography (CT) scan of the chest and of the upper abdomen is necessary in order to get

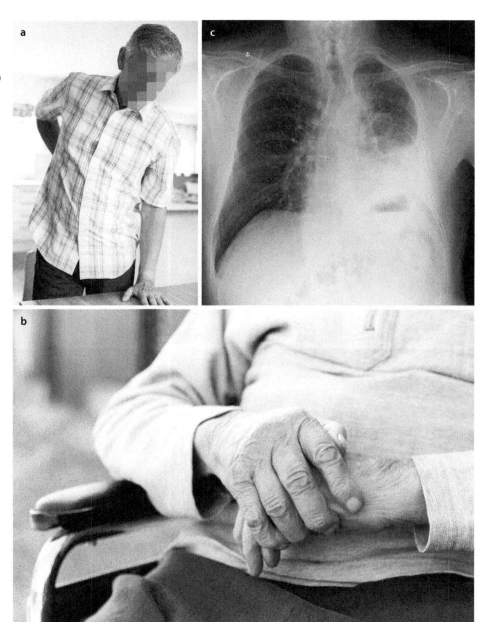

Fig. 33.4 Pleural effusion with shortness of breath, chest pain and weight loss are common symptoms for MPM. (Photo credit: Shutterstock, Inc.)

more details and to proceed with more invasive procedures and/or staging (■ Fig. 33.5).

CT scan findings, suggesting a MPM, include nodular pleural thickening, diffuse pleural thickening with circumferential extension, pleural thickness higher than 1 cm and mediastinal pleural involvement. These radiological findings do not differentiate MPM from a metastatic pleural disease, making the differential diagnosis for MPM a challenging work [12].

Cytological features of pleural effusion may permit the diagnosis of MPM, but the sensitivity of cytology alone ranges between 32% and 76%, and tissue biopsy is generally preferred [13]. A surgical thoracoscopy is often recommended to obtain adequate tissue for the histology through pleural biopsy, to proper stage the disease and to allow pleural fluid evacuation (with or without pleurodesis) [14]. This can be performed as a pleuroscopy or as video-assisted thoracic surgery (VATS).

33.7 The Role of Biomarkers

An ideal diagnostic biomarker should be able to discriminate between MPM and normal controls, but also between malignant and benign pleural effusions or lesions, especially in healthy asbestos-exposed patients.

To date, several circulating tumour biomarkers have been investigated, but none of them is currently validated in clinical practice as MPM biomarkers due to poor specificity [15].

33

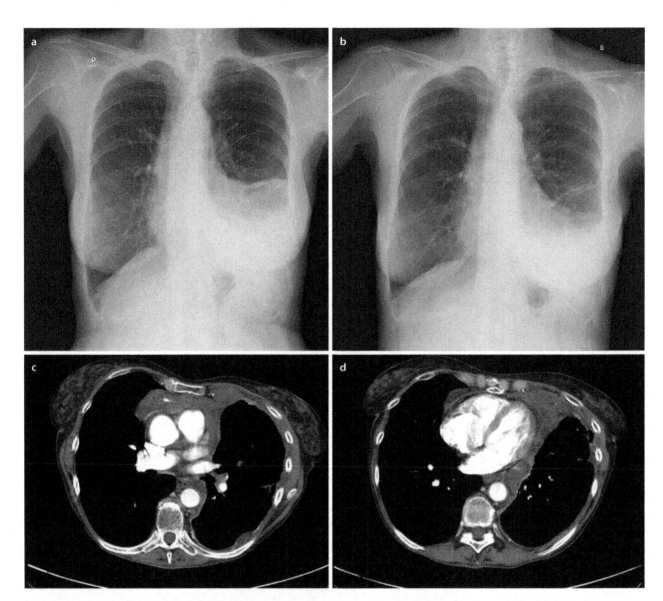

Fig. 33.5 Chest X-ray with left pleural effusion **a** and corresponding chest X-ray **b** and CT scan **c**, **d** after thoracentesis

The osteopontin protein, a mediator of the cell-matrix interactions, can result elevated in MPM when compared with healthy asbestos-exposed patients [16]. However, pleural or serum osteopontin cannot discriminate between MPM and other pleural effusions [17], having a limited role in diagnosis.

Mesothelin is an antigen of normally differentiated mesothelial cells. The entire protein is cleaved into a C-terminal membrane-bound fragment and an N-terminal fragment, released into the blood and called megakaryocyte potentiating factor (MPF). Also part of the membrane-bound C-terminal fragment is released into the blood (soluble mesothelin). Both MPF and soluble mesothelin have been studied as potential biomarkers; the MPF seems to distinguish MPM from healthy controls with history of asbestos exposure, benign pleural diseases and pleural effusions from metastatic disease, showing high specificity and low sensitivity [18, 19]. In any case, to date the use of MPF as diagnostic biomarker for MPM is not recommended by the international guidelines for MPM, and its use in the clinical practice is extremely rare.

Circulating proteomic, fibulin-3 and high mobility group box protein 1 (HMGB1) could represent important future biomarkers, but their role in MPM differential diagnosis is still uncertain [20, 21]. Similarly, changes in microRNA signatures may differentiate MPM from lung adenocarcinoma, and MPM from benign asbestos-related pleural effusions, but data are not still mature, and confirmatory evaluation is needed [22, 23].

33.8 Pathology

Differential diagnosis of MPM may be challenging being the pleura a common site of metastasis from other sites. Furthermore, inflammatory reactive changes of the pleura could be mistaken with a malignant disease. The term "atypical mesothelial proliferation" is often adopted to describe the atypical mesothelial hyperplasia found in the pleural effusion, which could accompany a MPM, but is not sufficient for a neoplastic malignant diagnosis. For the definitive diagnosis of MPM, it is necessary to have adequate tissue biopsies and to perform an adequate immunohistochemistry (IHC) panel. The larger the tissue biopsy and the more targeted the sampling approach, the more reliable and definitive the diagnosis [24].

The latest WHO classification of tumours of the pleura has been published in 2015 (Table 33.1) with a particular attention to the prognostic value of some histological subtypes and variants of MPM [1].

Diffuse malignant mesothelioma (DMM) in the new WHO classification is well distinguished from other forms with a better prognosis, such as localized malignant mesotheliomas (LMMs) and well-differentiated papillary mesotheliomas (WDPMs).

The commonest histological subtype of DMMs is the epithelioid (70% of cases). Tumours of pure epithelioid histology can have patterns prevalently described as papillary (cells growing along exophytic fronds with vascular cores), tubulopapillary (a mixture of small tubules and papillary structures with fibrovascular cores, often with clefts and trabeculae) and solid (nests and sheets of round or polygonal cells with abundant cytoplasm and vesicular nuclei with prominent nucleoli). Sarcomatoid DMM is composed of a fascicular proliferation of spindle cells with oval nuclei, scant cytoplasm and, occasionally, prominent nucleoli, usually displaying more atypia, mitotic activity and wide foci of necrosis. Desmoplastic MPM is a rare sarcomatoid MPM variant characterized by small atypical few neoplastic cells immersed in a dense collagen stroma. Biphasic (or mixed) DMM is characterized by a combination of epithelioid and sarcomatoid patterns together.

Patients with sarcomatoid and biphasic DMMs have a significantly poorer survival when compared to the other patients [25]. Within the group of pleural epithelioid DMMs, an aggressive behaviour of epithelioid MPM with pleomorphic features (with anaplastic or prominent giant cells, often multinucleated) has been repeatedly described in multiple studies, with a similar survival to that of patients with biphasic and sarcomatoid DMMs [26, 27]. The same studies show that the combined subgroup of tubulopapillary and trabecular MPM has a more favourable prognosis than the solid subtype and the combined solid/micropapillary group [27].

WDPM represents a distinct mesothelial tumour characterized histologically by superficial spreading of papillary formations with large fibrovascular cores and myxoid stroma. It's more frequently found in the peritoneal cavity, but it shows the same features also in the thorax. WDPMs usually are indolent and clinically benign if completely resected [28]. Differential diagnosis from the papillary form of conventional DMM may be difficult, especially in small biopsy specimen.

Table 33.1 WHO classification of tumours of the pleura

Mesothelial tumours	Mesenchymal tumours
Diffuse malignant mesothelioma (DMM)	*Epithelioid hemangioendothelioma*
— Epithelioid mesothelioma	*Angiosarcoma*
— Sarcomatoid mesothelioma	*Synovial sarcoma*
— Desmoplastic mesothelioma	*Solitary fibrous tumour*
— Biphasic mesothelioma	— Malignant solitary fibrous tumour
Localized malignant mesotheliomas (LMMs)	*Desmoid-type fibromatosis*
— Epithelioid mesothelioma	*Calcifying fibrous tumour*
— Sarcomatoid mesothelioma	*Desmoplastic round cell tumour*
— Biphasic mesothelioma	
Well-differentiated papillary mesotheliomas (WDPMs)	
Adenomatoid tumour	
Lymphoproliferative disorders	
Primary effusion lymphoma	
Diffuse large B-cell lymphoma associated with chronic inflammation	

33.9 The Role of Immunohistochemistry (IHC) in the Differential Diagnosis

Site-specific carcinoma marker panels have been introduced in the 2015 WHO classification for the differential diagnosis between MPM and other malignancies affecting the pleura. Their use is largely recommended [13] in order to enhance the specificity and sensitivity of the diagnosis [29]. These markers help to discriminate a MPM from a metastatic disease from other primary sites, including:

— TTF-1 and napsin A for adenocarcinoma of the lung
— PAX-8 for renal cell and thyroid carcinoma
— Prostate-specific antigen (PSA) and prostate-specific membrane antigen (PSMA) for adenocarcinoma of the prostate
— CDX2 and cytokeratin 20 for adenocarcinoma of the gastrointestinal tract
— PAX-8, PAX-2 and oestrogen receptor (ER) for serous papillary carcinoma of the ovary or peritoneum

Other useful markers in this context are CD45 and CD20 for differential diagnosis with haematogenous tumours and HMB45, melan A and SOX10 for melanoma [13].

The commonest and challenging differential diagnosis of MPM is done with primary lung adenocarcinoma. The use of at least two mesothelial markers and two carcinoma markers (including TTF-1 and CEA) is recommended to ameliorate the diagnosis [13, 29].

Immunohistochemistry has shown a limited role in the differentiation of sarcomatoid MPM from other sarcomas and sarcomatoid carcinoma of the lung with pleural involvement. Sarcomatoid MPMs often stain positive for a large spectrum of anti-cytokeratin antibodies, whereas most soft tissue sarcomas do not. Mesothelial markers used for the diagnosis of epithelioid MPM have showed limited utility for the sarcomatoid subtype, often negative for calretinin, cytokeratin 5/6 and WT-1. Sarcomatoid mesothelioma is typically positive for vimentin and may also show a positivity for S-100, actin or desmin, but these IHC markers have no diagnostic specificity [30].

Another challenging differential diagnosis for sarcomatoid mesothelioma is the differentiation from malignant solitary fibrous tumours of the pleura (SFTP), a rare mesenchymal tumour originating from the submesothelial tissue of the pleura, with a slow-growing rate and prevalently with benign histologic features. SFTPs stain positive for CD34 and bcl-2 and, usually, are keratin-negative. Recently, these tumours have been shown to be positive for STAT6 [31]. Solitary fibrous tumours of the pleura seem to have no relation to asbestos exposure, too.

Main criteria for separation of benign from malignant mesothelial proliferations are listed in ◘ Table 33.2.

Table 33.2 Reactive atypical mesothelial hyperplasia versus epithelioid malignant mesothelioma: main features

Histological features	Atypical mesothelial hyperplasia	Malignant mesothelioma
Major criteria		
Stromal invasion	Absent	Present
Cellularity	Confined to the pleural surface	Dense, with stromal reaction
Papillae	Simple, lined by single-cell layer	Complex, with cellular stratification
Growth pattern	Surface growth	Expansile nodules, disorganized pattern
Zonation	Process becomes less cellular towards chest wall	No zonation of process
Vascularity	Capillaries are perpendicular to the surface	Irregular and haphazard
Minor criteria		
Cytological atypia	Confined to areas of organizing effusion	Present in any area
Necrosis	Rare (necrosis may be within pleural exudates)	Necrosis is usually a sign of malignancy
Mitoses	Mitoses may be plentiful	Few mitoses (atypical mitoses favour malignancy)

33.10 Staging

In the oncologic field, staging always describes the anatomical extent of a tumour and plays a central role in the therapeutic decision-making process.

Historically, most staging systems for MPM have been based on single-institution databases with small retrospective surgical series. However, because of the small number of surgically resected MPMs, the main criticisms of most classifications are the discrepancy between clinical and pathological staging and the scant accuracy in describing the clinical tumour (T-) and nodal (N-) extension.

The latest developed and widely adopted staging system for MPM is the International Mesothelioma Interest Group (IMIG) classification and then approved by the Union for International Cancer Control (UICC) [32]. Details of the IMIG staging system for MPM are listed in ◘ Table 33.3.

The recent collaboration between IMIG and the International Association for the Study of Lung Cancer (IASLC) has developed an international prospective database in order to work out a data-driven revision of the current staging system: the database is geographically representative and includes thousand cases of MPM, irrespective of treatment, pathological subtype and stage.

The IASLC mesothelioma staging project is still ongoing with the aim to highlight the aspects that require further modifications in the upcoming eighth edition of the TNM classification for MPM, focusing the attention on factors, such as pleural thickness, nodal involvement and the invasion of the visceral pleura, that may influence prognosis [33, 34].

Computed tomography (CT) scan of the chest and upper abdomen still remains the only radiological assessment suggested for a proper staging of MPM non-candidate to surgical resection.

◻ Table 33.3 International Mesothelioma Interest Group staging system for malignant pleural mesothelioma

T	*Primary tumour*	*N*	*Regional lymph nodes*

T *Primary tumour*

Tx   Primary tumour cannot be assessed

T0   No evidence of primary tumour

T1   Tumour limited to the ipsilateral parietal pleura with or without mediastinal pleural and with or without diaphragmatic pleural involvement

T1a   No involvement of the visceral pleural

T1b   Tumour also involving the visceral pleura

T2   Tumour involving each of the ipsilateral pleural surfaces (parietal, mediastinal, diaphragmatic and visceral pleura) with at least one of the following:
Involvement of the diaphragmatic muscle
Extension of tumour from visceral pleura into the underlying pulmonary parenchyma

T3   Locally advanced but potentially resectable tumour. Tumour involving all of the ipsilateral pleural surfaces (parietal, mediastinal, diaphragmatic and visceral pleura), with at least one of the following:
Involvement of the endothoracic fascia
Extension into the mediastinal fat
Solitary, completely resectable focus of tumour extending into the soft tissue of the chest wall
Non transmural involvement of the pericardium

T4   Locally advanced technically unresectable tumour. Tumour involving all the ipsilateral pleural surfaces (parietal, mediastinal, diaphragmatic and visceral pleura) with at least one of the following:
Direct transdiaphragmatic extension of the tumour to the peritoneum
Diffuse extension or multifocal masses of tumour in the chest wall, with or without associated rib destruction
Direct extension of tumour to the contralateral pleura
Direct extension of the tumour to mediastinal organs
Direct extension of tumour into the spine Tumour extending through to the internal surface of the pericardium with or without a pericardial effusion or tumour involving the myocardium

N *Regional lymph nodes*

Nx   Regional lymph nodes cannot be assessed

N0   No regional lymph node metastasis

N1   Metastasis to the ipsilateral bronchopulmonary or hilar lymph nodes

N2   Metastases in the subcarinal lymph node or the ipsilateral mediastinal lymph nodes including the ipsilateral internal mammary and peridiaphragmatic node

N3   Metastasis in contralateral mediastinal, contralateral internal mammary, ipsilateral or contralateral supraclavicular lymph node

M *Distant metastasis*

M0   No distant metastasis

M1   Distant metastasis

Staging   *TNM*

Stage IA   T1aN0M0

Stage IB   T1bN0M0

Stage II   T2N0M0

Stage III   Any T3, any N1 or any N2, M0

Stage IV   Any T4, any N3 or any M1

Magnetic resonance imaging (MRI), using gadolinium, has resulted to be more accurate than CT scan in the delineation of the tumour border with regard to the surrounding tissues and in the evaluation of the diaphragmatic invasion, especially when surgical resection may be considered to be a part of the treatment plan [35].

The use of positron emission tomography (PET) scan in the staging process for MPM is still debated: false-positive findings may occur after pleurodesis, and the low spatial resolution may limit the characterization of the local growth and the nodal involvement. PET scan could be useful for the detection of distant metastases, even if rare [36].

33.11 Treatment

Treatment options for MPM potentially include surgery, radiation therapy (RT) and chemotherapy. Only selected patients with a surgically resectable disease (clinical stages I–III), good performance status and adequate respiratory function may be candidates for a multimodality treatment. For symptomatic pleural effusion in unresectable patients, pleurodesis with talc administered via tube thoracostomy represents the treatment of choice to reduce the frequency of thoracentesis and the related infective complications during chemotherapy [37].

33.11.1 Surgery

Surgical treatment with radical intent is occasionally performed in MPM patients with the aim to obtain a complete macroscopic resection.

After the establishment by the IASLC of a working group in order to recommend a uniform definition for surgical procedures [38], the main approaches to MPM are:

- Extrapleural pneumonectomy (EPP): complete en bloc removal of the involved parietal and visceral pleura including the whole ipsilateral lung. If required, the diaphragm and pericardium can also be resected.
- Extended pleurectomy/decortication (P/D): as the EPP, but with the lung left in situ.
- Pleurectomy/decortication (P/D): removal of all gross tumours, without resection of the lung, diaphragm or pericardium.

In P/D and EPP, mediastinal nodal dissection is always recommended.

The value of these procedures is extensively debated, because no definitive comparisons between EPP and P/D or between these procedures and nonsurgical treatment for MPMs are available. The only randomized clinical trial comparing the role of EPP in the context of a multimodal therapy is the Mesothelioma and Radical Surgery (MARS) trial. No difference has been observed with EPP after chemotherapy compared to chemotherapy alone. Results need to be considered with caution due to the low number of randomized patients and the mortality rate for the surgical arm, higher than expected [39].

Both surgical procedures have significant associated morbidity and mortality. P/D is resulted to be safer than EPP, with a perioperative mortality rate of about 1.5–5.4% [40]. In a large literature review including over 3700 MPM patients, perioperative mortality rates for EPP ranged from 0% to 11.8%, with major morbidities seen in 12–48% of patients (prevalently atrial arrhythmias, respiratory infections, respiratory failure, pulmonary embolus and myocardial infarction) [41].

33.11.2 Radiation Therapy (RT)

RT in MPM may have multiple indications: palliative care, preventive care or to be part of a multimodal treatment.

The purpose of RT with palliative intent is to reduce cancer pain due to chest wall invasion: this kind of treatment usually consists in short courses of RT with 10 grays (Gy) in a single fraction, or 8 Gy in three fractions [42]. However, there is no clinical evidence to support prescribing RT to reduce pain in MPM patients [43].

Preventive RT may be performed on the thoracoscopy scars and the drainage tracts to reduce the probability of seeding metastases. The efficacy of this strategy is still debated and currently is not part of the standard of care for MPM [24].

The introduction of intensity-modulated RT and 3D planning has improved the identification of the tumour border, increased the dose homogeneity and limited the normal tissue irradiation [44]. This kind of RT can be included in a multimodal strategy for the treatment of MPM, with or without chemotherapy, often after surgical approach. Data from many clinical trials suggest that RT after EPP may reduce local recurrence [45, 46]. In general, RT is not recommended as pre- or postoperative approach outside the setting of a clinical trial [24].

33.11.3 Chemotherapy

33.11.3.1 First-Line Chemotherapy and Targeted Agents

First-line chemotherapy is the only therapeutic option with proven survival benefit in patients with unresectable MPM. Chemotherapy doublets with cisplatin, in association with either pemetrexed or raltitrexed, have shown a higher median overall survival (OS) when compared to cisplatin alone (12.1 versus 9.3 months, $p = 0.02$, and 11.4 versus 8.8 months, $p = 0.04$, respectively) [47, 48]. The doublet of cisplatin/raltitrexed, however, showed a lower objective response rate compared to the other regimen, being not approved by regulatory agencies in many countries. For these reasons, to date front-line chemotherapy with cisplatin/pemetrexed represents the standard of care for unresectable MPM worldwide.

The optimum number of chemotherapy cycles is still debated. For patients with good clinical conditions, adequate organ function and radiological evidence of controlled disease, the current clinical practice is a maximum of six cycles of platinum/pemetrexed chemotherapy, even if it's not clear if four cycles would provide a similar benefit as already observed in the treatment of advanced non-small cell lung cancer patients [49]. Similarly, the use of maintenance treatment with pemetrexed as monotherapy, after induction with the combination regimen, or the switch maintenance treatment with a different agent, is uncertain and does not represent the standard of care for MPM.

The combination of carboplatin/pemetrexed is a reasonable alternative for those patients unable to receive cisplatin due to relevant clinical comorbidities. The median time to progression and the 1-year survival rate with this combination is similar to that described in patients treated with cisplatin/pemetrexed (7 versus 6.9 months and 63.1% and 64%, respectively) [50].

The use of gemcitabine, combined with a platinum agent, appears to be an active treatment in MPM; however, data coming from different studies are heterogeneous, with response rates ranging from 12% to 48% and median OS from 9.5 to 12 months [51, 52, 53].

With the attempt to improve survival for MPM patients, several targeted agents have been tested.

The role of angiogenesis is the field deeper explored: its relevance in MPM growth is demonstrated by the high levels of serum vascular endothelial growth factor (VEGF) found in MPM patients, which seem to be associated with poor prognosis [54].

A recent multicentre phase III trial has compared the addition of bevacizumab (a monoclonal antibody targeting the VEGF) to cisplatin/pemetrexed (with the possibility to be followed by the sole bevacizumab as maintenance therapy) with cisplatin/pemetrexed alone in unresectable MPM patients. This study has shown a statistically significant increase in the median OS for patients allocated in the bevacizumab-containing arm (18.8 versus 16.1 months, $p = 0.012$), reporting however a higher rate of drug-related adverse events, such as hypertension, proteinuria and arterial thrombotic events [55]. Based on this trial, the addition of bevacizumab to standard front-line chemotherapy seems to be feasible, but should be considered in selected group of patients due to the possible related adverse events.

Clinical trials are currently investigating the efficacy of small molecules, oral inhibitors of the angiogenesis, such as nintedanib, an intracellular tyrosine kinase inhibitor of the vascular endothelial growth factor receptor (VEGFR) 1-3, platelet derived growth factor receptor (PDGFR) -α and -β, and fibroblast growth factor receptor (FGFR)1-3. A recent phase II trial has reported an increased progression-free survival (PFS) for MPM patients treated with cisplatin/pemetrexed in association with nintedanib in comparison to patients treated with cisplatin/pemetrexed plus placebo (9.4 versus 5.7 months, $p = 0.0174$) [56]. A preliminary trend towards improved OS (18.3 versus 14.5 months, $p = 0.4132$) was also observed [56], but further investigations are needed and will be provided soon by the ongoing phase III trial (NCT01907100).

As previously described, the mesothelin is a potential biomarker for MPM, highly expressed in the epithelial and biphasic histology. Monoclonal antibodies, recombinant immunotoxins and antibody-drug conjugates targeting the mesothelin have been evaluated in clinical trials. The chimeric anti-mesothelin antibody amatuximab has been studied in a single-arm phase II trial in association with first-line platinum/pemetrexed chemotherapy for epithelial and epithelial-predominant biphasic MPM patients. The study did not meet its primary endpoint, the median PFS being lower than historical controls (6.1 months, 95% CI: 5.8–6.4) [57].

33.11.3.2 Second-Line Chemotherapy

To date there is no second-line standard of care for MPM patients.

In patients with good performance status, who relapse after a reasonable amount of time from front-line therapy, the retreatment with pemetrexed, used alone or in combination with a platinum salt, should be considered [58].

Many chemotherapy agents have demonstrated second-line activity in MPM, but none of them have been tested within a controlled randomized clinical trial. A phase II trial has assessed the safety and efficacy of the single-agent vinorelbine, demonstrating an objective response rate of 16% and a median OS of 9.6 months and favouring this agent as second-line treatment option in the clinical practice [59]. Similarly, on the basis of the demonstrated activity of cisplatin and gemcitabine in the front-line setting [60, 52], gemcitabine-based doublets appear to be an alternative second-line treatment as well [61].

Patients in good clinical condition should be recommended to join clinical trials in the second-line setting [24].

33.11.3.3 Immunotherapy

The immune compartment has proven to be a key component in the process of tumour initiation, progression and the response to treatment [62]. Targeting the molecular regulators of the immune function, such as cytotoxic lymphocyte antigen 4 (CTLA4) and programmed death-1/programmed death-ligand 1 (PD-1/PD-L1) signalling axis, has emerged as an effective therapeutic strategy in multiple cancers, including MPM, reported as a tumour with high infiltration of lymphocytes and macrophages and a significant T-cell inflammatory expression pattern. Preclinical studies have demonstrated that PD-1 and PD-L1 are expressed in a significant percentage of MPM and that the level of expression may characterize patients with a worse prognosis, especially in case of sarcomatoid histology [63, 64].

Tremelimumab, a fully human monoclonal antibody against CTLA-4, has been tested in a single-arm study in pretreated MPM patients, using the schedule of 10 mg/kg every 28 days. The study reported a disease control rate equal to 52%, a median OS of 11.3 months and a median immune-related PFS of 6.2 months [65]. Despite these first promising results, recent data from the phase II trial evaluating tremelimumab as second- or third-line treatment of MPM did not show a significantly longer OS compared to the placebo arm (7.7 versus 7.3 months, respectively, $p = 0.41$) [66].

A phase Ib trial that has enrolled previously treated patients with different solid tumours has evaluated the safety and efficacy of pembrolizumab, a humanized monoclonal antibody against PD-1 designed to block the interaction between PD-1 and its ligand, the PD-L1. Eligible patients presented with more than 1% positive membranous expression of PD-L1 on tumour or stromal cells. Pembrolizumab has appeared to be safe and tolerable for patients with MPM, conferring an objective response of 20% and durable response, but further investigation is needed to validate this treatment [67]. Thirty-eight patients with advanced MPM have been evaluated in a single-centre phase II study for the use of nivolumab, a human IgG4 monoclonal antibody targeting PD-1, as second-line treatment at the dose of 3 mg/kg every 2 weeks until progression or toxicity. This limited experience has shown a disease control rate of 50% at 12 weeks, suggesting, together with the data previously reported, that targeting the PD-1/PD-L1 axis in MPM appears promising [68].

Preliminary results from a phase II randomized study evaluating the efficacy of nivolumab versus the combination of nivolumab and ipilimumab, a monoclonal antibody targeting CTLA-4, for the second- or third-line treatment of MPM, have shown a higher disease control rate at 12 weeks and a longer median OS in favour of the combination arm (51.6% versus 39.7% and median OS not reached versus 10.5, respectively) after a follow-up period of about 10 months [69]. A phase III trial comparing nivolumab/ipilimumab versus standard platinum-based chemotherapy with pemetrexed for the front-line treatment of MPM is ongoing (NCT02899299).

33.11.4 Response Evaluation and Follow-Up

Response evaluation is performed with CT scan and the examinations performed at the time of presentation (PET scan for patients undergoing multimodal treatment).

Clinical and radiological follow-up of MPM patients will depend on the local recommendations or as specified by the protocol in case of participation in a clinical trial.

33.11.5 Screening

Routine screening tests with chest X-ray or CT scan did not demonstrate to be an effective tool for the early detection of MPM. To date, there are no sufficient data to suggest that a screening programme for MPM can reduce mortality, even in patients who had a clear occupational exposure to asbestos. In a large cohort of 1045 asbestos-exposed workers, no single case of pleural mesothelioma has been detected, confirming the previous statement [70].

Summary of Clinical Recommendations
ESMO (European Society for Medical Oncology) guidelines [24]
- Occupational history with emphasis on asbestos exposure is recommended.
- Large and targeted biopsy samples facilitate definitive diagnosis. Surgical-type samples should be preferred for diagnosis.
- A major subtype diagnosis (epithelioid, biphasic, sarcomatoid) should be given in all cases of MPM.
- Antifolate/platinum doublet is the only approved standard of care for advanced MPM.

NCCN (National Comprehensive Cancer Network) Malignant Pleural Mesothelioma guidelines (version 2.2017) [71]
- Management by a multidisciplinary team with experience in MPM is recommended.
- The addition of bevacizumab to platinum/pemetrexed front-line chemotherapy should be considered in selected MPM patients.
- Immunotherapy (nivolumab +/− ipilimumab or pembrolizumab) should be considered as a treatment option for pretreated MPM patients.

Case Study: A Rare Case of Metastatic MPM

Man, 52 years old
- Family history negative for malignancy
- No documented working exposure to asbestos
- APR: no relevant anamnestic data
- APP: shortness of breath and relevant chest wall pain
- Blood tests: no relevant abnormalities. Total leukocytes 11.7×10^9/L. Hb 13.0 g/dL. Adequate liver and kidney function

- Urgent CT scan of the chest and upper abdomen: modest pleural effusion in the lower part of the left thorax. Widespread pleural thickening, with prevalent involvement of the mediastinal pleura. Mediastinal nodal involvement, no distant metastasis (◘ Fig. 33.6)

Question
What action should be taken?
1. Radiological follow-up

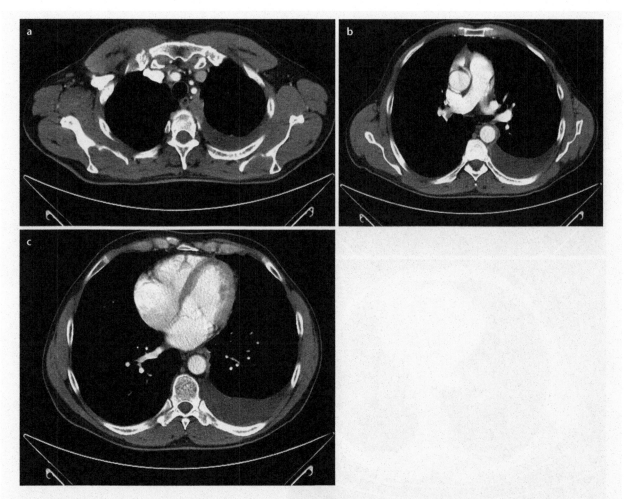

◘ Fig. 33.6 Effusion and widespread thickening of the pleura on CT scan

2. Ultrasound-guided biopsy of the mediastinal pleura
3. Surgical thoracoscopy for multiple pleural biopsies and pleurodesis

Answer

The patient performed a surgical pleural biopsy with pleurodesis with talc.

Histological report: malignant pleural mesothelioma with epithelioid features.

Question

What action should be taken?
1. Surgery
2. Chemotherapy
3. Radiotherapy

Answer

The patient has been enrolled in a randomized clinical trial and performed four chemotherapy cycles with cisplatin/pemetrexed plus nintedanib/placebo with no relevant side effects.

He reported a fast improvement of the shortness of breath and the chest wall pain.

CT scan of the chest and upper abdomen performed after four chemotherapy cycles: great reduction of the mediastinal pleural thickening, stable mediastinal nodal involvement. No distant metastasis, no pleural effusion (◘ Fig. 33.7). Global answer: partial response.

The widespread pleural involvement and the nodal infiltration did not indicate the possibility to perform a surgical resection. The patient started a regular clinical and radiological follow-up.

After 6 months, CT scan of the chest and upper abdomen showed a progression of the disease for the onset of multiple sub-centimetric bilateral lung nodes (◘ Fig. 33.8a).

PET scan confirmed the progression of the disease, showing hyperactivity not only on the pleural surface and the regional lymph nodes but also on the right iliac bone. No evidence of hyperactivity on the lung nodules because of their limited size (◘ Fig. 33.8b).

Good clinical conditions, no bone pain.

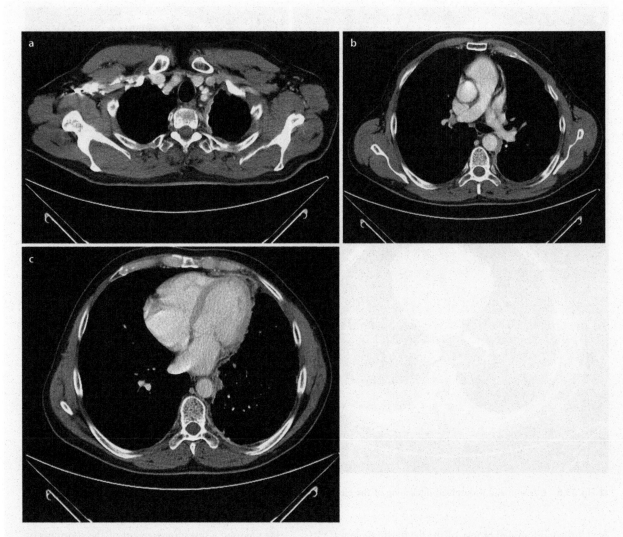

Fig. 33.7 Main radiological finding after first-line treatment

Question

What action should be taken?

1. Best supportive care
2. Single-agent chemotherapy
3. Enrollment in a clinical trial

Answer

No clinical trials available in our region. Patient began second-line chemotherapy with gemcitabine.

A deep genetic evaluation showed for this patient a germline mutation in the BAP1 gene, probably cause of the high predisposition to MPM in the absence of documented exposure to asbestos.

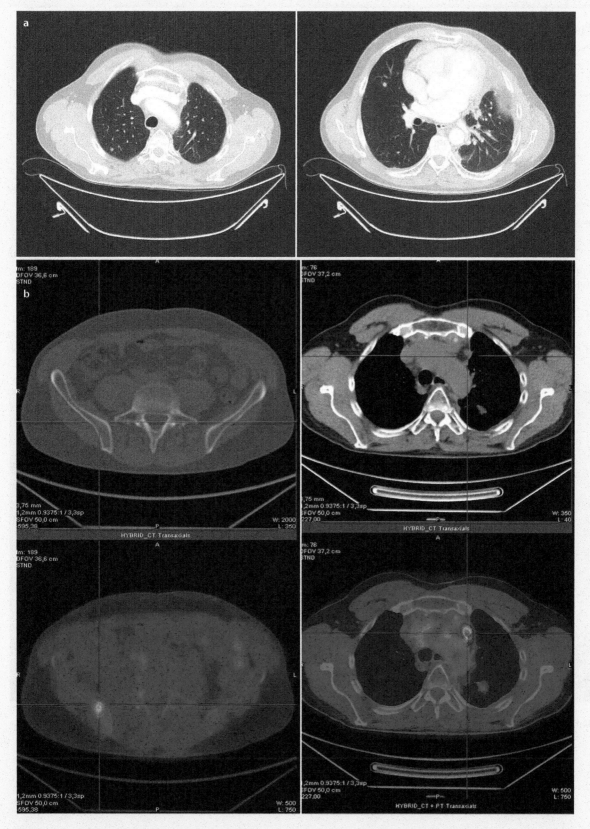

Fig. 33.8 CT scan of the chest showing multiple lung nodes, to be interpreted as of pulmonary metastases from MPM **a**. PET scan showing a bone metastasis from MPM on the right iliac bone **b**

Case Study: A Case of MPM with Aggressive Behaviour

Man, 58 years old
- Family history negative for malignancy
- Possible working exposure to asbestos (naval mechanical worker)
- Active smoker
- APR: no relevant anamnestic data
- APP: only modest chest wall pain (first assessments performed within a working prevention programme for respiratory diseases)
- Blood tests: no relevant abnormalities. Total leukocytes 7.5 × 109/L. Hb 15.4 g/dL. Adequate liver and kidney function
- Chest X-ray: right pleural effusion with apparent modest pleural thickening (■ Fig. 33.9)

Question
What action should be taken?
1. Medical treatment and radiological follow-up
2. Thoracentesis with cytological examination of the pleural effusion
3. Surgical thoracoscopy

Answer
The patient performed a thoracentesis with drainage of 2000 cc of pleural fluid.

Cytological examination of the pleural effusion: presence of neoplastic cells of mesothelial origin.

Question
What action should be taken?
1. Start chemotherapy.
2. Repeat thoracentesis.
3. Surgical thoracoscopy for multiple pleural biopsies and pleurodesis.

Answer
The patient performed a surgical pleural biopsy with pleurodesis with talc.

Histological report: Malignant pleural mesothelioma with sarcomatoid features.

CT scan of the chest and upper abdomen: circumferential pleural thickening with confluent mediastinal lymph nodes in the para-oesophageal region. Modest

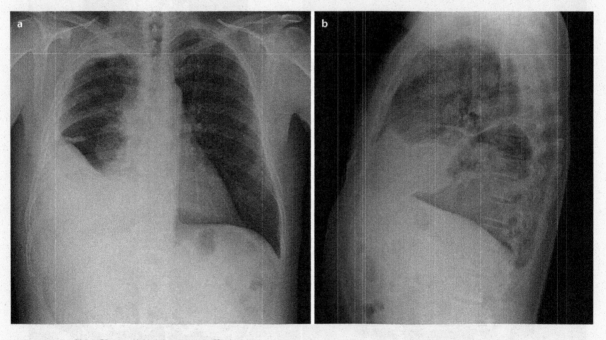

■ **Fig. 33.9**   Chest X-ray with right pleural effusion

residual right pleural effusion. No distant metastasis (■ Fig. 33.10).

Question

What action should be taken?

1. Surgery
2. Chemotherapy
3. Radiotherapy

Answer

The patient began chemotherapy with cisplatin/pemetrexed with rapid symptoms' deterioration in terms of chest pain, dyspnoea and weight loss.

Unscheduled CT scan of the chest and upper abdomen performed after two chemotherapy cycles: large increase of pleural thickenings with mediastinal infiltration. Stable pleural effusion. No distant metastasis (■ Fig. 33.11). Global answer: progression of disease.

The patient stopped chemotherapy in favour of the sole best supportive care and died after few weeks.

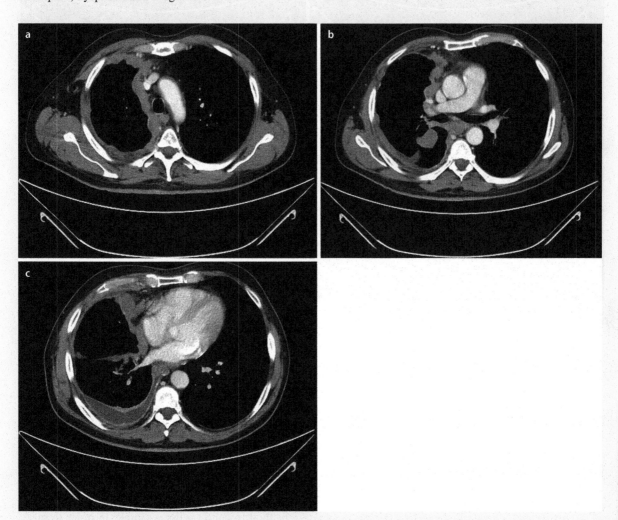

■ **Fig. 33.10** Circumferential pleural thickening with pathological mediastinal lymph nodes on CT scan

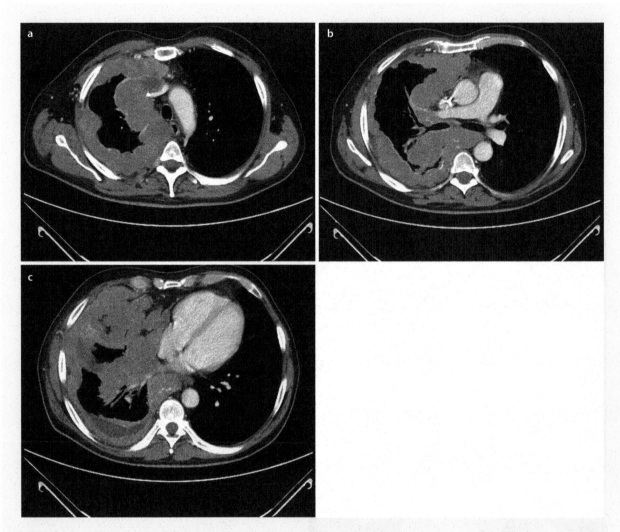

Fig. 33.11 Large circumferential pleural thickening with mediastinal infiltration

Expert Opinion

Federica Grosso

Mesothelioma Unit, Azienda Ospedaliera SS. Antonio e Biagio e Cesare Arrigo, Alessandria, Italy.

Key Points

1. Malignant pleural mesothelioma is a pleural cancer raising from mesothelial cells, often linked to a previous exposure to asbestos fibres.
2. It is considered as a rare disease even if its incidence is slowly growing worldwide with an expected peak in the following years between 2015 and 2025.
3. It is more common in 65–70 year-old men and the most frequent symptoms are dyspnoea, chest pain and weight loss.
4. Chest X-ray is the first imaging diagnostic technique; CT is used for staging while MRI can be useful to study the local involvement. Thoracoscopy is the best method to collect a tissue sample; in order to make a differential diagnosis between the various pleural malignancies it is recommended (WHO 2015) to use a marker panel including TTF1, napsin A, PAX8, PSA, CDX2, CD45, CD20, HMB45, melan-A and SOX10.
5. Surgery when possible is the most successful treatment; in case of unresectable disease, chemotherapy

with cisplatin/pemetrexed is recommended with a maximum of six cycles. There are no standard approaches for a second-line therapy. New drugs have been investigated such as bevacizumab or nintedanib, but more studies are required.

6. Some trials have showed hopeful results from immunotherapy (pembrolizumab-nivolumab), and it is likely that in the future they will represent the best approach to treat these patients.

Recommendations

- ESMO
  ▶ www.esmo.org/Guidelines/Lung-and-Chest-Tumours/Malignant-Pleural-Mesothelioma
- ASCO
  ▶ www.asco.org/practice-guidelines/quality-guidelines/guidelines/thoracic-cancer#/29376
- NCCN
  ▶ www.nccn.org

Hints for a Deeper Insight

The incidence of MPM is increasing worldwide, due to massive asbestos exposure, and a sort of epidemic is expected in developing countries where asbestos has not been banned yet [1]. In contrast with other solid tumours, overall survival has not been increased in recent years, reflecting the scarcity of improvements in our therapeutic capabilities.

Surgery and adjuvant radiotherapy in multimodal context are associated with survival advantage in retrospective studies, but this has never been confirmed in randomized studies, and only a minority of patients are diagnosed at early stages and candidate for surgery [2]. Of the two operations proposed pleurectomy/decortication (P/D) has lower morbidity and mortality compared to extrapleural pneumonectomy (EPP) and should be preferred whenever technically feasible, especially after the failure of MARS trial which concluded that EPP in trimodality setting offers no benefit [3]. The MARS2 trial is currently randomizing patients to define the impact on survival of P/D after induction chemotherapy [4]. In the meantime, evidence is being gathered about the feasibility of hemi-thoracic intensity modulated pleural RT after P/D [5]. Recently reported randomized clinical studies showed that prophylactic irradiation of thoracic intervention sites should not be used routinely [6, 7]. Conversely, radiotherapy is an effective treatment for pain control [8].

To date the cisplatin-pemetrexed doublet is the only evidence-based treatment, associated with better quality of life and clinically significant survival improvement [9]. Carboplatin may be an alternative to cisplatin in unfit

and elderly patients [10]. No predictive biomarker has a role in the everyday clinical practice. A lot of effort is ongoing to overcome the therapeutic limitations by increasing the knowledge of the molecular, biological and genetic aspects of this disease. MPM has no oncogenic driver, and future development of targeted therapies should be based on the exploration of pathways activated as a consequence of the loss of tumour suppressor genes or other targets associated with the disease phenotype [11]. Among targeted agents tested so far, only antiangiogenics in combination with standard chemotherapy showed promising results. Despite the survival benefit reported for bevacizumab plus cisplatin-pemetrexed in the phase III, randomized, open-label MAPS trial, EMA has not extended the label of the drug for this indication [12]. The phase II, randomized, placebo-controlled LUME-Meso study, testing the antiangiogenic nintedanib in combination with cisplatin-pemetrexed met its primary endpoint, and the results for the phase III part of the study are eagerly awaited [13].

Vinorelbine, rechallenge with pemetrexed and gemcitabine based chemotherapy are commonly resorted to in second-line setting, even if randomized evidence is lacking [14].

Novel immunotherapeutic approaches, including immune checkpoint inhibitors, are being explored and currently generate great expectation. Early clinical studies suggest activity in a small proportion of patients with some durable responses which constitute the proof of concept of its activity, but no clear biomarker has been found so far which is essential to exploit its full potential [15, 16].

Progresses in the MPM treatment claim appropriate designed studies, addressing the role of therapeutic/targeted agents selected on the molecular profiling of the tumour, and therefore the availability of adequate amounts of tumour tissue from each patient is critical. To warrant this, but also to satisfy other needs concerning diagnostic and staging challenges, MPM patients should be referred to centres where an expert multidisciplinary team exists. Whenever possible patients should be encouraged to enter available clinical trials in every setting of the treatment.

Suggested Reading

1. Yang H, Testa JR, Carbone M. Mesothelioma epidemiology, carcinogenesis, and pathogenesis. Curr Treat Options Oncol. 2008;9:147–57. ▶ https://doi.org/10.1007/s11864-008-0067-z

2. Nelson DB, Rice DC, Niu J, Atay S, Vaporciyan AA, Antonoff M, et al. Long-term survival outcomes of cancer-directed surgery for malignant pleural

mesothelioma: propensity score matching analysis. J Clin Oncol. 2017;35(29):3354–62. ► https://doi.org/10.1200/JCO.2017.73.8401.

3. Treasure T, Lang-Lazdunski L, Waller D, Bliss JM, Tan C, Entwisle J, et al. MARS trialists. Extra-pleural pneumonectomy versus no extra-pleural pneumonectomy for patients with malignant pleural mesothelioma: clinical outcomes of the Mesothelioma and Radical Surgery (MARS) randomised feasibility study. Lancet Oncol. 2011;12(8):763–72. ► https://doi.org/10.1016/S1470-2045(11)70149-8.

4. Trialists M, Lim E. Surgical selection in pleurectomy decortication for mesothelioma – an overview from screening and selection from MARS 2 pilot World Lung Cancer Conference 2017, abstract 10185.

5. Rimner A, Zauderer MG, Gomez DR, Adusumilli PS, Parhar PK, Wu AJ, et al. Phase II study of hemithoracic intensity-modulated pleural radiation therapy (IMPRINT) as part of lung-sparing multimodality therapy in patients with malignant pleural mesothelioma. J Clin Oncol. 2016;34(23):2761–8. ► https://doi.org/10.1200/JCO.2016.67.2675.

6. Clive AO, Taylor H, Dobson L, Wilson P, de Winton E, Panakis N, et al. Prophylactic radiotherapy for the prevention of procedure-tract metastases after surgical and large-bore pleural procedures in malignant pleural mesothelioma (SMART): a multicentre, open-label, phase 3, randomised controlled trial. Lancet Oncol. 2016;17(8):1094–104. ► https://doi.org/10.1016/S1470-2045(16)30095-X.

7. Neil Bayman, W. Appel, L. Ashcroft, David Raymond Baldwin, A. Bates, Liz Darlison, et al. Prophylactic irradiation of tracts (PIT) in patients with pleural mesothelioma: results of a multicentre phase III trial. World Lung Cancer Conference 2017, abstract 7980.

8. MacLeod N, Chalmers A, O'Rourke N, Moore K, Sheridan J, McMahon L, et al. Is Radiotherapy Useful for Treating Pain in Mesothelioma? A Phase II Trial. J Thorac Oncol. 2015;10(6):944–50. ► https://doi.org/10.1097/JTO.0000000000000499.

9. Vogelzang NJ, Rusthoven JJ, Symanowski J, Denham C, Kaukel E, Ruffie P, et al. Phase III study of pemetrexed in combination with cisplatin versus cisplatin alone in patients with malignant pleural mesothelioma. J Clin Oncol. 2003;21(14):2636–44.

10. Santoro A, O'Brien ME, Stahel RA, Nackaerts K, Baas P, Karthaus M, et al. Pemetrexed plus cisplatin or pemetrexed plus carboplatin for chemonaïve patients with malignant pleural mesothelioma: results of the International Expanded Access Program. J Thorac Oncol. 2008;3(7):756–63. ► https://doi.org/10.1097/JTO.0b013e31817c73d6.

11. Lo Iacono M, Monica V, Righi L, Grosso F, Libener R, Vatrano S, et al. Targeted next-generation sequencing of cancer genes in advanced stage malignant pleural mesothelioma: a retrospective study. J Thorac Oncol. 2015;10(3):492–9. ► https://doi.org/10.1097/JTO.0000000000000436.

12. Zalcman G, Mazieres J, Margery J, Greillier L, Audigier-Valette C, Moro-Sibilot D, et al. French Cooperative Thoracic Intergroup (IFCT). Bevacizumab for newly diagnosed pleural mesothelioma in the Mesothelioma Avastin Cisplatin Pemetrexed Study (MAPS): a randomised, controlled, open-label, phase 3 trial. Lancet. 2016;387(10026):1405–14. ► https://doi.org/10.1016/S0140-6736(15)01238-6.

13. Grosso F, Steele N, Novello S, Nowak AK, Popat S, Greillier L, et al. Nintedanib plus pemetrexed/cisplatin in patients with malignant pleural mesothelioma: phase II results from the randomized, placebo-controlled LUME-Meso trial. J Clin Oncol. 2017;35(31):3591–600. ► https://doi.org/10.1200/JCO.2017.72.9012.

14. Grosso F, Scagliotti GV. Systemic treatment of malignant pleural mesothelioma. Future Oncol. 2012;8(3):293–305. ► https://doi.org/10.2217/fon.12.14. Review.

15. Alley EW, Lopez J, Santoro A, Morosky A, Saraf S, Piperdi B, et al. Clinical safety and activity of pembrolizumab in patients with malignant pleural mesothelioma (KEYNOTE-028): preliminary results from a non-randomised, open-label, phase 1b trial. Lancet Oncol. 2017;18(5):623–30. ► https://doi.org/10.1016/S1470-2045(17)30169-9.

16. Ceresoli GL, Mantovani A. Immune checkpoint inhibitors in malignant pleural mesothelioma. Lancet Oncol. 2017;18(5):559–61. ► https://doi.org/10.1016/S1470-2045(17)30191-2.

33

References

1. Travis WD, Brambilla E, Burke AP, et al. WHO classification of tumours of the lung, pleura, thymus and heart. Lyon: International Agency for Research on Cancer; 2015.

2. SEER*Explorer: An interactive website for SEER cancer statistics [Internet]. Beta Version. Surveillance Research Program, National Cancer Institute. [Cited 2017 Apr 14]. Available from https://seer.cancer.gov/explorer/.

3. Carbone M, Ly VH, Dodson RF, et al. Malignant mesothelioma: facts, myths, and hypotheses. J Cell Physiol. 2012;227:44–58.

4. Carbone M, Bedrossian C. The pathogenesis of mesothelioma. Semin Diagn Pathol. 2006;23:53–60.

5. Robinson BM. Malignant pleural mesothelioma: an epidemiological perspective. Ann Cardiothorac Surg. 2012;1(4):491–6.

6. Chirieac LR, Barletta JA, Yeap BY, et al. Clinicopathologic characteristics of malignant mesotheliomas arising in patients with a history of radiation for Hodgkin and non-Hodgkin lymphoma. J Clin Oncol. 2013;31(36):4544–9.

7. Gibb H, Fulcher K, Nagarajan S, et al. Analyses of radiation and mesothelioma in the US Transuranium and Uranium Registries. Am J Public Health. 2014;103(4):710–6.

8. Cercek A, Zaderer M, Rimner A, et al. Confirmation of high prevalence of BAP1 inactivation in mesothelioma. J Clin Oncol. 2015;33(Suppl):Abstract 7564.

9. Testa JR, Cheung M, Pei J, et al. Germline BAP1 mutations predispose to malignant mesothelioma. Nat Genet. 2011;43:1022–5.

10. Cheung M, Talarchek J, Howard S, et al. Prevalence of BAP1 germline mutations in asbestos-exposed malignant mesothelioma cases and controls. Cancer Res. 2015;75(15 Suppl):Abstract 2752.

11. Bronte G, Incorvaia L, Rizzo S, et al. The resistance related to targeted therapy in malignant pleural mesothelioma: Why has not the target been hit yet?. Crit Rev Oncol Hematol. 2016;107: 20–32. https://doi.org/10.1016/j.critrevonc.2016.08.011.

12. Leung A, Muller N, Miller R. CT in differential diagnosis of diffuse pleural disease. AJR Am J Roentgenol. 1990;154:487–92.

13. Husain AN, Colby T, Ordonez N, et al. Guidelines for pathologic diagnosis of malignant mesothelioma: 2017 update of the consensus statement from the international mesothelioma interest group. Arch Pathol Lab Med. 2017;142:89–108.

14. Greillier L, Cavailles A, Fraticelli A, et al. Accuracy of pleural biopsy using thoracoscopy for the diagnosis of histologic subtype in patients with malignant pleural mesothelioma. Cancer. 2007;110:2248–52.

15. Greillier L, Baas P, Welch JJ, et al. Biomarkers for malignant pleural mesothelioma: current status. Mol Diagn Ther. 2008; 12:375–90.

16. Pass H, Lott D, Lonardo F, et al. Asbestos exposure, pleural mesothelioma, and serum osteopontin levels. N Engl J Med. 2005;353:1564–73.

17. Grigoriu B, Scherpereel A, Devos P, et al. Utility of osteopontin and serum mesothelin in malignant pleural mesothelioma diagnosis and prognosis assessment. Clin Cancer Res. 2007;13: 2928–35.

18. Creaney J, Yeoman D, Demelker Y, et al. Comparison of osteopontin, megakaryocyte potentiating factor, and mesothelin proteins as markers in the serum of patients with malignant mesothelioma. J Thorac Oncol. 2008;3:851–7.

19. Iwahori K, Osaki T, Serada S, et al. Megakaryocyte potentiating factor as a tumor marker of malignant pleural mesothelioma: evaluation in comparison with mesothelin. Lung Cancer. 2008;62:45–54.

20. Panou V, Vyberg M, Weinreich UM, et al. The established and future biomarkers of malignant pleural mesothelioma. Cancer Treat Rev. 2015;41(6):486–95.

21. Pass HI, Levin SM, Harbut MR, et al. Fibulin-3 as a blood and effusion biomarker for pleural mesothelioma. N Engl J Med. 2012;367(15):1417–27.

22. Ak G, Tomaszek S, Kosari F, et al. MicroRNA and mRNA features of malignant pleural mesothelioma and benign asbestos-related pleural effusion. Biomed Res Int. 2015;2015: 35748.

23. Benjamin H, Lebanony D, Rosenwald S, et al. A diagnostic assay based on microRNA expression accurately identifies malignant pleural mesothelioma. J Mol Diagn. 2010;12:771–9.

24. Baas P, Fennell D, Kerr KM, et al. Malignant pleural mesothelioma: ESMO Clinical Practice Guidelines for diagnosis, treatment and follow-up. Ann Oncol. 2015;26(Suppl 5):v31–9.

25. Meyerhoff RR, Yang CF, Speicher PJ, et al. Impact of mesothelioma histologic subtype on outcomes in the surveillance, epidemiology, and end results database. J Surg Res. 2015;196:23–32.

26. Brcic L, Jakopovic M, Brcic I, et al. Reproducibility of histological subtyping of malignant pleural mesothelioma. Virchows Arch. 2014;465:679–85.

27. Kadota K, Suzuki K, Sima CS, et al. Pleomorphic epithelioid diffuse malignant pleural mesothelioma: a clinicopathological review and conceptual proposal to reclassify as biphasic or sarcomatoid mesothelioma. J Thorac Oncol. 2011;6:896–904.

28. Galateau-Sallé F, Vignaud JM, Burke L, et al. Well differentiated papillary mesothelioma of the pleura: a series of 24 cases. Am J Surg Pathol. 2004;28:534–40.

29. Galateau-Salle F, Churg A, Roggli V, et al. The 2015 World Health Organization classification of tumors of the pleura: advances since the 2004 classification. J Thorac Oncol. 2015;11(2): 142–54.

30. Klebe S, Brownlee NA, Mahar A, et al. Sarcomatoid mesothelioma: a clinical-pathologic correlation of 326 cases. Mod Pathol. 2010;23:470–9.

31. Doyle LA, Vivero M, Fletcher CD, et al. Nuclear expression of STAT6 distinguishes solitary fibrous tumor from histologic mimics. Mod Pathol. 2014;27:390–5.

32. Rusch VW. A proposed new international TNM staging system for malignant pleural mesothelioma. From the International Mesothelioma Interest Group. Chest. 1995;108:122–1128.

33. Nowak AK, Chansky K, Rice DC, et al. The IASLC mesothelioma staging project: proposals for revisions of the T descriptors in the forthcoming eighth edition of the TNM classification for pleural mesothelioma. J Thorac Oncol. 2016;11(12):2089–99.

34. Rusch VW, Giroux D, Kennedy C, et al. Initial analysis of the international association for the study of lung cancer mesothelioma database. J Thorac Oncol. 2012;7:1631–9.

35. Heelan RT, Rusch VW, Begg CB, et al. Staging of malignant pleural mesothelioma: comparison of CT and MR imaging. AJR Am J Roentgenol. 1999;172:1039–47.

36. Armato SG, Labby ZE, Coolen J, et al. Imaging in pleural mesothelioma: a review of the 11th International Conference of the International Mesothelioma Interest Group. Lung Cancer. 2013;82:190–6.

37. Zarogoulidis K, Zarogoulidis P, Darwiche K. Malignant pleural effusion and algorithm management. J Thorac Dis. 2013;5(Suppl 4):S413–9.

38. Rice D, Rusch V, Pass H, et al. Recommendations for uniform definitions of surgical techniques for malignant pleural mesothelioma: a consensus report of the international association for the study of lung cancer international staging committee and the international mesothelioma interest group. J Thorac Oncol. 2011;6:1304–12.

39. Treasure T, Lang-Lazdunski L, Waller D, et al. Extra-pleural pneumonectomy versus no extra-pleural pneumonectomy for patients with malignant pleural mesothelioma: clinical outcomes

of the Mesothelioma and Radical Surgery (MARS) randomized feasibility study. Lancet Oncol. 2011;12(8):763–72.

40. Schipper PH, Nichols FC, Thomse KM, et al. Malignant pleural mesothelioma: surgical management in 285 patients. Ann Thorac Surg. 2008;85:257–64.

41. Cao CQ, Yan TD, Bannon PG, et al. A systematic review of extrapleural pneumonectomy for malignant pleural mesothelioma. J Thorac Oncol. 2010;5(10):1692–703.

42. Price A. What is the role of radiotherapy in malignant pleural mesothelioma? Oncologist. 2011;16:359–65.

43. Macleod N, Price A, O'Rouke N, et al. Radiotherapy for treatment of pain in malignant pleural mesothelioma: a systematic review. Lung Cancer. 2014;83:133–8.

44. Ahamad A, Stevens CW, Smyte WR, et al. Intensity-modulated radiation therapy: a novel approach to the management of malignant pleural mesothelioma. Int J Radiat Oncol Biol Phys. 2003;55(3):768–75.

45. Gomez DR, Hong DS, Allen PK, et al. Patterns of failure, toxicity, and survival after extrapleural pneumonectomy and hemithoracic intensity-modulated radiation therapy for malignant pleural mesothelioma. J Thorac Oncol. 2013;8:238–45.

46. Yajnik S, Rosenzweig KE, Mychalczak B, et al. Hemithoracic radiation after extrapleural pneumonectomy for malignant pleural mesothelioma. Int J Radiat Oncol Biol Phys. 2003;56:1319–26.

47. van Meerbeeck JP, Gaafar R, Manegold C, et al. Randomized phase III study of cisplatin with or without raltitrexed in patients with malignant pleural mesothelioma: an intergroup study of the European Organisation for Research and Treatment of Cancer Lung Cancer Group and the National Cancer Institute of Canada. J Clin Oncol. 2005;23:6881–9.

48. Vogezang NJ, Rusthoven JJ, Symanowski J, et al. Phase III study of pemetrexed in combination with cisplatin versus cisplatin alone in patients with malignant pleural mesothelioma. J Clin Oncol. 2003;21(14):2636–44.

49. Socinski M, Schell M, Peterman A, et al. Phase III trial comparing a defined duration of therapy versus continuous therapy followed by second-line therapy in advanced-stage IIIb/IV non-small-cell lung cancer. J Clin Oncol. 2002;20:1335–43.

50. Santoro A, O'Brien ME, Stahel RA, et al. Pemetrexed plus cisplatin or pemetrexed plus carboplatin for chemonaïve patients with malignant pleural mesothelioma: results of the international expanded access program. J Thorac Oncol. 2008;3(7):756–63.

51. Kalmadi SR, Rankin C, Kraut MJ, et al. Gemcitabine and cisplatin in unresectable malignant mesothelioma of the pleura: a phase II study of the Southwest Oncology Group (SWOG 9810). Lung Cancer. 2008;60:259–63.

52. Nowak AK, Byrne MJ, Williamson R, et al. A multicentre phase II study of cisplatin and gemcitabine for malignant mesothelioma. Br J Cancer. 2002;87:491–6.

53. van Haarst JM, Baas P, Manegold C, et al. Multicentre phase II study of gemcitabine and cisplatin in malignant pleural mesothelioma. Br J Cancer. 2002;86:342–5.

54. Yasumitsu A, Tabata C, Tabata R, et al. Clinical significance of serum vascular endothelia growth factor in malignant pleural mesothelioma. J Thorac Oncol. 2010;5:479–83.

55. Zalcman G, Mazières J, Margery J, et al. Bevacizumab 15mg/kg plus cisplatin-pemetrexed (CP) triplet versus CP doublet in Malignant Pleural Mesothelioma (MPM): results of the IFCT-GFPC-0701 MAPS randomized phase 3 trial. J Clin Oncol. 2015;33(suppl):400S.

56. Grosso F, Steele N, Novello S, et al. Nintedanib plus pemetrexed/cisplatin in patients with MPM: phase II findings from the placebo-controlled LUME-Meso trial. Vienna: 17th IASLC World Conference on Lung Cancer 2016: ID #4191.

57. Hassan R, Kindler HL, Jahan T, et al. Phase II clinical trial of amatuximab, a chimeric antimesothelin antibody with pemetrexed and cisplatin in advanced unresectable pleural mesothelioma. Clin Cancer Res. 2014;20:5927–36.

58. Ceresoli G, Zucali P, De Vincenzo F, et al. Retreatment with pemetrexed-based chemotherapy in patients with malignant pleural mesothelioma. Lung Cancer. 2011;72:73–7.

59. Stebbing J, Powles T, McPherson K, et al. The efficacy and safety of weekly vinorelbine in relapsed malignant pleural mesothelioma. Lung Cancer. 2009;63:94–7.

60. Castagneto B, Zai S, Dongiovanni D, et al. Cisplatin and gemcitabine in malignant pleural mesothelioma: a phase II study. Am J Clin Oncol. 2005;28:223–6.

61. Mutlu H, Gunduz S, Karaca C, et al. Second-line gemcitabine-based chemotherapy regimens improve overall 3-year survival rate in patients with malignant pleural mesothelioma: a multicenter retrospective study. Med Oncol. 2014;31:74.

62. Bersanelli M, Buti S. From targeting the tumor to targeting the immune system: transversal challenges in oncology with the inhibition of the PD-1/PD-L1 axis. World J Clin Oncol. 2017;8:37–53.

63. Cedrés S, Ponce-Aix S, Zugazagoitia J, et al. Analysis of expression of programmed cell death 1 ligand 1 (PD-L1) in malignant pleural mesothelioma (MPM). PLoS One. 2015;10(3):e0121071.

64. Mansfield AS, Roden AC, Peikert T, et al. B7-H1 expression in malignant pleural mesothelioma is associated with sarcomatoid histology and poor prognosis. J Thorac Oncol. 2014;9(7):1036–40.

65. Calabro L, Morra A, Fonsatti E, et al. Efficacy and safety of an intensified schedule of tremelimumab for chemotherapy-resistant malignant mesothelioma: an open-label, single-arm, phase 2 study. Lancet Respir Med. 2015;3:301–9.

66. Maio M, Scherpereel A, Calabrò L, et al. Tremelimumab as second-line or third-line treatment in relapsed malignant mesothelioma (DETERMINE): a multicentre, international, randomised, double-blind, placebo-controlled phase 2b trial. Lancet Oncol. 2017;18:1261–73.

67. Alley E, Lopez J, Santoro A, et al. Clinical safety and activity of pembrolizumab in patients with malignant pleural mesothelioma (KEYNOTE-028): preliminary results from a non-randomised, open-label, phase 1b trial. Lancet Oncol. 2017;18:623–30.

68. Quispel-Janssen J, Zago G, Schouten R, et al. A phase II study of nivolumab in malignant pleural mesothelioma (NivoMes): with translational research (TR) biopsies. J Thorac Oncol. 2017;12:S292–S3.

69. Scherpereel A, et al. Second- or third-line nivolumab (Nivo) versus nivo plus ipilimumab (Ipi) in malignant pleural mesothelioma (MPM) patients: results of the IFCT-1501 MAPS2 randomized phase II trial. J Clin Oncol. 2017;35(suppl):abstr LBA8507.

70. Fasola G, Belvedere O, Aita M, et al. Low-dose computed tomography screening for lung cancer and pleural mesothelioma in an asbestos exposed population: baseline results of a prospective, nonrandomized feasibility trial–an Alpe-adria Thoracic Oncology Multidisciplinary Group Study (ATOM 002). Oncologist. 2007;12(10):1215–24.

71. NCCN (National Comprehensive Cancer Network) Malignant Pleural Mesothelioma guidelines (version 2.2017).

33

Cancer of the Esophagus

Eugenio Fiorentino, Angelica Petrillo, Luca Pompella, Ina Macaione, and Ferdinando De Vita

Gastrointestinal Cancers

Contents

© Springer Nature Switzerland AG 2021
A. Russo et al. (eds.), *Practical Medical Oncology Textbook*, UNIPA Springer Series,
https://doi.org/10.1007/978-3-030-56051-5_34

Learning Objectives

By the end of the chapter the reader will:
- Be able to diagnose esophageal cancer
- Have learned the basic concepts of molecular classification of esophageal cancer
- Have reached in-depth knowledge of localized, inoperable locally advanced, and metastatic esophageal cancer treatment
- Be able to put acquired knowledge into daily clinical practice

34.1 Introduction and Epidemiology

Esophageal cancer (OC) is the ninth most common incident cancer in the world and the seventh leading cause of worldwide cancer-related mortality because of the its extremely aggressive nature and the poor survival rate of affected patients. The International Agency for Research on Cancer (IARC) estimates that there were about 450,000 cases of OC in 2012 [1, 2, 3, 4, 5].

Globally, esophageal squamous cell carcinoma (SCC) is the most common histological subtype of OC, particularly in high-incidence areas of eastern Asia and in eastern and southern Africa. In the highest-risk region, the so-called Asian Esophageal Cancer Belt, which extends from northern Iran, east to China, and north to Russia, presents an estimated SCC of more than 100 cases/100,000 person-years [6, 7]. Although the incidence of SCC has decreased in many regions, a marked increase in the incidence of esophageal adenocarcinoma (ADC), which appears to be sustained, has been observed in Europe, North America, and Australia during the past four decades. So, the incidence of ADC has surpassed that of SCC in many Western countries [8, 9, 3].

Historically, while most OC were derived from stratified epithelium of the middle and lower thirds of the esophagus and therefore named SCC, ADC derived from islands of columnar glandular cells near the gastroesophageal junction. Sarcomas and small cell carcinomas generally represent less than 1–2% of all esophageal cancers. On rare occasions, other carcinomas, melanomas, leiomyosarcomas, carcinoids, and lymphomas may develop in the esophagus as well [5, 10].

SCC and ADC are the two major histological types; they differ in biological features, geographic and demographic characteristics, risk factors, pathogenesis, patients' performance status, treatment, and HRQoL; and so they are discussed separately in the two following sections [3] (◻ Fig. 34.1).

34.2 Risk Factors

34.2.1 Squamous Cell Carcinoma

The pathophysiological pathway of SCC is typically initiated by carcinogenic compounds in direct contact with the esophageal mucosa. Mechanical injuries, such as achalasia, radiation therapy, or swallowing hot beverages or sodium hydroxide, increase susceptibility to carcinogenic compounds [3]. Transition models have described squamous epithelium undergoing inflammatory changes that progress to dysplasia and in situ carcinoma [5].

The etiology of SCC is multifactorial and strongly population dependent as a result of the following risk factors [11].

- Gender

In males the SCC incidence rates are two- to threefold higher than in females [12]. A global assessment indicated an overall male-to-female ratio of 4.4 which ranged from 1.7 in sub-Saharan Africa to 8.5 in North America [13].

- Smoking and Alcohol Drinking

Smoking and alcohol drinking are the main risk factors for SCC in Western countries [14], and the risk of SCC increases from threefold to sevenfold for smokers compared with non-smokers [15]. Tobacco smoke is known to contain polycyclic aromatic hydrocarbons, nitrosamines, and many other carcinogens. A commonly accepted interpretation of the synergy between ethanol and tobacco smoke is that ethanol dissolves and facilitates the transport of tobacco carcinogens to cells, making the cells more susceptible to carcinogenesis [12, 16]. Alcoholic beverage consumption has been linked causally to SCC because acetaldehyde, a class 1 carcinogen, is the first metabolite of ethanol metabolism. Microorganisms in oral cavity also produce acetaldehyde from ethanol and could contribute to the carcinogenic effects of alcohol [11].

- Diet and Hot Foods and Beverages

Dietary factors have also been suggested as etiological factors of SCC for US population, especially urban African Americans, whose intake of fruit and vegetables was lower than that of other ethnic groups [12]. Higher intake of fruit and vegetables probably decreases the risk of esophageal cancer; in fact each increment of 50 g/day of raw vegetables was associated with 31% decrease in the risk of esophageal cancer, while the same increment intake of fruit was associated with 22% decrease [17, 18]. Consumption of hot foods

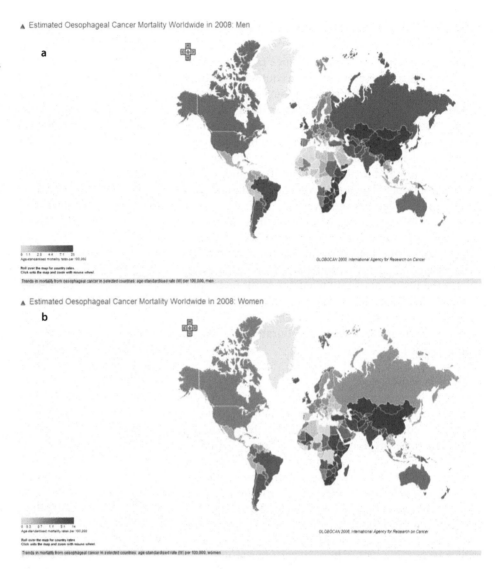

Fig. 34.1 Estimated esophageal cancer mortality worldwide in 2008. **a** Men. **b** Women. (Zhang Y. Risk factors of esophageal cancer)

and beverages has been associated with increased risk of SCC in subjects that drink the traditional herbal beverage maté, which is consumed at high temperature in large quantity (several liters per day) [11]. Other risk factors, such as micronutrients, PAHs (polycyclic aromatic hydrocarbons), BMI, medical conditions (such as Plummer-Vinson syndrome, Fanconi anemia), poor oral health, HPV infection, and mineral intakes, require confirmation with epidemiological studies in endemic areas.

Genetic Alteration

Dysplasia has been considered as a precancerous lesion of SCC with a significantly increased risk of developing into SCC. Therefore, identifying mutations occurring during SCC development could provide implications for early diagnosis and potential therapeutic strategies [16]. The genomic landscape of SCC,

which frequently shows mutations in TP53, CDKN2A, and PIK3CA, has been well characterized by whole-genome sequencing (WGS) and whole-exome sequencing (WES). However, most studies of precancerous lesions of SCC were limited to hotspot genes or the allelic loss of tumor-suppressor genes. The panoramic genetic architecture of the carcinogenesis process is unknown [19].

Recent research has provided evidence that chronic inflammation is a strong risk factor in the microenvironment for the development of digestive tumors and a close association between chronic inflammation and esophageal precancerous lesions from SCC patients exists. However, evidence to prove inflammation as a pathogenic factor in SCC development hasn't been found yet; beside the last events that promote intraepithelial neoplasia (IEN) into infiltrating carcinoma haven't been identified yet [19].

34.2.2 Adenocarcinoma

Esophageal adenocarcinoma incidence rates have been steadily increasing in several Western countries, although there are differences either between countries or between regions within the same country. The upward trends are in part due to the increased prevalence of recognized risk factors such as gastroesophageal reflux disease (GORD), obesity, and male sex, while *Helicobacter pylori* infection and dietary intake of fruit and vegetables, and possibly also non-steroidal anti-inflammatory drugs, are considered protective. The increasing prevalence of reflux and obesity, combined with a decreasing prevalence of *Helicobacter pylori* infection, probably contributes to the increasing incidence of esophageal adenocarcinoma. GORD and Barrett's esophagus are among the most commonly mentioned risk factors for ADC in epidemiological studies, and the existing meta-analyses reported a gradually increased risk of ADC with the increasing frequency and duration of GORD symptoms [20].

■ Gender and Race

The incidence of esophageal adenocarcinoma is eightfold more common in men than in women [21] and fivefold more common in whites than in blacks in the USA. The male predominance is not readily explained by sex differences in the exposure to the established risk factors for ADC, obesity, gastroesophageal reflux disease, *Helicobacter pylori* (*H. pylori*) infection (inverse association), or tobacco smoking. On the other hand, it has been hypothesized that sex hormones and reproductive factors might play a role in the development of ADC or its precancerous lesion Barrett's esophagus, although the existing evidence is far from conclusive [22].

■ Barrett's Esophagus

It is a condition in which the typical squamous epithelium of the esophageal mucosa is replaced with columnar intestinal epithelium. BO is a known precursor to the development of esophageal adenocarcinoma, which has a dramatically increasing incidence over the past 40 years. The risk of ADC among patients with BO is estimated to be 30–125-fold greater than that of the general population. Endoscopically, the prevalence of BO has been estimated at 1–2% in all patients receiving endoscopy for any indication and anywhere from 5% to 15% in patients with symptoms of GORD. The incidence of endoscopically detected BO appears to have increased dramatically over the past 30 years, a finding partially attributable to the increasing frequency of endoscopy during the same period. BO on average is diagnosed in the sixth to seventh decades of life, but may develop far earlier [23].

■ Obesity

Measured by BMI and central adiposity, obesity has been studied extensively as a risk factor for BO. The incidences of BO and esophageal ADC have risen dramatically in the past 40–50 years in Western societies, concurrent with rapid increases in the rate of obesity. From 1976 to 1991, the prevalence of obesity at all ages rose from 25% to 33%, and it now approaches 35% in adults.

Other risk factors, such as alcohol, nutritional deficit, and tobacco use, may be considered for their effects on both GORD and BO risk. On the other hand, the use of non-steroidal anti-inflammatory drugs (NSAIDs), proton pump inhibitors (PPIs), and statins in patients with BO reduced the progression to adenocarcinoma [23].

■ Genetic Aspects

Very recently, it has been demonstrated using GWAS (genome-wide association study) that the risk of BO and ADC is influenced by many germline genetic variants of small effect and that shared polygenic effects contribute to the risk of these two diseases. In fact, the genetic correlation between BO and ADC was high and estimated a statistically significant polygenic overlap between BO and esophageal adenocarcinoma. This strongly suggests that shared genes underlie the development of BO and ADC. GWAS-type studies have also been conducted to elucidate susceptibility loci. The most significant results were for cancer and pre-cancer combined, suggesting that much of the genetic basis for ADC lies in the development of BO, rather than to ADC. One of the novel regions is chromosome 3p13, near FOXP1, a gene encoding a transcription factor, which regulates esophageal development. Interestingly, two of the other regions (BARX1/9q22.32 and FOXF1/16q24.1) contain risk-associated SNPs which disrupt binding of FOXP1. Further dissection of these loci is likely to lead to insights into the etiology of this rapidly fatal cancer [22].

34.3 Clinical Features

Esophageal cancers are usually asymptomatic in the early stage and after they may cause different symptoms according to progression of tumor, leading to a diagnosis in a later stage.

Weight loss and dysphagia are the most common signs and symptoms at the diagnosis. The dysphagia arises typically when there is an involvement of more than one-third of the esophageal lumen. It can be limited to the liquids or can affect also the solids, leading to a complete dysphagia. Dysphagia, thoracic pain, regurgitation, hiccups, drooling, and odynophagia are common symptoms in the locally advanced disease with involvement of mediastinal structures. Dysphonia and cough at the deglutition may arise in case of involvement of recurrent laryngeal nerve or presence of esophagus-tracheal fistula, respectively.

The liver, peritoneum, lungs, and bones are the most common site of distant metastasis in case of esophageal cancer, whereas the involvement of the brain is rare. Liver involvement is predominant and can lead to hepatomegaly and jaundice, while dyspnea can appear in case of diffuse lung involvement, pleural effusion, or profuse ascites. Bone pain and neurologic signs and symptoms can appear in case of bone or different areas of the brain involvement, respectively. Peritoneal metastasis may cause different entity of peritoneal carcinomatosis with ascites or secondary implants.

34.4 Pathological Features

The subsequent histopathological pictures of the SCC and the ADC were taken from and based on the description made by [24].

34.4.1 Macroscopic Aspects

34.4.1.1 Squamous Cell Carcinoma

SCC occurs most commonly in the middle third of esophagus followed by lower one-third and upper one-third, respectively. Endoscopically, it can be polypoid, flat, or ulcerated. On endoscopic ultrasound (EUS), infiltrating SCC presents as a circumscribed diffuse wall thickening with echo-poor pattern due to destruction of layers of esophageal wall. Invasion of neoplastic squamous cells into lamina propria and deeper layers defines invasive SCC.

34.4.1.2 Adenocarcinoma

The main pathophysiological pathway of ADC is likely to be chronic gastroesophageal reflux disease, causing metaplasia from the native squamous cell mucosa to a specialized columnar epithelium, known as Barrett's esophagus (BO) [3]. Barrett's esophagus is a condition in which the normal squamous epithelial lining of the distal esophagus is replaced with specialized or intestinalized columnar epithelium. BO is a complication of chronic GORD although asymptomatic subjects might also be affected [25]. For the diagnosis of BO, which is considered the premalignant condition and the main risk factor of the esophageal adenocarcinoma, the presence of intestinal metaplasia is required because cur-

rently intestinal metaplasia is the only type of columnar epithelium that clearly predisposes toward development of this highly lethal disease [26]. Gastroesophageal reflux disease or just reflux [16, 27] can damage the lining of the esophagus, which causes BO, characterized by abnormal "tongues" of salmon-colored mucosa extending proximally from the squamo-columnar junction into the normal pale esophageal mucosa. BO develops in approximately 5–8 percent of patients with reflux disease and can progress to low-grade dysplasia, high-grade dysplasia, and invasive ADC [4].

34.4.2 Microscopic Aspects

34.4.2.1 Squamous Cell Carcinoma

Chronic Esophagitis: early studies suggested that mild to moderate chronic esophagitis was associated with family history of esophageal cancer and other risk factors of SCC [7]. Subsequently, systematic studies with endoscopic surveillance, biopsy evaluation, and follow-up to the development of SCC showed that esophagitis is nonspecific and the only true precursor lesion of SCC is squamous dysplasia [1, 11].

Squamous Dysplasia: It is a histologic lesion confined to the epithelium and is characterized by cytologic and architectural abnormalities. The cytologic abnormalities include nuclear enlargement, hyperchromasia, pleomorphism, and increased and/or abnormal mitosis. The architectural changes include loss of polarity and lack of surface maturation. The abnormality starts from the basal layer, and based on the extent of involvement of thickness of epithelium by atypical cells, the dysplasia was traditionally graded as mild (up to one-third), moderate (up to two-thirds), and severe (involving upper one-third). In 2000, the WHO adopted the term "intraepithelial neoplasia" (IEN) for dysplasia and classified IEN in a two-tier system as low-grade when less than half of thickness of the epithelium is involved with atypical cells (◘ Fig. 34.2a) and high-grade when greater than half of thickness is involved. Full-thickness involvement of the epithelium is called "squamous cell carcinoma in situ" (CIS).

Histologically, the tumor can show variable differentiation. Well-differentiated SCC show presence of keratin pearls, individual cell keratinization, and intercellular bridges. Poorly differentiated SCC lack these features and are determined to be squamous in origin based on pattern of infiltration and presence of IEN or in situ lesions in the adjacent squamous mucosa or with the help of immunohistochemical markers such as CK5/6 or p63. Moderately differentiated SCC show intermediate features.

34.4.2.2 Adenocarcinoma

ADC had copy number, RNA, and methylation patterns more similar to the chromosomally unstable subtype of gastric adenocarcinoma than to esophageal SCC.

The strongest predictor of progression to high-grade dysplasia (HGD) or ADC is baseline low-grade dysplasia. Dysplasia in BO is a histologic diagnosis suggesting that epithelial cells have acquired genetic or epigenetic alterations which predispose them to the development of malignancy. Dysplasia, when identified in a patient with BO, predicts a higher risk of ADC. The annual risk of progression in BO with low-grade dysplasia (LGD) is closer to 0.5–3%. Even among experienced pathologists, the extent of interobserver agreement, when diagnosing LGD, can be less than 50%, and this is in part due to the fact that inflammation can cause cytologic atypia in the bases of crypts that mimics dysplasia. Regression of LGD, or the failure to detect dysplastic changes on subsequent endoscopies, also may occur in half or more of patients with LGD. Incidence of ADC or HGD is estimated at 1.1–6% annually, but some estimates are as high as 13.4% per year. With HGD, interobserver agreement is better but is still less than 90%.

The risk of ADC is greater in longer segments of BO compared to shorter segments. The relationship between segment length and increased risk of AC is not always linear, but the preponderance of evidence suggests that greater surface area of columnar-lined mucosa correlates with increased cancer risk [23].

Low-Grade Dysplasia: Barrett's mucosa shows loss of surface maturation and architectural distortion with glandular crowding, in the absence of active inflammation. There is a sharp contrast between neoplastic and non-neoplastic mucosa. Nuclei in the surface mucosa show hyperchromasia, nuclear enlargement, stratification, and mucin loss. Mitotic figures can be seen on the surface (■ Fig. 34.2).

High-Grade Dysplasia: Barrett's mucosa shows loss of surface maturation (as in LGD) and glandular crowding. The nuclei show loss of polarity and are rounded, enlarged, and hyperchromatic with inconspicuous nucleoli. Mitoses are frequent. Inflammation is less in comparison to the architectural and cytologic atypia. Presence of ulceration, active inflammation, and prominent nucleoli are features indicative of reactive/reparative changes due to a benign process or are concerning for an associated invasive carcinoma. Additional features suggestive of invasive adenocarcinoma on biopsies include cribriform glandular architecture, luminal necrotic debris,

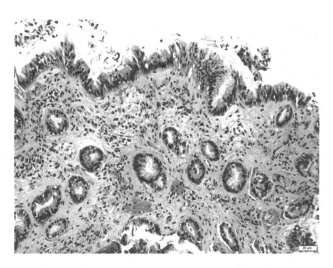

■ **Fig. 34.2**   Esophageal dysplasia: low grade; Dhingra, *MD, FACP, Associate Professor, Department of Pathology and Immunology, Baylor College of Medicine, Houston, TX* [24])

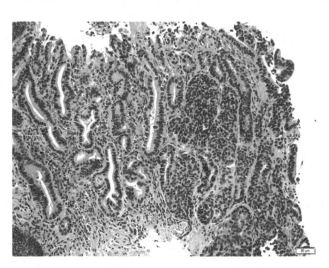

■ **Fig. 34.3**   Intramucosal adenocarcinoma. (From Dhingra, *MD, FCAP, Associate Professor, Departement of Pathology and Immunoly, Baylor College of Medicine, Houston, TX* [24])

ulceration, neutrophils within dysplastic glands, and pagetoid spread of neoplastic cells in the overlying squamous mucosa.

■ Intramucosal Adenocarcinoma

Intramucosal adenocarcinoma is defined by invasion of carcinoma into lamina propria but not beyond muscularis mucosae. The features of intramucosal adenocarcinoma are syncytial growth pattern with back-to-back glands, presence of single cells, and small clusters within lamina propria (■ Fig. 34.3). Desmoplasia may not be present, but if present, it is very subtle [24].

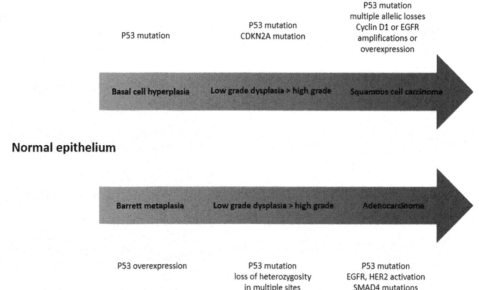

Fig. 34.4 Molecular alterations in esophageal cancers

■ **Esophageal Adenocarcinoma**

Endoscopically, if detected early, these tumors will present as mucosal irregularities. In later stages they appear as ulcerated/infiltrative or exophytic masses with obstruction. Histologically, these are gland-forming tumors with a tubular, tubulopapillary, or papillary growth pattern. A small subset of cases shows mucinous differentiation. A few cases of diffuse signet ring cell adenocarcinoma have also been reported. Foci of BO with high-grade dysplasia are commonly seen in epithelium adjacent to the tumor. The tumors show variable grades of differentiation based on the amount of gland formation, and the nuclear atypia generally follows the grade of differentiation.

Well-differentiated tumors show more than 95% gland formation, moderately differentiated tumors show 50–95% gland formation, and poorly differentiated tumors show <50% gland formation [24].

34.5 Molecular Biology

Esophageal cancer is characterized by alterations of some gene or molecules involved in different processes, such as cell proliferations, apoptosis, DNA repair, and signal transduction. In particular, loss of heterozygosis on chromosomes 1p, 3p, 5q, 9p, 9q, 13q, 17p, 17q, and 18 q, p53 mutations, Rb deletions, cyclin D1 and c-myc amplifications, NFκB hyperexpression, and bcl- 2, caspase 3, TRAIL, Fas, and Fas-L mutations are the most common alterations that can be found in these types of tumors.

RAS mutation is rare in case of esophageal tumors [28], while there is human epidermal growth factor receptor 2 (Her-2) amplification in 60% of cases of

Barrett's esophagus. Her-2/neu gene, located on chromosome 17q21, encodes the Her-2 protein that belongs to the epidermal growth factor receptor (EGFR) family pathway. In case of gene amplification, there is Her-2 receptor overexpression, resulting in a prolongation of transductional signals with uncontrolled cell growth and tumorigenesis. To date, the specific ligand of this receptor has not been identified, and it is considered a ligand-independent orphan receptor.

For many years, esophageal cancers were divided into two big groups according to histopathologic and epidemiologic aspects, as already mentioned: squamous cell carcinoma (SCC) and adenocarcinoma (ADC). Furthermore, these two types of tumors are distinguished also from a molecular point of view (■ Fig. 34.4). SCC, in fact, showed genomic amplifications of EGFR (19%), phosphatidylinositol 3-kinase (PI3K), and p63 pathway alterations, whereas ADC showed an increased E-cadherin signaling and common amplifications of Her-2 (32%), vascular endothelial growth factor A (VEGF-A), GATA 4, and GATA 6 [29].

Nevertheless, nowadays it is known that also into these two groups it can be distinguished different kind of tumors characterized by different features. These findings led to create a molecular classifications for esophageal cancers that could became important in the future in order to develop novel target therapies directed against specific molecular targets.

34.5.1 Molecular Classifications

The Cancer Genome Atlas Research (TGCA) network [29] reported the latest molecular classification for esophageal cancer based on the evaluation of genes

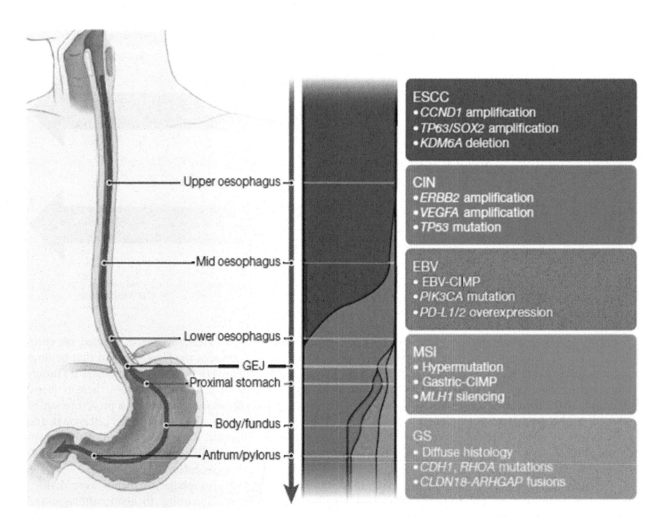

□ Fig. 34.5 Molecular subtypes of esophageal cancer [29]. ESCC esophageal squamous cell carcinoma, CIN chromosomal instability, EBV Epstein-Barr virus, MSI microsatellite instability, GS genomic stability

expression in 164 tumors (□ Fig. 34.5). According to this TGCA classification, esophageal cancer can be divided into two classical groups: SCC and ADC. Within SCC there are three molecular subtypes: SCC1, SCC2, and SCC3.

SCC1 represents the classical esophageal cancer subtype; it is predominant in Asiatic regions, and it is characterized by alterations in NRF2 pathway, involved in the regulation of response to oxidative stressors such as chemotherapy, and amplifications of SOX2 and/or p63. SCC2 is more frequent in Eastern Europe or South America; it is characterized by greater leukocyte infiltration and higher rates of PTEN inactivation and/or CDK6 amplification, whereas SCC3 is reported in the USA and Canada and shows activation of PI3K pathway. None of these subtypes was related to human papillomavirus (HPV), unlike the other types of SCC.

Esophageal ADC showed, in addition to the molecular features already mentioned, high rate of chromosomal instability (CIN) as well as gastric cancer subtype

one [30], suggesting that these two types of cancer might have the same origin and be considered as a single entity. Nevertheless, other molecular characteristics, such as DNA hypermethylation, distinguish the esophageal ADC from the gastric CIN one.

34.6 Esophageal Cancer Progression

Esophageal cancer can progress by different local and contiguity diffusion, lymphatic involvement, and hematic spread of metastasis. Among all, local infiltration and lymphatic spread represent the more frequent ways of diffusion. In the first case, tumor can involve all esophageal wall leading to a visceral stenosis, whereas in case of lymphatic diffusion the neoplasm can disseminate through the lymphatic vessels in the submucosa and muscular tunics leading to also different distant synchronous lesions, known as skip lesions. This peculiarity, in addition to the lack of a serosa around the esophagus and its close anatomical relationships with other mediastinum structures, such as the vessels, pericardium, or trachea, leads to an early diffusion of disease. Moreover, the lymphatic spread is according to the primary tumor site. In fact, there are a predominant involvement of cervical paratracheal and peribronchial lymph nodes in case of cancer of the upper third of the esophagus, a diffusion to the under-diaphragmatic stations in case of middle esophagus tumor, and involvement of the lymph nodes around the cardia in the third lower esophagus cancers.

The diffusion of disease by contiguity consists in the involvement of different organs around the primary tumor, such as the trachea and/or rachis in the upper cancers or the pericardium, diaphragm, or liver in the lower ones.

The hematic spread of tumor occurs at a later stage with frequent involvement of the liver and/or lung, whereas bone, brain, and adrenal metastases are rarer.

34.7 Diagnosis

A clinical and instrumental evaluation is mandatory in all patients with a risk condition or with new symptoms suspected for esophageal cancer. A first global clinical visit is recommended to evaluate risk factors, but specific assessment is needed to detect an esophageal tumor. Therefore, the endoscopy of the upper gastrointestinal tract is the most important exam to diagnose an esophageal cancer. The endoscopy gives a global view of esophageal mucosa and allows to obtain a biopsy on the suspected tumor lesions. In case of esophageal lesions, it is mandatory to obtain multiple biopsy on the mucosa of the lesion and around as well as a brushing of the lesion. Moreover, in case of stenosis, during the endoscopy the dilatation or the position of stents to palliate the dysphagia can be evaluated.

The radiological evaluation of the esophagus is not frequently used today. However, this study may help to define the presence, site, grade, and length of a stenosis or the presence of esophageal fistulas. The definition of length is important to plan the correct therapeutic strategy for these patients, because in case of length >5 cm, with or without distortion of the esophagus profile, there is a locally advanced disease and the upfront surgery is not recommended.

34.8 Differential Diagnosis

The most important differential diagnosis is between tumors and polyps, leiomyomas, or ulcers, because sometimes these lesions cause the same symptoms of cancer (heartburn, e.g.). In almost all cases, the endoscopy with biopsy or the morphologic characteristics at the radiological imaging of the esophagus are able to differentiate these benign lesions from the neoplastic ones.

34.9 Staging

An accurate staging is important to choose the appropriate approach to treat a patient with esophageal cancer. In order to obtain a correct staging of disease, it is important to define the site of primary tumor. In fact, it can distinguish tumors of the esophagus and tumors of the gastroesophageal junction.

The esophagus can be divided into cervical, thoracic, and abdominal, according to the following anatomical definitions [31]:

- Cervical: from the lower border of the cricoid cartilage (at the level of the sixth cervical vertebra) to the thoracic inlet (suprasternal notch); 18 cm from incisors.
- Upper thoracic: from the thoracic inlet to the level of tracheal bifurcation; 18–23 cm from incisors.
- Mid-thoracic: from the tracheal bifurcation midway to junction; 24–32 cm from incisors.
- Lower thoracic: from midway between tracheal bifurcation and gastroesophageal junction to gastroesophageal junction, including the abdominal esophagus; 32–40 cm from incisors.

The gastroesophageal junction is the point where the distal esophagus joins the proximal stomach, and it is divided from an anatomical point of view, according to Siewert classification, into [32]:

- Type I: adenocarcinoma of the distal esophagus, which usually arises from an area with specialized intestinal metaplasia of the esophagus (i.e., Barrett's esophagus) and may infiltrate the esophagogastric junction from above (center located within between 1 and 5 cm above the anatomic cardia).
- Type II: true carcinoma of the cardia arising at the esophagogastric junction (within 1 cm above and 2 cm below the cardia).
- Type III: subcardial gastric carcinoma that infiltrates the esophagogastric junction and distal esophagus from 2 to 5 cm below the cardia.

The stage is according to the American Joint Committee on Cancer (AJCC)/Union for International Cancer Control (UICC) TNM staging system (8th edition) (◘ Tables 34.1, 34.2, and 34.3) [33]. Like the previous one, the 8th edition distinguishes between SCC and ADC and includes the grading into the stage. Nevertheless, in this last edition, there are also three separate classifications for both ADC and SCC: the pathologic stage groups (pTNM), the newly introduced

■ Table 34.1 Clinical TNM staging (cTNM) for esophageal cancer, 8th edition [33]

Primary tumor (cT)

TX	Primary tumor cannot be assessed
T0	No evidence of primary tumor
T_{is}	Carcinoma in situ/high-grade dysplasia
T1	Tumor invades the lamina propria, muscularis mucosae, or submucosa
T1a	Tumor invades the mucosa or lamina propria or muscularis mucosae
T1b	Tumor invades the submucosa
T2	Tumor invades the muscularis propria
T3	Tumor invades the adventitia
T4	Tumor invades adjacent structures
T4a	Tumor invades the pleura, pericardium, diaphragm, or adjacent peritoneum
T4b	Tumor invades other adjacent structures such as the aorta, vertebral body, or trachea

Regional lymph nodes (cN)

Nx	Regional lymph nodes cannot be assessed
N0	No regional lymph node metastasis
N1	Metastasis in 1–2 regional lymph nodes
N2	Metastasis in 3–6 regional lymph nodes
N3	Metastasis in 7 or more regional lymph nodes

Distant metastasis (cM)

Mx	Distant metastasis cannot be assessed
M0	No distant metastasis
M1	Distant metastasis

Clinical stage groups

Squamous cell carcinoma			
	cT	cN	cM
0	Tis	N0	M0
I	T1	N0–1	M0
II	T2	N0–1	M0
	T3	N0	M0
III	T3	N1	M0
	T1–3	N2	M0
IVa	T4	N0–2	M0
IVb	T1–4	N0–3	M1

■ Table 34.1 (continued)

Adenocarcinoma			
0	Tis	N0	M0
I	T1	N0	M0
IIa	T1	N1	M0
IIb	T2	N0	M0
III	T2	N1	M0
	T3–4a	N0–1	M0
IVa	T1–4a	N2	M0
	T4b	N0–2	M0
	T1–4	N3	M0
IVb	T1–4	N1–3	M1

postneoadjuvant pathologic stage groups (ypTNM), and clinical stage groups (cTNM). Regarding the gastroesophageal junction adenocarcinoma, Siewert I and II with involvement of the esophagus are staged according to the esophageal cancer system, whereas type III and type II tumors with distal extension to the stomach are staged according to the gastric cancer system.

Staging should include a complete clinical examination, an endoscopic ultrasound (EUS), and a computed tomography (CT) scan of the neck, chest, and abdomen with contrast.

In particular, EUS is fundamental to evaluate the local invasion (T parameter) and nodal involvement (N parameter) with high precision than CT scan (96% sensitivity for T and 81% for N). Moreover, EUS can be able to perform biopsy of primary tumor and lymph nodes and for this reason is mandatory for all patients candidate to surgery, because the involvement of regional lymph nodes represents a clear indication to neoadjuvant treatment today. The main limitation of EUS is the frequent presence of esophageal stenosis that does not allow the exam.

CT scan allows to detect locoregional involvement of continuous organs, such as aorta and trachea, and distant metastasis. On the contrary, CT scan is not recommended to distinguish between T1 and T2 invasion.

18F-Fluorodeoxyglucose-positron emission tomography (18 FDG-PET alone or in combination with CT scan: PET-CT) is considered as a second-level exam able to identify undetected distant metastases, especially in patients candidate to esophagectomy in order to prevent a surgical non-curative procedure in IV stage setting. Moreover, 18 FDG-PET may be used to evaluate the

◻ Table 34.2 Pathological TNM staging (pTNM) for esophageal cancer, 8th edition [33]

Pathologic stage groups

Squamous cell carcinoma

	pT	pN	pM	pGRADE	pLOCATION
0	Tis	N0	M0	N/A	Any
Ia	T1a	N0	M0	G1, X	Any
Ib	T1b	N0	M0	G1, X	Any
	T1	N0	M0	G1–3	Any
	T2	N0	M0	G1	Any
IIa	T2	N0	M0	G2–3, X	Any
	T3	N0	M0	Any	Lower
	T3	N0	M0	G1	Upper/middle
IIb	T3	N0	M0	G2–3	Upper/middle
	T3	N0	M0	Any	Any
	T3	N0	M0	Any	Any
	T1	N1	M0	Any	Any
IIIa	T1	N2	M0	Any	Any
	T2	N1	M0	Any	Any
IIIb	T4a	N0–1	M0	Any	Any
	T3	N1	M0	Any	Any
	T2–3	N2	M0	Any	Any
IVa	T4a	N2	M0	Any	Any
	T4b	N0–3	M0	Any	Any
	T1–4	N3	M0	Any	Any
IVb	T1–4	N0–3	M1	Any	Any

Adenocarcinoma

0	Tis	N0	M0	N/A	
Ia	T1a	N0	M0	G1, X	
Ib	T1a	N0	M0	G2	
	T1b	N0	M0	G1–2, X	
Ic	T1	N0	M0	G3	
	T2	N0	M0	G1–2	
IIa	T2	N0	M0	G3,X	
IIb	T1	N1	M0	Any	
	T3	N0	M0	Any	
IIIa	T1	N2	M0	Any	
	T2	N1	M0	Any	
IIIb	T4a	N0–1	M0	Any	
	T3	N1	M0	Any	
	T2–3	N2	M0	Any	
IVa	T4a	N2	M0	Any	
	T4b	N0–2	M0	Any	
	T1–4	N3	M0	Any	
	T1–4	N0–3	M1	Any	

◻ Table 34.3 Postneoadjuvant treatment TNM staging (ypTNM) for esophageal cancer, 8th edition [33]

	ypT	ypN	ypM
I	T0–1	N0	M0
II	T3	N0	M0
IIIA	T0–2	N1	M0
IIIB	T4a	N0	M0
	T3	N1–2	M0
	T0–3	N2	M0
IVA	T4a	N1–2, Nx	M0
	T4b	N0–2	M0
	T1–4	N3	M0
IVB	Every T	Every N	M1

assessed by 18 FDG-PET could predict the pathologic response after surgery [34]. However, further confirmation is needed for this indication.

A tracheobronchoscopy should be carried out in the case of primary tumors located at thoracic esophagus in order to exclude tracheal invasion. Moreover, in the case of SCC related to chronic tobacco and alcoholism, an additional investigation of the aerodigestive tract is mandatory to exclude synchronous second cancer which is frequent in these conditions.

Ultrasonography is useful in case of cervical or upper thoracic tumor to evaluate the supraclavicular and cervical lymph nodes.

Laparoscopy can be done to detect peritoneal metastases in locally advanced ADC of the esophagus or gastroesophageal junction (15% at the diagnosis), even if this approach is not still considered mandatory.

Finally, in patients with esophageal cancer, it is important to assess the nutritional status and history of weight loss according to the European Society for Clinical Nutrition and Metabolism (ESPEN) guidelines [35], due to the primary site of tumor that leads to a difficult intake of food and subsequent weight loss. Weight loss confers an increased operative risk, worsens a patient's quality of life, and is associated with poor survival in advanced disease independent from the final body mass index. Therefore, nutritional support is mandatory at the diagnosis and during all treatment period for these patients.

34.10 Prognostic Factors

Despite the progression in knowledge and treatments for esophageal cancer, the prognosis of this type of tumor is still poor especially in case of locally advanced

response after a neoadjuvant treatment (restaging). In fact, some trials showed that an early metabolic response after the first cycle of neoadjuvant chemotherapy

or metastatic disease. The main prognostic factors for esophageal cancer are the depth of invasion, nodes, and distant metastasis that together represent the stage of disease. The median overall survival, therefore, is according to the stage, with less than 10% of patients alive at 5 years after the diagnosis.

The pathologic response to treatment represents another prognostic factor that may be considered in patients treated with a neoadjuvant approach. In fact, some trials showed that a complete pathological response (pCR) is related to better survival in these patients.

Finally, the performance status (PS) of patient can influence the prognosis by affecting the choice and the correct execution of treatments.

34.11   Treatment

Surgery represents the only curative approach in case of esophageal cancer. Unfortunately, only one-third of patients are candidate to surgery at the diagnosis, while the others showed a non-resectable locally advanced or metastatic disease. Nevertheless, the outcomes for these patients remain poor despite curative surgery, with a median overall survival from 11 to 18 months and a 5-year survival rate between 16% and 32%. In this context, an interdisciplinary planning of treatment becomes mandatory to evaluate the integration of different therapeutic approaches in addition to surgery in order to improve the prognosis [36]. The main factors for selecting primary therapy are tumor stage and location, histological type, and patient's PS, preferences, and comorbidities.

Response to systemic treatments should normally be assessed with interval imaging of the chest, abdomen, and pelvis, mostly with CT scan, although alternative imaging techniques may be used if required to monitor known sites of disease (e.g., magnetic resonance imaging for brain lesions or bone scintigraphy in case of bone lesions). The evaluation of response is according to standard radiologic criteria for solid tumor, also known as RECIST criteria, except in case of immunotherapy in which should be used the immune-modified RECIST (iRECIST). In case of neoadjuvant treatment, the restaging should comprise also a local evaluation of disease by EUS and 18FDG-PET to exclude the presence of distant metastasis before surgery.

34.11.1   Limited Disease

Surgery is the treatment of choice in limited disease (stages I and II). The goal of the surgical approach is to obtain a curative radical resection, also known as R0

resection, without macro- or microscopic residual disease. The presence of residual microscopic or macroscopic disease after surgery, known as R1 and R2 resections, respectively, represents an important bad prognostic factor for patients affected by esophageal cancer with a 5-year survival rate of 5–15% for R1 and 0% for R2.

In patients with ADC limited to the mucosa and submucosa (T1a and T1b), endoscopic therapy by endoscopic mucosal resection (EMR) and endoscopic submucosal dissection (ESD) is preferred. The endoscopic therapy is considered a curative approach as well as the esophagectomy in case of superficial ADC without risk factors (depth of invasion <500 μm, no ulceration, <20 mm diameter, well differentiated), whereas it is recommended a resection in case of presence of these ones.

In localized esophageal cancer beyond T1a N0, surgery is the current standard of care (◻ Fig. 34.6). It is important to refer to specialized and dedicated surgical centers to undergo this procedure due to the high postoperative mortality and the complexity of this surgery [37]. The type of surgical approach (transhiatal or transthoracic) depends on the tumor site without differences in survival between the different types [38]. Transthoracic esophagectomy by Ivor-Lewis procedure with two- or three-field lymphadenectomy is always the approach of choice because this type of resection makes possible to explore extensively the esophagus and to obtain a good lymphadenectomy.

Recently, the role of a minimally invasive approach to the thoracic and/or abdominal cavities is increasing in clinical practice compared to the open one. In fact, a newly randomized study in patients with esophageal cancer showed that hybrid minimally invasive esophagectomy (HMIO) reduces intra- and postoperative morbidity, especially pulmonary complications, if compared to an open esophagectomy and suggests a trend in improvement of survival [39].

Regarding the tumors of the gastroesophageal junction, the partial esophagectomy with gastroresection is the first choice in case of Siewert I tumors, whereas a total gastrectomy is reserved to patients with Siewert II or III neoplasms. A two-field lymphadenectomy is mandatory in all cases in addition to the surgery of primary tumor [40].

However, despite surgery, esophageal cancer shows high rate of locoregional relapses and early distant metastasization. For these reasons, a multimodal approach was evaluated also in these types of tumors in order to improve the outcome of patients.

A recent trial involving patients with stage I and stage II esophageal cancers showed that neoadjuvant chemoradiotherapy (CRT) with cisplatin and fluorouracil did not improve R0 resection rate or survival but enhances postoperative mortality if compared with surgery alone. Based on these results, surgery alone is recommended as the pri-

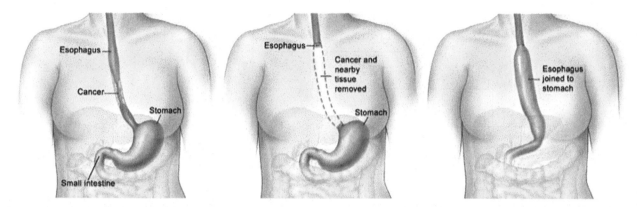

Fig. 34.6 Ivor-Lewis esophagectomy

mary treatment approach for cT2N0 esophageal cancer today [41], except in case of cervical carcinoma, in which definitive CRT represent the standard of care in localized and locally advanced disease. For these patients, in fact, the surgical approach is a total larynx-esophagectomy with high morbidity and mortality. However, his approach should be apply in cases of relapses or residual disease after multidisciplinary discussion.

In case of patients unable or unwilling to undergo surgery, combined CRT based on cisplatin/oxaliplatin and fluorouracil is superior to radiotherapy (RT) alone.

The adjuvant chemotherapy is currently limited in the esophageal disease, because the trials in this field did not show benefit with its use. All the studies, in fact, demonstrated a clear superiority for neoadjuvant approach, reserved the adjuvant RT in case of R1 or R2 resection.

34.11.2 Locally Advanced Disease

Surgery alone is not recommended as a curative approach in case of locally advanced disease (stage III), since the majority of patients cannot receive a complete R0 resection and, even after complete tumor resection, long-term survival is almost 20%. In this context, a multidisciplinary integrated neoadjuvant approach is mandatory to eradicate the micrometastatic disease and increase R0 resection and survival rates [42]. Therefore, preoperative treatment with chemotherapy or concomitant CRT is indicated in operable patients with locally advanced esophageal cancer according to the tumor's histotype. The global algorithm for treatment of non-metastatic esophageal cancer is reported in ☐ Fig. 34.6.

After a neoadjuvant treatment, all patients who did not progress during the therapy should be restaged in order to assess their response to treatment. Nowadays, pathological response is considered the only validated

Table 34.4 Tumor Regression Grade (TRG) score according to Mandard [43]

TRG1	No viable cancer cells, complete response
TRG2	Single cells or small groups of cancer cells
TRG3	Residual cancer outgrown by fibrosis
TRG4	Significant fibrosis outgrown by cancer
TRG5	No fibrosis with extensive residual cancer

factor that can predict the response to treatment, according to Mandard's Tumor Regression Grade (TRG) scale (☐ Table 34.4, [43]).

In fact, many trials demonstrated that patients who showed a pathologic complete response (pCR) had a significant survival benefit. Nevertheless, the evaluation of pathologic response is obviously obtained only on the surgical specimen of patients who underwent surgery. As already mentioned, a surrogate method that may predict the response is the evaluation of early metabolic response at 18-FDG-PET. The early metabolic response is the uptake reduction of 35% or more by PET after receiving one cycle of neoadjuvant chemotherapy [34]. Even if this represents a promising evaluation, further trials are needed to define its role as a prognostic marker, and it is not a standard in clinical practice today.

As shown in ☐ Fig. 34.7, there are two different algorithms according to histological subtypes of esophageal cancer. In case of SCC, it can be considered a neoadjuvant or a definitive approach. Regarding the neoadjuvant treatment, some trials demonstrated that patients with locally advanced disease benefit from preoperative chemo- or chemoradiotherapy with a high rate of R0 resection and better outcome [44]. The weekly administration of carboplatin and paclitaxel for 5 weeks and concurrent radiotherapy (41.4 Gy) followed by surgery represent the current standard of care

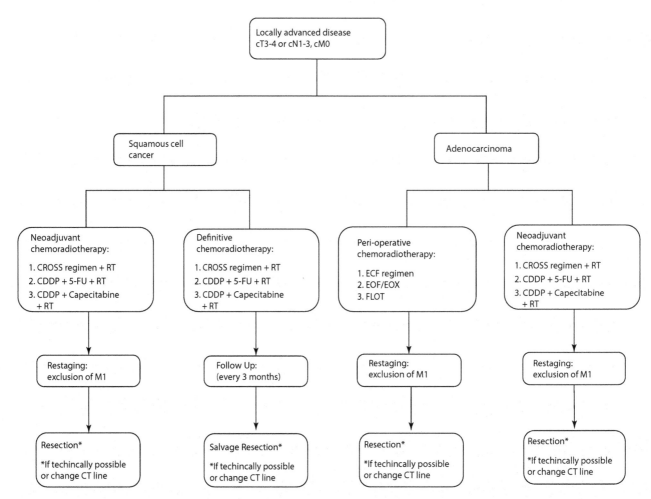

Fig. 34.7 Therapeutic algorithm for locally advanced disease

schedule for these patients [45]. However, also a cisplatin plus 5-fluorouracil schedule can be alternatively adopted. On the other hand, the comparison between definitive CRT without surgery and neoadjuvant CRT followed by surgery showed equivalent OS outcome [46, 47]. Therefore, both neoadjuvant chemoradiotherapy followed by surgery or definitive chemoradiotherapy with close surveillance and salvage surgery in case of local tumor persistence or progression can be considered for locally advanced SCC of the esophagus, except for cervical tumors in which a definitive approach is preferred. In case of response after neoadjuvant treatment, a follow-up program could be evaluated, reserved surgery at the relapse of disease.

Regarding the ADC, the standard treatment is represented by a perioperative chemotherapy with platinum- and fluoropyrimidine-based schedule or preoperative chemoradiotherapy (41.4–50.5 Gy). Moreover, in case of ADC of the gastroesophageal junction, the strongest

evidences suggest the use of a perioperative approach [48, 49, 50], while chemoradiotherapy did not show a clear OS benefit if compared to chemotherapy alone [51, 52, 53]. The perioperative chemotherapy consists of a preoperative treatment period of 3–4 cycles, followed by surgery and by 3–4 postoperative cycles. The preoperative period is well tolerated, whereas only few patients are able to complete the postoperative one with an higher rate of toxicity. The most common schedules used in this setting are ECX/ECF (epirubicin, cisplatin, capecitabine, or fluorouracil) and FLOT (fluorouracil, oxaliplatin, docetaxel) for perioperative chemotherapy or cisplatin/5-FU combined with 41.4–50.4 Gy oxaliplatin/5-FU or carboplatin/paclitaxel with radiotherapy for neoadjuvant concomitant approach. Pathological response represents the principal prognostic factor after neoadjuvant treatment also for ADC. Unlike the SCC, even after complete tumor response to treatment, in ADC surgery should be done anyway.

34.11.3 Metastatic Disease

34.11.3.1 Chemotherapy

More than 50% of patients show a metastatic disease at the diagnosis. The main goals in this setting are palliation of symptoms, improvement of quality of life, and survival. Polychemotherapy is the standard first-line treatment for patients with a good performance status, while best supportive care alone is recommended in case of poor conditions. Doublet combinations of platinum (cisplatin or oxaliplatin) and fluoropyrimidines (5-fluorouracil or capecitabine) or taxanes (paclitaxel) showed a benefit in response rate if compared to monochemotherapy and are generally used in SCC. In addition to these schedules, triplet combination based on platinum, fluorouracil, taxanes, or epirubicin could be used for ADC of the esophagus or gastroesophageal junction (GEJA) like in gastric cancer. In fact, the same algorithm for gastric cancer should be applied in case of GEJA, and the determination of Her-2 status is mandatory.

Approximately 40% of patients with metastatic esophageal cancer received a second-line therapy after failure of first line. Second-line treatment is recommended in patients with a progression of disease after a first-line treatment who conserved a good performance status. In fact, an active treatment, if possible, is associated with improvement in OS and quality of life compared with best supportive care. On the other hand, in case of worsening condition, the patient is candidate to best supportive care alone.

Among different chemotherapeutic agents and schedules investigated in this setting, taxanes and irinotecan [54], alone or in association with fluorouracil (FOLFIRI), showed a survival benefit with a good toxicity profile. In case of GEJA, the same algorithm for gastric cancer should be applied (see the description in metastatic gastric cancer chapter).

There is no clear evidence for a benefit beyond the second-line treatment, but a third line with active chemotherapy may be considered in patients with a good performance status who progressed after a second-line therapy. Generally, the choice of chemotherapy schedule beyond the second line is according to previous treatments and patient's preference and performance status.

34.11.3.2 Target and Immune Therapies

Strong data with biologically targeted therapies are limited in esophageal carcinoma. Trials in this field investigated drugs against epithelial growth factor receptors (EGFRs), vascular endothelial growth factor (VEGF) pathway, and programmed cell death 1 (PD-1).

EGFR is overexpressed in 50–70% SCC and correlates with a worse prognosis in this tumor. Cetuximab, a monoclonal chimeric antibody directed against EGFR, showed to improve the response rate and PFS if used in second-line treatment for esophageal cancers, alone or in association with chemotherapy [55]. The role of cetuximab in addition to chemoradiotherapy is still under debate.

The monoclonal anti-EGFR panitumumab did not show a benefit in addition to chemotherapy in first-line setting in a phase III international trial [56]. Moreover, other studies with different EGFR inhibitors, such as erlotinib or gefitinib, did not show survival benefit [57].

Her-2 is overexpressed in 24–32% of esophageal ADC or GEJA. For treating patients with ADC, the same algorithm of gastric cancer should be applied, and the determination of Her-2 status is mandatory. In the first-line treatment of Her-2-positive gastric cancer, the phase III ToGA trial demonstrated clinically and statistically significant improvements in response rate, progression-free survival (PFS), and OS with the addition of trastuzumab to cisplatin-fluoropyrimidine doublet [58] (median OS: 13.8 versus 11.1 months), especially in the subgroup with high expression of the protein (Her-2 3+ at IHC or 2+ IHC with FISH amplification).

Trastuzumab is a humanized antibody directed against the extracellular domain of Her-2 receptor that showed in preclinical models a selected inhibition of cancer cell growth that express the receptor on their surface. Based on the ToGA results, trastuzumab was approved in many countries in addition to cisplatin-fluoropyrimidine doublet as first-line standard of care in patients with Her-2-positive disease. Trastuzumab is currently used at the same dose for Her-2-positive breast cancer (8 mg/kg in the first induction dose and then 6 mg/kg every 21 days), even if today it is clear that Her-2-positive gastric cancer is biologically different from the breast one. However, the addition of trastuzumab with different schedule to chemotherapy did not show any benefit in patients with Her-2-positive metastatic gastric cancer and performance status 2 [59]. Moreover, trastuzumab is actually investigated in adjuvant and neoadjuvant setting for Her-2-positive gastric cancer.

Despite low evidence about the use of trastuzumab in esophageal cancer, a small phase I/II trial showed that the addition of trastuzumab to cisplatin, paclitaxel, and radiotherapy is feasible in locally advanced Her-2-positive tumors [60].

Regarding target therapies against VEGF pathway, no antiangiogenetic agents are currently used in metastatic or perioperative treatment [61] for esophageal and junctional cancer (see the chapter about metastatic gastric cancer) alone or in combination with chemo- or chemoradiotherapy.

Of particular relevance, over the last few years, we have seen in oncology a big explosion of immune-oriented therapies (mainly with immune checkpoint inhibitors) that completely changed the natural history of many awful malignancies, like melanoma, lung cancer, kidney cancer, urothelial cancer, and many others. Researchers mainly focused on immunological checkpoints like programmed cell death 1 (PD-1) and its ligands (PD-L1 and PD-L2) as well as CTLA-4 pathway. More in detail, PD-1 molecule is highly expressed on T-lymphocytes, and it acts as a co-inhibitory receptor, leading to a strong suppression of immunological T-cell-mediated response in tumor microenvironment, following the engagement with its ligands, PD-L1/PD-L2, which are mainly expressed on tumor cell surface.

Preliminary data from early phase clinical trials suggested that the use of immunotherapy could improve survival also in patients with esophageal cancer. Indeed, today we have positive results about two anti-PD1 drugs, nivolumab and pembrolizumab, emerging from two pivotal phase III clinical trials, one already published [62] and the other one only presented at 2019 ASCO Meeting [63]. The Attraction-3 study [62] randomized 419 advanced SCC PD-L1 unselected patients, already refractory to one previous platinum–/fluoropyrimidine-based chemotherapy, between the anti-PD1 nivolumab and investigator's choice chemotherapy (paclitaxel or docetaxel). Overall survival (primary endpoint) was consistently improved in experimental arm versus chemotherapy group (10.9 versus 8.4 months, HR: 0.77, $p = 0.019$), with a strong reduction of grade 3–4 adverse event (18% in nivolumab arm versus 63% in chemotherapy arm). Based on these results, nivolumab could really represent a new possible standard treatment for second-line treatment of SCC patients, although this drug is not yet registered in the EU with this indication.

On the other side, second-line Keynote-181 trial [63] analyzed also advanced patients with adenocarcinoma histology (in addition to SCC). This study enrolled 628 advanced esophageal adenocarcinoma (plus Siewert I GEJ adenocarcinoma) and SCC patients, already refractory to a previous line of therapy, who were randomized between the anti-PD1 pembrolizumab and investigator's choice chemotherapy (paclitaxel, docetaxel, irinotecan). Pembrolizumab, different from nivolumab in the Attraction-3 study, did not improve OS or PFS in the overall intention-to-treat (ITT) population, but the authors clearly showed a significant benefit obtained with pembrolizumab in PD-L1-positive patients with a CPS (combined positive score) > 10%. In fact, while in the overall ITT population mOS was 7.1 months in both treatment arms, in PD-L1 CPS-positive patients a mOS

of 9.3 months with pembrolizumab versus 6.7 months with conventional chemotherapy was observed. This trial strongly highlighted the necessity of PD-L1 CPS testing for metastatic patients with both adenocarcinoma and SCC refractory to a previous chemotherapy line, because for these subjects – especially for adenocarcinoma patients (not included in Attraction-3) – pembrolizumab could really make the difference, considering also the very good safety profile when compared with chemotherapy. However, to date, pembrolizumab is not registered by regulatory agencies in the EU for this indication, and we still wait for the full paper publication.

34.11.4 Supportive and Palliative Care

A multidisciplinary evaluation is important in every step of natural history of esophageal cancers due to the particular worsening of condition that these diseases could produce. In fact, a nutritional support should be evaluated after all lines of treatment as well as the palliation of dysphagia or pain. The correct choice of nutritional support (enteral, parenteral, etc.) should involve a specialist in nutrition supportive care [64].

Patients can be considered for different options of palliative treatment depending on the clinical situation. Single-dose brachytherapy may be a preferred option to treat dysphagia even after external radiotherapy with fewer complications than metal stent placement. Other possible options in case of dysphagia are the local expansion, the position of prosthesis, and the laser therapy. The local expansion is frequently used to prepare to a prosthesis placement. The use of prosthesis leads to a rapid resolution of dysphagia, but is not indicated in case of cervical or junctional tumors or in case of trachea involvement. Laser therapy is used also to obtain hemostasis in addition to treatment of dysphagia.

34.11.5 Follow-Up

There is no standardized follow-up program for esophageal cancers, because there is no evidence that regular follow-up has an impact on survival outcomes. However, follow-up should concentrate on symptoms, nutrition, and psychosocial support also by multidisciplinary evaluations. Imaging should be obtained only if clinically indicated. This program might be done every 3 months for 2 years and every 6 months for the next 3 years. In the case of complete response to definite chemoradiotherapy or after resection, a 3-month follow-up based on symptoms, endoscopy, biopsies, and CT scan may be recommended to detect early recurrence.

Case Study: An Unusual Histotype

Man, 62 years old
- *Family history*: negative for malignancy
- *APR*: no comorbidities
- *APP*: for nearly 2 months dysphagia
- *Objective examination*: negative. Performance status 0 according to ECOG
- *Blood tests*: Hb 12.1 g/dL.
- *Esophagogastroduodenoscopy*: presence of ulcerative area at the cardia (Siewert II)
- *Pathological report*: squamous cell carcinoma
- *TC chest and abdomen mdc*: lesion at the cardia with multiple perigastric lymphadenopathies. No distant metastasis
- *18-PDG-PET*: uptake at the cardia (SUV max 6.5) and perilesional lymph nodes (SUV max 7.4)

- *Diagnosis*: locally advanced SCC

Question

What action should be taken?

(1) Surgery. (2) Neoadjuvant chemotherapy. (3) Neoadjuvant chemoradiotherapy

Answer

Neoadjuvant chemoradiotherapy

The patient received treatment with carboplatin AUC 2+ weekly paclitaxel (VII courses) integrated with 45 Gy radiotherapy in 25 fractions of 1.8 Gy.

Question

After neoadjuvant treatment, what action should be taken?

(1) Surgery. (2) Restaging

Answer

Restaging
- *Esophagogastroduodenoscopy*: partial response to treatment with decrease of lesion diameter
- *TC chest and abdomen mdc*: response to treatment at the level of primary lesion. Nodular lesion at VI segment of the liver (metastatic lesion)

- *18-PDG-PET*: decrease in the uptake at the cardia (SUV max 3) and perilesional lymph nodes (SUV max 4.5). Uptake at the level of VI segment of the liver (SUV 9.4) and some bone districts (8.1, right scapula, left ribs, and right femur)
- *TC with bone window*: confirmation of the metastatic bone lesions showed at 18-FDG-PET.

- *Clinical evaluation*: arise of bone pain in the sites of metastasis.
- *Diagnosis*: progression of disease despite the partial response on the primary tumors

Question

What action should be taken?

(1) First-line chemotherapy. (2) Definition of Her-2 status. (3) Surgery

Answer

- *Revision of histotype and the definition of Her-2 status were performed.*

- Squamous cell carcinoma was confirmed. Her-2 status (IHC): 0. Microsatellite stable (MSS) and PD-L1 negative.
- *First-line chemotherapy with FOLFOX schedule after multidisciplinary evaluation*: ongoing.
- *Treatment with inhibitors of RANKL (denosumab) was evaluated.*
- *Palliative bone radiotherapy was evaluated to treat pain.*

Key Points
- The importance of a correct diagnosis even in the case of unusual histotype
- The importance of a correct choose of treatment based on the histotype
- Importance of re-staging after neoadjuvant treatment and multidisciplinary evaluation.

Case Study: A 35-Year-Old Woman with a Metastatic Esophageal Cancer

Woman, 32 years old
- *Family history:* negative for malignancy
- *APR:* negative
- *APP:* weight loss of 10 kg in the last 3 months, fatigue
- *Blood tests:* Hb 9.4 g/dL
- *Clinical evaluation:* dysphagia, weight loss, and lumbar pain
- *Esophagogastroduodenoscopy:* presence of lesion at the level of thoracic esophagus
- *Pathological report:* carcinoma with squamous aspects

Question

What action should be taken?
(1) Surgery. (2) Neoadjuvant treatment. (3) Staging

Answer

Staging
- *TC chest and abdomen mdc:* involvement of esophageal wall in the thorax part, perilesional lymph nodes. No liver or lung lesions. Osteolytic lesion at L3-L4 level, suggesting metastasis

- *Scintigraphy:* uptake at levels of L3–L4. Metastatic disease
- *Bronchoscopy:* no lesions or fistulas

Question

What action should be taken?
(1) First-line chemotherapy. (2) Multidisciplinary approach. (3) Neoadjuvant treatment

Answer

Multidisciplinary approach
- *First-line chemotherapy with FOLFOX, ongoing*
- *Palliative radiotherapy on L3–L4 to treat pain*
- *Treatment with inhibitors of RANKL, ongoing*

Key Points

- A correct and complete staging is mandatory before starting treatment.
- Importance of multidisciplinary approach.
- Importance of treatment according to primary site and histotype.

34

Summary of Clinical Recommendations and Key Points

- **AIOM**
  - All patients with new dysphagia, gastrointestinal bleeding or emesis, weight loss, and/or loss of appetite should undergo an upper intestinal endoscopy.
  - Endoscopy with ultrasonography (EUS) should be done in all patients candidate to neoadjuvant treatment.
  - 18-FDG-PET could be used to assess the response to neoadjuvant treatment in addition to CT scan and EUS, but nowadays it does not represent a standard.
- **ESMO**
  - Surgery is the treatment of choice in limited disease. In patients with T1a AC, endoscopic therapy is the preferred therapeutic approach.
  - Neoadjuvant CRT with planned surgery or definitive CRT with close surveillance and salvage surgery for local tumor persistence or progression can be considered as a recommended definitive treatment for locally advanced SCC of the esophagus. Definitive CRT is recommended for cervically localized tumors.
  - For patients with esophageal AC, perioperative chemotherapy should be considered standard

in locally advanced AC of the esophagus, including esophagogastric junctional cancers.
- **NCCN**
  - All patients with R1 or R2 resection may be treated with fluorouracil-based chemoradiotherapy.
  - Chemotherapy with supportive care represents the standard treatment for metastatic patients with good PS. On the other hand, in case of poor PS, only best supportive care should be considered.
  - Trastuzumab should be used in case of Her-2-positive ADC. Other target therapies are not currently used.

References

1. Arnold M, Soerjomataram I, Ferlay J, et al. Global incidence of oesophageal cancer by histological subtype in 2012. Gut. 2015;64:381–7.
2. Huang Y, Guo W, Shi S, et al. Evaluation of the 7(th) edition of the UICC-AJCC tumor, node, metastasis classification for esophageal cancer in a Chinese cohort. J Thorac Dis. 2016;8:1672–80.
3. Lagergren J, Smyth E, Cunningham D, et al. Oesophageal cancer. Lancet. 2017;390:2383–96.
4. Liang H, Fan J-H, Qiao Y-L. Epidemiology, etiology, and prevention of esophageal squamous cell carcinoma in China. Cancer Biol Med. 2017;14:33–41.

5. Zhang Y. Epidemiology of esophageal cancer. World J Gastroenterol. 2013;19:5598–606.

6. DeSantis CE, Lin CC, Mariotsto AB, et al. Cancer treatment and survivorship statistics, 2014. CA Cancer J Clin. 2014;64:252–71.

7. Glenn TF. Esophageal cancer. Facts, figures, and screening. Gastroenterol Nurs. 2001;24:271–3; quiz 274–5.

8. Global Burden of Disease Cancer Collaboration. Global, regional, and national cancer incidence, mortality, years of life lost, years lived with disability, and disability-adjusted life-years for cancer groups, 1990 to 2015. A systematic analysis for the global burden of disease study 2015. JAMA Oncol. 2017;3(4):524–48.

9. Hashemian M, Poustchi H, Abnet CC, et al. Dietary intake of minerals and risk of esophageal squamous cell carcinoma: results from the Golestan Cohort Study. Am J Clin Nutr. 2015;102:102–8.

10. Haidry RJ, Butt MA, Dunn JM, et al. Improvement over time in outcomes for patients undergoing endoscopic therapy for Barrett's Esophagus related neoplasia; 6-year experience from the rst 500 patients treated in the UK patient registry. Gut. 2015;64:1192–9.

11. Abnet CC, Arnold M, Wei WQ. Epidemiology of esophageal squamous cell carcinoma. Gastroenterology. 2018;154(2): 360–73.

12. Yang CS, Chen X, Tu S. Etiology and prevention of esophageal cancer. Gastrointest Tumors. 2016;3:3–16.

13. Abbas G, Krasna M. Overview of esophageal cancer. Ann Cardiothorac Surg. 2017;6:131–6.

14. Prabhu A, Obi KO, Lieberman D, et al. The race-specific incidence of esophageal squamous cell carcinoma in individuals with exposure to tobacco and alcohol. Am J Gastroenterol. 2016;111:1718–25.

15. Kamangar F, Chow WH, Abnet CC, et al. Environmental causes of esophageal cancer. Gastroenterol Clin N Am. 2009;38:27–57.

16. Prabhu A, Obi KO, Rubenstein JH. The synergistic effects of alcohol and tobacco consumption on the risk of esophageal squamous cell carcinoma: a meta-analysis. Am J Gastroenterol. 2014;109:822–7.

17. Engel LS, Chow WH, Vaughan TL, et al. Population attributable risks of esophageal and gastric cancers. J Natl Cancer Inst. 2003;95:1404–13.

18. Hongo M, Nagasaki Y, Shoji T. Epidemiology of esophageal cancer: Orient to Occident. Effects of chronology, geography and ethnicity. J Gastroenterol Hepatol. 2009;24:729–35.

19. Liu X, Zhang M, Ying S, et al. Genetic alterations in esophageal tissues from squamous dysplasia to carcinoma. Gastroenterology. 2017;153(1):166–77.

20. Castro C, Peleteiro B, Lunet N. Modifiable factors and esophageal cancer: a systematic review of published meta-analyses. J Gastroenterol. 2018;53(1):37–51.

21. Xie SH, Lagergren J. A global assessment of the male predominance in esophageal adenocarcinoma. Oncotarget. 2016;7: 38876–83.

22. Domper Arnal MJ, Ferrández Arenas Á, Lanas Arbeloa Á. Esophageal cancer: risk factors, screening and endoscopic treatment in western and eastern countries. World J Gastroenterol. 2015;21:7933–43.

23. Runge TM, Abrams JA, Shaheen NJ. Epidemiology of Barrett's esophagus and esophageal adenocarcinoma. Gastroenterol Clin N Am. 2015;44:203–31.

24. Jain S, Dhingra S. Pathology of esophageal cancer and Barrett's esophagus. Ann Thorac Surg. 2017;6(2):99–109.

25. Ronkainen J, Aro P, Storskrubb T, et al. Prevalence of Barrett's esophagus in the general population: an endoscopic study. Gastroenterology. 2005;129(6):1825–31.

26. Spechler SJ, Sharma P, Souza RF, et al. American Gastroenterological Association medical position statement on the management of Barrett's Esophagus. Gastroenterology. 2011;140:1084–91.

27. Islami F, Fedirko V, Tramacere I, et al. Alcohol drinking and esophageal squamous cell carcinoma with focus on light-drinkers and never-smokers: a systematic review and meta-analysis. Int J Cancer. 2011;129:2473–84.

28. Kuwano H, Kato H, Miyazaki T, et al. Genetic alterations in esophageal Cancer. Surg Today. 2005;35:7–18.

29. Cancer Genome Atlas Research Network. Integrated genomic characterization of oesophageal carcinoma. Nature. 2017;541(7636):169–75.

30. Cancer Genome Atlas Research Network. Comprehensive molecular characterization of gastric adenocarcinoma. Nature. 2014;513(7517):202–9.

31. SEER training modules, Anatomy of the esophagus. U. S. National Institutes of Health, National Cancer Institute. 2018. https://training.seer.cancer.gov.

32. Siewert JR, Stein HJ. Classification of carcinoma of the oesophagogastric junction. Br J Surg. 1998;85:1457–9.

33. Rice TW, Kelsen DP, Blackstone EH, et al. Esophagus and esophagogastric junction. In: Amin MB, Edge SB, Greene FL, et al., editors. AJCC cancer staging manual. 8th ed. New York: Springer; 2017. p. 185–202.

34. Zum Büschenfelde CM, Herrmann K, Schuster T, et al. (18) F-FDG PET-guided salvage neoadjuvant radiochemotherapy of adenocarcinoma of the esophagogastric junction: the MUNICON II trial. J Nucl Med. 2011;52(8):1189–96.

35. Arends J, Bachmann P, Baracos V, et al. ESPEN guidelines on nutrition in cancer patients. Clin Nutr. 2017;36(1):11–48.

36. Skynner DB. Esophageal malignancies: experiences with 110 cases. Surg Clin North Am. 1976;56:137–47.

37. Brusselaers N, Mattsson F, Lagergren J. Hospital and surgeon volume in relation to long-term survival after oesophagectomy: systematic review and meta-analysis. Gut. 2014;63:1393–400.

38. Hulscher JB, Tijssen JG, Obertop H, et al. Transthoracic versus transhiatal resection for carcinoma of the esophagus: a meta analysis. Ann Thorac Surg. 2001;72(1):306–13.

39. Mariette C, Markar S, Dabakuyo-Yonli TS, et al. Hybrid minimally invasive vs. open esophagectomy for patients with esophageal cancer: long-term outcomes of a multicenter, open-label, randomized phase III controlled trial, the MIRO trial. Ann Oncol. 2017;28(suppl_5):v605–49.

40. Von Rahden BHA, Stein HJ, Siewert JR. Surgical management of esophagogastric junction tumors. World J Gastroenterol. 2006;12:6608–13.

41. Markar SR, Gronnier C, Pasquer A, et al. Role of neoadjuvant treatment in clinical T2N0M0 oesophageal cancer: results from a retrospective multi-center European study. Eur J Cancer. 2016;56:59–68.

42. Allum WH, Stenning SP, Bancewicz J, et al. Long-term results of a randomized trial of surgery with or without preoperative chemotherapy in esophageal cancer. J Clin Oncol. 2009;27:5062–7.

43. Mandard AM, Dalibard F, Mandard JC, et al. Pathologic assessment of tumor regression after preoperative chemoradiotherapy of esophageal carcinoma. Clinicopathologic correlations. Cancer. 1994;73:2680–6.

44. Sjoquist KM, Burmeister BH, Smithers BM, et al. Survival after neoadjuvant chemotherapy or chemoradiotherapy for resectable oesophageal carcinoma: an updated meta-analysis. Lancet Oncol. 2011;12:681–92.

45. van Hagen P, Hulshof MC, van Lanschot JJ, et al. Preoperative chemoradiotherapy for esophageal or junctional cancer. N Engl J Med. 2012;366:2074–84.

46. Bedenne L, Michel P, Bouché O, et al. Chemoradiation followed by surgery compared with chemoradiation alone in squamous cancer of the esophagus: FFCD 9102. J Clin Oncol. 2007;25:1160–8.

47. Stahl M, Stuschke M, Lehmann N, et al. Chemoradiation with and without surgery in patients with locally advanced squamous cell carcinoma of the esophagus. J Clin Oncol. 2005;23:2310–7.

48. Al-Batran SE, Hofheinz RD, Pauligk C, et al. Histopathological regression after neoadjuvant docetaxel, oxaliplatin, fluorouracil, and leucovorin versus epirubicin, cisplatin, and fluorouracil or capecitabine in patients with resectable gastric or gastro-oesophageal junction adenocarcinoma (FLOT4-AIO): results from the phase 2 part of a multicentre, open-label, randomised phase 2/3 trial. Lancet Oncol. 2016;17(12):1697–708.

49. Cunningham D, Allum WH, Stenning SP, et al. Perioperative chemotherapy versus surgery alone for resectable gastroesophageal cancer. N Engl J Med. 2006;355:11–20.

50. Ychou M, Boige V, Pignon JP, et al. Perioperative chemotherapy compared with surgery alone for resectable gastroesophageal adenocarcinoma: an FNCLCC and FFCD multicenter phase III trial. J Clin Oncol. 2011;29:1715–21.

51. Klevebro F, Alexandersson von Döbeln G, Wang N, et al. A randomized clinical trial of neoadjuvant chemotherapy versus neoadjuvant chemoradiotherapy for cancer of the oesophagus or gastro-oesophageal junction. Ann Oncol. 2016;27:660–7.

52. Stahl M, Walz MK, Riera-Knorrenschild J, et al. Preoperative chemotherapy versus chemoradiotherapy in locally advanced adenocarcinomas of the oesophagogastric junction (POET): long-term results of a controlled randomised trial. Eur J Cancer. 2017;81:183–90.

53. Stahl M, Walz MK, Stuschke M. Phase III comparison of preoperative chemotherapy compared with chemoradiotherapy in patients with locally advanced adenocarcinoma of the esophagogastric junction. J Clin Oncol. 2009;27(6):851–6.

54. Thuss-Patience PC, Kretzschmar A, Bichev D, et al. Survival advantage for irinotecan versus best supportive care as second-line chemotherapy in gastric cancer--a randomised phase III study of the Arbeitsgemeinschaft Internistische Onkologie (AIO). Eur J Cancer. 2011;47(15):2306–14.

55. Reddy D, Wainberg ZA. Targeted therapies for metastatic esophagogastric cancer. Curr Treat Options in Oncol. 2011;12:46–60.

56. Waddell T, Chau I, Cunningham D, et al. Epirubicin, oxaliplatin, and capecitabine with or without panitumumab for patients with previously untreated advanced oesophagogastric cancer (REAL3): a randomised, open-label phase 3 trial. Lancet Oncol. 2013;4:481–9.

57. Ilson DH, Kelsen D, Shah M. A phase 2 trial of erlotinib in patients with previously treated squamous cell and adenocarcinoma of the esophagus. Cancer. 2011;117(7):1409–14.

58. Bang YJ, Van Cutsem E, Feyereislova A, et al. Trastuzumab in combination with chemotherapy versus chemotherapy alone for treatment of HER2-positive advanced gastric or gastro-oesophageal junction cancer (ToGA): a phase 3, open-label, randomised controlled trial. Lancet. 2010;376:687–97.

59. Shah MA, Xu RH, Bang YJ, et al. HELOISE: phase IIIb randomized multicenter study comparing standard-of-care and higher-dose trastuzumab regimens combined with chemotherapy as first-line therapy in patients with human epidermal growth factor receptor 2-positive metastatic gastric or gastro-esophageal junction adenocarcinoma. J Clin Oncol. 2017;35(22):2558–67.

60. Safran H, DiPetrillo T, Akerman P, et al. PhaseI/II study of trastuzumab, paclitaxel, cisplatin, and radiation for locally advanced, Her2 overexpressing, esophageal adenocarcinoma. Int J Radiat Oncol Biol Phys. 2007;67:405–9.

61. Cunningham D, Stenning SP, Smyth EC. Peri-operative chemotherapy with or without bevacizumab in operable oesophagogastric adenocarcinoma (UK Medical Research Council ST03): primary analysis results of a multicentre, open-label, randomised phase 2-3 trial. Lancet Oncol. 2017;18(3):357–70.

62. Kato K, Cho BC, Takahashi M, et al. Nivolumab versus chemotherapy in patients with advanced oesophageal squamous cell carcinoma refractory or intolerant to previous chemotherapy (ATTRACTION-3): a multicentre, randomised, open-label, phase 3 trial. Lancet Oncol. 2019;20(11):1506–17.

63. Kojima T, Muro K, Francois E, et al. Pembrolizumab versus chemotherapy as second-line therapy for advanced esophageal cancer: the phase 3 KEYNOTE-181 study. 2019 Gastrointestinal Cancers Symposium. Abstract 2. Presented January 17, 2019.

64. Lordick F, Mariette C, Haustermans K, et al. Oesophageaal cancer: ESMO clinical practice guidelines for diagnosis, treatment and follow-up. Ann Oncol. 2016;27(suppl 5):50–7.

34

Gastric Cancer: Locoregional Disease

General Section. Locoregional Disease

Valerio Gristina, Nadia Barraco, Antonio Galvano, Daniele Fanale, Maria La Mantia, Marc Peeters, Albert J. ten Tije, Antonio Russo, and Jhony Alberto De La Cruz Vargas

Gastrointestinal Cancers

Contents

Valerio Gristina and Nadia Barraco should be considered equally co-first authors.

© Springer Nature Switzerland AG 2021
A. Russo et al. (eds.), *Practical Medical Oncology Textbook*, UNIPA Springer Series,
https://doi.org/10.1007/978-3-030-56051-5_35

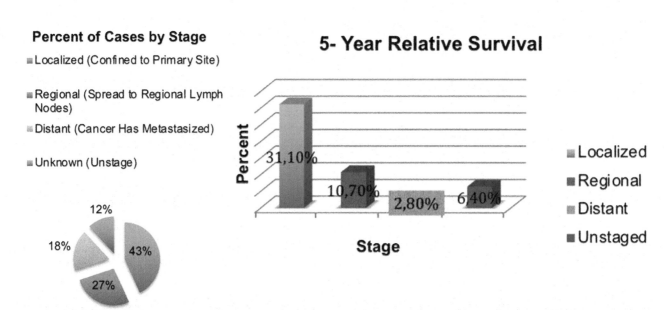

Learning Objectives

By the end of the chapter the reader will
- be able to apply diagnostic and therapeutic procedures
- have learned the basic concepts of gastric cancer
- have reached in depth knowledge of gastric cancer
- be able to put acquired knowledge into clinical practice.

35.1 Introduction

Gastric cancer (GC) is the fifth most common malignancy and the third most common cause of cancer-related death in both sexes with an incidence of about one million new cases worldwide [1].

Steady decline in incidence and mortality rates has been observed in most parts of the world [2], particularly limited to young patients affected by distal, sporadic, and intestinal type of GC [3]. Over the last few decades, while the incidence rate for cancers of cardia and gastroesophageal junction (GEJ) has been on a rapid upsurge and the incidence of distal GC has fallen in Western countries, the reverse occurred in Asian countries [4, 5].

By far, the large majority (about 90%) of all GCs belong to the group of adenocarcinomas, histologically classified into two major types (intestinal-type and diffuse-type) with distinct morphologic appearance, pathogenesis, and genetic profiles [6]. While diffuse-type GCs are more often determined by genetic abnormalities. Few cases (about <10%) of GCs are associated with inherited predisposition syndromes. Most of intestinal-type GCs are sporadic, mainly triggered by long-standing inflammatory conditions that result in a sequential progression from normal gastric mucosa through chronic gastritis, chronic atrophic gastritis, and intestinal metaplasia to dysplasia and carcinoma [7].

Prognosis remains dismal except in a few countries since this multifactorial tumor, with both environmental and genetic causative factors, often presents at an advanced stage of disease [8, 9] (◘ Fig. 35.1). Despite showing similar clinical-pathological characteristics and treatments, survival rates vary from 10% to 30% in European countries [10], whereas in Asian countries much higher 5-year overall survival rates have been achieved by screening endoscopic examinations and consecutive early tumor resection [11].

Moreover, notwithstanding different epidemiology and to a certain extent different histologic features, the clinical management of GC does not take differences into account with the only potentially curative treatment approach represented by surgical resection with adequate lymphadenectomy. Current evidence seems to support perioperative therapies to improve survival in patients affected by locally advanced disease. Finally, considering that unresectable or metastatic GC could solely and regrettably benefit only from life-prolonging palliative therapy regimens; prevention and early diagnosis are the most promising strategies for GC control.

35.2 Epidemiology

Anatomically, the stomach begins at the gastroesophageal junction or GEJ (so-called Z-line, a poorly defined anatomic area separating the lower esophagus from the

◘ **Fig. 35.1** Worldwide percentage of GC cases and 5-year survival rate by stage at diagnosis

cardia or proximal part of the stomach) and ends at the pylorus (the distal part of the stomach that connects to the duodenum).

The incidence and mortality rates for GC world wide have considerably changed over the past years, showing wide geographical variation (◙ Fig. 35.2).

— GC used to represent the most common neoplasm and the leading cause of cancer-related death through most of the twentieth century, now ranking third to lung and liver cancer [1] and showing an overall relative 5-year survival rate of approximately 30% in most parts of the world [12].

— More than 70% of cases chiefly occur in developing countries and half the world total appears to arise in Eastern Asia (mainly in China).

— Age-standardized incidence rates are about twice as high in men as in women [1].

— The highest estimated mortality rates are present in both sexes in Eastern Asia, Central and Eastern Europe, and in Central and South America, with lower rates in Western Europe and in Northern America [1] (◙ Fig. 35.3)

— In Japan, a mass screening program has been implemented since the 1960s, and early detection of

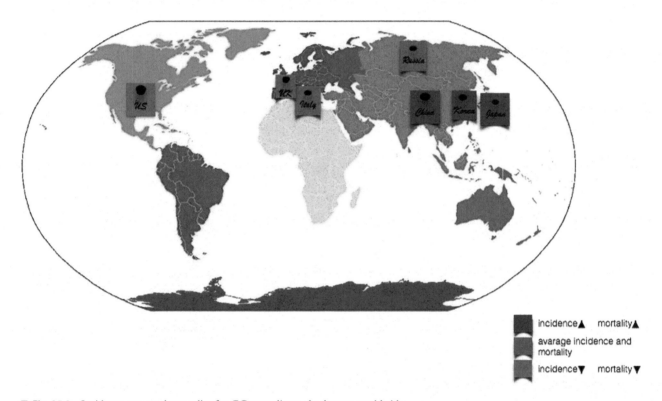

incidence▲   mortality▲

avarage incidence and mortality

incidence▼   mortality▼

◙ **Fig. 35.2** Incidence rates and mortality for GC according to both sexes worldwide

◙ **Fig. 35.3** Cancer-related deaths according to both sexes in the European Union

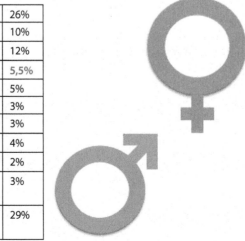

LUNG	26%
PROSTATE	10%
CRC	12%
STOMACH	5,5%
PANCREAS	5%
LEUKEMIA	3%
LIVER	3%
BLADDER	4%
KIDNEY	2%
NONH. LIMPHOMA	3%
OTHER SITES	29%

LUNG	13%
BREAST	17%
CRC	13%
PANCREAS	7%
OVARY	5%
STOMACH	5%
NONH LIMPHOMA	3%
UTERINE BODY	2%
MELANOMA	1%
OTHER SITES	35%

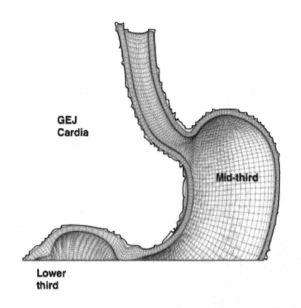

Subtypes	Risk factor		Incidence
GEJ, Cardia:	reflux, tobacco, fat diet	⬆	Western countries
Non-cardia intestinal-type:	HP	⬆	Asia, Russia and part of EU
		⬇	Western countries
Non-cardia diffuse-type:	loss of *CDH1*	⬇	Western countries

◘ Fig. 35.4   The heterogeneity of GC epidemiology

the disease combined with improved operative techniques has led to a significant decrease in mortality.

— In Western countries, the incidence of distal GC has steadily declined potentially because of changes in diet, improved food preparation, anti-*Helicobacter pylori* therapies and earlier diagnosis of smaller lesions; on the other hand, the incidence rates of proximal GC has strikingly increased since cardia lesions are not associated with *H. pylori* infection [13] (◘ Fig. 35.4).

— *H. pylori* accounts for at least 300,000 new cases of GC each year worldwide. Nonetheless, epidemiological studies report that only 2–3% of *H. pylori*-infected individuals eventually develop GC [14].

— Non cardia lesions seem to be more common in male, blacks, lower socioeconomic status and developing countries [15].

— Diffuse-type GC is more often seen in female and young individuals [16], while the intestinal-type adenocarcinoma is more often associated with intestinal metaplasia and Helicobacter pylori infection [17] (◘ Fig. 35.4).

— Death rate estimates for the year 2019 from gastric cancer show the most favorable declines, with a 17.1% decrease in men and a 13.7% in women since 2014 [18].

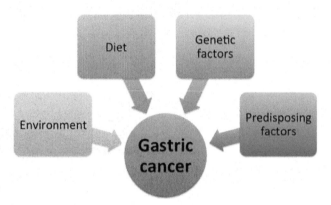

◘ Fig. 35.5   Multifactorial etiology in GC

35.3 Etiology and Prevention

The development of GC is a multifactor process associated with a large number of risk factors (◘ Fig. 35.5).

— Age was shown to be positively associated with a risk of gastric cancer (cardiac and non-cardiac) [19].

— Environmental exposure in early life together with the accumulation of specific genetic alterations and other cultural factors are essential in determining the risk and the predisposition to GC [20]. Several studies showed how immigrants gradually acquire the incidence rates of the country to which they move [21].

- Excessive intake of salt or salty food, low consumption of fresh fruits and vegetables likely contribute to the development of gastric cancer, while high intake of fresh fruits and vegetables, Mediterranean diet, a low-sodium diet, salt-preserved food, red and high cured meat, moderate alcohol drinking, and maintaining a proper body mass index might be significantly associated with a decreased risk of GC [22–24]. Low gastric acidity may additionally increase intraluminal formation of N-nitroso compounds (from preserved food or endogenous nitrates), which are recognized as mutagens and carcinogens [25] (◘ Fig. 35.6).
- Several studies have confirmed that tobacco smoking increases the risk of GC, both cardia and non-cardia subtypes, particularly in male [26, 27].
- Disparate data regarding occupational exposures suggested that coal and tin mining, metal processing (particularly steel and iron), and rubber manufacturing industries may lead to an increased risk of gastric cancer.
- *H. pylori* is a Gram-negative, flagellated, microaerophilic bacterium considered as a major predisposing factor for GC, increasing from three- to sixfold the risk for development of gastric carcinoma [28].
- Epstein-Barr virus (EBV) is a ubiquitous human herpes virus with oncogenic activity, which has been associated with about 10% of all gastric carcinoma cases. These EBV+ tumors are characterized by a diffuse-type histology with lymphoid infiltration (lymphoepithelioma-like carcinoma) and predominantly located in the non-antrum part of the stomach as superficial depressed (or ulcerated) lesions [29].
- Other predisposing factors, such as atrophic gastritis, gastric ulcer disease (sometimes related to *H. pylori* infection), partial gastrectomy, and Ménétrier's disease were additionally reported to increase the risk of GC [30]. In addition, adenomatous polyps of the fundic glands are considered dysplastic and most consistently associated with a cancerous transformation, mainly in the intestinal-type phenotype and in patients with familial adenomatous polyposis.
- Familiar studies have found that the risk of developing GC for relatives of cases is increased two- to threefold, suggesting a role of genetic factors [31,

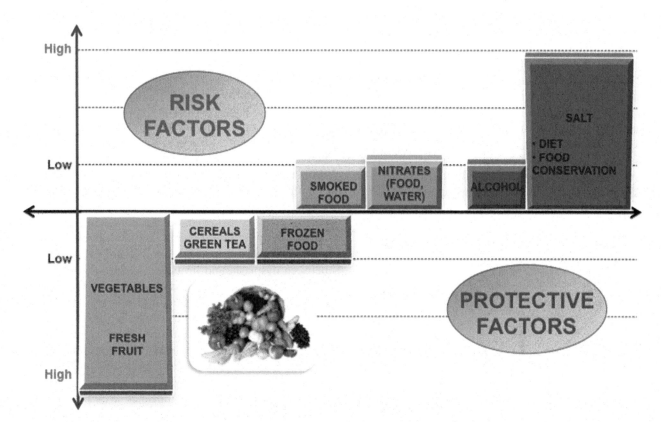

◘ **Fig. 35.6** Role of lifestyle and dietary habits in determining the risk of GC

32]. Nevertheless, an inherited genetic predisposition is found in a small proportion of cases with relevant syndromes, including hereditary non-polyposis colorectal cancer, familial adenomatous polyposis colorectal cancer, hereditary diffuse gastric cancer (HDGC), gastric adenocarcinoma and proximal polyposis of the stomach (GAPPS) and Peutz Jegher's syndrome.

Prevention is a key strategy to reduce GC-related mortality. The eradication of *H. pylori* infection and a healthy lifestyle appear to be the major primary preventive interventions, whereas mass screening programs (including also serum pepsinogen evaluation and endoscopic screening) have been strikingly successful in high-risk areas, especially in Japan [33]. Moreover, serological diagnostic tests are currently available, not only informing us of the presence of *H. Pylori* but also of the microenvironment of the gastric mucosa and its possible variations: normal mucosa, gastroesophageal reflux, *H. Pylori* infection, and gastric atrophy [34].

35.4 Carcinogenesis

GC is generally viewed as the consequence of a multifactorial and multistep process, involving the host responses, bacterial virulence, diet, environmental, and other predisposing factors.

According to the general hypothesis of sporadic carcinogenesis of intestinal-type GC proposed by Correa [7], the transition from normal mucosa to non-atrophic gastritis (triggered primarily by *H. pylori* infection but also by dietary factors, chemical agents, or autoimmune diseases), initiates precancerous lesions which may then progress to atrophic gastritis and intestinal metaplasia (◘ Fig. 35.7). Specifically, the basic components of the process are: chronic active non-atrophic gastritis, multi-

focal atrophy, intestinal metaplasia (first complete, then incomplete), dysplasia or advanced precancerous lesions (APLs; currently distinguished into low-grade [LG-IEN] and high-grade intraepithelial neoplasia [HG-IEN]), invasive carcinoma [35, 36].

H. pylori is not found in normal stomachs, but very frequently found in patients affected by chronic gastritis, even if only a minor proportion of individuals progress through the pre-neoplastic cascade [37]. *H. pylori* infection seems to play a causative role at the early phases of carcinogenesis in the intestinal-type of GC, as suggested by the significant regression of atrophic gastritis and initial precancerous lesions after antibiotic-mediated eradication of H. pylori [38]; however, no longer effective once the disease has progressed to the stage of intestinal metaplasia [39].

In the sporadic setting, the first stage of the neoplastic cascade consists of an active chronic inflammatory response to injury [40] (◘ Fig. 35.8). *H. pylori* infection, through the action of a variety of bacterial virulence factors (such as urease, vacuolating cytotoxin A [VacA], cag pathogenicity island, cytotoxin-associated gene A [CagA], bacterial gamma-glutamyl transpeptidase [GGT]) [41, 42] and higher level of production of free radicals, recruits inflammatory cells to the host gastric mucosa, promotes gastric cell apoptosis, and reduces epithelial cell turnover, thus resulting in superficial gastritis without atrophy and gastric atrophy (defined as loss of appropriate glands, such as mucosecreting and oxyntic glands in the antrum and in the corpus of the stomach, respectively) in the majority of infected cells. Furthermore, it has been hypothesized that the initial stages of inflammation and atrophy create an abnormal microenvironment favoring engraftment of bone marrow-derived cells (BMDCs) harboring an eventual neoplastic invasive behavior [43]. Additionally, loss of glandular structures may be subsequently replaced with glands inappropriate to the location (intestinal metaplasia), reflecting a sort of an adaption to a chronic injury, but conferring a high risk for the development of dysplasia and invasive gastric cancer. So far, the distinction between dysplasia and invasive GC relies essentially in the fact that fully-developed cancer shows histological evidence of stromal invasion/infiltration by neoplastic cells into the *lamina propria*, while the different grades of dysplasia have been recently redefined as an intraepithelial/intraglandular neoplasia confined by the basal membrane of the dysplastic glands and without any apparent metastatic potency [36].

Moreover, GEJ cancers appear to arise from foci of incomplete intestinal metaplasia that may be additionally triggered by gastroesophageal reflux disease (GERD) either in the distal esophagus or in the proximal stomach. In the distal esophagus of GERD patients, the chronic reflux causes inflammation of the squamous

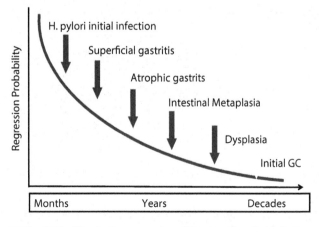

◘ **Fig. 35.7** Histologic progression of human *H. pylori* infection from the early stages of inflammation to invasive GC

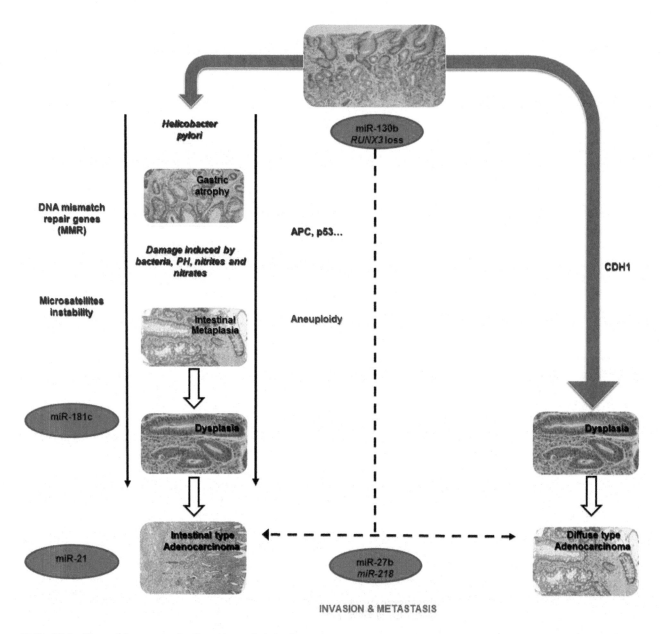

Fig. 35.8 The multi-step cascade of gastric carcinogenesis

epithelium, which is replaced by columnar epithelium as a result of metaplastic reaction, a condition known as Barrett's esophagus [44] that harbors a cumulative risk of progression to invasive cancer [45] (Fig. 35.9).

To a lesser extent, links of diffuse-type GC with atrophic gastritis or intestinal metaplasia are poor, or do not exist. Moreover, cell adhesion proteins (expressed at the adherence junctions of epithelial tissue and required for development, cell differentiation, and maintenance of epithelial architecture) seemed to act as suppressors of tumor invasion and metastasis. Indeed, a very small proportion of GCs (about 1–3%) can be caused by a specific germ-line mutation of the E-cadherin gene (*CDH1*) that harbors a 60–70% lifetime cumulative risk of advanced

diffuse GC clinically resulting in a cancer syndrome, the hereditary diffuse gastric cancer (HDGC) [46] (Fig. 35.8).

The pathogenesis of GC involves multi-step genetic and epigenetic alterations, which predispose cells to neoplastic transformation. Nevertheless, molecular mechanisms underlying disease tumorigenesis and progression are still not completely understood. MicroRNAs (miRNAs), a class of small noncoding RNAs with 18–24 nucleotides, which can cause mRNA degradation or translational inhibition, seem to play a role in inflammation, cell proliferation, apoptosis regulation, and differentiation. Given the importance of miRNAs in the regulation of cell growth and viability, miRNA dysregu-

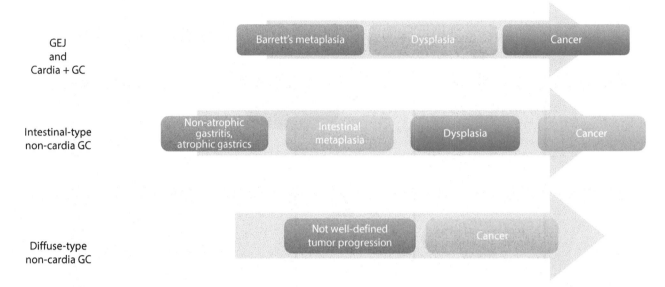

Fig. 35.9 Tumor progression models for GC

lation is believed to be closely correlated with the development and progression of gastric cancer [47]. Likewise most tumors, a growing body of evidence reveals how miRNAs influence the expression of tumor suppressor genes and oncogenes, possibly contributing to initiation and progression of GC (e.g., *miR-21* was found to be associated in the development of GC while *miR-130b* and *miR-301a* seemed to downregulate the expression of *RUNX3*, a known tumor suppressor silenced by promoter hypermethylation, leading to poor differentiated GC) [48] (◘ Fig. 35.8).

35.5 Clinical Presentation

Because of the lack of specific symptoms that could characterize GC, most of patients are commonly diagnosed with advanced disease, presenting with a combination of signs and symptoms that are not unequivocally suggestive for GC. Nonetheless, alarm symptoms, such as dysphagia, weight loss, and palpable abdominal mass appeared to be independently associated with survival and mortality [49].

Weight loss and abdominal pain are the most common symptoms at initial presentation and should not be underestimated, since weight loss seemed to be significantly associated with shorter survival [50]. Loss of appetite, fatigue, epigastric discomfort, postprandial fullness, heart burn, indigestion, nausea, and vomiting are often related to spread of disease. Dyspeptic symptoms, such as gastroesophageal reflux, peptic ulcer dis-

ease, and functional dyspepsia can be related to GC only in a few cases.

Occasionally, symptoms may be suggestive for a lesion at a specific site in some patients. As a matter of fact, a history of dysphagia or pseudoachalasia may correlate with a cancer of the cardia extending through the GEJ. Early satiety, even if not so frequent in GC patients, could be indicative of a loss of distensibility of the gastric wall due to a diffusely infiltrative tumor, whereas later satiety and vomiting may indicate pyloric involvement. Although gastrointestinal bleeding is uncommon, hematemesis and anemia do occur in approximately 10–15% of patients.

GCs can spread by local extension to adjacent structures and can develop lymphatic, peritoneal, and distant metastases. Diffuse peritoneal spread leading to a large ovarian mass (Krukenberg's tumor) or a large peritoneal implant in the pelvis (Blumer's shelf) can produce symptoms of colorectal obstruction. Ascites, jaundice, and palpable mass are sadly related to incurable disease. Furthermore, metastatic nodules to subcutaneous tissue around the umbilicus (Sister Mary Joseph's node) or supraclavicular lymph node (Virchow's node) traditionally suggest the status of an advanced disease.

35.6 Histopathology Overview

The term *gastric cancer* usually refers to adenocarcinoma of the stomach since most of these tumors (approximately 95%) represent malignant epithelial neo-

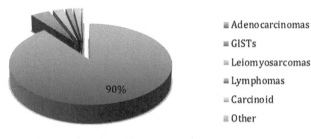

■ Adenocarcinomas
■ GISTs
■ Leiomyosarcomas
■ Lymphomas
■ Carcinoid
■ Other

Fig. 35.10 Histologic subtypes of gastric cancer

plasms, originating from glandular epithelium of the gastric mucosa. Other malignant tumors are rare and include carcinoid tumors, leiomyosarcomas, and gastrointestinal stromal tumors. Interestingly, the stomach is the most common site for lymphomas of the gastrointestinal tract in spite of the absence of lymphoid tissue in the normal gastric mucosa (■ Fig. 35.10).

Several schemes have been proposed based on the morphologic (the Japanese and the Paris classification for EGCs, the Borrmann classification for advanced GC) and pathologic features (Lauren's and the World Health Organization classification) of gastric tumors. On the other hand, other classifications based on a cellular level (such as Goseki's and Ming's) have not been proven to be superior to the preexisting systems [51].

35.6.1 Macroscopic Aspects

Concerning early gastric cancer (EGC), the neoplasms are grossly classified into Type I for the tumor with protruding growth, Type II with superficial growth (further

divided in elevated, flat, or depressed) and Type III with excavating growth, according to the Japanese Endoscopic Society [52] (■ Fig. 35.11). In addition, a more recent Paris classification, investigating also other superficial neoplastic lesions in the gastrointestinal tract, divided grossly and endoscopically the tumor as Type 0-I for polypoid growth (which is subcategorized to 0-Ip for pedunculated growth and 0-Is for sessile growth), Type 0-II for non-polypoid growth (which is subcategorized into Type 0-IIa for slightly elevated growth, Type 0-IIb for flat growth, and Type 0-IIc for slightly depressed growth) and Type 0-III for excavated growth [53].

Regarding more advanced tumors, the Borrmann classification divides GC into five types depending on macroscopic appearance and seems to be a valuable predictor for lymph node metastasis and survival [54]. Type I represents polypoid or fungating cancers (7–8%), Type II encompasses ulcerating lesions surrounded by elevated borders (30%), Type III represents ulcerated lesions infiltrating the gastric wall (30–40%), Type IV are diffusely infiltrating tumors (10–20%) and Type V are unclassifiable cancers.

35.6.2 Microscopic Aspects

Historically, the most widely used classification is by Laurén who first divided GC into either intestinal or diffuse form characterizing two varieties of tumors that distinctively present with different pathology, epidemiology, etiologies, and genetics [6] (■ Fig. 35.12); later, the indeterminate type was included to describe an uncommon histology. While the intestinal variety repre-

Fig. 35.11 Endoscopic classification of early gastric cancers. (Photos by courtesy of Prof. G. Genova, Surgical Oncology Unit-Department of Surgical, Oncological and Orals Sciences, University of Palermo)

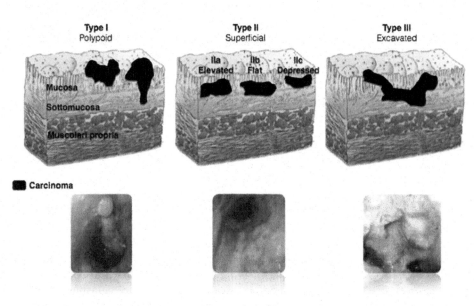

Fig. 35.12 The two histological subtypes of GC proposed by Lauren (1965). (Photos by courtesy of Prof. A. Martorana, Department of Health Promotion, Mother and Child Care, Internal Medicine and Medical Specialties, Pathologic Anatomy Unit-University of Palermo)

INTESTINAL-TYPE

✓ Older patients
✓ Most frequently in higher incidence areas
✓ Male
✓ Expansive growth pattern
✓ Intestinal metaplasia
✓ Better prognosis

DIFFUSE-TYPE

✓ Younger patients
✓ Most frequently in lower incidence areas
✓ Both sexes
✓ Infiltrative growth pattern
✓ Not intestinal metaplasia
✓ Worse prognosis

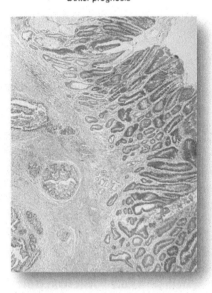

35

sents a differentiated cancer with a tendency to form glands (similarly to colon type), the diffuse form exhibits very little cell cohesion with a predilection for extensive submucosal spread and early metastases.

Even if all other GC types of lower frequency have been included (uncommon and mixed histologic variants), four major types are currently recognized by the WHO classification: papillary, tubular, mucinous adenocarcinoma, and poorly cohesive carcinoma (with or without signet ring cells) [55].

35.7 **Diagnosis and Staging**

Careful clinical staging is critical to ensure that patients are appropriately selected for treatment interventions, as outlined in the most recent international guidelines. As described below, the clinical stage in the 8th edition of TNM staging is defined prior to treatment based on endoscopy imaging (**Fig. 35.13a, b).**

Endoscopic ultrasound (EUS) provides evidence of depth and extension of tumoral invasion (T) and presence of abnormal or enlarged lymph nodes (N), which is crucial for deciding whether to administer preoperative therapy or to undergo potential endoscopic approaches in the light of an acceptable accuracy in distinguishing T1 from T2–T4 lesions; however, the diagnostic accuracy of EUS is operator-dependent, less useful in antral tumors, and only occasionally able to highlight signs of

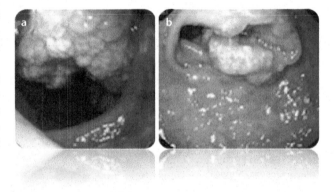

Fig. 35.13 **a**, **b** Diagnostic endoscopies are performed to determine the presence and the location of GC and biopsy for any suspicious lesions. (Photos by courtesy of Prof. G. Genova, Surgical Oncology Unit-Department of Surgical, Oncological and Oral Sciences, University of Palermo)

distant spread (M) [56]. Even if suboptimal in distant lymph nodes evaluation given the limited depth and visualization of the transducer, EUS readily identifies malignant perigastric lymph nodes (hypoechoic, round shape, smooth, distinct margin and size >1 cm). The combination of endoscopic nodal features, along with the use of fine needle-aspiration (FNA) biopsy for cytology assessment, significantly increases the accuracy of the diagnosis [57].

Contrast-enhanced computed tomography (CT) scan of thorax, abdomen, and pelvis is routinely used for preoperative staging showing a satisfactory overall accuracy for T staging. Nonetheless, CT is less consistently accurate than EUS for the diagnosis of malignant lymph nodes showing a variable sensitivity [58], even if eventually identifying some nodal characteristics suggestive for malignancy (short-axis diameter 6–8 mm in perigastric lymph nodes round shape, central necrosis, heterogeneous or high enhancement) [59].

Combined positron emission tomography (PET) – CT imaging may improve staging by showing an improved specificity in detecting involved lymph nodes or metastatic disease. However, PET may not be informative in patients with mucinous or diffuse tumors because of the low tracer accumulation.

Laparoscopy along with peritoneal washings is recommended to exclude radiologically occult metastatic disease for clinical stage higher than T1b when chemoradiation or surgery is indicated; the benefit may be greater for patients with T3/T4 disease [60].

35.8 Staging Systems, Classification, and Prognosis

Concerning GC patients surgically treated, two pathologic systems are currently used: the Japanese system and the American joint Committee on Cancer/Union for International Cancer Control (AJCC/UICC). While the former is more elaborate and based on anatomic involvement (particularly the lymph node stations), the latter is the system used in Western countries and more accurately estimates prognosis.

In the AJCC/UICC staging system, tumor (T) stage, which reflects the depth of tumor invasion into the gastric wall and extension into adjacent structures, is strictly related to survival rates (◘ Fig. 35.14).

Moreover, nodal (N) stage, which is determined by the number of involved lymph nodes (a minimum of 15 examined lymph nodes is recommended for adequate staging), appeared to predict outcome more accurately than the location of affected lymph nodes (◘ Fig. 35.15).

To date, the most important change made to the last 8th edition concerned stage III, detailing N3 staging into N3a (7–15 positive lymph nodes) and N3b (more than 15 lymph nodes) in the final pathologic stage, since they may represent diseases of differing severity (◘ Table 35.1). For example, involvement of ≥16 lymph nodes (N3b) was associated with worse outcomes than cases involving 7–15 positive nodes (N3a) according to 5-year survival rates.

Referring to Siewert's classification of GEJ cancers [61] (◘ Fig. 35.16), the current 8th American Joint Committee on Cancer (AJCC) classification has staged adenocarcinomas with epicenters no more than 2 cm into the gastric cardia as esophageal cancers, and those extending further as stomach cancers [62]. As opposed to the last AJCC classification system that ranks Siewert type 2 tumors with EGJ invasion as esophageal cancer whereas Siewert type 2 tumors without EGJ invasion and Siewert type 3 tumors as gastric cancer, the new stage grouping of the IGCA (The International Gastric

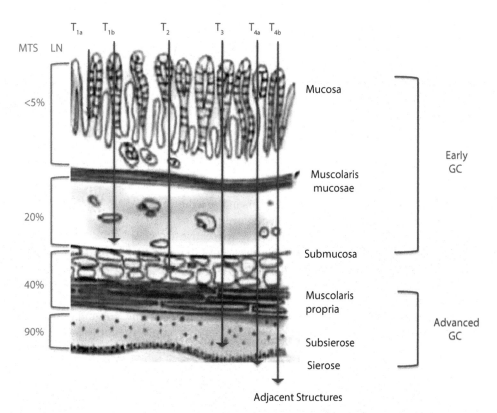

◘ **Fig. 35.14** Tumoral staging according to the 8th edition AJCC TNM system (2016)

◘ Fig. 35.15 Lymph node staging according to the 8th edition AJCC TNM system (2016)

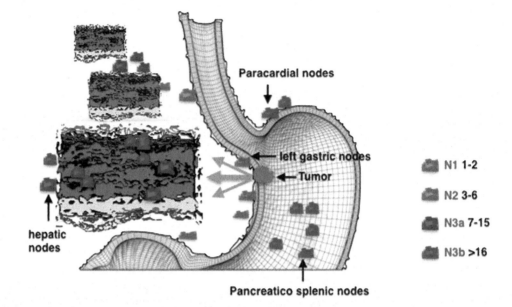

Paracardial nodes

left gastric nodes

Tumor

hepatic nodes

Pancreatico splenic nodes

N1 1-2

N2 3-6

N3a 7-15

N3b >16

◘ Table 35.1 AJCC stage and TNM subgroup distributions of the patients according to the 8th edition of the TNM classification

Stage	Subgroup
STAGE IA	T1N0M0
STAGE IB	T1N1M0, T2N0M0
STAGE IIA	T1N2M0, T2N1M0, T3N0M0
STAGE IIB	T1N3aM0, T2N2M0, T3N1M0, T4aN0M0
STAGE IIIA	T2N3aM0, T3N2M0, T4aN1M0, T4aN2M0, T4bN0M0
STAGE IIIB	T1N3bM0, T2N3bM0, T3/4N3aM0, T4bN1/2M0
STADIO IIIC	T4aN3bM0, T4bN3a/bM0
STADIO IV	any T, any N, M1

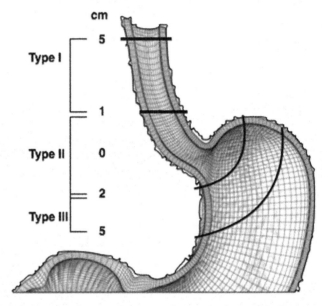

cm

5

Type I

1

Type II   0

2

Type III

5

◘ Fig. 35.16 According to Siewert's classification, cancers arising from the GEJ are anatomically classified in adenocarcinoma of the distal esophagus (type I: epicenter located within between 1–5 cm above the anatomic GEJ), true carcinoma of the cardia (type II: within 1 cm above and 2 cm below the junction) and subcardial carcinoma (type III: 2–5 cm below the junction)

Cancer Association) recommended the use of the GC staging for both Siewert type 2 and 3 tumors in the light of the not significantly different patients' overall survival and risk stratification [63]. Of note, a retrospective study suggested that cardiac carcinoma involving GEJ or distal esophagus could be more appropriately classified and staged as gastric rather than esophageal cancers, at least in the Chinese population [64]. However, more studies are warranted also in the light of the different molecular profiling and clinical follow-up data of both tumors.

35.9   Molecular Biology

GC patients can be classified according to clinical-pathological parameters together with the evaluation of serum CEA and CA-19-9 levels to predict prognosis [65] and to choose the therapeutic strategy. As regards patients with metastatic disease, the histological diagnosis should include the evaluation of HER-2 status from tumor tissues and plasma. Currently, the evaluation of HER-2 status in tumor tissues represents the only approved molecular biomarker taken into account by clinicians to decide the medical therapy and to predict its efficacy. Moreover, circulating tumor-derived cell-free DNA (the fraction of cell-free DNA that originates from primary tumors, metastases or from circulating tumor cells [66]) for HER2 analysis has been recently recommended in clinical practice as surrogate biomarker [67]. Nevertheless, the identification of new potential diagnostic, prognostic, and predictive molecular biomarkers represents a new challenge for current translational research. Recently, advances in next-generation sequencing technologies have enabled The Cancer Genome Atlas (TCGA) Research Network to classify GC tissue samples in four subtypes: chromosomal instability (CIN) GC (50%), microsatellite instability (MSI)+ GC (22%), genomically stable (GS) GC (20%), and Epstein-Barr Virus (EBV)+ GC (9%) [68]. These four distinct genomic subtypes appeared to differ for several genetic and epigenetic changes:

- The CIN tumors were found to be mainly located in the GEJ/cardia and show intestinal-type features. They exhibited higher prevalence of *TP53* mutations and elevated phosphorylation of epidermal growth factor receptor (*EGFR*). These tumors have a considerable number of genomic amplifications of cell cycle regulation genes, key receptor tyrosine kinases, and transcription factors [69, 70].
- The MSI+ tumors, characterized by genomic instability with high frequency of mutations due to malfunctioning in the DNA repair mechanisms. These types of GC showed to have targetable hotspot

mutations in *PIK3CA*, *ERBB2*, and *EGFR*, hypermethylation in the *MLH1* promoter region, and overexpression of PD-L1 [69].
- The GS tumors showed diffuse-type features and have been associated with expression changes of molecules such as *CDH1* and *RHOA* (Ras homolog gene family, member A) gene that proved to be involved in cell adhesion and angiogenesis-related signaling pathway, respectively. These alterations might contribute to lack of cellular cohesion, uncontrolled growth, and escape to programmed cell death [69].
- The EBV+ tumors are characterized by PIK3CA mutations, extreme DNA hypermethylation, amplification of JAK2 and overexpression of both PD-L1 and PD-L2. In EBV-associated gastric carcinoma (EBVaGC), tumor cells may evade immune reactions via the PD-1/PD-L1 immune check point pathway. The cellular DNA methylation status in EBVaGC is strictly regulated by EBV infection in epithelial gastric cells. In tumor cells, EBV infection alters the mRNA expression profile, including the expression of microRNAs and long non-coding RNAs (lncRNAs) [71].

These results represented an interesting contribution to research, which aims to further personalize the management and treatment of patients with GC (◘ Fig. 35.17).

Moreover, since the stomach harbors an abundant quantity of blood vessels, endothelial progenitor cells (EPCs), endothelial cells (ECs), vascular endothelial growth factor (VEGF), and microvessels density (MVD) may be used as candidate diagnostic and prognostic biomarkers for GC. Indeed, the evaluation of blood vessels

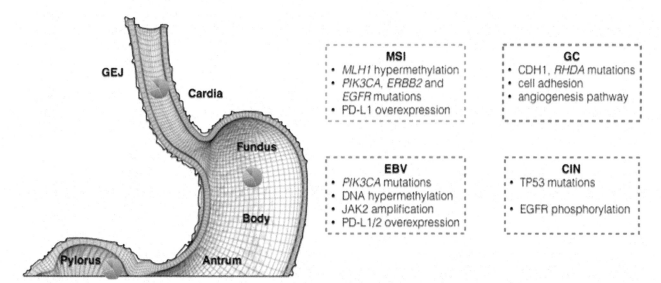

◘ **Fig. 35.17** Distribution of GC molecular subtypes according to The Cancer Genome Atlas (TCGA) Research Network

quantity and VEGF level expression along with EPCs and ECs number in patients' peripheral blood seemed to be significantly associated with TNM stage, invasion depth, and lymph node metastasis [72].

At last, the non-coding component seemed to play a key role in promoting cell growth, cell cycle progression and metastasis in GC. The TCGA analyzed miRNA expression profiles of GC tissues. Several miRNAs have shown deregulation in GC tissues and have been listed in TCGA data portal [65]. Among them, the *miR-196a*, *miR-21* (inhibiting the tumor-suppressor genes *PDCD4* that encodes a protein involved in the control of cell growth and invasion) and *miR-106a* (that positively regulates the G1-to-S transition) were revealed to be significantly overexpressed, while *miR-101* (activating *COX2* which stimulates cell proliferation) and *let-7a* appeared to be down-regulated in GC tumor samples when compared to normal tissues [73]. The expression of miRNAs seemed to be epigenetically regulated by the methylation status in gastric cancer cells [74]. A growing body of evidence has recently demonstrated that high expression levels of circulating miRNAs, evaluated in pre-operative serum and other body fluids samples, are consistent with GC tissues and turned out to be significantly reduced following surgery. Thus, miRNAs are emerging as possible noninvasive biomarkers for GC diagnosis and treatment [65]. Recent data have also shown that other emerging classes of non-coding RNA, such as lncRNA, could represent a new, valid, and largely unexplored field of investigation. LncRNAs have been arbitrarily defined according to their size, as transcribed RNA molecules greater than 200 nucleotides in length. LncRNAs regulate gene expression through mechanisms that are mostly poorly understood [75, 76]. Higher expression levels of circulating *H19*, *HOTAIR*, *MALAT1*, *HULC*, *UCA1* lncRNAs have been detected in plasma of GC patients compared to healthy controls. Overexpression of these lncRNAs was associated with proliferation, tumor metastasis, apoptosis, worse survival among GC specimens, indicating that the lncRNAs could be useful diagnostic and prognostic biomarkers [74].

In addition, immunotherapeutic agents, targeting new biological molecules, such as PD-1 and PD-L1 that would lead to immune suppression, have been recently used for treating GC patients. This strategy is showing promising results in on-going randomized clinical trials [77] (Fig. 35.18).

35.10 Treatment

GC is clinically classified as early or advanced stage to help determine appropriate intervention. Surgical resection remains the main form of curative treatment whenever feasible. However, despite advances made in

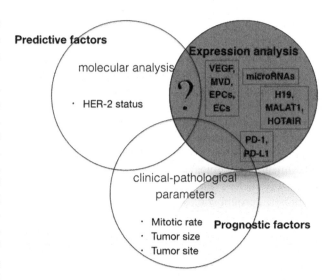

Fig. 35.18 The Diagram of Venn aims to link predictive factors with prognostic factors to assess the potential prognostic or predictive role of microRNAs, lncRNAs, or other molecular biology expression levels

treatment strategies over past decades, the majority of patients are diagnosed at advanced stages, reflecting poor overall survival rates. In Western countries, 55–65% of patients present with locally advanced or metastatic disease. This is in contrast to Japan, where diagnosis usually occurs at an earlier stage and the majority of patients (68%) present with resectable disease. Consequently, there is an East–West division in both the surgical and medical management of gastric cancer (Fig. 35.19).

The extent of resection along with lymphadenectomy could be potentially curative and strictly depends on the assessment of the preoperative stage. Presence of comorbidities, nutritional status, and geriatric frailty should be evaluated and taken into account in the surgical risk assessment [78]. Over the past decades, not only surgical efforts have been implemented to improve patients' survival but medical oncology has also contributed a great deal with neoadjuvant and adjuvant chemotherapeutic regimens.

35.10.1 Endoscopic Therapies

EGC is defined as invasive carcinoma confined to mucosa and/or submucosa, with or without lymph node involvement and irrespective of the tumor size. Most EGCs are small (measuring 1 to 5 cm in size) and often located at lesser curvature around angularis.

There are two forms of endoscopic resection widely accepted as standard treatment for clearly confined to the mucosa, well differentiated, ≤2 cm and non-ulcerated EGCs: endoscopic mucosal resection (EMR) and

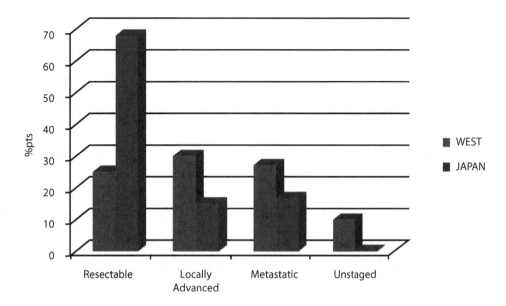

Fig. 35.19 Differences between Western and Japanese GC stage at first diagnosis

Table 35.2 Survival rates and lymph node involvement incidence in EGCs

EGC subtype	N+ incidence	5 year survival rates	
Intramucosal	3–4%	N+	90%
		N–	93%–95%~
Submucosal	19–22%	N+	80%
		N-	~90%

endoscopic submucosal dissection (ESD) have been used as valid alternatives to surgery for selected patients in medical centers with extensive experiences. According to the European Society of Gastrointestinal Endoscopy, very early gastric cancers smaller than 10–15 mm with a very low probability of advanced histology may undergo EMR since the associated lymph node metastatic risk in this group is quite low, even though ESD is strongly recommended as first-line treatment for all gastric superficial neoplastic lesions since it allows high rates of en bloc R0 curative resection with a good safety profile [79]. Thus, while EMR is minimally invasive, cost effective, and well tolerated but associated with a high local recurrence rate for incomplete resection, ESD results in higher rates of en bloc resection and histologically complete resection with low local recurrence rates but also showing higher rates of perforation and extended operation time [80]. After all, long-term survival does not appear to be compromised by the chosen technique and showed an excellent prognosis with high 5-year survival rates and very low metastatic risk (**Table 35.2**).

35.10.2 Surgery

Surgery is the cornerstone treatment for gastric malignancy, representing the only chance for cure in patients with localized resectable disease. Gastrectomy with complete margin resection of macro/microscopic tumor (R0) along with systematic lymphadenectomy is considered to be the only curative treatment, especially in early-stage disease with favorable prognosis (stage IB-III). As described below, perioperative therapies should be evaluated for these patients.

The extent of gastric resection depends on the site and size of the primary tumor, mainly considering that surgical morbidity was reported to be as high as about 30–40% [81] and complications after curative surgery showed a negative effect on overall and disease specific survival [82]. Therefore, subtotal gastrectomy for mid-distal third GC showed similar long-term survival results compared to total gastrectomy, with lower morbidity and mortality rates and improved postoperative quality of life as well as higher calorie intake and better nutritional status [83–85]. Hence, when the general goal of a macroscopic proximal margin of 5 cm between the tumor and the EGJ can be achieved without any microscopic (R1) or gross residual disease (R2) by a gastric-preserving approach, partial gastrectomy is preferred over total gastrecomy, especially for distal GCs (for diffuse-type cancers, a margin of 8 cm is advocated).

Nonetheless, total gastrectomy should be indicated in poorly differentiated tumors located in the angularis portion of the stomach (at high risk of microscopic invasion of the GEJ), in patients affected by multicentric disease, and/or distally located cancers with multiple lymph node metastases (in order to allow an extended lymph node dissection). Moreover, distal pancreatectomy with splenectomy for gastric cancer was found to be related to high morbidity and poor prognosis and should not be performed, except when the primary tumor directly invades spleen and/or pancreas or definite gross lymph node metastases are present [86]. Additionally, total gastrectomy has also been advocated as a prophylactic treatment in the event of hereditary diffuse gastric cancer [87].

Concerning localized tumors of proximal stomach, the optimal surgical procedure would consist of proximal gastrectomy or total gastrectomy that seemed to be both associated with postoperative nutritional impairment.

Of interest, laparoscopic gastrectomy proved to be a safe and technically feasible procedure with a shorter hospital stay and fewer complications than open surgery. Even if associated with increased likelihood of receiving adjuvant systemic therapy when indicated and not apparently affecting lymph node staging, a higher incidence of microscopic margin positivity (above all in diffuse-type GC) was reported and long-term survival rates are yet to be determined [88, 89]. Similarly, future prospective studies and long-term results are needed to better evaluate the oncological adequacy of robotic gastric resection that was revealed not to be inferior to laparoscopic gastrectomy, except for the longer operation time and higher costs [90].

■ **Lymph Node Dissection**
Unlike the extent of resection of the primary tumor, lymph node status and ratio are considered the most important surgical prognostic factor in advanced GC [91–93].

There has been intense debate surrounding the extent of lymphadenectomy suggesting that a more extensive dissection with the removal of an adequate number of nodes (15 or greater) may be both beneficial for staging purposes (to assign a final N pathologic stage) and associated with improved long-term survival [94, 95]. Depending on the mapped location and resection of metastatic lymph nodes, the Japanese Research Society for Gastric Cancer briefly classified the lymph node dissection at the time of gastrectomy as D1 (removal of the perigastric lymph nodes), D2 (D1 plus removal of those nodes along the left gastric, common hepatic and splenic arteries and the coeliac axis) and D0 (incomplete removal of perigastric lymph nodes) [96]. The benefits of a more extended D3 (D2 plus para-aortic nodal dissection) dissection had not been clearly demonstrated in the light of similar survival rates and higher incidence of complications when compared to D2 resection [97].

Whereas in Asian countries D2 dissection is deemed to be a standard treatment because of superior outcomes observed in randomized trials when compared to D1, none of the prospective randomized clinical trials executed in the West initially demonstrated survival advantage for more extensive lymphadenectomy. Nonetheless, fewer loco-regional recurrences and gastric cancer-related deaths were reported with D2 resection in spite of higher postoperative mortality, morbidity, and re-operation rates. However, subgroup analyses from these European trials appeared to suggest that D2 resection might be a better choice in patients affected by an advanced disease with lymph node metastases, as confirmed by long-term follow-up data [98–100]. Moreover, recent findings from an Italian systematic review and meta-analysis supported the superiority of D2 versus D1 dissection in terms of survival benefit, even if mainly limiting the advantage to the disease-specific survival and also not considering the interaction with other factors affecting patients' survival (such as complementary medical therapy) [101]. In addition, two other studies from Western countries reported longer 5-year and 10-year survival rates in the D2 group [102–104].

In summary, in the Western countries, medically fit patients affected by localized resectable GC should undergo D2 dissection that is carried out in specialized, high-volume centers with appropriate surgical expertise and postoperative care, as stated by the American and European guidelines. Notably, considering that the number of metastatic lymph nodes increases with the depth of tumor invasion through the gastric wall and EGCs showed a very low rate of lymph node involvement, a less extensive dissection could be considered in patients with T1 cancer and clinical node-negative disease (D1+, with removal of local N2 nodes according to the site of cancer).

35.10.3 Combined Modality Treatment

As stated before, many patients regrettably present with locally advanced tumors at diagnosis. In this setting, perioperative (pre- and postoperative) or neoadjuvant treatments have been considered in the last decade as attractive concepts for primary tumor downstaging, improving R0 resection rates and treating micrometastatic disease early.

Thus, considering the poor 5-year survival rate for advanced stages of GC [105] and the increasing likelihood of local recurrence or distant metastases even after macroscopic resection of the primary tumor [106], a multimodality approach, including perioperative chemotherapy or chemoradiation, has been suggested as the standard treatment for locally advanced GCs in most oncological centers today and recommended in several national guidelines (☐ Figs. 35.20 and 35.21).

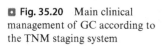

■ **Fig. 35.20** Main clinical management of GC according to the TNM staging system

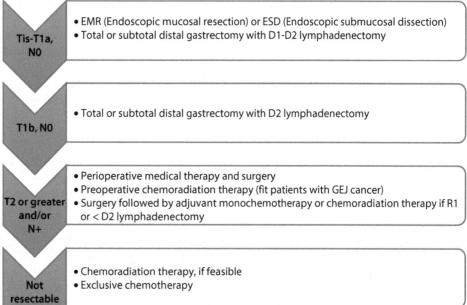

Tis-T1a, N0
- EMR (Endoscopic mucosal resection) or ESD (Endoscopic submucosal dissection)
- Total or subtotal distal gastrectomy with D1-D2 lymphadenectomy

T1b, N0
- Total or subtotal distal gastrectomy with D2 lymphadenectomy

T2 or greater and/or N+
- Perioperative medical therapy and surgery
- Preoperative chemoradiation therapy (fit patients with GEJ cancer)
- Surgery followed by adjuvant monochemotherapy or chemoradiation therapy if R1 or < D2 lymphadenectomy

Not resectable patients
- Chemoradiation therapy, if feasible
- Exclusive chemotherapy

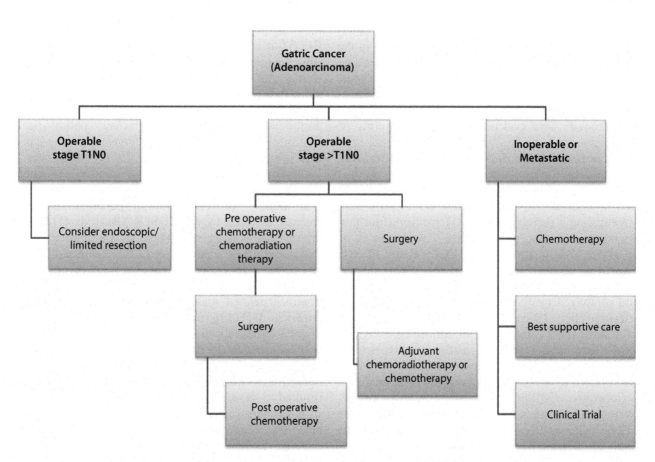

■ **Fig. 35.21** Overview of GC treatment algorithm

■ **Perioperative Treatment**

The use of perioperative chemotherapy with a platinum/fluoropyrimidine combination has been supported by the results of the MAGIC [107] and FNCLCC-FFCD [108] randomized clinical trials that documented both an improvement in 5-year overall survival rate and a disease-free survival benefit after a median of six cycles of perioperative chemotherapy (three preoperative and three postoperative 3-week cycles of epirubicin, cisplatin, and 5-fluorouracil [5-FU] or cisplatin and 5-FU, respectively) compared to surgery alone, mostly in case of a clinically suspected lymph node involvement (cN+) or a clinical TNM stage 3 or higher (cT3+). Notwithstanding, in both trials the 5-year survival rate of chemotherapy-arms appeared to be even lower than those reported in international series after only adequate curative surgery with extended lymph node dissection. In addition, perioperative chemotherapy effects seemed to be much more evident for GEJ cancers, therefore claiming for further high-volume sample-size multicenter randomized clinical trials.

Capecitabine-containing regimens and other platinum/fluoropyrimidine doublets or triplets can also be suggested in the perioperative setting (as ECX [epirubicin, cisplatin, capecitabine] or EOX [epirubicin, oxaliplatin, capecitabine], in preference to ECF), since, in the advanced disease, capecitabine and oxaliplatin resulted not to be inferior to 5-fluorouracil and cisplatin, respectively [109]. However, dose intensification with taxanes or with prolonged ECX regimen in the perioperative setting showed some evidence of benefit in terms of progression-free survival, disease-free survival, and tumor regression at resection, but this did not translate into an overall survival improvement [110].

More recently, results from the German randomized, multicenter, open-label phase 2/3 FLOT4 trial, investigating a perioperative FLOT regimen (four preoperative and four postoperative 2-week cycles of docetaxel, oxaliplatin, and 5-FU) versus ECX/F, showed significantly higher proportion of pathological complete response, increased rate of curative surgery, and prolonged median survival rates in patients with advanced clinical stage cT2 or higher and/or nodal positive stage (cN+), intestinal- or diffuse-type GC. In locally advanced, resectable gastric or gastroesophageal junction adenocarcinoma, perioperative FLOT has revealed to improve overall survival compared with perioperative ECF/ECX (50 vs. 35 months, respectively), rates in patients with advanced clinical stage cT2 or higher and/or nodal positive stage (cN+), intestinal- or diffuse-type GC. In locally advanced, resectable gastric or gastroesophageal junction adenocarcinoma, perioperative FLOT has revealed to improve overall survival compared with perioperative

ECF/ECX, reporting an acceptable drug-specific toxicity profile with no increase in surgical morbidity and mortality [111]. Accordingly, FLOT4 should be considered the new standard of care in the perioperative treatment of GC patients with a good performance status. Nonetheless, any platinum/fluoropyrimidine doublet or triplet before surgery may be reasonable with the belief that the choice of the compound should be only addressed according to the side effect profile of the cytostatic agents. In any case, the duration should be 2–3 months each for the neoadjuvant and for the adjuvant part [112].

Of interest, the novel fluoropyrimidine S-1 containing tegafur (an inactive 5-FU prodrug) and the two enzyme inhibitors, gimeracil and oteracil, proved to be effective as infusional 5-FU with an improved safety profile [113]. Data on S-1, licensed only in combination with cisplatin in advanced GC, are limited to Asian patients since this drug appeared to be curiously more toxic in western patients requiring the administration of lower doses. Finally, no evidence in the perioperative setting supported the use of those targeted therapies which significantly improved the palliative treatment of advanced GC. Furthermore, the ongoing phase III FLOT5/Renaissance and FLOT6 trials from the German AIO group will possibly answer the question whether additional surgery would confer a survival benefit over chemotherapy alone in GC patients with oligometastatic disease and if the addition of trastuzumab and pertuzumab to perioperative FLOT would affect pathological response and survival in HER2-overexpressing cancers, respectively.

Considering radiation therapy as an integral part of the treatment, the value of preoperative chemoradiation therapy for resectable GC patients has been recently assessed by the TOPGEAR study [114], an international prospective phase III randomized trial that underlined the advantage of delivering radiotherapy in the preoperative rather than postoperative setting. As a matter of fact, unlike the potential late treatment-related toxic effects showed in the North American INT0116 trial where adjuvant fluoropyrimidine-based therapy was administered in combination with conventionally fractionated RT [115], interim results of the TOPGEAR trial demonstrated that preoperative chemoradiation added to perioperative ECF resulted to be safe and feasible, not adversely affecting surgical compliance and morbidity while not increasing hematologic and non-hematologic toxicities. Further ongoing randomized trials investigating the uncertain role of preoperative chemoradiation are under evaluation in order to select the most promising strategy, especially in resectable GC (the CRITICS II trial).

■ **Adjuvant Treatment**

The use of chemoradiation in the postoperative setting is somewhat controversial. Although currently considered as standard therapy in the USA, this treatment approach has not been widely accepted in Europe due to concerns regarding toxicity. As supported by both the subgroup analyses of the INT0116 and the retrospective data from the Dutch Gastric Cancer Group trial [116], postoperative chemoradiation seemed to compensate mainly for suboptimal surgery reducing local recurrence rate after D1 resection, whereas not providing any benefit following D2 resection. So far, no strong evidence of survival benefit of chemoradiation over chemotherapy alone was demonstrated in the ARTIST trial [117], even though interim results of a phase III study (the ARTIST II trial) have recently shown that adjuvant chemotherapy (S-1 plus oxaliplatin) and/or chemoradiotherapy (S-1 plus oxaliplatin and RT) are effective in prolonging disease-free survival, when compared to S-1 monotherapy, in Asian patients with curatively resected D2, stage II/III, node-positive GC. While significantly reducing mortality and risk of tumor recurrence in terms of overall and relapse-free survival improvement when compared to surgery alone [115], the combination of radiotherapy with chemotherapeutic agents entailed a higher rate of hematologic and gastrointestinal toxicities and did not highlight a clear advantage over chemotherapy alone [118]. Hence, other alternative postoperative chemoradiation regimens have been evaluated suggesting the use of capecitabine with concurrent radiation therapy as a safe and well-tolerated option in resected GC patients. In addition, the randomized phase III CRITICS trial concluded that the addition of postoperative radiation therapy did not add any benefit in patients who have undergone preoperative chemotherapy [119].

Postoperative chemotherapy following D2 resection has not been historically associated with significant survival benefit [120–122], considering also that this approach is less well tolerated than neoadjuvant treatment. Interestingly, curative surgery alone showed very good survival rates in patients with T1 cancer [123]. However, two large randomized phase III trials conducted in Asia changed the landscape of postsurgical chemotherapy for resectable GC, reporting an improved survival benefit after curative D2 lymph node dissection in patients affected by stage II and III gastric cancer. Specifically, while the Japanese ACTS-GC trial evaluated S-1 showing the greatest survival benefit for node-negative disease [124], the Korean CLASSIC trial investigated a capecitabine-oxaliplatin doublet indicating the greatest survival benefit in N1-2 disease [125]. Moreover, results from the randomized phase III POST Trial have recently suggested that an S-1 based doublet (with cisplatin or docetaxel) could be an effective and tolerable option in Asian patients with curatively

resected stage III gastric cancer [126]. In a large individual patient-level meta-analysis [127], chemotherapy based on fluorouracil regimens was associated with a 6% absolute benefit compared with surgery alone and could be consequently recommended in stage II and III GC patients who have undergone optimal surgery without the administration of preoperative treatment.

35.11 Follow-Up

Mainly considering that an improvement in survival outcomes has not been demonstrated for all types of cancers and no randomized controlled trials have been published for GC patients, the role of follow-up is still controversial and no real consensus exists. The main goal of a regular follow-up program is to diagnose local or metachronous cancer recurrence early, promptly detecting any adverse effects or treatment-related complications, while collecting data concerning cancer history and treatment outcomes.

Most relapses used to occur within the first 2–3 years, and nearly all relapses occurring by 5 years are not surgically curable. Specifically, recurrence patterns may be generally classified into locoregional recurrence (at the proximal/distal resection margin or in the adjacent tissue of the surgical bed), distant or hematogenous metastases, peritoneum implanting, and nodal recurrence (within the regional and distant lymph nodes) [128, 129] (◘ Fig. 35.22).

Due to the lack of strong evidence, several regimens have been proposed and international guidelines slightly differ from each other. However, follow-up strategies should be always tailored to both the individual patient and the stage of the disease. The follow-up surveillance panel should be generally based on an interim history and physical examination, repeated every 3 to 6 months for the first postoperative 2 years and every 6 to 12 months for at least 5 years, thereafter annually. Complete blood chemistry lab tests along with tumor marker assays, such as CEA and Ca 19.9, are simple and inexpensive to perform, often occur earlier than imaging abnormalities, but specificity and sensitivity are quite low. Either abdominal ultrasonography or CT could be considered every 6 months, while endoscopic surveillance, especially after the endoscopic treatment of early gastric cancer, should be performed annually [130]. Likewise, endoscopic surveillance should be offered to precancerous lesions according to risk factors for progression toward gastric cancer. In case of suspected relapse/disease progression or significant clinical deterioration, physical examination along with direct blood tests and radiologic investigations should be carried out. *HER-2* testing is only recommended in metastatic or advanced disease (◘ Fig. 35.23).

Fig. 35.22 Most frequent sites of disease recurrence in GC

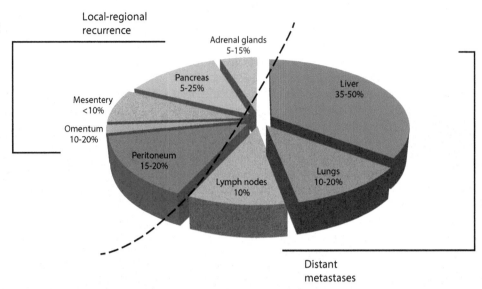

Fig. 35.23 Follow-up, long-term implications and survivorship

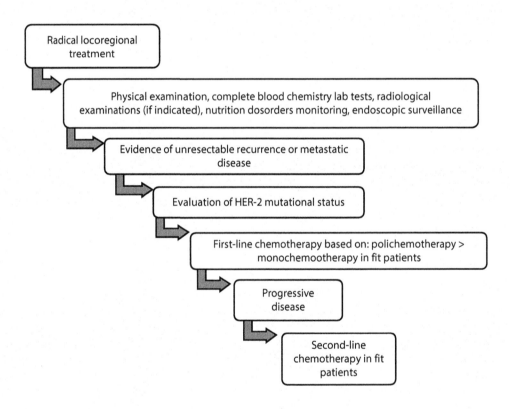

In addition, a proper follow-up program should allow the detection and the prompt treatment of long-term adverse effects following the primary therapy, such as digestive problems (dyspepsia, nausea, vomiting, early satiety, reflux, anorexia), post-gastrectomy syndromes (dumping syndrome, bile reflux, Roux-en-Y stasis syndrome, and afferent and efferent loop syndromes), malabsorption (iron deficiency or megaloblastic anemia in approximately 30% of patients, osteopenia, or osteoporosis) or psychological disorders. Similarly, a dietary support for patients on either a radical treatment or palliative pathway with reference to vitamin and mineral deficiencies is recommended.

Finally, further studies are warranted to better characterize the expression of vascular endothelial growth factors along with the role of several microRNAs (miRNA-328) [131] and various genes (E-cadherin [132] and cyclin E [133]) as potential biomarkers for recurrence after curative resection, allowing personalization of follow-up according to the individual risk of relapse.

Case Study: Management of a Patient Affected by Early Gastric Cancer

Male, 65 years old

- *Family history* negative for malignancies
- *PMH:* former tobacco smoker, systemic arterial hypertension
- *RMH:* Complaints of severe fatigue and nausea
- *Objective examination:* normal physical examination, except pale oral and scleral mucosa
- *Blood tests:* low hemoglobin (9.8 mg/dL) and ferritin (3.9 mg/dL) level, normal biochemical tests

Question

What action should be taken?

(1) Abdominal ultrasound. (2) Upper gastrointestinal endoscopy. (3) Abdominal computed tomography scan with contrast

Answer

Upper gastrointestinal endoscopy (for determining the etiology of the iron deficiency anemia)

An 8 mm erythematous, flat-elevated area was seen in the cardia and biopsy was obtained from the lesion. Histopathological examination confirmed well-differentiated adenocarcinoma from biopsy material, pT1Nx.

Question

What will be the next step?

(1) Endoscopic mucosal resection (EMR). (2) Subtotal gastrectomy + lymphadenectomy. (3) Endoscopic submucosal dissection (ESD)

Answer

Very early gastric cancers smaller than 10–15 mm with a very low probability of advanced histology may undergo *endoscopic mucosal resection (EMR)* since the associated lymph node metastatic risk in this group is quite low. ESD results in higher rates of en bloc resection and histologically complete resection with low local recurrence rates but also showing higher rates of perforation and extended operation time.

Question

What action should be taken after endoscopic resection?

(1) Chemotherapy. (2) Radiation therapy. (3) Endoscopic surveillance

Answer

The role of biannual or annual *endoscopic surveillance* has been well established since patients who undergo endoscopic treatment of EGC are at risk for synchronous and metachronous multiple cancers. To the contrary, however, the role of computed tomographic (CT) surveillance has not yet been well determined.

Key Points

- Start with medical history, physical examination, and diagnostic work-up.
- Endoscopic approaches remain the cornerstone of early gastric cancer initial treatment.
- Early detection and treatment contribute to decreased mortality rates.
- Follow-up strategies should be always tailored to both the individual patient and the stage of the disease.

Case Study: Management of Locally Advanced Gastric Cancer Successfully Treated by Combined Modality Treatment

Male, 54 years old.

- *Family history* positive for malignancy (mother's history of colon cancer).
- *PMH:* occupational exposure to iron processing, active tobacco smoker, no prior GI-tract disease, no drugs.
- *RMH:* a 4-month history of upper abdominal discomfort, mild nausea, anorexia, and weight loss.
- *Physical examination:* all normal findings.
- *Laboratory tests:* no abnormalities except for an increased CA 19-9 to 108 U/ml (normal range up to 39 U/ml).

- *Staging:* esophagogastroduodenoscopy revealed a 4 × 8 cm mass along the lesser curvature of the stomach, extending into the EGJ. The mass was confirmed on endoscopic ultrasound (EUS) and was staged as cT3N1 based on the presence of gastrohepatic lymphadenopathy measuring up to 1.2 cm in maximum diameter. A biopsy confirmed a poorly differentiated invasive adenocarcinoma with signet ring features. Additionally, computed tomography (CT) of the chest, abdomen, and pelvis showed no hepatic lesions and/or involvement of other organs.

Question

What action should be taken?

(1) Subtotal gastrectomy + lymphadenectomy. (2) Laparoscopy with peritoneal washings. (3) PET-FDG

Answer

Laparoscopy along with peritoneal washings is recommended to exclude radiologically occult metastatic disease for clinical stage higher than T1b when chemoradiation or surgery is indicated; the benefit may be greater for patients with T3/T4 disease since positive cytology can be present in about a third of cases and denotes M1 disease, which portends a poor prognosis, even if this is the only site of metastasis.

The preoperative peritoneal washing cytology produced a negative result.

Question

What action should be taken?

(1) Subtotal gastrectomy + lymphadenectomy. (2) Perioperative FLOTx4. (3) Perioperative ECF

Answer

In locally advanced, resectable gastric, or gastroesophageal junction adenocarcinoma, *perioperative FLOT* has revealed to improve overall survival compared with perioperative ECF/ECX (50 vs. 35 months, respectively), reporting an acceptable drug-specific toxicity profile with no increase in surgical morbidity and mortality [111]. Accordingly, FLOTx4 should be now considered the new standard of care in the perioperative treatment of GC patients with a good performance status.

Question

What will be the next step?

(1) Total gastrectomy + D2 lymphadenectomy. (2) Partial gastrectomy + lymphadenectomy. (3) Total gastrectomy + distal pancreasectomy and splenectomy

Answer

Total gastrectomy should be indicated in poorly differentiated tumors located in the angularis portion of the stomach (at high risk of microscopic invasion of the GEJ). *D2 lymphadenectomy* might be a better choice in patients affected by an advanced disease with lymph node metastases. Distal pancreatectomy with splenectomy for gastric cancer was found to be related to high morbidity and poor prognosis.

Final pathology revealed a tumor staged as yT2N0 with negative margins and 0/16 lymph nodes positive for metastatic disease, Stage IIA. The patient's postoperative staging did not show any evidence of disease and he was closely followed with adjuvant treatment.

Key Points

- The importance of proper clinical management in locally advanced GC.
- Consider imaging techniques for an appropriate preoperative staging.
- Multidisciplinary treatment is crucial for locally advanced GC.
- Understand the role of surgery along with lymphadenectomy as a part of both staging and treatment strategy.
- The choice of the most effective and tailored perioperative treatment is crucial for the patients' clinical outcome.

Expert Opinion
Antonio Russo

Key Points
- The global incidence of GC shows a wide geographical variation with the highest rates occurring in East Asia, while decreasing incidence and mortality in the vast majority of the developed world have been observed for non cardiac GC.
- Classification based on anatomic location and histologic subtypes has significant implications for therapy,
- New staging recommendations according to the 8th edition of the American Joint Committee on Cancer (AJCC) dramatically affects prognosis and treatment decisions.
- A multimodal approach has been implemented into the clinical practice to refine the management of locoregional disease with perioperative chemotherapy representing the standard therapy in curatively intended disease.

- Radical gastrectomy with D2 lymph node dissection has become the standard surgery in most high-volume centers

Summary of Clinical Recommendations

- Prevention and early diagnosis may be the most promising strategies for cancer control and key strategies to reduce mortality.
- Most of patients are commonly diagnosed with advanced disease, presenting with a combination of signs and symptoms that are not unequivocally suggestive for GC. Weight loss and abdominal pain are the most common symptoms at initial presentation.
- Careful clinical staging is critical to ensure that patients are appropriately selected for treatment interventions.
- Endoscopic resection is a curative option for early gastric neoplastic lesions. Surgery is the cornerstone treatment for gastric malignancy, representing the only chance for cure in patients with localized resectable disease. Lymph node status and ratio are considered the most important surgical prognostic factor in advanced GC.
- A multimodality approach including perioperative chemotherapy or chemoradiation has been suggested as the standard treatment for locally advanced GCs in most oncological centers today and recommended in several national guidelines.

Hints for Deeper Insight

Based on the exciting results reported in the metastatic setting, targeted agents and immunotherapy have been investigated in the perioperative approach in order to improve survival rates of such patients.

HER-2 status has not shown to be either predictive or prognostic in the neoadjuvant setting, even if ongoing clinical trials are currently investigating the role of trastuzumab together with pertuzumab in addition to FLOT- and XELOX-based regimens (PETRARCA and INNOVATION trials). As concerns antiangiogenic agents, bevacizumab was not associated with OS benefit when added to chemotherapy as perioperative treatment (UK MRC ST03 trial), whereas the RAMSES trial is currently evaluating ramucirumab in the perioperative treatment of Her-2 negative gastric and GEJ adenocarcinomas. Furthermore, the Phase III KEYNOTE-585

and the Phase I/II ICONIC trials are currently investigating the efficacy and the safety of pembrolizumab plus chemotherapy or FLOT and avelumab plus FLOT, respectively, in the perioperative management of gastric cancer.

To date, the most important and debated issue is the research of prognostic and predictive factors that might affect the efficacy of perioperative treatments, enabling the appropriate and prompt selection of patients for surgery and/or multimodality approach. In this field, the use of 18-fluorodeoxyglucose positron emission tomography (18-FDG-PET) scan as a predictor of early response to neoadjuvant treatment has been associated with a prognostic meaning rather that predictive, highlighting the biological aggressiveness of the tumors in non-responder patients and finally leading to a worse outcome.

The use of next-generation sequencing (NGS) has not been clearly supported by sufficient data at the time of initial diagnosis for the clinical decision-making process in the locoregional disease. The genomic and molecular characterization of gastric cancer (TCGA) has not found applications in daily clinical practice and further studies are needed to translate these findings for the management of patients. The prognostic and predictive roles of both microsatellites (MSI) and programmed cell death ligand-1 (PD-L1) are implicated in the management of the metastatic disease.

Suggested Reading

1. Al-Batran S-E, Homann N, Pauligk C, et al. Perioperative chemotherapy with fluorouracil plus leucovorin, oxaliplatin, and docetaxel versus fluorouracil or capecitabine plus cisplatin and epirubicin for locally advanced, resectable gastric or gastro-oesophageal junction adenocarcinoma (FLOT4): a randomised, phase 2/3 trial. Lancet 2019

2. Tirino G, Pompella L, Petrillo A, Laterza MM, Pappalardo A, Caterino M, Orditura M, Ciardiello F, Galizia G, De Vita F. What's new in gastric cancer: the therapeutic implications of molecular classifications and future perspectives. Int J Mol Sci. 2018;7:19

3. Ilson DH. Advances in the treatment of gastric cancer: 2019. Curr Opin Gastroenterol. 2019 Nov;35(6): 551–554

References

1. Torre LA, Bray F, Siegel RL, Ferlay J, Lortet-Tieulent J, Jemal A. Global cancer statistics, 2012. CA Cancer J Clin. 2015;65:87–108.
2. Bertuccio P, Chatenoud L, Levi F, et al. Recent patterns in gastric cancer: a global overview. Int J Cancer. 2009;125:666–73.
3. Kaneko S, Yoshimura T. Time trend analysis of gastric cancer incidence in Japan by histological types, 1975-1989. Br J Cancer. 2001;84:400–5.
4. Jemal A, Bray F, Center MM, Ferlay J, Ward E, Forman D. Global cancer statistics. CA Cancer J Clin. 2011;61:69–90.
5. Norouzinia M, Asadzadeh H, Shalmani HM, Al Dulaimi D, Zali MR. Clinical and histological indicators of proximal and distal gastric cancer in eight provinces of Iran. Asian Pac J Cancer Prev. 2012;13:5677–9.
6. Lauren P. The two histological main types of gastric carcinoma: diffuse and so-called intestinal-type carcinoma. An attempt at A HISTO-clinical classification. Acta Pathol Microbiol Scand. 1965;64:31–49.
7. Correa P. Human gastric carcinogenesis: a multistep and multifactorial process--first American Cancer Society award lecture on cancer epidemiology and prevention. Cancer Res. 1992;52:6735–40.
8. Carcas LP. Gastric cancer review. J Carcinog. 2014;13:14.
9. Karimi P, Islami F, Anandasabapathy S, Freedman ND, Kamangar F. Gastric cancer: descriptive epidemiology, risk factors, screening, and prevention. Cancer Epidemiol Biomark Prev. 2014;23:700–13.
10. Parkin DM, Bray F, Ferlay J, Pisani P. Global cancer statistics, 2002. CA Cancer J Clin. 2005;55:74–108.
11. Stock M, Otto F. Gene deregulation in gastric cancer. Gene. 2005;360:1–19.
12. Park JY, von Karsa L, Herrero R. Prevention strategies for gastric cancer: a global perspective. Clin Endosc. 2014;47:478–89.
13. Yu X, Hu F, Li C, Yao Q, Zhang H, Xue Y. Clinicopathologic characteristics and prognosis of proximal and distal gastric cancer. Onco Targets Ther. 2018;11:1037–44.
14. Herrera V, Parsonnet J. Helicobacter pylori and gastric adenocarcinoma. Clin Microbiol Infect. 2009;15:971–6.
15. Crew KD, Neugut AI. Epidemiology of gastric cancer. World J Gastroenterol. 2006;12:354–62.
16. Caldas C, Carneiro F, Lynch HT, et al. Familial gastric cancer: overview and guidelines for management. J Med Genet. 1999;36:873–80.
17. Parsonnet J, Vandersteen D, Goates J, Sibley RK, Pritikin J, Chang Y. Helicobacter pylori infection in intestinal- and diffuse-type gastric adenocarcinomas. J Natl Cancer Inst. 1991;83:640–3.
18. Malvezzi M, Carioli G, Bertuccio P, et al. European cancer mortality predictions for the year 2019 with focus on breast cancer. Ann Oncol. 2019;30:781–7.
19. Tran GD, Sun XD, Abnet CC, et al. Prospective study of risk factors for esophageal and gastric cancers in the Linxian general population trial cohort in China. Int J Cancer. 2005;113:456–63.
20. Kim Y, Park J, Nam BH, Ki M. Stomach cancer incidence rates among Americans, Asian Americans and Native Asians from 1988 to 2011. Epidemiol Health. 2015;37:e2015006.
21. Kamineni A, Williams MA, Schwartz SM, Cook LS, Weiss NS. The incidence of gastric carcinoma in Asian migrants to the United States and their descendants. Cancer Causes Control. 1999;10:77–83.
22. Buckland G, Travier N, Huerta JM, et al. Healthy lifestyle index and risk of gastric adenocarcinoma in the EPIC cohort study. Int J Cancer. 2015;137:598–606.
23. Lin SH, Li YH, Leung K, Huang CY, Wang XR. Salt processed food and gastric cancer in a Chinese population. Asian Pac J Cancer Prev. 2014;15:5293–8.
24. Massarrat S, Stolte M. Development of gastric cancer and its prevention. Arch Iran Med. 2014;17:514–20.
25. Wiseman M. The second World Cancer Research Fund/American Institute for Cancer Research expert report. Food, nutrition, physical activity, and the prevention of cancer: a global perspective. Proc Nutr Soc. 2008;67:253–6.
26. Nishino Y, Inoue M, Tsuji I, et al. Tobacco smoking and gastric cancer risk: an evaluation based on a systematic review of epidemiologic evidence among the Japanese population. Jpn J Clin Oncol. 2006;36:800–7.
27. Ladeiras-Lopes R, Pereira AK, Nogueira A, et al. Smoking and gastric cancer: systematic review and meta-analysis of cohort studies. Cancer Causes Control. 2008;19:689–701.
28. Suerbaum S, Michetti P. Helicobacter pylori infection. N Engl J Med. 2002;347:1175–86.
29. Iizasa H, Nanbo A, Nishikawa J, Jinushi M, Yoshiyama H. Epstein-Barr Virus (EBV)-associated gastric carcinoma. Viruses. 2012;4:3420–39.
30. Forman D, Burley VJ. Gastric cancer: global pattern of the disease and an overview of environmental risk factors. Best Pract Res Clin Gastroenterol. 2006;20:633–49.
31. Choi YJ, Kim N. Gastric cancer and family history. Korean J Intern Med. 2016;31:1042–53.
32. Choi YJ, Kim N, Jang W, et al. Familial clustering of gastric cancer: a retrospective study based on the number of first-degree relatives. Medicine (Baltimore). 2016;95:e3606.
33. Yamaguchi S, Sakata Y, Iwakiri R, et al. Increase in endoscopic and laparoscopic surgery regarding the therapeutic approach of gastric cancer detected by cancer screening in Saga Prefecture, Japan. Intern Med. 2016;55:1247–53.
34. Syrjänen K, Eskelinen M, Peetsalu A, et al. GastroPanel® biomarker assay: the most comprehensive test for. Anticancer Res. 2019;39:1091–104.
35. Correa P, Houghton J. Carcinogenesis of Helicobacter pylori. Gastroenterology. 2007;133:659–72.
36. Rugge M, Capelle LG, Cappellesso R, Nitti D, Kuipers EJ. Precancerous lesions in the stomach: from biology to clinical patient management. Best Pract Res Clin Gastroenterol. 2013;27:205–23.
37. Peek RM, Blaser MJ. Helicobacter pylori and gastrointestinal tract adenocarcinomas. Nat Rev Cancer. 2002;2:28–37.
38. Mera R, Fontham ET, Bravo LE, et al. Long term follow up of patients treated for Helicobacter pylori infection. Gut. 2005;54:1536–40.
39. Massarrat S, Haj-Sheykholeslami A, Mohamadkhani A, et al. Precancerous conditions after H. pylori eradication: a randomized double blind study in first degree relatives of gastric cancer patients. Arch Iran Med. 2012;15:664–9.
40. Valenzuela MA, Canales J, Corvalán AH, Quest AF. Helicobacter pylori-induced inflammation and epigenetic changes during gastric carcinogenesis. World J Gastroenterol. 2015;21:12742–56.
41. Polk DB, Peek RM. Helicobacter pylori: gastric cancer and beyond. Nat Rev Cancer. 2010;10:403–14.
42. Valenzuela M, Bravo D, Canales J, et al. Helicobacter pylori-induced loss of survivin and gastric cell viability is attributable to secreted bacterial gamma-glutamyl transpeptidase activity. J Infect Dis. 2013;208:1131–41.
43. Varon C, Dubus P, Mazurier F, et al. Helicobacter pylori infection recruits bone marrow-derived cells that participate in gastric preneoplasia in mice. Gastroenterology. 2012;142:281–91.
44. Forman D. Re: the role of overdiagnosis and reclassification in the marked increase of esophageal adenocarcinoma incidence. J Natl Cancer Inst. 2005;97:1013–1014; author reply 1014.

35

45. Jung KW, Talley NJ, Romero Y, et al. Epidemiology and natural history of intestinal metaplasia of the gastroesophageal junction and Barrett's esophagus: a population-based study. Am J Gastroenterol. 2011;106:1447–1455; quiz 1456.

46. Hansford S, Kaurah P, Li-Chang H, et al. Hereditary diffuse gastric cancer syndrome: CDH1 mutations and beyond. JAMA Oncol. 2015;1:23–32.

47. Hwang J, Min BH, Jang J, et al. MicroRNA expression profiles in gastric carcinogenesis. Sci Rep. 2018;8:14393.

48. Libânio D, Dinis-Ribeiro M, Pimentel-Nunes P. Helicobacter pylori and microRNAs: relation with innate immunity and progression of preneoplastic conditions. World J Clin Oncol. 2015;6:111–32.

49. Maconi G, Manes G, Porro GB. Role of symptoms in diagnosis and outcome of gastric cancer. World J Gastroenterol. 2008;14:1149–55.

50. Dewys WD, Begg C, Lavin PT, et al. Prognostic effect of weight loss prior to chemotherapy in cancer patients. Eastern Cooperative Oncology Group. Am J Med. 1980;69:491–7.

51. Berlth F, Bollschweiler E, Drebber U, Hoelscher AH, Moenig S. Pathohistological classification systems in gastric cancer: diagnostic relevance and prognostic value. World J Gastroenterol. 2014;20:5679–84.

52. Murakami T. Early cancer of the stomach. World J Surg. 1979;3:685–92.

53. The Paris endoscopic classification of superficial neoplastic lesions: esophagus, stomach, and colon: November 30 to December 1, 2002. Gastrointest Endosc. 2003;58:S3–43.

54. Li C, Oh SJ, Kim S, et al. Macroscopic Borrmann type as a simple prognostic indicator in patients with advanced gastric cancer. Oncology. 2009;77:197–204.

55. Fléjou JF. WHO classification of digestive tumors: the fourth edition. Ann Pathol. 2011;31:S27–31.

56. Bentrem D, Gerdes H, Tang L, Brennan M, Coit D. Clinical correlation of endoscopic ultrasonography with pathologic stage and outcome in patients undergoing curative resection for gastric cancer. Ann Surg Oncol. 2007;14:1853–9.

57. Bhutani MS, Hawes RH, Hoffman BJ. A comparison of the accuracy of echo features during endoscopic ultrasound (EUS) and EUS-guided fine-needle aspiration for diagnosis of malignant lymph node invasion. Gastrointest Endosc. 1997;45:474–9.

58. Kwee RM, Kwee TC. Imaging in assessing lymph node status in gastric cancer. Gastric Cancer. 2009;12:6–22.

59. Chen CY, Hsu JS, Wu DC, et al. Gastric cancer: preoperative local staging with 3D multi-detector row CT--correlation with surgical and histopathologic results. Radiology. 2007;242:472–82.

60. Leake PA, Cardoso R, Seevaratnam R, et al. A systematic review of the accuracy and indications for diagnostic laparoscopy prior to curative-intent resection of gastric cancer. Gastric Cancer. 2012;15(Suppl 1):S38–47.

61. Stein HJ, Feith M, Siewert JR. Cancer of the esophagogastric junction. Surg Oncol. 2000;9:35–41.

62. Rice TW, Patil DT, Blackstone EH. 8th edition AJCC/UICC staging of cancers of the esophagus and esophagogastric junction: application to clinical practice. Ann Cardiothorac Surg. 2017;6:119–30.

63. Sano T, Coit DG, Kim HH, et al. Proposal of a new stage grouping of gastric cancer for TNM classification: International Gastric Cancer Association staging project. Gastric Cancer. 2017;20:217–25.

64. Huang Q, Shi J, Feng A, et al. Gastric cardiac carcinomas involving the esophagus are more adequately staged as gastric cancers by the 7th edition of the American Joint Commission on Cancer Staging System. Mod Pathol. 2011;24:138–46.

65. Wu HH, Lin WC, Tsai KW. Advances in molecular biomarkers for gastric cancer: miRNAs as emerging novel cancer markers. Expert Rev Mol Med. 2014;16:e1.

66. Nordgård O, Tjensvoll K, Gilje B, Søreide K. Circulating tumour cells and DNA as liquid biopsies in gastrointestinal cancer. Br J Surg. 2018;105:e110–20.

67. Wang H, Li B, Liu Z, et al. HER2 copy number of circulating tumour DNA functions as a biomarker to predict and monitor trastuzumab efficacy in advanced gastric cancer. Eur J Cancer. 2018;88:92–100.

68. Network CGAR. Comprehensive molecular characterization of gastric adenocarcinoma. Nature. 2014;513:202–9.

69. Kankeu Fonkoua L, Yee NS. Molecular characterization of gastric carcinoma: therapeutic implications for biomarkers and targets. Biomedicine. 2018;6:32.

70. Charalampakis N, Economopoulou P, Kotsantis I, et al. Medical management of gastric cancer: a 2017 update. Cancer Med. 2018;7:123–33.

71. Nishikawa J, Iizasa H, Yoshiyama H, et al. The role of epigenetic regulation in Epstein-Barr virus-associated gastric cancer. Int J Mol Sci. 2017;18:1606.

72. Li B, Nie Z, Zhang D, et al. Roles of circulating endothelial progenitor cells and endothelial cells in gastric carcinoma. Oncol Lett. 2018;15:324–30.

73. Ishiguro H, Kimura M, Takeyama H. Role of microRNAs in gastric cancer. World J Gastroenterol. 2014;20:5694–9.

74. Puneet KHR, Kumari S, Tiwari S, Khanna A, Narayan G. Epigenetic mechanisms and events in gastric cancer-emerging novel biomarkers. Pathol Oncol Res. 2018;24:757.

75. Mirabella AC, Foster BM, Bartke T. Chromatin deregulation in disease. Chromosoma. 2016;125:75–93.

76. Wilusz JE, Sunwoo H, Spector DL. Long noncoding RNAs: functional surprises from the RNA world. Genes Dev. 2009;23:1494–504.

77. Verma R, Sharma PC. Next generation sequencing-based emerging trends in molecular biology of gastric cancer. Am J Cancer Res. 2018;8:207–25.

78. Tegels JJ, De Maat MF, Hulsewé KW, Hoofwijk AG, Stoot JH. Improving the outcomes in gastric cancer surgery. World J Gastroenterol. 2014;20:13692–704.

79. Pimentel-Nunes P, Dinis-Ribeiro M, Ponchon T, et al. Endoscopic submucosal dissection: European Society of Gastrointestinal Endoscopy (ESGE) guideline. Endoscopy. 2015;47:829–54.

80. Zhao Y, Wang C. Long-term clinical efficacy and perioperative safety of endoscopic submucosal dissection versus endoscopic mucosal resection for early gastric cancer: an updated meta-analysis. Biomed Res Int. 2018;2018:3152346.

81. Bösing NM, Goretzki PE, Röher HD. Gastric cancer: which patients benefit from systematic lymphadenectomy? Eur J Surg Oncol. 2000;26:498–505.

82. Kubota T, Hiki N, Sano T, et al. Prognostic significance of complications after curative surgery for gastric cancer. Ann Surg Oncol. 2014;21:891–8.

83. Bozzetti F, Marubini E, Bonfanti G, et al. Total versus subtotal gastrectomy: surgical morbidity and mortality rates in a multicenter Italian randomized trial. The Italian Gastrointestinal Tumor Study Group. Ann Surg. 1997;226:613–20.

84. Bozzetti F, Marubini E, Bonfanti G, Miceli R, Piano C, Gennari L. Subtotal versus total gastrectomy for gastric cancer: five-year survival rates in a multicenter randomized Italian trial. Italian Gastrointestinal Tumor Study Group. Ann Surg. 1999;230:170–8.

85. Ji X, Yan Y, Bu ZD, et al. The optimal extent of gastrectomy for middle-third gastric cancer: distal subtotal gastrectomy is superior to total gastrectomy in short-term effect without sacrificing long-term survival. BMC Cancer. 2017;17:345.

86. Cuschieri A, Fayers P, Fielding J, et al. Postoperative morbidity and mortality after D1 and D2 resections for gastric cancer: preliminary results of the MRC randomised controlled surgical trial. The Surgical Cooperative Group. Lancet. 1996;347:995–9.

87. Lewis FR, Mellinger JD, Hayashi A, et al. Prophylactic total gastrectomy for familial gastric cancer. Surgery. 2001;130:612–617; discussion 617-619.

88. Viñuela EF, Gonen M, Brennan MF, Coit DG, Strong VE. Laparoscopic versus open distal gastrectomy for gastric cancer: a meta-analysis of randomized controlled trials and high-quality nonrandomized studies. Ann Surg. 2012;255:446–56.

89. Kelly KJ, Selby L, Chou JF, et al. Laparoscopic versus open gastrectomy for gastric adenocarcinoma in the west: a case-control study. Ann Surg Oncol. 2015;22:3590–6.

90. Chen K, Pan Y, Zhang B, Maher H, Wang XF, Cai XJ. Robotic versus laparoscopic gastrectomy for gastric cancer: a systematic review and updated meta-analysis. BMC Surg. 2017;17:93.

91. Spanknebel KA, Brennan MF. Is D2 lymphadenectomy for gastric cancer a staging tool or a therapeutic intervention? Surg Oncol Clin N Am. 2002;11:415–430, xii.

92. Karpeh MS, Leon L, Klimstra D, Brennan MF. Lymph node staging in gastric cancer: is location more important than number? An analysis of 1,038 patients. Ann Surg. 2000;232:362–71.

93. Kim JP, Lee JH, Kim SJ, Yu HJ, Yang HK. Clinicopathologic characteristics and prognostic factors in 10 783 patients with gastric cancer. Gastric Cancer. 1998;1:125–33.

94. Schwarz RE, Smith DD. Clinical impact of lymphadenectomy extent in resectable esophageal cancer. J Gastrointest Surg. 2007;11:1384–1393; discussion 1393-1384.

95. Biondi A, D'Ugo D, Cananzi FC, et al. Does a minimum number of 16 retrieved nodes affect survival in curatively resected gastric cancer? Eur J Surg Oncol. 2015;41:779–86.

96. Kajitani T. The general rules for the gastric cancer study in surgery and pathology. Part I. clinical classification. Jpn J Surg. 1981;11:127–39.

97. Sasako M, Sano T, Yamamoto S, et al. D2 lymphadenectomy alone or with Para-aortic nodal dissection for gastric cancer. N Engl J Med. 2008;359:453–62.

98. Bonenkamp JJ, Hermans J, Sasako M, et al. Extended lymph-node dissection for gastric cancer. N Engl J Med. 1999;340: 908–14.

99. Cuschieri A, Weeden S, Fielding J, et al. Patient survival after D1 and D2 resections for gastric cancer: long-term results of the MRC randomized surgical trial. Surgical Co-operative Group. Br J Cancer. 1999;79:1522–30.

100. Degiuli M, Sasako M, Ponti A, et al. Randomized clinical trial comparing survival after D1 or D2 gastrectomy for gastric cancer. Br J Surg. 2014;101:23–31.

101. Mocellin S, Nitti D. Lymphadenectomy extent and survival of patients with gastric carcinoma: a systematic review and meta-analysis of time-to-event data from randomized trials. Cancer Treat Rev. 2015;41:448–54.

102. Jatzko GR, Lisborg PH, Denk H, Klimpfinger M, Stettner HM. A 10-year experience with Japanese-type radical lymph node dissection for gastric cancer outside of Japan. Cancer. 1995;76:1302–12.

103. Paul TO, Hoyt WF. Funduscopic appearance of papilledema with optic tract atrophy. Arch Ophthalmol. 1976;94:467–8.

104. Sierra A, Regueira FM, Hernández-Lizoáin JL, Pardo F, Martínez-Gonzalez MA, A-Cienfuegos J. Role of the extended lymphadenectomy in gastric cancer surgery: experience in a single institution. Ann Surg Oncol. 2003;10:219–26.

105. Xu AM, Huang L, Liu W, Gao S, Han WX, Wei ZJ. Neoadjuvant chemotherapy followed by surgery versus surgery alone for gastric carcinoma: systematic review and meta-analysis of randomized controlled trials. PLoS One. 2014;9:e86941.

106. Sant M, Allemani C, Santaquilani M, et al. EUROCARE-4. Survival of cancer patients diagnosed in 1995-1999. Results and commentary. Eur J Cancer. 2009;45:931–91.

107. Cunningham D, Allum WH, Stenning SP, et al. Perioperative chemotherapy versus surgery alone for resectable gastroesophageal cancer. N Engl J Med. 2006;355:11–20.

108. Ychou M, Boige V, Pignon JP, et al. Perioperative chemotherapy compared with surgery alone for resectable gastroesophageal adenocarcinoma: an FNCLCC and FFCD multicenter phase III trial. J Clin Oncol. 2011;29:1715–21.

109. Cunningham D, Okines AF, Ashley S. Capecitabine and oxaliplatin for advanced esophagogastric cancer. N Engl J Med. 2010;362:858–9.

110. Alderson D, Cunningham D, Nankivell M, et al. Neoadjuvant cisplatin and fluorouracil versus epirubicin, cisplatin, and capecitabine followed by resection in patients with oesophageal adenocarcinoma (UK MRC OE05): an open-label, randomised phase 3 trial. Lancet Oncol. 2017;18:1249–60.

111. Al-Batran SE, Hofheinz RD, Pauligk C, et al. Histopathological regression after neoadjuvant docetaxel, oxaliplatin, fluorouracil, and leucovorin versus epirubicin, cisplatin, and fluorouracil or capecitabine in patients with resectable gastric or gastro-oesophageal junction adenocarcinoma (FLOT4-AIO): results from the phase 2 part of a multicentre, open-label, randomised phase 2/3 trial. Lancet Oncol. 2016;17: 1697–708.

112. Smyth EC, Verheij M, Allum W, et al. Gastric cancer: ESMO clinical practice guidelines for diagnosis, treatment and follow-up. Ann Oncol. 2016;27:v38–49.

113. Ajani JA, Buyse M, Lichinitser M, et al. Combination of cisplatin/S-1 in the treatment of patients with advanced gastric or gastroesophageal adenocarcinoma: results of noninferiority and safety analyses compared with cisplatin/5-fluorouracil in the first-line advanced gastric cancer study. Eur J Cancer. 2013;49:3616–24.

114. Leong T, Smithers BM, Haustermans K, et al. TOPGEAR: a randomized, phase III trial of perioperative ECF chemotherapy with or without preoperative chemoradiation for resectable gastric cancer: interim results from an International, Intergroup Trial of the AGITG, TROG, EORTC and CCTG. Ann Surg Oncol. 2017;24:2252–8.

115. Macdonald JS, Smalley SR, Benedetti J, et al. Chemoradiotherapy after surgery compared with surgery alone for adenocarcinoma of the stomach or gastroesophageal junction. N Engl J Med. 2001;345:725–30.

116. Dikken JL, Jansen EP, Cats A, et al. Impact of the extent of surgery and postoperative chemoradiotherapy on recurrence patterns in gastric cancer. J Clin Oncol. 2010;28:2430–6.

117. Lee J, Lim DH, Kim S, et al. Phase III trial comparing capecitabine plus cisplatin versus capecitabine plus cisplatin with concurrent capecitabine radiotherapy in completely resected gastric cancer with D2 lymph node dissection: the ARTIST trial. J Clin Oncol. 2012;30:268–73.

118. Wang MJ, Li C, Sun Y, Shen FJ, Wang CB. Prognostic effect of adjuvant chemoradiotherapy for patients with gastric cancer: an updated evidence of randomized controlled trials. Oncotarget. 2017;8:102880–7.

119. Dikken JL, van Sandick JW, Maurits Swellengrebel HA, et al. Neo-adjuvant chemotherapy followed by surgery and chemotherapy or by surgery and chemoradiotherapy for patients with resectable gastric cancer (CRITICS). BMC Cancer. 2011; 11:329.

120. Di Costanzo F, Gasperoni S, Manzione L, et al. Adjuvant chemotherapy in completely resected gastric cancer: a randomized phase III trial conducted by GOIRC. J Natl Cancer Inst. 2008;100:388–98.

35

121. De Vita F, Giuliani F, Orditura M, et al. Adjuvant chemotherapy with epirubicin, leucovorin, 5-fluorouracil and etoposide regimen in resected gastric cancer patients: a randomized phase III trial by the Gruppo Oncologico Italia Meridionale (GOIM 9602 Study). Ann Oncol. 2007;18:1354–8.

122. Bouché O, Ychou M, Burtin P, et al. Adjuvant chemotherapy with 5-fluorouracil and cisplatin compared with surgery alone for gastric cancer: 7-year results of the FFCD randomized phase III trial (8801). Ann Oncol. 2005;16:1488–97.

123. Nakajima T, Nashimoto A, Kitamura M, et al. Adjuvant mitomycin and fluorouracil followed by oral uracil plus tegafur in serosa-negative gastric cancer: a randomised trial. Gastric Cancer Surgical Study Group. Lancet. 1999;354:273–7.

124. Sakuramoto S, Sasako M, Yamaguchi T, et al. Adjuvant chemotherapy for gastric cancer with S-1, an oral fluoropyrimidine. N Engl J Med. 2007;357:1810–20.

125. Noh SH, Park SR, Yang HK, et al. Adjuvant capecitabine plus oxaliplatin for gastric cancer after D2 gastrectomy (CLASSIC): 5-year follow-up of an open-label, randomised phase 3 trial. Lancet Oncol. 2014;15:1389–96.

126. Lee CK, Jung M, Kim HS, et al. S-1 based doublet as an adjuvant chemotherapy for curatively resected stage III gastric cancer: results from the randomized phase III POST trial. Cancer Res Treat. 2018;51:1.

127. Paoletti X, Oba K, Burzykowski T, et al. Benefit of adjuvant chemotherapy for resectable gastric cancer: a meta-analysis. JAMA. 2010;303:1729–37.

128. Liu D, Lu M, Li J, et al. The patterns and timing of recurrence after curative resection for gastric cancer in China. World J Surg Oncol. 2016;14:305.

129. Barchi LC, Yagi OK, Jacob CE, et al. Predicting recurrence after curative resection for gastric cancer: external validation of the Italian Research Group for Gastric Cancer (GIRCG) prognostic scoring system. Eur J Surg Oncol. 2016;42:123–31.

130. Aurello P, Petrucciani N, Antolino L, Giulitti D, D'Angelo F, Ramacciato G. Follow-up after curative resection for gastric cancer: is it time to tailor it? World J Gastroenterol. 2017;23:3379–87.

131. Xue HG, Yang AH, Sun XG, Lu YY, Tian ZB. Expression of microRNA-328 functions as a biomarker for recurrence of Early Gastric Cancer (EGC) after endoscopic submucosal dissection (ESD) by modulating CD44. Med Sci Monit. 2016;22:4779–85.

132. Li Y, Liang J, Hou P. Hypermethylation in gastric cancer. Clin Chim Acta. 2015;448:124–32.

133. Tenderenda M. A study on the prognostic value of cyclins D1 and E expression levels in resectable gastric cancer and on some correlations between cyclins expression, histoclinical parameters and selected protein products of cell-cycle regulatory genes. J Exp Clin Cancer Res. 2005;24:405–14.

Gastric Cancer: Advanced/ Metastatic Disease

Ferdinando De Vita, Giuseppe Tirino, Luca Pompella, and Angelica Petrillo

Gastrointestinal Cancers

Contents

© Springer Nature Switzerland AG 2021
A. Russo et al. (eds.), *Practical Medical Oncology Textbook*, UNIPA Springer Series,
https://doi.org/10.1007/978-3-030-56051-5_36

Learning Objectives

By the end of the chapter, the reader will:

- Be able to choose the correct treatment algorithm for inoperable locally advanced and metastatic gastric cancer
- Have learned the basic concepts of molecular classification of gastric cancer
- Have reached in-depth knowledge of inoperable locally advanced and metastatic stomach cancer treatment
- Be able to put acquired knowledge into daily clinical practice

36.1 Introduction

Gastric cancer (GC) is the fifth most common tumor and the second leading cause of cancer-related death worldwide. Nowadays, we know that gastric cancers can be divided into two different clinical entities, gastroesophageal junction and stomach (body/antrum) tumors, that showed different features from epidemiologic, biologic, genetic, and clinical points of view.

In this chapter, only relevant aspects for the evaluation and treatment of unresectable locally advanced and metastatic disease are reported. For a complete description of the general features of gastric cancer, see the previous chapter.

36.2 Epidemiology

Gastric cancer shows significant global differences in incidence worldwide. Indeed, the highest rates are recorded in Eastern Asia, South America, and Eastern Europe while the lowest in North America and Western Europe. In particular, in Europe, the highest rates are reported in Portugal in addition to the eastern countries, while the lower incidence is described in Denmark [1]. According to this global view, a gradual decline of the incidence of GC has been observed in Western Europe and North America in the last decades due to the improvement of life conditions and due to an epidemiologic shift that lead to the decrease of distal gastric cancer and the increase of the junctional disease [2]:

- Globally, gastric cancer had an estimated unadjusted incidence of around 18 and 9/100,000/year for men and women, respectively.
- Gastric cancer is frequently diagnosed in men with an age between 60 and 80 years.
- More than 60% of patients are older than 65 years, with an age-related increase of the risk (from 15 new diagnosis/100,000/year in under 30 years patients to 140/100,000/year in over 75 years old patients)
- 90% of gastric cancer are sporadic, while only 1–3% are hereditary.

36.3 Clinical Features

Gastric cancers are usually asymptomatic in the early stage, and they may cause specific and faded symptoms afterward, leading to a late diagnosis.

Weight loss, anorexia, dysphagia, and heartburn are the most common signs and symptoms at the diagnosis. Specific symptoms may arise in more advanced stage due to the growth of tumor that could lead to significant stenosis or hemorrhages. Dysphagia and vomit may appear in case of a stenosis located at the gastroesophageal junction or if a prominent stenosis is located at the antrum. Hematemesis, melena, or sign and symptoms of chronic anemia (malaise, fatigue, or exertional dyspnea) are the most common clinical manifestation of active bleeding.

During the natural history of these tumors, lymphonodal involvement is frequent and represents an early step in metastatic spread. The most common signs of superficial lymphonodal involvement are Troisier's sign due to the left supraclavicular lymphadenopathy (Virchow's lymph node), Sister Joseph's nodule at the navel, and Irish's sign, which is a left axillar lymphadenopathy.

The liver, peritoneum, retroperitoneal lymph nodes, and lung are the most common sites of metastasis. Bones and brain metastasis are less common but possible. Liver involvement is predominant through celiac vessels and can lead to hepatomegaly and jaundice, while dyspnea can appear in case of diffuse lung involvement, pleural effusion, or profuse ascites. Bone pain and neurologic signs and symptoms can appear in case of bone and brain involvement, respectively. Peritoneal involvement is frequent in case of GC with a signet-ring cell component or in case of undifferentiated or diffuse-type tumors (according to Lauren classification). It spreads through lymphatic vessels on the gastric wall and cause different entity of peritoneal carcinomatosis with ascites, secondary ovary involvement (Krukenberg tumor), or nodules in the pouch of Douglas, also known as a sign of Blumer's shelf.

As other tumors, also in metastatic gastric cancer, some paraneoplastic syndromes can occur, such as acanthosis nigricans, diffuse intravascular coagulation, venous thrombosis (Trousseau syndrome), and many others, due to the secretion of different active substances (cytokines, hormones, etc.) by the tumor.

36.4 Pathological Features

36.4.1 Microscopic Aspects and Immunohistochemical

In case of locally advanced, recurrent, or metastatic GC, pathological report should include not only the classical microscopic parameters, such as the histological subtypes and Lauren's classification, but also the evaluation of human epidermal growth factor receptor 2 (HER2) status.

Still today, HER2 determination represents the only validated biomarker in GC, able to influence the treatment choices. HER2 positivity is determined by quantification of the HER2 cell surface receptors by immunohistochemistry (IHC) and/or by measuring the number of HER2 gene copy numbers using fluorescence in situ hybridization (FISH). Determination of HER2 status via IHC is distinct for gastric and breast cancer, because an incomplete basolateral or lateral staining alone in gastric cancer is considered positive in addition to complete membrane staining. This difference results in tumor heterogeneity and potential inaccuracy determination of the HER2 positivity, and multiple biopsies of different sites of neoplastic lesion are recommended

to overcome this risk (at least five to six biopsies are usually required).

In GC, HER2 positivity is defined by 3+ scoring on IHC or 2+ on IHC with a FISH amplification (HER2/CEP 17 ratio $\geq$ 2.0), according to an IHC scoring criteria specific for HER2 overexpression in gastric cancer. HER2 status is considered negative in case of results 0 or 1+ by IHC [3]. Another relevant issue in this field is that the IHC staining pattern that determines the highest level of HER2 expression by IHC (IHC 3+) depends on whether a surgical specimen or biopsy is tested. As a matter of fact, basolateral or lateral membranous reactivity in $\geq$10% of tumor cells represents an IHC 3+ staining pattern in a surgical specimen, while an IHC 3+ staining pattern on a tumor biopsy is determined by tumor cell clusters with a strong complete, basolateral, or lateral membranous reactivity irrespective of percentage of tumor cell stained (◘ Fig. 36.1). Tumors with equivocal IHC scores (2+) should be tested further using FISH or other in situ methods (ISH (immunofluorescence in situ hybridization)) in order to evaluate gene amplification(◘ Fig. 36.2).

Even if different trials have investigated the role of mesenchymal-epithelial transition factor (c-Met) in gastric cancer, the results are still controversial, and there is

Score	Staining pattern (biopsy)	Staining pattern (resection)	Classification	IHC
0	No reactivity or no membranous reactivity in any tumor cell	No reactivity or membranous reactivity in < 10% of cells	Negative	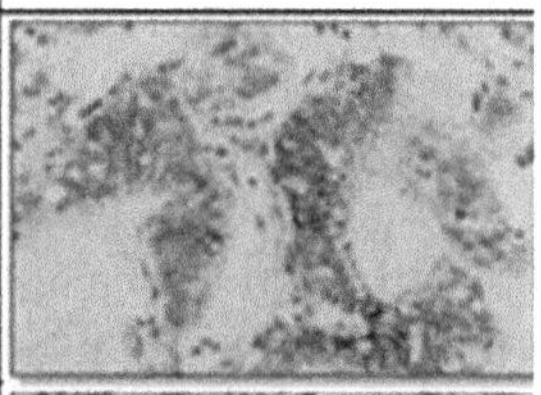
1+	Tumor cell cluster with a faint/barely perceptible membranous reactivity irrespective of percentage of tumor cells stained	Faint/barely perceptible membranous reactivity in >10% of cells; cells are reactive only in part of their membrane	Negative	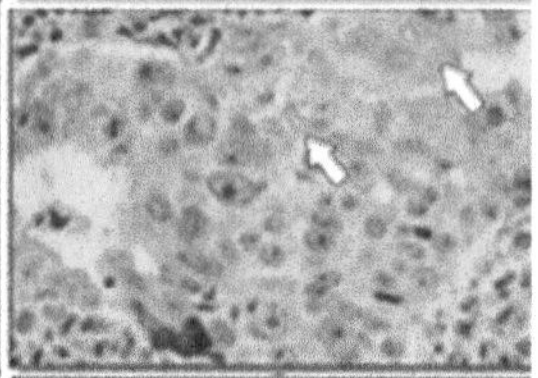
2+	Tumor cell cluster with a weak to moderate complete, basolateral or lateral membranous reactivity irrespective of percentage of Tumor cells stained	Weak o moderate complete or basolateral membranous reactivity in > 10% of tumor cells	Equivocal	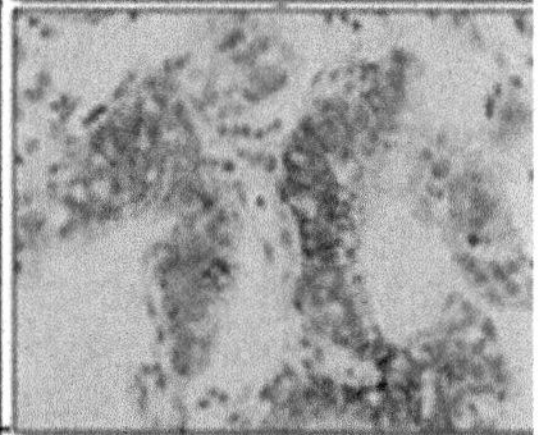
3+	Tumor cell cluster with a strong complete, basolateral or lateral membranous reactivity irrespective of percentage of tumor cells stained	Moderate to strong complete or basolateral membranous reactivity in > 10% of tumor cells	Positive	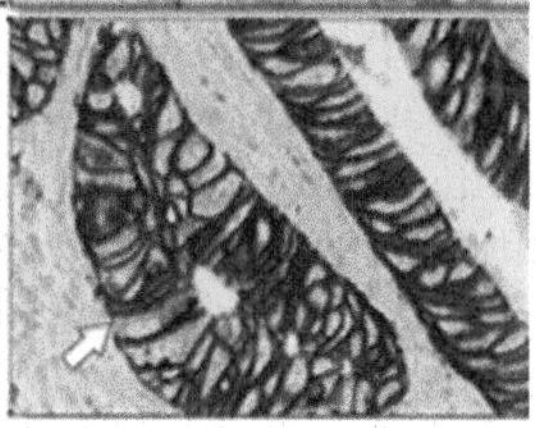

◘ **Fig. 36.1** HER2 scoring system in gastric cancer

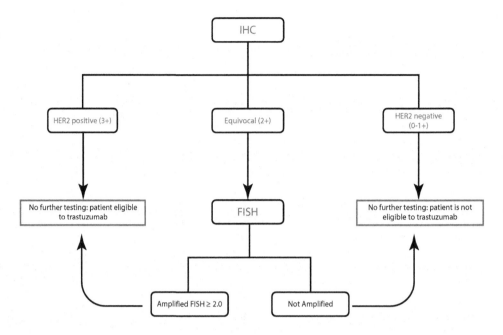

◻ Fig. 36.2 Algorithm of HER2 status determination by IHC and FISH

not yet a validated method to assess Met amplification and overexpression. Furthermore, Met evaluation is not recommended in daily clinical practice.

With the development of immunotherapy, further biomarkers have been investigated and validated during the last years. Microsatellite instability (MSI) evaluates the genetic mutability condition. In case of impaired DNA mismatch repair (MMR), the normal function of these mechanisms leads to a genetic hypermutability and a kind of mutation accumulation that result in a high neoantigen production and a consequent sensitivity to immunotherapeutic agents. This condition is called "high microsatellite instability" (MSI-H). MMR status can also be determined by the immunohistochemical analysis of some protein expression (such as MLH1, PMS2, MSH2, MSH6).

Another possible predictive factor for immunotherapy is the programmed death-ligand 1 (PD-L1).

PD-L1 is a transmembrane protein involved in the suppressing signaling of the immune response and in the "self-tolerance," acting as an inhibition factor (coinhibitor) for T-cell activity. It is a part of those regulators that constitute the so-called immune checkpoints. The "immune checkpoint inhibitors" are the drugs mainly use as immunotherapy against cancer, thanks to their blocking action on these receptors or their ligands. A high PD-L1 expression, assessed via IHC, is considered a positive predictive factor for immunotherapy across many tumor types. Its evaluation may be carried out according to tumor proportion score (TPS) or, more effectively, according to combined positive score (CPS) analysis of not only the viable tumor cells but also the other PD-L1 staining cells in the microenvironment (lymphocytes and macrophages).

In addition to these biomarkers, also the Epstein-Barr virus (EBV) status may be a useful tool for treatment selection. Its evaluation can be done by ICH or by Epstein-Barr encoding region (EBER) in situ hybridization, even if its role is still debated and far from being already validated for GC.

36.5 Molecular Biology and Main Therapeutic Targets in Advanced Gastric Cancer

For many years, GC was considered as a single disease: however, we know that it should be considered as a collection of very different molecular entities, each characterized by different clinical and molecular features. A first attempt to define GC heterogeneity was performed by Lauren P [4], who identified two types of GC on histological bases: the first one called "intestinal," because it displayed feature characteristic of the intestinal mucosa (in fact, it arises from intestinal metaplasia), and the other one called "diffuse," because the cancer cells, often poorly cohesive, diffusely infiltrated the gastric wall. On the other side, the World Health Organization (WHO) Classification of Tumors of the Digestive System (2019) classifies GC, according to their histological appearance, in "tubular adenocarcinomas," "papillary adenocarcinomas," "mucinous adenocarcinomas," and "signet-ring cell adenocarcinomas," the latter one resembling those that are classified as "diffuse-type" in the Lauren classification. Moreover, in addition to classic histological features, we can now classify these neoplasms also by their molecular profile. In particular, many studies have shown that gastric cancer can be driven by different genetic and/or epigenetic abnormalities: these findings led us to create robust molecular classifications that could become important especially in metastatic setting in order to develop novel target therapies.

36.5.1 Molecular Classifications

One of the first molecular GC classifications was by Patrick Tan et al. [5]: they classified GC into two distinct intrinsic subgroups – G-INT (genomic intestinal) and G-DIF (genomic diffuse). The authors used a panel of 37 GC cell lines and identified a "gene expression signature" of 171 genes that is able to distinguish between these two intrinsic subtypes, the first one called "G-INT" because more related to Lauren's intestinal subtype and the other one "G-DIF" because more related to diffuse subtype. The classification was then validated in a clinical cohort of 270 GC patients, showing that these two intrinsic classes really exist. Moreover, useful predictive information came out from in vitro experiments on 28 cell lines, with relevant implications for patient's care: G-INT cell lines were found to be more sensitive to 5-fluorouralcil and oxaliplatin, while G-DIF resulted to be more sensitive to cisplatin.

The same research group reported 2 years later [6] another GC classification based on the evaluation of gene expression in 248 tumors. According to this classification, GC can be divided into three subgroups: proliferative, metabolic, and mesenchymal. Proliferative subtypes are characterized by genomic instability, p53 mutations, and DNA hypomethylation; in the metabolic type, there is an increased activity of spasmolytic polypeptide-expressing metaplasia (SPEM metaplasia), while the mesenchymal type shows an epithelial mesenchymal transition (EMT) signature with high level of N-cadherin and low level of E-cadherin that leads to poorly differentiated tumors. Again, some interesting translational implications emerged: metabolic subtype seems more sensitive to 5-fluorouracil than the other two, while the mesenchymal subtype (probably due to "oncogenic addiction" to PI3K-AKT-mTOR pathway) seems to be more sensitive to drugs that block PI3K or mTOR, opening the way for a more precise therapy for GC.

In 2014, the Cancer Genome Atlas (TCGA) investigators published the most important and comprehensive study that we have to date on molecular GC classification. Four subtypes of gastric cancer have been described: Epstein-Barr virus (EBV)-positive, 9% of cases; microsatellite instability (MSI-H), 22% of cases; genomically stable (GS), 20% of cases; and chromosomal instability (CIN), 50% of cases ([7]; ◘ Fig. 36.3).

Each subtype shows different features and it is enriched for selected molecular abnormalities. In particular, the EBV-positive type is characterized by the posi-

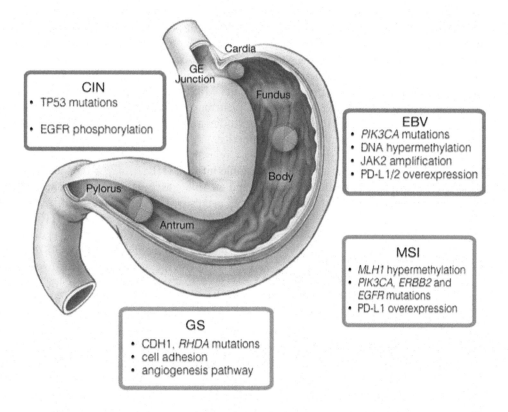

◘ **Fig. 36.3** Molecular subtypes of gastric cancer as emerged from TCGA. See the text for more information

CIN
- TP53 mutations
- EGFR phosphorylation

EBV
- *PIK3CA* mutations
- DNA hypermethylation
- JAK2 amplification
- PD-L1/2 overexpression

MSI
- *MLH1* hypermethylation
- *PIK3CA*, *ERBB2* and *EGFR* mutations
- PD-L1 overexpression

GS
- CDH1, *RHDA* mutations
- cell adhesion
- angiogenesis pathway

Cardia
GE Junction
Fundus
Body
Pylorus
Antrum

tivity for EBV, mutations, or amplifications of PI3K, PD-L1, and JAK2; these cancers can mostly arise in the fundus or gastric body and are more frequent in men.

MSI-H tumors are more frequent in older women and comprise especially intestinal-type cancers. From a molecular point of view, this group is characterized by mutations of p53, EGFR, HER2, HER3, PTEN, or silencing of the promoter of MLH1, a gene involved in the mismatch repair process.

GS gastric cancers are frequently diffuse and arise in younger age: they lack somatic copy number aberrations and are more related to Lauren's diffuse histology than the other ones. A pathway frequently destroyed in this subtype is that related to "cell adhesion," with the most relevant genes mutated CDH1, RHOA, and chromosomal translocation involving CLDN18 and ARHGAP.

Finally, the CIN subtype is enriched for copy number changes in key receptor tyrosine kinase oncogenes such as HER2, EGFR, fibroblast growth factor receptor 2 (FGFR2), and MET. This type is composed mostly of intestinal tumors, and it involves predominantly the gastroesophageal junction. These findings have potentially important therapeutic implications in order to improve the founding of target therapies against the specific key pathways driving the tumor in each individual patient.

Recently, the Asian Cancer Research Group [8] proposed a third molecular classification based on molecular and genetic alterations in gastric cancer. According to this one, it can distinguish four groups of gastric cancer: MSI (23%), microsatellite stable with intact (MSS/TP53-, 36%), microsatellite stable with p53 mutations (MSS/TP53+, 26%), and microsatellite stable with epithelial-mesenchymal transition (MSS/EMT, 15%) [8]. Unlike the TGCA classification, the ACRG reported different outcomes for each gastric cancer's subgroup. In particular, MSI had a better prognosis, whereas MSS/EMT had a worse prognosis with high rate of recurrence and peritoneal involvement. However, further studies are needed to translate these results in clinical practice.

In the next sections, we describe the most relevant therapeutic targets in gastric cancer with notable information about pivotal clinical trials conducted in this area and some resistance mechanisms to targeted agents.

36.5.2 Human Epidermal Growth Factor Receptor 2 (HER2)-Related Pathways: Therapeutic Targeting and Resistance Mechanisms

One of the first molecular pathways studied in gastric cancer was the epidermal growth factor receptor (EGFR) family pathway, which includes EGFR/HER1, HER2/neu, HER3, and HER4 receptors. Each receptor consists of an extracellular ligand-binding domain, an intracellular domain with kinase activity, and a short, lipophilic, transmembrane domain. The binding of ligands to their own receptor leads to homodimerization or heterodimerization with other members of the EGFR family, phosphorylation of intracellular domain, and activation of downstream pathways including the Ras/Raf/mitogen-activated protein kinase (MAPK) and phosphatidylinositol 3-kinase/protein kinase B/mammalian target of rapamycin (PI3K/Akt/mTOR) pathways. Stimulation of these pathways influences many aspects of tumor cell biology, such as proliferation, differentiation, migration, and apoptosis (◘ Fig. 36.4). Among these receptors, HER2 plays a key role in gastric cancer.

HER2, encoded at chromosome 17q21, acts as proto-oncogene in many human cancers: its main oncogenic mechanism is represented by gene amplification (determining protein overexpression) or, less commonly, by activating mutations.

HER2 lacks of a known exogenous ligand, and it is transactivated by the interaction with other HER family members (EGFR or HER3 overall) or other tyrosine kinase receptors: its activation leads to a complex signaling cascade already described above. In GC, HER2 overexpression is mainly due to gene amplification: it occurs more frequently in proximal tumors (more than 30% of cases), than in distal cancers (less than 20%). Furthermore, Lauren intestinal subtype shows a higher expression of HER2 (up to 34%) than diffuse subtype (6%), while, concerning to TCGA classification, CIN tumors more often express HER2 as consequence of gene amplification. Different strategies to target HER2 were developed over the years: monoclonal antibodies (like trastuzumab) that bind to the extracellular domain of the receptor and TKIs (tyrosine kinase inhibitors). The pivotal phase III ToGA trial [3] showed that in HER2-positive GCs, the addition of trastuzumab to standard platinum-based first-line treatment was effective, with a median overall survival (mOS) of about 13.8 months in the experimental arm versus 11.1 in the standard one (HR: 0.74; $p = 0.0046$). This OS still represents the highest ever reached in a phase III trial recruiting GC patients. The greatest benefit was observed in high HER2-expressing patients (IHC3+ or IHC2+/FISH+), with an mOS of 16 months versus 11.8 in low HER2-expressing patients (IHC0-1+/FISH+). Therefore, this trial led to the approval of trastuzumab in HER2-positive GC, in the first-line setting for patients with IHC3+ or IHC2+/FISH+ (see ◘ Fig. 36.2). Next, it has been speculated that in GC, the addition of pertuzumab (another monoclonal antibody targeting a different HER2 domain than trastuzumab) to trastuzumab itself and platinum-based chemotherapy could improve the ToGA survival rates, leading to JACOB trial design. Unfortunately, this study [10] was negative, because mOS was 17.5 months

Fig. 36.4 EGFR pathways. (Used with permission from Apicella et al. [9]. See the references for the original source of this material)

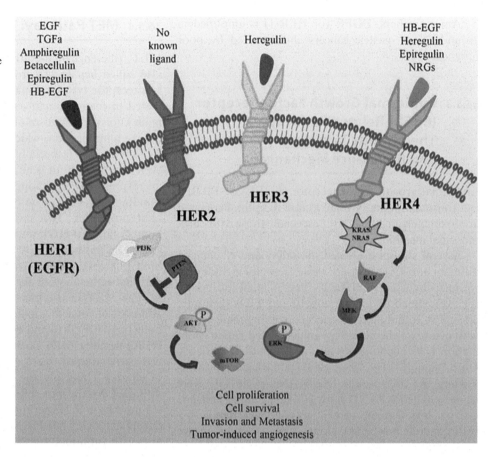

in experimental arm versus 14.2 in the standard (HR: 0.84; $p = 0.0565$), a difference that did not find statistical significance. Moreover, trastuzumab emtansine (TDM-1), an antibody-drug conjugate, was studied in second-line therapy of HER2-positive GC (previously treated with trastuzumab) within the GATSBY phase III trial [11]: unfortunately, TDM-1 therapy was not superior to standard taxanes (mOS 7.9 months versus 8.6, respectively, HR: 1.15, $p = 0.86$).

Due to the disappointing results of these trials (JACOB, GATSBY), many researchers began to study mechanisms of targeted therapy resistance in GC, considering that also patients who achieved a significant response to first-line trastuzumab-based treatment can develop resistance within a few months. In fact, one main bias of the second-line trials, especially the GATSBY trial, seems to be the absence of tumor re-biopsy (e.g., at one metastatic site) at screening, taking for granted that the tumor was still HER2-positive on the basis of the "historical" diagnostic biopsy. The study by Pietrantonio et al. [12] clearly showed that a possible acquired resistance mechanism to trastuzumab-based first-line treatment could be the loss of HER2 receptor, especially for patients with dubious immunohistochemistry (IHC2+/FISH+). In that way, the negative results of the GATSBY study could be

related to the fact that in a significant proportion of cases, the authors have treated with TDM-1 patients who had become HER2-negative de facto at the beginning of the second line.

More important, even primary resistance to first-line anti-HER2 drugs seems to exist: in fact, objective response rates to trastuzumab plus chemotherapy in ToGA trial was about 50% only, which implies that at least 50% of HER2-positive tumors could have coexisting molecular alterations that confer resistance. In support of this hypothesis, the group lead by Adam Bass [13] clearly showed that almost 50% of HER2-amplified gastroesophageal cancers have preexisting co-amplifications or co-mutations in key oncogenes (others than HER2), for example, cell cycle-related genes (CCNE1, CDK6, and CCND1), RTK-related genes (EGFR, HER3, MET, FGFR2), or PI3K-related genes (PIK3CA, PIK3R1, PTEN). These amplifications/mutations confer resistance to anti-HER2-targeted drugs in cell line experiments. This preliminary report was then confirmed by Pietrantonio et al. [14], who showed that mutations of EGFR, MET, KRAS, PIK3CA, and PTEN or amplifications of EGFR, MET, and KRAS can co-occur in HER2-positive GC and could explain the lack of trastuzumab efficacy and/or the appearance of primary resistance.

Among others, EGFR (or HER-1) is amplified in around 5% of gastric cancers characterized by poor prognosis.

36.5.3 Epidermal Growth Factor Receptor (EGFR)-Related Pathways: Therapeutic Targeting and Resistance Mechanisms

Epidermal growth factor receptor (EGFR) or ERBB1 is a transmembrane tyrosine kinase receptor, expressed approximately in 30% of GC, especially those with chromosomal instability.

Several studies evaluated the safety and efficacy of different anti-EGFR drugs: these therapies include – as we just discussed for HER2 – monoclonal antibodies (like cetuximab or panitumumab) and TKIs (gefitinib, erlotinib). Initial phase II trials combining these agents with cytotoxic chemotherapy in unselected patient population have encouraging results for first-line patients. Unfortunately, all of the phase III published trials investigating the role of anti-EGFR therapy in GC were negative. The EXPAND study [15] randomized first-line GC patients between cetuximab plus capecitabine/cisplatin and chemotherapy alone, showing no advantage for cetuximab arm. However, the patient recruitment was unselected for EGFR positivity, and in a post hoc analysis, the highest survival benefit was observed in a small subset of patients with high EGFR expression. The REAL-III trial [16] demonstrates that adding panitumumab to epirubicin-oxaliplatin-capecitabine was even detrimental, as the mOS for the experimental arm was 8.8 months versus 11.3 months for the standard one (HR: 1.37, $p = 0.013$).

The shocking failure of all anti-EGFR drugs in gastric cancer could be explained with the lack of a proper patient selection. In fact, a recent work by Catenacci et al. [17] showed that EGFR amplified tumors (almost 5% in this study) seem very prone to respond to cetuximab or ABT-806 (an investigational anti-EGFR drug), with an ORR of 58%, a DCR of 100%, and an mPFS of about 10 months. Thanks to the next-generation sequencing (NGS) and circulating tumor DNA (ctDNA) studies, the authors also showed the mechanisms of resistance to anti-EGFR drugs, such as the presence of EGFR-negative tumor clones, KRAS mutation/amplifications, PTEN deletion, and NRAS/HER2/MYC amplifications. This study definitively demonstrates that EGFR amplification is able to predict response to anti-EGFR therapies, despite the negative results in prior unselected phase III trials (EXPAND and REAL-III), but also showed crucial mechanisms of resistance.

36.5.4 MET Pathway: Therapeutic Targeting

MET (mesenchymal-epithelial transition) oncogene, also called hepatocyte growth factor receptor (HGF), is a receptor tyrosine kinase that appears to be deregulated in many human cancers, included in GC. The main known mechanism of MET overexpression in GC is gene amplification, which occurs in about 6% of the TCGA dataset (especially in CIN tumors). However, even tumors without gene amplification can express (or overexpress) MET, although it is not clear whether these tumors really depend on MET for survival and malignant properties. Two monoclonal antibodies, rilotumumab (an anti-HGF antibody) and onartuzumab (an anti-MET antibody), were tested in clinical trials in GC: both phase III clinical trials evaluating onartuzumab and rilotumumab were negative.

The METGastric phase III trial [18] evaluated the addition of onartuzumab to a chemotherapy backbone (mFOLFOX6) and enrolled 562 GC patients with HER2-negative/MET-positive tumors. The enrollment was early stopped due to sponsor decision, for a lack of efficacy. Unluckily, the addition of onartuzumab to mFOLFOX6 did not result in an improvement of OS (11 months in the experimental arm versus 11.3 in standard, HR: 0.82, $p = 0.24$). Negative results were obtained also with rilotumumab within the RILOMET-1 phase III trial [19], which used a different chemotherapy backbone (epirubicin plus cisplatin and capecitabine). As for the previous trial, results were clearly negative with a detrimental effect (mOS was 8.8 in experimental arm versus 10.7 in the placebo group, HR: 1.34, $p = 0.003$), and, again, study treatment was stopped early, because an independent data monitoring found a higher number of deaths in the rilotumumab group. Probably the main limit of RILOMET and METGastric trials is to have included mostly patients in whom MET was not a clear "driver" of the disease, since the highest expressing tumors (MET gene amplification) are underrepresented, which can explain the negative results described.

36.5.5 VEGF Pathway: Therapeutic Targeting

In the TCGA "CIN" subtype, vascular endothelial growth factor (VEGF), a crucial mediator of normal and pathogenic angiogenesis, is frequently amplified (up to 7% of cases). However, initial studies with bevacizumab (a monoclonal antibody targeting VEGF-A) were negative, such as the AVAGAST trial [20] and the Asiatic AVATAR trial [21], in which bevacizumab was combined with platinum-based chemotherapy in the first-line setting. Subsequently, ramucirumab, a fully human monoclonal antibody directed against VEGFR2 (vascular endothelial growth factor receptor 2), the main receptor of the VEGF system, has been used in the second-line setting alone [22] or in combination with weekly paclitaxel [23]. Both studies were positive, with the REGARD trial showing a significant improvement in OS with ramucirumab alone versus BSC (mOS 5.2 months versus 3.8, respectively, HR: 0.776, $p = 0.047$) and the RAINBOW trial showing a significant superiority of combination arm (ramucirumab plus paclitaxel) versus paclitaxel alone (mOS 9.63 months versus 7.36 months, respectively, HR: 0.807, $p = 0.017$).

On that positive basis, ramucirumab has been tested in first-line setting in combination with cisplatin-based standard chemotherapy within the RAINFALL trial [24]: although the study formally met its primary endpoint, with an improvement in mPFS from 5.4 months (placebo arm) to 5.7 months (ramucirumab arm) (HR: 0.75, $p = 0.011$), there was no survival benefit for patients in the experimental arm, making the results negative de facto and not significant for clinical practice. Therefore, the role of antiangiogenic agents seems to be essential in second-line setting, but in the first line, like the AVAGAST and AVATAR trial, showed for bevacizumab, probably we need to better understand the patients who really benefit from this strategy.

36.5.6 Tumor Microenvironment: The Biological Basis of Immune Checkpoint Usage in Metastatic Gastric Cancer

Immunotherapy deeply changed the therapeutic landscape for several malignancies (advanced melanoma, lung, urothelial, kidney cancer, etc.) determining a completely unexpected improvement of survival by boosting the body's natural defenses to fight cancer.

As already reported, comprehensive molecular characterization performed by the TGCA group showed a relatively high mutational load (up to 10–15 mutations per megabase) in about 34% of gastric adenocarcinomas analyzed and a subset of tumors with microsatellite instability-high (MSI-H, 22%) or with an ideally favorable immune environment (the "EBV-related" subgroup that shows molecular hallmarks of sensitivity to immunotherapy, such as intratumoral or peritumoral immune cell infiltration and PD-L1/PD-L2 expression), suggesting that also gastric cancer could be a promising "fertile soil" for immunotherapy, especially based on immune checkpoint inhibitors [25].

36.6 Prognostic Factors

Despite the expanding knowledge about molecular mechanisms that lead to a better comprehension of GC, the prognosis of this tumor is still poor, especially in case of locally advanced or metastatic disease. In this context, the research for prognostic and predictive factors became particularly relevant.

Diffuse histotype, performance status, and number and location of distant metastasis are the principal prognostic factors in the metastatic setting. According to these and other biochemical factors, different prognostic scores have been validated over the past years. The Royal Marsden prognostic score [26, 27] divides GC patients into three risk groups on the bases of four parameters: performance status, liver metastasis, peritoneal metastasis, and serum alkaline phosphatase. Patients with peritoneal metastasis, performance status ≥ 2, and serum alkaline phosphatase ≥ 100 U/L had the worse prognosis, with a 1-year survival of 11% compared to 25.7% and 48.5% in the moderate- and low-risk groups, respectively.

In addition to these parameters, many trials showed that tumor prognosis may be influenced not only by tumor features themselves but also by tumor microenvironment. In this context, the neutrophil/lymphocyte ratio (NLR) in venous peripheral blood has been highly investigated in order to find a possible simple and quick prognostic factor. A recent research [28] showed that in a clinical cohort of 151 metastatic gastric cancer patients, NLR obtained before starting first-line chemotherapy is a strong independent predictor of poor survival, suggesting its utility for a quick and cheap patient prognostic stratification.

Regarding prognostic scores for mGC patients receiving a second-line treatment, an Italian model (Gastric life nomogram) showed to predict 12-week life expectancy for these patients [29]. However, all these promising factors need to be further validated in prospective clinical trials.

36.7 Treatment

Chemotherapy represents the standard treatment for unresectable locally advanced and metastatic gastric cancer, showing improvement of survival and quality of life compared with best supportive care [30]. ◘ Figure 36.5 summarizes the current "state of the art" for treatment selection in metastatic GC patients.

Despite of the term "advanced gastric cancer" comprising also patients with inoperable locally advanced tumors, it is important to distinguish this group of patients from the metastatic one, because in this case patients have not distant metastasis and tumor could be

◻ Fig. 36.5 Biomarker-driven therapy for advanced gastric cancer in 2020

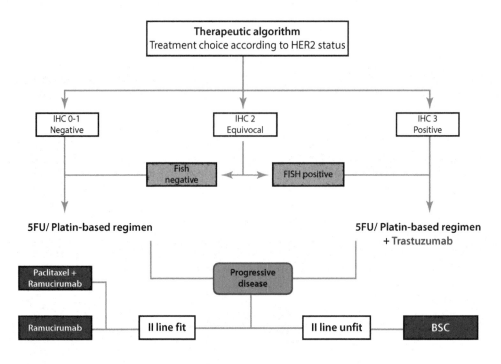

converted into an operable disease after a chemotherapy response. Therefore, more aggressive and active chemotherapy schedules are recommended for these patients as a conversion therapy in order to obtain a tumor downsizing and downstaging. On the other hand, it is important to consider that the target of treatment in case of metastatic disease is the palliation, because we still do not have sufficient evidence to support the recommendation of tumor resection in this population, and surgery does not prolong survival and can even produce a detrimental effect (see below for more details). Moreover, the general clinical condition of these patients are frequently poor so a multidisciplinary evaluation of different aspects of disease, comprising a nutritional and toxicity evaluation as well as the palliation of symptoms, is fundamental to improve the efficacy of active treatments.

The nutritional assessment is crucial since the first take charge in order to prevent malnutrition and to avoid the poor compliance and tolerability caused by nutritional condition decline.

Because of tumor locations (cardia or antrum) and possible luminal obstruction, it is necessary sometimes to resort to parenteral nutrition.

Response to systemic treatments should normally be assessed with interval imaging of the chest, abdomen, and pelvis, mostly with computer tomography (CT) scan, although alternative imaging techniques may be used if required to monitor known sites of disease (e.g., magnetic resonance imaging for brain lesions). The evaluation of response is according to standard radiologic criteria for solid tumor, also known as RECIST criteria, except in case of immunotherapy in which the immune-modified RECIST (iRECIST) should be used.

36.7.1 First Line

The determination of HER2 status is essential before starting a first-line therapy in order to distinguish HER2-negative and HER2-positive gastric cancer, selecting patients for appropriate treatment with trastuzumab (an anti-HER2 monoclonal antibody). However, a more complete molecular dissection before starting a first-line chemotherapy is today highly desirable, considering the promising results of the recently presented KEYNOTE-062 trial [31], in which first-line metastatic GC patients with a MSI-H disease or a high expression of PD-L1 received greater benefit from anti-PD-1 pembrolizumab compared to standard chemotherapy arm (HR: 0.29, 95% IC 0.11–0.81). For this reason, MSI testing is absolutely recommended, although immune checkpoint inhibitors are not yet approved for this indication in EU nowadays.

No anti-HER2 agent showed a survival benefit beyond the first-line setting indeed.

36.7.1.1 Chemotherapy

In patients with HER2-negative disease, the only effective therapeutic option we have to date is chemotherapy. However, despite the use of the most modern regimens, the survival of these patients remains overall poor (median OS: 11 months), even if a correct "continuum of care" strategy and molecular selection is starting to lead to less rare longer survivals.

Polichemotherapy is still the standard first-line treatment for patients with a good performance status, while best supportive care alone is recommended in cases with poor clinical conditions considered "unfit" for active treatments.

Doublet combinations of platinum (either cisplatin or oxaliplatin) and fluoropyrimidines (5-fluorouracil or capecitabine) showed greater benefit if compared to mono-chemotherapy and are generally used in fit patients as standard regimens [30].

On the other side, the utility of triplet regimens as first-line therapy is still under debate, and their use should be evaluated, in the context of a multidisciplinary discussion, only in selected cases. For example, triplet regimen utility could be speculated in GC patients with:

1. Locally advanced disease, in which a more active regimen (like a triplet one) could lead to tumor downstaging and to a possible rescue to radical surgery on primary tumor
2. High tumor burden disease with severe symptoms, in which a rapid clinical response (such as that obtainable with triplet regimen) could be required to improve patient general clinical conditions and to achieve a more rapid symptom recovery (i.e., for severe dysphagia)
3. Oligo-metastatic diseases, in which a triplet-based "neoadjuvant" approach (e.g., with a taxane-based regimen such as "FLOT") could be followed by primary plus metastatic lesion(s) surgical resections, according to preliminary results of the phase II AIO FLOT 3 trial [32]

Triplets containing taxanes (DCF, FLOT) showed survival benefits in first-line setting, while schedules containing anthracyclines, although initially associated with better outcomes, today must not be used anymore, as we later explain.

In the phase III randomized trial TAX-325 [33], the addition of docetaxel to 5-FU/cisplatin in a three weekly regimen named DCF was associated with improved overall survival in first-line therapy (OS: 9.2 versus 8.6 months) but at the cost of significantly more toxic effects, including increased rates of febrile neutropenia. For this reason, other studies have examined the efficacy of alternative taxane-based triplets, like FLOT regimen (docetaxel, fluoropyrimidine, and oxaliplatin), with positive results both in terms of efficacy and tolerability [34].

With regard to anthracycline-based triplets, the REAL-II trial [35] demonstrated non-inferiority between ECF, ECX, EOF (epirubicin, oxaliplatin, 5-FU), and EOX (epirubicin, oxaliplatin, and capecitabine), making the substitution of 5-FU with capecitabine and cisplatin with oxaliplatin possible. However, as already anticipated, anthracycline-containing regimens should not be considered anymore for GC patient treatment: in fact, according also to a famous editorial by Jaffer Ajani, only three drugs have demonstrated an OS improvement in first-line setting – forming level I of evidence – and they are docetaxel, cisplatin, and trastuzumab, while epirubicin has never gained this "honor." As a matter of fact, a standard doublet has been demonstrated to be as effective as an anthracycline-base triplet but with significant less toxicity. For this reason and for the increased cardiac risk that is associated with these drugs, we can assert that today no GC patient should continue to receive epirubicin-based triplet.

To reinforce this concept, we refer to a fundamental study lead by Guimbaud R et al.: in this trial, the FOLFIRI regimen (irinotecan plus leucovorin and infusional 5-FU) was compared to the anthracycline-based ECX regimen in first-line setting. The authors showed a non-inferiority of doublet versus triplet regimen combination, supporting once more the necessity to avoid anthracycline from gastric cancer therapy, because it cannot add nothing to survival benefit.

Furthermore, in a different setting (neoadjuvant) the taxane-based triplet FLOT showed its superiority, in terms of responses and survival, over the epirubicin-based triplet [36].

The S1 fluoropyrimidine is an another orally choice to be evaluated in association with cisplatin in first-line setting in Asiatic population, while it is not recommended in the Caucasian due to high rate of toxicity in this population [37].

In conclusion, data are not supporting the use of triplet regimens in all patients with metastatic gastric cancer, but only in selected patients (see above), even if an increase of side effects should be considered.

36.7.1.2 Chemotherapy for HER2-Positive Disease

In the first-line treatment of HER2-positive gastric cancer, the phase III ToGA trial demonstrated clinically and statistically significant improvements in response rate, progression-free survival (PFS), and OS with the addition of trastuzumab to cisplatin/fluoropyrimidine doublet [3], especially in patients with higher expression of the protein (HER2 3+ at IHC or 2+ IHC with FISH amplification).

Based on the ToGA results, trastuzumab was approved in many countries in addition to cisplatin-fluoropyrimidine doublet as first-line standard of care in patients with HER2-positive disease. This drug is currently used at the same dose of HER2-positive breast cancer (8 mg/Kg in the first induction dose and then 6 mg/Kg every 21 days), even if today it is clear that HER2-positive gastric cancer is biologically different from the breast one. However, the addiction of trastuzumab with different schedule to chemotherapy did not show any benefit in patients with HER2-positive metastatic gastric cancer [18, 38]. Moreover, trastuzumab is actually investigated in adjuvant and neoadjuvant setting for HER2-positive gastric cancer.

Unfortunately, trastuzumab remains the only anti HER2 target therapy approved in the first-line setting.

Lapatinib, an oral inhibitor of tyrosine kinase domain of EGFR and HER2, failed to add the same efficacy as trastuzumab in addiction to capecitabine and oxaliplatin.

Similarly, negative results were achieved by Pertuzumab within the Jacob trial [10], as already reported in the previous section. For this reason, pertuzumab is not actually approved in addition to standard first-line treatment.

Anti-HER2 strategy beyond first-line setting is actually not recommended. The TDM-1 (an "antibody-drug conjugate" in which the molecule of trastuzumab is combined with a cytotoxic drug) did not show a survival benefit in the second-line treatment of patients previously treated with trastuzumab [11].

36.7.2 Second Line

Approximatively 40% of patients (and even more in high-volume centers) with metastatic gastric cancer patients receive a second-line treatment after the first-line failure. Second-line treatment is recommended in patients with a progressive disease and with a good performance status. An active treatment is associated with an improvement in OS and quality of life compared with best supportive care.

Among different chemotherapy agents and schedules investigated in this setting, taxanes, irinotecan [39], and ramucirumab (alone or in association with paclitaxel) showed a survival benefit with a good toxicity profile.

In particular, the COUGAR trial showed a benefit in OS for docetaxel if compared to best supportive care (median OS: 5.2 vs 3.6 months) [40], and the randomized phase III trial by Hironaka directly compared weekly paclitaxel with irinotecan and demonstrated similar efficacy and feasibility for both regimens [41].

In 2014, two randomized phase III clinical trials [22, 23] demonstrated the efficacy of ramucirumab (alone or in combination with weekly paclitaxel, respectively) in second-line setting. To note, until this moment, no target agents have shown a benefit in second line in association with chemotherapy with the exception of this drug. Ramucirumab is in fact a fully humanized monoclonal antibody that binds the extracellular domain of vascular endothelial growth factor receptor 2 (VEGFR2). Its mechanism of action prevents the binding with VEGF-A, VEGF-C, and VEGF-D leading to a strong antiangiogenetic property. As a single agent in the REGARD trial [22], ramucirumab was associated with a survival benefit versus best supportive care alone (median OS: 5.2 versus 3.8 months). Moreover, in addition to paclitaxel in RAINBOW trial [23], it was reported a survival benefit compared with paclitaxel alone of 2.2 months (median OS: 9.6 versus 7.4 months), with improvement also in PFS and objective response rate.

In patients with disease progression >6 months following first-line chemotherapy, the evaluation of a rechallenge with the same drug combination used in first line may be also appropriate.

Ramucirumab remains the only biological agent approved in second-line treatment for HER2-positive and HER2-negative gastric cancer today, while specific anti-HER2 drugs, such as lapatinib and TDM-1, did not improve survival in HER2-positive gastric cancer that progressed after a first-line treatment containing trastuzumab. In particular, TDM1, as already mentioned above, was studied in the GATSBY trial [11] and compared to taxanes showing no superiority in patients with previously treated, HER2-positive advanced gastric cancer. Similar results were reported for lapatinib associated with paclitaxel in the TYTAN phase III study [42], without significant difference in OS and PFS compared to paclitaxel alone.

Other targeted therapies investigated in this setting, such as sorafenib and sunitinib, did not show clinical benefit. Due to these reasons, the actual second-line treatment in HER2-positive gastric cancer is not different from HER2-negative one.

36.7.3 Third-Line Therapy and Beyond

Thanks to the novel drugs and the improvement of supportive care (especially nutritional support), a biggest amount of patient (20–25% approximately) is arriving in good clinical condition beyond a second line of treatment.

This is why a correct "continuum of care strategy" should be always supposed and tailored on the single patient features.

Current European guidelines do not recommend any specific treatment for patients with disease refractory to two or more previous regimens.

Despite this assumption, a third-line strategy with active chemotherapy should be taken into account for selected patients, if we consider the positive results of the recently published TAGS trial [43].

This was the first phase III clinical trial to evaluate GC patients who had received at least two previous chemotherapy lines: subjects were randomly assigned to receive oral trifluridine/tipiracil (TAS102) or placebo. The study met its primary endpoint, and in fact, median OS was considerably better in the experimental arm compared to placebo arm (5.7 months versus 3.6 months, HR: 0.69, $p = 0.00029$), and the treatment was well tolerated, with manageable adverse events (the most common in the TAS102 arm were neutropenia and anemia, compared to abdominal pain and deterioration of clinical condition in the placebo arm). So for the first time ever, the TAGS trial paved the way to a real "con-

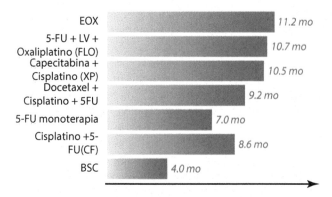

Fig. 36.6 Median OS in patients with advanced/metastatic gastric cancer. The "continuum of care" (see next in the text) has greatly improved quantity and quality of life

tinuum of care" concept even in GC, because we now have effective first-, second-, and third-line therapies, and their sequential usage could greatly expand the survival of GC patients (see ☐ Fig. 36.6) as well as their quality of life.

Moreover, a multidisciplinary evaluation is crucial in every step of natural history of gastric cancer due to the particular worsening of clinical condition that this disease produces. For example, as already reported, a nutritional support should be evaluated after all lines of treatment as well as the palliation of dysphagia or pain. After the third line, if the patient is still in good clinical conditions, the choice of new chemotherapy schedule should be done according to previous treatments, patient's preference, performance status, and clinical trials eventually available.

As reported below, in this setting of treatment, there is also a possible place for immunotherapy.

36.7.4 Immunotherapy

Emerging data from early-phase trials have suggested that the use of immunotherapy may improve survival in patients with advanced gastric cancer. In particular, the research focused on immune checkpoint of programmed cell death 1 and its ligands (PD-1/PD-L1). PD-1 is a receptor expressed on the surface of tumor cells, macrophages, activated dendritic cells, and T and B lymphocytes. As mentioned above, this receptor acts as a coinhibitor, leading to suppression of immunological T-lymphocyte-mediated response in tumor microenvironment. The TCGA molecular classification identified elevated PD-L1 expression especially in the EBV subtype.

Cancer cells use these factors and other mechanisms in order to elude the immune system reaction.

Monoclonal antibodies that target either PD-1 or PD-L1, such as pembrolizumab, nivolumab, and ave-

lumab, can block this checkpoint inhibition and stimulate the immune response against tumor.

In a certain way, the immune system is "remodulated" in order to fight the cancer cells itself.

The phase III trial ONO-4538-12 "ATTRACTION-2" represents the current milestone for the development of immunotherapy with nivolumab (anti-PD-1 antibody) in the chemotherapy-refractory molecularly unselected population. In this entirely Asian trial, surprising survival rates of 27.3 and 10.6% at 1 year and 2 years, respectively, have been achieved in the nivolumab arm. Responders to immunotherapy had a 12-month survival rate of 86.7%, suggesting the presence of a subset of patients who greatly benefit from "checkpoint inhibition" strategy.

This trial is the only phase III positive one to date.

Immunotherapy is quickly evolving also for GC, and the correct patient selection is going to be clarified, even if the results of trials available are controversial and often negative across the different settings of treatment.

As a matter of fact, in first- and second-line setting, immunotherapy did not significantly improve survival compared to standard chemotherapy both in Asian and Western patients in two recent phase III randomized trials: KEYNOTE-062 and KEYNOTE-061.

However, although these trials have been formally negative on the whole unselected population, they have been able to recognize a subgroup of patients who benefited most from immunotherapy. Exploratory analyses identified MSI-H status and PD-L1 positivity (with CPS >1% and especially 10%) as strong positive predictor factor for immunotherapy with pembrolizumab, leading to regulatory agency approval in the USA (as previously in some Asian countries according to ATTRACTION-2 trial).

At current time, European guidelines do not recommend immunotherapy in the routine clinical practice, but the future perspectives for these drugs are promising also for GC, thanks to brilliant results in well-selected population.

36.7.5 Particular Conditions

36.7.5.1 Surgery of Primary Tumor and Metastasectomy

Surgery of primary tumor in case of metastatic disease is recommended only in the event of bleeding or luminal obstruction with a palliative intent.

Patients with metastatic cancer in fact do not benefit from addition of gastrectomy to chemotherapy as demonstrated by the randomized phase III REGATTA trial [44]. Furthermore, the surgical approach may determine a detrimental effect delaying the systemic treatment, favoring immunosuppression and aggravating the nutritional status of the patient [45].

Anyway the REGATTA trial had a number of limitations (first of all, it did not provide for the resection of the metastatic lesions, while a good surgery has always to be radical in oncology), and further trials are investigating the possible role of surgery in the "oligometastatic" population, in order to give a survival benefit in selected patients and not only a palliative meaning [46].

The most important one is currently the phase II FLOT-3 trial [32].

This trial demonstrated a possible role of surgery (both primary and metastatic lesions resection) in patients with limited metastatic disease who received neoadjuvant chemotherapy and had a good response. In patients with only retroperitoneal lymph node involvement, liver or lung involvement, and localized peritoneal involvement (all with a significant change of margin-free resection of the primary tumor and at least a macroscopic complete resection of the metastatic lesions at the posttreatment restaging), surgery showed a favorable survival (median overall survival of 31.3 months, while survival in unresected patients was 15.9 months).

This data needs a further validation and a dedicated phase III trial is ongoing at current time [47].

36.7.5.2 Peritoneal Involvement

The role of specific peritoneal treatment using hyperthermic intraperitoneal chemotherapy (HIPEC) is still controversial. Several small randomized trials in Asian patients have demonstrated a significant survival benefit for adjuvant HIPEC after cytoreductive surgery, but actually there are no solid data in non-Asian population [48–50]. For these reasons, the HIPEC is currently considered an experimental approach that should not be used in daily clinical practice, as well as the more modern PIPAC (pressurized intraperitoneal aerosol chemotherapy) [51–53].

Summary of Clinical Recommendations
- *AIOM*
  - Polichemotherapy should be considered in the first-line treatment of fit patients with advanced gastric cancer.
  - Trastuzumab in combination with platinum and fluorouracil should be considered the standard treatment for first-line HER2-positive gastric cancer patients.
  - Anti-EGFR drugs, such as cetuximab and panitumumab, are not recommended in treatment of gastric cancer.
- *ESMO*
  - Doublet or triplet platinum/fluoropyrimidine combinations are recommended for fit patients with advanced gastric cancer.
  - Trastuzumab is recommended in conjunction with platinum- and fluoropyrimidine-based chemotherapy for patients with HER2-positive advanced gastric cancer.
  - Second-line chemotherapy with a taxane (docetaxel, paclitaxel), or irinotecan, or ramucirumab as a single agent or in combination with paclitaxel is recommended for patients who are of PS 0–1.
- *NCCN*
  - Trastuzumab should be added to first-line chemotherapy for HER2 overexpressing metastatic adenocarcinoma.
  - Trastuzumab is not recommended for use with anthracyclines.
  - Two drug cytotoxic regimens are preferred because of lower toxicity, while three-drug regimens should be reserved for medically fit patients.

Case Study: An Unusual Clinical Progression

Man: 54 years old
- *Family history*: Negative for malignancy
- *APR*: Hypertension, psoriasis
- *APP*: For nearly 2 months fatigue and epigastralgia
- *Objective examination*: Negative. Performance status 0 according to ECOG
- *Blood tests*: Hb 7.1 g/dl
- *Esofagogastroduodenoscopy*: Presence of ulcerative area in the antrum of the stomach
- *Pathological report*: Gastric adenocarcinoma (diffuse type according to Lauren's classification)
- *TC chest and abdomen mdc*: Lesion at the antrum of the stomach with multiple perigastric lymphadenopathies. No distant metastasis

⇩

- *Surgery*: Partial gastrectomy with D2 lymphadenectomy
- *Pathological report*: Diffuse gastric adenocarcinoma limited to the mucosa with involvement of 4/20 lymph nodes resected. No margins or perivascular invasion
- *Pathological stage*: pT1N2
- Stage: pT1N2cM0 (stage IIA)

Question

What action should be taken?

(1) Follow-up (2) Adjuvant chemotherapy (3) Adjuvant chemoradiotherapy

Answer

Adjuvant Chemotherapy

Patient received 12 cycles of FOLFOX chemotherapy

⇩

Follow-up according to international guidelines for 5 years

- *After 3 years from the last follow-up visit*: Appearance of the right eyelid swelling with ptosis, cutaneous nodules at the neck and in the frontal region

Question

What action should be taken?

(1) Dermatologic visit (2) Cutaneous biopsy

Answer

Cutaneous biopsy

Tumor cells with an upper gastrointestinal origin. In consideration of the clinical history of patient, this record is in line with a cutaneous progression of disease.

⇩

- *Clinical evaluation*: Presence of nodules with increased consistency, no defined margins. Performance status 0 according to ECOG. No weight loss
- *CT scan*: No distant metastasis
- *Diagnosis*: Progression of disease (cutaneous non-resectable metastasis)

Question

What action should be taken?

(1) First-line chemotherapy upfront (2) Definition of HER2 status

Answer

Definition of HER2 status

HER2 status (IHC): 0

⇩

- *First-line chemotherapy with 12 cycles of Xelox schedule*: Major cutaneous response with reduction of all nodules and reduction of consistence
- *Clinical and instrumental follow-up every 3 months*: Maintenance of response
- *After PFS of 9 months*: Increase of known cutaneous lesions

Question

What action should be taken?

(1) Second-line chemotherapy upfront (2) Re-biopsy with definition of HER2 status

Answer

Re-biopsy with definition of HER2 status

Tumor cells with an upper gastrointestinal origin. HER2 status (IHC): 0

Question

What action should be taken?

(1) Rechallenge of Xelox (2) Taxolo + Ramucirumab (3) Ramucirumab (4) Irinotecan

Answer

Second-line with Taxolo + Ramucirumab. The decision was based on time of oxaliplatin exposure

Good performance status (0 according to ECOG)

Multidisciplinary evaluation

Key Points

- The importance of a correct diagnosis even in case of unusual clinical presentation
- The importance of a correct choose of treatment based on HER2 status of tumor
- Importance of re-biopsy after progression to evaluate changes in tumor characteristic

---

Case Study: A 32-Year-Old Man with a Metastatic Gastric Cancer

Man: 32 years old
- *Family history*: Negative for malignancy
- *APR*: Negative
- *APP*: Weight loss of 12 Kg in the last 3 months, fatigue
- *Blood tests*: Hb 10.2 g/dl
- *Esofagogastroduodenoscopy*: Presence of ulcerative area in the body of the stomach. Diffuse involvement of all stomach's wall
- *Pathological report*: Gastric adenocarcinoma (diffuse type according to Lauren's classification)
- *TC chest and abdomen mdc*: Diffuse involvement of stomach, perigastric and lombo-aorthic lymph nodes.

Presence of multiple liver metastases with a maximum diameter of 12 cm

Question

What action should be taken?

(1) Surgery (2) First-line chemotherapy (3) Multidisciplinary group evaluation

Answer

Multidisciplinary group evaluation

Nutritional assessment

Pain evaluation

Oncological assessment → stage IV, performance status 1 according to ECOG

Question

What action should be taken?

(1) First-line chemotherapy upfront (2) Definition of HER2 status

Answer

Definition of HER2 status. HER2 status (IHC): 0

- *First-line chemotherapy with cisplatin/fluorouracil schedule*, ongoing
- *First instrumental assessment after three cycles*: Stable disease

Key Points

- Surgery is not recommended in case of metastatic disease at the diagnosis even in case of young patient
- Importance of multidisciplinary approach
- Importance of evaluation of performance status and HER2 status before starting treatment

Expert Opinion

Clara Montagut

Medical Oncology Department, Hospital del Mar, Barcelona, Spain.

Key Points

1. The prognosis of this neoplasm is still poor above all in case of locally advanced or metastatic disease. Diffuse histotype, performance status, and number and site of distant metastasis are the principal prognostic factors in the metastatic setting. The Royal Marsden prognostic score individualizes three risk groups of patients on the base of four parameters: performance status, liver metastasis, peritoneal metastasis, and serum alkaline phosphatase.

2. In the metastatic setting, the research of prognostic and predictive factors is more than relevant in order to select patients to treat. Other important aspects are tumor microenvironment, immunological state of the patient, and molecular features of the neoplasm.

3. Polichemotherapy (doublet or triplet platinum/fluoropyrimidine) should be considered in the first-line treatment of fit patients with advanced gastric cancer.

4. Trastuzumab in combination with platinum and fluorouracil should be considered the standard treatment for first-line HER-2-positive gastric cancer patients.

5. Anti-EGFR drugs, such as cetuximab and panitumumab, are not recommended in treatment of gastric cancer.

6. Second-line chemotherapy with a taxane (docetaxel, paclitaxel), or irinotecan, or ramucirumab as a single agent or in combination with paclitaxel is recommended for patients who are of PS 0–1.

7. Trastuzumab is not recommended for use with anthracyclines.

8. Two-drug cytotoxic regimens are preferred because of lower toxicity, while three-drug regimens should be reserved for medically fit patients.

Recommendations

- *ESMO*
  ▶ https://www.esmo.org/Guidelines/Gastrointestinal-Cancers/Pan-Asian-adapted-ESMO-Clinical-Practice-Guidelines-for-the-management-of-patients-with-metastatic-gastric-cancer
- *ASCO*
  ▶ https://www.asco.org/practice-guidelines/quality-guidelines/guidelines/gastrointestinal-cancer#/14446

Hints for a Deeper Insight

- Progress in the treatment of advanced gastric cancer: ▶ https://www.ncbi.nlm.nih.gov/pubmed/28671042
- Expression Profile of Markers for Targeted Therapy in Gastric Cancer Patients: HER-2, Microsatellite Instability and PD-L1: ▶ https://www.ncbi.nlm.nih.gov/pubmed/31595457
- From Tumor Immunology to Immunotherapy in Gastric and Esophageal Cancer: ▶ https://www.ncbi.nlm.nih.gov/pubmed/30577521
- Prognostic value and association of Lauren classification with VEGF and VEGFR-2 expression in gastric cancer: ▶ https://www.ncbi.nlm.nih.gov/pubmed/31611999

36

References

1. Torre LA, Bray F, Siegel RL, et al. Global cancer statistics, 2012. CA Cancer J Clin. 2015;65:87–108.

2. Arnold M, Karim-Kos HE, Coebergh JW, et al. Recent trends in incidence of five common cancers in 26 European countries since 1988: analysis of the European Cancer Observatory. Eur J Cancer. 2015;51:1164–87.

3. Bang YJ, Van Cutsem E, Feyereislova A, et al. Trastuzumab in combination with chemotherapy versus chemotherapy alone for treatment of HER2-positive advanced gastric or gastro-oesophageal junction cancer (ToGA): a phase 3, open-label, randomised controlled trial. Lancet. 2010;376:687–97.

4. Lauren P. The two histological main types of gastric carcinoma: diffuse and so-called intestinal-type carcinoma. An attempt at a histo-clinical classification. Acta Pathol Microbiol Scand. 1965;64:31–49.

5. Tan IB, Ivanova T, Lim KH, Ong CW, Deng N, Lee J, Tan SH, Wu J, Lee MH, Ooi CH, et al. Intrinsic subtypes of gastric cancer, based on gene expression pattern, predict survival and respond differently to chemotherapy. Gastroenterology. 2011;141:476–85.

6. Lei Z, Tan IB, Das K, et al. Identification of molecular subtypes of gastric cancer with different responses to PI3-kinase inhibitors and 5-fluorouracil. Gastroenterology. 2013;145(3):554–65.

7. Cancer Genome Atlas Research Network. Comprehensive molecular characterization of gastric adenocarcinoma. Nature. 2014;513(7517):202–9.

8. Cristescu R, Lee J, Nebozhyn M, et al. Molecular analysis of gastric cancer identifies subtypes associated with distinct clinical outcomes. Nat Med. 2015;21(5):449–56.

9. Apicella M, Corso S, Giordano S. Targeted therapies for gastric cancer: failures and hopes from clinical trials. Oncotarget. 2017;8(34):57654–69.

10. Tabernero J, Hoff PM, Shen L, et al. Pertuzumab plus trastuzumab and chemotherapy for HER2-positive metastatic gastric or gastro-oesophageal junction cancer (JACOB): final analysis of a double-blind, randomised, placebo-controlled phase 3 study. Lancet Oncol. 2018;19(10):1372–84. https://doi.org/10.1016/S1470-2045(18)30481-9.

11. Thuss-Patience PC, Shah MA, Ohtsu A, et al. Trastuzumab emtansine versus taxane use for previously treated HER2-positive locally advanced or metastatic gastric or gastro-oesophageal junction adenocarcinoma (GATSBY): an international randomised, open-label, adaptive, phase 2/3 study. Lancet Oncol. 2017;18(5):640–53. https://doi.org/10.1016/S1470-2045(17)30111-0.

12. Pietrantonio F, Caporale M, Morano F, et al. HER2 loss in HER2-positive gastric or gastroesophageal cancer after trastuzumab therapy: implication for further clinical research. Int J Cancer. 2016;139(12):2859–64. https://doi.org/10.1002/ijc.30408.

13. Adam Bass. Preexisting oncogenic events impact trastuzumab sensitivity in ERBB2-amplified gastroesophageal adenocarcinoma. J Clin Invest. 2014;124(12):5145–58. https://doi.org/10.1172/JCI75200.

14. Pietrantonio F, Fucà G, Morano F, et al. Biomarkers of primary resistance to trastuzumab in HER2-positive metastatic gastric cancer patients: the AMNESIA case-control study. Clin Cancer Res. 2018;24(5):1082–9. https://doi.org/10.1158/1078-0432.CCR-17-2781.

15. Lordick F, Kang YK, Chung HC, et al. Capecitabine and cisplatin with or without cetuximab for patients with previously untreated advanced gastric cancer (EXPAND): a randomised, open-label phase 3 trial. Lancet Oncol. 2013;14:490–9.

16. Waddell T, Chau I, Cunningham D, et al. Epirubicin, oxaliplatin, and capecitabine with or without panitumumab for patients with previously untreated advanced oesophagogastric cancer (REAL3): a randomised, open-label phase 3 trial. Lancet Oncol. 2013;14:481–9.

17. Catenacci et al. Genomic Heterogeneity as a Barrier to Precision Medicine in Gastroesophageal Adenocarcinoma. 2018;8(1):37–48. https://doi.org/10.1158/2159-8290.CD-17-0395.

18. Shah MA, Bang YJ, Lordick F, Alsina M, Chen M, Hack SP, Bruey JM, Smith D, McCaffery I, Shames DS, et al. Effect of fluorouracil, leucovorin, and oxaliplatin with or without onartuzumab in, H.E.R2-negative, MET-positive gastroesophageal adenocarcinoma: the METGastric randomized clinical trial. JAMA Oncol. 2017;3:620–7.

19. Catenacci DVT, Tebbutt NC, Davidenko I, et al. Rilotumumab plus epirubicin, cisplatin, and capecitabine as first-line therapy in advanced MET-positive gastric or gastro-oesophageal junction cancer (RILOMET-1): a randomised, double-blind, placebo-controlled, phase 3 trial. Lancet Oncol. 2017;18(11):1467–82. pii: S1470-2045(17)30566-1.

20. Ohtsu A, Shah MA, Van Cutsem E, Rha SY, Sawaki A, Park SR, Lim HY, Yamada Y, Wu J, Langer B, et al. Bevacizumab in combination with chemotherapy as first-line therapy in advanced gastric cancer: a randomized, double-blind, placebo-controlled phase III study. J Clin Oncol. 2011;29:3968–76.

21. Shen L, Li J, Xu J, Pan H, Dai G, Qin S, Wang L, Wang J, Yang Z, Shu Y, et al. Bevacizumab plus capecitabine and cisplatin in Chinese patients with inoperable locally advanced or metastatic gastric or gastroesophageal junction cancer: randomized, double-blind, phase III study (AVATAR study). Gastric Cancer. 2015;18:168–76.

22. Fuchs CS, Tomaek J, Yong CJ, et al. Ramucirumab monotherapy for previously treated advanced gastric or gastro-oesophageal junction adenocarcinoma (REGARD): an international, randomised, multicenter, placebo-controlled, phase 3 trial. Lancet Oncol. 2014;383:31–9.

23. Wilke H, Muro K, Van Cutsem E, et al. RAINBOW Study Group. Ramucirumab plus paclitaxel versus placebo plus paclitaxel in patients with previously treated advanced gastric or gastro-oesophageal junction adenocarcinoma (RAINBOW): a double-blind, randomized phase 3 trial. Lancet Oncol. 2014;15(11):1224–35.

24. Fuchs CS, Shitara K, Di Bartolomeo M, et al. Ramucirumab with cisplatin and fluoropyrimidine as first-line therapy in patients with metastatic gastric or junctional adenocarcinoma (RAINFALL): a double-blind, randomised, placebo-controlled, phase 3 trial. Lancet Oncol. 2019;20(3):420–35. https://doi.org/10.1016/S1470-2045(18)30791-5.

25. Russo A, Incorvaia L, Malapelle U, et al. The tumor-agnostic treatment for patients with solid tumors: a position paper on behalf of the AIOM-SIAPEC/IAP-SIBIOC-SIF italian scientific societies [published online ahead of print, 2021 Aug 6]. Crit Rev Oncol Hematol. 2021;103436. https://doi.org/10.1016/j.critrevonc.2021.103436.

26. Chau I, Norman AR, Cunningham D, Waters JS, Oates J, Ross PJ. Multivariate prognostic factor analysis in locally advanced and metastatic esophago-gastric cancer--pooled analysis from

three multicenter, randomized, controlled trials using individual patient data. J Clin Oncol. 2004;22:2395–403.

27. Chau I, Ashley S, Cunningham D. Validation of the Royal Marsden hospital prognostic index in advanced esophagogastric cancer using individual patient data from the REAL 2 study. J Clin Oncol. 2009;27:e3–4.

28. Petrillo A, Laterza MM, Tirino G, Pompella L, et al. Systemic-inflammation-based score can predict prognosis in metastatic gastric cancer patients before first-line chemotherapy. Future Oncol. 2018;14(24):2493–505. https://doi.org/10.2217/fon-2018-0167.

29. Pietrantonio F, Barretta F, Fanotto V, et al. Estimating 12-weeks life expectancy in metastatic gastric cancer (mGC) patients (pts) candidates for second-line treatment: the "Gastric Life" nomogram. Ann Oncol. 2017;28(suppl_5):v209–68.

30. Wagner AD, Grothe W, Haerting J, et al. Chemotherapy meta-analysis based on aggregate data. J Clin Oncol. 2006;24:2903–9.

31. Shitara K, Van Cutsem E, Bang Y-J, et al. Pembrolizumab with or without chemotherapy vs chemotherapy in patients with advanced G/GEJ cancer (GC) including outcomes according to microsatellite instability-high (MSI-H) status in KEYNOTE-062. Ann Oncol. 2019;30:v878–9.

32. Al-Batran SE, Homann N, Pauligk C, et al. Effect of neoadjuvant chemotherapy followed by surgical resection on survival in patients with limited metastatic gastric or gastroesophageal junction cancer: the AIO-FLOT3 trial. JAMA Oncol. 2017;3(9):1237–44. https://doi.org/10.1001/jamaoncol.2017.0515.

33. Van Cutsem E, Moiseyenko VM, Tjulandin S, et al. V325 Study Group. Phase III study of docetaxel and cisplatin plus fluorouracil compared with cisplatin and fluorouracil as first-line therapy for advanced gastric cancer: a report of the V325 Study Group. J Clin Oncol. 2006;24(31):4991–7.

34. Al-Batran SE, Hartmann JT, Hofheinz R, et al. Biweekly fluorouracil, leucovorin, oxaliplatin, and docetaxel (FLOT) for patients with metastatic adenocarcinoma of the stomach or esophagogastric junction: a phase II trial of the Arbeitsgemeinschaft Internistische Onkologie. Ann Oncol. 2008;19:1882–7.

35. Cunningham D, Starling N, Rao S, et al. Capecitabine and oxaliplatin for advanced esophagogastric cancer. N Engl J Med. 2008;358:36–46.

36. Al-Batran SE, Homann N, Pauligck C, et al. Perioperative chemotherapy with fluorouracil plus leucovorin, oxaliplatin, and docetaxel versus fluorouracil or capecitabine plus cisplatin and epirubicin for locally advanced, resectable gastric or gastro-oesophageal junction adenocarcinoma (FLOT4): a randomised, phase 2/3 trial. Lancet. 2019;393(10184):1948–57.

37. Ajani JA, Rodriguez W, Bodoky G, et al. Multicenter phase III comparison of cisplatin/S-1 with cisplatin/infusional fluorouracil in advanced gastric or gastroesophageal adenocarcinoma study: the FLAGS trial. J Clin Oncol. 2010;28(9):1547–53.

38. Shah MA, Xu RH, Bang YJ, et al. HELOISE: phase IIIb randomized multicenter study comparing standard-of-care and higher-dose trastuzumab regimens combined with chemotherapy as first-line therapy in patients with human epidermal growth factor receptor 2-positive metastatic gastric or gastroesophageal junction adenocarcinoma. J Clin Oncol. 2017;35(22):2558–67.

39. Thuss-Patience PC, Kretzschmar A, Bichev D, et al. Survival advantage for irinotecan versus best supportive care as second-line chemotherapy in gastric cancer – a randomised phase III study of the Arbeitsgemeinschaft Internistische Onkologie (AIO). Eur J Cancer. 2011;47:2306–14.

40. Ford HE, Marshall A, Bridgewater JA, et al. Docetaxel versus active symptom control for refractory oesophagogastric adeno-

carcinoma (COUGAR-02): an open-label, phase 3 randomised controlled trial. Lancet Oncol. 2014;15:78–86.

41. Hironaka S, Ueda S, Yasui H, et al. Randomized, open-label, phase III study comparing irinotecan with paclitaxel in patients with advanced gastric cancer without severe peritoneal metastasis after failure of prior combination chemotherapy using fluoropyrimidine plus platinum: WJOG 4007 trial. J Clin Oncol. 2013;31:4438–44.

42. Satoh T, Xu RH, Chung HC, et al. Lapatinib plus paclitaxel versus paclitaxel alone in the second-line treatment of HER2-amplified advanced gastric cancer in Asian populations: TyTAN--a randomized, phase III study. J Clin Oncol. 2014;32(19):2039–49.

43. Shitara K, Doi T, Dvorkin M, et al. Trifluridine/tipiracil versus placebo in patients with heavily pretreated metastatic gastric cancer (TAGS): a randomised, double-blind, placebo-controlled, phase 3 trial. Lancet Oncol. 2018;19(11):1437–48. https://doi.org/10.1016/S1470-2045(18)30739-3.

44. Fujitani K, Yang HK, Mizusawa J, et al. Gastrectomy plus chemotherapy versus chemotherapy alone for advanced gastric cancer with a single non-curable factor (REGATTA): a phase 3, randomised controlled trial. Lancet Oncol. 2016;17:309–18.

45. Shah MA, Janjigian YY, Stoller R, et al. Randomized multicenter phase II study of modified docetaxel, cisplatin, and fluorouracil (DCF) versus DCF plus growth factor support in patients with metastatic gastric adenocarcinoma: a study of the US Gastric Cancer Consortium. J Clin Oncol. 2015;33:3874–9.

46. Shitara K, Ozguroglu M, Bang YJ, et al. Pembrolizumab versus paclitaxel for previously treated, advanced gastric or gastro-oesophageal junction cancer (KEYNOTE-061): a randomised, open-label, controlled, phase 3 trial. Lancet. 2018;392(10142):123–33.

47. Pinto et al. Carcinoma della giunzione gatro-esofagea e dello stomaco. Pensiero scientifico editore; 2015.

48. Yang XJ, Huang CQ, Suo T, et al. Cytoreductive surgery and hyperthermic intraperitoneal chemotherapy improves survival of patients with peritoneal carcinomatosis from gastric cancer: final results of a phase III randomized clinical trial. Ann Surg Oncol. 2011;18:1575–81.

49. Kang YK, Boku N, Satoh T, et al. Nivolumab in patients with advanced gastric or gastro-oesophageal junction cancer refractory to, or intolerant of, at least two previous chemotherapy regimens (ONO-4538-12, ATTRACTION-2): a randomised, double-blind, placebo-controlled, phase 3 trial. Lancet. 2017;390(10111):2461–71.

50. Kim J, Fox C, Peng S, et al. Preexisting oncogenic events impact trastuzumab sensitivity in ERBB2-amplified gastroesophageal adenocarcinoma. J Clin Invest. 2014;124(12):5145–58. https://doi.org/10.1172/JCI75200.

51. Maron SB, Alpert L, Kwak HA, Lomnicki S, Chase L, Xu D, O'Day E, Nagy RJ, Lanman RB, Cecchi F, et al. Targeted therapies for targeted populations: anti-EGFR treatment for EGFR-amplified gastroesophageal adenocarcinoma. Cancer Discov. 2018;8:696–713.

52. Muro K, Chung HC, Shankaran V, et al. Pembrolizumab for patients with PD-L1-positive advanced gastric cancer (KEYNOTE-012): a multicentre, open-label, phase 1b trial. Lancet Oncol. 2016;17(6):717–72636.

53. Nagtegaal ID, Odze RD, Klimstra D, Paradis V, Rugge M, Schirmacher P, Washington KM, Carneiro F, Cree IA, WHO Classification of Tumours Editorial Board. The 2019 WHO classification of tumours of the digestive system. Histopathology. 2020;76(2):182–8. https://doi.org/10.1111/his.13975.

36

Colorectal Cancer: Locoregional Disease

Erika Martinelli, Claudia Cardone, and Giulia Martini

Gastrointestinal Cancers

Contents

© Springer Nature Switzerland AG 2021
A. Russo et al. (eds.), *Practical Medical Oncology Textbook*, UNIPA Springer Series,
https://doi.org/10.1007/978-3-030-56051-5_37

⊜ **Learning Objectives**

By the end of the chapter, the reader will:

- Have learned the basic concepts of CRC carcinogenesis
- Be able to apply CRC screening procedures
- Have reached in-depth knowledge of CRC clinical presentation and diagnostic work-up
- Have learned the key role of MTDs in CRC work-up
- Be able to put acquired knowledge into early CRC treatment

37.1 Introduction

Colorectal cancer (CRC) is the third most common tumour in men and the second in women, accounting for 10% of all tumour types worldwide; incidence is higher in males (ratio, 1:4). Country-specific incidence rates are available through the World Health Organization (WHO) GLOBOCAN database. Despite mortality has declined progressively due to effective screening strategies and better treatment procedures, CRC remains the fourth most common cancer-related cause of death in the world [1–3].

Risk factors for developing CRC are:

- Lifestyle or behavioural factors (smoking, high red meat consumption, obesity, low physical activity)
- Personal history (previous polyps, inflammatory bowel disease)
- Genetically determinant factors

Screening tests should be offered to average population (range according to screening programme, 50–74 years old) (◻ Table 37.1) and high-risk subjects (◻ Table 37.2) in order to detect precancerous conditions and early-stage disease, susceptible of a curative treatment [4–6]:

- Personal history of adenoma, previous CRC, inflammatory bowel disease (Crohn's disease and ulcerative colitis).
- Family history of CRC or polyps.

◻ **Table 37.1** Screening procedures to be offered to average risk for CRC developing population

Screening method (average-risk population)	Frequency
Faecal occult blood test (FOBT) (immunochemical test> guaiac-based test)	Yearly
Flexible sigmoidoscopy (FS)	5 years
Colonoscopy	10 years
Computed tomography colonography Circulating methylated SEPT9 DNA	Currently not recommended in guidelines

◻ **Table 37.2** Screening procedure to be offered to high risk for CRC developing population

Screening method (high-risk population)	Initiation of screening	Frequency of colonoscopy
Familial polyposis	Teen age	Every 1–2 years
Lynch syndrome	20–25 years or 5 years before the youngest case in the family	
Family history of colorectal cancer or polyps (first degree relative ≤60 years)	40 years or 10 years before the youngest case in the family	Every 5 years
Crohn's colitis/ ulcerative colitis	After 8 years of chronic disease	Every 2 years
Personal history of colorectal cancer	One year from baseline colonoscopy	
High-risk adenoma	After 3 years from baseline colonoscopy	
Low-risk adenoma	After 5 years from baseline colonoscopy	

- Genetic syndromes: familial adenomatous polyposis (FAP) coli and its variants, Lynch-associated syndromes and associated polyposis syndromes (MUTYH; Turcot; Peutz-Jeghers). In case of suspicious of genetic syndromes, it is recommended a genetic counselling.

37.2 Carcinogenesis

CRC is a heterogeneous disease, developed by complex multistep genetic and environmental influences. Three mechanisms often in overlap are implicated in CRC carcinogenesis (◻ Fig. 37.1) [7, 8].

- Fearon and Vogelstein proposed a stepwise genetic model to explain the traditional transition from adenoma to carcinoma, initiated by mutations in *APC* (*adenomatous polyposis coli*) followed by mutations in *KRAS* and *TP53*, in the context of genomic instability, aneuploidy and loss of heterozygosity (LOH). This pathway, mainly related to chromosomal instability (CIN), constitutes most of the sporadic tumours (85%) and is associated with familial adenomatous polyposis caused by germline mutations in the *APC*.
- The microsatellite instability (MSI) pathway is caused by the loss of DNA mismatch repair (MMR) activity. MSI phenotype is detected in about 15% of CRC: in 3% is associated with familial Lynch syndrome (mutations in MMR genes, more fre-

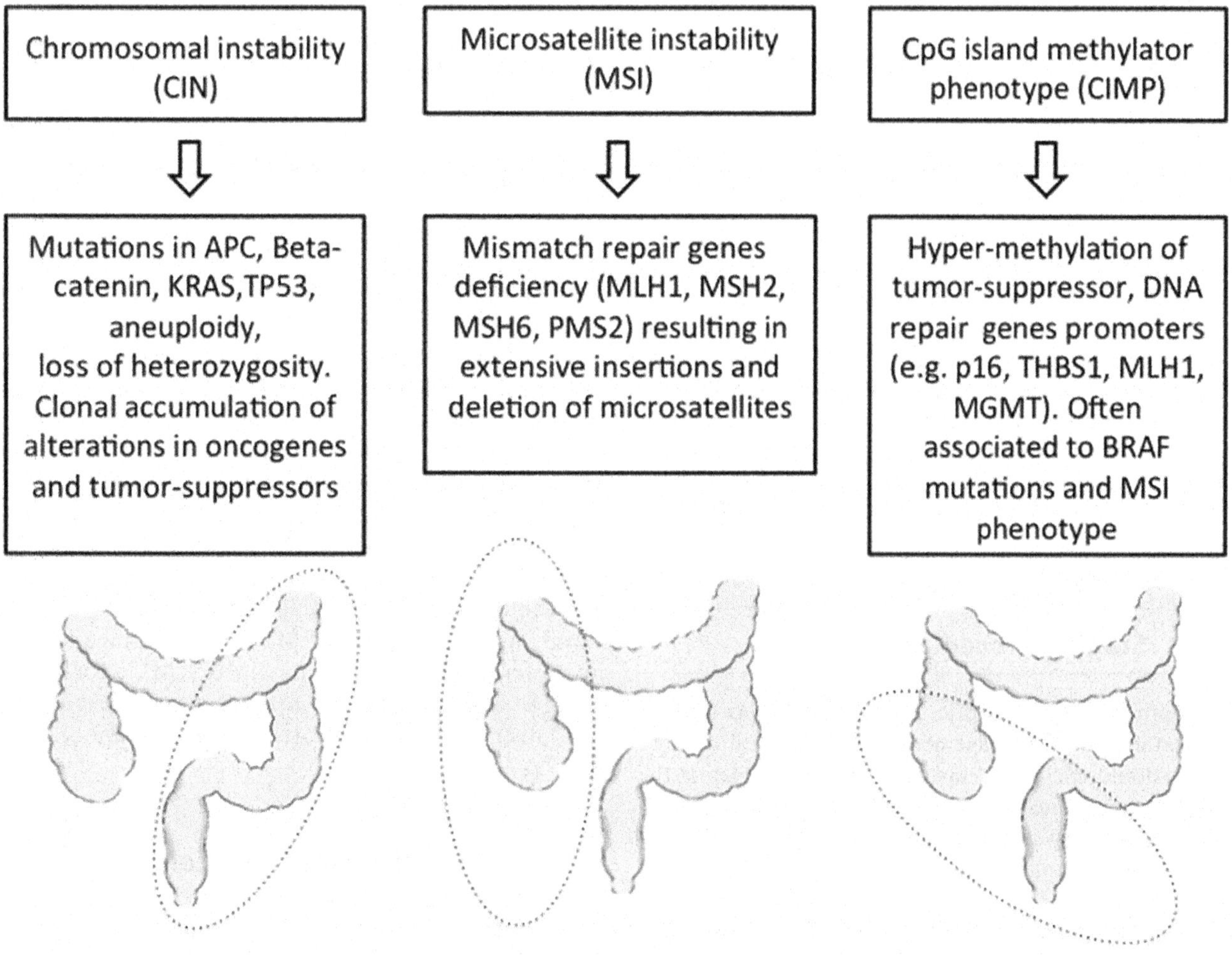

Chromosomal instability (CIN)	Microsatellite instability (MSI)	CpG island methylator phenotype (CIMP)
⇩	⇩	⇩
Mutations in APC, Beta-catenin, KRAS,TP53, aneuploidy, loss of heterozygosity. Clonal accumulation of alterations in oncogenes and tumor-suppressors	Mismatch repair genes deficiency (MLH1, MSH2, MSH6, PMS2) resulting in extensive insertions and deletion of microsatellites	Hyper-methylation of tumor-suppressor, DNA repair genes promoters (e.g. p16, THBS1, MLH1, MGMT). Often associated to BRAF mutations and MSI phenotype

Fig. 37.1 Three pathways involved in colorectal carcinogenesis

quently in *MLH1* and *MSH2*) and in 12% with sporadic cases (mostly due to the acquired promoter hyper-methylation of *MLH1* inducing expression silencing) [9].

- The CpG island methylator phenotype (CIMP) is characterized by promoter hyper-methylation of tumour suppressor genes, such as *MGMT* and *MLH1*. It is commonly associated with serrate adenoma, BRAF mutation and microsatellite instability.

37.3 Clinical Features

Symptoms associated with CRC are usually non-specific: weakness, change in appetite, weight loss without other specific causes, general or localized abdominal pain and change in bowel habits.

In the case of right-sided tumours, clinical presentation is often insidious; iron deficiency and micro-normocytic anaemia are the most common symptoms; in left-sided tumours or rectal cancer, lower gastrointestinal bleeding and obstructive symptoms may occur.

The most frequent complications of localized CRC are acute gastrointestinal bleeding and bowel obstruction, with perforation and subsequent peritonitis and sepsis.

Synchronous CRC tumours may occur in 2.5% of cases, with identical or different histological patterns and stages of development.

As other gastrointestinal cancers, also CRC may be rarely associated with paraneoplastic syndromes (i.e. acanthosis nigricans, Leser-Trelat syndrome, dermatomyositis and thrombophlebitis migrans).

37.4 Diagnosis

Physical examinations may reveal an abdominal palpable mass in case of locally advanced disease. Digital rectal examination (DRE) is the first exam to be performed in case of suspected low rectal tumours.

Laboratory exams may reflect iron deficiency anaemia and raised inflammatory markers. The carcinoembryonic antigen (CEA), an oncofoetal antigen described in 1965 by Gold and Freedman, is often associated with CRC, and it represents a useful tool during postoperative follow-up. An increased preoperative CEA (values >5 ng/mL indicate poor prognosis), not normalized after 4 weeks after surgery, is suspicious of persistent disease.

The main procedure for diagnosis is endoscopy, to be preferably carried out as a complete colonoscopy to the caecal pole. During endoscopic exam all suspicious lesions should undergo multiple tumour biopsies, in order to obtain definitive diagnosis. If not carried out before, a complete colonoscopy should be performed within 3–6 months after surgery.

Computed tomography (CT) colonography (virtual colonoscopy) is useful to identify tumour location and to detect synchronous lesions or polyps in case colonoscopy is contraindicated.

37.5 Staging

37.5.1 Staging Procedures

An appropriate diagnostic work-up is important to define therapeutic management. Preoperative staging of CRC should exclude metastatic disease and define the exact tumour location (right colon/left colon/rectum) and nodal involvement. A dedicated multidisciplinary team should manage patients, especially in the case of rectal neoplasia.

Tumours with distal extension to >15 cm from anal margin by using rigid sigmoidoscopy are classified as colon cancer. Tumours with distal extension ≤15 cm from anal margin by using rigid sigmoidoscopy are classified as rectal cancer and defined as low (≤5 cm), middle (>5–10 cm) and high (>10–15 cm).

Abdominal ultrasound (US) is a useful approach to exclude visceromegaly, ascites not evaluable at physical examination and, in most of cases, liver metastasis.

CT scan plays a key role in CRC staging, detecting the exact tumour site, usually defined as bowel wall thickening, tumour size, the degree of wall invasion, involvement of adjacent structures, tumour extension into the mesentery, the presence of lymph node, distant metastases and abdominal tumour-related complications. Bone scan and brain imaging should only be carried out if symptoms warrant.

However, in the case of rectal cancers, endorectal ultrasound (ERUS) and magnetic resonance imaging (MRI) are gold standard procedures. ERUS is helpful to define treatment for the earliest tumours, detecting mucosal or submucosal invasion. Pelvic MRI is useful to evaluate tumour size, tumour location, lymph node involvement and specific prognostic parameters used in rectal cancer imaging, such as the relationship between tumour and mesorectal fascia (MRF), extramural vascular invasion (EMVI) and distance to the circumferential resection margin (CRM). Moreover, MRI is indicated in the assessment of suspicious CRC liver metastasis and peritoneal implants [2, 3] (◘ Fig. 37.2).

37.5.2 TNM Classification for Colon and Rectal Cancer

The pathological stage must be reported according to the American Joint Cancer Committee (AJCC)/Union for International Cancer Control (UICC) tumour node metastasis (TNM) staging classification system (8th edition) (◘ Tables 37.3 and 37.4) [2, 3].

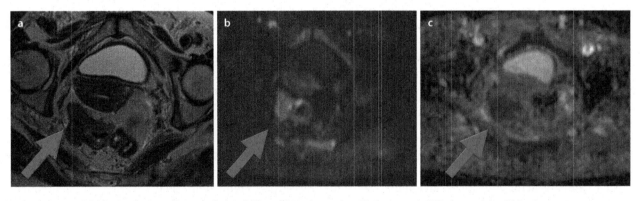

◘ **Fig. 37.2** MRI imaging for rectal tumour (lesion indicated by red arrow). **a** T2 sequence; **b** diffusion-weighted imaging sequence; **c** apparent diffusion coefficients (ADC map) sequence

■ **Table 37.3**   TNM classification for colon and rectal cancer

T	*Primary tumour*
TX	Primary tumour cannot be assessed
T0	No evidence of primary tumour
Tis	Carcinoma in situ: invasion of the lamina propria
T1	Tumour invades the submucosa
T2	Tumour invades the muscularis propria
T3	Tumour invades the subserosa/non-peritoneal pericolic or perirectal tissues
T4	Tumour invades other organs/structures and perforates the visceral peritoneum
T4a	Tumour perforates the visceral peritoneum
T4b	Tumour invades other organs/structures
N	*Regional nodes*
NX	Regional lymph nodes cannot be assessed
N0	No metastasis in regional lymph nodes
N1	Metastasis in 1–3 regional lymph nodes
N1a	Metastasis in 1 regional lymph node
N1b	Metastasis in 2–3 regional lymph nodes
N1c	Tumour deposit(s) in the subserosa/non-peritoneal pericolic or perirectal soft tissues without metastasis in regional lymph nodes
N2	Metastasis in 4 or more regional lymph nodes
N2a	Metastasis in 4–6 regional lymph nodes
N2b	Metastasis in 7 or more regional lymph nodes
M	*Distant metastasis*
M0	No distant metastasis
M1a	Metastasis confined to one organ (liver, lung, ovary, non-regional lymph nodes) without peritoneal metastases
M1b	Metastasis in more than one organ
M1c	Metastasis to the peritoneum with or without other organ involvement

Note: in case of rectal cancer, T3 tumours should be subclassified according to depth of invasion in the muscularis propria observed with MRI (T3a, <1 mm; T3b, 1–5 mm; T3c, 6–15 mm; T3d, >15 mm)

■ **Table 37.4**   Staging grouping of colon and rectal cancer

Stage 0	Tis N0 M0
Stage I	T1–2 N0 M0
Stage II	T3–4 N0 M0
Stage IIA	T3 N0 M0
Stage IIB	T4a N0 M0
Stage IIC	T4b N0 M0
Stage III	Any T N1–2 M0
Stage IIIA	T1–2 N1 M0; T1 N2a M0
Stage IIIB	T1–2 N2b M0; T2–3 N2a M0; T3–T4a N1 M0
Stage IIIC	T3–4a N2b M0; T4a N2a M0; T4b any N M0
Stage IV	Any T any N M1
Stage IVA	Any T any N M1a
Stage IVB	Any T any N M1b
Stage IVC	Any T any N M1c

37.6 Pathological Features

37.6.1 Histological Features

Around 90% of CRC are adenocarcinomas originating from epithelial cells of the mucosa, characterized by glandular formation and graded according to deviation from normal glandular tissue (ranging from more differentiated Grade 1 to undifferentiated Grade 4).

Other histologic types (i.e. neuroendocrine, squamous cell, adenosquamous, spindle cell, undifferentiated carcinomas, lymphomas) are rarely observed. According to the World Health Organization (WHO) classification, there are several histologic variants of CRC, such as mucinous, signet ring cell, medullary, micropapillary, serrated, cribriform comedo-type, adenosquamous, spindle cell and undifferentiated.

In particular, mucinous adenocarcinoma, characterized by a worse prognosis, is diagnosed when mucus occurs in >50% of the tumour tissue. In case mucinous component is <50%, they are usually termed adenocarcinoma with mucinous features or mucinous differentiation.

The most used immunohistochemical markers for colorectal adenocarcinoma are cytokeratin (CK)20, CK7 and CDX2. Usually CRC adenocarcinoma displays positivity for CK20 and negativity for CK7. CDX2 is a marker of enteric differentiation and is positive in around 90% of colorectal adenocarcinomas [10].

37.6.2 Pathological Assessment

Several information should be included in the pathological report: the morphologic description and type of surgery; presence of tumour perforation; tumour location size and invasion into adjacent structures; tumour histology and grading; status of margin; presence of tumour deposits; vascular, lymphatic, perineural invasion; tumour budding; and site and number of regional lymph nodes, considering that an adequate lymphadenectomy should include at least 12 lymph nodes.

In the case of rectal cancers, CRM distance and extranodal extension should be comprised in the pathological report.

37.7 Treatment

37.7.1 Colon Cancer

Treatment of colon cancer is based on the stage of the disease.

Stage 0 (Tis N0 M0) disease treatment options are local excision, polypectomy and segmentary en bloc resections if lesions are too large to be amenable for local excision. Colonoscopic polypectomy can be considered curative for malignant peduncolated polyps if high-risk factors as Grade 3 differentiation, level 4 Haggitt invasion (invasion of the submucosa of the bowel wall below the polyp), involved margins of excision and lymphatic or vascular invasion are excluded. Sessil polyps are graded using Kikuchi classification (involvement of submucosae, sm1, sm2 and sm3, involves the superficial, middle and deep thirds of the submucosa, respectively) and considered as a level 4 Haggitt invasion. Sm1 and sm2 lesions can be treated with polypectomy alone; otherwise, all sm3 sessile polyps and sm2 lesions with unfavourable histology should be considered for surgical resection.

For Stage I (T1–2N0M0, old staging: Dukes' A or modified Astler-Coller A and B1) surgical resection with anastomosis alone represents the standard, without adjuvant chemotherapy.

Regarding Stage II A, B and C (T3N0M0, T4 a-b N0 M0), adjuvant therapy after surgery is not recommended, but patients presenting at least one of the high-risk features (lymph nodes sampling <12, poorly differentiated tumours, vascular or lymphatic or perineural invasion, tumour presentation with obstruction or tumour perforation and pT4 stage) should receive

adjuvant treatment [11]. MSI/MMR status may be useful to identify a 10–15% subset of Stage II patients who are at a very low risk of recurrence and should not receive chemotherapy [12].

Standard treatment options for Stage III (any T, N1-N2, M0) colon cancer are represented by surgical resection and anastomosis followed by chemotherapy with a doublet schedule of oxaliplatin and a fluoropyrimidine. When oxaliplatin is contraindicated, fluoropyrimidines are selected as treatment.

In the last years, several clinical trials have demonstrated the benefit of combining cytotoxic drugs. Results from the MOSAIC trial evidenced the superiority of FOLFOX4 regimen, compared with LV-5FU2, in terms of reduction in the risk of recurrence and disease-free survival (DFS) at 3 years, confirmed at 6-year follow-up 8 [13]. XELOXA phase III study assessed the safety and efficacy of adjuvant capecitabine (CPC) + oxaliplatin vs 5FU2/LV in Stage III patients, and capecitabine was defined as a well-tolerated compared with i.v. fluoropyrimidine. The X-ACT trial showed the favourable toxicity profile of capecitabine in Stage III patients and confirmed the equivalence with intravenous (i.v.) 5FU in terms of DFS.

Other agents have been studied in the adjuvant setting, but trials showed no improvement in OS when irinotecan was added to a treatment with 5-FU/LV (CALGB-89803) or LV5FU2 or AIO regimen (PETACC-3). Moreover, regarding the evaluation of targeted agents associated with chemotherapy (CT) in the adjuvant setting, all trials resulted negative, due to a different biology of early and metastatic disease.

Recently, the optimal duration of adjuvant treatment of Stage III patients has been studied by six randomized trials forming a big international collaboration called "IDEA" trial. Statistically, 3 months of treatment with FOLFOX or CAPOX was slightly inferior to 6 months in the overall study population of Stage III patients, but additional analysis of subgroups demonstrated that selected low-risk patients could be treated with CT for 3 months, given the reduction in neurotoxicity, while a 6-month treatment is reserved for those patients with a high risk of relapse (T4 or N2). Future goals are the validation of prognostic/predictive markers leading to a more personalized therapy also in the adjuvant setting [14].

37.7.2 Rectal Cancer

Rectal cancers represent approximately one third of all colorectal malignancies and have a different behaviour from colonic tumours. In fact, early and locally advanced rectal adenocarcinomas require a specific multimodal approach. Several years ago, high recurrence rates led to an evaluation of the role of postoperative RT and adjuvant therapy with 5-fluorouracil (5FU) as the backbone in several clinical trials [15]. In the last years the role of neoadjuvant treatment with chemo-radiation (45 GY followed by surgery after 6–8 weeks) has been investigated in several clinical trials and resulted in a better local disease control, minimizing toxicity from RT and chemotherapy and eliminating local recurrence. Neoadjuvant chemo-radiation treatment has been found to determine more conservative surgery and sphincter preservation in 60–90% of cases, with a pathological complete response (pCR) in 10–25% of patients.

The choice of a preoperative treatment is based on staging and magnetic resonance imaging (MRI) or transrectal endoscopic ultrasound (EUS) that allows to a better study of pelvic structures and an involvement of nodes.

Stage I (T1, T2 N0) Early-stage tumours, defined as T1–2N0, are usually treated with surgery alone. Local excisional procedures as TEM (transanal endoscopic microsurgery) are reserved for those patients with a very early disease (cT1 N0, G1, sm1, EMVI) or for patients with a more advanced disease but with a high risk to undergo surgery. In the case of unfavourable pathological features after local excision, as the role of adjuvant CRT is not proven in preventing local recurrence, the standard treatment remains a TME (total mesorectal excision), which includes the removal of mesorectal fascia (MRF) and lymph nodes. Local RT and CRT could be used as an alternative option. TME is the chosen strategy also in those patients with tumours that are early rectal cancers but not suitable for local excision as cT1–T2 with adverse histopatologic assessment (G3, sm2–3, V1, L1) [16].

Stage II (T3–T4N0) cT3 a/b without involvement of (MRF), when located above the levators, could be treated with TME alone, only if a good-quality TME can be reached.

T3 tumours with mesorectal fat infiltration <5 mm (uT3a) should be treated with CRT followed by radical TME within 6–8 weeks. Radiation treatment consists in a traditional dose of 40–50 Gy in 25–28 fractions and concomitant treatment of infusional 5-FU or oral capecitabine. A short-course radiation treatment with high daily doses (5 × 5 Gy), followed by surgery within 10 days, could be considered as an alternative when it is not necessary to achieve a tumour-free CRM or to preserve the sphincter activity. A recent approach is represented by the use of a SCPRT not followed by immediate surgery, to avoid the risk of postoperative complications [17].

T3 tumours with mesorectal fat infiltration >5 mm (uT3b) or T4 tumours are treated with preoperative CRT followed by radical TME and adjuvant CT with infu-

sional 5-FU or capecitabine for 4 months. SCPRT is not indicated for patients with cT4 or large bulky tumours. However, some trials are evaluating the effect of SCPRT followed by a consolidation oxaliplatin-based chemotherapy treatment prior to surgery. Results are promising, even if not yet considered as a standard of care.

Stage III (any T N+) treatment consists in preoperative CRT, followed by radical TME and adjuvant CT with oxaliplatin plus infusional 5-FU or oral capecitabine (FOLFOX or XELOX). For patients with CRM and MRF involvement, neoadjuvant treatment is necessary to shrink the cancer back away from the threatened margin, and CRT has increased the percentage of patients achieving a R0 surgery.

A different new strategy is the "watch-and-wait approach" for those patients achieving a clinical complete response (cCR) after induction treatment (10–40%). Even if several clinical trials report a similar outcome for patients not undergoing surgery, compared with operated patients, results are controversial and depend from the initial stage and unknown molecular features. Until well-designed clinical trials, longer follow-up analysis and larger numbers of patients will be able to give additional data, surgical approach remains the standard of care [18].

The role of postoperative chemotherapy in patients with locally advanced rectal cancer receiving preoperative radiation or chemoradiotherapy has been studied in clinical trials but results are not consistent, and tolerance and compliance with postoperative chemotherapy are consistently dismal [19]. Moreover, it also remains unclear which parameter choose to define the risk/benefit of an adjuvant treatment, between initial clinical (yc) and pathological (yp) stage [20].

37.8 Follow-Up

Even if surgery represents the cornerstone of early colorectal cancer treatment, a big portion of patients relapses, and, nowadays, this event is unpredictable. In the last years, four meta-analyses have showed an improvement in survival for those patients receiving a more intense follow-up, due to the possibility to detect earlier isolated locoregional recurrences. After curative resection of the cancer, patients should undergo colonoscopy 1, 3 and 5 years after the initial colonoscopy, looking for metachronous adenomas and cancers, if findings on these surveillance colonoscopies remain normal. Intervals may be shortened after the 1-year examination based on adenomatous findings or hereditary causes of colon cancer. A computer tomography of the chest and abdomen should be performed every year (abdominal CT scan could be substituted by CEUS), together with a physical examination and a evaluation of carcinoembryonic antigen (CEA) every 3–6 months for the first 3 years and every 6 months during years 4 and 5 and subsequently at the discretion of the physician. Other laboratory and radiological examinations are of unproven benefit and should be reserved for symptomatic patients.

Despite data showed a benefit of 12% in OS in patients undergoing intensive clinical and instrumental follow-up, there is still a low adherence to physicians' recommendations, giving also the heterogeneity of the trials included in the meta-analyses and the absence of an exact optimal strategy of surveillance [21–25].

Case Study: A Suspect Case of Asthenia

Man, 56 years old
- *Family history* positive for CRC
- *APR*: Essential hypertension
- *APP*: diffuse abdominal pain; change in bowel habits, asthenia
- *Objective examination*: mild tenderness on deep palpation (lower quadrants)
- *Blood tests*: Hb 9.0 g/dL; iron deficiency

Question

What action should be taken?
   (1) Barium enema. (2) Sigmoidoscopy with biopsy. (3) Complete colonoscopy with biopsy

Answer

Complete colonoscopy with biopsy
   An ulcerative mass is observed in the right colon. Histological examination: adenocarcinoma, moderate differentiation (G2)

Question

What action should be taken?
   (1) Thorax and abdomen CT scan. (2) Abdomen MRI. (3) Others

Answer

Thorax and abdomen CT scan. Revealed bowel wall circumferential thickening and lymph node regional metastasis. No evidence of distant metastasis

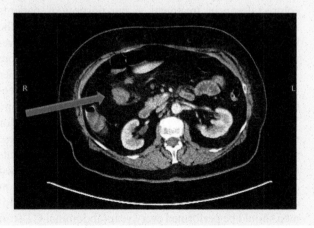

Question

What action should be taken?
   (1) Surgery. (2) Medical therapy. (3) Others

Answer

Surgery (right hemicolectomy) was performed. Histological examination: adenocarcinoma, G2 stage pTa N2a cM0

Question

What action should be taken?
   (1) Follow-up. (2) Medical therapy. (3) Others

Answer

Patient received medical therapy: 6 months adjuvant chemotherapy XELOX capecitabine 2000 mg/mq G1 –> G14 q21 + oxaliplatin 130 mg/mq q21.

Key Points

- Right colon cancer presentation is often insidious.
- Symptoms are often non-specific.
- Perform a complete colonoscopy to the caecal pole with biopsy.
- Perform adequate surgery and, if indicated, adjuvant chemotherapy.

Female, 55 years old
- *Family history* negative for malignancy
- *APR*: negative, smoker 1 pack/day
- *APP*: rectorrhagia
- *Blood tests*: Hb 9.9 g/dL
- *FOBT*: positive. *DRE*: positive
- *Sigmoidoscopy with biopsy*: Ulcerative rectal mass. Histological examination: adenocarcinoma

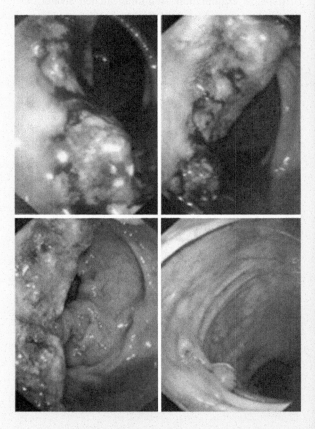

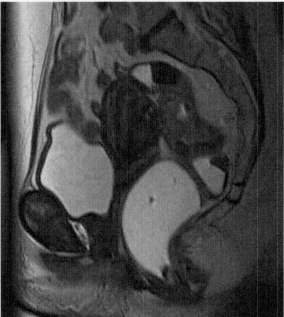

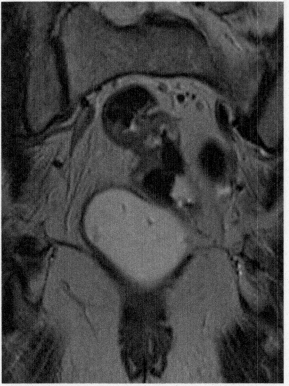

- *TC Abdomen mdc*: lower bowel wall circumferential thickening, multiple perirectal lymph nodes. No evidence of distance metastasis.

Question

What action should be taken?
(1) Perform ERUS. (2) Perform MRI. (3) Others

Answer

Perform MRI: rectal wall circumferential thickening, thickening of the mesorectal fascia; multiple perirectal lymph nodes, EMVI present; stage cT3 N+. The case was discussed within the multidisciplinary team.

Question

What action should be taken?
(1) Surgery. (2) Neoadjuvant CRT. (3) Others

Answer

Neoadjuvant CRT: radiotherapy (total 50 Gy) + capecitabine 825 mg/mq bis in die (bid)

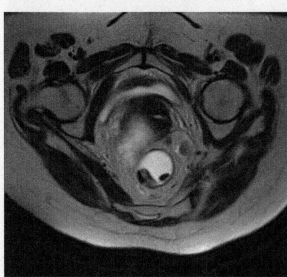

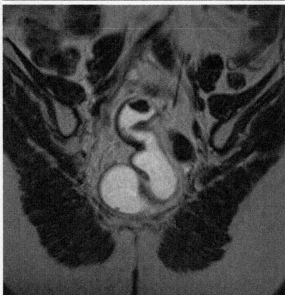

MRI shows tumour and lymph node regression

Question

What action should be taken?
(1) Surgery. (2) Follow-up. (3) Others

Answer

Surgery: Total mesorectal Excision (TME) was performed. Histological examination: well-differentiated adenocarcinoma G1. stage ypT1 N0 (0/15) cM0; TRG: 2

Key Points

- Importance of proper work-up.
- Rectal cancer cases should always be discussed with the multidisciplinary team.
- ERUS and MRI are the appropriate procedures to locally stage rectal cancer.

Expert Opinion

Marc Peeters

- Colorectal cancer (CRC) is the third most common neoplasm in men and the second in women. Risk factors are represented by smoking, high red meat consumption, obesity, low physical activity, personal history such as previous polyps or IBDs and genetically determinant factors.

- Three theories are used to explain the multimodal onset of CRC: Fearon and Vogelstein model, the microsatellite instability and the cpG island methylator phenotype. These three models involve different genes such as APC, KRAS, Tp53, MLH1, MSH2 and MGMT.

- Symptoms of CRC are usually non-specific and they can vary in dependence of cancer localization in the colon: weight loss, general or localised abdominal pain, diarrhoea or constipation, weakness and lower gastro-intestinal bleeding.

- In case of suspicious of a lower rectal tumour, digital anal examination must be done. Physical examination can give useful information such as the presence of a mass in the abdomen; blood test can show iron deficiency anaemia and if investigated, increased levels of CEA (a tumour marker associated also to CRC). A colonoscopy must be performed taking tissue samples in case of suspicious masses. CT allows a correct staging with the evidence of possible metastases. For rectal cancers, MRI is the golden standard procedure.

- The most frequent histological type is adenocarcinoma; other forms are neuroendocrine, squamous cell, adenosquamous, spindle cell, undifferentiated carcinomas and lymphomas. WHO classification identifies different subtypes of CRC such as mucinous, signet ring cell, medullary, etc.

- Treatments differ from types and stage of CRC: for colon cancers, they can consist in locoregional procedures or surgery alone (0-I stages) and adjuvant chemotherapy (in some cases of II stage and in III stage) with oxaliplatin and fluoropyrimidine. For early and locally advanced rectal cancers, a neoadjuvant approach with chemo-radiation (CRT) is usually chosen; stage III tumours with mesorectal fat infiltration >5 mm or T4 tumours are treated with preoperative CRT followed by radical total mesorectal excision (TME) and adjuvant chemotherapy.

- Follow-up strategies consist in colonoscopy, CEA evaluations and CT scan in order to identify early relapses or late metastases.

Recommendations

- AIOM
  - ▶ https://www.aiom.it/wpcontent/uploads/2020/10/2020_LG_AIOM_Colon.pdf
- ESMO
  - ▶ www.esmo.org/Guidelines/Gastrointestinal-Cancers/Rectal-Cancer
  - ▶ www.esmo.org/Guidelines/Gastrointestinal-Cancers/Early-Colon-Cancer
- ASCO
  - ▶ www.asco.org/practice-guidelines/quality-guidelines/guidelines/gastrointestinal-cancer#/10251
  - ▶ www.asco.org/practice-guidelines/quality-guidelines/guidelines/gastrointestinal-cancer#/34946
  - ▶ www.asco.org/practice-guidelines/quality-guidelines/guidelines/gastrointestinal-cancer#/34951

Hints for a Deeper Insight

- Understanding the role of primary tumour localisation in colorectal cancer treatment and outcomes: ▶ https://www.ncbi.nlm.nih.gov/pubmed/28787661
- Transanal total mesorectal excision (taTME) for rectal cancer: beyond the learning curve: ▶ https://www.ncbi.nlm.nih.gov/pubmed/31602515
- Identification of the Risk Factors for Recurrence of Stage III Colorectal Cancer: ▶ https://www.ncbi.nlm.nih.gov/pubmed/31570473
- Postoperative XELOX therapy for patients with curatively resected high-risk stage II and stage III rectal cancer without preoperative chemoradiation: a prospective, multicenter, open-label, single-arm phase II study: ▶ https://www.ncbi.nlm.nih.gov/pubmed/31533662
- Long-term Transanal Excision Outcomes in Patients With T1 Rectal Cancer: Comparative Analysis of Radical Resection: ▶ https://www.ncbi.nlm.nih.gov/pubmed/31487767

References

1. Ferlay J, Soerjomataram I, Dikshit R, Eser S, Mathers C, Rebelo M, Parkin DM, Forman D, Bray F. Cancer incidence and mortality worldwide: sources, methods and major patterns in GLOBOCAN 2012. Int J Cancer. 2015;136(5):E359–86. https://doi.org/10.1002/ijc.29210. PMID: 25220842. Published online 9 October 2014.

2. Labianca R, Nordlinger B, Beretta GD, Mosconi S, Mandalà M, Cervantes A, D. Arnold on behalf of the ESMO Guidelines Working Group Early colon cancer. ESMO clinical practice guidelines for diagnosis, treatment and follow-up. Ann Oncol. 2013;24(Supplement 6):vi64–72.

3. Glynne-Jones R, Wyrwicz L, Tiret E, Brown G, Rodel C, Cervantes A, Arnold D, on behalf of the ESMO Guidelines Committee. Rectal cancer: ESMO clinical practice guidelines for diagnosis, treatment and follow-up. Ann Oncol. 2017;28(Supplement 4):iv22–40.

4. Inadomi JM. Screening for colorectal neoplasia. N Engl J Med. 2017;376:149–56.

5. Balmaña J, Balaguer F, Cervantes A, Arnold D, on behalf of the ESMO. Familial risk-colorectal cancer: ESMO Clinical Practice Guidelines. Ann Oncol. 2013;24(Supplement 6):vi73–80.

6. Lieberman D, Ladabaum U, Cruz-Correa M, Ginsburg C, Inadomi JM, Kim LS, Wender RC. Screening for colorectal cancer and evolving issues for physicians and patients: a review. JAMA. 2016;316(20):2135–45.

7. Tariq K, Ghias K. Colorectal cancer carcinogenesis: a review of mechanisms. Cancer Biol Med. 2016;13(1):120–35. https://doi.org/10.28092/j.issn.2095-3941.2015.0103.

8. Fredericks E, Dealtry G, Roux S. Molecular aspects of colorectal carcinogenesis: a review. J Cancer Biol Res. 2015;3(1):1057.

9. Russo A, Incorvaia L, Malapelle U, et al. The tumor-agnostic treatment for patients with solid tumors: a position paper on behalf of the AIOM-SIAPEC/IAP-SIBIOC-SIF italian scientific societies [published online ahead of print, 2021 Aug 6]. Crit Rev Oncol Hematol. 2021;103436. https://doi.org/10.1016/j.critrevonc.2021.103436.

10. Fleming M, Ravula S, Tatishchev SF, Wang HL. Colorectal carcinoma: pathologic aspects. J Gastrointest Oncol. 2012;3(3):153–73.

11. Tournigand C, André T, Bonnetain F, et al. Adjuvant therapy with fluorouracil and oxaliplatin in stage II and elderly patients (between ages 70 and 75 years) with colon cancer: subgroup analyses of the Multicenter International Study of oxaliplatin, Fluorouracil and leucovorin in the Adjuvant Treatment of Colon Cancer trial. J Clin Oncol. 2012;30:3353–60.

12. Tejpar S, Saridaki Z, Delorenzi M, et al. Microsatellite instability, prognosis and drug sensitivity of stage II and III colorectal cancer: more complexity to the puzzle. J Natl Cancer Inst. 2011;103:841–4.

13. Andre T, Boni C, Navarro M, et al. Improved overall survival with oxaliplatin, fluorouracil, and leucovorin as adjuvant treatment in stage II or III colon cancer in the MOSAIC trial. J Clin Oncol. 2009;27:3109–16.

14. André T, Iveson T, Labianca R, et al. The IDEA (International Duration Evaluation of Adjuvant Chemotherapy) collaboration: prospective combined analysis of phase III trials investigating duration of adjuvant therapy with the FOLFOX (FOLFOX4 or modified FOLFOX6) or XELOX (3 versus 6 months) regimen for patients with stage III colon cancer: trial design and current status. Curr Colorectal Cancer Rep. 2013;9:261–9.

15. Bosset JF, Collette L, Calais G, et al. Chemotherapy with preoperative radiotherapy in rectal cancer. N Engl J Med. 2006;355:1114–23.

16. Junginger T, Goenner U, Hitzler M, et al. Long-term oncologic outcome after transanal endoscopic microsurgery for rectal carcinoma. Dis Colon Rectum. 2016;59:8–15.

17. Ngan SY, Burmeister B, Fisher RJ, et al. Randomized trial of shortcourse radiotherapy versus long-course chemoradiation comparing rates of local recurrence in patients with T3 rectal cancer: TransTasman Radiation Oncology Group Trial 01.04. J Clin Oncol. 2012;31:3827–33.

18. Glynne-Jones R, Hughes R. Critical appraisal of the 'wait and see' approach in rectal cancer for clinical complete responders after chemoradiation. Br J Surg. 2012;99:897–909.

19. Bosset JF, Calais G, Mineur L, et al. Fluorouracil-based adjuvant chemotherapy after preoperative chemoradiotherapy in rectal cancer: long-term results of the EORTC 22921 randomised study. Lancet Oncol. 2014;15:184–90.

20. Sauer R, Becker H, Hohenberger W, et al. Preoperative versus postoperative chemoradiotherapy for rectal cancer. N Engl J Med. 2004;351:1731–40.

21. Rosen M, Chan L, Beart RW Jr, et al. Follow-up of colorectal cancer: a metaanalysis. Dis Colon Rectum. 1998;41:1116–26.

22. Renehan AG, Egger M, Saunders MP, et al. Impact on survival of intensive follow up after curative resection for colorectal cancer: systematic review and metaanalysis of randomised trials. BMJ. 2002;324:813–9.

23. Tjandra JJ, Chan MK. Follow-up after curative resection of colorectal cancer: a meta-analysis. Dis Colon Rectum. 2007;50:1783–99.

24. Jeffery GM, Hickey BE, Hider P. Follow-up strategies for patients treated for nonmetastatic colorectal cancer. Cochrane Database Syst Rev. 2007;1:CD002200.

25. Renehan AG, Egger M, Saunders MP, et al. Mechanisms of improved survival from intensive follow-up in colorectal cancer: a hypothesis. Br J Cancer. 2005;92:430–3.

37

Colorectal Cancer: Metastatic Disease

Antonio Galvano, Aurelia Ada Guarini, Valerio Gristina, Nadia Barraco, Maria La Mantia, Marta Castiglia, and Antonio Russo

Gastrointestinal Cancers

Contents

Antonio Galvano and Aurelia Ada Guarini should be considered equally co-first authors.

© Springer Nature Switzerland AG 2021
A. Russo et al. (eds.), *Practical Medical Oncology Textbook*, UNIPA Springer Series,
https://doi.org/10.1007/978-3-030-56051-5_38

⊜ Learning Objectives

By the end of the chapter the reader will:

- Be able to apply molecular, diagnostic, and therapeutic procedures in metastatic colorectal cancer
- Have learned the basic concepts of metastatic colorectal cancer
- Have reached in-depth knowledge of colon and rectal cancer
- Be able to put newly acquired knowledge into clinical practice

38.1 Introduction

While approximately one-fourth of patients diagnosed with metastatic colorectal cancer (mCRC) most frequently present with liver metastases at the initial diagnosis (synchronous metastases) and seem to be associated with a more disseminated disease state along with a worse prognosis, the majority of them would develop metastases during the disease course after the resection of locoregional colorectal cancer (metachronous metastases). To date, the liver represents the most common site of metastatic involvement [1], with the lung also occurring almost as frequently in the specific case of rectal cancer, whereas peritoneal, bone, ovarian, and central nervous system metastatic sites are less common.

Although several different biological and clinical hallmarks exist between the colon and rectum (different embryological origin, anatomy and function) [2] along with different (neo)adjuvant treatment and surgical approaches advocated in the locoregional setting, mCRC requires similar staging procedures and systemic treatment strategies (first and subsequent lines) in terms of a multimodal approach treatment as a part of a "continuum of care."

Moreover, patients affected by oligometastatic disease confined to a single or a few organs (most frequently the liver and, secondly, the lung) should undergo an upfront evaluation by a multidisciplinary team for assessing a disease which could be initially resectable or may become completely resectable following treatment ("conversion therapy"), achieving a potentially curative approach with improved long-term survival rates.

So far, the standard of care for treatment of mCRC has been built on the backbone of 5-fluorouracil (5-FU)-based chemotherapy, including first-line combination treatment with either oxaliplatin or irinotecan (FOLFOX and FOLFIRI, respectively), plus a monoclonal antibody (bevacizumab versus cetuximab or panitumumab). In the era of personalized medicine, genotyping of tumor tissue (either primary tumor or metastasis) for *RAS* and *BRAF* testing in all patients with mCRC has been associated with significant prognostic and predictive implications and therefore is strongly recommended. In addition, primary tumor location appeared to impact both prognosis and prediction of responsiveness to targeted therapy in advanced disease.

However, despite major advances in a more tailored approach to systemic treatment and a substantial rise in survival rates over the last two decades, mortality from CRC remains high with a huge number of patients who would eventually succumb to disease progression.

38.2 Molecular Biology

Colorectal cancer (CRC) exhibits differences in incidence, pathogenesis, molecular pathways, and outcome depending on tumor location. Indeed, recent epidemiological and scientific studies have showed that proximal (right-sided) and distal (left-sided) colon cancers are biologically different regarding both genetic and immunologic factors. Moreover, it has been shown that primary tumor location has a relevant prognostic value in both earlier and advanced stages of disease, and it should be acknowledged before taking important clinical decision, such as choosing between first-line or palliative treatment [3].

More than 1000 genes are differentially expressed in adult ascending versus descending colon, and biopsies of the adult colonic epithelium can be correctly classified as proximal or distal by gene expression profile, with almost 100% concordance [4]. According to their different embryological origin, the right colon and left colon have a different vascular supply; the proximal colon receives its main blood supply from the superior mesenteric artery, while the distal colon is perfused by inferior mesenteric artery. Interestingly the proximal and distal colon are exposed to different pro-carcinogenic factors that may contribute in determining the epidemiological and biological differences that characterize right and left colon cancer. The right colon and left colon differ in the expression of several antigens, but also in bile acid concentration and in the composition of the bacterial population [5–7]. Indeed, mucosal microbiota organization is a critical factor, and it is associated with a specific subset of CRC. Invasive polymicrobial bacterial biofilms have been reported in 89% of right-sided tumors but in only 12% of left-sided tumors [7].

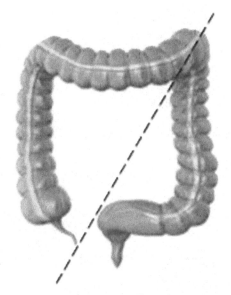

Right-sided (proximal) colon cancer

Common in women

Derived from midgut

MSI-high; CIMP+; CIN-

BRAF (more frequently) and KRAS (less frequently) mutations

Polymicrobial biofilms

CMS 1 and 3

Worse prognosis

Resistance to anti-EGFR mAb

Left-sided (distal) colon cancer

Common in men

Derived from hindgut

CIN+; MSI-low

KRAS mutations

No polymicrobial biofilms

CMS 2 e 4

HER2 amplification

Better prognosis

Response to anti-EGFR mAb

Perhaps one of the most important discoveries in mCRC has been the recognition that mutations of the gene encoding for KRAS (a signal transduction protein which is a crucial intermediate in transmission of growth and survival signals from the EGFR to the nucleus) are early events in colorectal cancer formation, with a very tight correlation between mutation status in the primary tumor and metastases. A growing body of literature has shown that mutations in KRAS exon 2 (occurring in approximately 40% of mCRCs) are predictive of lack of response to targeted therapy, in the light of a constitutive activation of this signaling pathway which renders blocking of the EGFR binding site on the surface useless. Subsequently, update analyses from several retrospective studies have investigated the role of NRAS (exons 2, 3, and 4) and other KRAS (exons 3 and 4) mutations, resulting that targeted therapy likely has a detrimental effect in patients with *KRAS* or *NRAS* mutations [8, 9] (see ▪ Figs. 38.1 and 38.2). Moreover, approximately 8–12% of colorectal cancers have resulted to be characterized by a specific mutation in the *BRAF* gene (V600E), downstream of EGFR and mutually exclusive of *RAS* mutations, which is responsible for the constitutive activation of the MAPK pathway and postulated as a possible additional predictive biomarker of lack of response to targeted therapy [10].

BRAF-mutated (10%) mCRCs are often linked to negative prognostic implications, such as right-sided tumors. MSI results from a deficient mismatch repair system (dMMR), responsible for correcting nucleotide base mispairings which occurred during DNA replication. Immunohistochemistry (IHC) tests for MMR proteins orPCR tests for microsatellite instability (MSI) in metastatic disease setting could assist clinicians in genetic counseling and should be considered a predictive biomarker in the use of immunotherapy in mCRC, as discussed below (see ▪ Table 38.1).

Furthermore, experimental approaches have been conducted to investigate the overexpression of HER2 (human epidermal growth factor receptor 2) in mCRCs, whose prevalence is higher in *RAS/BRAF* wild-type tumors (5–14%). Preliminary findings demonstrate the use of HER2 as a potential predictive biomarker for refractory *HER-2* positive mCRC, yet further studies are needed. Several retrospective analyses have shown a possible prognostic or predictive role of PTEN or PIK3CA because of their relationships with EGFR pathways. Lastly, other genes like ALK, ROS1, RET, and NTRK are under investigation as predictive factors. Recent data suggested how well NTRK inhibitors work in patients carrying NTRK 1, 2, or 3 genes involving other partners.

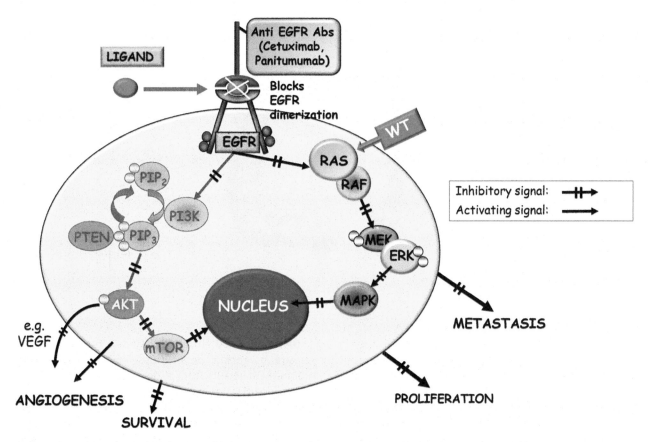

Fig. 38.1 Anti-EGFR mechanism in a wild-type KRAS scenario

38.3 Clinical Presentation and Diagnosis of Metastatic Disease

Clinical presentation of a metastatic disease can be asymptomatic and unspecific.

CRC can spread via lymphatic and hematogenous dissemination, as well as by contiguous and transperitoneal routes. The venous drainage of the intestinal tract is via the portal system; the first site of hematogenous dissemination is usually the liver, followed by the lungs, bone, and many other sites. Patients may present with signs or symptoms referable to any of these areas. It has been shown that patients with liver metastases at initial diagnosis of colon cancer have a more aggressive disease than patients with metachronous metastases. A retrospective study led by Tsai et al. showed that patients with synchronous metastases had bilobar metastases and a more aggressive disease than patients with metachronous metastases [11].

Liver metastases can be detected by CT scan, which is the first imaging technique useful for staging. Liver MRI performs better than CT scan in term of sensitivity; thus MRI is the modality preferred for liver metastases detection [12].

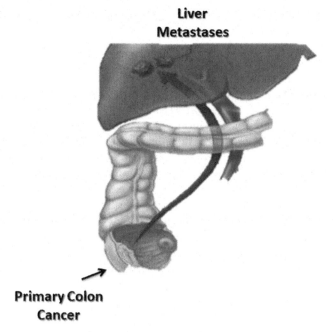

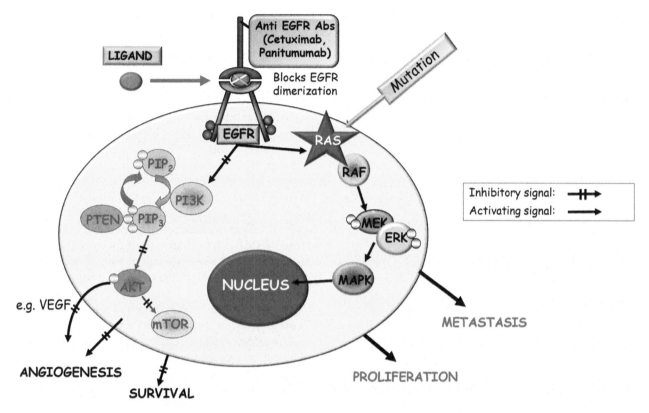

◘ **Fig. 38.2** Anti-EGFR mechanism in a KRAS-mutated scenario

38.4 Principles of Management of Metastatic Disease

As endorsed by all the international guidelines, the choice of a treatment strategy in mCRC should be evaluated as part of "continuum of care," based on consideration of the tumor- and disease-related characteristics (the mutational profile and the clinical presentation of the tumor), the goals of therapy (cytoreduction vs disease control), the type and timing of prior therapy, the patient-related factors (performance status, motivation, and expectations), and the treatment-related features (toxicity profiles of drugs).

38.4.1 Surgical Management of Colorectal Metastases

ESMO and other groups have established guidelines for the management and treatment of metastatic colorectal cancer. For selected patients, liver metastases removal

and a cure are possible; this perspective should be the goal of our practice. The definition of resectable colorectal liver metastases (CLM) evolved in the past few years. There is a consensus proposing that disease should be considerable "resectable" as long as the procedure can be technically performed and the remaining liver should be at least 30%.

For technically resectable liver metastases, oncological prognostic factors should be considered since surgery upfront and perioperative chemotherapy are both feasible.

The oncological criteria provide prognostic information on DFS. These criteria are summarized by a score designed by Fung et al., and they include elements, such as number of lesions, presence of extrahepatic disease, long-term metachronous disease, and vessel relationship [13].

According to the EPOC trial, patients who have unfavorable oncological criteria but a technically resectable disease should undergo a perioperative chemotherapy: 3 months before surgery and 3 months after surgery. CAPOX and FOLFOX should be considered in this set-

Table 38.1 Summary of mCRC molecular testing recommendations

Molecular pathology and biomarkers

Extended RAS testing

RAS mutational status is a predictive biomarker for therapeutic choices involving EGFR antibody therapies in the metastatic disease setting

RAS testing should be carried out on all patients at the time of diagnosis of mCRC

RAS testing is mandatory before treatment with the EGFR-targeted monoclonal antibodies cetuximab and panitumumab

Primary or metastatic colorectal tumour tissue can be used for RAS testing (see also Recommendation 3)

RAS analysis should include at least KRAS exons 2, 3 and 4 (codons 12, 13, 59, 61, 117 and 146) and NRAS exons 2, 3 and 4 (codons 12, 13, 59, 61 and 117)

BRAF testing	*MSI (MMR) testing*
Tumor BRAF mutation status (V600E) should be assessed alongside the assessment of tumor RAS mutational status for prognostic assessment	Immunohistochemistry (IHC) tests for MMR proteins or PCR tests for microsatellite instability (MSI) in the metastatic disease setting can assist clinicians in genetic counseling. Tumor MMR testing has strong predictive value for the use of immune check-point inhibitors in the treatment of patients with mCRC

ting of patients, while anti-EGFR and bevacizumab are not recommended, as demonstrated in the new EPOC trial [14].

38.4.2 "Conversion": Strategic Treatment Goal for Unresectable Liver Metastases

Patients with limited liver/lung metastases unresectable upfront might receive a systemic therapy in order to render the disease surgically resectable. This strategy is defined as "conversion." The main limitation of trials investigating this complex therapeutic area is due to the definition of upfront unresectable liver metastases.

The CELIM trial has been one of the first trials aiming to evaluate two groups of KRAS wild-type patients, both with upfront unresectable liver metastases, who underwent two different preoperative protocols: FOLFOX6 + Cetuximab and FOLFIRI+Cetuximab. The study demonstrated that a tumor RR ranging around 60–70% was achieved in both groups and 30–40% underwent a R0 liver resection. No data on the more effective chemotherapy protocol, albeit the oxali-

platin backbone strategy, seemed to be more efficient than treatment with irinotecan [15].

Besides, the OLIVIA phase II randomized prospective trial evaluated the FOLFOX6 plus bevacizumab regimen compared to the same strategy with the addition of Irinotecan for patients with initially unresectable colorectal liver metastases. Resection rates were 49% and 61%, respectively, although it is still unknown the benefit of a third chemotherapy addition since FOLFOXIRI alone achieved high RR, as demonstrated in the phase II trial by Masi et al. [16].

Furthermore, anti-EGFR combinations were investigated to downsize colorectal liver metastases from colorectal cancer. Particularly, the PLANET-TTD [17] and the PRIME [18] trials overall efficacy results showed that panitumumab in association with FOLFOX or FOLFIRI regimens should be considered a good option in this setting.

Nevertheless, no robust data suggest a real clear advantage regarding the addition of anti-VEGF or anti-EGFR strategy, despite results from clinical trials on liver resection rate and overall response rate supposed their impact on prognosis.

Other data from the CALGB 80405 [Elez, 2015, First-Line Treatment of Metastatic Colorectal Cancer: Interpreting FIRE-3`, PEAK`, and CALGB/SWOG 80405] and FIRE-3 [19] trial showed that a doublet of chemotherapeutic agents (FOLFOX6 or FOLFIRI) plus anti-EGFR or anti-VEGF in KRAS wild-type patients was associated with higher RRs compared to bevacizumab, yet these data have not shown higher resection rates. In particular, in CALGB 80405 a subgroup of 180 pts. containing liver-only disease were converted to surgery reaching median survival times around 64 and 67 months for anti-EGFR and anti VEGF combinations.

The response after chemotherapy may be evaluated with some response parameters: early tumor shrinkage (ETS) and depth of response (DpR).

The ETS is associated with a long-term outcome, and this parameter has been first used as a response parameter in a study designed by Piesseaux et al. in patients treated with chemotherapy plus cetuximab in first line. ETS was evaluated according to cutoff values decided by the investigators (radiological tumor size at 8 weeks) [20]. However, it is still unclear the role of the antibodies post-surgery.

Local therapies like intra-arterial chemotherapy or chemoembolization might be used to shrink a large tumor as evaluated in a small study, the DEBIRI, where 296 patients among 600 patients with unresectable liver metastases had undergone hepatic arterial drug-eluting irinotecan bead (DEBIRI) therapy. Patients treated with DEBIRI achieved higher resection rates and R0 resections [21] (see Table 38.2).

Table 38.2 Conversion chemotherapy approach

Study	Chemotherapy	Liver resection rate %
Vie-LM-Bev	CAPOX + bevacizumab	93
CELIM	FOLFOX6/FOLFIRI + cetuximab	33
GONO	FOLFOXIRI + bevacizumab	40
POCHER	Chrono-IFLO + cetuximab	60
BOXER	CAPOX + bevacizumab	40
OLIVIA	FOLFOXIRI + bevacizumab versus FOLFOX + bevacizumab	49 versus 23 (RO)
Ye et al.	FOLFIRI/FOLFOX ± cetuximab	26 versus 7 (RO)

38.4.3 Local and Ablative Treatments

The goal of an ablation treatment is not curative as surgery, since the prognosis of these patients is poor due to the spread of the disease and the sites of metastases. The ablation of visible metastases could be combined with systemic therapy in order to improve the survival rate of a patient in a stage IV.

Many data for stereotactic body radiation therapy (SBRT) have been reported, assessing this technique as an optimal tool, combined with systemic therapy, in selected patients with unresectable liver metastases [22].

The CLOCC phase II trial showed radiofrequency ablation (RFA) and chemotherapy combination treatment improvement in OS [23].

38.4.3.1 Thermal Ablation

Treatments like RFA, using temperatures ranging from 55 °C to 100 °C, could be used for unresectable liver metastases with comorbidities and liver dysfunction as shown in the phase II CLOCC trial. Notably, patients underwent to RFA + FOLFOX +/− bevacizumab or FOLFOX +/− bevacizumab showing a significant improvement in overall survival in the RFA strategy.

Moreover, these thermal ablation techniques have been established to be effective in lung metastases. Petre et al. presented that RFA on the lung could improve the local tumor progression (LTP) and the survival rates by sparing the lung parenchyma. LTP-free survival rates achieved 77% at 3 years [24]. Despite these encouraging results, some limitations affected the routine use of RFA in clinical practice because of dissemination or incomplete ablation rendering this topic as controversial and limited for patients with comorbidities, unresectable lesions, or extrahepatic lesions.

38.4.3.2 Chemoembolization

Transarterial chemoembolization (TACE) is a potential option in this setting, although evidences are limited in respect to TARE. A 2013 Cochrane review has not recommended the use of TACE outside clinical trials, according to the results of a trial comparing TACE versus FOLFIRI chemotherapy regimen. A recent study by Martin et al. comparing TACE with irinotecan-loaded drug-eluting beads (DEBIRI) in addition to FOLFOX plus bevacizumab has evaluated an improvement in PFS of DEBIRI arm (15.3 vs 7.6 month)[Martin, 2015, Randomized controlled trial of irinotecan drug-eluting beads with simultaneous FOLFOX and bevacizumab for patients with unresectable colorectal liver-limited metastasis].

Notwithstanding, notably chemoembolization is still not recommended. There are few data available based on small series, like the DEBIRI [21].

Several trials based on chemotherapy-loaded particles (beads) are still ongoing.

38.4.3.3 Radioembolization

Radioembolization [selective internal radiation therapy (SIRT) or transarterial radioembolization (TARE)] is indicated in patients who have failed prior chemotherapies, and it consists in a single delivery of yttrium-90 connected to either resin or glass particles into the hepatic artery with the therapeutic effect limited to irradiation. Many trials evaluated the role of this technique as first-line or salvage approach. For chemo-refractory disease, progression-free survival and overall survival were 8.8 and 2.9, respectively [25]. In chemo-naive setting, TARE efficacy was evaluated in two randomized phase III studies in association with fluorouracil infusion (SIRFLOX and FOXFIRE), showing no clear benefit in overall survival, but only in liver-specific progression-free survival and response rates (Harpreet W, Guy V, Volker H, et al. Overall survival analysis of the FOXFIRE-SIRFLOX-FOXFIRE global prospective randomized studies of first-line selective internal radiotherapy (SIRT) in patients with liver metastases from colorectal cancer). In the same year, Garlipp B. et al. at the ASCO Annual Meeting discussed the results of the addition of TARE to chemotherapy alone in the

SIRFLOX study reaching a significant improvement in resection rate (38% vs 29%) [26]. According to these results, today this procedure should be considered as a valid option for chemotherapy-refractory liver-limited selected mCRC patients [27].

38.4.3.4 HIPEC

Hyperthermic intraperitoneal chemotherapy (HIPEC) could be considered as a valid option in patients with isolated and resectable peritoneal carcinomatosis. As shown by Elias D. et al., median survival can be prolonged in patients with resectable PC followed by HIPEC [26]. This treatment may be effective if the peritoneal dissemination is scored as "low volume," using the peritoneal cancer index (PCI). A PCI under 12 is always suggested [28].

It is still unclear whether to use oxaliplatin or mitomycin C for HIPEC; nevertheless this combination is going to become a valid standard for patients with peritoneal metastases from CRC [29].

38.4.4 Palliative Treatment

Systemic chemotherapy has been established as the main treatment approach for most patients with unresectable mCRC [30]. For decades, 5-fluorouracil (5-FU)-based chemotherapy was the only treatment option for mCRC patients, resulting in a median overall survival (mOS) of up to 12 months. Over the past 10 to 15 years, the therapeutic landscape has markedly evolved with the approval of irinotecan, oxaliplatin, capecitabine, and monoclonal antibodies [acting against vascular endothelial growth factor (bevacizumab, aflibercept, and ramucirumab) or the epidermal growth factor receptor (cetuximab and panitumumab) and are largely dependent by *RAS* and BRAF status], achieving a mOS of about 30 months. More recently, the oral multi-targeted kinase inhibitor regorafenib and TAS-102, combining trifluridine and tipiracil, have shown to be effective, reporting an improvement in OS rates in chemo-refractory setting; moreover, the use of immunotherapy checkpoint inhibitors (ICIs) is actually under evaluation within phase II or phase III trials after their investigations in preclinical and first-stage clinical trials in which their responses were associated with immunological disease status in special subgroups of mCRC patients (MSI-H).

In the specific case of advanced/metastatic rectal cancer with no surgically treated primary tumor, the treatment strategy differed since chemotherapy alone may be insufficient requiring the addition of radiotherapy for local palliation of local symptoms.

38.4.4.1 First-Line Treatment

A number of randomized clinical studies have compared two-drug regimens (FOLFOX and FOLFIRI) to the combination of 5-FU and leucovorin (5-FU/LV) as first-line therapy, showing the addition of both oxaliplatin and irinotecan offered to patients a statistically significant advantage in terms of progression-free survival (PFS), (partly) OS, and response rates (RRs) over 5-FU/LV regimens [31]. While trends appeared to favor combined chemotherapy versus serial sequential single agents, the toxicity profiles differed with oxaliplatin-based protocols leading to more neutropenia and neuropathy and irinotecan-based causing more gastrointestinal impairment and alopecia. Therefore, the choice of therapy should be considered on a patient-by-patient approach. The oral fluoropyrimidine capecitabine, less frequently used in combination with irinotecan due to early gastrointestinal toxicity concerns [32], could be used as an alternative to 5-FU/leucovorin alone [33] and in combination with oxaliplatin [34]. Moreover, the triplet combination chemotherapy regimen FOLFOXIRI has been compared with FOLFIRI as initial therapy for mCRC patients, showing to maintain long-term outcomes with statistically significant improvements in PFS (9.8 vs 6.9 months) and median OS (21.5 vs 19.5 months), albeit with some increased toxicity but no differences in the rate of toxic death [35].

Cetuximab and panitumumab, two monoclonal antibodies directedagainst EGFR inhibiting its downstream signaling pathways, have resulted to be effective either alone as salvage or in combination with FOLFIRI and FOLFOX as initial therapy options, providing a clear clinical benefit (in terms of RRs, PFS, and OS) that is limited to patients with *RAS* wild-type metastatic colorectal cancer, as demonstrated by several randomized clinical trials [36–38] and recent meta-analyses. To date, a growing body of literature has shown that expanded RAS (KRAS/NRAS) mutational analysis of tumors (either primary or metastasis) is able to predict which patients are unlikely to benefit from EGFR antibody therapy (negative predictive factor). Therefore, it should be carried out at initial diagnosis including at least detection of mutations of KRAS exons 2, 3, and 4 (codons 12, 13, 59, 61, 117, and 146) and NRAS exons 2, 3, and 4 (codons 12, 13, 59, 61, and 117) (see ◘ Fig. 38.3) in terms of a proper first-line treatment plan, as recommended by all the current guidelines. As regards BRAF mutational status, it should be assessed alongside the RAS analysis for prognostic assessment (and/or potential selection for clinical trials), in the light of a strong evidence for its use as a prognostic factor compared to its predictive value. BRAF-mutated patients have been significantly associated with more aggressive clinical features and poorer survival rates. For a long time, the addition

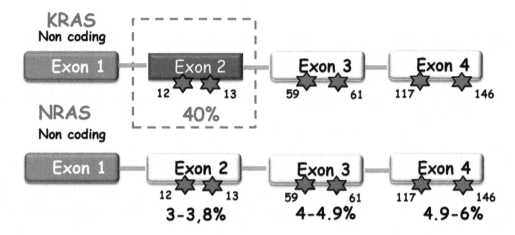

Trial	Sample	Technique	Evaluable for RAS (N)	New RAS mt (N)	New RAS Mutation (%)
CRYSTAL	Extracted DNA	BEAMing	430	63	15
PRIME	Macrodissection (<50% tumor cells)	Sanger Sequencing	620	108	17

◻ **Fig. 38.3** Mutation hotspot in metastatic CRC: from KRAS to Pan-RAS

of EGFR agents did not appear to increase the benefit of standard therapy in terms of PFS and OS in the BRAF-mutated group when compared to BRAF wild-type counterpart [39]. Recent data from the randomized phase III BEACON trial suggest a potential role of the binimetinib (anti-MEK), encorafenib (anti-BRAF), and cetuximab association if compared to the doublet regimen (encorafenib + cetuximab) as salvage therapy reaching a mOS of 9.0 months (vs 5.4 months) [40].

Side effects of both anti-EGFR inhibitors include severe infusion reactions (including anaphylaxis) along with the most common skin reactions which have been shown to be predictive of increased response and survival [41].

Bevacizumab, a humanized monoclonal antibody which blocks the angiogenic activity of circulating vascular endothelial growth factor (VEGF)-A, has proved to enhance activity (in terms of PFS, RR, and/or OS) in combination with FOLFIRI [42] and to be safe and effective, especially in unfit or elderly patients, when added to 5-FU/LV [43] (or capecitabine [44]). On the other hand, the addition of bevacizumab to oxaliplatin-based regimens was associated with a more modest increase of PFS with the difference in RR and OS not reaching statistical significance in a large phase III study [45]. In addition, the phase III TRIBE trial tested the possibility of adding bevacizumab to FOLFOXIRI showing significantly increased PFS and response rate when compared to FOLFIRI/bevacizumab in the first-line treatment of very selected patients with unresectable mCRC [46]. Hence, taking into account the toxicity profile of this drug (most frequently hypertension with higher risk of gastrointestinal hemorrhage, perforation, and venous thromboembolism), no validated predictive marker currently exists for bevacizumab which is therefore indicated in combination with any cytotoxic agent until disease progression or unacceptable toxicity.

As previously discussed, the location of the primary tumor (sidedness) exhibits some important prognostic and predictive implications which significantly impact on the response to targeted therapy as well as on the treatment plan strategy, especially in the first-line setting. According to recent meta-analysis results [47, 48], considering that right-sided mCRCs seem to be associated with more frequently BRAF-mutated tumors, lower response to anti-EGFR antibodies, and poorer outcomes, the initial use of anti-EGFR agents is somewhat controversial when the treatment goal regards prolongation of survival rates along with disease control and palliation of tumor-related symptoms, even in RAS wild-type cancers; on the other hand, it is strongly recommended to initiate first-line chemotherapy in combination with an anti-EGFR antibody in RAS wild-type left-sided mCRCs, which show a markedly greater benefit from anti-EGFR therapy (see ◘ Fig. 38.4).

Although in the FIRE-3 [49] and PEAK studies (but not in the CALGB 80905 study) improved RR and OS rates have favored the addition of EGFR antibody to combination chemotherapy as first-line treatment, when compared with bevacizumab therapy that however shows similar PFS rates, no unequivocal evidence between classes superiority (bevacizumab versus the EGFR antibody therapies) in the first-line treatment of patients with RAS wild-type mCRC can be drawn. Thus, the choice of therapy should be considered depending on the individualization of the treatment approach and the therapeutic goal.

As demonstrated in the CAIRO3 [50] and AIO 0207 trials [51], fluoropyrimidine plus bevacizumab may be considered as the preferable maintenance treatment for patients receiving a first-line "induction therapy" based on the combination of fluoropyrimidine, oxaliplatin, and bevacizumab (◘ Fig. 38.5). In the first-line setting of mCRC patients presenting with tumors deficient in DNA mismatch repair (dMMR) resulting in the phenotype of high microsatellite instability (MSI-H), the PD-1 inhibitor pembrolizumab as monotherapy has recently proved to double time to disease progression when compared to the approved treatment based on chemotherapy plus the targeted drugs bevacizumab or cetuximab. After being approved for MSI-H or dMMR solid tumors progressing on treatment and without satisfactory alternative treatment options, interim findings from the KEYNOTE-177 trial seem to offer a new standard of care as first-line therapy in such patients in the very next future, confirming a clinically meaningful and statistically significant improvement in PFS in favor of upfront pembrolizumab comparing to chemotherapy (16.5 versus 8.2 months) with fewer treatment-related adverse events [52].

38.4.4.2 Second-Line Treatment Setting

Despite the fact that few studies have addressed the sequencing of therapies in mCRC, decisions concerning therapy after progression of metastatic disease depend

---

B-RAF gene

❑ Proto-oncogene on chromosome 7 (7q34), 18 codifying exons

❑ Protein is member of Serine/Threonine Kinase Family and of the RAF Subfamily (together with the ARAF and RAF1 proteins)

❑ Mutational hot-spot: V600E on exon 15 (80% CRC cases)

❑ K-RAS and B-RAF gain-of-function mutations are mutually exclusive

❑ B-RAF mutation rate in CRC: 3-15%

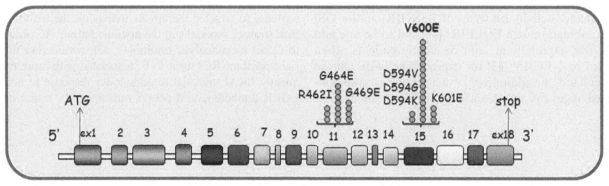

◘ Fig. 38.4   B-RAF gene

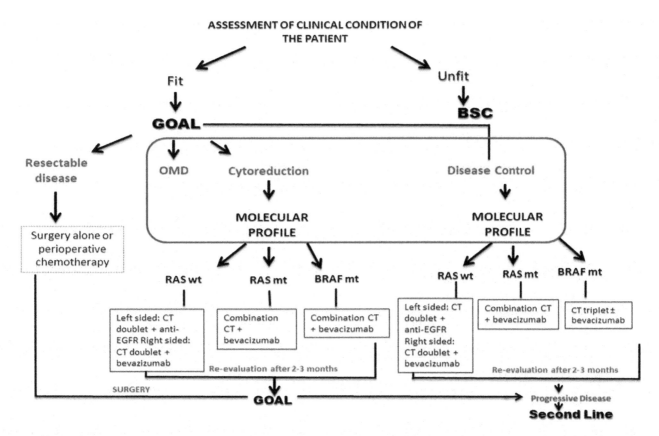

Fig. 38.5 Treatment algorithm of mCRC. *BSC* best supportive care, *CT* chemotherapy, *EGFR* epidermal growth factor receptor, *mt* mutant, *OMD* oligometastatic disease, *wt* wild-type

on upfront strategy. Second-line treatment should be offered to well-motivated patients in good performance status and adequate organ function and strictly depends on the first-line treatment choice. When considering a new treatment option, biological agents and predictive markers (e.g., tumor RAS mutation status for EGFR antibody therapy) together with a proper balance between potential treatment toxicity and efficacy should be considered in the decision-making process.

The chemotherapy backbone should be changed whenever failing in the first-line treatment. Importantly, while both EGFR antibodies have been associated with increased PFS and RR rates (but not OS) when added to irinotecan-based chemotherapy in the second-line setting [53, 54] and have shown a similar relative benefit in later lines compared with the second line of RAS wt mCRCs [55], bevacizumab has confirmed to improve OS rates in both patients who are bevacizumab naïve [56] and, albeit modestly, beyond progression in patients previously treated with bevacizumab [57], suggesting that these patients could benefit from subsequent therapies which target VEGF [58]. Hence, the anti-angiogenic fusion protein aflibercept (designed to function as a VEGF trap to prevent activation of VEGF receptors 1 and 2) has been tested in the VELOUR trial [59], result-

ing in survival advantage when added to FOLFIRI in patients previously progressed on a prior oxaliplatin containing regimen compared with FOLFIRI plus placebo and also in patients who are "fast progressors" on first-line bevacizumab therapy. Likewise, another anti-angiogenic agent, ramucirumab (a human monoclonal antibody that targets the extracellular domain of VEGF receptor 2), has reported a similar OS and PFS benefit, also in association with FOLFIRI, in patients whose disease progressed on first-line therapy with fluoropyrimidine/oxaliplatin/bevacizumab [60].

38.4.5 Third and Subsequent Lines

Both cetuximab and panitumumab can be used in the third line as single agents. Moreover, it has been demonstrated that cetuximab plus irinotecan is even more effective than cetuximab alone in irinotecan refractory patients [61].

Regorafenib is a multi-targeted kinase inhibitor; its activity is more effective than placebo in two trials. The CORRECT phase III trial achieved its primary endpoint OS. Patients who had progressed after all standard treatments were treated with regorafenib. The median overall survival was 6.4 months in the regorafenib group versus 5 months in the placebo group. The main issue of this treatment remains the safety: several side effects were reported during this trial. Hypertension, diarrhea, fatigue, and hand-foot syndrome were the most common grade 3 side effects.

Another valid option in the third line is a molecule that combines trifluridine and tipiracil hydrochloride, *TAS-102*. TAS-102 reported less toxicities than regorafenib. Also, it has been shown to be effective in the refractory mCRC. A randomized trial showed an improvement in OS of the TAS group compared to the placebo, with a median OS that was, respectively, 7.1 months versus 5.3 months [62].

Even if remaining less immunogenic than other types of tumors, a small subset of mCRC patients (about 4–5%) with microsatellite instability (MSI) and deficient mismatch repair (dMMR) chemo-refractory disease seem to benefit from the novel immunotherapy checkpoint inhibitors (ICIs), nivolumab and pembrolizumab, when compared to proficient mismatch repair (pMMR) chemo-refractory patients. In recent open-label phase II studies [63, 64], these two PD-1 inhibitors have been associated with increased immune-related objective response rate in

their respective dMMR arm, with pembrolizumab not still reaching median PFS and OS rates and nivolumab (also in combination with ipilimumab) showing significant PFS and OS rates at 1 year, indicating that MSI could be a predictive marker of response to ICIs independently of RAS/BRAF mutational status (see ◙ Fig. 38.6) [65].

> **Summary of Clinical Recommendations**
> - *AIOM*
>   - ▶ https://www.aiom.it/wp-content/uploads/2018/11/2018_LG_AIOM_Colon.pdf
>   - ▶ https://www.aiom.it/linee-guida/linee-guida-aiom-2018-neoplasie-del-retto-e-ano/
> - *ESMO*
>   - ▶ https://www.esmo.org/Guidelines/Gastrointestinal-Cancers
> - *NCCN*
>   - ▶ https://www.nccn.org/professionals/physician_gls/pdf/colon_blocks.pdf
>   - ▶ https://www.nccn.org/professionals/physician_gls/pdf/rectal_blocks.pdf

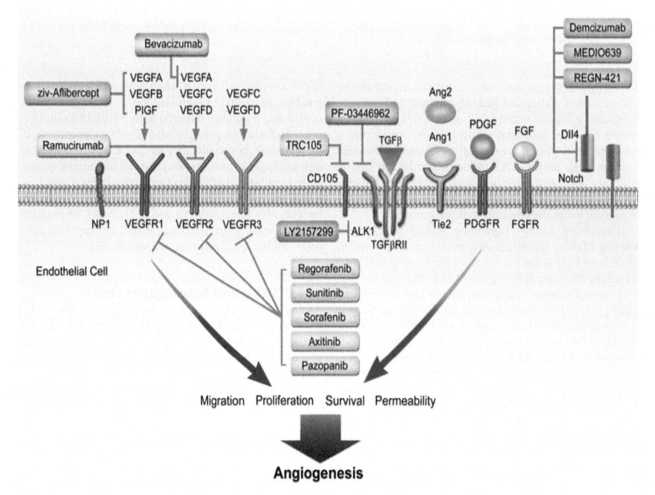

◙ **Fig. 38.6**   Mechanism of selected anti-VEGF agents

Case Study: Metastatic Colon Cancer, RAS wt

Man, 70 years old
- *Family history* negative for malignancy
- *APR*: nothing to report
- *APP*: left flank pain
- *Blood tests*: Hb 12.1 g/dL; mild increased level of gammaGT, ALT, and AST

Question

What action should be taken?
(1) Surgery. (2) Colonoscopy + biopsy. (3) Others

Answer

- *Colonoscopy*: bleeding ulcerative lesion in the left colon. Biopsies were performed.
- *Histological examination*: "Colon adenocarcinoma, G2"

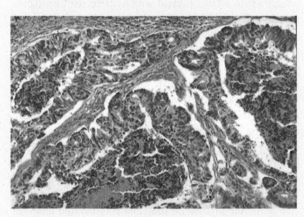

Question

What action should be taken?
(1) CT scan. (2) Medical therapy. (3) Others

Answer

Clinical staging → with chest-abdominal CT scan: bilobar liver metastases

Question

What would you do next?
(1) Surgery. (2) Medical therapy. (3) Others

Answer

n-RAS and k-RAS are not mutated.
  Medical therapy: FOLFOX bevacizumab and FOLFOX cetuximab are both options.

Case Study: Metastatic Colon Cancer, RAS Mutated

Woman, 65 years old
- *Family history* negative for malignancy
- *APR*: negative
- *APP*: asthenia, dyspepsia, change in bowel habit
- *Blood tests*: Hb 9.2 g/dL
- *Colonoscopy and biopsies*: bleeding mass at the right colon. "Colon adenocarcinoma."
- *Chest and abdominal CT scan*: multiple bilobar liver lesions
- *RAS mutated*

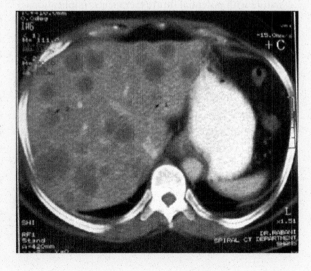

Question

What action should be taken?
 (1) Surgery. (2) Biopsy. (3) Chemotherapy

Answer

Chemotherapy with FOLFOXIRI plus bevacizumab

Question

Is therapy with panitumumab recommended?
 (1) Yes, if there is a progression disease. (2) No it is not.
(3) Yes, combined with bevacizumab.

Answer

Anti-EGFR therapy is not recommended in RAS mutated colon cancer.

Key Points

- The importance of a correct diagnosis
- The importance of administering the right chemotherapy combination

Expert Opinion

Marc Peeters

- Metastatic colorectal cancer (mCRC) is the second most common cause of cancer-related death in both sexes, and, despite major advances in treatment, mortality remains high.
- A multidisciplinary team approach effort that considers patients' characteristics, tumor genomics, and treatment goals is crucial for the best treatment selection of mCRC patients.
- Treatment intensification strategies should be considered to improve response and resectability in potentially resectable mCRC.
- An upfront molecular testing (RAS/BRAF/MSI) has become of paramount importance to best determine the most effective therapeutic intervention. Likewise, the widespread use of next-generation sequencing paves the way for a more comprehensive molecular signature with potential future therapeutic implications.
- Although the optimal use and sequencing of chemotherapeutic and targeted agents across multiple lines of treatment remains unclear, the proper choice of an effective first-line therapy has resulted to be a key determinant for successful treatment outcomes.
- The impact of primary tumor location (sidedness) on the biological and clinical outcome of mCRC has recently resulted to be prognostic as well as predictive of response and survival in patients receiving biological therapies.

Hints for a Deeper Insight

Despite a substantial rise in survival over the last two decades *due* to the success of molecularly *targeted therapies,* both clinical and molecular data have shown that patients with mCRC present with heterogeneous prognosis and response to treatment.

Unfortunately, a single tissue biopsy often underestimates the dynamic molecular landscape of the disease with a limited ability to understand intra- and inter-tumoral heterogeneity, which is considered one of the major reasons for treatment failure and drug resistance. In the era of precision oncology, the noninvasive evaluation of tumor-derived biomarkers (including circulating tumor cells [CTCs], circulating tumor DNA [ctDNA], and exosomes) more frequently isolated from the peripheral blood (liquid biopsy) is a viable alternative to tissue-based genotyping, providing a comprehensive real-time picture of the tumor-associated changes in terms of a serial assessment of the clonal tumor dynamics and a meticulous characterization of drug tailoring and response in an individual cancer patient. Although the use of liquid biopsy has resulted in limited and mixed success while being still extremely limited in mCRC clinical practice, recent data demonstrate that tumor clonal evolution can be detected and longitudinally monitored in circulating ctDNA, revealing that mutant RAS clones arise in blood during EGFR blockade and exponentially decline upon withdrawal of treatment. Hence, several ongoing and future studies investigating the molecular characterization of mCRC by ctDNA detection trigger an interest in anti-EGFR retreatment and will elucidate how the dynamic clonal competition would likely impact on this therapeutic strategy (either by rechallenge strategy or by switching to alternative EGFR-targeted drugs or to new-generation agents targeting other specific subclones upon resistance), mostly considering that no phase 3 data are currently available.

BRAF mutant tumors have poorer prognosis and limited therapeutic options.

Recently, new pharmacological approaches to treat BRAF-mutated mCRC patients have shown survival benefit in a randomized phase III trial. Upon BRAF inhibition, upregulation of EGFR occurs as an escape molecular mechanism. A novel pharmacological approach that includes combination of a selective BRAF inhibitor with an anti-EFGR drug (with or without a MEK inhibitor) has shown to improve survival compared to standard arm with chemotherapy plus anti-EGFR drug. This is the first chemo-free regimen that shows efficacy in mCRC and brings hope for BRAF the very aggressive BRAF mutant tumors.

In the near future, both the emerging genome-wide gene expression analyses and the clinical proteomics will help promote personalized medicine with the identification and the refinement of new targets and signature biomarkers for combination therapy strategies.

Immunotherapy has shown striking results in the subset of mCRC tumor with microsatellite instability (MSI-H) or mismatch repair deficiency (dMMR), which accounts for approximately 5% of all mCRC. Despite these promising results and tangible advances, uncovering the molecular mechanisms responsible for primary and acquired resistance to immune checkpoint inhibitors will be crucial to develop more reliable predictive biomarkers and new potential treatment strategies, hopefully for a larger subset of mCRC patients.

Suggested Reading

1. Punt CJA, Koopman M, Vermeulen L. From tumour heterogeneity to advances in precision treatment of colorectal cancer. Nat Rev Clin Oncol. 2017;14: 235–46.
2. Peeters M, et al. Effect of primary tumor location on second- or later-line treatment outcomes in patients with RAS wild-type metastatic colorectal cancer and all treatment lines in patients with RAS mutations in four randomized panitumumab studies. Clin Colorect Cancer. 2018;17(3):170–8.
3. Chen DS, Mellman I. Elements of cancer immunity and the cancer–immune set point. Nature. 2017;541:321–30.
4. Russo A, Giordano A, Rolfo C. Liquid biopsy in cancer patients. Curr Clin Pathol. 2017:117–24.
5. Dienstmann R, Salazar R, Tabernero J. Molecular subtypes and the evolution of treatment decisions in metastatic colorectal cancer. ASCO Educ Book. 2018;38:231–8.

References

1. De Greef K, Rolfo C, Russo A, et al. Multisciplinary management of patients with liver metastasis from colorectal cancer. World J Gastroenterol. 2016;22:7215–25.
2. Li FY, Lai MD. Colorectal cancer, one entity or three. J Zhejiang Univ Sci B. 2009;10:219–29.
3. Baguley E, Hughes GR. Antiendothelial cell antibodies. J Rheumatol. 1989;16:716–7.
4. Sakai K, Nakagawa M, Hosoda S, Nakano K, Koyanagi H. Changes in the treatment procedures for mitral stenosis. Jpn Circ J. 1992;56 Suppl 5:1369–72.
5. Bufill JA. Colorectal cancer: evidence for distinct genetic categories based on proximal or distal tumor location. Ann Intern Med. 1990;113:779–88.
6. Distler P, Holt PR. Are right- and left-sided colon neoplasms distinct tumors? Dig Dis. 1997;15:302–11.
7. Dejea CM, Wick EC, Hechenbleikner EM, et al. Microbiota organization is a distinct feature of proximal colorectal cancers. Proc Natl Acad Sci U S A. 2014;111:18321–6.
8. Douillard JY, Oliner KS, Siena S, et al. Panitumumab-FOLFOX4 treatment and RAS mutations in colorectal cancer. N Engl J Med. 2013;369:1023–34.
9. Heinemann V, von Weikersthal LF, Decker T, et al. FOLFIRI plus cetuximab versus FOLFIRI plus bevacizumab as first-line treatment for patients with metastatic colorectal cancer (FIRE-3): a randomised, open-label, phase 3 trial. Lancet Oncol. 2014;15:1065–75.
10. Russo A, Incorvaia L, Del Re M, et al. The molecular profiling of solid tumors by liquid biopsy: a position paper of the AIOM-SIAPEC-IAP-SIBioC-SIC-SIF italian scientific societies. ESMO Open. 2021;6(3):100164. https://doi.org/10.1016/j.esmoop.2021.100164.
11. Tsai MS, Su YH, Ho MC, et al. Clinicopathological features and prognosis in resectable synchronous and metachronous colorectal liver metastasis. Ann Surg Oncol. 2007;14:786–94.
12. Floriani I, Torri V, Rulli E, et al. Performance of imaging modalities in diagnosis of liver metastases from colorectal cancer: a systematic review and meta-analysis. J Magn Reson Imaging. 2010;31:19–31.
13. Fong Y, Fortner J, Sun RL, Brennan MF, Blumgart LH. Clinical score for predicting recurrence after hepatic resection for metastatic colorectal cancer: analysis of 1001 consecutive cases. Ann Surg. 1999;230:309–18; discussion 18–21.
14. Primrose J, Falk S, Finch-Jones M, et al. Systemic chemotherapy with or without cetuximab in patients with resectable colorectal liver metastasis: the new EPOC randomised controlled trial. Lancet Oncol. 2014;15:601–11.
15. Folprecht G, Gruenberger T, Bechstein WO, et al. Tumour response and secondary resectability of colorectal liver metastases following neoadjuvant chemotherapy with cetuximab: the CELIM randomised phase 2 trial. Lancet Oncol. 2010;11:38–47.
16. Bruera G, Ricevuto E. Intensive chemotherapy of metastatic colorectal cancer: weighing between safety and clinical efficacy: evaluation of Masi G, Loupakis F, Salvatore L, et al. Bevacizumab with FOLFOXIRI (irinotecan, oxaliplatin, fluorouracil,

and folinate) as first-line treatment for metastatic colorectal cancer: a phase 2 trial. Lancet Oncol 2010;11:845–52. Expert Opin Biol Ther. 2011;11:821–4.

17. Carrato A, Abad A, Massuti B, et al. First-line panitumumab plus FOLFOX4 or FOLFIRI in colorectal cancer with multiple or unresectable liver metastases: a randomised, phase II trial (PLANET-TTD). Eur J Cancer. 2017;81:191–202.

18. Douillard JY, Siena S, Cassidy J, et al. Final results from PRIME: randomized phase III study of panitumumab with FOLFOX4 for first-line treatment of metastatic colorectal cancer. Ann Oncol. 2014;25:1346–55.

19. Stintzing S, Modest DP, Rossius L, et al. FOLFIRI plus cetuximab versus FOLFIRI plus bevacizumab for metastatic colorectal cancer (FIRE-3): a post-hoc analysis of tumour dynamics in the final RAS wild-type subgroup of this randomised open-label phase 3 trial. Lancet Oncol. 2016;17:1426–34.

20. Piessevaux H, Buyse M, Schlichting M, et al. Use of early tumor shrinkage to predict long-term outcome in metastatic colorectal cancer treated with cetuximab. J Clin Oncol. 2013;31:3764–75.

21. Bhutiani N, Akinwande O, Martin RC. Efficacy and toxicity of hepatic intra-arterial drug-eluting (Irinotecan) bead (DEBIRI) therapy in irinotecan-refractory unresectable colorectal liver metastases. World J Surg. 2016;40:1178–90.

22. Scorsetti M, Arcangeli S, Tozzi A, et al. Is stereotactic body radiation therapy an attractive option for unresectable liver metastases? A preliminary report from a phase 2 trial. Int J Radiat Oncol Biol Phys. 2013;86:336–42.

23. Rusthoven KE, Kavanagh BD, Cardenes H, et al. Multi-institutional phase I/II trial of stereotactic body radiation therapy for liver metastases. J Clin Oncol. 2009;27:1572–8.

24. Petre EN, Jia X, Thornton RH, et al. Treatment of pulmonary colorectal metastases by radiofrequency ablation. Clin Colorectal Cancer. 2013;12:37–44.

25. Benson AB, Geschwind J-F, Mulcahy MF, et al. Radioembolisation for liver metastases: results from a prospective 151 patient multi-institutional phase II study. Eur J Cancer. 2013;49:3122–30.

26. Garlipp B, Gibbs P, Van Hazel GA, et al. REsect: blinded assessment of amenability to potentially curative treatment of previously unresectable colorectal cancer liver metastases (CRC LM) after chemotherapy ± RadioEmbolization (SIRT) in the randomized SIRFLOX trial. J Clin Oncol. 2017;35:3532.

27. Hendlisz A, Van den Eynde M, Peeters M, et al. Phase III trial comparing protracted intravenous fluorouracil infusion alone or with yttrium-90 resin microspheres radioembolization for liver-limited metastatic colorectal cancer refractory to standard chemotherapy. J Clin Oncol. 2010;28:3687–94.

28. Elias D, Mariani A, Cloutier AS, et al. Modified selection criteria for complete cytoreductive surgery plus HIPEC based on peritoneal cancer index and small bowel involvement for peritoneal carcinomatosis of colorectal origin. Eur J Surg Oncol. 2014;40:1467–73.

29. Turaga K, Levine E, Barone R, et al. Consensus guidelines from the American Society of Peritoneal Surface Malignancies on standardizing the delivery of hyperthermic intraperitoneal chemotherapy (HIPEC) in colorectal cancer patients in the United States. Ann Surg Oncol. 2014;21:1501–5.

30. Cremolini C, Schirripa M, Antoniotti C, et al. First-line chemotherapy for mCRC—a review and evidence-based algorithm. Nat Rev Clin Oncol. 2015;12:607–19.

31. de Gramont A, Figer A, Seymour M, et al. Leucovorin and fluorouracil with or without oxaliplatin as first-line treatment in advanced colorectal cancer. J Clin Oncol. 2000;18:2938–47.

32. Fuchs CS, Marshall J, Mitchell E, et al. Randomized, controlled trial of irinotecan plus infusional, bolus, or oral fluoropyrimidines in first-line treatment of metastatic colorectal cancer: results from the BICC-C study. J Clin Oncol. 2007;25:4779–86.

33. Van Cutsem E, Hoff PM, Harper P, et al. Oral capecitabine vs intravenous 5-fluorouracil and leucovorin: integrated efficacy data and novel analyses from two large, randomised, phase III trials. Br J Cancer. 2004;90:1190–7.

34. Cassidy J, Clarke S, Díaz-Rubio E, et al. Randomized phase III study of capecitabine plus oxaliplatin compared with fluorouracil/folinic acid plus oxaliplatin as first-line therapy for metastatic colorectal cancer. J Clin Oncol. 2008;26:2006–12.

35. Falcone A, Ricci S, Brunetti I, et al. Phase III trial of infusional fluorouracil, leucovorin, oxaliplatin, and irinotecan (FOLFOXIRI) compared with infusional fluorouracil, leucovorin, and irinotecan (FOLFIRI) as first-line treatment for metastatic colorectal cancer: the Gruppo Oncologico Nord Ovest. J Clin Oncol. 2007;25:1670–6.

36. Van Cutsem E, Köhne C-H, Láng I, et al. Cetuximab plus Irinotecan, fluorouracil, and Leucovorin as first-line treatment for metastatic colorectal Cancer: updated analysis of overall survival according to tumor KRAS and BRAF mutation status. J Clin Oncol. 2011;29:2011–9.

37. Bokemeyer C, Bondarenko I, Makhson A, et al. Fluorouracil, leucovorin, and oxaliplatin with and without cetuximab in the first-line treatment of metastatic colorectal cancer. J Clin Oncol. 2009;27:663–71.

38. Douillard J-Y, Siena S, Cassidy J, et al. Randomized, phase III trial of Panitumumab with Infusional fluorouracil, Leucovorin, and Oxaliplatin (FOLFOX4) versus FOLFOX4 alone as first-line treatment in patients with previously untreated metastatic colorectal cancer: the PRIME study. J Clin Oncol. 2010;28:4697–705.

39. Pietrantonio F, Petrelli F, Coinu A, et al. Predictive role of BRAF mutations in patients with advanced colorectal cancer receiving cetuximab and panitumumab: a meta-analysis. Eur J Cancer. 2015;51:587–94.

40. Shahjehan F, Kamatham S, Chandrasekharan C, Kasi PM. Binimetinib, encorafenib and cetuximab (BEACON trial) combination therapy for patients with BRAF V600E-mutant metastatic colorectal cancer. Drugs Today. 2019;55:683.

41. Petrelli F, Borgonovo K, Barni S. The predictive role of skin rash with cetuximab and panitumumab in colorectal cancer patients: a systematic review and meta-analysis of published trials. Target Oncol. 2013;8:173–81.

42. Hurwitz H, Fehrenbacher L, Novotny W, et al. Bevacizumab plus irinotecan, fluorouracil, and leucovorin for metastatic colorectal cancer. N Engl J Med. 2004;350:2335–42.

43. Kabbinavar F, Irl C, Zurlo A, Hurwitz H. Bevacizumab improves the overall and progression-free survival of patients with metastatic colorectal cancer treated with 5-fluorouracil-based regimens irrespective of baseline risk. Oncology. 2008;75:215–23.

44. Cunningham D, Lang I, Marcuello E, et al. Bevacizumab plus capecitabine versus capecitabine alone in elderly patients with previously untreated metastatic colorectal cancer (AVEX): an open-label, randomised phase 3 trial. Lancet Oncol. 2013;14:1077–85.

45. Saltz LB, Clarke S, Díaz-Rubio E, et al. Bevacizumab in combination with oxaliplatin-based chemotherapy as first-line therapy in metastatic colorectal cancer: a randomized phase III study. J Clin Oncol. 2008;26:2013–9.

46. Loupakis F, Cremolini C, Masi G, et al. Initial therapy with FOLFOXIRI and bevacizumab for metastatic colorectal cancer. N Engl J Med. 2014;371:1609–18.

47. Holch JW, Ricard I, Stintzing S, Modest DP, Heinemann V. The relevance of primary tumour location in patients with metastatic colorectal cancer: a meta-analysis of first-line clinical trials. Eur J Cancer. 2017;70:87–98.

48. Arnold D, Lueza B, Douillard JY, et al. Prognostic and predictive value of primary tumour side in patients with RAS wild-

38

type metastatic colorectal cancer treated with chemotherapy and EGFR directed antibodies in six randomized trials. Ann Oncol. 2017;28:1713–29.

49. Holch JW, Ricard I, Stintzing S, et al. Relevance of baseline carcinoembryonic antigen for first-line treatment against metastatic colorectal cancer with FOLFIRI plus cetuximab or bevacizumab (FIRE-3 trial). Eur J Cancer. 2019;106:115–25.

50. Simkens LH, van Tinteren H, May A, et al. Maintenance treatment with capecitabine and bevacizumab in metastatic colorectal cancer (CAIRO3): a phase 3 randomised controlled trial of the Dutch Colorectal Cancer Group. Lancet. 2015;385:1843–52.

51. Hegewisch-Becker S, Graeven U, Lerchenmüller CA, et al. Maintenance strategies after first-line oxaliplatin plus fluoropyrimidine plus bevacizumab for patients with metastatic colorectal cancer (AIO 0207): a randomised, non-inferiority, open-label, phase 3 trial. Lancet Oncol. 2015;16:1355–69.

52. Sobrero AF, Maurel J, Fehrenbacher L, et al. EPIC: phase III trial of cetuximab plus irinotecan after fluoropyrimidine and oxaliplatin failure in patients with metastatic colorectal cancer. J Clin Oncol. 2008;26:2311–9.

53. Peeters M, Oliner KS, Price TJ, et al. Analysis of KRAS/NRAS mutations in a phase III study of panitumumab with FOLFIRI compared with FOLFIRI alone as second-line treatment for metastatic colorectal cancer. Clin Cancer Res. 2015;21:5469–79.

54. Cascinu S, Rosati G, Nasti G, et al. Treatment sequence with either irinotecan/cetuximab followed by FOLFOX-4 or the reverse strategy in metastatic colorectal cancer patients progressing after first-line FOLFIRI/bevacizumab: an Italian Group for the Study of Gastrointestinal Cancer phase III, randomised trial comparing two sequences of therapy in colorectal metastatic patients. Eur J Cancer. 2017;83:106–15.

55. Giantonio BJ, Catalano PJ, Meropol NJ, et al. Bevacizumab in combination with oxaliplatin, fluorouracil, and leucovorin (FOLFOX4) for previously treated metastatic colorectal cancer: results from the Eastern Cooperative Oncology Group Study E3200. J Clin Oncol. 2007;25:1539–44.

56. Masi G, Salvatore L, Boni L, et al. Continuation or reintroduction of bevacizumab beyond progression to first-line therapy in metastatic colorectal cancer: final results of the randomized BEBYP trial. Ann Oncol. 2015;26:724–30.

57. Tabernero J, Van Cutsem E, Lakomý R, et al. Aflibercept versus placebo in combination with fluorouracil, leucovorin and irinotecan in the treatment of previously treated metastatic colorectal cancer: prespecified subgroup analyses from the VELOUR trial. Eur J Cancer. 2014;50:320–31.

58. Galvano A, Taverna S, Badalamenti G, et al. Detection of RAS mutations in circulating tumor DNA: a new weapon in an old war against colorectal cancer. A systematic review of literature and meta-analysis. Ther Adv Med Oncol. 2019;11:1758835919874653. Published 2019 Sep 10. https://doi.org/10.1177/1758835919874653.

59. Tabernero J, Yoshino T, Cohn AL, et al. Ramucirumab versus placebo in combination with second-line FOLFIRI in patients with metastatic colorectal carcinoma that progressed during or after first-line therapy with bevacizumab, oxaliplatin, and a fluoropyrimidine (RAISE): a randomised, double-blind, multicentre, phase 3 study. Lancet Oncol. 2015;16:499–508.

60. Cunningham D, Humblet Y, Siena S, et al. Cetuximab monotherapy and cetuximab plus irinotecan in irinotecan-refractory metastatic colorectal cancer. N Engl J Med. 2004;351:337–45.

61. Mayer RJ, Van Cutsem E, Falcone A, et al. Randomized trial of TAS-102 for refractory metastatic colorectal cancer. N Engl J Med. 2015;372:1909–19.

62. Le DT, Uram JN, Wang H, et al. PD-1 blockade in tumors with mismatch-repair deficiency. N Engl J Med. 2015;372:2509–20.

63. Overman MJ, Lonardi S, Wong KYM, et al. Durable clinical benefit with Nivolumab plus Ipilimumab in DNA mismatch repair-deficient/microsatellite instability-high metastatic colorectal Cancer. J Clin Oncol. 2018;36:773–9.

64. PD-1 Inhibitor Bests Chemo for Colorectal Cancer. Cancer Discov. 2020 Jul;10(7):OF2. https://doi.org/10.1158/2159-8290.CD-NB2020-051. Epub 2020 Jun 1. PMID: 32482631.

65. Russo A, Incorvaia L, Malapelle U, et al. The tumor-agnostic treatment for patients with solid tumors: a position paper on behalf of the AIOM-SIAPEC/IAP-SIBIOC-SIF italian scientific societies [published online ahead of print, 2021 Aug 6]. Crit Rev Oncol Hematol. 2021;103436. https://doi.org/10.1016/j.critrevonc.2021.103436.

Anal Cancer

*Antonio Galvano, Aurelia Ada Guarini, Valerio Gristina,
Maria La Mantia, and Antonio Russo*

Gastrointestinal Cancers

Contents

© Springer Nature Switzerland AG 2021
A. Russo et al. (eds.), *Practical Medical Oncology Textbook*, UNIPA Springer Series,
https://doi.org/10.1007/978-3-030-56051-5_39

Learning Objectives

By the end of the chapter the reader will:

1. Have learned the basic concepts of epidemiology, histological subtype, and clinical manifestation of anal neoplasms
2. Be able to define staging strategies, diagnostic, and therapeutic procedures
3. Be able to put acquired knowledge into clinical practice
4. Be able to realize future perspectives of anal neoplasms

39.1 Introduction

The anal canal is the terminal part of the digestive canal, between the rectum and the skin of the anal margin, approximately 3–4 cm long. The anal carcinoma is considered to be a rare type of cancer. The squamous forms of tumor of the anus consist in about 95% of the tumors of the anal canal, and only a small portion of these (about 10%) begins at an advanced stage. Conditions that increase the risk of HPV infection and/or modulate host response and persistence of infection appear to influence the epidemiology of this tumor. In particular, anal intercourse and a high number of sexual partners increase the risk of persistent HPV infection, both in men and women, with consequent development of neoplasia. Among the subtypes, HPV-16 is responsible for the infection in 73% of all HPV-related tumors and is the most commonly found variant. The importance of HPV is in its role as a potential risk factor for the development of precancerous lesions (AIN, anal intraepithelial neoplasia) and therefore neoplastic (SCCA, squamous cell carcinoma). Other important risk factors include HIV infection, immunosuppressive therapy in transplant patients, the use of immunosuppressant such as high-dose steroid therapy, a history of other HPV-related neoplasms, disadvantaged socioeconomic conditions and cigarette smoking. Smoking may also be important in modulating the persistence of HPV infection with a possible impact on treatment outcomes. Also consider the number of sexual partners, a history of anal warts, previous dysplasia or genital tract carcinomas, and smoking [1–3].

39.2 Epidemiology

The annual incidence rate is approximately 1/100,000 inhabitants per year, and its incidence is increased in developing countries: there are approximately 27,000 new cases of anal carcinoma per year.

The incidence rate is three- to sixfold for women, but men with HIV infection have a greater risk to be infected by HPV. Other risk factors are represented by a history of cervical, vulvar, or vaginal carcinoma and persistent infection with high-risk form of HPV (e.g., HPV-16, HPV-18).

Sexually transmitted diseases and certain autoimmune disorders are considered to be other important risk factors.

Most primary cancers of the anal canal are of squamous cell histology. There are other common anal canal tumors that have different histological features: adenocarcinoma, small-cell carcinoma, undifferentiated cancers, and melanomas.

The incidence rate of anal carcinoma associated with HPV infection is 88%. HPV-16 is the genotype that is most involved in the anal carcinoma HPV-related.

A 9-valent HPV vaccine is available, protecting against HPV-6, HPV-11, HPV-16, HPV-18, HPV-31, HPV-33, HPV-45, HPV-52, and HPV-58. It is predicted that this new vaccine will prevent additional 464 cases of anal cancer annually.

HPV is responsible for precancerous lesion, called anal intraepithelial neoplasia (AIN), that can be divided into low-grade and high-grade.

High-grade AIN can be a precursor of anal carcinoma, and its treatment can prevent the development of cancer. AIN can be identified by HPV testing, cytology, digital rectal examination (DRE), and high-resolution anoscopy and/or biopsy. The regression of high-grade AIN is unknown, and it is estimated to be very low in men that have sex with men [1, 2].

High-risk patients are known to be those with HIV infection. Routine screening for AIN lesions is controversial, although few guidelines recommend screening programs for HIV-positive people (◘ Fig. 39.1) [3–6].

39.3 Anatomy, Histology, and Pathology

The anal region is made of the anal canal and the anal margin, so that we can distinguish two different types of anal cancer.

The anal canal is the most proximal part of the anal region.

Histologically, the mucosal lining of the anal canal is composed of squamous epithelium, while the mucosa of the rectum is lined with glandular epithelium.

The anal margin is lined with skin.

The most superior aspect of the anal canal is a 1–2 cm zone between the anal and rectal epithelium. The most inferior aspect of the anal canal corresponds to the area where the mucosa, lined with modified squamous epithelium, transitions to an epidermis-lined anal margin. The anatomic anal canal begins at the anorectal ring and extends to the anal verge (i.e., squamous mucocutaneous junction with the perianal skin)

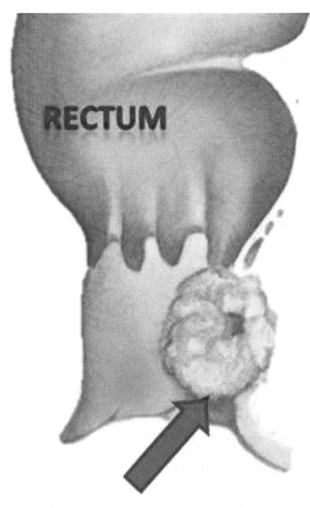

The squamous cell histology is the most common type of cancer. There are many other variants, recognized by the WHO, as large cell keratinizing, large cell non-keratinizing, and basaloid. All these subtypes are included in a single definition of squamous cell carcinoma.

Other less common anal canal cancers are adenocarcinomas, small-cell (anaplastic) carcinoma, undifferentiated carcinoma, and melanomas [7].

Anal carcinoma can be well differentiated (G1) and poorly differentiated (G4) [8, 9].

39.4 Staging and Prognostic Factors

The TNM staging for anal carcinoma is developed by the American Joint Committee on Cancer (7th edition).

Current recommendations do not involve a surgical excision, and most tumors are staged clinically by direct examination and microscopic confirmation. A biopsy

is always required. Rectal ultrasound, to determine the size and the extension of the tumor, is not required during this phase.

The prognosis of anal carcinoma is related to the size of the primary tumor and the lymph node involvement.

Lymph node staging is based on location of involved lymph nodes:

1. N1, one or more perirectal nodes
2. N2, unilateral internal iliac nodes and/or inguinal nodes
3. N3, perirectal and inguinal nodes and/or bilateral internal iliac nodes and/or bilateral inguinal nodes

Surgery excision is not considered to be the initial therapy, and the lymph nodes status should be determined clinically and radiologically.

Fine needle aspiration (FNA) biopsy of inguinal nodes can be considered if node involvement is suspected. PET CT and CT scans alone are not recommended to investigate node involvement. In a series of patient that underwent abdominoperineal resection (APR), it was noted that pelvic nodal metastases were often less than 5 mm and PET and CT scans were not reliable to determinate their involvement.

Size, sex, and lymph node involvement are considered to be prognostic factors. Multivariate analysis of data from the RTOG 98-11 showed that male sex and positive nodes were independent prognostic factors for disease-free survival in patient with anal cancer treated with 5FU and radiation and either mitomycin or cisplatin. Male sex, node positivity, and tumor size greater than 5 cm were independent prognostic factors for worse overall survival.

In the EORTC 22861 trial, it has been noted that male sex, node positivity, and skin ulceration were prognostic factors for worse survival and local control (◘ Tables 39.1 and 39.2) [13].

39.5 Clinical Presentation and Evaluation

The most common clinical presentation of anal carcinoma is represented by rectal bleeding, pain, and sensation of a rectal mass.

A clinical examination is recommended: DRE, anoscopic examination, and inguinal lymph nodes palpation.

MRI and CT scan are recommended for the evaluation of the pelvic lymph nodes. A FNA, when feasible, is always recommended to investigate lymph node involvement.

CT scan and MRI pelvis are always important to determine whether the tumor involves other abdominal/pelvic organs; however a T stage assessment is performed

Table 39.1 TNM classification for anal cancer. (American Joint Committee on Cancer, 8th edition)

Primary tumor (T)

TX	Primary tumor cannot be assessed
T0	No evidence of primary tumor
Tis	Carcinoma in situ (Bowen disease, high-grade squamous intraepithelial lesion [H-SIL], anal intraepithelial neoplasia II–III (AIN II–III)
T1	Tumor 2 cm or less in greatest dimension
T2	Tumor more than 2 cm but not more than 5 cm in greatest dimension
T3	Tumor more than 5 cm in greatest dimension
T4	Tumor of any size invades adjacent organ(s) (e.g., vagina, urethra, bladder); direct invasion of the rectal wall, perirectal skin, subcutaneous tissue, or the sphincter muscle(s) is not classified as T4

Regional lymph nodes (N)

NX	Regional lymph nodes cannot be assessed
N0	No regional lymph node metastasis
N1	*N1a* metastases in inguinal, mesorectal, and/or internal iliac nodes
	N1b metastases in external iliac nodes
	N1c metastases in external iliac and in inguinal, mesorectal, and/or internal iliac nodes

Distant metastasis (M)

M0	No distant metastasis
M1	Distant metastasis

Table 39.2 Anatomic stage/prognostic group

Stage		T	N	M
0		Tis	N0	M0
I		T1	N0	M0
II	*IIa*	T2	N0	M0
	IIb	T3	N0	M0
III	*IIIa*	T1	N1	M0
	IIIa	T2	N1	M0
	IIIb	T4	N0	M0
	IIIc	T3	N1	M0
I	*IIIc*	T4	N1	M0
IV		Any T	Any N	M1

through clinical examination. Chest CT scan is recommended to evaluate pulmonary metastasis.

HIV testing and measurement of CD4 levels can be performed since the anal cancer has been reported to have a higher incidence rate in HIV-positive patients.

A gynecologic examination is also suggested, including cervical cancer screening, since HPV is also associated with cervical cancer.

The staging before any treatment should be performed through PET and CT scan. PET/CT should be performed also in patients who have normal-sized lymph node at the CT scan [21–24].

Clinical presentation

↓

Anal canal cancer→ | Biopsy: Squamous Cell Carcinoma | Work up→

- Digital rectal examination (DRE)
- Inguinal lymph node evaluation (consider biopsy or FNA)
- Chest and abdominal CT and abdominal MRI
- Anoscopy
- Consider PET/CT scan
- Gynecologic examination and HPV testing
- HIV testing

39.6 Management

39.6.1 Primary Treatment of Non Metastatic Anal Carcinoma

In the past, patients with invasive carcinoma were treated with abdominoperineal resection (APR), but local recurrence rates were high, and the 5-year survival rate is about 40%.

Many non-randomized studies demonstrated that the administration of chemotherapy and radiation therapy had a higher efficacy (in terms of local recurrence) than surgery (APR).

Currently concurrent chemoRT is the recommended primary treatment for locally advanced anal canal cancer.

(a) *Chemotherapy and Radiation Therapy (chemoRT):* A phase III study from the EORTC compared radiation therapy (RT) alone versus chemotherapy (5FU and mitomycin) and radiation therapy (chemoRT). The second option (chemoRT arm) showed more local control than RT alone.

A few studies have addressed the safety and efficacy of many chemotherapeutic agents. In a phase III intergroup study, patients receiving chemoRT with the combination of 5FU and mitomycin had a lower colostomy rate and a higher DFS compared to patients receiving chemoRT with 5FU alone, indicating that mitomycin is important in the treatment of anal carcinoma.

Capecitabine is a good alternative to 5FU in the treatment of the anal carcinoma.

Cisplatin, as a substitute to 5FU was evaluated in a phase II trial, and results suggest that cisplatin or 5FU may be comparable for treatment of locally advanced anal cancer.

The phase III UK ACT II trial compared 5FU/mitomycin and 5FU/cisplatin, RT was also administered, and a maintenance therapy with 5FU or cisplatin was administered in one of the two arms. Results showed that mitomycin can be replaced by cisplatin because this will not affect the complete response; on the other hand, it was also demonstrated that maintenance therapy did not decrease the rate of disease recurrence.

It has also been discussed the role of induction therapy, prior to a chemoRT.

The results of a recent study, the ACCORD 03, showed that there was no benefit in patients that had received induction chemotherapy prior to chemoRT. In this study patients with locally advanced anal cancer were randomized to receive induction therapy with 5FU/cisplatin or no induction therapy followed by chemoRT.

Cetuximab is an epidermal growth factor receptor (EGFR) inhibitor that works very well when RAS family genes status (KRAS and NRAS above all) is wild type. Since RAS mutations in anal cancer are very rare, cetuximab has been considered to be a promising avenue of investigation. Few studies evaluated toxicity and efficacy of chemoRT and cetuximab. The ACCORD 16 phase II trial was designed to assess response rate after chemoRT with cisplatin/5FU and cetuximab was terminated because of many adverse events. Other studies are still ongoing [17–20, 25].

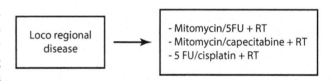

1. *Surgery:* it is recommended in a few cases:
2. *Recurrence after chemoRT:* an abdominoperineal resection is recommended in patients that present a recurrence after a concurrent chemoRT.
3. *T1, N0 (well-differentiated, <1.0 cm):* a local excision is recommended for patients with a T1, N0 well-differentiated and small lesion. It is important that margins are not involved. If margins are inadequate a re-excision is a preferred treatment. If a re-excision cannot be performed, local RT with or without chemotherapy is recommended [14, 15, 16].

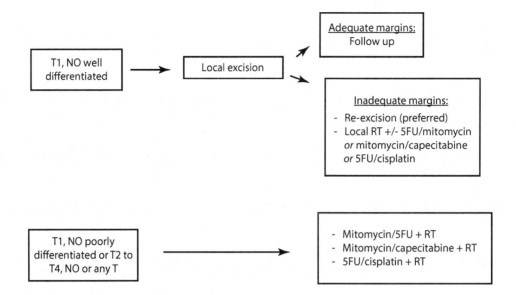

39.7 Metastatic Disease

It has been reported that the most common sites of metastasis outside the pelvis are the liver, lungs, and lymph nodes. Since anal carcinoma is a rare cancer, only 10–20% of patients present extra pelvic metastasis. Despite this fact, some evidences suggested that chemotherapy with fluoropyrimidine-based regimen plus cisplatin has some benefit in patients with metastatic anal carcinoma [25–28].

No evidence supports resection of metastatic disease. Recently, the INTERAACT trial results were published. This is an open-label randomized phase II trial that was aimed to compare cisplatin (CDDP) plus 5-fluorouracil (5FU) versus carboplatin (CBDCA) plus weekly paclitaxel (PTX) in patients with inoperable locally recurrent (ILR) or metastatic disease and 5FU. Patients with metastatic squamous cell carcinoma of the anus were randomly assigned to receive cisplatin and 5FU or weekly carboplatin and paclitaxel. The primary endpoint was ORR, and it was reached in the group treated with cisplatin and 5FU (59% versus 57%) [29].

39.7.1 Treatment of Recurrent Anal Carcinoma

Despite the effectiveness of chemoRT as primary treatment for locally advanced anal cancer, rates of 10–30% of local recurrence are reported. When recurrence occurs, APR is indicated. A recent retrospective analysis showed that patients who received intra-operatory RT during APR had improved local recurrence. Inguinal node dissection is reserved for recurrence in that area and can be performed without an APR in cases where recurrence is limited at inguinal nodes. Patients that presented inguinal recurrence without APR could receive chemoRT with RT to the groin, if no prior RT to the groin was given [26].

39.8 Screening

Routine screening for AIN lesions is controversial, although few guidelines recommend screening programs for HIV-positive people. Gynecologic examination, HPV testing, and cytology in high-risk patients can be performed even if it is not recommended.

High-grade AIN can be a precursor of anal carcinoma. The spontaneous regression of AIN is possible but the regression rate is unknown [9].

Anal canal lesions, according to their cytology, can be classified (Bethesda Classification 2001) into:

1. AIN: anal intraepithelial neoplasia
2. ASCUS: atypical squamous cell of undetermined significance
3. ASC-H: atypical squamous cell suspicious for H-SIL
4. L-SIL: low-grade squamous intraepithelial lesion
5. H-SIL: high-grade squamous intraepithelial lesion
6. SCC: squamous cell carcinoma

If the cytology indicates ASCUS, L-SIL, or H-SIL, the patients will perform high-resolution anoscopy and/or biopsy:

7. AIN 1 (L-SIL): a clinical assessment should be performed every 6–12 months.
8. AIN 2/3 (H-SIL): should be treated and/or clinical assessment after 6 months [9–12].

39.9 Summary: Conclusion

Anal carcinoma is a rare type of cancer but its incidence rate is increasing.

The treatment of this disease should be approached by a multidisciplinary team including physicians from GI, medical oncology, surgical oncology, and radiology.

Recommendations for the primary treatment of locally advanced anal cancer are very similar and include chemoRT.

The treatment for T1, N0 well-differentiated cancers is represented by local excision with adequate margins.

Following complete remission, patients with local recurrence should be treated with APR.

A 5FU/mitomycin or 5FU/cisplatin regimen is associated to RT. Since RAS mutations are very rare in the anal cancer, cetuximab is a promising agent, although toxicity still represents a big issue.

Case Study: Locally Advanced Anal Carcinoma

Man: 55 years old
- *Family history*: negative for malignancy
- *APR*: nothing to report
- APP: pain, bleeding, and poor bowel function unresponsive to laxative treatment of 5 months' duration.
- *Objective examination*: EDAR → depressed hard area in the anal canal with blood on the glove.
- *Blood tests*: Hb 12.1 g/dL; mild increased level of gammaGT

Question

What action should be taken?
(1) Surgery. (2) Biopsy. (3) Others

Answer

- *Anoscopy*: ulcer in the anterior anal canal and biopsies were taken.
- *Histological examination:* "Squamous cell carcinoma of the anus (SCCA)"

Question

What action should be taken?
(1) Surgery. (2) Medical therapy. (3) Clinical staging

Answer

Clinical Staging → with pelvic MRI: pelvic lymph nodes not involved. The patient was staged as *cTNM, T4, N0 → Chest and abdominal CT scan with and without contrast*: no distant metastases

Question

What would you do next?
(1) Surgery. (2) Medical therapy. (3) Others

Answer

Medical Therapy: RT and 5FU + cisplatin

Key Points

1. The importance of a correct diagnosis: attention to rectal masses
2. Symptoms often nonspecific
3. The importance of the management of a locally advanced disease

---

Case Study: Metastatic SCCA

Man: 70 years old
- *Family history*: negative for malignancy
- *APR*: negative
- *APP*: asthenia, dyspepsia, change in bowel habit
- *Blood tests*: Hb 9.2 g/dL
- *Objective examination*: EDAR → hard and bleeding area in the anal canal
- *Anoscopy and biopsies*: SCCA
- *Chest and Abdominal CT scan*: multiple liver lesions

Question

What action should be taken?
(1) Surgery. (2) Biopsy. (3) Chemotherapy

Answer

Chemotherapy with 5FU and cisplatin

Question

Is metastasectomy on liver lesions recommended?
(1) Yes, after four cycles of chemotherapy. (2) Surgery is not indicated for the metastatic setting. (3) Others

Answer

No evidence supports resection of metastatic disease.

Expert Opinion

Marc Peeters

- Anal canal neoplasms are a group of diseases with a low incidence but a relative increase in the most industrialized countries. The main risk factors are HPV and HIV infection, immunosuppressive therapy in transplant patients, the use of immunosuppressant such as high-dose steroid therapy, a history of other HPV-related neoplasms, disadvantaged socioeconomic conditions, and cigarette smoking.
- The instrumental diagnostic approach in case of suspected disease is represented by clinical examination and endoscopic evaluation. More specific evaluation must be carried out using the TC and the MRI using in some circumstances PET integration.
- Local stage: currently concurrent chemoRT (using 5FU and/or mitomycin) is the recommended primary treatment for locally advanced anal canal cancer, and capecitabine is a good alternative to 5FU. Surgery could be a valid option in those superficially minimal invasive squamous cell carcinomas.
- Local recurrence/persistence: APR represents a fundamental moment.
- Advanced stage: chemotherapy with fluoropyrimidine-based regimen plus cisplatin has some benefit in patients with metastatic anal carcinoma.

Hints for a Deeper Insight

In the era of personalized medicine, the treatment of anal squamous cell carcinoma (ASCC) is changing, and several therapeutic options are going to be explored.

The development and introduction of immunotherapeutic agents have brought new possibilities in the treatment of metastatic ASCC. HPV-positive ASCC is associated with more immunogenicity, and thus immunotherapy is going to represent an intriguing alternative. Several trials indicate that immunotherapy combined with chemoradiotherapy (CRT) might be a valid option: RT can activate the immune system and promote tumor infiltration of CD8+ TILs. Immunotherapies can enhance TILs cytotoxic function and motility. Further-more, the introduction of vaccines is bringing new hope in the treatment of ASCC; the live-attenuated listeria monocytogenes cancer vaccine ADXS11-001 targeting HPV-positive is going to be tested in combination with standard CRT in patients with ASCC treated for curative intent. For this reason, the use of immunotherapeutics need a patient stratification since the HPV infection plays an important role in predicting the treatment response.

Besides immunotherapy, efforts are being made to reduce the CRT-related toxicity CRT: the PLATO trial is testing the concept of stage-dependent RT dose adaptation. Since the dose modulations are small, the oncological outcome should not change. In this respect, data from the Danish Head and Neck Cancer Association (DAHANCA) have showed that the use of 5 fractions per week instead of 6 led to higher acute toxicity, while no differences in late toxicities were reported. Interestingly, there was an improvement in DFS.

In conclusion, although 5FU/MMC CRT still constitutes the standard of care, new approaches are currently being explored. The "dose adaptation" concept can avoid unnecessary toxicity, and the HPV status can help to stratify patients for immunotherapy.

New clinical trials are needed to test the combination between immunotherapy and CRT in the primary and metastatic setting; all these new perspectives could have an important impact on the way physicians can treat patients with ASCC in the near future.

Suggested Reading

- ▶ https://www.aiom.it/wp-content/uploads/2019/10/2019_LG_AIOM_Retto_ano.pdf
- Glynne-Jones R, Nilsson PJ, Aschele C, et al. Anal cancer: ESMO-ESSO-ESTRO clinical practice guidelines for diagnosis, treatment and follow-up. Radiother Oncol. 2014;111(3):330–9. ▶ https://doi.org/10.1016/j.radonc.2014.04.013
- NCCN Clinical Practice Guidelines in Oncology (NCCN Guidelines) Anal Carcinoma Version 2.2017 — April 20, 2017, ▶ NCCN.org

References

1. Siegel RL, Miller KD, Jemal A. Cancer statistics, 2016. CA Cancer J Clin. 2016;66(1):7–30. https://doi.org/10.3322/caac.21332. Epub 2016 Jan 7.

2. de Martel C, Ferlay J, Franceschi S, Vignat J, Bray F, Forman D, Plummer M. Global burden of cancers attributable to infections in 2008: a review and synthetic analysis. Lancet Oncol. 2012;13(6):607–15. https://doi.org/10.1016/S1470-2045(12)70137-7. Epub 2012 May 9. Review.

3. D'Souza G, Wiley DJ, Li X, Chmiel JS, Margolick JB, Cranston RD, Jacobson LP. Incidence and epidemiology of anal cancer in the multicenter AIDS cohort study. J Acquir Immune Defic Syndr. 2008;48(4):491–9. https://doi.org/10.1097/QAI.0b013e31817aebfe. PubMed Central PMCID: PMC3991563.

4. Patel P, Hanson DL, Sullivan PS, Novak RM, Moorman AC, Tong TC, Holmberg SD, Brooks JT, Adult and Adolescent Spectrum of Disease Project and HIV Outpatient Study Investigators. Incidence of types of cancer among HIV-infected persons compared with the general population in the United States, 1992-2003. Ann Intern Med. 2008;148(10):728–36.

5. Piketty C, Selinger-Leneman H, Grabar S, Duvivier C, Bonmarchand M, Abramowitz L, Costagliola D, Mary-Krause M, FHDH-ANRS CO 4. Marked increase in the incidence of invasive anal cancer among HIV-infected patients despite treatment with combination antiretroviral therapy. AIDS. 2008;22(10):1203–11. https://doi.org/10.1097/QAD.0b013e3283023f78.

6. Franceschi S, De Vuyst H. Human papillomavirus vaccines and anal carcinoma. Curr Opin HIV AIDS. 2009;4(1):57–63. https://doi.org/10.1097/COH.0b013e32831b9c81. Review.

7. Salati SA, Al Kadi A. Anal cancer – a review. Int J Health Sci (Qassim). 2012;6(2):206–30. PubMed Central PMCID: PMC3616949.

8. Glynne-Jones R, Nilsson PJ, Aschele C, Goh V, Peiffert D, Cervantes A, Arnold D, European Society for Medical Oncology (ESMO); European Society of Surgical Oncology (ESSO); European Society of Radiotherapy and Oncology (ESTRO). Anal cancer: ESMO-ESSO-ESTRO clinical practice guidelines for diagnosis, treatment and follow-up. Eur J Surg Oncol. 2014;40(10):1165–76. https://doi.org/10.1016/j.ejso.2014.07.030.

9. De Vuyst H, Clifford GM, Nascimento MC, Madeleine MM, Franceschi S. Prevalence and type distribution of human papillomavirus in carcinoma and intraepithelial neoplasia of the vulva, vagina and anus: a meta-analysis. Int J Cancer. 2009;124(7):1626–36. https://doi.org/10.1002/ijc.24116.

10. Bosch FX, Broker TR, Forman D, Moscicki AB, Gillison ML, Doorbar J, Stern PL, Stanley M, Arbyn M, Poljak M, Cuzick J, Castle PE, Schiller JT, Markowitz LE, Fisher WA, Canfell K, Denny LA, Franco EL, Steben M, Kane MA, Schiffman M, Meijer CJ, Sankaranarayanan R, Castellsagué X, Kim JJ, Brotons M, Alemany L, Albero G, Diaz M, de Sanjosé S, authors of ICO Monograph Comprehensive Control of HPV Infections and Related Diseases Vaccine Volume 30, Supplement 5, 2012. Comprehensive control of human papillomavirus infections and related diseases. Vaccine. 2013;31(Suppl 7):H1–31. https://doi.org/10.1016/j.vaccine.2013.10.003.

11. Watson AJ, Smith BB, Whitehead MR, Sykes PH, Frizelle FA. Malignant progression of anal intra-epithelial neoplasia. ANZ J Surg. 2006;76(8):715–7.

12. Nyitray AG, Smith D, Villa L, Lazcano-Ponce E, Abrahamsen M, Papenfuss M, Giuliano AR. Prevalence of and risk factors for anal human papillomavirus infection in men who have sex with women: a cross-national study. J Infect Dis. 2010;201(10):1498–508. https://doi.org/10.1086/652187. PubMed Central PMCID: PMC2856726.

13. Edge SB, Compton CC. The American Joint Committee on Cancer: the 7th edition of the AJCC cancer staging manual and the future of TNM. Ann Surg Oncol. 2010;17(6):1471–4. https://doi.org/10.1245/s10434-010-0985-4.

14. Mitra S, Crane L. Diagnosis, treatment, and prevention of anal cancer. Curr Infect Dis Rep. 2012;14(1):61–6. https://doi.org/10.1007/s11908-011-0227-3.

15. Wietfeldt ED, Thiele J. Malignancies of the anal margin and perianal skin. Clin Colon Rectal Surg. 2009;22(2):127–35. https://doi.org/10.1055/s-0029-1223845. PubMed Central PMCID: PMC2780245.

16. Scholefield JH, Castle MT, Watson NF. Malignant transformation of high-grade anal intraepithelial neoplasia. Br J Surg. 2005;92(9):1133–6.

17. Pineda CE, Berry JM, Jay N, Palefsky JM, Welton ML. High-resolution anoscopy targeted surgical destruction of anal high-grade squamous intraepithelial lesions: a ten-year experience. Dis Colon Rectum. 2008;51(6):829–35; discussion 835–7. https://doi.org/10.1007/s10350-008-9233-4. Epub 2008 Mar 25.

18. Eng C, Chang GJ, You YN, Das P, Rodriguez-Bigas M, Xing Y, Vauthey JN, Rogers JE, Ohinata A, Pathak P, Sethi S, Phillips JK, Crane CH, Wolff RA. The role of systemic chemotherapy and multidisciplinary management in improving the overall survival of patients with metastatic squamous cell carcinoma of the anal canal. Oncotarget. 2014;5(22):11133–42. PubMed Central PMCID: PMC4294384.

19. Gnanajothy R, Warren GW, Okun S, Peterson LL. A combined modality therapeutic approach to metastatic anal squamous cell carcinoma with systemic chemotherapy and local therapy to sites of disease: case report and review of literature. J Gastrointest Oncol. 2016;7(3):E58.

20. Marks DK, Goldstone SE. Electrocautery ablation of high-grade anal squamous intraepithelial lesions in HIV-negative and HIV-positive men who have sex with men. J Acquir Immune Defic Syndr. 2012;59(3):259–65. https://doi.org/10.1097/QAI.0b013e3182437469.

21. Ghosn M, Kourie HR, Abdayem P, Antoun J, Nasr D. Anal cancer treatment: current status and future perspectives. World J Gastroenterol. 2015;21(8):2294–302. https://doi.org/10.3748/wjg.v21.i8.2294. Review. PubMed Central PMCID: PMC4342904.

22. Solomon D, Davey D, Kurman R, Moriarty A, O'Connor D, Prey M, Raab S, Sherman M, Wilbur D, Wright T Jr, Young N, Forum Group Members; Bethesda 2001 Workshop. The 2001 Bethesda system: terminology for reporting results of cervical cytology. JAMA. 2002;287(16):2114–9. Review.

23. Scott-Sheldon LA, Huedo-Medina TB, Warren MR, Johnson BT, Carey MP. Efficacy of behavioral interventions to increase condom

use and reduce sexually transmitted infections: a meta-analysis, 1991 to 2010. J Acquir Immune Defic Syndr. 2011;58(5):489–98. https://doi.org/10.1097/QAI.0b013e31823554d7.

24. Watson RA. Human papillomavirus: confronting the epidemic-a urologist's perspective. Rev Urol. 2005;7(3):135–44. PubMed Central PMCID: PMC1477576.

25. Deutsch E, Lemanski C, Pignon JP, Levy A, Delarochefordiere A, Martel-Lafay I, Rio E, Malka D, Conroy T, Miglianico L, Becouarn Y, Malekzadeh K, Paris E, Juzyna B, Ezra P, Azria D. Unexpected toxicity of cetuximab combined with conventional chemoradiotherapy in patients with locally advanced anal cancer: results of the UNICANCER ACCORD 16 phase II trial. Ann Oncol. 2013;24(11):2834–8. https://doi.org/10.1093/annonc/mdt368. Epub 2013 Sep 11.

26. Gilbert DC, Williams A, Allan K, Stokoe J, Jackson T, Linsdall S, Bailey CM, Summers J. p16INK4A, p53, EGFR expres-sion and KRAS mutation status in squamous cell cancers of the anus: correlation with outcomes following chemo-radiotherapy. Radiother Oncol. 2013;109(1):146–51. https://doi.org/10.1016/j.radonc.2013.08.002. Epub 2013 Sep 7.

27. Welton ML, Varma MG. Anal cancer. In: Fleshman JW, Wolff BG, editors. The ASCRS textbook of colon and rectal surgery. New York: Springer; 2007. p. 82–500.

28. Fenger DF, Marti MC, editors. Tumors of the anal canal. Pathology and genetics of tumors of the digestive system. Lyon: IARC Press; 2000.

29. InterAACT: An international multicenter open label randomized phase II advanced anal cancer trial comparing cisplatin (CDDP) plus 5-fluorouracil (5-FU) versus carboplatin (CBDCA) plus weekly paclitaxel (PTX) in patients with inoperable locally recurrent (ILR) or metastatic disease.

Cancer of Exocrine Pancreas

Daniele Fanale, Giorgio Madonia, Antonio Galvano, Marc Peeters, Albert J. ten Tije, Juan Lucio Iovanna, and Antonio Russo

Gastrointestinal Cancers

Contents

Daniele Fanale and Giorgio Madonia should be considered equally co-first authors.

© Springer Nature Switzerland AG 2021
A. Russo et al. (eds.), *Practical Medical Oncology Textbook*, UNIPA Springer Series,
https://doi.org/10.1007/978-3-030-56051-5_40

Learning Objectives

By the end of the chapter, the reader will

- Have reached a good knowledge of the epidemiology and risk factors of pancreatic adenocarcinoma
- Have learned the most important pathogenic mechanisms at the basis of pancreatic cancer development
- Be able to identify signs and symptoms that can raise suspect of pancreatic cancer
- Have a good knowledge of the different diagnostic tools available in diagnosis and staging of pancreatic cancer
- Be able to understand the difference between resectable, borderline resectable, unresectable, and metastatic pancreatic cancer, learning the criteria that drive the clinician in this classification
- Have gained a better understanding of well-established and innovative therapeutic algorithms

40.1 Introduction

Pancreatic cancer is one of the most lethal and aggressive human malignancies, accounting for the fourth leading cause of cancer-related death in United States of America and causing approximately 350,000 deaths world wide every year [1]. Pancreatic ductal adenocarcinoma (PDAC) is a malignant disease of the exocrine pancreas with poor prognosis and a 5-year survival rate lower than 5%. The risk of developing this tumor is equal both for men and women [2]. Many risk factors, both environmental and genetic, have been identified, the most important of which are: excessive body weight, diabetes and smoking [3]. Although, in the last few years, attempts have been made to develop early detection methods, such as spiral TC, MRCP, and EUS, and innovative therapeutic strategies in order to prolong survival and improve patient life quality, these efforts have met limited success, and surgical resection remains the only possible successful treatment option when resection margins remain negative [4, 5]. However, only a small percentage of patients (about 15%) with localized pancreatic tumors is candidate for surgical resection, since most of them, instead, exhibits a locally advanced or metastatic disease with unresectable lesions at the diagnosis. Indeed, pancreatic cancer is a silent disease, with few or no symptoms and signs until late stages [6]. Because most of surgically resected patients rapidly develop new locoregional lesions or exhibit metastatic disease progression, surgery alone appears to be inadequate and insufficient in eradicating the disease and improving prognosis [7, 8]. Therefore, along with surgery, chemo- and radiotherapy represent other treatment options, though the current therapeutic regimens provide only some small benefit for PDAC patients. Unfortunately, pancreatic cancer is inherently resistant to most currently available therapies, and, unlike other cancers, few progresses have been achieved with radio- or chemotherapy [9, 10]. Moreover, many patients with pancreatic cancer suffer from rapidly declining performance status, anorexia, and cachexia, which make it challenging to treat them. The cellular and molecular characteristics of ductal pancreatic cancer it is aggressive, with multiple levels of therapeutic resistance determined by reduced vascular density, stromal proliferation, and immune suppression. Indeed, the development and selection of pancreatic cancer cells resistant to therapies is one of the major hurdles for the clinical management of PDAC patients, leading to tumor recurrence and, consequently, a poor prognosis [11]. Therefore, adopting adequate strategies capable of overcoming the resistance which patients may develop during chemo- or radiotherapy is the main goal of clinical research. Understanding the molecular mechanisms underlying the therapy resistance and identifying new targets able to improve efficacy of therapeutic treatment may help oncologists to favor the development of personalized therapies for PDAC patients [12]. Since pancreatic cancer shows a multifactorial nature, early detection strategies or specific disease biomarkers are difficult to identify. The identification of new diagnostic, prognostic, and predictive biomarkers could represent an important tool to select patients who may benefit from a specific treatment and a crucial step toward a tailored therapy. Improvements in early screening strategies, the development of new therapies, and further progress in understanding the genetic and molecular basis of PDAC are needed in order to greatly reduce high mortality rates [13].

In this chapter, we will discuss the genetic, molecular, and clinical aspects of pancreatic cancer, by describing the alterations involved in carcinogenesis process and providing an overview of current therapeutic options and potential reasons of their failure.

40.2 Epidemiology

About 338.000 people develop pancreatic cancer every year, making it the 11th most common cancer worldwide [14]. Incidence can vary from 7.4/100.000 in the western world, where more than half of new cases are diagnosed to 2/100.000 in developing countries. These differences can be attributed to lifestyle and environment factors but, in a smaller proportion, also to differences in the accuracy of the diagnosis [15–18]. The

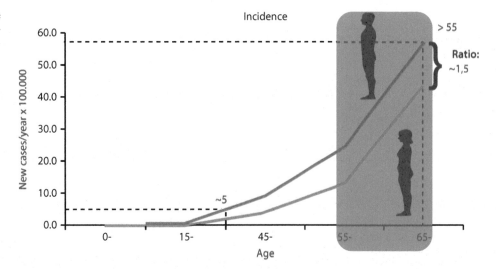

■ **Fig. 40.1** Difference in male and female incidence of pancreatic cancer according to age

risk is higher in males, with a man/woman rate of 1.5:1, and greatly increases with aging, the highest peak being in patients older than 70 years and more than 90% of cases being diagnosed after the age of 55. On the contrary, this disease is very rare under the age of 45 (■ Fig. 40.1) [19–21].

Even though PDAC is not among the most frequent kinds of cancer, it certainly is one of the deadliest: PDAC is the seventh cause of death among cancers globally, both in men and women, with a total of more than 331.000 death per year, and it can be held accountable for the 6% of all cancer-related deaths [14]. In developed countries such as Europe and United States, it represents the fifth and fourth cancer-related cause of death, respectively [1, 22]. Incidence can also differ on the basis of the ethnicity of the patient, being higher in Afro-Americans, but the reasons for this are still unclear: differences in dietary habits, smoking, and obesity rates play important roles, but genetic factors are also involved [23, 24].

Notably mortality and incidence rates are very similar: due to the extremely low survival rates for this tumor, around 5% at 5 years, one of the lowest among all cancers [11, 14, 25, 26]. This data has remained stable in the last 20 years, with little progresses obtained for the prognosis of these patients [27, 28]. Incidence and mortality of pancreatic cancer are also rising globally, especially in Western world (+19% deaths in Europe from 2009 to 2014) [19, 21]: it is expected that in 2030, the number of patients affected by PDAC will have increased more than twofold over the current global rate. Considering these data, the number of deaths will probably exceed those of breast and colorectal cancer, and pancreatic cancer will be the second tumor for mortality worldwide, being surpassed only by lung cancer [17].

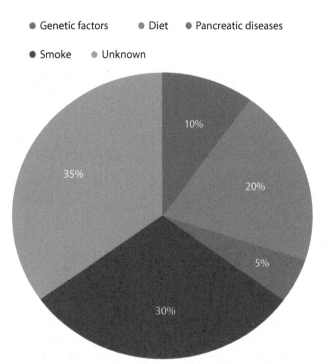

■ **Fig. 40.2** Most important causes of pancreatic cancer

40.3 Risk factors

40.3.1 Environmental risk factors

Most of PDAC are caused by environmental causes, by lifestyle, or by other, non-oncological, reasons (80–90% of total) (■ Fig. 40.2) [16, 29]. Of these factors, the most important can undoubtedly be considered cigarette smoking [30–32]: chronic intake of nitro derivatives contained in tobacco can cause genetic mutations such as the activation of K-Ras and the subsequent

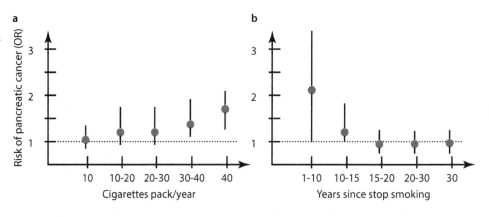

■ **Fig. 40.3** Risk of pancreatic cancer, on the basis of the number of cigarettes smoked **a** and of the years passed since smoking has been stopped **b**

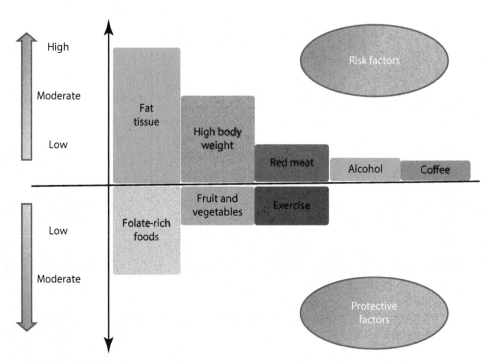

■ **Fig. 40.4** Most important risk factors and protective factors in pancreatic cancer

development of pancreatic adenocarcinoma. Autopsies provided data that demonstrate how nitro derivatives damage pancreatic tissue. Smoking has been related up to 30% of all cases. The overall risk increases up to 2–5 times, and it keeps growing steadily with the number of cigarettes consumed, while it decreases with the number of years since smoking has been stopped, being comparable to that of nonsmokers after 15 years (■ Fig. 40.3) [33]. Passive smoking too has been associated with a higher risk [34, 35].

Other important environmental risk factors are, in order of importance (■ Fig. 40.4 and ■ Table 40.1):

— Body fat tissue, particularly abdominal fat tissue, probably by contributing to the development of an abnormal glucose metabolism mechanism, can increase the risk of pancreatic cancer [36, 37].

— Obesity (BMI > 30): 20–40% higher risk of death by pancreatic cancer [37–39].
— Red or processed meat [40–42].
— Alcohol consumption [43].

■ **Table 40.1** Risk factors for pancreatic

Aquired risk factors	Pathologies
Abdominal fat tissue	Diabetes mellitus
Obesity	Chronic Pancreatitis
Red or processed meat	Hereditary pancreatitis
Alcool consumption	*H. pylori*, HCV or HIV infection

Foods rich in folate (while not folate dietary supplements), fruit, vegetables, and exercise are instead considered protective factors (▶ Box 40.1) [44, 45]. It is still unclear if coffee regular consumption can increase the risk of pancreatic cancer [42, 46].

Diabetes mellitus has been linked to pancreatic cancer:

> **Box 40.1   Protective factors for pancreatic cancer**
> − Folate-rich foods
> − Fruit and vegetables
> − Aerobic Physical exercise

both type I and II can increase the chance of developing pancreatic cancer, with a relative risk, respectively of 2 and of 1.8 (◘ Fig. 40.5) [47–49].

The risk decreases with the duration of diabetes, and insulin and oral antidiabetic drugs have been associated with a reduction of this risk [35, 50, 51].

Chronic pancreatitis can account for 5% of all pancreatic cancer, probably because of the role that chronic inflammation can have in the genesis of cancer. Patients with chronic pancreatitis have a 26-fold increased risk, which keeps growing with the disease duration: 4% of patients affected by chronic pancreatitis for at

least 20 years will develop this tumor, and the main cause of this disease, alcohol consumption, is also an independent risk factor for pancreatic cancer. Patients with hereditary pancreatitis have an extremely high risk of developing this tumor, up to 50–60 times greater than expected [17].

Infection diseases have been related to an increased risk of pancreatic cancer, even though data are not conclusive: *H. pylori* infection, human hepatitis B virus infection, and human immunodeficiency virus infection [35, 45].

Occupational risk factors are considered working in mines (especially carbon mines) or in a sawmill and being employed in the metallurgical, petrochemical, or rubber industry. All these jobs can increase the risk of pancreatic carcinoma up to fivefold [52].

40.3.2 Genetic Risk Factors

Sporadic pancreatic cancer accounts for 70% of total, and 17% more, diagnosed before the age of 60, can be considered as early-onset sporadic pancreatic cancers.

Familial pancreatic cancers are defined by the presence of at least two first-degree relatives with pancreatic cancer (◘ Fig. 40.6 and ◘ Table 40.2) and can be held accountable for no more than 10–13% of all cases. Moreover, in less than 25–30% of familiar pancreatic cancer (3% of all pancreatic cancers), an inherited germline mutation can be found, and, therefore, a genetic syndrome can be identified (◘ Fig. 40.7) [35, 53].

Clinical features that can suggest a hereditary cancer syndrome are:
− Young age at diagnosis (<60 years)
− Multiple cases of pancreatic cancer within the same family
− Cancer clusters that can be part of a defined genetic syndrome
− Multiple tumors in the same individual

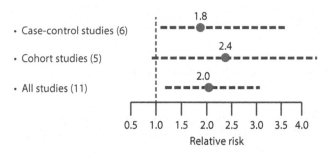

- Case-control studies (6)   1.8
- Cohort studies (5)   2.4
- All studies (11)   2.0

Relative risk

◘ **Fig. 40.5** Diabetes-related risk of pancreatic cancer, according to different studies

◘ **Fig. 40.6** A family tree in case of sporadic pancreatic cancer **a** and a family tree in case of familial pancreatic cancer be associated with a hereditary genetic mutation **b**

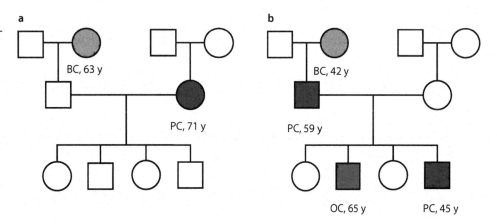

◘ Table 40.2 Risk of pancreatic cancer based on the number of affected relatives

Affected relatives	Relative risk	Lifelong risk (%)
1 first-degree relative	4.6	6
2 first-degree relatives	6.4–9	8–12
3 or more first-degree relatives	32	40

◘ Table 40.3 Most common symptoms in pancreatic cancer

Syndrome	Genes	Relative risk
HBOC	BRCA1	3.5–10
	BRCA2	2.3
HNPCC	MSH2, MLH1, MSH6, PMS, PMS2	4.7
FAP	APC	4.5
FAMM	CDKN2A/P16	34–39
PJS	LKB1/STK11	132

● Sporadic cancer ● Young onset sporadic cancer (<60)
● Familiar cancer ● Genetic syndromes

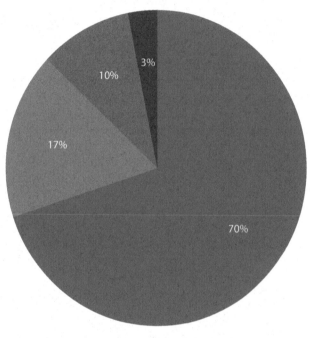

◘ Fig. 40.7 Weight of familial and hereditary cancers on the total of pancreatic cancers

As said, specific genetic syndromes can be defined in only a third of all familial pancreatic cancers (◘ Table 40.3). Different germline mutations are associated with varying risk of pancreatic cancer [54], and, of these, the most common are the BRCA1/2 gene mutations, cause of the hereditary breast and ovarian cancer syndrome (HBOC) [55, 56].

Other genes involved are:
- APC, whose mutation causes familial adenomatous polyposis (FAP), primarily associated with colorectal cancer
- Mismatch repair genes (MMR), whose mutations cause the Lynch syndrome, also associated with colon, endometrial, ovarian, and gastric cancer [57]
- CDKN2a and P16, associated with the hereditary melanoma syndrome
- VHL Gene

- LKB1 and STK11, associated with the Peutz-Jeghers syndrome, characterized by small bowel hamartomatosis and pigmented spots on the lips

40.4 Carcinogenesis of Pancreatic Adenocarcinoma

In recent years, thanks to progress in the fields of genomics, biotechnology, and molecular pathology, a large number of molecular, genetic, and epigenetic alterations related to proliferation and survival of pancreatic tumor cell and therapy response were found, unfortunately these have not shown utility as biomarkers for clinical use [58, 59]. Also, several studies revealed that response to treatment can be affected by epigenetic mechanisms involving a gene expression regulation [60].

Other studies showed that pancreatic carcinogenesis occurs through a gradual multistep process which determinates the progression from intraepithelial neoplasia to invasive cancer, increasing the extent of cytological and morphological atypia [61, 62]. Onset of infiltrating carcinoma in patients with intraductal mucinous tumor not resected, frequent presence of ductal lesions in pancreases of infiltrating carcinoma patients and increase in the degree of atypia of lesions adjacent to infiltrating carcinoma are suggestive for the hypothesis of a multistep carcinogenesis which leads to PDAC [63]. An accurate classification of the PDAC precursor lesions was suggested only at the beginning of the 2000s, despite their discovery goes back to more than a century ago [64, 65]. Thanks to morphological analyses performed on pancreatic cancers resected from PDAC patients, three different types of histologically defined PDAC precursor lesions have been described: pancreatic intraepithelial neoplasia (PanIN), intraductal papillary mucinous neoplasm (IPMN) and mucinous cystic neoplasm (MCN) [66–68] (◘ Fig. 40.8).

40

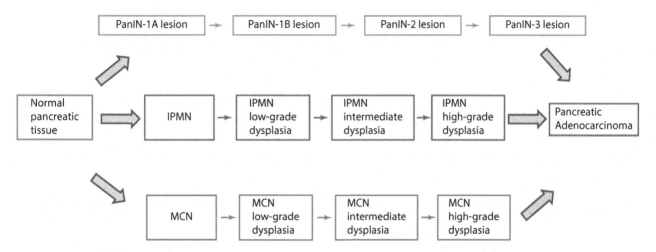

Fig. 40.8 Model of three distinct pancreatic cancer progression pathways from preneoplastic lesions to invasive pancreatic carcinoma

Nowadays, the major aim of scientific research is to early detect and genetically characterize these precancerous lesions, especially PanIN-3, before an invasive pancreatic cancer may develop. Unlike IPMNs and MCNs which are macroscopically detectable rare precancerous pancreatic lesions, PanINs are the most frequently detected microscopic lesions located in the smaller pancreatic ducts. PanIN lesions were classified in 2001 by Hruban and colleagues [65, 68] based on the degree of epithelial atypia and divided into three subtypes ranging from low-grade lesions with minimal cytological and architectural atypia (PanIN-1) to intermediate-grade lesions (PanIN-2) to in situ carcinomas (PanIN-3). These generally asymptomatic noninvasive lesions are supposed to occur before the invasion of the surrounding stroma [66, 69]. In turn, the PanIN-1 lesions have been further categorized into two different subtypes, PanIN-1A (flat) and PanIN-1B (papillary). Immunohistochemical characterization of PanINs showed that apomucin MUC1 is mainly expressed in high-grade lesions (PanIN-2/PanIN-3) and invasive PDAC as well as in the normal pancreatic ducts, whereas MUC5AC is detected in all PanIN lesions [70]. The accumulation of genetic and molecular alterations underlying these lesions has been shown to be correlated with the histological progression of PanINs. Understanding these genetic changes may allow us to early detect the transition mechanism from precancerous to malignant lesions [71–74]. One of the earliest events in pancreatic carcinogenesis is represented by overexpression of *ERBB2* oncogene encoding a tyrosine kinase growth factor receptor. The *ERBB2* activation promotes cell proliferation and was found in 82% of PanIN-1A lesions and in 100% of PanIN-3 lesions [75, 76]. Several animal models proved that the multistep progression for pancreatic cancer always involves activating mutations in *KRAS* onco-

gene as early event driving the carcinogenesis process [77–80]. Generally, over 90% of PDACs harbor activating point mutations mainly located in codons 12 and 13 of *KRAS* exon 2 [81, 82]. *KRAS* mutations induce cell cycle progression through activation of the MAP and AKT kinase signaling pathways [83] and were detected in 36% of PanIN-1A lesions, 44% of PanIN-1B and PanIN-2 lesions, and 87% of PanIN-3 lesions [81]. Other *HRAS* and *NRAS* mutations were not detected in PDAC patients [84].

Other early genetic events include the loss of activity of tumor suppressor gene cyclin-dependent kinase inhibitor *CDKN2A/p16*, involved in regulation of the G1/S transition of cell cycle, and telomere shortening, which determines abnormal fusion of chromosomes at the ends, resulting in the chromosome instability and induction of neoplastic progression of the cells [85, 86]. Indeed, increased cell proliferation and formation of PanIN lesions are induced by occurrence of *KRAS* mutations that alone are not sufficient for the malignant transformation process [87], which instead requires the inactivation of tumor suppressor genes, such as *CDKN2A/p16*, *SMAD4/DPC4* or others involved in the TGF-b and TP53 signaling pathways [88–93], or chronic pancreatic inflammation [94]. The loss of function of *p16/CDKN2A* can be already detected in the early PanIN stages of almost all pancreatic carcinomas with increasing frequency according to histological progression of PanINs (30% for PanIN-1A, 55% for PanIN-1B, about 90% for PanIN-2/3) [63, 95], whereas the *SMAD4/DPC4* and *TP53* inactivation occurs in the later stages of the tumorigenesis model (30% and 12% in PanIN-3, respectively) [96–98]. Since p53 modulates the cell cycle control, G2/M arrest, and apoptosis, its loss of function, detected in more than 50% of pancreatic adenocarcinomas, induces alterations in cell death and cell division processes. The mechanism that leads

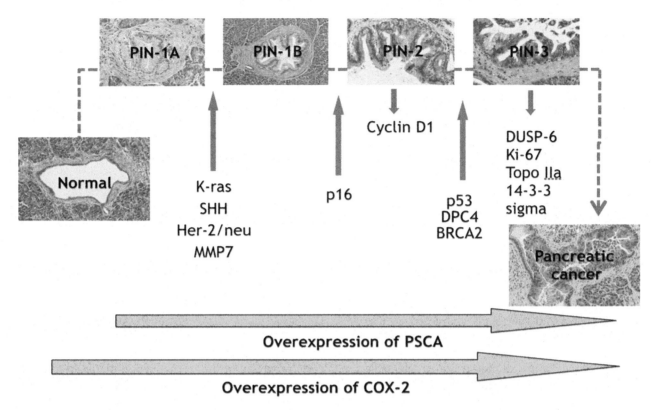

● **Fig. 40.9** Genetic alterations involved in the PanIN-progression model

to its inactivation involves the deletion of one allele and an inactivating mutation in the second allele [99, 100]. *SMAD4* is involved in TGF-b signaling pathway, and its inactivation promotes an abnormal cancer cell growth [83]. PanIN lesions deriving from chronic pancreatitis show *p16* inactivation with lower frequency. Three different mechanisms may cause the *p16* inactivation, such as promoter hypermethylation, homozygous deletion of the *CDKN2A/INK4A* locus, and intragenic mutation causing loss of the second allele [101–104]. Among the epigenetic events causing gene silencing, the hypermethylation of CpG islands at the level of the promoter of several genes is the mechanism more observed in patients with pancreatic cancer [105–107]. Using a microarray analysis, Sato and colleagues [108] demonstrated that early PanIN stages exhibit an aberrant CpG island hypermethylation which gradually enhances during neoplastic transformation. Recently, a genome-wide DNA methylation analysis has allowed to identify different molecular subtypes of pancreatic cancer [109].

In addition, the stepwise progression toward malignant transformation involves the overexpression of other molecules, such as Ki-67, topoisomerase II, and cyclin D1. The Ki-67 overexpression, correlated with cell proliferation, is more often observed in nuclei of high-grade PanIN lesions (PanIN-3) [110, 111], whereas that of cyclin D1 is detected in 30% of PanIN-2, 50% of PanIN-3, and 80% of pancreatic adenocarcinoma [112, 113]. The progressive accumulation of previously

described genomic alterations determines evolution from PanIN-1A to PanIN-3 then to pancreatic adenocarcinoma (● Fig. 40.9).

IPMNs are tumors of the duct epithelium characterized by ductal cystic dilatation deriving from papillary epithelial proliferation and mucin production [114, 115]. Genetic alterations identified in IPMN involves three oncogenes, such as *KRAS*, *ERBB2*, and *AKT*, and five tumor suppressor genes, such as *CDKN2A/p16*, *TP53*, *SMAD4*, *LKB1*, and *DUSP6*. *KRAS* mutations have been detected in about 70% of IPMN lesions both at low-grade and high-grade and seem to be responsible for the IPMN development [116]. According to the hypothesis of Yoshizawa and collaborators [117], high-grade lesions arise from low-grade lesions through a clonal pathway, whereas low-grade lesions derive by a polyclonal mechanism. Also, like PanIN lesions, IPMN lesions show the *ERBB2* overexpression as early genetic event in approximately 60% of cases [118, 119]. *AKT* activation, involved in cell growth and survival, was observed in 63% of IPMN lesions with a slightly higher frequency in high-grade than in low-grade forms [120, 121]. About 50% of all IPMN lesions shows loss of function in *CDKN2A/p16*, mainly caused by hypermethylation of its promoter, which increases concomitantly with the grade of dysplasia [122]. Loss of p53 function is also detected in 50% of IPMN lesions, especially in the high-grade forms, inducing defects in the genome integrity and, in turn, determining malignant transfor-

40

mation [123]. The *SMAD4* inactivation, instead, is considered a rare and late event in the IPMN development [124]. *LKB1* alterations were observed in 25% of IPMN lesions of patients without Peutz-Jeghers syndrome [125], while DUSP6 expression is lost or greatly reduced in some IPMN lesions [126]. A small percentage of IPMNs shows also other genetic alterations in *PIK3CA* and *BRAF* genes [127–129]. Additionally, several studies showed that almost all IPMNs harbor a mutation in *GNAS* complex gene locus (*GNAS*) or *KRAS*, and more of 50% of them is carrier of both mutations, with a higher prevalence of *GNAS* mutations in the intestinal subtype and a higher frequency of *KRAS* mutations in the pancreatobiliary subtype [130–132]. Since mutations in *GNAS*, *KRAS*, and *TP53* represent early genetic events in the IPMN onset, these alterations are not useful for identifying individuals with high-grade dysplasia or invasive disease.

MCNs are rare mucin-producing and septated cyst-forming precursor lesions of pancreatic cancer, generally asymptomatic, with favorable prognosis, and mainly observed in women [133]. Although not yet completely clear, the molecular alterations underlying MCN development and progression involve *KRAS* mutations at codon 12 observed as early event in low-grade MCNs and with increased frequency in the advanced stages, and mutations in *TP53*, *p16*, and *SMAD4/DPC4* genes mainly detected in high-grade MCNs and invasive disease. Since no *GNAS* mutations have been observed in MCNs, these may be used as useful genetic markers to discriminate between MCN and IPMN [134–136].

Furthermore, a familial predisposition for PDAC may be observed in about 10% of patients, some of which carry germline mutations in *BRCA2*, *P16/CDKN2A*, *STK11/LKB1*, and *PRSS1* genes, or, infrequently, also in DNA mismatch repair genes [137, 138].

40.5 Clinical Features

Pancreatic cancer is considered a silent disease, characterized by only vague and unspecific symptoms, with up to 4 months passing since their presentation to a defined diagnosis and only a third of all patients diagnosed within 2 months since the first symptoms have occurred. Moreover, often these symptoms only occur at late stages of disease. Because of this, delayed diagnosis is the most common problem in these patients.

Approximately 60–70% of pancreatic cancer occurs in the head of the pancreas, 20–25% in the body and the tail, and the remaining 10–20% diffusely involve the whole pancreatic gland [139].

Diagnosis is usually earlier for the head cancers, because of the jaundice that usually occur at early stages: in these cases, the most common symptoms are body weight loss (90%), epigastric pain (80%), and

icterus (75%) (■ Table 40.4). Body and tail pancreatic cancers, instead, are not diagnosed until late stages, with the most common symptoms being weight loss (100%) and pain (85%), while jaundice only occurs in 5% of the cases (■ Table 40.5) [140, 141].

Overall, the most common symptoms and signs of pancreatic adenocarcinoma are (■ Table 40.6):

- Body weight loss (observed in 75% of cases), mainly caused by a combination of anorexia, subclinical malabsorption syndrome, and dyspeptic disorders.
- Epigastric pain (70%): usually severe, dull, variously radiating to the left or right ipochondria or at the back. It usually begins at early stages as a discontinu-

■ **Table 40.4** Most common symptoms and signs at admission to hospital (pancreatic head cancer)

Signs and symptoms at admission to hospital (pancreatic head)	Frequency (%)
Body weight loss	100
Epigastric pain	85
Anorexia	35
Jaundice	5
Constipation	25
Asthenia	40
Nausea and Vomit	45

■ **Table 40.5** Most common symptoms and signs at admission to hospital (body and tail cancer)

Signs and symptoms at admission to hospital (body and tail)	Frequency (%)
Body weight loss	90
Epigastric pain	80
Jaundice	75
Courvoisier law	25
Itching and scratching lesions	40–60

■ **Table 40.6** Most common symptoms in pancreatic cancer

Symptom	Frequency (%)
Excessive body weight loss (8–10 kg)	75
Epigastric pain	70
Anorexia	50
Jaundice	25

Pain: Pathogenesis

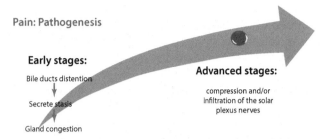

Early stages:

Bile ducts distention

Secrete stasis

Gland congestion

Advanced stages:

compression and/or
infiltration of the solar
plexus nerves

◘ **Fig. 40.10** Causes of pain in pancreatic cancer at different disease stages

ous, postprandial pain and is due to the obstruction of the pancreatic ducts, which causes ductal distention, secretes stasis, and gland congestion; at the later stages, pain can become continuous and is often caused by infiltration or compression of the celiac ganglion by the tumor (◘ Fig. 40.10) [142].

- Anorexia (50%)
- Obstructive icterus (jaundice, 25%), usually only present in tumors occurring at the pancreatic head, is caused by compression or infiltration of the common bile duct. Signs of this event, besides jaundice, are a progressive increase of both direct and total bilirubin, together with dark urines and acholic stools.
- Courvoisier law: sometimes, at the physical examination, can be identified a palpable, enlarged and not painful cholecystitis: this is due to compression of the common bile duct.
- Trousseau syndrome: this syndrome is a cutaneous migrant thrombophlebitis, and it may be the first sign of the disease. It reflects the state of hypercoagulability often present in pancreatic cancer [143].
- Recent development of diabetes mellitus: even though this sign is not common, a rapid onset of atypical diabetes should raise suspects of pancreatic cancer [144, 145].
- Deep vein thrombosis [146].
- Nonbacterial thrombotic endocarditis, which can be easily confused with a subacute bacterial endocarditis [147].
- Ascites.
- Hepatomegaly, usually caused by hepatic metastases.
- Splenomegaly, caused by a thrombosis of the portal vein.
- Virchow sign: left over-clavicular lymph node: pancreatic cancer is the cause of 25% of metastases at cervical lymph nodes from a cancer of unknown origin.
- Sister Mary Joseph sign: palpable umbilical mass; pancreatic cancer is the cause of a metastatic umbilical lesion in 9% of cases [148].
- Blumer's shelf: presence of metastatic mass at the digital rectal examination.
- Local invasion of the duodenum can result in an upper gastro-duodenal obstruction.

Occasionally, fever, nausea, vomit, and diarrhea may occur. Itching, caused by increased bile acids in blood, may not be the most serious symptom, but can be the most distressful for the patient [141].

40.6 Diagnosis and Staging

40.6.1 Laboratory Findings

40.6.1.1 Molecular Biology

The most common laboratory tests utilized in the diagnosis of pancreatic cancer are (► Box 40.2):
- Alkaline phosphatases
- Fasting blood glucose
- Amylases and lipase

However, all these tests have proved to have low sensitivity and specificity rates, and so their usefulness is scarce [139].

> **Box 40.2   Laboratory testing in diagnosis of pancreatic cancer**
> - Alkaline phosphatase
> - Fasting blood glucose
> - Amylases and lipase
> - CEA
> - CA19.9

40.6.1.2 Biomarkers

CEA (carcinoembryonic antigen) is a glycoprotein involved in cell adhesion, expressed only in fetal gastrointestinal tissue: in adults, serum levels are usually very low but can raise in many types of cancers, especially gastrointestinal tumors, including pancreatic adenocarcinoma. However, it has low sensitivity (45%) and specificity and can increase in many non-oncological diseases or conditions such as in heavy smokers. For these reasons, it is of no use in the diagnosis of pancreatic cancer. It is instead quite useful during the follow-up in patients who had high CEA levels at diagnosis, allowing to monitor an ongoing therapy or identify a recurrent disease.

CA19.9 (also called GICA, gastrointestinal cancer antigen) has a sensitivity of 70–92% and a specificity of 68–92%, but these data can vary a lot, depending on tumor size: its levels are increased in 80% of pancreatic cancers, but it has limited sensitivity for small cancers is undetectable in patients who don't express the Lewis blood group antigen (5–10% of general population) [149]. On the other hand, it increases together with the bilirubin levels, and high values can be found in many cholestasis-inducing conditions. Because of this, as for CEA, its usefulness in diagnosis of pancreatic cancer is limited. Ca19.9 has instead a very important prognostic value and can be used to evaluate disease burden and in follow-up, in monitoring the efficacy of a therapy or disease recurrence; level > 500 UI/ml indicates a worse prognosis after surgery [139].

40.6.2 Imaging

40.6.2.1 Transabdominal Ultrasonography

The first imaging test usually used in case of jaundice, of abdominal pain, or of clinical suspect of pancreatic cancer is transabdominal ultrasonography, because of its low cost and diffuse availability. It is performed with a low-frequency probe (2–5 MHz) and can easily study the liver and bile ducts, helping excluding other causes of jaundice. However, the pancreas is often difficult to visualize with this technique, because of constitutional factors of the patient, such as bowel gas, abdominal fat, or surgical scars: transabdominal ultrasonography has low sensitivity for pancreatic lesions (60–70%, with more than 40% of false-negative rate for tumors smaller than 3 cm), and its accuracy varies greatly depending on the operator's expertise (◘ Table 40.7) [139].

◘ **Table 40.7** Features of the most relevant imaging techniques utilized in diagnosis and staging of pancreatic cancer

		Contrast	Biopsy	Ionizing radiations
Noninvasive imaging techniques	Ecography	No	No	No
	CT	Yes	Yes	Yes
	MRI	Yes	No	No
	MRCP	No	No	No
	PET/ PET-CT	No/yes	No/yes	No/yes
Invasive imaging techniques	EUS	No	Yes	No
	ERCP	Yes	Yes	Yes

40.6.2.2 CT, MRI, and PET

Contrast CT, thanks to its diffusion and to the capability to acquire whole body images, represents the first imaging technique used in case of high suspection of pancreatic cancer. It is also the most common second level test after ultrasound, being used to confirm diagnosis or to complete staging. It can both study local vessels infiltration and perineural invasion, together with the presence of metastatic lesions. Pancreatic cancer appears as an hypodense, homogeneous lesion with indistinct margins (◘ Fig. 40.11). Calcifications are very rare, while cystic formations can be found more frequently, especially in tumors derived from cystic lesions, and an obstruction or compression of the common bile duct (with or without dilatation) is commonly found for tumors located in the pancreatic head. Contrast CT allows to evaluate a pancreatic lesion in three different phases (◘ Fig. 40.12):

- Before contrast: can study the presence or absence of pathological calcifications.
- Arterial phase: can study the primitive tumor and arterial involvement.
- Venous phase: can study the presence of liver metastases and venous involvement.

Maximum contrast between tumor and normal pancreatic tissue can be obtained after the enhancement peak of the arterial phase but before that of the venous phase (this is sometimes defined as "pancreatic phase") [150, 151]. Triple-phase spiral TC is capable of obtaining very thin slices (2–3 mm), increasing test sensitivity (90%), and tumor tissue samples can be obtained through percutaneous CT-guided fine needle aspiration (FNA), even though the risk of contamination has not been established yet [139].

MRI has shown no superiority to CT in diagnosis of pancreatic cancer but is useful to solve problems such as the detection of hepatic lesions that cannot be characterized by CT [152].

PET utilizes 18FDG to visualize the primitive tumor and metastatic sites and is usually used to confirm diagnosis and to evaluate nodal involvement or the presence of concealed metastases, by measuring the metabolic activity of the lesions (◘ Fig. 40.13). It can also be used to evaluate the response to neoadjuvant therapy or to detect a relapsing disease. Anyway, this technique is particularly useful in combination with CT, enabling to correctly classify as resectable 16% of cancers considered unresectable by previous CT evaluation (◘ Table 40.7).

◘ **Fig. 40.11** Role of CT phases in the diagnosis and staging of pancreatic cancer

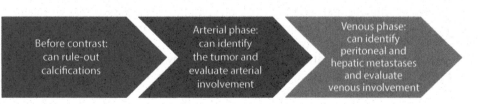

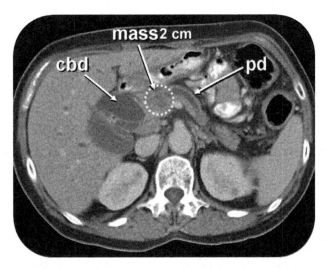

◧ Fig. 40.12 TC scanning of pancreatic cancer. CBD common bile duct, PD pancreatic duct

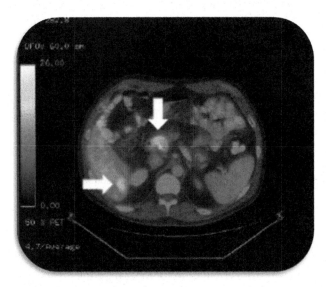

◧ Fig. 40.13 PET imaging of a primitive pancreatic cancer and of liver metastases

40.6.2.3 ERCP and MRCP

Endoscopic retrograde cholangiopancreatography (ERCP) has high sensitivity (90–95%) and can help in diagnosis of uncommon forms of pancreatic cancers such as mucinous intraductal pancreatic cancers. It also allows for histological and cytological diagnosis throughout FNA or brushing, even though cytological examination has very low sensitivity (50%). However, ERCP is of little or no help in regard to disease staging and is an invasive technique, having a high risk of complications, the most common of which is acute pancreatitis (5–10%); other side effects can be infections, hemorrhages, or intestinal perforation. Because of that, today, ERCP is mostly used for therapeutic purposes, such as stenting of obstructed bile ducts with metal or plastic

stents [139]. Nowadays, magnetic resonance cholangiopancreatography (MRCP), despite the lack of ability to perform biopsies, is preferred to ERCP because of the lower rate of complications and the similar sensitivity, and may also be preferred to CT for cystic neoplasms of the pancreas and to evaluate biliary anatomy. It doesn't use ionizing radiation or contrasts, but secretin can be utilized to induce pancreatic secretion: this can be used as an endogenous contrast agent to better visualize the Wirsung duct or substenoses and allows to evaluate pancreatic function by measuring the pancreatic secrete produced (◧ Table 40.7) [139].

40.6.2.4 EUS

Endoscopic ultrasonography (EUS) is today a largely used technique for pancreatic cancer staging and diagnosis: it uses a 7.5–12 MHz high-frequency probe mounted on an endoscope that can reach the stomach and the duodenum and is considered superior to CT in identifying lesion smaller than 2 cm, having a sensitivity of almost 100%, while it is able to assess the vascular and lymph node involvement with an 80% sensitivity. It is comparable to ERCP and MRCP in regard to the bile duct imaging. It also allows histological diagnosis on tumor samples through transparietal FNA, having a lower risk of contamination than percutaneous CT-guided FNA [153]. However, it still has issues with high cost, lack of operator expertise, and equipment availability. Also, different from CT and MRI, it can't evaluate distant metastases, and sedation is needed for this technique (◧ Table 40.7) [154].

40.6.2.5 Pancreatic Incidentalomas

Pancreatic incidentaloma are more and more frequently diagnosed, because of the increasing number of radiological exams performed for other reasons. When found, upfront surgery should not be the first option; instead, histological diagnosis should be obtained first, if feasible [139].

40.7 Cancer Diffusion and Resectability Evaluation

The pancreas has not a capsule and is in close proximity of other abdominal organs and of important vascular and nervous structures, such as the portal vein or the superior mesenteric artery and vein; moreover, pancreatic cancer usually shows great local aggressiveness. Because of this, at the time of diagnosis, pancreatic cancer has often already infiltrated important structures. Lymphatic diffusion occurs earlier than blood diffusion, with 40–50% of patients presenting nodal metastases at diagnosis, while instead 30–50% of patients present with hepatic metastases. Less common metastatic sites are (▶ Box 40.3):

Box 40.3   Most common metastatic sites in pancreatic cancer, ordered by frequencies:
- Nodes
- Liver
- Lung
- Bones
- Brain
- Skin

- Lung
- Skin, usually painful nodules
- Bones
- Brain, usually in the form of meningeal carcinomatosis [139]

Complete staging classification is reported in ◘ Tables 40.8 and 40.9.

Localized pancreatic cancer can be classified, on the basis of staging and vascular invasion, as (◘ Tables 40.10 and 40.11) [155, 156]:
- Resectable: I–II stage (T1–3 Nx M0), without involvement of major blood vessels such as the celiac trunk, common hepatic artery, superior mesenteric vein, and artery and portal vein.

◘ **Table 40.9**   Pancreatic cancer staging (2)

0	Tis, N0, M0
IA	T1, N0, M0
IB	T2, N0, M0
IIA	T3, N0, M0
IIB	T1, N1, M0 T2, N1, M0 T3, N1, M0
III	T4, any N, M0
IV	Any T, any N, M0

◘ **Table 40.10**   Resectability criteria for localized pancreatic cancer according to staging and vascular invasion

	Stage	Arterial invasion	Venous invasion
Resectable	I–II (T1–3)	No	No
Borderline resectable	II–III (T3–4)	<50%	Reconstructable
Unresectable	III (T4)	>50%	Unreconstructable

◘ **Table 40.8**   Pancreatic cancer staging

Primary tumor (T)	TX	*Primary tumor not assessable*
	T0	No evidence of primary tumor
	Tis	In situ carcinoma
	T1	Tumor limited to the pancreas, <2 cm in maximum diameter
	T2	Tumor limited to the pancreas, >2 cm in maximum diameter
	T3	Tumor extended beyond the pancreas but without involvement of the celiac axis or of the superior mesenteric artery
	T4	Involvement of the celiac axis or of the superior mesenteric artery
Regional lymph nodes (N)	NX	Regional lymph nodes are unassessable
	N0	No regional lymph nodes involvement
	N1	Regional limph nodes involvement
Distant metastasis (M)	M0	No distant metastasis
	M1	Presence of distant metastasis

◘ **Table 40.11**   Therapeutic options based on cancer resectability and on the presence/absence of metastatic lesions

	Surgery	Chemotherapy	Radiotherapy
Resectable	+	+	+
Borderline resectable	+	+	+
Locally advanced	–	+	?
Metastatic	–	+	–

- Borderline resectable: II–III stages (T3–4 Nx M0), with marginal arterial involvement (<50% of circumference) or reconstructable invasion of the superior mesenteric vein and portal vein.
- Locally advanced or unresectable: III stage (T4 Nx M0), with major arterial involvement (>50% of circumference) or not-reconstructable vein invasion; mesenteric or para-aortic node invasion is considered an absolute unresectability criteria.

Extrapancreatic disease precludes curative resection, and surgery may have only palliative purposes this case.

☐ Fig. 40.14 Patient distribution according to tumor stage at diagnosis and their relative mean survival

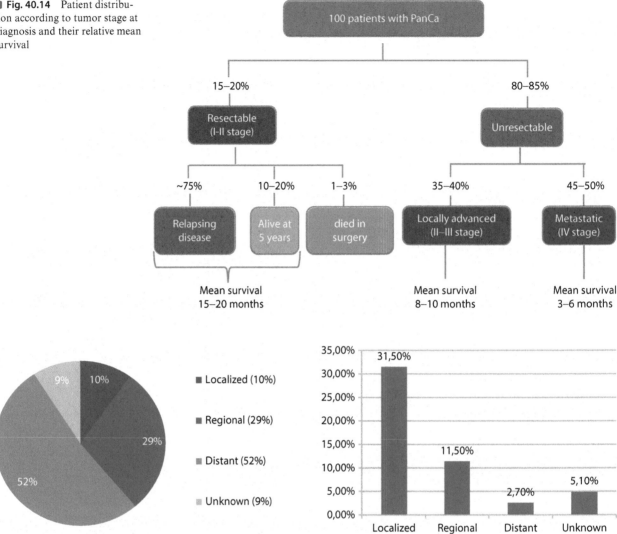

☐ **Fig. 40.15** Percentage of cases and 5-year-survival rates by stage

Historically, vascular involvement has been considered a contraindication to resective cure, but nowadays, the invasion of the superior mesenteric or portal vein is not an absolute contraindication. These veins can be partially resected, and, also, complete reconstruction is possible, using native veins as replacement. Nonetheless, invasion of the superior mesenteric, celiac, and hepatic arteries still presents a barrier to resection.

Inclusion in the borderline resectable category also depends on surgeon's expertise, on the clinical status, and personal choice of the patient [139].

Only 15–20% of pancreatic carcinomas are considered resectable at diagnosis, and, moreover, while CT or MRI can assess non-resectability with a positive predictive value of more than 90%, the positive predictive value for resectability is lower than 50% [157]. The remaining 80–85% of cancers are unresectable (35–40%) or metastatic (45–50%) and will not undergo curative surgery

but only palliative chemotherapy and/or radiotherapy (☐ Figs. 40.14 and 40.15). Medical comorbidities, performance, and nutritional status must be considered before evaluating any of these treatment modalities, whereas age alone must never be considered as an absolute contraindication [139].

40.8 Treatment

40.8.1 Resectable cancer

40.8.1.1 Surgery

Surgery is the only curative treatment for pancreatic adenocarcinoma: to this date, open surgery remains the gold standard, and data on laparoscopic surgery are still scarce [158]. The main goal is to obtain microscopically negative margins (R0); R1 is defined by the presence of microscopically positive margins, while R2 corresponds to macroscopically positive margins or unresected positive nodes [159].

After complete preoperative evaluation, surgical approach must be chosen on the basis of tumor's size, localization, and aggressiveness; the most common kind of resection are:

— Head: Whipple pancreatoduodenectomy (preserving the body and tail, with or without conservation of the pylorus) [160]
— Body/tale: Pancreatectomy (preserving the head) and splenectomy [161].

Standard node dissection, with at least 15 lymph nodes removed, should always be performed to allow proper staging, but extended lymphadenectomy is not recommended [162]. Considering the higher complication risk, preoperatory bile drainage should not be performed routinely but only in patients with active cholangitis or bilirubin serum levels higher than 250 micromoloes/L [163]. An open question remains whether or not radical pancreatectomy can improve prognosis, especially in patients with macroscopically positive margins (R2).

R1 or R2 margins are also considered independent negative surgical prognostic factors, together with surgeon's expertise and the entity of blood loss. Pathological or molecular prognostic factors are (◘ Table 40.12):

— Staging (tumor size, node involvement)
— Vascular and perineurial invasion
— Location
— Proliferation indexes
— Chromosomal abnormalities

40.8.1.2 Adjuvant and Neoadjuvant Therapies

Chemotherapy, with or without radiotherapy, is essential to improve outcomes in patients with pancreatic cancer eligible for surgical treatment [164, 165]. Adjuvant regi-

mens achieve this result by eliminating possible micrometastasis, thus reducing the risk of relapsing disease and increasing survival rates. Therapy should ideally be initiated within 8 weeks after surgery.

Standard regimens are considered single-drug chemotherapy with up to 6 cycles of gemcitabine or of 5-fluorouracil plus leucovorin [166]. Other options may include 5-FU in continuous infusion (CI 5-FU) or capecitabine monotherapy, if other options are not feasible. Of note, recent evidence have showed that combination regimen could represent innovative strategies to achieve significant improvements. In particular, gemcitabine plus capecitabine [167] or modified FOLFIRINOX (ASCO Annual meeting 2018) represent the new standard regimens in this setting of patients with an acceptable toxicity profile. The gemcitabine + nab-paclitaxel combination treatment has been studied against standard gemcitabine monotherapy in the adjuvant setting in the APACT study, presented at the 2019 annual ASCO meeting [168]. In this study, even though overall survival and investigator-assessed disease-free survival showed an advantage for gemcitabine + nab-paclitaxel, the primary endpoint, independent reviewer disease-free survival, was not reached.

Radiotherapy can be added for patients at a high risk for local recurrence (i.e., positive resection

margins and/or lymph nodes) but has shown no improvement in disease-free survival rates outside of these subsets of patients and therefore is not routinely utilized in clinical practice for all of pancreatic cancer cases.

Sadly, only 25% of patients who could possibly undergo surgery, and 50% of those who obtain complete macroscopic resection (R0 or R1), can initiate adjuvant chemotherapy (◘ Fig. 40.16). This is because of various reasons:

— The poor performance status of many patients with pancreatic cancer (after surgery)
— An inadequate recover from surgery
— Because previously unnoticed metastases are found at the postoperative restaging

These problems could be overcome by using a neoadjuvant chemotherapy regimen: in this case, therapy is administered before surgery and allows for an earlier treatment of micrometastases and a higher chance to obtain complete resection. It also increases the number of patients that can receive chemotherapy or radiations, and, moreover, surgery appears to be safe, with a possible reduction of the risk of tumor spread during surgery. Finally, it allows to stratify patients on the basis of their response to chemotherapy to better select those who may benefit from surgery (◘ Fig. 40.17) (NCCN guidelines, Version 2.2019). The downside is the risk of a progression of the disease in patients who will not

◘ **Table 40.12** Main surgical, pathological and molecular prognostic factors in pancreatic cancer

Surgical	Anatomical/ pathological	Biomolecular
Surgeon and surgical equipe	Primitive tumor size	Proliferation index
Resection margins	Tumor site (worse at body tail)	Chromosomal abnormalities
Blood loss during surgery	LN involvement or metastasis	
	Neural or vascular invasion	

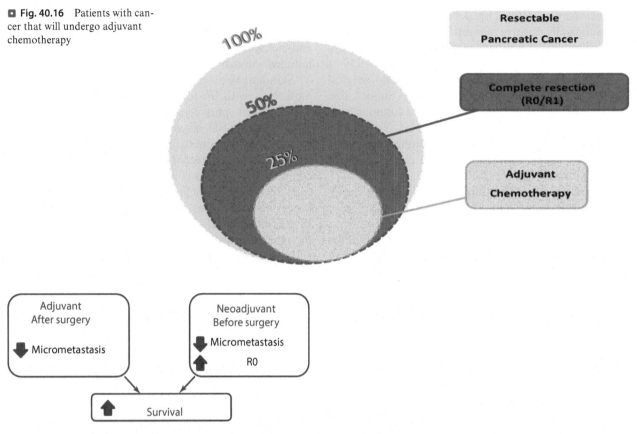

Fig. 40.16 Patients with cancer that will undergo adjuvant chemotherapy

Fig. 40.17 Advantages of both adjuvant and neoadjuvant chemotherapy

Fig. 40.18 Therapeutic algorithm in resectable cancer

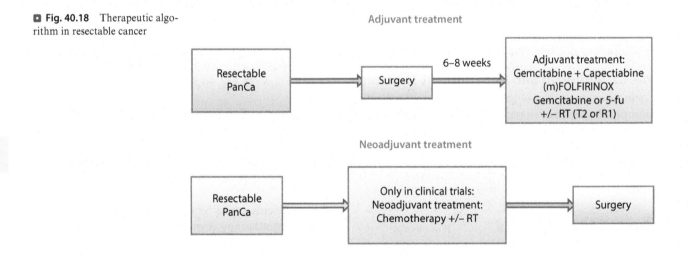

respond to neoadjuvant treatment: this can result in a poorer surgical outcome for these subjects or even in the progression to a stage in which surgery is no longer an option. However, at the present day, in the setting of resectable disease, this regimen, as well as neoadjuvant chemoradiation therapy with standard 50Gy fractionation, is not part of clinical practice and is not recommended outside of clinical trials (■ Fig. 40.18) [159].

40.8.2 Borderline Resectable and Unresectable Cancer

Borderline resectable disease represents up to 50% of all pancreatic cancers. Nowadays, surgery is no more considered the upfront treatment for this disease. However, no standard chemotherapy/chemoradiation treatment has been identified for these patients, and many options are available, with reported resectability ranging around 30–90% rates. Probably the major limitation is due to the absence of randomized phase III trials comparing sequences and combinations and from the high heterogeneity of studies.

Acceptable treatments involve FOLFIRINOX (or modified FOLFIRINOX) and gemcitabine-based multiagent chemotherapy (i.e., gemcitabine + albumin-bound paclitaxel).

The patient may also be scheduled to receive a multimodal induction therapy [169], usually using 3 or 4 cycles of a gemcitabine-based multi-agent chemotherapy or FOLFIRINOX regimen (if good performance status) as a first step. This is usually followed by a low-dose 5-fluorouracil monotherapy infusion at a dose of 200–250 mg/mq or oral capecitabine treatment, together with radiotherapy at a dose of at least 50Gy [170]. Gemcitabine monotherapy can be associated to radiations instead of fluoropyrimidine-based chemotherapy [171].

Despite no differences in long-term survival rates have been demonstrated, multimodal regimens have been associated with better response rates than chemotherapy alone. In particular, gemcitabine-based drug combinations reached up to about 90% of response rates if compared to fluoropyrimidine-based (25–70%), accounting for an increased rate in toxicities and worse quality of life [172].

Upfront chemoradiation is not usual in this setting, but it may represent an option for patients presenting with poorly controlled pain or local invasion with bleeding (NCCN guidelines, Version 2.2019).

Independently from the kind of treatment that has been used, the subsequent steps depend on the results of the neoadjuvant treatment: if downstaging has been obtained and the tumor can now be considered resectable, the patient will undergo potentially curative surgical treatment. If, otherwise, the disease is progressed to locally advanced or metastatic disease, palliative chemotherapy will be initiated (◨ Fig. 40.19) [156, 159]. In the latter case, the choice of the subsequent treatment will depend on the patient's PS and on the kind of drugs previously administered. Anyway, retrospective studies [173, 174] suggest that radiographic response doesn't always correlate with pathological response: if no apparent tumor shrinkage is observed after neoadjuvant treatment and no extrapancreatic progressive disease is evident, surgery could still be attempted.

According to guidelines, locally advanced cancers classified as unresectable will never undergo curative surgery. Standard treatment nowadays is represented by 6-month gemcitabine-based chemotherapy (i.e., gemcitabine + albumin-bound paclitaxel) or FOLFIRINOX / modified FOLFIRINOX. Gemcitabine monotherapy, 5-fluorouracil plus leucovorin, 5-FU in continuous infusion (CI 5-FU) or capecitabine monotherapy may also be used (NCCN guidelines, Version 2.2019).

A new, common approach to this disease is a multistep combination of chemotherapy and radiotherapy. After 2 or 3 months of chemotherapy alone (any of the aforementioned regimens may be used), the patient will be restaged to evaluate if objective response or, at least, stable disease have been achieved, and progression has not occurred [175–177]. If so, and if the patient's performance status is good enough, chemoradiation therapy can be started; this usually consists in a 5-fluorouracil, capecitabine or, alternatively, gemcitabine monotherapy, associated with radiotherapy [169, 170]. If disease has progressed, the patient will undergo palliative chemotherapy without radiation, using a different drug than the one that has been used previously. In any case, standard durations and drugs for this regimen have not been defined yet, and recent evidence are questioning the effectiveness of this approach (◨ Fig. 40.20) [178].

40.8.3 Metastatic Disease

Patients with metastatic disease at diagnosis have a mean survival of only about 6 months, and standard therapy have not achieved satisfying results in improving survival. On the other hand, quality of life is of

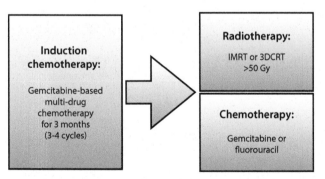

◨ **Fig. 40.19** Therapeutic algorithm in borderline resectable pancreatic cancer

◨ **Fig. 40.20** Therapeutic algorithm in unresectable pancreatic cancer

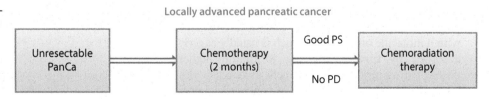

great relevance for these subjects, and the most common symptoms such as pain, weight loss, nausea, or anorexia should be properly handled [179]. Therefore, in pancreatic cancer, the role of palliative treatment is not only to increase survival but also:

- To improve quality of life
- To obtain an adequate control of symptoms

These factors are difficult to evaluate through objective measurements but can be measured through the analysis of clinical benefit. This is an efficacy criteria created to evaluate response when therapy achieves minimal or no results in terms of standard criteria (such as overall survival or progression-free survival). It can be achieved by satisfying at least one of the following four main goals:

- 50% or more reduction of pain, measured daily with visual analogue scale (VAS), for at least 4 weeks
- At least 50% reduction of opioid drugs administration, expressed in mg morphine equivalent, for at least 4 weeks
- Karnofsky PS score improvement of 20% or more for at least 4 weeks
- At least 7% of body weight gain

Clinical benefit evaluation has received both great praise and great criticism. The first because it allows to keep in count factors other than life expectancy, which were previously dismissed but can be very important in the everyday life of an oncological patient; the latter for the lack of reproducibility of the results: even though body weight and opioid consumption can be objectively measured, clinical benefit still is a criteria prone to subjective evaluation from the patient (pain evaluation) and from the physician (PS analysis) [139].

Until recent times, gemcitabine monotherapy has been considered the standard of care in metastatic pancreatic cancer, having shown better results than 5-fluorouracil, both in clinical benefit, and overall survival improvements [180]. However, new data have shown the benefits of combination regimens, at least in selected patients [181]:

- FOLFIRINOX is a multi-agent chemotherapy combining 5-fluorouracil, irinotecan, and oxaliplatin. It is more effective than gemcitabine, improving overall survival of about 4 months in mean, but at the cost of higher toxicity (i.e., higher risk of febrile neutropenia): its use is limited to patients with good performance status (0–1 ECOG performance status and normal or subnormal levels of serum bilirubin), who can tolerate these side effects [182].
- Nab-paclitaxel is a drug that combines a taxane with a molecule of albumin, which is usually eagerly absorbed by tumors, allowing to obtain higher doses of drug inside the cancer cells associated with lower toxicity. It has been used in pancreatic cancer

together with gemcitabine, proving itself superior to gemcitabine alone (2 months of median improvement in overall survival) with slightly lower activity but also a more favorable toxicity profile than FOLFIRINOX [183].

- As regards to target therapy, the efficacy of erlotinib, an EGFR inhibitor, in addition to gemcitabine has been evaluated too. However, although statistically significant, improvements in terms of overall survival have been very limited (median overall survival benefit of only 12 days), and so its role in advanced pancreatic cancer management is arguable [178, 184].
- 5-fluorouracil plus leucovorin, 5-FU in continuous infusion (CI 5-FU) or capecitabine monotherapy may also be considered (NCCN guidelines, Version 2.2019).

The current standard of care can be summarized as follows (Tables 40.13 and 40.14) [139]:

- Patients with 0–1 ECOG performance status, no comorbidities and bilirubin levels lower than 1.5× ULN: FOLFIRINOX should be considered.
- Patients with ECOG performance status 2 or minor comorbidities: nab-paclitaxel plus gemcitabine regimen can be used.

Table 40.13 Main factors involved in the decision of the right therapeutic regimen in patients affected by metastatic pancreatic cancer

Patient	Disease	Treatment
Age	Stenting	Toxicity
Performance status	Bilirubin serum levels	Quality of life
Comorbidities	Aggressiveness of the disease	Cost
Patient's choice		Clinical experience of the oncologist

Table 40.14 Choice of chemotherapy regimen based on PS, comorbidities, and bilirubin level

PS	Comorbidities	Bilirubin levels	Regimen
0–1	None/minor	<1.5 × ULN	FOLFIRINOX
2	Minor	<1.5 × ULN	Nab-paclitaxel+ gemcitabine
2	Yes	>1.5 × ULN	Gemcitabine alone
3–4	Severe	>1.5 × ULN	Only BSC

- Patients with performance status 2, comorbidities, or bilirubin serum levels higher than 1.5× ULN: gemcitabine monotherapy remains the standard.
- Patients with poor performance status, many comorbidities, or high levels of serum bilirubin: only best supportive cares (BSC) should be administered.

Second-line treatments are currently undefined, and their suitability must be evaluated case by case. However, in progressive, gemcitabine refractory, metastatic pancreatic cancer, the most commonly used regimens are 5-fluorouracil and leucovorin alone or in combination with oxaliplatin or irinotecan (FOLFOX and FOLFIRI regimens) [185] (NCCN guidelines, Version 2.2019). On the basis of the recently published NAPOLI-1 phase III trial, the NALIRI regimen (nanoliposomal Irinotecan with 5-FU and leucovorin) is now considered a new II line treatment option for these patients [186].

Gemcitabine monotherapy can be considered in patients previously treated with fluoropyrimidine-based first-line therapy.

Pembrolizumab has been approved in the United States as a second-line treatment option in patients with MSI-H or dMMR tumor without other satisfactory treatment options [187].

40.8.4 BRCA-Mutated Pancreatic Cancer

BRCA-mutated pancreatic cancer has been associated to better response to platinum-based treatments and could be good candidate to FOLFIRINOX or 5-fluorouracil and cisplatin regimens [183].

The POLO trial, presented at the 2019 annual ASCO meeting, evaluated the role of Olaparib, a PARP-inhibitor, vs placebo as maintenance therapy in BRCA1/2 germline-mutated patients with metastatic pancreatic adenocarcinoma who did not progressed after at least 16 weeks of first-line platinum-based chemotherapy. The results have shown a doubling of the median progression-free survival (7.4 months in the olaparib group vs 3.8 months in the placebo group), with a statistically significant hazard ratio of 0.53 [188].

40.8.5 Palliative Treatments

Palliative surgery plays an important role in the management of patients with pancreatic adenocarcinoma. Approximately 65–75% of patients with pancreatic cancer develop symptomatic biliary obstruction [189]. In this case, the best palliative option consists is the endoscopical insertion of a biliary stent. Metallic covered stents should be preferred to plastic or uncovered stents, having a lower biliary obstruction recurrence rate. If endoscopic management is not feasible, it is possible to surgically perform a biliopancreatic or gastric derivation [190]. Symptomatic gastric outlet obstruction occurs in 10–25% of patients with pancreatic cancer [189]. Similar to biliary obstruction management, duodenal obstruction can be handled endoscopically, positioning an expandable metallic stent or, as a second choice, surgically, positioning a percutaneous endoscopic gastrostomy (PEG) tube or performing a gastrojejunostomy [190].

Endoscopic surgery can also be used to reduce pain in pancreatic cancer, by blocking the coeliac plexus by performing a celiac plexus neurolysis: this method is safer than percutaneous insertion and equally effective [190]. Palliative radiotherapy can be used to relieve pain, bleeding, and/or local obstructive symptoms (NCCN guidelines, Version 2.2019).

Oral pancreatic exocrine enzyme replacement therapy can be administered to patients with pancreatic cancer with symptoms of pancreatic enzyme deficiency. This therapy may be initiated without diagnostic tests, considering the high frequency of this deficiency (94%) [191, 192] (NCCN guidelines, Version 2.2019).

40.9 Surveillance

NCCN guidelines recommend history and physical examination every 3–6 months with 2 years and then every 6–12 months in patients for resected pancreatic adenocarcinoma without evidence of active disease. CA19.9 measurement and chest-abdomen-pelvis CT scans every 3–6 months for 2 years can be performed, even though no significant survival benefit for patients who received regular CT scans surveillance has been shown [193].

Case Study: Pancreatic Cancer Diagnosis and Treatment

Man, 47 years old
- *Family history* positive for malignancy: maternal grandmother with gastric cancer.
- *PMH*: Diabetes mellitus type II, smoker of 1 pack/day for 20 years.
- *RMH*: development of jaundice in the last 2 months, with *ECOG PS*: 0.
- *Blood tests*: high blood levels of bilirubin, mostly direct (5 mg/dL).

Question

What imaging technique should be chosen?
   (1) PET. (2) Abdominal contrast CT. (3) ERCP

Answer

Contrast CT

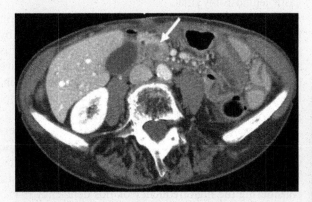

- *Abdominal contrast CT*: hyperdense lesion at the head of the pancreas (maximum diameter 2.5 cm) in the context of a modest increase in the dimensions of the pancreatic head (3 cm). No lymphadenopathies.

Question

No thoracic lesions at the CT evaluation. What action should be taken?
   (1) Surgery. (2) CT-guided FNA biopsy. (3) Chemotherapy

Answer

CT-guided FNA biopsy
- *Cytological examination*: compatible with pancreatic adenocarcinoma.

Question

Which one is the right treatment?
   (1) Surgery. (2) Radiotherapy. (3) Chemotherapy

Answer

Surgery
- *Whipple pancreatoduodenectomy without preservation of the pylorus.*
- *Histology*: Pancreatic adenocarcinoma, pT3N0M0, G2, R0.

Question

What to do now?
   (1) Palliative chemotherapy. (2) Adjuvant radiotherapy. (3) Adjuvant chemotherapy

Answer

Adjuvant chemotherapy
- *Patient underwent adjuvant chemotherapy*: single-drug gemcitabine schedule for 6 months (7 cycles).
- *CT follow-up*: 2 years after surgery, detection of local pancreatic recurrence (maximum diameter 2.1 cm), infiltrating the splenic and mesenteric vein, together with their confluence and part of the portal vein.

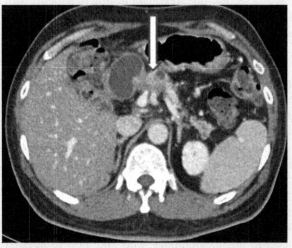

- *EUS FNA biopsy*: diagnosis confirmed through cytological examination

Question

How to treat this local recurrence?
   (1) New surgery. (2) Radiotherapy. (3) Palliative chemotherapy

Answer

- *Palliative chemotherapy*: the entity of vascular invasion contraindicates both surgery and radiotherapy.

— *Clinical evaluation*: The patient has very good performance status (0) and no relevant comorbidities.

Question

Which therapy?

(1) FOLFIRINOX. (2) Gemcitabine. (3) Gemcitabine + nab-paclitaxel

Answer

FOLFIRINOX: Considering the very good PS of the patient, he underwent six cycles of FOLFIRINOX, with partial response, and relevant, but incomplete regression of venous involvement.

— *New evaluation of the case*, considering the high compliance of the patient and his will to undergo surgery or radiotherapy.

Question

What action should be taken?

(1) New surgery. (2) Radiotherapy. (3) Follow-up

Answer

Palliative radiotherapy: Vascular invasion still forbids surgery, but considering patients' will and good PS radiotherapy is, though risky, the selected option.

Key Points

— Consider with suspect a gradually developing, direct bilirubin jaundice
— Importance of appropriate diagnosis and staging
— Carefully choose the right therapeutic option
— How to treat local relapse
— Importance of patient's will in clinical decisions

Case Study: Pancreatic Cancer Diagnosis and Treatment

Woman, 70 years old
— *Family history*: negative for malignancies
— *PMH*: HCV-positive hepatitis (treated in 2017 with new oral antiviral therapy), recurrent lung and bladder infections, ascending aortic aneurysm, and moderate mitral regurgitation
— *RMH*: occurrence of recurrent abdominal pain in the last 3 months, investigate with abdominal echotomography that showed nothing relevant.
— *ECOG PS*: 1/2.

Question

How would you proceed?

(1) Diagnostic laparoscopy. (2) Abdominal contrast CT. (3) New echography

Answer

Abdominal contrast CT: hyperdense lesion at the body of the pancreas (maximum diameter 1.5 cm), apparently infiltrating the peripancreatic fat tissue.

Question

What action should be taken?

(1) Surgery. (2) EUS with FNA biopsy. (3) Chemotherapy

Answer

EUS with FNA biopsy
— *Cytological examination*: compatible with pancreatic adenocarcinoma.

Question

How would you complete staging?

(1) PET. (2) Chest contrast CT. (3) EUS

Answer

Chest contrast CT: no signs of metastatic lesions.

Question

Which one is the right treatment?

(1) Whipple pancreatoduodenectomy. (2) Radiotherapy. (3) Pancreatectomy and splenectomy

Answer

Pancreatectomy and splenectomy (with preservation of pancreatic head)
— *Histology*: Pancreatic adenocarcinoma, pT1N1M0, (5/22 nodes positive for metastases) G2, R0, presence of vascular and neural infiltration, no infiltration of the adipose tissue.

Question

What to do now?

(1) Palliative chemotherapy. (2) Adjuvant radiotherapy. (3) Adjuvant chemotherapy

Answer

Adjuvant chemotherapy
— *Patient underwent adjuvant chemotherapy*: single-drug gemcitabine schedule (6 cycles), with dose reduction

because of the scarce PS and many comorbidities of the patient.

- *MRI follow-up*: 3 years after surgery, detection of local pancreatic recurrence (maximum diameter 2.1 cm), not infiltrating any major arterial or venous vessel, and local nodal metastases, confirmed with PET-CT.

Question

How to treat this local recurrence?

(1) New surgery. (2) Radiotherapy. (3) Palliative chemotherapy

Answer

Radiotherapy: the PS of the patient doesn't allow for a new surgical procedure, but, considering the absence of vascular involvement, RT is a possible option.

- *Stereotaxic helical RT* is performed in five sessions, for a total of 50 Gy. The treatment is well tolerated by the patient, and partial response is obtained.
- After 6 months, at follow-up MRI, detection of new *peritoneal and hepatic metastatic lesions*, confirmed at PET-CT.

Question

What action should be taken?

(1) New surgery. (2) I line palliative chemotherapy. (3) Best supportive cares

Answer

I line palliative chemotherapy

Question

Which therapy?

(1) FOLFIRINOX. (2) Gemcitabine. (3) Gemcitabine + nab-paclitaxel

Answer

Gemcitabine: considering the low PS of the patient and the many comorbidities, gemcitabine alone is the most suitable regimen.

- After four cycles of gemcitabine, RMI detection of peritoneal and hepatic *progressive disease*.

Question

What action should be taken?

(1) Best supportive cares. (2) FOLFIRINOX. (3) Capecitabine

Answer

II line palliative chemotherapy with capecitabine

Key Points

- Intermittent abdominal pain, in the absence of jaundice, can be a sign of body-tail pancreatic cancer.
- Always consider PS and comorbidities when selecting a treatment.
- Role of II line chemotherapy.

Expert Opinion
Marc Peeters

Key Points

Pancreatic cancer represents one of the deadliest among all cancers, with extremely low survival rates. Because of the lack of early symptoms and the not-so-high sensitivity of first-line diagnostic techniques such as abdominal US, diagnosis is often retarded, being reached when it is already too late and there are no more chances of curative treatments.

In case of local disease, proper staging and arterial and venous involvement evaluation are essential to appropriately evaluate the best therapeutic path and to select between immediate surgery, neoadjuvant chemo- or chemoradioterapy or definitive chemo- or chemoradiotherapy. Modern imaging techniques such as MRCP and EUS are thus fundamental for proper staging, and all patients should be referred to hub centers which dispose of them.

In contrast to other cancers, where targeted therapies and immunotherapy have revolutionized treatments, offering a significant improvement in life expectancy, the backbone of pancreatic cancer treatment is still based on chemotherapy, with few or no improvements in survival until recently. The introduction of new drugs (nab-paclitaxel, nanoliposomal irinotecan) or combination schedules (FOLFIRINOX, adjuvant gemcitabine and capecitabine combination) have shown significant results, but the overall prognosis of the patient have not changed much. Interesting results have been shown by the recently published POLO trial in patients harboring germline BRCA 1 or 2 mutations, demonstrating the efficacy of adding olaparib as maintenance therapy after

40

first-line platinum-based chemotherapy in this subgroup of patients. This trial showed a statistically and clinically significant progression risk reduction opening the way to the use of PARPi as a new class of targeted therapies in pancreatic adenocarcinoma.

However, more efforts must be put in place to better understand the genetic and biological bases of this pathology, to develop and select drugs that can be active against it, and to find those subgroups of patients that could benefit the most from these treatments.

- Main risk factors are tobacco and excessive body weight; pancreatic cancer is usually asymptomatic in early stages, and the most frequent symptoms are jaundice (pancreatic head), abdominal pain, and weight loss.
- In case of high suspect of pancreatic cancer, contrast CT is the first imaging technique to consider. PET, MRI, EUS, ERCP, and MRCP could be needed to complete staging; CA19.9 is the most utilized biomarker in pancreatic cancer, even though its usefulness for diagnosis is limited;
- Resectable stage: pancreatoduodenectomy and pancreatectomy+splenectomy with preservation of the head are the two main surgical procedures performed; adjuvant chemotherapy with 5-FU or gemcitabine should be carried out.
- Borderline stage: tumors should be treated with a multimodal chemoradiation therapy, followed by surgery if feasible; the actual standard of care for unresectable cancer is 6 month of gemcitabine, but chemo-radiotherapy schedules should be considered.
- Advanced cancer: in selected patients, with very good performance status FOLFIRINOX is an option, while in patients with good performance status nab-paclitaxel should be considered; other patients should be treated with gemcitabine alone or only BSC.

Recommendations

- Ducreux M, Chuna AS, Caramella C, et al. Cancer of the pancreas: ESMO Clinical Practice Guidelines for diagnosis, treatment and follow-up. Ann Oncol. 2015;26(Supplement 5):v56–68. ▶ https://doi.org/10.1093/annonc/mdv295;
- Balaban EP, Mangu PB, Khorana AA, et al. Locally advanced, unresectable pancreatic cancer: American Society of Clinical Oncology Clinical Practice Guideline. J Clin Oncol. 2016;34(22):2654–68. ▶ https://doi.org/10.1200/JCO.2016.67.5561. Epub 2016 May 31;
- Khorana AA, Mangu PB, Berlin J, et al. Potentially curable pancreatic cancer: American Society of Clinical Oncology Clinical Practice Guideline update. J Clin Oncol. 2017;35(20):2324–8. ▶ https://doi.org/10.1200/JCO.2017.72.4948. Epub 2017 Apr 11;
- Sohal DPS, Kennedy EB, Khorana A, et al. Metastatic pancreatic cancer: ASCO Clinical Practice Guideline update. J Clin Oncol. 2018:JCO2018789636. ▶ https://doi.org/10.1200/JCO.2018.78.9636;
- NCCN Clinical Practice Guidelines in Oncology (NCCN Guidelines®): Pancreatic Adenocarcinoma.
- ▶ https://www.aiom.it/wp-content/uploads/2019/10/2019_LG_AIOM_Pancreas.pdf

Hints for a Deeper Insight

- Golan T, Hammel P, Reni M, et al. Maintenance olaparib for germline BRCA-mutated metastatic pancreatic cancer. N Engl J Med. 2019;381(4):317–27. ▶ https://doi.org/10.1056/NEJMoa1903387
- McGuigan A, Kelly P, Turkington RC, Jones C, Coleman HG, McCain RS. Pancreatic cancer: a review of clinical diagnosis, epidemiology, treatment and outcomes. World J Gastroenterol. 2018;24(43):4846–61. ▶ https://doi.org/10.3748/wjg.v24.i43.4846
- APACT: phase III, multicenter, international, open-label, randomized trial of adjuvant nab-paclitaxel plus gemcitabine (nab-P/G) vs gemcitabine (G) for surgically resected pancreatic adenocarcinoma. J Clin Oncol. 2019;37(15_suppl):4000–4000. Published online May 26, 2019. ▶ https://doi.org/10.1200/JCO.2019.37.15_suppl.4000.
- Macarulla Mercadé T, Chen LT, Li CP, et al. Liposomal Irinotecan +5-FU/LV in metastatic pancreatic cancer: subgroup analyses of patient, tumor, and previous treatment characteristics in the pivotal NAPOLI-1 trial [published correction appears in Pancreas. 2020;49(3):e27]. Pancreas. 2020;49(1):62–75. ▶ https://doi.org/10.1097/MPA.0000000000001455
- Conroy T, Ducreux M. Adjuvant treatment of pancreatic cancer. Curr Opin Oncol. 2019;31(4):346–53. ▶ https://doi.org/10.1097/CCO.0000000000000546
- Lai E, Puzzoni M, Ziranu P, et al. New therapeutic targets in pancreatic cancer. Cancer Treat Rev. 2019;81:101926. ▶ https://doi.org/10.1016/j.ctrv.2019.101926

References

1. Siegel RL, Miller KD, Jemal A. Cancer statistics, 2018. CA Cancer J Clin. 2018;68(1):7–30. https://doi.org/10.3322/caac.21442.

2. Vincent A, Herman J, Schulick R, Hruban RH, Goggins M. Pancreatic cancer. Lancet. 2011;378(9791):607–20. https://doi.org/10.1016/s0140-6736(10)62307-0.

3. Lowenfels AB, Maisonneuve P. Risk factors for pancreatic cancer. J Cell Biochem. 2005;95(4):649–56. https://doi.org/10.1002/jcb.20461.

4. Bachmann J, Michalski CW, Martignoni ME, Büchler MW, Friess H. Pancreatic resection for pancreatic cancer. HPB. 2006;8(5):346–51. https://doi.org/10.1080/13651820600803981.

5. Torgeson A, Garrido-Laguna I, Tao R, Cannon GM, Scaife CL, Lloyd S. Value of surgical resection and timing of therapy in patients with pancreatic cancer at high risk for positive margins. ESMO Open. 2018;3(1):e000282. https://doi.org/10.1136/esmoopen-2017-000282.

6. Katz MHG, Wang H, Fleming JB, Sun CC, Hwang RF, Wolff RA, et al. Long-term survival after multidisciplinary management of resected pancreatic adenocarcinoma. Ann Surg Oncol. 2009;16(4):836–47. https://doi.org/10.1245/s10434-008-0295-2.

7. Rahbari NN, Mollberg N, Koch M, Neoptolemos JP, Weitz J, Büchler MW. Surgical resection for pancreatic cancer. In: Pancreatic cancer. 2010. p. 971–96. https://doi.org/10.1007/978-0-387-77498-5_39.

8. Boeck S, Heinemann V. Improving post-surgical management of resected pancreatic cancer. Lancet. 2017;390(10097):847–8. https://doi.org/10.1016/s0140-6736(17)31806-8.

9. Wang F, Kumar P. The role of radiotherapy in management of pancreatic cancer. J Gastrointest Oncol. 2011;2(3):157–67. https://doi.org/10.3978/j.issn.2078-6891.2011.032.

10. Neoptolemos JP, Kleeff J, Michl P, Costello E, Greenhalf W, Palmer DH. Therapeutic developments in pancreatic cancer: current and future perspectives. Nat Rev Gastroenterol Hepatol. 2018. https://doi.org/10.1038/s41575-018-0005-x.

11. Oberstein PE, Olive KP. Pancreatic cancer: why is it so hard to treat? Ther Adv Gastroenterol. 2013;6(4):321–37. https://doi.org/10.1177/1756283x13478680.

12. Hurtado M, Sankpal UT, Ranjan A, Maram R, Vishwanatha JK, Nagaraju GP, et al. Investigational agents to enhance the efficacy of chemotherapy or radiation in pancreatic cancer. Crit Rev Oncol Hematol. 2018;126:201–7. https://doi.org/10.1016/j.critrevonc.2018.03.016.

13. Ansari D, Tingstedt B, Andersson B, Holmquist F, Sturesson C, Williamsson C, et al. Pancreatic cancer: yesterday, today and tomorrow. Future Oncol. 2016;12(16):1929–46. https://doi.org/10.2217/fon-2016-0010.

14. Ferlay J, Soerjomataram I, Dikshit R, Eser S, Mathers C, Rebelo M, et al. Cancer incidence and mortality worldwide: Sources, methods and major patterns in GLOBOCAN 2012. Int J Cancer. 2015;136(5):E359–E86. https://doi.org/10.1002/ijc.29210.

15. Bosetti C, Bertuccio P, Negri E, La Vecchia C, Zeegers MP, Boffetta P. Pancreatic cancer: overview of descriptive epidemiology. Mol Carcinog. 2012;51(1):3–13. https://doi.org/10.1002/mc.20785.

16. Parkin DM, Boyd L, Walker LC. The fraction of cancer attributable to lifestyle and environmental factors in the UK in 2010. Br J Cancer. 2011;105(S2):S77–81. https://doi.org/10.1038/bjc.2011.489.

17. Ilic M, Ilic I. Epidemiology of pancreatic cancer. World J Gastroenterol. 2016;22(44):9694. https://doi.org/10.3748/wjg.v22.i44.9694.

18. Ferlay J, Steliarova-Foucher E, Lortet-Tieulent J, Rosso S, Coebergh JWW, Comber H, et al. Cancer incidence and mortality patterns in Europe: estimates for 40 countries in 2012. Eur J Cancer. 2013;49(6):1374–403. https://doi.org/10.1016/j.ejca.2012.12.027.

19. Malvezzi M, Carioli G, Bertuccio P, Rosso T, Boffetta P, Levi F, et al. European cancer mortality predictions for the year 2016 with focus on leukaemias. Ann Oncol. 2016;27(4):725–31. https://doi.org/10.1093/annonc/mdw022.

20. Qiu D, Katanoda K, Marugame T, Sobue T. A Joinpoint regression analysis of long-term trends in cancer mortality in Japan (1958-2004). Int J Cancer. 2009;124(2):443–8. https://doi.org/10.1002/ijc.23911.

21. Wang L. Pancreatic cancer mortality in China (1991-2000). World J Gastroenterol. 2003;9(8):1819. https://doi.org/10.3748/wjg.v9.i8.1819.

22. Malvezzi M, Bertuccio P, Levi F, La Vecchia C, Negri E. European cancer mortality predictions for the year 2014. Ann Oncol. 2014;25(8):1650–6. https://doi.org/10.1093/annonc/mdu138.

23. Silverman DT, Hoover RN, Brown LM, Swanson GM, Schiffman M, Greenberg RS, et al. Why do Black Americans have a higher risk of pancreatic cancer than White Americans? Epidemiology. 2003;14(1):45–54.

24. Jemal A, Simard EP, Xu J, Ma J, Anderson RN. Selected cancers with increasing mortality rates by educational attainment in 26 states in the United States, 1993–2007. Cancer Causes Control. 2012;24(3):559–65. https://doi.org/10.1007/s10552-012-9993-y.

25. Coleman MP, Forman D, Bryant H, Butler J, Rachet B, Maringe C, et al. Cancer survival in Australia, Canada, Denmark, Norway, Sweden, and the UK, 1995–2007 (the International Cancer Benchmarking Partnership): an analysis of population-based cancer registry data. Lancet. 2011;377(9760):127–38. https://doi.org/10.1016/s0140-6736(10)62231-3.

26. Levi F, Lucchini F, Negri E, La Vecchia C. Pancreatic cancer mortality in Europe: the leveling of an epidemic. Pancreas. 2003;27(2):139–42.

27. Lambe M, Eloranta S, Wigertz A, Blomqvist P. Pancreatic cancer; reporting and long-term survival in Sweden. Acta Oncol. 2011;50(8):1220–7. https://doi.org/10.3109/0284186x.2011.599338.

28. Hiripi E, Gondos A, Emrich K, Holleczek B, Katalinic A, Luttmann S, et al. Survival from common and rare cancers in Germany in the early 21st century. Ann Oncol. 2011;23(2):472–9. https://doi.org/10.1093/annonc/mdr131.

29. Hidalgo M. Pancreatic cancer. N Engl J Med. 2010;362(17):1605–17. https://doi.org/10.1056/NEJMra0901557.

30. Jarosz M, Sekuła W, Rychlik E. Influence of diet and tobacco smoking on pancreatic cancer incidence in Poland in 1960–2008. Gastroenterol Res Pract. 2012;2012:1–9. https://doi.org/10.1155/2012/682156.

31. Iodice S, Gandini S, Maisonneuve P, Lowenfels AB. Tobacco and the risk of pancreatic cancer: a review and meta-analysis. Langenbeck's Arch Surg. 2008;393(4):535–45. https://doi.org/10.1007/s00423-007-0266-2.

32. Ezzati M, Henley SJ, Lopez AD, Thun MJ. Role of smoking in global and regional cancer epidemiology: Current patterns and data needs. Int J Cancer. 2005;116(6):963–71. https://doi.org/10.1002/ijc.21100.

33. Weiss W, Benarde MA. The temporal relation between cigarette smoking and pancreatic cancer. Am J Public Health. 1983;73(12):1403–4.

34. Vrieling A, Bueno-de-Mesquita HB, Boshuizen HC, Michaud DS, Severinsen MT, Overvad K, et al. Cigarette smoking, environmental tobacco smoke exposure and pancreatic cancer risk in the European Prospective Investigation into Cancer and Nutrition. Int J Cancer. 2010. https://doi.org/10.1002/ijc.24907.

40

35. Yeo TP. Demographics, epidemiology, and inheritance of pancreatic ductal adenocarcinoma. Semin Oncol. 2015;42(1):8–18. https://doi.org/10.1053/j.seminoncol.2014.12.002.

36. Aune D, Greenwood DC, Chan DSM, Vieira R, Vieira AR, Navarro Rosenblatt DA, et al. Body mass index, abdominal fatness and pancreatic cancer risk: a systematic review and non-linear dose–response meta-analysis of prospective studies. Ann Oncol. 2012;23(4):843–52. https://doi.org/10.1093/annonc/mdr398.

37. Genkinger JM, Spiegelman D, Anderson KE, Bernstein L, van den Brandt PA, Calle EE, et al. A pooled analysis of 14 cohort studies of anthropometric factors and pancreatic cancer risk. Int J Cancer. 2011;129(7):1708–17. https://doi.org/10.1002/ijc.25794.

38. Zhang J, Zhao Z, Berkel HJ. Animal fat consumption and pancreatic cancer incidence: evidence of interaction with cigarette smoking. Ann Epidemiol. 2005;15(7):500–8. https://doi.org/10.1016/j.annepidem.2004.11.005.

39. Calle EE, Rodriguez C, Walker-Thurmond K, Thun MJ. Overweight, obesity, and mortality from cancer in a prospectively studied cohort of U.S. adults. N Engl J Med. 2003;348(17):1625–38. https://doi.org/10.1056/NEJMoa021423.

40. Anderson KE, Mongin SJ, Sinha R, Stolzenberg-Solomon R, Gross MD, Ziegler RG, et al. Pancreatic cancer risk: associations with meat-derived carcinogen intake in the Prostate, Lung, Colorectal, and Ovarian Cancer Screening Trial (PLCO) cohort. Mol Carcinog. 2012;51(1):128–37. https://doi.org/10.1002/mc.20794.

41. Appleby PN, Crowe FL, Bradbury KE, Travis RC, Key TJ. Mortality in vegetarians and comparable nonvegetarians in the United Kingdom. Am J Clin Nutr. 2016;103(1):218–30. https://doi.org/10.3945/ajcn.115.119461.

42. Larsson SC, Wolk A. Red and processed meat consumption and risk of pancreatic cancer: meta-analysis of prospective studies. Br J Cancer. 2012;106(3):603–7. https://doi.org/10.1038/bjc.2011.585.

43. Michaud DS, Vrieling A, Jiao L, Mendelsohn JB, Steplowski E, Lynch SM, et al. Alcohol intake and pancreatic cancer: a pooled analysis from the pancreatic cancer cohort consortium (PanScan). Cancer Causes Control. 2010;21(8):1213–25. https://doi.org/10.1007/s10552-010-9548-z.

44. Wu Q-J, Wu L, Zheng L-Q, Xu X, Ji C, Gong T-T. Consumption of fruit and vegetables reduces risk of pancreatic cancer. Eur J Cancer Prev. 2016;25(3):196–205. https://doi.org/10.1097/cej.0000000000000171.

45. Maisonneuve P, Lowenfels AB. Risk factors for pancreatic cancer: a summary review of meta-analytical studies. Int J Epidemiol. 2014;44(1):186–98. https://doi.org/10.1093/ije/dyu240.

46. Willett WC. Diet and cancer. Oncologist. 2000;5(5):393–404.

47. Rosato V, Polesel J, Bosetti C, Serraino D, Negri E, La Vecchia C. Population attributable risk for pancreatic cancer in Northern Italy. Pancreas. 2015;44(2):216–20. https://doi.org/10.1097/mpa.0000000000000251.

48. Batabyal P, Vander Hoorn S, Christophi C, Nikfarjam M. Association of diabetes mellitus and pancreatic adenocarcinoma: a meta-analysis of 88 studies. Ann Surg Oncol. 2014;21(7):2453–62. https://doi.org/10.1245/s10434-014-3625-6.

49. Stevens RJ, Roddam AW, Beral V. Pancreatic cancer in type 1 and young-onset diabetes: systematic review and meta-analysis. Br J Cancer. 2007;96(3):507–9. https://doi.org/10.1038/sj.bjc.6603571.

50. Bosetti C, Rosato V, Li D, Silverman D, Petersen GM, Bracci PM, et al. Diabetes, antidiabetic medications, and pancreatic cancer risk: an analysis from the International Pancreatic Cancer Case-Control Consortium. Ann Oncol. 2014;25(10):2065–72. https://doi.org/10.1093/annonc/mdu276.

51. Li D, Tang H, Hassan MM, Holly EA, Bracci PM, Silverman DT. Diabetes and risk of pancreatic cancer: a pooled analysis of three large case–control studies. Cancer Causes Control. 2010;22(2):189–97. https://doi.org/10.1007/s10552-010-9686-3.

52. Ojajarvi IA, Partanen TJ, Ahlbom A, Boffetta P, Hakulinen T, Jourenkova N, et al. Occupational exposures and pancreatic cancer: a meta-analysis. Occup Environ Med. 2000;57(5):316–24.

53. Jacobs EJ, Chanock SJ, Fuchs CS, LaCroix A, McWilliams RR, Steplowski E, et al. Family history of cancer and risk of pancreatic cancer: A pooled analysis from the Pancreatic Cancer Cohort Consortium (PanScan). Int J Cancer. 2010;127(6):1421–8. https://doi.org/10.1002/ijc.25148.

54. Slebos RJC, Hoppin JA, Tolbert PE, Holly EA, Brock JW, Zhang RH, et al. K-ras and p53 in pancreatic cancer: association with medical history, histopathology, and environmental exposures in a population-based study. Cancer Epidemiol Biomarkers Prev. 2000;9(11):1223–32.

55. Greer JB, Whitcomb DC, Brand RE. Genetic predisposition to pancreatic cancer: a brief review. Am J Gastroenterol. 2007;102(11):2564–9. https://doi.org/10.1111/j.1572-0241.2007.01475.x.

56. Bono M, Fanale D, Incorvaia L, et al. Impact of deleterious variants in other genes beyond BRCA1/2 detected in breast/ovarian and pancreatic cancer patients by NGS-based multi-gene panel testing: looking over the hedge [published online ahead of print, 2021 Aug 6]. ESMO Open. 2021;6(4):100235. https://doi.org/10.1016/j.esmoop.2021.100235.

57. Russo A, Incorvaia L, Malapelle U, et al. The tumor-agnostic treatment for patients with solid tumors: a position paper on behalf of the AIOM-SIAPEC/IAP-SIBIOC-SIF italian scientific societies [published online ahead of print, 2021 Aug 6]. Crit Rev Oncol Hematol. 2021;103436. https://doi.org/10.1016/j.critrevonc.2021.103436.

58. Fanale D, Iovanna JL, Calvo EL, Berthezene P, Belleau P, Dagorn JC, et al. Germline copy number variation in theYTHDC2gene: does it have a role in finding a novel potential molecular target involved in pancreatic adenocarcinoma susceptibility? Expert Opin Ther Targets. 2014;18(8):841–50. https://doi.org/10.1517/14728222.2014.920324.

59. Fanale D, Iovanna JL, Calvo EL, Berthezene P, Belleau P, Dagorn JC, et al. Analysis of germline gene copy number variants of patients with sporadic pancreatic adenocarcinoma reveals specific variations. Oncology. 2013;85(5):306–11. https://doi.org/10.1159/000354737.

60. Paradise B, Barham W, Fernandez-Zapico M. Targeting epigenetic aberrations in pancreatic cancer, a new path to improve patient outcomes? Cancers. 2018;10(5):128. https://doi.org/10.3390/cancers10050128.

61. Koorstra J-BM, Hustinx SR, Offerhaus GJA, Maitra A. Pancreatic carcinogenesis. Pancreatology. 2008;8(2):110–25. https://doi.org/10.1159/000123838.

62. Petersen GM, Boffetta P. Carcinogenesis of pancreatic cancer: challenges, collaborations, progress. Mol Carcinog. 2012;51(1):1–2. https://doi.org/10.1002/mc.20876.

63. Gnoni A, Licchetta A, Scarpa A, Azzariti A, Brunetti A, Simone G, et al. Carcinogenesis of pancreatic adenocarcinoma: precursor lesions. Int J Mol Sci. 2013;14(10):19731–62. https://doi.org/10.3390/ijms141019731.

64. Kozuka S, Sassa R, Taki T, Masamoto K, Nagasawa S, Saga S, et al. Relation of pancreatic duct hyperplasia to carcinoma. Cancer. 1979;43(4):1418–28. https://doi.org/10.1002/1097-0142(197904)43:4<1418::aid-cncr2820430431>3.0.co;2-o.

65. Hruban RH, Adsay NV, Albores-Saavedra J, Compton C, Garrett ES, Goodman SN, et al. Pancreatic Intraepithelial Neoplasia. Am J Surg Pathol. 2001;25(5):579–86. https://doi.org/10.1097/00000478-200105000-00003.

66. Singh M, Maitra A. Precursor lesions of pancreatic cancer: molecular pathology and clinical implications. Pancreatology. 2007;7(1):9–19. https://doi.org/10.1159/000101873.

67. Hruban RH, Takaori K, Canto M, Fishman EK, Campbell K, Brune K, et al. Clinical importance of precursor lesions in the pancreas. J Hepato-Biliary-Pancreat Surg. 2007;14(3):255–63. https://doi.org/10.1007/s00534-006-1170-9.

68. Hruban RH, Takaori K, Klimstra DS, Adsay NV, Albores-Saavedra J, Biankin AV, et al. An illustrated consensus on the classification of pancreatic intraepithelial neoplasia and intraductal papillary mucinous neoplasms. Am J Surg Pathol. 2004;28(8): 977–87. https://doi.org/10.1097/01.pas.0000126675.59108.80.

69. Stelow EB, Adams RB, Moskaluk CA. The prevalence of pancreatic intraepithelial neoplasia in pancreata with uncommon types of primary neoplasms. Am J Surg Pathol. 2006;30(1):36–41. https://doi.org/10.1097/01.pas.0000180440.41280.a5.

70. Nagata K, Horinouchi M, Saitou M, Higashi M, Nomoto M, Goto M, et al. Mucin expression profile in pancreatic cancer and the precursor lesions. J Hepato-Biliary-Pancreat Surg. 2007;14(3):243–54. https://doi.org/10.1007/s00534-006-1169-2.

71. Koorstra J-BM, Feldmann G, Habbe N, Maitra A. Morphogenesis of pancreatic cancer: role of pancreatic intraepithelial neoplasia (PanINs). Langenbeck's Arch Surg. 2008;393(4):561–70. https://doi.org/10.1007/s00423-008-0282-x.

72. Zamboni G, Hirabayashi K, Castelli P, Lennon AM. Precancerous lesions of the pancreas. Best Pract Res Clin Gastroenterol. 2013;27(2):299–322. https://doi.org/10.1016/j.bpg.2013.04.001.

73. Kong B, Bruns P, Behler NA, Chang L, Schlitter AM, Cao J, et al. Dynamic landscape of pancreatic carcinogenesis reveals early molecular networks of malignancy. Gut. 2018;67(1):146–56. https://doi.org/10.1136/gutjnl-2015-310913.

74. Takaori K. Current understanding of precursors to pancreatic cancer. J Hepato-Biliary-Pancreat Surg. 2007;14(3):217–23. https://doi.org/10.1007/s00534-006-1165-6.

75. Chou A, Waddell N, Cowley MJ, Gill AJ, Chang DK, Patch A-M, et al. Clinical and molecular characterization of HER2 amplified-pancreatic cancer. Genome Med. 2013;5(8):78. https://doi.org/10.1186/gm482.

76. Komoto M, Nakata B, Amano R, Yamada N, Yashiro M, Ohira M, et al. HER2 overexpression correlates with survival after curative resection of pancreatic cancer. Cancer Sci. 2009;100(7):1243–7. https://doi.org/10.1111/j.1349-7006.2009.01176.x.

77. Aichler M, Seiler C, Tost M, Siveke J, Mazur PK, Da Silva-Buttkus P, et al. Origin of pancreatic ductal adenocarcinoma from atypical flat lesions: a comparative study in transgenic mice and human tissues. J Pathol. 2012;226(5):723–34. https://doi.org/10.1002/path.3017.

78. Shi C, Hong SM, Lim P, Kamiyama H, Khan M, Anders RA, et al. KRAS2 mutations in human pancreatic acinar-ductal metaplastic lesions are limited to those with PanIN: implications for the human pancreatic cancer cell of origin. Mol Cancer Res. 2009;7(2):230–6. https://doi.org/10.1158/1541-7786.mcr-08-0206.

79. Murtaugh LC. Pathogenesis of pancreatic cancer. Toxicol Pathol. 2013;42(1):217–28. https://doi.org/10.1177/0192623313508250.

80. Hingorani SR, Petricoin EF, Maitra A, Rajapakse V, King C, Jacobetz MA, et al. Preinvasive and invasive ductal pancreatic cancer and its early detection in the mouse. Cancer Cell. 2003;4(6):437–50. https://doi.org/10.1016/s1535-6108(03)00309-x.

81. Löhr M, Klöppel G, Maisonneuve P, Lowenfels AB, Lüttges J. Frequency of K-ras mutations in pancreatic intraductal neoplasias associated with pancreatic ductal adenocarcinoma and chronic pancreatitis: a meta-analysis. Neoplasia. 2005;7(1):17–23. https://doi.org/10.1593/neo.04445.

82. Hingorani SR, Wang L, Multani AS, Combs C, Deramaudt TB, Hruban RH, et al. Trp53R172H and KrasG12D cooperate to promote chromosomal instability and widely metastatic pancreatic ductal adenocarcinoma in mice. Cancer Cell. 2005;7(5):469–83. https://doi.org/10.1016/j.ccr.2005.04.023.

83. Cicenas J, Kvederaviciute K, Meskinyte I, Meskinyte-Kausiliene E, Skeberdyte A, Cicenas J. KRAS, TP53, CDKN2A, SMAD4, BRCA1, and BRCA2 mutations in pancreatic cancer. Cancers. 2017;9(12):42. https://doi.org/10.3390/cancers9050042.

84. Hruban RH, Wilentz RE, Kern SE. Genetic progression in the pancreatic ducts. Am J Pathol. 2000;156(6):1821–5. https://doi.org/10.1016/s0002-9440(10)65054-7.

85. van Heek NT, Meeker AK, Kern SE, Yeo CJ, Lillemoe KD, Cameron JL, et al. Telomere shortening is nearly universal in pancreatic intraepithelial neoplasia. Am J Pathol. 2002;161(5):1541–7. https://doi.org/10.1016/s0002-9440(10)64432-x.

86. Lustig AJ, Matsuda Y, Ishiwata T, Izumiyama-Shimomura N, Hamayasu H, Fujiwara M, et al. gradual telomere shortening and increasing chromosomal instability among PanIN grades and normal ductal epithelia with and without cancer in the pancreas. PLoS One. 2015;10(2):e0117575. https://doi.org/10.1371/journal.pone.0117575.

87. Guerra C, Mijimolle N, Dhawahir A, Dubus P, Barradas M, Serrano M, et al. Tumor induction by an endogenous K-ras oncogene is highly dependent on cellular context. Cancer Cell. 2003; 4(2):111–20. https://doi.org/10.1016/s1535-6108(03)00191-0.

88. Aguirre AJ. Activated Kras and Ink4a/Arf deficiency cooperate to produce metastatic pancreatic ductal adenocarcinoma. Genes Dev. 2003;17(24):3112–26. https://doi.org/10.1101/gad.1158703.

89. Bardeesy N, Aguirre AJ, Chu GC, Cheng K, Lopez LV, Hezel AF, et al. Both p16Ink4a and the p19Arf-p53 pathway constrain progression of pancreatic adenocarcinoma in the mouse. Proc Natl Acad Sci. 2006;103(15):5947–52. https://doi.org/10.1073/pnas.0601273103.

90. Ijichi H, Chytil A, Gorska AE, Aakre ME, Fujitani Y, Fujitani S, et al. Aggressive pancreatic ductal adenocarcinoma in mice caused by pancreas-specific blockade of transforming growth factor-beta signaling in cooperation with active Kras expression. Genes Dev. 2006;20(22):3147–60. https://doi.org/10.1101/gad.1475506.

91. Izeradjene K, Combs C, Best M, Gopinathan A, Wagner A, Grady WM, et al. KrasG12D and Smad4/Dpc4 haploinsufficiency cooperate to induce mucinous cystic neoplasms and invasive adenocarcinoma of the pancreas. Cancer Cell. 2007;11(3):229–43. https://doi.org/10.1016/j.ccr.2007.01.017.

92. Kojima K, Vickers SM, Adsay NV, Jhala NC, Kim HG, Schoeb TR, et al. Inactivation of Smad4 accelerates KrasG12D-mediated pancreatic neoplasia. Cancer Res. 2007;67(17):8121–30. https://doi.org/10.1158/0008-5472.can-06-4167.

93. Sharpless NE, Ramsey MR, Balasubramanian P, Castrillon DH, DePinho RA. The differential impact of p16 INK4a or p19 ARF deficiency on cell growth and tumorigenesis. Oncogene. 2004;23(2):379–85. https://doi.org/10.1038/sj.onc.1207074.

94. Guerra C, Schuhmacher AJ, Cañamero M, Grippo PJ, Verdaguer L, Pérez-Gallego L, et al. Chronic pancreatitis is essential for induction of pancreatic ductal adenocarcinoma by K-Ras oncogenes in adult mice. Cancer Cell. 2007;11(3):291–302. https://doi.org/10.1016/j.ccr.2007.01.012.

95. Kanda M, Matthaei H, Wu J, Hong SM, Yu J, Borges M, et al. Presence of somatic mutations in most early-stage pancreatic intraepithelial neoplasia. Gastroenterology. 2012;142(4):730–3. e9. https://doi.org/10.1053/j.gastro.2011.12.042.

96. Xia X, Wu W, Huang C, Cen G, Jiang T, Cao J, et al. SMAD4 and its role in pancreatic cancer. Tumor Biol. 2014;36(1):111–9. https://doi.org/10.1007/s13277-014-2883-z.

97. Ahmed S, Bradshaw A-D, Gera S, Dewan M, Xu R. The TGF-β/Smad4 signaling pathway in pancreatic carcinogenesis and its clinical significance. J Clin Med. 2017;6(1):5. https://doi.org/10.3390/jcm6010005.

98. Mello SS, Valente LJ, Raj N, Seoane JA, Flowers BM, McClendon J, et al. A p53 super-tumor suppressor reveals a tumor suppressive p53-Ptpn14-Yap axis in pancreatic cancer. Cancer Cell. 2017;32(4):460–73.e6. https://doi.org/10.1016/j.ccell.2017.09.007.

99. Deb S, Lu L, Zeng J. Evaluation of K-ras and p53 expression in pancreatic adenocarcinoma using the cancer genome atlas. PLoS One. 2017;12(7):e0181532. https://doi.org/10.1371/journal.pone.0181532.

100. Casey G, Yamanaka Y, Friess H, Kobrin MS, Lopez ME, Buchler M, et al. p53 Mutations are common in pancreatic cancer and are absent in chronic pancreatitis. Cancer Lett. 1993;69(3):151–60. https://doi.org/10.1016/0304-3835(93)90168-9.

101. Caldas C, Hahn SA, da Costa LT, Redston MS, Schutte M, Seymour AB, et al. Frequent somatic mutations and homozygous deletions of the p16 (MTS1) gene in pancreatic adenocarcinoma. Nat Genet. 1994;8(1):27–32. https://doi.org/10.1038/ng0994-27.

102. Ueki T, Toyota M, Sohn T, Yeo CJ, Issa JP, Hruban RH, et al. Hypermethylation of multiple genes in pancreatic adenocarcinoma. Cancer Res. 2000;60(7):1835–9.

103. Maitra A, Kern SE, Hruban RH. Molecular pathogenesis of pancreatic cancer. Best Pract Res Clin Gastroenterol. 2006;20(2):211–26. https://doi.org/10.1016/j.bpg.2005.10.002.

104. Wilentz RE, Argani P, Hruban RH. Loss of heterozygosity or intragenic mutation, which comes first? Am J Pathol. 2001;158(5):1561–3. https://doi.org/10.1016/s0002-9440(10)64109-0.

105. Clark SJ. Action at a distance: epigenetic silencing of large chromosomal regions in carcinogenesis. Hum Mol Genet. 2007;16(R1):R88–95. https://doi.org/10.1093/hmg/ddm051.

106. Tan AC, Jimeno A, Lin SH, Wheelhouse J, Chan F, Solomon A, et al. Characterizing DNA methylation patterns in pancreatic cancer genome. Mol Oncol. 2009;3(5–6):425–38. https://doi.org/10.1016/j.molonc.2009.03.004.

107. House MG, Herman JG, Guo MZ, Hooker CM, Schulick RD, Lillemoe KD, et al. Aberrant hypermethylation of tumor suppressor genes in pancreatic endocrine neoplasms. Trans Meet Am Surg Assoc. 2003;121:117–26. https://doi.org/10.1097/01.sla.0000086659.49569.9e.

108. Sato N, Fukushima N, Hruban RH, Goggins M. CpG island methylation profile of pancreatic intraepithelial neoplasia. Mod Pathol. 2007;21(3):238–44. https://doi.org/10.1038/modpathol.3800991.

109. Mishra NK, Guda C. Genome-wide DNA methylation analysis reveals molecular subtypes of pancreatic cancer. Oncotarget. 2017;8(17). https://doi.org/10.18632/oncotarget.15993.

110. Klein WM, Hruban RH, Klein-Szanto AJP, Wilentz RE. Direct correlation between proliferative activity and dysplasia in pancreatic intraepithelial neoplasia (PanIN): additional evidence for a recently proposed model of progression. Mod Pathol. 2002;15(4):441–7. https://doi.org/10.1038/modpathol.3880544.

111. Karamitopoulou E, Zlobec I, Tornillo L, Carafa V, Schaffner T, Brunner T, et al. Differential cell cycle and proliferation marker expression in ductal pancreatic adenocarcinoma and pancreatic intraepithelial neoplasia (PanIN). Pathology. 2010;42(3):229–34. https://doi.org/10.3109/00313021003631379.

112. Chung DC, Brown SB, Graeme-Cook F, Seto M, Warshaw AL, Jensen RT, et al. Overexpression of cyclin D1 occurs frequently in human pancreatic endocrine tumors. J Clin Endocrinol Metabol. 2000;85(11):4373–8. https://doi.org/10.1210/jcem.85.11.6937.

113. Kornmann M, Ishiwata T, Itakura J, Tangvoranuntakul P, Beger HG, Korc M. Increased cyclin D1 in human pancreatic cancer is associated with decreased postoperative survival. Oncology. 1998;55(4):363–9. https://doi.org/10.1159/000011879.

114. Grutzmann R, Niedergethmann M, Pilarsky C, Kloppel G, Saeger HD. Intraductal papillary mucinous tumors of the pancreas: biology, diagnosis, and treatment. Oncologist. 2010;15(12):1294–309. https://doi.org/10.1634/theoncologist.2010-0151.

115. Brugge WR, Lauwers GY, Sahani D, Fernandez-del Castillo C, Warshaw AL. Cystic neoplasms of the pancreas. N Engl J Med. 2004;351(12):1218–26. https://doi.org/10.1056/NEJMra031623.

116. Schönleben F, Qiu W, Bruckman KC, Ciau NT, Li X, Lauerman MH, et al. BRAF and KRAS gene mutations in intraductal papillary mucinous neoplasm/carcinoma (IPMN/IPMC) of the pancreas. Cancer Lett. 2007;249(2):242–8. https://doi.org/10.1016/j.canlet.2006.09.007.

117. Yoshizawa K, Nagai H, Sakurai S, Hironaka M, Morinaga S, Saitoh K, et al. Clonality and K-ras mutation analyses of epithelia in intraductal papillary mucinous tumor and mucinous cystic tumor of the pancreas. Virchows Arch. 2002;441(5):437–43. https://doi.org/10.1007/s00428-002-0645-6.

118. Shibata W, Kinoshita H, Hikiba Y, Sato T, Ishii Y, Sue S et al. Overexpression of HER2 in the pancreas promotes development of intraductal papillary mucinous neoplasms in mice. Sci Rep. 2018;8(1). https://doi.org/10.1038/s41598-018-24375-2.

119. Ohira G, Kimura K, Yamada N, Amano R, Nakata B, Doi Y, et al. MUC1 and HER2 might be associated with invasive phenotype of intraductal papillary mucinous neoplasm. Hepato-Gastroenterology. 2013;60(125):1067–72. https://doi.org/10.5754/hge121268.

120. Kuboki Y, Shimizu K, Hatori T, Yamamoto M, Shibata N, Shiratori K, et al. Molecular biomarkers for progression of intraductal papillary mucinous neoplasm of the pancreas. Pancreas. 2015;44(2):227–35. https://doi.org/10.1097/mpa.0000000000000253.

121. Semba S, Moriya T, Kimura W, Yamakawa M. Phosphorylated Akt/PKB controls cell growth and apoptosis in intraductal papillary-mucinous tumor and invasive ductal adenocarcinoma of the pancreas. Pancreas. 2003;26(3):250–7. https://doi.org/10.1097/00006676-200304000-00008.

122. House MG, Guo MZ, Iacobuzio-Donahue C, Herman JG. Molecular progression of promoter methylation in intraductal papillary mucinous neoplasms (IPMN) of the pancreas. Carcinogenesis. 2003;24(2):193–8. https://doi.org/10.1093/carcin/24.2.193.

123. Lubezky N, Ben-Haim M, Marmor S, Brazowsky E, Rechavi G, Klausner JM, et al. High-throughput mutation profiling in intraductal papillary mucinous neoplasm (IPMN). J Gastrointest Surg. 2011;15(3):503–11. https://doi.org/10.1007/s11605-010-1411-8.

124. Xiao S-Y. Intraductal papillary mucinous neoplasm of the pancreas: an update. Scientifica. 2012;2012:1–20. https://doi.org/10.6064/2012/893632.

125. Sahin F, Maitra A, Argani P, Sato N, Maehara N, Montgomery E, et al. Loss of Stk11/Lkb1 expression in pancreatic and biliary neoplasms. Mod Pathol. 2003;16(7):686–91. https://doi.org/10.1097/01.mp.0000075645.97329.86.

126. Furukawa T. Molecular genetics of intraductal papillary–mucinous neoplasms of the pancreas. J Hepato-Biliary-Pancreat Surg. 2007;14(3):233–7. https://doi.org/10.1007/s00534-006-1167-4.

127. Morales-Oyarvide V, Fong ZV, Fernández-del Castillo C, Warshaw AL. Intraductal papillary mucinous neoplasms of the pancreas: strategic considerations. Visc Med. 2017;33(6):466–76. https://doi.org/10.1159/000485014.

128. Schönleben F, Qiu W, Remotti HE, Hohenberger W, Su GH. PIK3CA, KRAS, and BRAF mutations in intraductal papillary mucinous neoplasm/carcinoma (IPMN/C) of the pancreas. Langenbeck's Arch Surg. 2008;393(3):289–96. https://doi.org/10.1007/s00423-008-0285-7.

129. Schonleben F. PIK3CA mutations in intraductal papillary mucinous neoplasm/carcinoma of the pancreas. Clin Cancer Res. 2006;12(12):3851–5. https://doi.org/10.1158/1078-0432.ccr-06-0292.

130. Wu J, Matthaei H, Maitra A, Dal Molin M, Wood LD, Eshleman JR, et al. Recurrent GNAS mutations define an unexpected pathway for pancreatic cyst development. Sci Transl Med. 2011;3(92):92ra66. https://doi.org/10.1126/scitranslmed.3002543.

131. Furukawa T, Kuboki Y, Tanji E, Yoshida S, Hatori T, Yamamoto M, et al. Whole-exome sequencing uncovers frequent GNAS mutations in intraductal papillary mucinous neoplasms of the pancreas. Sci Rep. 2011;1(1) https://doi.org/10.1038/srep00161.

132. Dal Molin M, Matthaei H, Wu J, Blackford A, Debeljak M, Rezaee N, et al. Clinicopathological correlates of activating gnas mutations in intraductal papillary mucinous neoplasm (IPMN) of the pancreas. Ann Surg Oncol. 2013;20(12):3802–8. https://doi.org/10.1245/s10434-013-3096-1.

133. Crippa S, Salvia R, Warshaw AL, Domínguez I, Bassi C, Falconi M, et al. Mucinous cystic neoplasm of the pancreas is not an aggressive entity. Ann Surg. 2008;247(4):571–9. https://doi.org/10.1097/SLA.0b013e31811f4449.

134. Wu J, Jiao Y, Dal Molin M, Maitra A, de Wilde RF, Wood LD, et al. Whole-exome sequencing of neoplastic cysts of the pancreas reveals recurrent mutations in components of ubiquitin-dependent pathways. Proc Natl Acad Sci. 2011;108(52):21188–93. https://doi.org/10.1073/pnas.1118046108.

135. Fujikura K, Akita M, Abe-Suzuki S, Itoh T, Zen Y. Mucinous cystic neoplasms of the liver and pancreas: relationship between KRAS driver mutations and disease progression. Histopathology. 2017;71(4):591–600. https://doi.org/10.1111/his.13271.

136. Conner JR, Marino-EnrIquez A, Mino-Kenudson M, Garcia E, Pitman MB, Sholl LM, et al. Genomic characterization of low- and high-grade pancreatic mucinous cystic neoplasms reveals recurrent KRAS alterations in "high-risk" lesions. Pancreas. 2017;46(5):665–71. https://doi.org/10.1097/Mpa.0000000000000805.

137. Klein AP. Genetic susceptibility to pancreatic cancer. Mol Carcinog. 2012;51(1):14–24. https://doi.org/10.1002/mc.20855.

138. Ghiorzo P. Genetic predisposition to pancreatic cancer. World J Gastroenterol. 2014;20(31):10778. https://doi.org/10.3748/wjg.v20.i31.10778.

139. Ducreux M, Cuhna AS, Caramella C, Hollebecque A, Burtin P, Goéré D, et al. Cancer of the pancreas: ESMO Clinical Practice Guidelines for diagnosis, treatment and follow-up. Ann Oncol. 2015;26(suppl 5):v56–68. https://doi.org/10.1093/annonc/mdv295.

140. Bakkevold KE, Arnesjo B, Kambestad B. Carcinoma of the pancreas and papilla of Vater: presenting symptoms, signs, and diagnosis related to stage and tumour site. A prospective multicentre trial in 472 patients. Norwegian Pancreatic Cancer Trial. Scand J Gastroenterol. 1992;27(4):317–25.

141. Porta M, Fabregat X, Malats N, Guarner L, Carrato A, de Miguel A, et al. Exocrine pancreatic cancer: symptoms at presentation and their relation to tumour site and stage. Clin Transl Oncol. 2005;7(5):189–97.

142. Furukawa H, Okada S, Saisho H, Ariyama J, Karasawa E, Nakaizumi A, et al. Clinicopathologic features of small pancreatic adenocarcinoma. A collective study. Cancer. 1996;78(5):986–90.

143. Khorana AA, Fine RL. Pancreatic cancer and thromboembolic disease. Lancet Oncol. 2004;5(11):655–63. https://doi.org/10.1016/s1470-2045(04)01606-7.

144. Chari S, Leibson C, Rabe K, Ransom J, Deandrade M, Petersen G. Probability of pancreatic cancer following diabetes: a population-based study. Gastroenterology. 2005;129(2):504–11. https://doi.org/10.1016/j.gastro.2005.05.007.

145. Aggarwal G, Kamada P, Chari ST. Prevalence of diabetes mellitus in pancreatic cancer compared to common cancers. Pancreas. 2013;42(2):198–201. https://doi.org/10.1097/MPA.0b013e3182592c96.

146. Pinzon R, Drewinko B, Trujillo JM, Guinee V, Giacco G. Pancreatic carcinoma and Trousseau's syndrome: experience at a large cancer center. J Clin Oncol. 1986;4(4):509–14. https://doi.org/10.1200/jco.1986.4.4.509.

147. Chen L, Li Y, Gebre W, Lin JH. Myocardial and cerebral infarction due to nonbacterial thrombotic endocarditis as an initial presentation of pancreatic adenocarcinoma. Arch Pathol Lab Med. 2004;128(11):1307–8.

148. Galvan VG. Sister Mary Joseph's nodule. Ann Intern Med. 1998;128(5):410.

149. Tempero MA, Uchida E, Takasaki H, Burnett DA, Steplewski Z, Pour PM. Relationship of carbohydrate antigen 19-9 and Lewis antigens in pancreatic cancer. Cancer Res. 1987;47(20):5501–3.

150. Fletcher JG, Wiersema MJ, Farrell MA, Fidler JL, Burgart LJ, Koyama T, et al. Pancreatic malignancy: value of arterial, pancreatic, and hepatic phase imaging with multi–detector row CT. Radiology. 2003;229(1):81–90. https://doi.org/10.1148/radiol.2291020582.

151. Lu DS, Vedantham S, Krasny RM, Kadell B, Berger WL, Reber HA. Two-phase helical CT for pancreatic tumors: pancreatic versus hepatic phase enhancement of tumor, pancreas, and vascular structures. Radiology. 1996;199(3):697–701. https://doi.org/10.1148/radiology.199.3.8637990.

152. Bipat S, Phoa SSKS, van Delden OM, Bossuyt PMM, Gouma DJ, Lameris JS, et al. Ultrasonography, computed tomography and magnetic resonance imaging for diagnosis and determining resectability of pancreatic adenocarcinoma: a meta-analysis. J Comput Assist Tomogr. 2005;29(4):438–45.

153. Ngamruengphong S, Swanson KM, Shah ND, Wallace MB. Preoperative endoscopic ultrasound-guided fine needle aspiration does not impair survival of patients with resected pancreatic cancer. Gut. 2015;64(7):1105–10. https://doi.org/10.1136/gutjnl-2014-307475.

154. Nawaz H, Fan CY, Kloke J, Khalid A, McGrath K, Landsittel D, et al. Performance characteristics of endoscopic ultrasound in the staging of pancreatic cancer: a meta-analysis. JOP. 2013;14(5):484–97.

155. Callery MP, Chang KJ, Fishman EK, Talamonti MS, William Traverso L, Linehan DC. Pretreatment assessment of resectable and borderline resectable pancreatic cancer: expert consensus statement. Ann Surg Oncol. 2009;16(7):1727–33. https://doi.org/10.1245/s10434-009-0408-6.

156. Bockhorn M, Uzunoglu FG, Adham M, Imrie C, Milicevic M, Sandberg AA, et al. Borderline resectable pancreatic cancer: a consensus statement by the International Study Group of Pancreatic Surgery (ISGPS). Surgery. 2014;155(6):977–88. https://doi.org/10.1016/j.surg.2014.02.001.

157. Wong JC, Lu DSK. Staging of pancreatic adenocarcinoma by imaging studies. Clin Gastroenterol Hepatol. 2008;6(12):1301–8. https://doi.org/10.1016/j.cgh.2008.09.014.

158. Ricci C, Casadei R, Taffurelli G, Toscano F, Pacilio CA, Bogoni S, et al. Laparoscopic versus open distal pancreatectomy for ductal adenocarcinoma: a systematic review and meta-analysis. J Gastrointest Surg. 2015;19(4):770–81. https://doi.org/10.1007/s11605-014-2721-z.

40

159. Abrams RA, Lowy AM, O'Reilly EM, Wolff RA, Picozzi VJ, Pisters PWT. Combined modality treatment of resectable and borderline resectable pancreas cancer: expert consensus statement. Ann Surg Oncol. 2009;16(7):1751–6. https://doi.org/10.1245/s10434-009-0413-9.

160. Delpero JR, Bachellier P, Regenet N, Le Treut YP, Paye F, Carrere N, et al. Pancreaticoduodenectomy for pancreatic ductal adenocarcinoma: a French multicentre prospective evaluation of resection margins in 150 evaluable specimens. HPB. 2014;16(1):20–33. https://doi.org/10.1111/hpb.12061.

161. Mitchem JB, Hamilton N, Gao F, Hawkins WG, Linehan DC, Strasberg SM. Long-term results of resection of adenocarcinoma of the body and tail of the pancreas using radical antegrade modular pancreatosplenectomy procedure. J Am Coll Surg. 2012;214(1):46–52. https://doi.org/10.1016/j.jamcollsurg.2011.10.008.

162. Tol JAMG, Gouma DJ, Bassi C, Dervenis C, Montorsi M, Adham M, et al. Definition of a standard lymphadenectomy in surgery for pancreatic ductal adenocarcinoma: a consensus statement by the International Study Group on Pancreatic Surgery (ISGPS). Surgery. 2014;156(3):591–600. https://doi.org/10.1016/j.surg.2014.06.016.

163. van der Gaag NA, Rauws EAJ, van Eijck CHJ, Bruno MJ, van der Harst E, Kubben FJGM, et al. Preoperative biliary drainage for cancer of the head of the pancreas. N Engl J Med. 2010;362(2):129–37. https://doi.org/10.1056/NEJMoa0903230.

164. Neoptolemos JP, Dunn JA, Stocken DD, Almond J, Link K, Beger H, et al. Adjuvant chemoradiotherapy and chemotherapy in resectable pancreatic cancer: a randomised controlled trial. Lancet. 2001;358(9293):1576–85.

165. Oettle H, Post S, Neuhaus P, Gellert K, Langrehr J, Ridwelski K, et al. Adjuvant chemotherapy with gemcitabine vs observation in patients undergoing curative-intent resection of pancreatic cancer. JAMA. 2007;297(3):267. https://doi.org/10.1001/jama.297.3.267.

166. Neoptolemos JP, Stocken DD, Bassi C, Ghaneh P, Cunningham D, Goldstein D, et al. Adjuvant chemotherapy with fluorouracil plus folinic acid vs gemcitabine following pancreatic cancer resection. JAMA. 2010;304(10):1073. https://doi.org/10.1001/jama.2010.1275.

167. Neoptolemos JP, Palmer DH, Ghaneh P, Psarelli EE, Valle JW, Halloran CM, et al. Comparison of adjuvant gemcitabine and capecitabine with gemcitabine monotherapy in patients with resected pancreatic cancer (ESPAC-4): a multicentre, open-label, randomised, phase 3 trial. Lancet. 2017;389(10073):1011–24. https://doi.org/10.1016/S0140-6736(16)32409-6.

168. Tempero MA, Cardin DB, Goldstein D, O'Reilly EM, Philip PA, Riess H, et al. APACT: phase III randomized trial of adjuvant treatment with nab-paclitaxel (nab-P) plus gemcitabine (Gem) versus Gem alone in patients (pts) with resected pancreatic cancer (PC). J Clin Oncol. 2016;34(4_suppl):TPS473–TPS. https://doi.org/10.1200/jco.2016.34.4_suppl.tps473.

169. Denost Q, Laurent C, Adam JP, Capdepont M, Vendrely V, Collet D, et al. Pancreaticoduodenectomy following chemoradiotherapy for locally advanced adenocarcinoma of the pancreatic head. HPB. 2013;15(9):716–23. https://doi.org/10.1111/hpb.12039.

170. Landry J, Catalano PJ, Staley C, Harris W, Hoffman J, Talamonti M, et al. Randomized phase II study of gemcitabine plus radiotherapy versus gemcitabine, 5-fluorouracil, and cisplatin followed by radiotherapy and 5-fluorouracil for patients with locally advanced, potentially resectable pancreatic adenocarcinoma. J Surg Oncol. 2010;101(7):587–92. https://doi.org/10.1002/jso.21527.

171. Seiler C, Gillen S, Schuster T, Meyer zum Büschenfelde C, Friess H, Kleeff J. Preoperative/neoadjuvant therapy in pancreatic cancer: a systematic review and meta-analysis of response and resection percentages. PLoS Med. 2010;7(4):e1000267. https://doi.org/10.1371/journal.pmed.1000267.

172. Hurt CN, Mukherjee S, Bridgewater J, Falk S, Crosby T, McDonald A, et al. Health-related quality of life in SCALOP, a randomized phase 2 trial comparing chemoradiation therapy regimens in locally advanced pancreatic cancer. Int J Radiat Oncol Biol Phys. 2015;93(4):810–8. https://doi.org/10.1016/j.ijrobp.2015.08.026.

173. Dholakia AS, Hacker-Prietz A, Wild AT, Raman SP, Wood LD, Huang P, et al. Resection of borderline resectable pancreatic cancer after neoadjuvant chemoradiation does not depend on improved radiographic appearance of tumor–vessel relationships. J Radiat Oncol. 2013;2(4):413–25. https://doi.org/10.1007/s13566-013-0115-6.

174. Katz MHG, Fleming JB, Bhosale P, Varadhachary G, Lee JE, Wolff R, et al. Response of borderline resectable pancreatic cancer to neoadjuvant therapy is not reflected by radiographic indicators. Cancer. 2012;118(23):5749–56. https://doi.org/10.1002/cncr.27636.

175. Shinchi H, Takao S, Noma H, Matsuo Y, Mataki Y, Mori S, et al. Length and quality of survival after external-beam radiotherapy with concurrent continuous 5-fluorouracil infusion for locally unresectable pancreatic cancer. Int J Radiat Oncol Biol Phys. 2002;53(1):146–50.

176. Sultana A, Tudur Smith C, Cunningham D, Starling N, Tait D, Neoptolemos JP, et al. Systematic review, including meta-analyses, on the management of locally advanced pancreatic cancer using radiation/combined modality therapy. Br J Cancer. 2007;96(8):1183–90. https://doi.org/10.1038/sj.bjc.6603719.

177. Loehrer PJ, Feng Y, Cardenes H, Wagner L, Brell JM, Cella D, et al. Gemcitabine alone versus gemcitabine plus radiotherapy in patients with locally advanced pancreatic cancer: an Eastern Cooperative Oncology Group trial. J Clin Oncol. 2011;29(31):4105–12. https://doi.org/10.1200/jco.2011.34.8904.

178. Hammel P, Huguet F, van Laethem J-L, Goldstein D, Glimelius B, Artru P, et al. Effect of chemoradiotherapy vs chemotherapy on survival in patients with locally advanced pancreatic cancer controlled after 4 months of gemcitabine with or without erlotinib. JAMA. 2016;315(17):1844. https://doi.org/10.1001/jama.2016.4324.

179. Ripamonti CI, Santini D, Maranzano E, Berti M, Roila F. Management of cancer pain: ESMO Clinical Practice Guidelines. Ann Oncol. 2012;23(suppl 7):vii139–vii54. https://doi.org/10.1093/annonc/mds233.

180. Burris HA, Moore MJ, Andersen J, Green MR, Rothenberg ML, Modiano MR, et al. Improvements in survival and clinical benefit with gemcitabine as first-line therapy for patients with advanced pancreas cancer: a randomized trial. J Clin Oncol. 1997;15(6):2403–13. https://doi.org/10.1200/jco.1997.15.6.2403.

181. Ciliberto D, Botta C, Correale P, Rossi M, Caraglia M, Tassone P, et al. Role of gemcitabine-based combination therapy in the management of advanced pancreatic cancer: a meta-analysis of randomised trials. Eur J Cancer. 2013;49(3):593–603. https://doi.org/10.1016/j.ejca.2012.08.019.

182. Conroy T, Desseigne F, Ychou M, Bouché O, Guimbaud R, Bécouarn Y, et al. FOLFIRINOX versus gemcitabine for metastatic pancreatic cancer. N Engl J Med. 2011;364(19):1817–25. https://doi.org/10.1056/NEJMoa1011923.

183. Saltz LB, Bach PB. Albumin-bound paclitaxel plus gemcitabine in pancreatic cancer. N Engl J Med. 2014;370(5):478.

184. Moore MJ, Goldstein D, Hamm J, Figer A, Hecht JR, Gallinger S, et al. Erlotinib plus gemcitabine compared with gemcitabine alone in patients with advanced pancreatic cancer: a

phase iii trial of the National Cancer Institute of Canada Clinical Trials Group. J Clin Oncol. 2007;25(15):1960–6. https://doi.org/10.1200/jco.2006.07.9525.

185. Citterio C, Baccini M, Orlandi E, Di Nunzio C, Cavanna L. Second-line chemotherapy for the treatment of metastatic pancreatic cancer after first-line gemcitabine-based chemotherapy: a network meta-analysis. Oncotarget. 2018;9(51):29801–9. https://doi.org/10.18632/oncotarget.25639.

186. Wang-Gillam A, Li C-P, Bodoky G, Dean A, Shan Y-S, Jameson G, et al. Nanoliposomal irinotecan with fluorouracil and folinic acid in metastatic pancreatic cancer after previous gemcitabine-based therapy (NAPOLI-1): a global, randomised, open-label, phase 3 trial. Lancet. 2016;387(10018):545–57. https://doi.org/10.1016/s0140-6736(15)00986-1.

187. Le DT, Durham JN, Smith KN, Wang H, Bartlett BR, Aulakh LK, et al. Mismatch repair deficiency predicts response of solid tumors to PD-1 blockade. Science. 2017;357(6349):409–13. https://doi.org/10.1126/science.aan6733.

188. Golan T, Hammel P, Reni M, Van Cutsem E, Macarulla T, Hall MJ, et al. Maintenance olaparib for germline BRCA-mutated metastatic pancreatic cancer. N Engl J Med. 2019; https://doi.org/10.1056/NEJMoa1903387.

189. House MG, Choti MA. Palliative therapy for pancreatic/biliary cancer. Surg Clin N Am. 2005;85(2):359–71. https://doi.org/10.1016/j.suc.2005.01.022.

190. Stark A, Hines OJ. Endoscopic and operative palliation strategies for pancreatic ductal adenocarcinoma. Semin Oncol. 2015;42(1):163–76. https://doi.org/10.1053/j.seminoncol.2014.12.014.

191. Domínguez-Muñoz JE. Pancreatic exocrine insufficiency: Diagnosis and treatment. J Gastroenterol Hepatol. 2011;26:12–6. https://doi.org/10.1111/j.1440-1746.2010.06600.x.

192. Lemaire E, O'Toole D, Sauvanet A, Hammel P, Belghiti J, Ruszniewski P. Functional and morphological changes in the pancreatic remnant following pancreaticoduodenectomy with pancreaticogastric anastomosis. Br J Surg. 2000;87(4):434–8. https://doi.org/10.1046/j.1365-2168.2000.01388.x.

193. Witkowski ER, Smith JK, Ragulin-Coyne E, Ng S-C, Shah SA, Tseng JF. Is it worth looking? Abdominal imaging after pancreatic cancer resection: a national study. J Gastrointest Surg. 2011;16(1):121–8. https://doi.org/10.1007/s11605-011-1699-z.

Biliary Cancer

Giuseppe Tonini, Michele Iuliani, Giulia Ribelli, Sonia Simonetti, and Francesco Pantano

Gastrointestinal Cancers

Contents

© Springer Nature Switzerland AG 2021
A. Russo et al. (eds.), *Practical Medical Oncology Textbook*, UNIPA Springer Series,
https://doi.org/10.1007/978-3-030-56051-5_41

41.1 Epidemiology and Risk Factors

Biliary tract cancers (BTCs) comprise a heterogeneous group of neoplasms including cholangiocarcinoma (CCA), classified as intrahepatic (iCCA), perihilar or extrahepatic (eCCA) and gallbladder cancer. CCA is the second most common primary hepatic malignancy accounting for 10–20% of primary liver cancers [1]. The epidemiology of CCA and its subtypes display enormous geographic differences reflecting the distribution of different risk factors, both environmental and genetic alike [2, 3, 4]. eCCA represents the most common form of CCA; whereas in East Asian countries, iCCA is more the common form [5]. Globally, CCA is exceptionally common in Chile, Bolivia, South Korea and North Thailand, while it is a rare cancer (incidence less than 6 cases per 100,000) in Western countries [6].

Several conditions have been linked to CCA carcinogenesis. Some are considered established risk factors such as primary sclerosing cholangitis (PSC), while some have a weak association and are therefore considered possible risk factors. Several studies have demonstrated that individuals with PSC have a high risk of developing CCA [7, 8, 9, 10]. Liver fluke infestation is also strongly associated with CCA [11]. Indeed, prevalence rates of CCA are maximum in regions with higher prevalence rates of liver fluke infestations [5, 12] caused by *Opisthorchis viverrini* and *Clonorchis sinensis* species acquired by oral ingestion of undercooked fish [13, 14]. Choledochal cysts [15] especially type I (solitary, extrahepatic) and type IV (extrahepatic and intrahepatic) cysts are also associated with a high risk for cholangiocarcinogenesis. In addition, Caroli's disease, a rare congenital disorder characterized by nonobstructive dilatation of segmental intrahepatic bile duct, has been linked with intrahepatic CCA [16]. Other common risk factors is the presence of gallstones in the intrahepatic biliary tree, known as hepatolithiasis [17] and toxic agents like thorotrast and dioxin [18, 19]. Recent evidences have demonstrated a correlation between hepatitis B virus (HBV) and HCV infections with cholangiocarcinogenesis [20, 21]. Finally, other pathological conditions as cirrhosis [22], obesity [23, 24] and diabetes [25] have been associated to CCA incidence even if they need to be further validated.

41.2 Classification and Histological Types

Cholangiocarcinomas (CCA) can develop anywhere along the biliary tree and are anatomically classified as intrahepatic (10%), perihilar (50–60%) and distal CCA (20–30%) [6]. Lesions can be defined as mass-like, periductal, intraductal or mixed based on clinical presentation and site of origin. Most cholangiocarcinomas are well or moderately differentiated tumours with a locally aggressive behaviour. They present mainly with infiltration of contiguous structures (liver, hepatic artery and portal vein), nodal involvement (up to 30% at diagnosis), invasive spread with neural, perineural and lymphatic involvement and subepithelial extension [26]. In particular, iCCAs arise from the small bile ducts in the liver and can be divided into mass-forming, periductal infiltrating and intraductal growth types [27]; pCCAs originate in the main hepatic ducts or at the bifurcation of the common biliary tract, and they can have exophytic (forming-mass) or intraductal macroscopic growth patterns; dCCAs arise from the extrahepatic tract comprehending the cystic duct up to the ampulla of Vater. Macroscopic subtypes are: sclerosing tumours, nodular (often both) and papillary.

41.3 Screening and Diagnosis

The prevention of underlying liver disease and the identification of high risk patients is the best choice to improve clinical outcome. It is important pay attention to the potential symptoms of the disease, even if clinical presentation of CCA is unspecific. Patients with CCA could present several symptoms such as malaise, abdominal pain, loss of weight and appetite as well as obstructive jaundice, common also with other pathologies (i.e. hepatocellular cancer, pancreatic cancer, biliary stones) [28, 29, 30]. CCA screening cannot be performed with any degree of reliability in individuals who are not experiencing symptoms. Moreover, there are not effective lab tests that can identify biliary cancers at early stage and the disease is usually diagnosed late.

Since CCA recommended screening methods are not available in clinical practice, the surveillance of risk patients is crucial for early diagnosis at resectable stage.

Patients with hepatolithiasis, PSC, cholangitis, hepatobiliary flukes and choledochal cysts could be the best candidates for the screening [31, 32]. Nevertheless, patients with hepatolithiasis usually develop several complications that make the diagnosis of CCA more difficult; thus patients' prognosis is significantly worst.

It is known that PSC patients have an increased risk to develop CCA, but given the low annual incidence, it is difficult to identify a high-risk group within those patients that could benefit from a screening program. In particular, the current technologies used for CCA screening and diagnosis (ultrasound (US), magnetic resonance imaging (MRI/MRCP), computed tomography (CT) scan, cholangiography and endoscopic retrograde cholangiopancreatography (ERCP), as well as serum and bile markers for cancer) lack of efficacy, cost-effectiveness and reliability.

41

Carbohydrate antigen 19-9 (CA 19-9), a glycolipid expressed by cancer cells, is the most common circulated marker associated with CCA. Nevertheless, it cannot be considered a screening marker, given its variability of sensitivity and specificity. Indeed its serum levels increased after several inflammatory processes common in different types of cancer and in infectious conditions (i.e. cholangitis). At contrary, patients who are negative for Lewis antigen do not produce CA 19-9 neither in presence of CCA [33]. Recently, novel molecular markers have been introduced to differentiate CCA from other biliary diseases like angiopoietin-2 secreted by tumour cells [34, 35].

Imaging studies allow a noninvasive examination of the biliary tree, but they are inadequate when used alone. For example, US is not recommended for screening or diagnosis of CCA given its limited resolution [36].

CT and MRI are useful for the distinction of CCA from hepatocellular carcinoma for tumours >2 cm. In particular, CT has a high accuracy for evaluating portal vein and arterial involvement, even if it has low sensitivity in detecting lymph node metastases.

Another imaging technique used for CCA detection is MRI with magnetic resonance cholangiopancreatography (MRCP), especially to evaluate pCCAs with an accuracy up to 95% [37].

When these imaging systems are inadequate to diagnose CCA, positron emission tomography (PET) can be used. PET-CT has high sensitivity and specificity to detect primary tumours and metastasis of iCCA, even if its sensitivity and specificity decrease in pCCA evaluation [38].

Another imaging system used for the evaluation of CCAs is cholangiography performed by percutaneous transhepatic cholangiography (PTC), MRCP or endoscopically using endoscopic retrograde cholangiopancreatography (ERCP). ERCP is useful to diagnose perihilar and distal extrahepatic CCA and, with PTC, allows biliary stent placement when biliary obstruction occurs. Moreover, ERCP with brush cytology is used to sample tissue biopsies thanks to the advantage of wire guidance with high specificity of CCA diagnosis. Nevertheless, meta-analysis study showed that the sensitivity of ERCP is around 40–50%, and thus it cannot be used as diagnostic method for early diagnosis [38, 39]. To increase the sensitivity of cytology, fluorescent in situ hybridization can be used [40].

41.4 Staging and Prognosis

The previous edition of the American Joint Committee on Cancer (AJCC) staging system staged intrahepatic tumours as hepatocarcinoma and extrahepatic CCAs

Table 41.1 The AJCC/UICC staging of intrahepatic cholangiocarcinoma

Primary Tumor (T)

Tx	Primary tumor cannot be assessed
T0	No evidence of primary tumor
Tis	Carcinoma *in situ*
T1	Tumor confined to the bile duct, with extension up to
T2A	the muscle layer or fibrous tissue
T2B	Tumor invades beyond the wall of the bile duct to the
T3	surrounding adipose tissue
T4	Tumor invades the adjacent hepatic parenchyma
	Tumor invades unilateral branches of the portal vein or the hepatic artery
	Tumor invades the main portal vein or its branches bilaterally; or the common hepatic artery; or the second-order biliary radicals bilaterally; or unilateral second-order biliary radicals with contralateral portal vein or hepatic artery involvement

Regional lymph nodes (N)

Nx	Regional lymph nodes cannot be assessed
N0	No regional lymph node metastasis
N1	Regional lymph node metastasis (including nodes
N2	along the cystic duct, common bile duct, hepatic artery and portal vein)
	Metastasis to periaortic, pericaval, superior mesenteric artery and/or coeliac artery lymph nodes

Distant Metastasis (M)

M0	No distant metastases
M1	Distant metastases present

(perihilar and distal) considered as unique entity. The new classification for iCCAs focuses on tumour extension, vascular invasion and extrahepatic structures infiltration, representing a useful prognostic factor (Table 41.1). The classification for eCCAs includes separate TNM for perihilar and distal carcinomas [41] (Tables 41.2 and 41.3).

Surgical treatment represents the only curative treatment option. If radical surgery is performed, prognosis is not influenced by cancer primary site and extension of resection. Patients with unresectable iCCA have a life expectancy <5% at 5 years that increases to 20–44% for patients with early stage disease (T1–T2). Survival is related to the presence of multiple tumours, vascular invasion, regional nodal involvement and large tumour size [42], and it is also linked to the macroscopic subtype (better for papillary) and tumour differentiation grading (better if well-differentiated). In particular, vascular invasion and the presence of multiple tumour sites are poor prognostic factors only in N0 stage disease, while regional nodal involvement has an important prognostic value just in localized disease (M0). For extrahepatic neoplasms, the depth of tumour invasion has been identified as an independent predictor of outcome. Recently

Table 41.2 The AJCC/UICC staging of perihilar cholangiocarcinoma

Primary Tumor (T)

Tx	Primary tumor cannot be assessed
T0	No evidence of primary tumor
Tis	Carcinoma *in situ* (intraductal tumor)
T1a	Solitary tumor without vascular invasion (maximum
T1b	diameter < 5 cm)
T2a	Solitary tumor without vascular invasion (maximum
T2b	diameter > 5 cm)
T3	Solitary tumor with vascular invasion
T4	Multiple tumors, with or without vascular invasion
	Tumor perforating the visceral peritoneum or involving the local extrahepatic structures by direct invasion
	Tumor with periductal invasion

Regional lymph nodes (N)

Nx	Regional lymph nodes cannot be assessed
N0	No regional lymph node metastasis
N1	Regional lymph node metastasis present

Distant Metastasis (M)

M0	No distant metastases
M1	Distant metastases present

Table 41.3 The AJCC/UICC staging of distal cholangiocarcinoma

Primary Tumor (T)

Tx	Primary tumor cannot be assessed
T0	No evidence of primary tumor
Tis	Carcinoma *in situ*
T1	Tumor depth of invasion <5 mm
T2	Tumor depth of invasion between 5 and 12 mm
T3	Tumor depth of invasion >12 mm
T4	Tumor involves the coeliac axis, or the superior mesenteric artery

Regional lymph nodes (N)

Nx	Regional lymph nodes cannot be assessed
N0	No regional lymph node metastasis
N1	Regional lymph node metastasis

Distant Metastasis (M)

M0	Non distant metastasis
M1	Distant metastasis present

other prognostic factors have been identified in advanced unresectable BTC including poor performance status (ECOG ≥ 2), high neutrophils and bilirubin serum levels, low haemoglobin and disease stage (metastatic vs locally advanced) associated with worse outcome [43]. Finally, high levels of neutrophil/lymphocyte ratio (NLR) are correlated with poor outcome [44, 45].

41.5 Treatment

The therapeutic strategies include surgery, adjuvant and neoadjuvant treatments and palliative therapies. A detailed treatment algorithm is shown in ■ Fig. 41.1.

41.6 Surgery

Surgical resection of CCA remains the only potentially curative treatment associated with long-term survival [46]. Unfortunately, the surgical approach is feasible in only about 20–40% of patients because of they often present advanced unresectable tumours. For this reason, it is important to select patients who can really benefit from surgery, considering the tumour's anatomical site and the extent of local and metastatic spread [47].

Radical resection with clear pathological margins is crucial to achieve a long survival as well as the absence of vascular invasion, lymph node metastasis and adequate functional liver [42, 48]. Hepatic resection is usually performed as standard treatment of CCA. In particular, resection of intrahepatic and extrahepatic bile ducts and affected segments or lobe is recommended for iCCA, pancreatoduodenectomy for dCCA and resection of the involved intrahepatic and extrahepatic bile ducts, the gallbladder and regional lymph nodes for pCCA [42]. The cholecystectomy is the treatment for gallbladder cancer at early stage, while reoperation is indicated in advance stages (liver resection and nodal dissection) [49].

CCA has a median overall survival at 5 years of 20–36 months, while in patients undergone to complete pathological resection, overall survival increases to 65 months [50, 51]. After surgery, some complications occur including hepatic failure, cholangitis, wound infection and sepsis which lead to a significant decrease in survival rates. Several co-morbidities could affect patients' survival such as hypoalbuminemia and jaundice in the preoperative period, even if mortality is similar to those of extended resection (with or without vascular resection) patients [50–53].

Although the recent advances in surgical treatment, about 60% of patients have a recurrent disease after resection within 2 years. Nevertheless, the mortality after recurrence is worst in patients treated with standard therapies compared to those undergone to pathological resection (3-year overall survival 32% vs 3%; $p < 0.0001$) [54].

Liver transplantation is not recommended as treatment for unresectable CCA, because it is associated with rapid tumour recurrence and low survival. A best novel approach for CCA is preoperative chemoradiotherapy followed by liver transplantation [55].

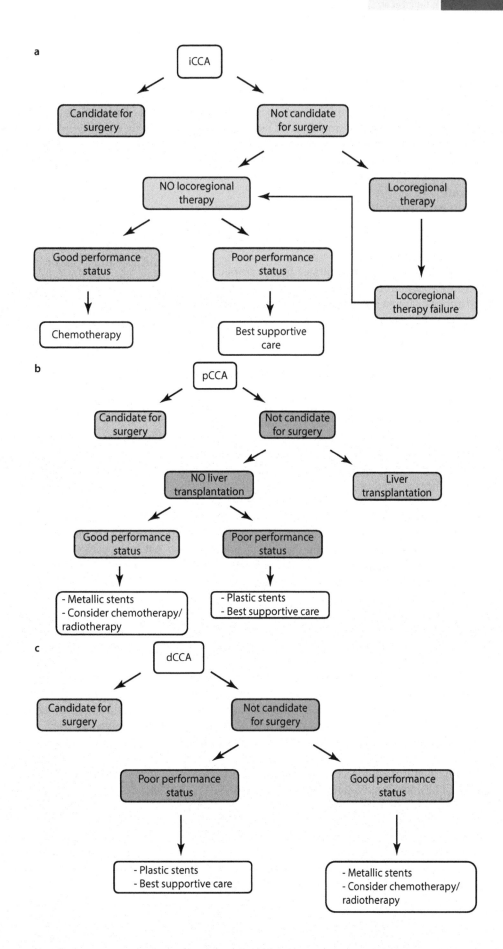

Fig. 41.1 Clinical management algorithms for adult patients with **a** iCCA; **b** pCCA; **c** dCCA

Data supporting the benefit of this treatment in iCCA are controversial, due to the small number of sample size and the heterogeneity of perioperative treatment. Moreover, some factors contraindicate this procedure including multiple tumour, perineural, vascular and liver infiltration and lack of adjuvant and/or neoadjuvant therapy [56, 57] (Fu et al. 2011). A recent multicentre study reported that 73% of patients with cirrhosis and early iCCA have a high actuarial survival at 5 years [58].

In early stage of pCCA, the rate of recurrence-free survival at 5 years is about 65–68% in patients undergone liver transplantation previously treated with neoadjuvant therapy [59].

Based on promising results of liver transplantation, this approach needs to further investigations and could be applied only in specific groups of patients in specialized centres.

41.7   Adjuvant and Neoadjuvant Treatment

Both radiation and chemotherapy have been analysed in the adjuvant setting (either apart or concomitantly). In particular, a large meta-analysis performed by Horgan et al. [60] evaluating 6712 patients, among which 1792 received adjuvant treatment (both radiotherapy and chemotherapy) demonstrated no survival benefit of the overall population. Anyway, authors observed that adjuvant chemotherapy is associated with improved survival among patients with R1 resection and N1 stage [60]. Therefore, adjuvant chemotherapy should not be considered a standard in BTC but could be discussed in patients with high risk of tumour recurrence.

Similarly, retrospective analysis suggested that adjuvant radiation therapy can achieve survival advantage just in selected patients' subgroups, especially in R1 resection [61, 62], but no randomized trials assessing are available.

The main data assessing the role of adjuvant chemoradiotherapy derive only from retrospective analysis. The most commonly used concomitant chemotherapeutic agents were 5-fluorouracil and gemcitabine. Although several evidences suggest that adjuvant concomitant chemoradiotherapy could achieve survival advantage mainly in R1–R2 and N1 stage disease [63, 64, 65], it cannot be considered a standard of treatment.

Regarding neoadjuvant setting, a novel optional treatment for CCA is preoperative chemoradiotherapy followed by liver transplantation [66]. Promising results were obtained treating patients affected by hilar CCA with stereotactic radiotherapy followed by chemotherapy and liver transplantation [55]. Further studies are needed to confirm the efficacy of this therapy, which, at the moment, should be proposed only in selected cases.

41.8   Palliative Therapy

41.8.1   Chemoradiotherapy in Locally Advanced Disease

Concomitant chemoradiotherapy has been largely investigated in locally advanced CCA showing survival benefit. A retrospective analysis evaluated the activity of concomitant treatment in patients receiving capecitabine and cisplatin alone or in combination with radiotherapy. Data showed that overall survival and progression free survival were significantly longer in the chemoradiotherapy group and concurrent treatment achieved a higher (but no statistically significant) disease control rate [67]. These results should be confirmed in prospective randomized trials in order to define a standard of treatment.

41.8.2   Chemotherapy in Advanced Disease

For patients with unresectable or metastatic CCA, systemic chemotherapy remains the mainstay palliative treatment modality. Unfortunately, advanced CCA is often associated with liver function impairment, jaundice, weight loss, pain and poor performance status which contraindicate chemotherapy. The most active cytotoxic chemotherapy agents in the management of BTCs are gemcitabine and platinum agents [68, 69].

The role of chemotherapy in improving patient outcome and quality of life was reported in 1996, and gemcitabine was established as reference treatment in advanced disease [70]. Many following trials have been performed [68], but they were negative or lacked the statistical power to change clinical practice.

In 2010, ABC-02 study phase III trial defined gemcitabine and cisplatin (GEMCIS) combination as standard treatment for advanced CCA [71]. This combination showed an improvement in overall survival compared to gemcitabine alone (11.7 months versus 8.1 months). The following studies confirmed these findings [72, 73]. A large meta-analysis comparing oxaliplatin (GEMOX) and cisplatin (GEMCIS) combination with gemcitabine found a longer survival in patients treated with GEMCIS (11.7 vs 9.7 months), although a higher toxicity rate [74]. Other potentially active regimens, such as gemcitabine and capecitabine combination [75], or triplets comprehending fluoropyrimidines, gemcitabine and platinum compound [76, 77] need to further investigations.

41.8.3 Second-Line Chemotherapy

Failure of first-line treatment is often associated with rapidly worsening performance status, and only a small number of patients may be suitable for further treatments. In addition, patients often have the inherent problems of biliary obstruction and sepsis associated with BTC, which may contraindicate further chemotherapy. Considering the low number of patients able to undergo to second-line, very limited literature data are available in this setting.

Small prospective and retrospective studies have shown potential benefit in selected patients (good performance status, long PFS after first-line chemotherapy (>6 months), resected primary tumour and low CA 19.9 value) [78, 79]. A British trial (ABC-06), comparing second-line chemotherapy with oxaliplatin and 5-fluorouracil versus best supportive care is currently ongoing (NCT01926236).

41.8.4 Locoregional Treatment

Locoregional treatment is indicated in the patients where surgical resection is not to be performed. This approach includes transarterial chemoembolization (TACE), intraarterial chemotherapy and radiofrequency ablation (RFA). Retrospective and prospective analyses demonstrated that TACE [80, 81] and intraarterial chemotherapy [82, 83] are associated with a good disease control rate.

Moreover, photodynamic therapy is another treatment option in locally advanced hilar and perihilar CCA that gives a good locoregional tumour control. Recent data demonstrated that photodynamic therapy with concomitant biliary stenting is associated with improved survival and quality of life compared to biliary stenting alone [84].

41.9 Key Genomic Alterations and Emerging Therapies

Advances in molecular medicine allowed the identification of a wide range of mutations, amplifications and deletions in BTC, many of which have targetable options. Several studies have documented important driver mutations reported in other tumours including the epidermal growth factor (EGF) pathway with EGF receptor (EGFR), k-ras and b-raf mutations or overexpression and alteration in the mitogen-activated protein kinase and PI3K/mammalian target of rapamycin pathways. More recently, recurrent translocation events involving fibroblast growth factor receptor (FGFR) loci and mutations in the metabolic pathway involving isocitrate dehydrogenase 1 (IDH1) and isocitrate dehydrogenase 2 (IDH2) have been reported. Finally, mutations in chromatin-remodelling genes BAP1 (encoding a nuclear deubiquitinase), ARID1A (encoding a subunit of the SWI/SNF chromatin-remodelling complexes) and PBRM1 (encoding a subunit of the ATP-dependent SWI/SNF chromatin remodelling complexes) have been described [85].

41.9.1 EGFR Pathway

The EGFR family comprises four tyrosine kinase receptors (ERBB1–4) that regulate cell proliferation, survival, angiogenesis and invasion through ligand binding and subsequent activation of signal transduction cascades involving the MAPK pathway (Ras-Raf-MEK-ERK) and the PI3K/AKT pathway [86].

EGFR amplifications are seen in 8% of BTC cases, while mutations in 13–15% [87, 88, 89].

Despite encouraging results from early studies [90, 91], randomized trials of EGFR antagonists erlotinib and cetuximab, each added to gemcitabine and oxaliplatin, showed no improvement in survival outcomes in advanced BTC [92, 93].

HER2 (v-ERB-B2, erythroblastic leukaemia viral oncogene homolog-2) overexpression and gene amplification are also described in BTCs with a higher incidence in gallbladder cancer (19%) [94]. Similarly to EGFR inhibitors, HER2 antagonists, trastuzumab, lapatinib and afatinib have demonstrated no clinical benefit in advanced BTC [95, 96].

41.9.2 MAPK Pathway

Aberrations in cell-surface receptors and their ligands (e.g. EGFR, VEGF) can lead to constitutive activation of downstream cascades, including the MAPK signalling (RAS-RAF-MEK-ERK). KRAS mutations are very common in BTCs, with highest rates seen in eCCA, followed by iHCC, and lowest in GBC (Li et al. 2014; [85, 97]). KRAS mutations have been associated with perineural invasion, advanced stage and poor prognosis [98].

Principal BRAF mutation (V600E) was reported also in CCA with varying frequency [99]. Despite the recognized frequency of KRAS and BRAF mutations, targeting this pathway remains challenging. A phase II study of selumetinib, a MEK inhibitor, showed a disease control rate of 80% and median overall survival of

9.8 months in patients with advanced biliary tract cancer [100]. Conversely, clinical trials of sorafenib, a multikinase inhibitor targeting the MAPK axis, failed to show clinical benefit in BTC [101, 102].

41.9.3 PI3K Pathway

The phosphoinositide-3-kinase (PI3K), signalling pathway involved in cell proliferation, is upregulated in CCA, and its activation was associated both with poor and good prognosis in BTC patients [103]. Several studies have reported PIK3CA hotspot mutations in BTC [104], mostly in GBC (Jeffrey et al. 2015; [105, 106]). Clinical trials are lacking except for an early study of everolimus, a mTOR inhibitor acting downstream of the PI3K signal. This study showed evidence of antitumour activity with a median overall survival of 9.5 months in 27 advanced BTC patients [107]. Moreover, a phase II trial using a PI3K inhibitor, copanlisib, in combination with gemcitabine and cisplatin as first-line therapy is ongoing (NCT02631590).

41.9.4 FGF Pathway

The fibroblast growth factor (FGF) ligands and receptors (FGFR1-4) are involved in cancer development and progression via activation of mitogenic and mesenchymal signals [108]. Genome-wide structural analyses in BTCs showed recurrent translocation events that involved the FGFR2 locus [109]. In particular, chromosomal fusions occur between FGFR2 and various genomic partners (e.g. AHCYL1, BICC1, PARK2, KCTD1, MGEA5, TACC3, TXLNA) ([110, 111]; Nakamura et al. 2014).

FGFR translocations were reported in 13% of iCCA with improved survival in these cases [110]. The recent discovery of recurrent FGFR2 fusions has opened a promising therapeutic avenue. Multitargeted tyrosine kinase inhibitor (TKIs) that also inhibits FGFR (such as ponatinib, nintedanib, dovitinib and brivanib) and FGFR antibodies and FGFR trap molecules have been developed. These FGF inhibitors are currently in their early phases, and few trials focusing on BTC are underway to investigate their potential clinical utility.

41.9.5 IDH Pathway

The IDH family of enzymes comprises the proteins IDH1, IDH2 and IDH3 that are involved in different cellular processes, including mitochondrial oxidative phosphorylation, glutamine metabolism, lipogenesis, glucose sensing and regulation of cellular redox status [112]. Mutations in IDH1 and IDH2 genes lead to accumulation of metabolites that result in altered intracellular processes including DNA methylation and hypoxia responses, ultimately leading to oncogenesis [113].

Mutations in IDH1 and IDH2 have been identified in BTC, especially in iCC, but the prognostic significance remains conflicting. Indeed, several studies have demonstrated that IDH mutations were correlated with decreased overall survival [114], while other studies reported that IDH alterations were not associated with survival [115] or associated with longer time to disease recurrence [116].

A large recent genomic profiling analysis identified IDH mutations in 20% of iCCA cases but none in eCCA or GBC. Pharmacologic IDH inhibitors have been developed and some clinical trials are underway. Early results from studies of oral IDH1 (AG-120) and IDH2 (AG-221) inhibitors have shown encouraging results in acute myeloid leukaemia setting [117, 118]. Trials with these agents are being expanded to solid tumours including BTC patients (NCT02073994, NCT02273739).

41.9.6 Chromatin Modifiers

Chromatin remodelling allows genomic DNA to access regulatory transcriptional proteins and thereby controls gene expression. Genetic alterations in ARID, BAP1 and PBRM, responsible for chromatin remodelling, have been implicated in BTC. In particular, ARID1A, encoding a subunit of the SWI/SNF chromatin-remodelling complex, seems to act as a tumour suppressor gene, and its inactivation is linked to multiple malignancies [119]. Exome sequencing analysis identified ARID1A mutations in 19% of iCCA [114].

BAP1 and PBRM1 are also involved in chromatin remodelling, and their alterations are described in 7–25% of cases of BTC and associated to worse survival in iCCA [120]. Histone deacetylase inhibitors such as vorinostat and panobinostat may offer new therapeutic chances in this setting [121].

41.9.7 Other Molecular Pathways

The WNT/β-CATENIN pathway is involved in the regulation of cell invasion and migration. Preclinical evidences demonstrated that WNT pathway activation is associated with chemo-resistance and metastatic spread [122, 123]. High levels of activated β-CATENIN into the nucleus has been described in iCCA (15%) [124]. Although multiple WNT pathway inhibitors are currently under development in solid tumours [125], only few clinical trial have been reported for BTC as yet.

The Hedgehog pathway may also be involved in the development of BTC [126, 127, 128, 129]. Indeed, suppression of Hedgehog pathway reduced tumour volume in preclinical BTC models [130, 131]; in addition, BTC patients with activated Hedgehog pathway had a more aggressive behaviour and worse outcome [132, 133].

c-MET tyrosine kinase plays a key role in carcinogenesis by promoting angiogenesis, tumour invasion and metastasis. c-MET overexpression has been reported in CCA patients associated with a poor prognosis [89, 134, 135], while c-MET amplification is very rare. HGF/c-MET pathway promotes the invasive progression of gallbladder carcinoma cell lines [136] and data from human tissue confirmed the higher c-MET expression in cancer cells compared to normal gallbladder tissue [137].

41.10 Conclusion

BTCs are a group of devastating heterogeneous tumours difficult to diagnose and associated with poor outcome. The incidence of iCCA is increasing worldwide due to a complex interplay between predisposing genetic factors and environmental triggers. Surgery with complete resection is the only chance for cure, but this approach is applicable in few patients and, often, is associated with a high percentage of disease recurrence. Recent evidences suggest that liver transplantation combined with neoadjuvant chemoradiotherapy could offer long-term benefit in selected patients. Unfortunately, the most part of BTCs are diagnosed at advanced unresectable stage, and the chemotherapy remains the only treatment available to improve symptoms palliation but with a poor impact on patients survival. To achieve improved outcomes, better understanding of tumour biology, combined with the development of novel diagnostic and treatment strategies, is crucial. Several genomic alterations have been identified in BTCs, and newer targeted therapies acting on these pathways are being tested in clinical trials.

Expert Opinion
Marc Peeters
1. Biliary tract cancers are a group of heterogeneous neoplasms that comprise gallbladder cancer and cholangiocarcinoma (CCA) which can be classified in an intrahepatic, perihilar and extrahepatic form, actually the most frequent type (50–60%).
2. Different risk factors (such as primary sclerosing cholangitis and liver fluke infestation) and a genetic predisposition account for the various worldwide diffusion of this neoplasm, more common in the southwest of Asia and South America than in Western countries. Although the awareness about the risk factors for the low incidence of this neoplasm and for the lack of efficacy, cost-effectiveness and reliability no screening programs can be adopted.
3. No specific symptoms are present at the diagnosis, and frequently they consist in jaundice, abdominal pain and weight loss.
4. Just a multimodal diagnostic approach can give the necessary information about the neoplasm: CT scan is quite useful for masses >2 cm in order to study the portal vein and arterial involvement; magnetic resonance cholangiopancreatography (MRCP), has an important role in evaluating perihilar CCAs with an accuracy up to 95%. Moreover, ERCP with brush cytology can be used to sample tissue biopsies thanks to the advantage of wire guidance.
5. Surgery is the only curative treatment (20–40% of patients); furthermore, in selected patients with high risk of recurrence after surgery, adjuvant chemoradiotherapy can be evaluated. New studies have shown that liver transplantation combined with neoadjuvant chemoradiotherapy could offer long-term benefit in selected patients.
6. In case of unresectable cancer, chemotherapy with platinum agents and gemcitabine is the most recommended treatment even if it is linked to a poor prognosis (<5% at 5 years). There is not a standard recommended second-line chemotherapy, so more studies are needed; locoregional treatments (TACE, RFA) must be considered in this setting of patients.
7. Innovative drugs (such as MEK or mTOR inhibitors), have shown interesting results and more trials are ongoing in order to verify the efficacy of these drugs. More evidences will be obtained continuing the study of biological features of these neoplasms in order to obtain new therapies.

Recommendations

- AIOM
  - ▶ https://www.aiom.it/linee-guida-aiom-tumori-delle-vie-biliari/
- ESMO
  - ▶ https://www.esmo.org/Guidelines/Gastrointestinal-Cancers/Biliary-Cancer
- ASCO
  - ▶ https://ascopubs.org/doi/abs/10.1200/JCO.18.02178

Hints for a Deeper Insight

- Randomized clinical trial of adjuvant gemcitabine chemotherapy versus observation in resected bile duct cancer: ▶ https://www.ncbi.nlm.nih.gov/pubmed/29405274
- Salvage radiotherapy for locoregionally recurrent extrahepatic bile duct cancer after radical surgery: ▶ https://www.ncbi.nlm.nih.gov/pubmed/28937265
- Karnofsky Performance Score Is Predictive of Survival After Palliative Irradiation of Metastatic Bile Duct Cancer: ▶ https://www.ncbi.nlm.nih.gov/pubmed/28179357
- Race, ethnicity, and socioeconomic factors in cholangiocarcinoma: What is driving disparities in receipt of treatment? ▶ https://www.ncbi.nlm.nih.gov/pubmed/31301148
- Smoking, Alcohol, and Biliary Tract Cancer Risk: A Pooling Project of 26 Prospective Studies. ▶ https://www.ncbi.nlm.nih.gov/pubmed/31127946

References

1. Shaib Y, El-Serag HB. The epidemiology of cholangiocarcinoma. Semin Liver Dis. 2004;24:115–25.
2. Alvaro D, Crocetti E, Ferretti S, Bragazzi MC, Capocaccia R. AISF Cholangiocarcinoma committee. Descriptive epidemiology of cholangiocarcinoma in Italy. Dig Liver Dis. 2010;42:490–5.
3. Bergquist A, von Seth E. Epidemiology of cholangiocarcinoma. Best Pract Res Clin Gastroenterol. 2015;29:221–32.
4. Cardinale V, Semeraro R, Torrice A, Gatto M, Napoli C, Bragazzi MC, et al. Intra-hepatic and extra-hepatic cholangiocarcinoma: new insight into epidemiology and risk factors. World J Gastrointest Oncol. 2010;2:407–16.
5. Bragazzi MC, Bragazzi MC, Cardinale V, Carpino G, Venere R, Semeraro R, et al. Cholangiocarcinoma: epidemiology and risk factors. Transl Gastrointest Cancer. 2012;1:21–32.
6. Rizvi S, Gores GJ. Pathogenesis, diagnosis, and management of cholangiocarcinoma. Gastroenterology. 2013;145:1215–29.
7. Burak K, Angulo P, Pasha TM, Egan K, Petz J, Lindor KD. Incidence and risk factors for cholangiocarcinoma in primary sclerosing cholangitis. Am J Gastroenterol. 2004;99:523–6.
8. Kerr SE, Barr Fritcher EG, Campion MB, Voss JS, Kipp BR, Halling KC, et al. Biliary dysplasia in primary sclerosing cholangitis harbors cytogenetic abnormalities similar to cholangiocarcinoma. Hum Pathol. 2014;45:1797–804.
9. Liu R, Cox K, Guthery SL, Book L, Witt B, Chadwick B, et al. Cholangiocarcinoma and high-grade dysplasia in young patients with primary sclerosing cholangitis. Dig Dis Sci. 2014;59:2320–4.
10. Morris-Stiff G, Bhati C, Olliff S, Hübscher S, Gunson B, Mayer D, et al. Cholangiocarcinoma complicating primary sclerosing cholangitis: a 24-year experience. Dig Surg. 2008;25:126–32.
11. Watanapa P, Watanapa WB. Liver fluke-associated cholangiocarcinoma. Br J Surg. 2002;89:962–70.
12. Shin HR, Oh JK, Masuyer E, Curado MP, Bouvard V, Fang YY, et al. Epidemiology of cholangiocarcinoma: an update focusing on risk factors. Cancer Sci. 2010;101:579–85.
13. Jang KT, Hong SM, Lee KT, Lee JG, Choi SH, Heo JS, et al. Intraductal papillary neoplasm of the bile duct associated with Clonorchis sinensis infection. Virchows Arch. 2008;453:589–98.
14. Kurathong S, Lerdverasirikul P, Wongpaitoon V, Pramoolsinsap C, Kanjanapitak A, Varavithya W, et al. Opisthorchis viverrini infection and cholangiocarcinoma. A prospective, case-controlled study. Gastroenterology. 1985;89:151–6.
15. Lipsett PA, Pitt HA, Colombani PM, Boitnott JK, Cameron JL. Choledochal cyst disease. A changing pattern of presentation. Ann Surg. 1994;220:644–52.
16. Lazaridis KN, Gores GJ. Cholangiocarcinoma. Gastroenterology. 2005;128:1655–67.
17. Chen MF, Jan YY, Wang CS, Hwang TL, Jeng LB, Chen SC, et al. A reappraisal of cholangiocarcinoma in patient with hepatolithiasis. Cancer. 1993;71:2461–5.
18. Liu D, Momoi H, Li L, Ishikawa Y, Fukumoto M. Microsatellite instability in thorotrast-induced human intrahepatic cholangiocarcinoma. Int J Cancer. 2002;102:366–71.
19. Walker NJ, Crockett PW, Nyska A, Brix AE, Jokinen MP, Sells DM, et al. Dose-additive carcinogenicity of a defined mixture of "dioxin-like compounds". Environ Health Perspect. 2005;113:43–8.
20. Matsumoto K, Onoyama T, Kawata S, Takeda Y, Harada K, Ikebuchi Y, et al. Hepatitis B and C virus infection is a risk factor for the development of cholangiocarcinoma. Intern Med. 2014;53:651–4.
21. Wu Y, Wang T, Ye S, Zhao R, Bai X, Wu Y, et al. Detection of hepatitis B virus DNA in paraffin-embedded intrahepatic and extrahepatic cholangiocarcinoma tissue in the northern Chinese population. Hum Pathol. 2012;43:56–61.
22. Palmer WC, Patel T. Are common factors involved in the pathogenesis of primary liver cancers? A meta-analysis of risk factors for intrahepatic cholangiocarcinoma. J Hepatol. 2012;57:69–76.
23. Li JS, Han TJ, Jing N, Li L, Zhang XH, Ma FZ, et al. Obesity and the risk of cholangiocarcinoma: a meta-analysis. Tumour Biol. 2014a;35:6831–8.
24. Li M, Zhang Z, Li X, Ye J, Wu X, Tan Z, et al. Whole-exome and targeted gene sequencing of gallbladder carcinoma identifies recurrent mutations in the ErbB pathway. Nat Genet. 2014b;46:872–6.
25. Jing W, Jin G, Zhou X, Zhou Y, Zhang Y, Shao C, et al. Diabetes mellitus and increased risk of cholangiocarcinoma: a meta-analysis. Eur J Cancer Prev. 2012;21:24–31.

41

26. Weinbren K, Mutum SS. Pathological aspects of cholangiocarcinoma. J Pathol. 1983;139:217–38.

27. Yamasaki S. Intrahepatic cholangiocarcinoma: macroscopic type and staging classification. J Hepato-Biliary-Pancreat Surg. 2003;10:288–91.

28. Chen HW, Lai EC, Pan AZ, Chen T, Liao S, Lau WY. Preoperative assessment and staging of hilar cholangiocarcinoma with 16-multidetector computed tomography cholangiography and angiography. Hepato-Gastroenterology. 2009;56:578–83.

29. Manfredi R, Barbaro B, Masselli G, Vecchioli A, Marano P. Magnetic resonance imaging of cholangiocarcinoma. Semin Liver Dis. 2004;24:155–64.

30. Masselli G, Manfredi R, Vecchioli A, Gualdi G. MR imaging and MR cholangiopancreatography in the preoperative evaluation of hilar cholangiocarcinoma: correlation with surgical and pathologic findings. Eur Radiol. 2008;18:2213–21.

31. Blechacz B, Gores GJ. Cholangiocarcinoma: advances in pathogenesis, diagnosis, and treatment. Hepatology. 2008;48: 308–21.

32. Razumilava N, Gores GJ, Lindor KD. Cancer surveillance in patients with primary sclerosing cholangitis. Hepatology. 2011;54:1842–52.

33. Konstadoulakis MM, Roayaie S, Gomatos IP, Labow D, Fiel MI, Miller CM, et al. Fifteen-year, single-center experience with the surgical management of intrahepatic cholangiocarcinoma: operative results and long-term outcome. Surgery. 2008;143: 366–74.

34. Lang H, Sotiropoulos GC, Sgourakis G, Schmitz KJ, Paul A, Hilgard P, et al. Operations for intrahepatic cholangiocarcinoma: single-institution experience of 158 patients. J Am Coll Surg. 2009;208:218–28.

35. Nagino M, Ebata T, Yokoyama Y, Igami T, Sugawara G, Takahashi Y, et al. Evolution of surgical treatment for perihilar cholangiocarcinoma: a single-center 34-year review of 574 consecutive resections. Ann Surg. 2013;258:129–40.

36. Kluge R, Schmidt F, Caca K, Barthel H, Hesse S, Georgi P, et al. Positron emission tomography with [(18)F]fluoro-2-deoxy-D-glucose for diagnosis and staging of bile duct cancer. Hepatology. 2001;33:1029–35.

37. Navaneethan U, Njei B, Venkatesh PG, Vargo JJ, Parsi MA. Fluorescence in situ hybridization for diagnosis of cholangiocarcinoma in primary sclerosing cholangitis: a systematic review and metaanalysis. Gastrointest Endosc. 2014;79:943–950.e3.

38. Trikudanathan G, Navaneethan U, Njei B, Vargo JJ, Parsi MA. Diagnostic yield of bile duct brushings for cholangiocarcinoma in primary sclerosing cholangitis: a systematic review and meta-analysis. Gastrointest Endosc. 2014;79:783–9.

39. Njei B, McCarty TR, Varadarajulu S, Navaneethan U. Systematic review with meta-analysis: endoscopic retrograde cholangiopancreatography-based modalities for the diagnosis of cholangiocarcinoma in primary sclerosing cholangitis. Aliment Pharmacol Ther. 2016;44:1139–51.

40. Kalaitzakis E, Webster GJ, Oppong KW, Kallis Y, Vlavianos P, Huggett M, et al. Diagnostic and therapeutic utility of single-operator peroral cholangioscopy for indeterminate biliary lesions and bile duct stones. Eur J Gastroenterol Hepatol. 2012;24: 656–64.

41. Edge SB, Byrd DR, Compton CC, Fritz AG, Greene FL, Trotti A. AJCC cancer staging manual. 7th ed. New York: Springer; 2010.

42. Endo I, Gonen M, Yopp AC, Dalal KM, Zhou Q, Klimstra D, et al. Intrahepatic cholangiocarcinoma: rising frequency, improved survival and determinants of outcome after resection. Ann Surg. 2008;248:84–96.

43. Bridgewater J, Lopes A, Wasan H, Malka D, Jensen L, Okusaka T, et al. Prognostic factors for progression-free and overall survival in advanced biliary tract cancer. Ann Oncol. 2016;27: 134–40.

44. Grenader T, Nash S, Plotkin Y, Furuse J, Mizuno N, Okusaka T, et al. Derived neutrophil lymphocyte ratio may predict benefit from cisplatin in the advanced biliary cancer: the ABC-02 and BT-22 studies. Ann Oncol. 2015;26:1910–6.

45. McNamara MG, Templeton AJ, Maganti M, Walter T, Horgan AM, McKeever L, et al. Neutrophil/lymphocyte ratio as a prognostic factor in biliary tract cancer. Eur J Cancer. 2014;50: 1581–9.

46. Akamatsu N, Sugawara Y, Hashimoto D. Surgical strategy for bile duct cancer: advances and current limitations. World J Clin Oncol. 2011;2:94–107.

47. Cho MS, Kim SH, Park SW, Lim JH, Choi GH, Park JS, et al. Surgical outcomes and predicting factors of curative resection in patients with hilar cholangiocarcinoma: 10-year single-institution experience. J Gastrointest Surg. 2012;16:1672–9.

48. Zaydfudim VM, Rosen CB, Nagorney DM. Hilar cholangiocarcinoma. Surg Oncol Clin N Am. 2014;23:247–63.

49. Shih SP, Schulick RD, Cameron JL, Lillemoe KD, Pitt HA, Choti MA, et al. Gallbladder cancer: the role of laparoscopy and radical resection. Ann Surg. 2007;245:893–901.

50. Gerhards MF, van Gulik TM, de Wit LT, Obertop H, Gouma DJ. Evaluation of morbidity and mortality after resection for hilar cholangiocarcinoma a single center experience. Surgery. 2000;127:395–404.

51. Kondo S, Hirano S, Ambo Y, Tanaka E, Okushiba S, Morikawa T, et al. Forty consecutive resections of hilar cholangiocarcinoma with no postoperative mortality and no positive ductal margins: results of a prospective study. Ann Surg. 2004;240: 95–101.

52. Ebata T, Nagino M, Kamiya J, Uesaka K, Nagasaka T, Nimura Y. Hepatectomy with portal vein resection for hilar cholangiocarcinoma: audit of 52 consecutive cases. Ann Surg. 2003;238: 720–7.

53. Neuhaus P, Jonas S, Settmacher U, Thelen A, Benckert C, Lopez-Hänninen E, et al. Surgical management of proximal bile duct cancer: extended right lobe resection increases resectability and radicality. Langenbeck's Arch Surg. 2003;388:194–200.

54. Takahashi Y, Ebata T, Yokoyama Y, Igami T, Sugawara G, Mizuno T, et al. Surgery for recurrent biliary tract cancer: a single-center experience with 74 consecutive resections. Ann Surg. 2015;262:121–9.

55. Rea DJ, Heimbach JK, Rosen CB, Haddock MG, Alberts SR, Kremers WK, et al. Liver transplantation with neoadjuvant chemoradiation is more effective than resection for hilar cholangiocarcinoma. Ann Surg. 2005;242:451–8.

56. Bridgewater J, Galle PR, Khan SA, Llovet JM, Park JW, Patel T, et al. Guidelines for the diagnosis and management of intrahepatic cholangiocarcinoma. J Hepatol. 2014;60:1268–89.

57. Sotiropoulos GC, Kaiser GM, Lang H, Molmenti EP, Beckebaum S, Fouzas I, et al. Liver transplantation as a primary indication for intrahepatic cholangiocarcinoma: a single-center experience. Transplant Proc. 2008;40:3194–5.

58. Sapisochin G, Facciuto M, Rubbia-Brandt L, Marti J, Mehta N, Yao FY, et al. iCCA International Consortium. Liver transplantation for "very early" intrahepatic cholangiocarcinoma: international retrospective study supporting a prospective assessment. Hepatology. 2016;64:1178–88.

59. Darwish Murad S, Kim WR, Harnois DM, Douglas DD, Burton J, Kulik LM, et al. Efficacy of neoadjuvant chemoradiation, followed by liver transplantation, for perihilar cholangiocarcinoma at 12 US centers. Gastroenterology. 2012;143:88–98.e3.

60. Horgan AM, Amir E, Walter T, Knox JJ. Adjuvant therapy in the treatment of biliary tract cancer: a systematic review and meta-analysis. J Clin Oncol. 2012;30:1934–40.

61. Cheng Q, Luo X, Zhang B, Jiang X, Yi B, Wu M. Predictive factors for prognosis of hilar cholangiocarcinoma: post resection radiotherapy improves survival. Eur J Surg Oncol. 2007;33: 202–7.

62. Todoroki T, Ohara K, Kawamoto T, Koike N, Yoshida S, Kashiwagi H, et al. Benefits of adjuvant radiotherapy after radical resection of locally advanced main hepatic duct carcinoma. Int J Radiat Oncol Biol Phys. 2000;46:581–7.

63. Ben-Josef E, Guthrie KA, El-Khoueury AB, Corless CL, Zalupski MM, Lowy AM, et al. SWOG S0809: a phase II intergroup trial of adjuvant capecitabine and gemcitabine followed by radiotherapy and concurrent capecitabine in extrahepatic cholangiocarcinoma and gallbladder carcinoma. J Clin Oncol. 2015;33:2617–22.

64. Kim S, Kim SW, Bang YJ, Heo DS, Ha SW. Role of post operative radiotherapy in the management of extrahepatic bile duct cancer. Int J Radiat Oncol Biol Phys. 2002;54:414–9.

65. Lim KH, Oh DY, Chie EK, Jang JY, Im SA, Kim TY, et al. Adjuvant concurrent chemoradiation therapy (CCRT) alone versus CCRT followed by adjuvant chemotherapy: which is better in patients with radically resected extrahepatic biliary tract cancer? A non-randomized single center study. BMC Cancer. 2009;9:345.

66. Zhu GQ, Shi KQ, You J, Zou H, Wang LR, Braddock M, et al. Systematic review with network meta-analysis: adjuvant therapy for resected biliary tract cancer. Aliment Pharmacol Ther. 2014;40:759.

67. Kim YI, Park JW, Kim BH, Woo SM, Kim TH, Koh YW, et al. Outcomes of concurrent chemoradiotherapy versus chemotherapy alone for advanced-stage unresectable intrahepatic cholangiocarcinoma. Radiat Oncol. 2013;8:292.

68. Eckel F, Schmid RM. Chemotherapy in advanced biliary tract carcinoma: a pooled analysis of clinical trials. Br J Cancer. 2007;96:896–902.

69. Tsavaris N, Kosmas C, Gouveris P, Gennatas K, Polyzos A, Mouratidou D, et al. Weekly gemcitabine for the treatment of biliary tract and gallbladder cancer. Invest New Drugs. 2004;22:193–8.

70. Raderer M, Hejna MH, Valencak JB, Kornek GV, Weinlander GS, Bareck E, et al. Two consecutive phase II studies of 5-fluorouracil/leucovorin/mitomycin C and of gemcitabine in patients with advanced biliary cancer. Oncology. 1999;56: 177–80.

71. Valle J, Wasan H, Palmer DH, Cunningham D, Anthoney A, Maraveyas A, et al. Cisplatin plus gemcitabine versus gemcitabine for biliary tract cancer. N Engl J Med. 2010;362: 1273–81.

72. Okusaka T, Nakachi K, Fukutomi A, Mizuno N, Ohkawa S, Funakoshi A, et al. Gemcitabine alone or in combination with cisplatin in patients with biliary tract cancer: a comparative multicentre study in Japan. Br J Cancer. 2010;103:469–74.

73. Valle JW, Furuse J, Jitlal M, Beare S, Mizuno N, Wasan H, et al. Cisplatin and gemcitabine for advanced biliary tract cancer: a meta-analysis of two randomised trials. Ann Oncol. 2014;25: 391–8.

74. Fiteni F, Nguyen T, Vernerey D, Paillard MJ, Kim S, Demarchi M, et al. Cisplatin/gemcitabine or oxaliplatin/gemcitabine in the treatment of advanced biliary tract cancer: a systematic review. Cancer Med. 2014;3:1502–11.

75. Iyer RV, Gibbs J, Kuvshinoff B, Fakih M, Kepner J, Soehnlein N, et al. A phase II study of gemcitabine and capecitabine in advanced cholangiocarcinoma and carcinoma of the gallbladder: a single-institution prospective study. Ann Surg Oncol. 2007;14:3202–9.

76. Cereda S, Passoni P, Reni M, Viganò MG, Aldrighetti L, Nicoletti R, et al. The cisplatin, epirubicin, 5-fluorouracil, gemcitabine (PEFG) regimen in advanced biliary tract adenocarcinoma. Cancer. 2010;116:2208–14.

77. Yamashita Y, Taketomi A, Itoh S, Harimoto N, Tsujita E, Sugimachi K, et al. Phase II trial of gemcitabine combined with 5-fluorouracil and cisplatin (GFP) chemotherapy in patients with advanced biliary tree cancers. Jpn J Clin Oncol. 2010;40: 24–8.

78. Fornaro L, Cereda S, Aprile G, Di Girolamo S, Santini D, Silvestris N, et al. Multivariate prognostic factors analysis for second-line chemotherapy in advanced biliary tract cancer. Br J Cancer. 2014;110:2165–9.

79. Hyder O, Marques H, Pulitano C, Marsh JW, Alexandrescu S, Bauer TW, et al. A nomogram to predict long-term survival after resection for intrahepatic cholangiocarcinoma: an Eastern and Western experience. JAMA Surg. 2014;149:432–8.

80. Hyder O, Marsh JW, Salem R, Petre EN, Kalva S, Liapi E, et al. Intra-arterial therapy for advanced intrahepatic cholangiocarcinoma: a multi-institutional analysis. Ann Surg Oncol. 2013;20:3779–86.

81. Vogl TJ, Naguibi NN, Nour-Eldin NE, Bechstein WO, Zeuzem S, Trojan J, et al. Transarterial chemoembolization in the treatment of patients with unresectable cholangiocarcinoma: results and prognostic factors governing treatment success. Int J Cancer. 2012;131:733–40.

82. Hayashi T, Ishiwatari H, Yoshida M, Sato T, Miyanishi K, Sato Y, et al. A phase I trial of arterial infusion chemotherapy with gemcitabine and 5-fluorouracil for unresectable biliary tract cancer. Int J Clin Oncol. 2012;17:491–7.

83. Sinn M, Nicolau A, Gebauer B, Podrabsky P, Seehofer D, Ricke J, et al. Hepatic arterial infusion with oxaliplatin and 5-FU/folinic acid for advanced biliary tract cancer: a phase II study. Dig Dis Sci. 2013;58:2399–405.

84. Leggett CL, Gorospe EC, Murad MH, Montori VM, Baron TH, Wang KK. Photodynamic therapy for unresectable cholangiocarcinoma: a comparative effectiveness systematic review and meta-analyses. Photodiagnosis Photodyn Ther. 2012;9: 189–95.

85. Nakamura H, Arai Y, Totoki Y, Shirota T, Elzawahry A, Kato M, et al. Genomic spectra of biliary tract cancer. Nat Genet. 2015;47:1003–10.

86. Scaltriti M, Baselga J. The epidermal growth factor receptor pathway: a model for targeted therapy. Clin Cancer Res. 2006;12:5268–72.

87. Gwak GY, Yoon JH, Shin CM, Ahn YJ, Chung JK, Kim YA, et al. Detection of response-predicting mutations in the kinase domain of the epidermal growth factor receptor gene in cholangiocarcinomas. J Cancer Res Clin Oncol. 2005;131:649–52.

88. Leone F, Cavalloni G, Pignochino Y, Sarotto I, Ferraris R, Piacibello W, et al. Somatic mutations of epidermal growth factor receptor in bile duct and gallbladder carcinoma. Clin Cancer Res. 2006;12:1680–5.

89. Nakazawa K, Dobashi Y, Suzuki S, Fujii H, Takeda Y, Ooi A. Amplification and overexpression of c-erbB-2, epidermal growth factor receptor, and c-met in biliary tract cancers. J Pathol. 2005;206:356–65.

90. Hezel AF, Noel MS, Allen JN, Abrams TA, Yurgelun M, Faris JE, et al. Phase II study of gemcitabine, oxaliplatin in combination with panitumumab in KRAS wild-type unresectable or metastatic biliary tract and gallbladder cancer. Br J Cancer. 2014;111:430–6.

91. Philip PA, Mahoney MR, Allmer C, Thomas J, Pitot HC, Kim G, Donehower RC, et al. Phase II study of erlotinib in patients with advanced biliary cancer. J Clin Oncol. 2006;24: 3069–74.

92. Lee J, Park SH, Chang HM, Kim JS, Choi HJ, Lee MA, et al. Gemcitabine and oxaliplatin with or without erlotinib in advanced biliary-tract cancer: a multicentre, open-label, randomised, phase 3 study. Lancet Oncol. 2012;13:181–8.

41

93. Malka D, Cervera P, Foulon S, Trarbach T, de la Fouchardière C, Boucher E, Fartoux L, Faivre S, et al. BINGO investigators. Gemcitabine and oxaliplatin with or without cetuximab in advanced biliary-tract cancer (BINGO): a randomised, open-label, non-comparative phase 2 trial. Lancet Oncol. 2014;15: 819–28.

94. Galdy S, Lamarca A, McNamara MG, Hubner RA, Cella CA, Fazio N, et al. HER2/HER3 pathway in biliary tract malignancies; systematic review and meta-analysis: a potential therapeutic target? Cancer Metastasis Rev. 2016;36:141–57.

95. Kaseb A. A phase II study trastuzumab (NSC 688097) in Her2/Neu positive cancer of the gallbladder or biliary tract (NCI 7756). In: Clinicaltrials.gov. National Cancer Institute (NCI); 2014.

96. Peck J, Wei L, Zalupski M, O'Neil B, Villalona Calero M, Bekaii-Saab T. HER2/neu may not be an interesting target in biliary cancers: results of an early phase II study with lapatinib. Oncology. 2012;82:175–9.

97. Ross JS, Wang K, Gay L, Al-Rohil R, Rand JV, Jones DM, et al. New routes to targeted therapy of intrahepatic cholangiocarcinomas revealed by next-generation sequencing. Oncologist. 2014;19:235–42.

98. Chen TC, Jan YY, Yeh TS. K-ras mutation is strongly associated with perineural invasion and represents an independent prognostic factor of intrahepatic cholangiocarcinoma after hepatectomy. Ann Surg Oncol. 2012;19(Suppl 3):S675–81.

99. Tannapfel A, Sommerer F, Benicke M, Katalinic A, Uhlmann D, Witzigmann H, et al. Mutations of the BRAF gene in cholangiocarcinoma but not in hepatocellular carcinoma. Gut. 2003;52:706–12.

100. Bekaii-Saab T, Phelps MA, Li X, Saji M, Goff L, Kauh JS, O'Neil BH, et al. Multi-institutional phase II study of selumetinib in patients with metastatic biliary cancers. J Clin Oncol. 2011;29:2357–63.

101. El-Khoueiry AB, Rankin CJ, Ben-Josef E, Lenz HJ, Gold PJ, Hamilton RD, et al. SWOG 0514: a phase II study of sorafenib in patients with unresectable or metastatic gallbladder carcinoma and cholangiocarcinoma. Invest New Drugs. 2012;30:1646–51.

102. Moehler M, Maderer A, Schimanski C, Kanzler S, Denzer U, Kolligs FT, et al. Working Group of Internal Oncology. Gemcitabine plus sorafenib versus gemcitabine alone in advanced biliary tract cancer: a double-blind placebo-controlled multicentre phase II AIO study with biomarker and serum programme. Eur J Cancer. 2014;50:3125–35.

103. Herberger B, Puhalla H, Lehnert M, Wrba F, Novak S, Brandstetter A, et al. Activated mammalian target of rapamycin is an adverse prognostic factor in patients with biliary tract adenocarcinoma. Clin Cancer Res. 2007;13:4795–9.

104. Riener MO, Bawohl M, Clavien PA, Jochum W. Rare PIK3CA hotspot mutations in carcinomas of the biliary tract. Genes Chromosomes Cancer. 2008;47:363–7.

105. Deshpande V, Nduaguba A, Zimmerman SM, Kehoe SM, Macconaill LE, Lauwers GY, et al. Mutational profiling reveals PIK3CA mutations in gallbladder carcinoma. BMC Cancer. 2011;11:60.

106. Simbolo M, Fassan M, Ruzzenente A, Mafficini A, Wood LD, Corbo V, et al. Multigene mutational profiling of cholangiocarcinomas identifies actionable molecular subgroups. Oncotarget. 2014;5:2839–52.

107. Yeung YH, Chionh FJM, Price TJ, Scott AM, Tran H, Fang G, et al. Phase II study of everolimus monotherapy as first-line treatment in advanced biliary tract cancer: RADichol. J Clin Oncol. 2014;32(suppl):5s. abstr 4101.

108. Turner N, Grose R. Fibroblast growth factor signalling: from development to cancer. Nat Rev Cancer. 2010;10:116–29.

109. Borad MJ, Champion MD, Egan JB, Liang WS, Fonseca R, Bryce AH, et al. Integrated genomic characterization reveals novel, therapeutically relevant drug targets in FGFR and EGFR pathways in sporadic intrahepatic cholangiocarcinoma. PLoS Genet. 2014;10:e1004135.

110. Arai Y, Totoki Y, Hosoda F, Shirota T, Hama N, Nakamura H, et al. Fibroblast growth factor receptor 2 tyrosine kinase fusions define a unique molecular subtype of cholangiocarcinoma. Hepatology. 2014;59:1427–34.

111. Graham RP, Barr Fritcher EG, Pestova E, Schulz J, Sitailo LA, Vasmatzis G, et al. Fibroblast growth factor receptor 2 translocations in intrahepatic cholangiocarcinoma. Hum Pathol. 2014;45:1630–8.

112. Reitman ZJ, Yan H. Isocitrate dehydrogenase 1 and 2 mutations in cancer: alterations at a crossroads of cellular metabolism. J Natl Cancer Inst. 2010;102:932–41.

113. Saha SK, Parachoniak CA, Ghanta KS, Fitamant J, Ross KN, Najem MS, et al. Mutant IDH inhibits HNF-4α to block hepatocyte differentiation and promote biliary cancer. Nature. 2014;513:110–4.

114. Jiao Y, Pawlik TM, Anders RA, Selaru FM, Streppel MM, Lucas DJ, et al. Exome sequencing identifies frequent inactivating mutations in BAP1, ARID1A and PBRM1 in intrahepatic cholangiocarcinomas. Nat Genet. 2013;45:1470–3.

115. Kipp BR, Voss JS, Kerr SE, Barr Fritcher EG, Graham RP, Zhang L, et al. Isocitrate dehydrogenase 1 and 2 mutations in cholangiocarcinoma. Hum Pathol. 2012;43:1552–8.

116. Wang P, Dong Q, Zhang C, Kuan PF, Liu Y, Jeck WR, et al. Mutations in isocitrate dehydrogenase 1 and 2 occur frequently in intrahepatic cholangiocarcinomas and share hypermethylation targets with glioblastomas. Oncogene. 2013;32:3091–100.

117. Pollyea DA, De Botton S, Fathi AT, et al. Clinical safety and activity in a phase I trial of AG-120, a first in class, selective, potent inhibitor of theIDH1-mutant protein, in patients with IDH1 mutant positive advanced hematologic malignancies. In: EORTC-NCI-AACR symposium. Barcelona: European Cancer Organisation; 2014.

118. Stein EM, Altman JK, Collins R, et al. AG-221, an oral, selective, first-in-class, potent inhibitor of the IDH2 mutant metabolic enzyme, induces durable remissions in a phase I study in patients with IDH2 mutation positive advanced hematologic malignancies. San Francisco: American Society of Hematology (ASH); 2014.

119. Wu RC, Wang TL, Shih Ie M. The emerging roles of ARID1A in tumor suppression. Cancer Biol Ther. 2014;15:655–64.

120. Churi CR, Shroff R, Wang Y, Rashid A, Kang HC, Weatherly J, et al. Mutation profiling in cholangiocarcinoma: prognostic and therapeutic implications. PLoS One. 2014;23:e115383.

121. Chong DQ, Ax Z. The landscape of targeted therapies for cholangiocarcinoma: current status and emerging targets. Oncotarget. 2016;7:46750–67.

122. Shen DY, Zhang W, Zeng X, Liu CQ. Inhibition of Wnt/beta-catenin signaling downregulates P-glycoprotein and reverses multi-drug resistance of cholangiocarcinoma. Cancer Sci. 2013;104:1303–8.

123. Wang W, Zhong W, Yuan J, Yan C, Hu S, Tong Y, et al. Involvement of Wnt/beta-catenin signaling in the mesenchymal stem cells promote metastatic growth and chemoresistance of cholangiocarcinoma. Oncotarget. 2015;6:42276–89.

124. Settakorn J, Kaewpila N, Burns GF, Leong AS. FAT, E-cadherin, beta catenin, HER 2/neu, Ki67 immuno-expression, and histological grade in intrahepatic cholangiocarcinoma. J Clin Pathol. 2005;58:1249–54.

125. Rosenbluh J, Wang X, Hahn WC. Genomic insights into WNT/beta-catenin signaling. Trends Pharmacol Sci. 2014;35:103–9.

126. Fingas CD, Bronk SF, Werneburg NW, Mott JL, Guicciardi ME, Cazanave SC, et al. Myofibroblast-derived PDGF-BB promotes Hedgehog survival signaling in cholangiocarcinoma cells. Hepatology. 2011;54:2076–88.

127. Fingas CD, Mertens JC, Razumilava N, Sydor S, Bronk SF, Christensen JD, et al. Polo-like kinase 2 is a mediator of hedgehog survival signaling in cholangiocarcinoma. Hepatology. 2013;58:1362–74.

128. Mertens JC, Fingas CD, Christensen JD, Smoot RL, Bronk SF, et al. Therapeutic effects of deleting cancer-associated fibroblasts in cholangiocarcinoma. Cancer Res. 2013;73:897–907.

129. Xie F, Xu X, Xu A, Liu C, Liang F, Xue M, et al. Aberrant activation of sonic hedgehog signaling in chronic cholecystitis and gallbladder carcinoma. Hum Pathol. 2014;45:513–21.

130. Matsushita S, Onishi H, Nakano K, Nagamatsu I, Imaizumi A, Hattori M, et al. Hedgehog signaling pathway is a potential therapeutic target for gallbladder cancer. Cancer Sci. 2014;105:272–80.

131. Riedlinger D, Bahra M, Boas-Knoop S, Lippert S, Bradtmoller M, Guse K, et al. Hedgehog pathway as a potential treatment target in human cholangiocarcinoma. J Hepatobiliary Pancreat Sci. 2014;21:607–15.

132. Li J, Wu T, Lu J, Cao Y, Song N, Yang T, et al. Immunohistochemical evidence of the prognostic value of hedgehog pathway components in primary gallbladder carcinoma. Surg Today. 2012;42:770–5.

133. Tang L, Tan YX, Jiang BG, Pan YF, Li SX, Yang GZ, et al. The prognostic significance and therapeutic potential of hedgehog signaling in intrahepatic cholangiocellular carcinoma. Clin Cancer Res. 2013;19:2014–24.

134. Miyamoto M, Ojima H, Iwasaki M, Shimizu H, Kokubu A, Hiraoka N, et al. Prognostic significance of overexpression of c-met onco protein in cholangiocarcinoma. Br J Cancer. 2011;105:131–8.

135. Terada T, Nakanuma Y, Sirica AE. Immunohistochemical demonstration of MET overexpression in human intrahepatic cholangiocarcinoma and in hepatolithiasis. Hum Pathol. 1998;29:175–80.

136. Li H, Shimura H, Aoki Y, Date K, Matsumoto K, Nakamura T, et al. Hepatocyte growth factor stimulates the invasion of gallbladder carcinoma cell lines in vitro. Clin Exp Metastasis. 1998;16:74–82.

137. Yang L, Guo T, Jiang S, Yang Z. Expression of ezrin, HGF and c-met and its clinicopathological significance in the benign and malignant lesions of the gallbladder. Hepato-Gastroenterology. 2012;59:1769–75.

41

Hepatocellular Cancer

Riccardo Memeo, Patrick Pessaux, Nicola Silvestris, Oronzo Brunetti, Antonio Giovanni Solimando, and Andrea Casadei Gardini

Gastrointestinal Cancers

Contents

© Springer Nature Switzerland AG 2021
A. Russo et al. (eds.), *Practical Medical Oncology Textbook*, UNIPA Springer Series,
https://doi.org/10.1007/978-3-030-56051-5_42

42.1 Introduction

Hepatocellular carcinoma (HCC) is the most common type of primary liver cancer in adults. Even if improvements in prevention and diagnosis have been done in recent years, HCC still remains the third leading cause of cancer death [1].

It occurs in the setting of chronic liver inflammation, mostly linked to chronic viral hepatitis B or C. Exposure to toxins such as alcohol or aflatoxin could conceivably be causes of HCC. Also metabolic syndrome and nonalcoholic steatohepatitis (NASH) are increasingly recognized as risk factors for HCC. Hemochromatosis and α1-antitrypsin deficiency could increase the risk of developing HCC.

Often, but not always, HCC develops through a fibrotic degenerative process with the formation of nodules called cirrhosis. So far, HCC is the most common cause of death in people affected by cirrhosis [2].

Most patients affected by HCC have signs and symptoms of chronic liver disease (jaundice, ascites, abnormalities of blood coagulation, hyporexia, weight loss, abdominal pain, nausea, and vomiting). Sometimes they do not show any symptoms. In some cases, HCC patients could present worsening of the symptoms.

42.2 Epidemiology

In the US surveillance, epidemiology, and outcome (SEER) database program, HCC accounts for 65 % of all cases of liver cancer [3, 4]. The incidence rate of HCC increased from 1.4/100,000 cases/year in the 1980s to 6.2/100,000 cases in 2011 [3, 5]. HCC is more frequent in men than in women, with a ratio of about 2.4:1 [6]. It is generally diagnosed between 50 and 70 years of age [7], is predominant in Asian and African countries, and is not very common in Northern Europe and North America [4]. The main risk factors are hepatotropic viruses infection, such as HBV and HCV, and alcohol abuse. About 80–90 % of HCCs occur within the context of cirrhosis [8]. In recent years an increase in the number of cases associated with metabolic syndrome has been observed.

42.3 Physiopathology

Hepatitis B virus is the principal cause of hepatocellular carcinoma. There are clear evidences of such an association, accumulated from biological studies in patients with chronic liver disease degenerated into neoplastic disease and from prospective and retrospective epidemiological studies conducted on populations from Africa, Malaysia, Japan [9, 10], China [11], Europe [12], and the USA [13]. Hepatitis C is also strongly associated with the risk of primitive HCC [14, 15], with a relative risk estimated up to more than a 20%, which is a figure similar to the one of hepatitis B.

Alcohol abuse is another risk factor for the development of this tumor type.

In recent years it has been shown as in developed countries there is a correlation between the metabolic syndrome (NASH and NAFLD) and HCC. However, the above form is still poorly studied.

In the world, the principal liver carcinogen aflatoxin content in food is a product of the metabolism of the fungus *Aspergillus flavus* that contaminates foods (usually the produce of grain stored in hot and humid environment) in many tropical countries, particularly in Southern Africa and Southeast Asia. Experimentally, it is among the most potent liver carcinogen known for certain animal species, and it is likely that it is a potential carcinogen also for men. In addition, the incidence of primitive HCC in some areas of Southern Africa (where this cancer is particularly prevalent) is positively correlated with the content of aflatoxin in the diet [16]. In developed countries, food is less contaminated by *Aspergillus flavus*, and this fungus is not involved in the carcinogenesis of HCC.

There is also a difference in the incidence of hepatitis B infection between developed and developing countries. In developing countries infection with hepatitis B, it is more common, while in developed countries hepatitis C infection is more frequent. The hepatitis B virus is a direct carcinogenic, while the hepatitis C virus is an indirect carcinogen: hepatitis C exerts its carcinogenic action through the inflammatory process and the resulting cirrhosis that develops in the liver. These etiological differences are reflected in a different biological behavior of HCC: the majority of Caucasian patients have a slow-growing and expansive cancer [17], whereas South African patients have a rapid-growing cancer [18]. As a consequence, there are significant different etiologies between primary HCC in Africans and Europeans and North Americans.

In turn, even among Europeans there are pathway and genetic differences between patients with HCC related to hepatitis and HCC patients related to metabolic syndrome.

Being a major player in the inflammation in carcinogenesis of this tumor, the expression of hepatitis virus-related proteins very likely reflects the differences between the various types of HCC.

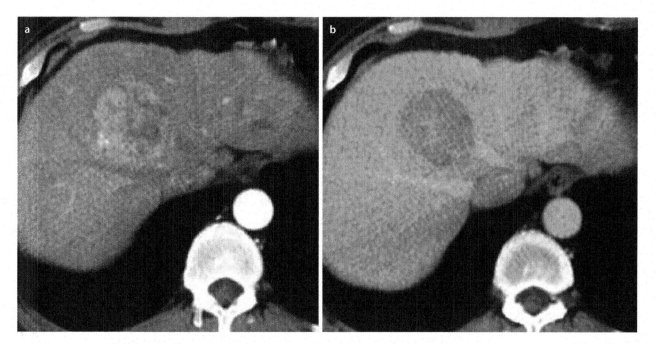

Fig. 42.1 HCC CT-scan. **a** Arterial phase sequence with wash in and **b** washout

42.4 Diagnosis

42.4.1 Radiological Criteria

The presence of small nodules in a cirrhotic liver is normal, making the differential diagnosis between regeneration nodules and neoplastic nodules often difficult. A "focal lesion," i.e., a lesion measuring at least 5 mm detected by ultrasound or another method is first identified [19]. Hepatic carcinogenesis occurs in stages in 90% of cases: the lesion progresses from regenerative micronodule to regenerative macronodule, with histological changes that lead from mild to severe dysplasia to carcinoma, extending to the entire nodule and beyond.

From a histological point of view, the transformations that occur during carcinogenesis are generally accompanied by a progressive formation of anomalous arterial vessels (tumor neoangiogenesis) and loss of the portal component [20]. The imbalance between the components of the vascular support gives HCC a unique behavior in the different contrast phases that enables imaging techniques to identify the tumor, i.e., an increase in the arterial phase signal in the lesion compared to the surrounding parenchyma (commonly called arterial hypervascularization or wash-in), followed by a reduction in the venous phase that makes the lesion appear moderately less contrast-enhanced than the parenchyma (appearance defined as premature washing or washout). In the presence of wash-in followed by washout, a 10-mm lesion in a cirrhotic liver can be fairly confidently diagnosed as HCC.

Suspicious nodules should be evaluated with contrast-enhanced MRI and/or CT scan to identify a diagnostic pattern typical of HCC (hypervascularization in the arterial phase and washout in the venous/late phase) and to carry out staging in order to define prognosis and the most suitable therapy if malignancy is confirmed (Fig. 42.1). The role of contrast-enhanced ultrasound (CEUS) in the diagnosis of HCC has been questioned due to its poor ability to differentiate intrahepatic cholangiocarcinoma from HCC [21].

In the case of a typical MRI and/or CT (with wash-in and washout) appearance of lesions exceeding 10 mm, a diagnosis of HCC can be considered confirmed. Conversely, for lesions with an atypical appearance (lack of arterial hypervascularization and/or washout), further evaluation with an alternative contrastographic technique (MRI or CT) or CEUS is performed, or it may be decided to proceed directly to biopsy, if technically feasible [21] (Fig. 42.2).

42.4.2 Role of Alpha-Fetoprotein

Alpha-fetoprotein is the most commonly used serum marker for HCC. Alpha-fetoprotein is no longer recommended as a diagnostic test because of the low sensitivity of its threshold value (about 20%), especially in small nodules, and also because of its lack of specificity when lower limits are used, e.g., >20 ng/dL). Thus, diagnosis of HCC is based on the results from typical imaging of malignancy in a cirrhotic liver or histological confirmation. High values of alpha-fetoprotein have a clear negative prognostic significance [21].

Fig. 42.2 Diagnostic flow chart

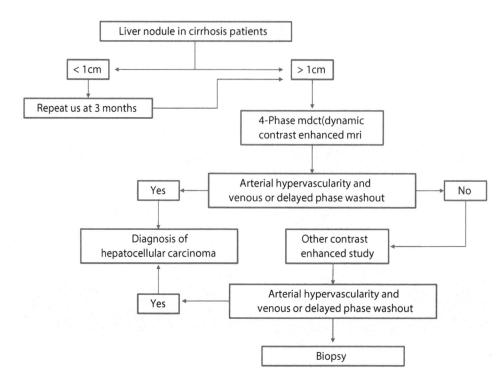

42.4.3 Histological Criteria and Classification

42.4.3.1 Liver Biopsy

Even if instrumental investigations could be able to achieve a diagnosis, sometimes HCC should be investigated by the histological examination of the lesion through ultrasound- or CT-guided percutaneous biopsy usually when radiological examinations lead to diagnostic doubts.

42.4.3.2 Pathology
Macroscopic Features

Macroscopic characteristics of HCC are related to both the size of the tumor and the presence or absence of liver cirrhosis. In fact, HCCs associated with liver cirrhosis show fibrous capsule and intratumoral septa, while the ones without cirrhosis tend to be massive and nonencapsulated (■ Fig. 42.3). HCC could occasionally present itself as a pedunculated lesion. Surrounding intrahepatic metastases are frequent in advanced phases.

Due to its significant angiogenesis features (Longo et al.), macrovascular invasion of portal vein could be present in more than 70% of advanced HCC. Furthermore, intrahepatic metastases are caused mostly by tumor spread in the portal vein branches. Less frequently, tumor invades the major bile ducts. Extrahepatic metastases are mostly hematogenous (i.e., liver, lung and less frequently bone). Regional lymph node metastases are frequent.

Microscopic Features

Neoplastic cells resemble polygonals with distinct cell membranes and abundant granular eosinophilic cytoplasm with a nucleus/cytoplasm ratio which is higher than normal. Moreover, the nucleus is round with coarse chromatin and a thickened nuclear membrane. The presence of sinusoidal vessels surrounding tumor cells is an important diagnostic feature. Common characteristics are portal vein thrombosis and microvascular invasion with presence of mitotic figures. The presence of abundant fat or bile canaliculi, copper, intracellular hyaline bodies, and intranuclear pseudoinclusions could be less frequent (■ Fig. 42.4). HCC is immunohistochemically positive for HepPar-1 and AFP, even if these markers may be negative in high-grade tumors. Also glypican-3 may be positive in both cytoplasm and membrane. Unlike the sinusoidal endothelial cells in normal liver tissue, those in HCC are immunohistochemically positive for CD34 and factor-VIII-related antigen.

A variable number of macrophages with similar features of well-differentiated tumors Kupffer cells are present in the sinusoidal blood spaces. They bear an immunohistochemical positivity for CD68 and antilysozyme [22].

Different Histological Patterns

The trabecular (plate-like) pattern is the most common in well- and moderately differentiated HCCs. Neoplastic cells are grouped in cords of variable thickness which are separated by sinusoid-like blood spaces. Sinusoid-like blood spaces often show varying degrees of dilata-

Fig. 42.3 Macroscopic aspect of hepatocellular carcinoma on cirrhotic liver

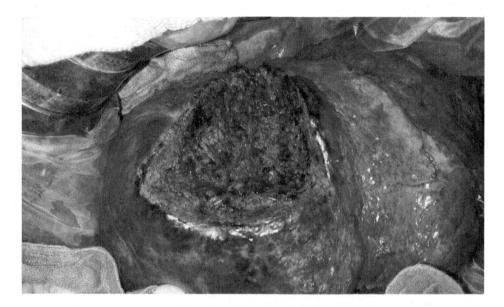

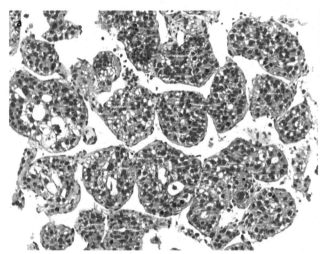
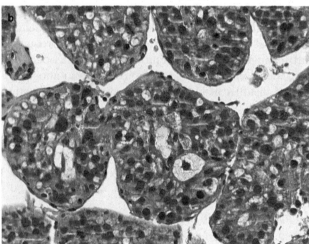

Fig. 42.4 **a** Well-differentiated HCC. Typical roll-off appearance due to the capillaryization of sinusoids. 20× (H/E). **b** Greater magnification (40×). Endothelins continuously delimit the aggregates of atypical hepatocytes (H/E)

tion, and peliosis hepatis-like changes are occasionally observed in advanced HCCs (◘ Fig. 42.5).

Pseudoglandular and acinar variants of HCC frequently show a glandular pattern, usually admixed with the trabecular pattern.

An uncommon HCC subtype is scirrhous. It is characterized by marked fibrosis along the sinusoid-like blood spaces with varying degrees of atrophy of tumor trabeculae. The scirrhous type must not be confused with cholangiocarcinoma or fibrolamellar carcinoma.

The term "sclerosing hepatic carcinoma" has been used to designate a variety of tumors arising in non-cirrhotic livers. This variant is often associated with hypercalcemia, but it doesn't constitute a distinct histopathological entity [23].

Cell Variants

*Pleomorphic HCC*s show marked variation in cellular and nuclear size, shape, and staining. Multinucleated or mononuclear giant cells are often present, appearing as osteoclast-like giant cells. They are frequently observed as common in poorly differentiated tumors. In clear cell HCC, cancer cells present clear cytoplasm due to the presence of abundant glycogen. Those features make the differential diagnosis from metastatic clear cell type renal carcinoma challenging.

Sarcomatoid HCC is a subtype with sarcomatous change which is characterized by the proliferation of spindle cells or bizarre giant cells. It is more frequent in patients who have undergone TACE. Most of them are positive for vimentin or desmin.

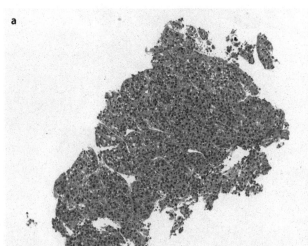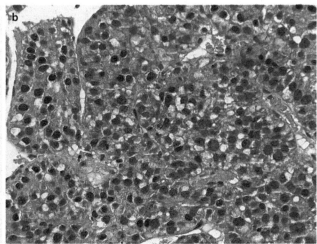

◻ Fig. 42.5 **a** Moderately differentiated trabecular hepatocarcinoma. 20× hematoxylin/eosin. **b** Greater magnification (40×). Evident nuclear dysmetries with hypercromasia (H/E)

Fatty change HCC is most frequent in early-stage tumors with a diameter lower than 2 cm. Its frequency declines as tumor size increases, with rather infrequent fatty changes in advanced tumors. It could be associated with metabolic disorders related to hepatocarcinogenesis and insufficient blood supply in the early neoplastic stages.

Bile production HCC is occasionally observed, usually as plugs in dilated biliary ducts, with a prominent bile production. It is interesting to see that cancer cells turn green after formalin fixation. Mallory hyaline bodies are intracytoplasmic, irregular in shape, eosinophilic, and PAS-negative.

Fibrolamellar HCC is usually observed in noncirrhotic livers with a higher incidence in adolescents or young adults. Cancer cells are grouped in sheets or small trabeculae which are divided by hyalinized collagen bundles with a characteristic lamellar pattern. These cells contain deeply eosinophilic and coarsely granular cytoplasm and distinct nucleoli. Pale bodies are present, and stainable copper, usually in association with bile, can occasionally be shown.

Undifferentiated carcinoma represents about 2% of epithelial liver tumors. Its characteristics resemble those of all the undifferentiated cancers, with poorly differentiated small cells and a high mitotic cell rate. Its prognosis is worst compared to other HCC variants [23].

Grading

According to the histological grade of differentiation, HCC can be divided into well-differentiated, moderately differentiated, and poorly differentiated.

Well-differentiated HCC cells present minimal atypia and increased nuclear/cytoplasmic ratio. They are organized in trabecular patterns: pseudoglandular or acinar structures are frequently observed.

Moderately differentiated HCC is the most common in tumors which are larger than 3 cm in diameter. Cells show abundant eosinophilic cytoplasm and round nuclei. A pseudoglandular pattern is also frequent with bile or proteinaceous fluid. Cancer cells are organized in trabeculae.

In *poorly differentiated HCC*, cancer cells show an increased nuclear/cytoplasmic ratio, frequent pleomorphism, and high proliferation rate. Poorly differentiated HCC is frequent in late stages of the disease [23].

42.5 Staging

One of the most important moments in the onset of an HCC is the possibility to achieve a correct staging of the cancer to choose the best therapeutic option. Currently, the most common staging system for HCC is the Barcelona Clinic Liver Cancer (BCLC) system, which determines cancer stage and patient's prognosis based on tumor burden, severity of the diseases, and patient's performance status [24].

We identify very early and early stage (BCLC 0 and BCLC A) in patients with solitary lesion or up to three nodules ≤3 cm (no macrovascular invasion or extrahepatic disease). In this case patients can benefit from potentially curative treatment (resection, transplant, or ablation). In case of intermediate stage HCC (BCLC B), in asymptomatic patients with multifocal HCC, without vascular invasion or extrahepatic disease, patients could be candidate for transarterial chemoembolization (TACE). In case of multifocal HCC with vascular invasion or extrahepatic disease, systemic treatment with tyrosine kinase inhibitor (sorafenib) currently offers the best therapeutic option. Patients with end-stage liver disease (BCLC D) have a very poor prognosis and require supportive care alone.

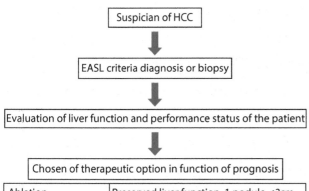

Ablation	Preserved liver function, 1 nodule <2cm
Resection	Preserved liver function, 1 nodule
TACE	Internmediate liver fuction, multiple nodules
Transplant	Any liver function, 1 nodule <5 cm or 3 nodules >3cm
Systemic therapy	Preserved liver function, and in rarecase intermediate liver function, advanced and metastatic stages
Bestsupportive care	Terminal stages

■ **Fig. 42.6** Therapeutic algorithm

42.6 Treatment

Considering the multifactorial evaluation of cirrhotic patient with HCC, different therapeutical options are available to treat cancer (■ Fig. 42.6).

42.6.1 Surgery

In order to achieve a correct diagnosis of HCC in cirrhotic patients, the EASL panel of experts and the American Association for the Study of Liver Disease (AASLD) [1] adopted the definition of HCC radiological hallmark, considering radiological criteria for diagnosis, based on typical contrast uptake of the nodule in arterial phase and washout in the late phase. In case of >1 cm nodule, one radiological technique (CT, MRI, US-contrast) could be sufficient for diagnosis. If the diagnosis is uncertain, a second radiological exam could integrate the result. In case of further doubts, a specimen biopsy is necessary. The AFP value might be useful for diagnosis but in practice it will not affect the treatment strategy.

42.6.1.1 Liver Resection

With a 50% 5-year overall survival (OS), liver resection is considered the only therapy which seems to cure the disease while maintaining liver function. Liver resection remains the most accessible treatment for liver malignancies, because a limited availability of graft limits

transplantation in selected cases. There has been some progress recently which has aimed at improving the results of liver resection. Better patient selection and preoperative studies, associated with the improvement of surgical tools and techniques including laparoscopic [25] and robotic surgery [26], have enhanced postoperative outcome. Unfortunately, only 20–30% of patients have resectable disease at diagnosis. The ideal resection candidate is a patient with a single nodule, Child-Pugh A, without satellite nodules or vascular invasion, and the possibility to perform an anatomical resection to reduce the risk of untreated satellite nodules. Bilobar pathology is usually a surgery contraindication, and more conservative strategies are preferred in order to control the pathology.

42.6.1.2 Preoperative Assessment of the Patient Plays a Key Role

The main risks related to liver resection are hepatic insufficiency and failure [27]. This risk is heightened in case of an excessively large amount of hepatic parenchyma liver resection [28]. For that reason, the preoperative risk assessment is a fundamental process before liver resection. In case of liver resection, we should consider two fundamental evaluations: a quantitative evaluation based on the percentage of hepatic parenchyma [29] that could be resected and a qualitative evaluation [30] involving functional reserve of the whole liver. For liver resection in cirrhotic patients, a minimal amount of 40% of liver should be preserved to avoid liver failure. For qualitative measurement, the main test is the evaluation of the indocyanine green at 15 min retention rate. Another feature evaluated before liver resection is portal hypertension [31], which should be absent in order to achieve better postoperative course and Child-Pugh classification, which allows the calculation of a score based on biological tests and clinical evidence to estimate the cirrhosis severity [32]. This classification is used to assess the prognosis of chronic liver disease, mainly in cirrhotic patients. It is based on the analysis of five items and divides patients in three classes in function according to the cumulative score. Analyzed items are total bilirubin, serum albumin, prothrombin time or INR, ascites and hepatic encephalopathy. The combination of these factors could minimize the risk of liver failure.

The ECOG (Eastern Cooperative Oncology Group) [33] (■ Table 42.1) scale of performance status is a scale which helps to understand how the disease can impact the patient's daily life. It measures the patients' level of functioning in terms of their ability to take care of themselves in terms of daily activity and physical ability. Grade 0 and 1 describe patients who are able to perform the same activity before disease or patients, who, although with restrictions in performing physical activ-

Table 42.1 ECOG performance status

ECOG	ECOG performance status
0	Fully active, able to carry on all pre-disease performance without restriction
1	Restricted in physically strenuous activity but able to move and to carry out tasks of a light or sedentary nature, e.g., light house work, office work
2	Able to move and capable of any personal tasks but unable to carry out any work activities; up and about for more than 50% of waking hours
3	Capable of only limited self-care; confined to bed or chair for more than 50% of waking hours
4	Completely disabled; unable to carry on any self-care; totally confined to bed or chair
5	Dead

ity, could nonetheless perform simple tasks. These categories are the ideal categories of patients who could undergo treatment, with a low risk of posttreatment complications.

Firstly, a CT scan of abdomen and thorax is mandatory to exclude major parenchymal involvement or distal metastases. The role of the CT can facilitate both the definition of a correct diagnosis and the evaluation of the relationship between nodules and both vascular and biliary structures. In case of major resection, it is mandatory to calculate the amount of theoretical future remnant liver (FRL) through a CT 3D reconstruction [34]. FRL corresponds to the quantity of liver which should be preserved after surgery in order to be sufficient to guarantee a normal liver function. In case of insufficient FRL, portal vein embolization [35] (selective occlusion of monolateral portal flow to obtain contralateral hypertrophy of the liver) could be useful for its increase. In case of major resection, at least 40 % of FRL should be preserved in cirrhotic patients.

The most important aspect related to liver resection is the identification of appropriate candidates who could stand liver resection. A correct assessment of the patient's general status and liver function must be performed to reduce the risk of an uneventful postoperative course to a minimum. One of the main concepts in liver resection is the necessity to preserve a quantity of functional liver parenchyma after surgery to avoid postoperative liver failure. This quantity of functional liver is called FRL, and it is calculated before surgery with an appropriate software. According to Couinaud's classification and the division of the anatomy of the liver in eight segments [36], minor liver resection is the definition used when ≤3 segments are resected, or there is a major resection involving >3 segments. According to these classifications, patients that can be considered for

minor resection should be Child A with bilirubin levels ≤2 mg/dL and an absence of ascites and with more than 100.000/mm^3 platelets. If major resection indicated, criteria for minor resection should be respected with the addition of bilirubin levels ≤1 mg/dL, the absence of portal hypertension, and portal vein embolization for future remnant liver of <40 %.

Surgical Technique

The aim of liver resection is to offer the best treatment with adequate resection margins [37]. A tumor-free margin of at least 1 cm should be guaranteed, with better results when there are more than 2 cm of margins. This is due to the necessity to remove the zone in which satellite nodule could be present and therefore inducing an early pathology recurrence. For the same reason, anatomical resection is preferred to nonanatomical resection [38] due to intrahepatic diffusion following portal vein pedicle, which could be ideal in patients with inadequate liver function, in order to reduce the liver failure risk.

Liver resection needs an initial intraoperative ultrasound, in order to identify liver lesions and anatomical relation among liver lesion and vascular and biliary structure. Once assessed the resection feasibility and identified a surgical plan, liver resection could be performed using different techniques and devices, to reduce blood loss and perform an easier hepatectomy [39]. In the majority of liver resections, a tape is passed around the round ligament in order to clamp the inflow (Pringle maneuver) of the liver and to control a possible intraoperative bleeding, even if the duration of pedicle clamping is limited in time. More measures could be adopted to achieve a better control of bleeding, including vascular exclusion of the liver with pedicle clamping associated to caval and hepatic vein clamping, along with an important hemodynamic impact.

42.6.1.3 Laparoscopic Liver Surgery

In last 20 years, the improved accuracy and diffusion of laparoscopic liver surgery in combination with the development of new surgical tools have made liver resection easier and increasingly less invasive. Apart from the advantage of minimally invasive access on postoperative pain, laparoscopic liver surgery has been demonstrated to reduce intraoperative bleeding, leading to faster recovery and with the same short- and long-term oncological results [40]. It is possible to associate liver resection and radiofrequency ablation. Recently, robotic surgery has increased the number and reproducibility of liver resection. In terms of percentage with robotic surgery a 5-year disease-free survival is almost 45%, compared with a 25% disease-free survival due to the high rate of recurrence and the presence of vascular invasion or microsatellite nodules, most of the time with the presence of liver cirrhosis.

◘ Fig. 42.7 Surgery: flow chart

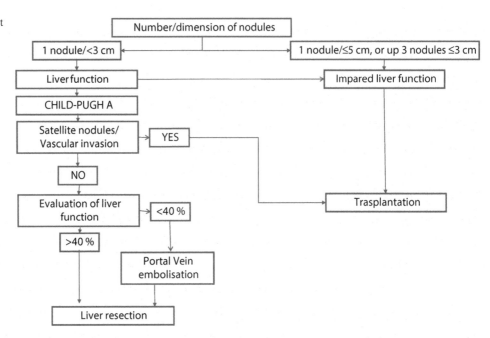

42.6.1.4 Liver Transplant

Liver transplant offers a better (OS) (70 % at 5 years); it is limited by strict selection criteria and organ shortage. It's indicated especially for HCC patients with impaired liver function.

HCC often onsets on a pathological liver condition. Even if viral hepatitis reduced its frequency after the development of antiviral therapies, other causes including fatty liver disease and alcohol still represent a fertile ground on which HCC can easily develop, compared to a non-pathological liver [41]. Transplant offers the possibility to treat both the cancer and the underlying disease. Unfortunately, not all patients with liver disease and HCC could benefit from liver transplant, due to organ shortage and to limited benefit of treatment for patients with advanced liver disease. For this reason, to optimize transplant benefits, some criteria have been established. The most common criteria are "Milan criteria" [42], which consider the presence of any solitary HCC ≤5 cm, or up to three lesions ≤3 cm each, without vascular invasion or metastasis as the ideal candidate for liver transplant.

In order to treat patients who are beyond transplant criteria, it is possible to treat liver nodules in order to reduce tumor load, for example, with liver resection [43], or locoregional therapies, allowing the patients to fill translatability criteria. This strategy allows the HCC downstaging within Milan criteria in 40 % of patients outside criteria; however, posttransplant HCC recurrence rates are high at 16 % [44].

In order to allow more patients to be transplanted, some strategies have been considered to expand donor pools [45]: partial graft, deriving from living donor, or donor after cardiac death and recently, some tools as

perfusion machine are used to improve the quality of grafts and to prolong their viability before being transplanted to recipient patients.

Even if transplant centers are trying to expand the donor pool, one of the main problems of liver transplant remains the dropout [46] of those patients waiting for liver transplant, in whom liver disease progresses.

Nowadays, surgery represents the only change of long-term survival in these patients. ◘ Figure 42.7 is a summary of the characteristics of HCC patients able to underwent to surgery (◘ Fig. 42.7).

42.6.2 Locoregional Procedures

42.6.2.1 Ablation

HCC locoregional treatment [47] is gaining increasing treatment interest. Even if surgical resection guarantees the possibility to ablate the tumor and eventually satellite nodules, recent studies demonstrate that locoregional treatment leads to equivalent results. It could also be considered as a palliative treatment for patients who can't undergo other treatments for HCC.

The most common ablation treatments are percutaneous ethanol injection (PEI), radiofrequency ablation (RFA), and microwave ablation (MWA). All these approaches are image-guided procedures, in most cases performed through ultrasound.

42.6.2.2 PEI

This procedure [48] needs to monitor the distribution of alcohol in the nodule to achieve the best results. The particularity of this procedure is the low cost of the material. It is feasible and safe, especially for lesions

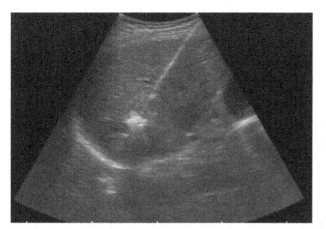

Fig. 42.8 Ultrasound guided ablation of liver lesion

close to the bile duct or to the bowel, due to the non-transmission of energy during the procedure. In fact, alcohol is easily diffused in hyper vascularized HCC. Furthermore, it can be performed in patients with portal thrombosis.

42.6.2.3 RFA and MWA

RF [49, 50, 51] is considered the gold-standard ablation technique. Even if transplantation and liver resection represents the best chance for patients concerning long-term survival, RF represents a valid alternative, and it could be used in association with resection or could be part of a downstaging treatment before liver transplant. Based on constant radiofrequency, energy-generated heat, it transmits the energy to the lesion and to surrounding tissue. It can be performed in sedation or general anesthesia. Under ultrasound control (Fig. 42.8), the needle is placed in the middle of the lesion, to transmit energy uniformly in and around the lesion. In case of more than one lesion, simultaneous treatment could be performed.

In literature, the best results are described for HCC Child A patients with lesions <3 cm, with long-term 5-year OS (50–60 %) comparable to surgical resection and liver transplantation. Small solitary HCC can achieve 5-year OS of 85 %. It is associated with a shorter postoperative stay and lower mortality rate compared to resection [50].

MWA [52, 53] is a recent technique which proposes faster and more extensive ablation areas, allowing the treatment of larger lesions closer to large vessels and biliary structures.

42.6.3 TACE

TACE is a radiological technique which combines inflow occlusion of feeding artery tumor inflow with

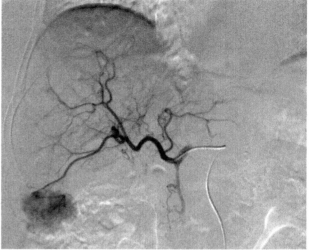

Fig. 42.9 TACE of HCC of right liver

the locoregional therapy directly in the tumor area [35] (Fig. 42.9). This treatment induces the local necrosis of the tumor associated with high intratumor concentration of chemotherapy.

TACE could allow the treatment either of multiple nodules or a selective treatment of a single nodule. Moreover, when during the radiological evaluation of tumor response, the treatment results incomplete, it can be repeated, since it is well tolerated by liver function, due to the low impact on liver function. It is indicated for patients with liver disease associated with impaired liver function.

Herein (Fig. 42.10), it is represented the summary of HCC patients features able to underwent to locoregional approaches.

42.6.4 Systemic Treatments

Even if for the last 10 years, sorafenib was the only therapeutic strategy, nowadays new tyrosine kinase inhibitors [54] and immune checkpoint inhibitors [55] improved the survival of HCC patients.

42.6.4.1 Sorafenib

The efficacy of sorafenib, a small-molecule multitarget kinase inhibitor, in the treatment of advanced HCC has been demonstrated in two randomized phase III trials, the SHARP [56] study and the Asia-Pacific study [57]. Both studies enrolled patients not eligible for locoregional treatment (at diagnosis or after failure of any previous treatment) but with good hepatic function (Child-Pugh A). In both trials, sorafenib treatment (400 mg twice daily up to instrumental and clinical progression or unacceptable toxicity) resulted in a significant prolongation of OS and time to progression (TTP).

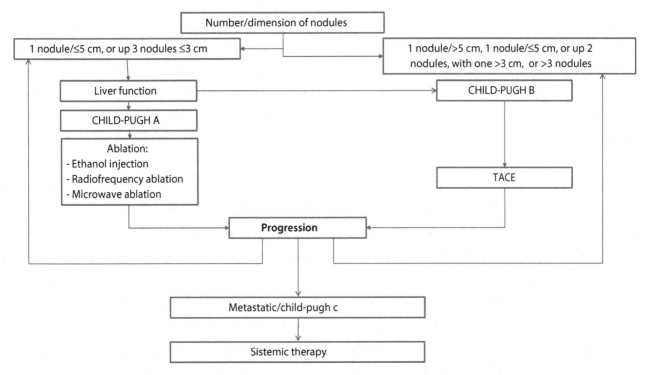

Fig. 42.10 Locoregional procedures: flow chart

In absolute terms, the median survival prolongation was approximately 3 months in the SHARP study and approximately 2 months in the Asian study, but findings are only comparable in relative terms (hazard ratio 0.69 and 0.68, 95 % CI 0.55–0.87, and 0.50–0.93, respectively). On the basis of these results, sorafenib was approved by the EMA for the treatment of HCC in October 2007 (Table 42.2).

The main adverse events of sorafenib are hand-foot skin reaction, hypertension, and diarrhea. Numerous studies have focused on the role of factors and biomarkers predictive and/or prognostic to response to sorafenib, but currently no marker is used in current clinical trials. The most interesting factors studied are the correlation between toxicity and response [58, 59], immune inflammation indicators, and level of lactate dehydrogenase [60, 61, 62].

42.6.4.2 Lenvatinib

Recently, the results from a multicenter randomized non-inferiority phase 3 study comparing lenvatinib and sorafenib were published [63]. Patients with advanced HCC or HCC not recommendable for locoregional treatment and who had never received systemic treatment were recruited and randomized to receive lenvatinib (12 mg/day (body weight ≥ 60 kg) or 8 mg/day (body weight < 60 kg) or sorafenib (400 mg twice daily for 28-day cycles). The primary endpoint was OS,

Table 42.2 Main TKI in use for HCC, lines of indication, survival, side effects

Drug	Lines of indication	Overall survival in phase 3 trial [Months (95 % CI)]	Adverse events
Sorafenib	First	10.7 (9.4–13.3)	Hand-foot skin reaction, hypertension, and diarrhea
Lenvatinib	First	13.6 (12.1–14.9)	Hypertension, fatigue, diarrhea, joint and muscle pain
Regorafenib	Second	10.6 (9.1–12.1)	Breathlessness and looking pale, bruising, bleeding gums or nosebleeds, fatigue, hand-foot skin reaction
Cabozantinib	Second	10.2 (9.1–12.0)	Severe bleeding (hemorrhage), emesis, blood red or black tarry stool

measured from the date of randomization to the date of death from any cause. Median survival time for lenvatinib was 13.6 months (95 % CI 12.1–14.9), therefore not lower than sorafenib (12.3 months, 10.4–13.9; HR 092, 95 % CI 0.79–1.06). Among secondary endpoints (progression-free survival [PFS] and TTP), although lenvatinib was superior to sorafenib, in the study design, the evaluation of the radiological response according to mRECIST was not centralized. Among adverse events of any grade, hypertension occurred more frequently in lenvatinib-arm patients (42 % vs. 30 %), while palmar-plantar erythrodysesthesia syndrome was more frequent in those treated with sorafenib, as expected. In conclusion, lenvatinib did not result inferior to sorafenib in terms of OS in untreated advanced HCC. The safety and tolerability profiles of lenvatinib were consistent with those previously observed (◧ Table 42.2).

42.6.4.3 Atezolizumab Plus Bevacizumab

IMbrave150 trial [64], a randomized double-blind phase III trial, evaluated the efficacy of atezolizumab plus bevacizumab versus sorafenib in first-line chemotherapy. Study meets the co-primary endpoint for OS and PFS. Atezolizumab plus bevacizumab improved OS (hazard ratio [HR] 0.58; 95 % CI 0.42–0.79, $p = 0.0006$) and PFS (hazard ratio [HR] 0.59; 95 % CI 0.47–0.76, $p < 0.0001$) with respect to sorafenib. mOS was not reach in atezolizumab plus bevacizumab arm compared to 13.2 months for sorafenib arm; PFS was 6.8 months in atezolizumab plus bevacizumab arm compared to 4.3 months for sorafenib arm.

42.6.4.4 Regorafenib

In the RESORCE study [65], a randomized double-blind phase III study, Child-Pugh A patients with advanced or intermediate HCC (the latter was not eligible for locoregional treatment) who had tolerated first-line sorafenib at a dose of at least 400 mg/day for at least 20 of the 28 days prior to discontinuation but had progressed during treatment were randomized to receive the best supportive therapy (BSC) in combination with oral regorafenib (160 mg once a day for 21 days of each 4-week cycle) vs. BSC and placebo. The primary endpoint was OS (defined as the time from randomization to death from any cause). Regorafenib improved OS (HR 0.63; 95 % CI 0.50–0.79, $p < 0.0001$). Median OS was 10.6 months (95 % CI 9.1–12.1) for regorafenib compared to 7.8 months (6.3–8.8) for placebo. Adverse events (AEs) were reported in all patients treated with regorafenib. In particular, the AEs with the highest grade (3 or 4) were hypertension (15 % in the regorafenib group vs. 5 % in the placebo group), hemorrhagic fever with renal syndrome (HFRS) (13 % vs.1 %), fatigue (9 % vs. 5 %), and diarrhea (3 % vs. no patient in the placebo group). In all additional efficacy endpoints (PFS, TTP, response rate [RR] and disease control rate [DCR]), regorafenib was statistically superior to placebo (◧ Table 42.2).

42.6.4.5 Cabozantinib

The CELESTIAL study [66], a randomized double-blind phase III trial, evaluated the efficacy of cabozantinib in patients progressing on sorafenib. Cabozantinib improved OS (hazard ratio [HR] 0.76; 95 % CI 0.63–0.92, $p = 0.0049$). mOS was 10.2 months (95 % CI 9.1–12.0) for cabozantinib compared to 8 months (95 % CI 6.8–9.4) for placebo. In addition to being statistically superior to placebo in terms of PFS, TTP, RR, and DCR, cabozantinib was also superior in terms of PFS and ORR (◧ Table 42.2).

42.6.4.6 Ramucirumab

REACH-2 trial [67], a randomized double-blind phase III trial, evaluated the efficacy of ramucirumab versus placebo sorafenib in patients progressing on sorafenib with α-fetoprotein concentrations of 400 ng/mL or higher. Study meets the primary endpoint for OS. Ramucirumab improved OS (hazard ratio [HR] 0.71; 95% CI 0.53–0.95, $p = 0.0199$). mOS was 8.5 months (95% CI 7.0–10.6) for ramucirumab compared to 7.3 months (95% CI 5.4–9.1) for placebo. In addition, to confirm the better results compared to placebo in terms of PFS, no difference was found in terms of DCR.

42

Case Study

Man: 55 years old
- Family history: negative for malignancies
- APR: treated HCV infection, cirrhosis

- Blood test: normal liver function test, Child A, Meld 8, Afp 200 ng/mL
- TC abdomen and MRI: lesion of 24 × 20 × 22 mm in segment 4, confirmed for HCC

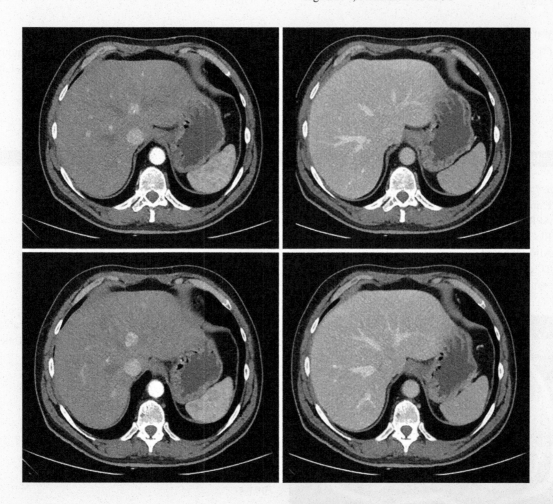

Question

What action should be taken?
1. Surgery
2. RFA
3. Others

Answer

A. Liver resection, if possible laparoscopy

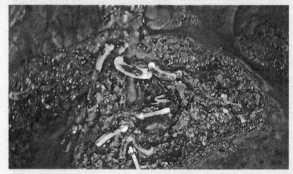

Question

Which is the best follow-up?
1. CT scan every 3 months
2. Nexavar
3. Others

Answer

1. CT scan

Question

Which is the best treatment in case of recurrence?
1. Liver resection
2. Liver transplant
3. Others

Answer

2. In case of recurrence, treatment of choice should be liver transplant, which guarantees best overall and disease-free survival.

Case Study

Man: 75 years old
- Family history: negative for malignancies
- APR: treated HCV infection, cirrhosis, PS 2
- Blood test: normal liver function test, Child A, Meld 8, Afp 500 ng/mL
- TC abdomen and MRI: lesion of $15 \times 10 \times 12$ mm in segment 6, confirmed for HCC

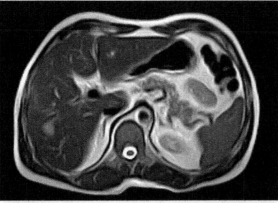

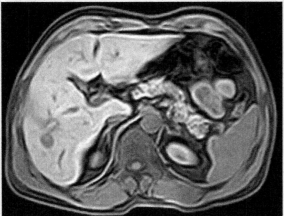

Question

Which is the best treatment of choice?
1. Resection
2. RFA
3. Others

Answer

1. RFA in consideration of performance status of patient and small size of the lesion. Results are comparable to liver resection, with better postoperative outcome in such a fragile patient.

Question

Which is the best treatment in case of recurrence?
1. Liver resection
2. RFA
3. Others

Answer

2. In case of recurrence, treatment of choice should be radiofrequency ablation or TACE in case of multinodular lesions

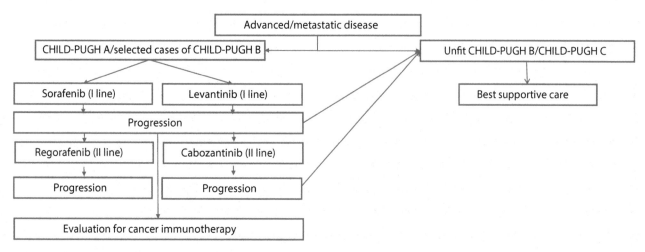

Fig. 42.11 Systemic therapy: flow chart

42.7 Future Perspectives

Even if new molecular approaches have been experimented, only slightly significant improvements have been achieved in survival. Therefore, clinicians need to both identify new therapeutic approaches and select patients suitable for these treatments.

Moreover, it must be pointed out that cancer immunotherapy is the new open option for solid treatments. Different clinical trials evaluating the role of immunotherapy in treating HCC have been conducted. Initial promising results have been obtained among cytokine-induced killer cells and immune checkpoint inhibitors in the adjuvant setting and advanced stages, respectively. Anyway, there are several ongoing trials, the results of which appear intriguing. Conclusively, since the liver immune system the plays an important role in immune tolerance, the possibility of unmasking these mechanisms can be a winning weapon in HCC, so immunotherapy [68] will represent the future therapy in this cancer (◘ Fig. 42.11).

42.8 Highlights

Hepatocellular carcinoma (HCC) is the most common type of primary liver cancer in adults.

It occurs in the setting of chronic liver inflammation, mostly linked to chronic viral hepatitis B or C.

Hepatic carcinogenesis occurs in stages in 90% of cases: the lesion progresses from regenerative micronodule to regenerative macronodule.

Suspicious nodules should be evaluated with contrast-enhanced MRI and/or CT scan to identify a diagnostic pattern typical of HCC

One of the most important moments in the onset of an HCC is the possibility to achieve a correct staging of the cancer to choose the best therapeutic option. Currently, the most common staging system for HCC is the Barcelona Clinic Liver Cancer (BCLC) system, which determines cancer stage and patient's prognosis based on tumor burden, severity of the diseases, and patient's performance status

Very early and early stage (BCLC 0 and BCLC A) in patients with solitary lesion or up to three nodules ≤3 cm (no macrovascular invasion or extrahepatic disease). In this case patients can benefit from potentially curative treatment (resection, transplant, or ablation).

In case of intermediate stage HCC (BCLC B), in asymptomatic patients with multifocal HCC, without vascular invasion or extrahepatic disease, patients could be candidate for transarterial chemoembolization (TACE).

In case of multifocal HCC with vascular invasion or extrahepatic disease, systemic treatment with tyrosine kinase inhibitor (sorafenib/lenvatinib) or in the next future with atezolizumab plus bevacizumab it could be suggested.

Different clinical trials evaluating the role of immunotherapy, antiangiogenic, and TKI or their combinations in treating HCC have been conducted.

Expert Opinion

Vito Di Marco

1. Hepatocellular carcinoma is one of the leading causes of cancer on cirrhotic patients.

2. Many different approaches are available, depending on tumor diffusion and status of the patient.

3. To date, sorafenib and regorafenib are the approved therapies in advanced HCC. Levantinib and cabozantinib could represent other therapies that have shown efficacy in advanced HCC. Even if new molecular approaches have been experimented, only slightly significant improvements have been achieved in survival. Therefore, clinicians need to both identify new therapeutic approaches and select patients suitable for these treatments.

4. Moreover, it must be pointed out that cancer immunotherapy is the new open option for solid treatments.

Different clinical trials evaluating the role of immunotherapy in treating HCC have been conducted. Initial promising results have been obtained among cytokine-induced killer cells and immune checkpoint inhibitors in the adjuvant setting and advanced stages, respectively. However, there are several ongoing trials, the results of which appear intriguing. Conclusively, since the liver immune system plays an important role in immune tolerance, the possibility of unmasking these mechanisms can be a winning weapon in HCC, so immunotherapy will represent the future therapy in this cancer.

Recommendations

- ESMO
  ▸ https://www.esmo.org/Guidelines/Gastrointestinal-Cancers/Hepatocellular-Carcinoma

References

1. Llovet JM, Ducreux M, Lencioni R, et al. EASL-EORTC clinical practice guidelines: management of hepatocellular carcinoma. Eur J Cancer. 2012;48:599–641.

2. Forner A, Llovet JM, Bruix J. Hepatocellular carcinoma. Lancet. 2012;379:1245–55.

3. El-Serag HB. Hepatocellular carcinoma. N Engl J Med. 2011;365:1118–27.

4. Mittal S, El-Serag HB. Epidemiology of hepatocellular carcinoma: consider the population. J Clin Gastroenterol. 2013;47:S2–6.

5. El-Serag HB, Mason AC. Rising incidence of hepatocellular carcinoma in the United States. N Engl J Med. 1999;340:745–50.

6. Parkin DM, Bray F, Ferlay J, et al. Global cancer statistics, 2002. CA Cancer J Clin. 2005;55:74–108.

7. Kumar V, Abbas AK, Fausto N, et al. Robbins and cotran pathologic basis of disease. 7th ed. Philadelphia: Elsevier Saunders; 2004.

8. Zhang DY, Friedman SL. Fibrosis-dependent mechanisms of hepatocarcinogenesis. Hepatology. 2012;56:769–75.

9. Nomura A, Stemmermann GN, Wasnich RD. Presence of hepatitis B surface antigen before primary hepatocellular carcinoma. JAMA. 1982;247:2247–9.

10. Tsukuma H, Hiyama T, Oshima A, et al. A case-control study of hepatocellular carcinoma in Osaka. Japan. Int J Cancer. 1990;45:231–6.

11. Beasley RP, Hwang LY, Lin CC, et al. Hepatocellular carcinoma and hepatitis B virus. A prospective study of 22707 men in Taiwan. Lancet. 1981;2:1129–33.

12. Trichopoulos D. Hepatitis B virus and hepatocellular carcinoma. Lancet. 1979;8127:1192.

13. Tabor E. Hepatitis C virus and hepatocellular carcinoma. AIDS Res Hum Retrovir. 1992;5:793–6.

14. Tabor E, Kobayashi K. Hepatitis C virus, a causative infectious agent of non-A, non-B hepatitis: prevalence and structure--summary of a conference on hepatitis C virus as a cause of hepatocellular carcinoma. J Natl Cancer Inst. 1992;84:86–90.

15. Zavitsanos X, Hatzakis A, Kaklamani E, et al. Association between hepatitis C virus and hepatocellular carcinoma using assays based on structural and nonstructural hepatitis C virus peptides. Cancer Res. 1992;52:5364–7.

16. Peers FG, Linsell CA. Dietary aflatoxins and human primary liver cancer. Ann Nutr Aliment. 1977;31:1005–17.

17. Franco D, Capussotti L, Smadja C, et al. Resection of hepatocellular carcinomas. Results in 72 European patients with cirrhosis. Gastroenterology. 1990;98:733–8.

18. Anthony PP. Primary carcinoma of the liver: a study of 282 cases in Ugandan Africans. J Pathol. 1973;110:37–48.

19. Bolondi L, Sofia S, Siringo S, et al. Surveillance programme of cirrhotic patients for early diagnosis and treatment of HCC: a cost effectiveness analysis. Gut. 2001;48:251–9.

20. Sangiovanni A, Del Ninno E, Fasani P, et al. Increased survival of cirrhotic patients with a hepatocellular carcinoma detected during surveillance. Gastroenterology. 2004;126:1005–14.

21. Forner A, Reig M, Bruix J. Hepatocellular carcinoma. Lancet. 2018;391:1301–14.

22. Tanaka M, Nakashima O, Wada Y, Kage M, Kojiro M. Pathomorphological study of Kupffer cells in hepatocellular carcinoma and hyperplastic nodular lesions in the liver. Hepatology. 1996;24:807–12.

23. Hamilton SR, Aaltonen LA. Pathology and genetics of tumours of the digestive system. Lyon: IARC Press; 2000.

24. Bruix J, Reig M, Sherman M. Evidence-based diagnosis, staging, and treatment of patients with hepatocellular carcinoma. Gastroenterology. 2016;150:836–53.

25. Wakabayashi G, Cherqui D, Geller DA, et al. Recommendations for laparoscopic liver resection: a report from the second international consensus conference held in Morioka. Ann Surg. 2015;261:619–29.

26. Giulianotti PC, Bianco FM, Daskalaki D, et al. Robotic liver surgery: technical aspects and review of the literature. Hepatobiliary Surg Nutr. 2016;5:311–21.

27. Rahnemai-Azar AA, Cloyd JM, Weber SM, et al. Update on liver failure following hepatic resection: strategies for prediction and avoidance of post-operative liver insufficiency. J Clin Transl Hepatol. 2018;6:1–8.

28. Chan J, Perini M, Fink M, et al. The outcomes of central hepatectomy versus extended hepatectomy: a systematic review and meta-analysis. HPB. 2018;20:487–96.

29. Cieslak KP, Huisman F, Bais T, et al. Future remnant liver function as predictive factor for the hypertrophy response after portal vein embolization. Surgery. 2017;162:37–47.

30. de Baere T, Teriitehau C, Deschamps F, et al. Predictive factors for hypertrophy of the future remnant liver after selective portal vein embolization. Ann Surg Oncol. 2010;17:2081–9.

31. Rhaiem R, Piardi T, Chetboun M, et al. Portal inflow modulation by somatostatin after major liver resection. Ann Surg. 2017;276:e101–3.

32. Okajima C, Arii S, Tanaka S, et al. Prognostic role of Child-Pugh score 5 and 6 in hepatocellular carcinoma patients who underwent curative hepatic resection. Am J Surg. 2015;209:199–205.

33. Oken MM, Creech RH, Tormey DC, et al. Toxicity and response criteria of the Eastern Cooperative Oncology Group. Am J Clin Oncol. 1982;5:649–55.

34. Cieslak KP, Runge JH, Heger M, et al. New perspectives in the assessment of future remnant liver. Dig Surg. 2014;31:255–68.

35. Memeo R, De Blasi V, Adam R, et al. Parenchymal-sparing hepatectomies (PSH) for bilobar colorectal liver metastases are associated with a lower morbidity and similar oncological results: a propensity score matching analysis. HPB. 2016;18:781–90.

36. Pauli EM, Staveley-O'Carroll KF, Brock MV, et al. A handy tool to teach segmental liver anatomy to surgical trainees. Arch Surg. 2012;147:692–3.

37. Memeo R, De'Angelis N, Compagnon P, et al. Laparoscopic vs. open liver resection for hepatocellular carcinoma of cirrhotic liver: a case-control study. World J Surg. 2014;38:11.

38. Huang X, Lu S. A meta-analysis comparing the effect of anatomical resection vs. non-anatomical resection on the long-term outcomes for patients undergoing hepatic resection for hepatocellular carcinoma. HPB. 2017;19:843–9.

39. Appéré F, Piardi T, Memeo R, et al. Comparative study with propensity score matching analysis of two different methods of transection during hemi-right hepatectomy: Ultracision Harmonic Scalpel versus Cavitron Ultrasonic Surgical Aspirator. Surg Innov. 2017;24:5.

40. Sotiropoulos GC, Prodromidou A, Kostakis ID, et al. Meta-analysis of laparoscopic vs open liver resection for hepatocellular carcinoma. Updat Surg. 2017;69:291–311.

41. Byam J, Renz J, Millis JM. Liver transplantation for hepatocellular carcinoma. Hepatobiliary Surg Nutr. 2013;2:22–30.

42. Silva MF, Sherman M. Criteria for liver transplantation for HCC: what should the limits be? J Hepatol. 2011;55:1137–47.

43. Cherqui D, Laurent A, Mocellin N, et al. Liver resection for transplantable hepatocellular carcinoma: long-term survival and role of secondary liver transplantation. Ann Surg. 2009;250:5.

44. Parikh ND, Waljee AK, Singal AG, et al. Downstaging hepatocellular carcinoma: a systematic review and pooled analysis. Liver Transpl. 2015;21:1142–52.

45. deLemos AS, Vagefi PA. Expanding the donor pool in liver transplantation: extended criteria donors. Clin Liver Dis. 2013;2:156–9.

46. Salvalaggio PR, Felga GE, Guardia BD, et al. Time of dropout from the liver transplant list in patients with hepatocellular carcinoma: clinical behavior according to tumor characteristics and severity of liver disease. Transplant Proc. 2016;48:2319–22.

47. Facciorusso A, Serviddio G, Muscatiello N. Local ablative treatments for hepatocellular carcinoma: an updated review. World J Gastrointest Pharmacol Ther. 2016;7:477.

48. Luo W, Zhang Y, He G, et al. Effects of radiofrequency ablation versus other ablating techniques on hepatocellular carcinomas: a systematic review and meta-analysis. World J Surg Oncol. 2017;15:126.

49. Rhim H, Lim HK. Radiofrequency ablation of hepatocellular carcinoma: pros and cons. Gut Liver. 2010;1(Suppl 1):S113–8.

50. Yang W, Yan K, Goldberg SN, et al. Ten-year survival of hepatocellular carcinoma patients undergoing radiofrequency ablation as a first-line treatment. World J Gastroenterol. 2016;22:2993–3005.

51. Lee S, Kang TW, Cha DI, et al. Radiofrequency ablation vs. surgery for perivascular hepatocellular carcinoma: propensity score analyses of long-term outcomes. J Hepatol. 2018;69:70–8.

52. Dou J-P, Yu J, Yang X-H, et al. Outcomes of microwave ablation for hepatocellular carcinoma adjacent to large vessels: a propensity score analysis. Oncotarget. 2017;8:28758–68.

53. Vietti Violi N, Duran R, Guiu B, et al. Efficacy of microwave ablation versus radiofrequency ablation for the treatment of hepatocellular carcinoma in patients with chronic liver disease: a randomised controlled phase 2 trial. Lancet Gastroenterol Hepatol. 2018;3:317–25.

54. Gnoni A, Santini D, Scartozzi M, et al. Hepatocellular carcinoma treatment over sorafenib: epigenetics, microRNAs and microenvironment. Is there a light at the end of the tunnel? Expert Opin Ther Targets. 2015;19:1623–35.

55. Longo V, Brunetti O, Gnoni A, et al. Angiogenesis in pancreatic ductal adenocarcinoma: a controversial issue. Oncotarget. 2016;7:58649–58.

56. Llovet JM, Ricci S, Mazzaferro V, et al. Sorafenib in advanced hepatocellular carcinoma. N Engl J Med. 2008;359:378–90.

57. Cheng AL, Kang YK, Chen Z, et al. Efficacy and safety of sorafenib in patients in the Asia-Pacific region with advanced hepatocellular carcinoma: a phase III randomised, double-blind, placebo-controlled trial. Lancet Oncol. 2009;10:25–34.

58. Casadei Gardini A, Scarpi E, Marisi G, et al. Early onset of hypertension and serum electrolyte changes as potential predictive factors of activity in advanced HCC patients treated with sorafenib: results from a retrospective analysis of the HCC-AVR group. Oncotarget. 2016a;12:15243–51.

59. Di Costanzo GG, Casadei Gardini A, Marisi G, et al. Validation of a simple scoring system to predict sorafenib effectiveness in patients with hepatocellular carcinoma. Target Oncol. 2017;6:795–803.

60. Brunetti O, Gnoni A, Licchetta A, et al. Predictive and prognostic factors in HCC patients treated with sorafenib. Medicina (Kaunas). 2019;55:pii: E707.

61. Casadei Gardini A, Scarpi E, Faloppi L, et al. Immune inflammation indicators and implication for immune modulation strategies in advanced hepatocellular carcinoma patients receiving sorafenib. Oncotarget. 2016b;41:67142–9.

62. Faloppi L, Bianconi M, Memeo R, et al. Lactate dehydrogenase in hepatocellular carcinoma: something old, something new. Biomed Res Int. 2016;2016:7196280.

63. Kudo M, Finn RS, Qin S, et al. Lenvatinib versus sorafenib in first-line treatment of patients with unresectable hepatocellular carcinoma: a randomised phase 3 non-inferiority trial. Lancet. 2018;391:1163–73.

64. Cheng A-L, Qin S, Ikeda M, et al. IMbrave150: efficacy and safety results from a Ph 3 study evaluating ATEZOLIZUMAB (atezo) + bevacizumab (bev) vs sorafenib (sor) as first treatment (tx) for patients (pts) with unresectable hepatocellular carcinoma (HCC). Ann Oncol. 2019;30(9):ix186–7.

65. Bruix J, Qin S, Merle P, Granito A, et al. Regorafenib for patients with hepatocellular carcinoma who progressed on sorafenib treatment (RESORCE): a randomised, double-blind, placebo-controlled, phase 3 trial. Lancet. 2017;389:56–66.

66. Abou-Alfa GK, Cheng A-L, et al. Phase 3 randomized, double-blind, controlled study of cabozantinib (XL184) versus placebo in subjects with hepatocellular carcinoma who have received prior sorafenib (CELESTIAL; NCT01908426). J Clin Oncol. 2014;32(5s (suppl)):abstr TPS4150.

67. Zhu AX, Kang YK, Yen CJ, et al. Ramucirumab after sorafenib in patients with advanced hepatocellular carcinoma and increased α-fetoprotein concentrations (REACH-2): a randomised, double-blind, placebo-controlled, phase 3 trial. Lancet Oncol. 2019;20:282–96.

68. Longo V, Gnoni A, Casadei Gardini A, et al. Immunotherapeutic approaches for hepatocellular carcinoma. Oncotarget. 2017;8:33897–910.

Head and Neck Cancers

Carlo Resteghini, Donata Galbiati, Giuseppina Calareso,
Nicola Alessandro Iacovelli, Alberto Paderno, Cesare Piazza,
Silvana Sdao, and Laura Deborah Locati

Head and Neck Cancers

Contents

© Springer Nature Switzerland AG 2021
A. Russo et al. (eds.), *Practical Medical Oncology Textbook*, UNIPA Springer Series,
https://doi.org/10.1007/978-3-030-56051-5_43

By the end of this chapter, the reader will:
- Be able to correctly apply diagnostic and staging procedures
- Have learned the basic concepts of treatments and supportive care
- Have reached the basic knowledge for the management of HNC patients
- Be able to apply the knowledge in clinical practice

43.1 Introduction

Head and neck cancers (HNCs) represent a heterogeneous group of tumors arising from the epithelial tissue of the upper aerodigestive track. Oral cavity, oropharynx, larynx, and hypopharynx carcinoma are classically included in the defintion of HNCs. Although these cancers share some risk factors (e.g., smoking and alcohol exposure, human papilloma virus infection, premalignant lesions) and histotype (squamocellular carcinoma in at least 90% of the cases), the disease management (e.g., surgery, external beam radiation, and systemic therapy alone or combined) and natural history differ quite significantly in the curative setting. On the other hand, squamocellular carcinomas of the head and neck area are generally considered altogether in the recurrent/metastatic setting.

Epithelial malignant tumors originating from other sites, such as nasopharynx, paranasal sinuses, and salivary glands (majors and minors) have different risk factors (e.g., Epstein-Barr virus infection; exposure to leather and wood dust), histologies (e.g., in the last WHO classification, more than 20 different histotypes have been described for salivary gland carcinomas), and treatment approaches (e.g., surgery; external beam radiotherapy with photons or particles). This chapter focuses only on classical squamous cell carcinoma (SCC) of the HN (SCCHN).

43.2 Epidemiology and Risk Factors

43.2.1 Epidemiology

SCCHNs are rare malignancies, according to RARECARE definition (incidence <6/100,000 year) [1]. Worldwide, the incidence rates of SCCHNs exhibit a wide geographical heterogeneity, reflecting variability in the prevalence of risk factors [2]. In the United States, it is estimated that about 64,690 new cases of SCCHN will occur in 2018 (33,950 oral cavity, 17,590 pharyngeal, and 13,150 laryngeal), which will account for about 3.7% of new cancer cases [3]. In Europe, new cases are expected to affect approximately 151,000 patients in 2020 [2].

Over the last decades, in economically developed countries, a trend toward increased incidence of human papillomavirus (HPV)-related oropharyngeal cancers has been detected, especially and among men. Conversely, the incidence of HPV negative cancers has been decreasing [4, 5].

European data showed improvement in survival for most HNCs, with the highest 5-year relative survival detected for larynx (59%) and the poorest for hypopharynx (25%). Results for other subsites were intermediate (oropharynx, 39%; tongue, 43%; oral cavity, 45%) [6].

43.2.2 Risk Factors

Tobacco consumption and alcohol intake are the main recognized risk factors for SCCHNs. Smoke from tobacco combustion contains several harmful chemicals able to cause DNA damage leading to mutations. Alcohol has an intrinsic transforming action via its metabolite, acetaldehyde, and heavy consumption of alcohol is recognized as an independent risk factor for SCCHN, especially for hypopharynx. Furthermore, alcohol has the ability to magnify the effect of tobacco smoke in a synergistic manner: the risk of cancer development among heavy smokers and drinkers is much higher than expected based on the additive effects of the individual risks [7]. The ability of alcohol to potentiate the effects of smoking more likely resides in its nature as a chemical solvent, enhancing and prolonging mucosal exposure to the carcinogens present in tobacco smoke. The entire aerodigestive track epithelium and other organs are continuously exposed to these carcinogens, thus their transforming effects act synergically on the whole mucosal complex. Therefore, patients diagnosed and treated for SCCHN are at risk of developing second primary tumors, both in the same region and elsewhere (i.e., lung, bladder, esophagus). The estimated risk is 12%, but it is thought to be lower for HPV-related disease [8].

These agents act altering the normal activity of immune system, inducing a state of immunosuppression through different mechanisms. The host defense impairment as well as the inflammation environment caused by smoking and alcohol consumption increase the risk of cancer development.

High-risk HPV oral infection is an established risk factor for oropharyngeal SCC, with no or limited effect on other subsites of the region [9]. More than 200 HPV genotypes have been identified and categorized by their risk of inducing malignancies; among these 12 HPV types are considered oncogenic by the International Agency for research on cancer (IARC). HPV16 is the most frequent "high-risk" virus involved in head and neck carcinogenesis, followed by HPV18. Whereas other genotypes are much less frequent (HPV 33, HPV 35, HPV 58) [10].

HPV-positive patients tend to be younger compared to HPV-negative patients; they also have less exposure to tobacco and alcohol. HPV infections are mainly transmitted by oral sex, although other factors have been implicated, such as marijuana consumption, dietary factors, and genetic polymorphisms. It should be noted that, even if HPV infection represents a causal factor for tumor occurrence, it is also a positive prognostic factor [11]. In fact, HPV-associated oropharyngeal carcinomas (OPCs) are more responding to both chemotherapy (CT) and radiotherapy (RT), therefore higher survival rates are recorded after curative treatments of patients with HPV-associated OPC compared to those with a HPV-negative OPC. A longer survival is also observed in HPV-related OPCs in the recurrent/metastatic setting, which again illustrates a different natural history of this disease entity. Even though a different metastatic pattern has been suggested, this data is controversial and it might reflect the longer survival time observed in this subset of patients [12].

Other factors may also contribute to the development of HNC in selected patients, such as poor oral hygiene, oral cavity infections, as well as betel nut chewing, a widespread habit in certain regions of Asia [13]. Some dietary measures may have a role in protecting individuals from HNC, such as using a diet high in fruit and vegetable and low in red meat intake [14].

43.3 Clinical Features

Specific signs and symptoms, related to the anatomy, the local lymphatic system and the innervations of primary involved sites, characterized SCCHN. Dysphonia, pharyngodynia, dysphagia, lump in the neck, etc., are frequently reported. Although unspecific, the persistence of these symptoms for a long period (>3 weeks), requires a prompt clinical evaluation with an otolaryngologist or ear-nose-throat (ENT) surgeon. Common signs and symptoms usually present at diagnosis of SCCHNC are listed in ◻ Table 43.1.

Clinical history (e.g., smoking history; alcohol exposure; HPV infection; comorbidities) and physical examination play an essential role in both treatment planning and follow-up. The primary purpose is to define the locoregional tumor extension (T and N categories according to tumor staging [15]), to exclude second primaries, evaluate airway patency or quantify alterations

◻ **Table 43.1** Signs and symptoms at presentation and presumptive correlated with primary site

Signs and symptoms	Primary tumor subsite
Lingual pain, persistent ulceration, leukoplakia erythroplakia; bleeding lesions	Oral cavity; oropharynx
Odynophagia	Oral cavity, oropharynx, hypopharynx
Pharyngodynia	Oropharynx, hypopharynx, larynx
Dysphonia	Larynx, hypopharynx
Swollen neck lymph nodes	Each subsite, depending on the nodes levels (see ◻ Fig. 43.1)

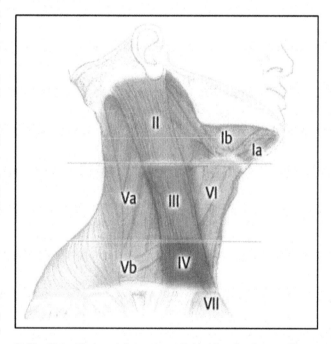

◻ **Fig. 43.1** Neck nodal structures divided into levels according to Robbins

related to previous treatments. Inspection of the entire upper aerodigestive tract (UADT) and bilateral neck is mandatory. Digital palpation may add further information, for example, in the evaluation of the deep extension of lesions involving the oral cavity and/or oropharynx or in assessing the nature of neck nodes. Palpable nodes with increased consistency, poorly defined margins, reduced mobility on superficial or deep planes should be always considered as suspicious. The clinical evidence of a "fixed lymph node" should be remarked and taken into account in the treatment plan. All suspicious neck lymph nodes have to be evaluated by

43

an imaging technique, such as ultrasonography, contrast-enhanced computer tomography scan (CECT) or magnetic resonance imaging (MRI).

43.3.1 Clinical Issues According to the Anatomic Subsite

Evaluation of SCCHNs is still primarily based on simple mucosal inspection [16], even though several adjunctive visual aids have been introduced in the past decades to provide deeper insight into the specific biological behavior of such lesions [17]. As a consequence, the concept of "optical biopsy" has been gradually developed to designate a non-invasive, real-time diagnostic approach aimed at a more accurate early diagnosis of (pre)malignant lesions, and to avoid unnecessary biopsies or incomplete surgical removal. Narrow Band Imaging (NBI) has been already proven to be a useful diagnostic tool in identifying early-stage mucosal SCCHNs [18]. It applies optical filters to enhance visualization of the mucosal and submucosal microvascular pattern. These filters enhance blue and green light (wavelengths of 415 and 540 nm, respectively), corresponding to the peaks of hemoglobin absorption, thus penetrating superficial mucosal layers and highlighting the underlying capillary network without scattering in the deeper layers. Therefore, it is thus possible to identify specific neoangiogenic patterns suggestive of premalignant and neoplastic transformation (see also ◘ Fig. 43.2). Apart

from NBI, a number of other biologic endoscopy tools have been widely described and adopted in the head and neck clinical examination (e.g., supravital stainings by toluidine blue, autofluorescence, confocal microendoscopy, optical coherence tomography, and others). However, clinical examination of each head and neck region needs to consider its specific characteristics and is therefore presented separately.

43.3.2 Oral Cavity

The oral cavity is the entrance of the digestive tube. It spans between the oral fissure (anteriorly), and the oropharyngeal isthmus (posteriorly) and includes the following subsites: buccal mucosa, upper and lower alveolar ridge, anterior two-thirds of the tongue, retromolar trigone, floor of the mouth, and hard palate [19].

Inspection of the oral cavity can be performed by direct visualization or employing video-endoscopes that allow image magnification and application of filters such as NBI.

Superficial premalignant/malignant lesions of oral cavity may appear as leukoplakia (white patch), erythroplakia (red patch), or erythroleukoplakia (mixed or speckled, white, and red patch). These are merely descriptive terms, just referring to the whitish or erythematous appearance of the lesion at the mucosal level that may be the presentation of a number of different benign and malignant diseases. In fact, oral leukopla-

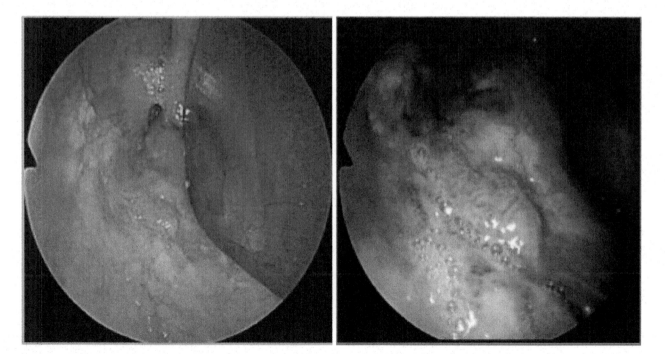

◘ **Fig. 43.2** Buccal mucosa aspect upon inspection with normal light (left) and NBI (right), highlighting the underlying capillary network with neoangiogenic patterns, indicating a neoplastic lesion

kias may present a malignant transformation rate from 0.13% to 17.5%, while erythroplakias, although rarer, may harbor severe dysplasia or invasive carcinoma. According to different experiences, the transformation rate of oral dysplasia is approximately 8% [20], while for erythroplakia it might range from 14% to 60% [21–23]. The indication for a biopsy is dependent on the characteristics of the lesion and the patient's clinical history (previous SCCHNs or inflammatory diseases of the UADT). Irregular margins, prominent vascularity, increased consistency, and signs of deep infiltration are typical factors that increase the risk of malignancy, requiring a biopsy or a closer follow-up.

All subsites should be carefully examined, taking care of those where direct visualization is naturally impaired, such as the oral vestibule, floor of the mouth, and alveolar ridge. The presence and state of dentition should be always evaluated given its influence on the risk of mandibular invasion. In tumors reaching the alveolar crest, the likelihood of bone infiltration is significantly increased in edentulous patients. In fact, in the presence of teeth, tumors invade the mandible by extending through the dental sockets and advance into the cancellous part of the bone after overcoming the natural barrier represented by the dental ligaments. Conversely, in the edentulous subjects, tumors extend up to the alveolar process and infiltrate the dental pores to extend to the cancellous part of the mandible. Moreover, in this situation, the mandible and maxilla are usually much more limited in their vertical height and, therefore, the distance between the bony cancellous portion and the mucosal surface of the gum is greatly reduced. Bone infiltration has to be assessed by bimanual palpation of the lesion that appears to be fixed to the alveolus. However, local evaluation by imaging techniques is always needed.

In tongue tumors, critical points are represented by the depth of infiltration and the extension beyond the median line. It is difficult to obtain a fine evaluation of the deep extension by palpation alone. However, it is often possible to assess if the tumor reaches the median septum of the tongue or if it deeply infiltrates the floor of the mouth. These are fundamental anatomic boundaries that help in giving a better definition of tumor extension inside the hemi-tongue (and hemi-floor of the mouth) compartment. This is a key concept that results in marked differences in the surgical approach.

43.3.3 Oropharynx

The oropharynx extends from the plane of the hard palate superiorly to the plane of the hyoid bone inferiorly. It communicates with the nasopharynx above, the hypo-pharynx inferiorly, and the oral cavity anteriorly. Oropharyngeal subsites are the base of the tongue, the tonsils and the tonsillar pillars, the soft palate, and the posterior pharyngeal wall [19].

Most of the oropharynx can be visualized transorally, while the base of tongue usually requires a transnasal flexible endoscope or a transoral rigid 70°/90° endoscope to be examined. While the concepts of superficial examination are similar to those described for the oral cavity, palpation and examination of the deep extent of the tumor are focused on different critical sites. In particular, in tonsillar tumors, trismus (inability to completely open the mouth) and pain during mastication are suggestive of infiltration of the medial pterygoid muscle. This can be verified by palpation of the tonsillar lesion and the surrounding structures. When the tumor appears to be fixed to the deep plane, an infiltration of the medial pterygoid muscle or the mandible is more likely.

In tumors of the base of tongue, a critical sign suggesting deep infiltration is hypoglossal nerve palsy. At rest, if the nerve is injured, a tongue may have the appearance of a "bag of worms" (fasciculations) or wasting (atrophy). The nerve is then tested by extruding the tongue that will deviate toward the palsy side, in case of nerve palsy.

Finally, a superficial or deep extension to nearby regions should also be considered, since it is a significant factor influencing the treatment choice.

43.3.4 Larynx

The larynx (voice box) is a component of the respiratory tract located in the anterior neck. It is a complex organ whose primary function is to protect the lower airway from the entry of foreign matter, but it has also other important functions, such as phonation and swallowing. The larynx is divided into three regions: supraglottis, glottis, and sublottis [19].

Clinical examination of the larynx is mainly dependent on endoscopic instruments (fibro- or video-laryngoscopes) that allow to completely visualize all laryngeal subsites (i.e., supraglottic, glottic, and subglottic regions). The vocal folds are the primary site of origin of laryngeal cancer, followed by the supraglottis. Tumors rarely originate from the subglottis that is generally involved in case of secondary extension of glottic tumors.

In glottic tumors, the superficial extension over the glottic plane (up to the anterior commissure and contralateral vocal fold, T1b) to different subsites (supraglottis or subglottis, T2) and the motility of vocal folds are critical factors to be ascertained before making any ther-

43

apeutic decision. Furthermore, high-definition videoendoscopes may help in better defining the tumor's superficial spread, also thanks to adjunctive techniques, such as NBI. Concerning the tumor's depth of invasion, the clinical examination is capable of giving precise information, especially in early and intermediate tumors. This is especially important when a transoral laser cordectomy is planned. In fact, in such a conservative approach, type of cordectomy is dependent on the deep tumor extension (i.e., mucosa, vocal ligament, vocal muscle, paraglottic space, cartilage). A first step is to evaluate the mucosal wave by laryngostroboscopy. This exam allows visualizing the vocal fold's mucosal wave during phonation. In case of invasion through the epithelium into the vocal ligament, the mucosal wave progression is altered. It is also possible to confirm this evidence by an intraoperative evaluation thanks to the saline injection into the Reinke space: when a complete "ballooning" of the mucosa is not possible due to tumor adhesions to the vocal ligament, this should be considered an indirect sign of infiltration. Finally, vocal muscle and/or cricoarytenoid joint involvement should be assessed considering the vocal fold and arytenoid motility. In case of deep muscle infiltration, the vocal cord motility is impaired, while the arytenoid motility is normal ("impaired vocal cord motility", T2). Conversely, in case of arytenoid and cricoarytenoid joint infiltration, both vocal cord and arytenoid motility are impaired ("fixed vocal fold", T3). Concerning supraglottic carcinomas, early-stage lesions are significantly less frequent in view of their non-specific symptom profile. The deep extension is mainly represented by upper paraglottic and pre-epiglottic spaces involvement. Spread to neck lymph nodes is more common than in other larynx subsites. However, the primary role of clinical examination is visualizing the superficial tumor spread, while imaging techniques give a better view of deep laryngeal compartments.

43.3.5 Hypopharynx

Hypopharynx is the anatomical region that connects the oropharynx superiorly with both the larynx and esophagus inferiorly. It extends from the superior border of the hyoid bone to the lower border of the cricoid cartilage and comprises posterolateral pharyngeal wall, pyriform sinuses, and pharyngo-oesophageal junction (postcricoid area) [19].

As in supraglottic tumors, early diagnosis is infrequent in hypopharyngeal cancers due to a lack of notable symptoms in the initial phases of disease. Transnasal laryngoscopy is the main clinical examination for such tumors and should be focused on determining their superficial extension and quantifying laryngeal involvement. The Valsalva maneuver and phonation may help in distending the piriform sinus mucosa, further improving visualization. When considering the inferior extension, the Betz fold (created by the superior border of the cricopharyngeus muscle), located at the apex of the piriform sinus, delineates the junction with the esophageal inlet. Tumor spreading below this anatomical boundary should dictate a better evaluation of the upper esophagus to adequately delineate its inferior margin of extension. Similarly, each hypopharyngeal subsite harbors different challenges and critical issues.

Tumors frequently arise from the piriform sinus and can superficially spread to the entire hypopharyngeal mucosa. The medial wall is in direct connection with the larynx; thus, deep infiltration may present as impairment or fixation of the ipsilateral hemilarynx. As previously mentioned, this may be related to vocal muscle (and paraglottic space) infiltration or extension to the arytenoid and cricoarytenoid joint. This is possible even without radiologic signs of cartilage infiltration. Conversely, deep infiltration from the lateral wall of the piriform sinus may lead to involvement of lateral neck structures. In particular, relationships with the carotid artery should be thoroughly clarified before the treatment planning. Finally, in case of bulky or deeply infiltrating disease at the level of the posterior wall of the hypopharynx, it is mandatory to clarify its relationship with the prevertebral fascia and prevertebral muscles. The infiltration of these structures evaluated by CT or MRI (better) contraindicates a surgical approach.

Ultimately, postcricoid carcinomas are significantly less frequent in the general population. In these cases, a precise evaluation of laryngeal subsites and motility gives important information on their superficial and deep extension. However, the inferior spread should also be considered in view of their aggressive biologic behavior.

Hypopharynx tumor has the worse prognosis within the SCCHN subsites (10-year survival 10% in locally advanced cases). Distant metastasis (lung) can be present also at diagnosis. A complete disease staging (locoregional plus distant) is recommended at diagnosis.

43.3.6 Occult Primary Head and Neck Cancer

A tumor is defined as occult or unknown primary cancer (CUP) when it presents in metastatic stage without an identifiable primary site after appropriate investigation. This category includes tumors with different histologies (SCC, adenocarcinoma, melanoma, anaplastic tumors). SCCs account for 5% of all CUPs and are most frequently detected in cervical lymph nodes [24]. The neck level site of metastases is indicative of the possible origin of the neoplasm: tumor involving upper or mid-level cervical nodes (levels I–III, VA) likely originates from the head and neck district. Conversely, a primary site beneath the clavicles (tracheal-bronchial, lung, esophagus) or skin cancer should be suspected in those cases with lower cervical lymph nodes (supraclavicular area, levels IV and Vb), although a head and neck primary is still possible. Thyroid neoplasms can metastasize to all nodal levels.

Patients presenting with a neck mass should have a complete H&N examination using fiber-optic endoscopy, as well as a careful examination of the skin and skin appendages of the entire cervico-cephalic region. A detailed anamnesis of risk factors, previous history of malignancy or resection of cutaneous lesions should be collected.

In the absence of a suspected primary lesion, fine needle aspiration biopsy (FNAB) is the preferred pathological assessment. Core or open biopsy should be avoided, because they may alter the physiological cervical lymphatic drainage and expose the patient to tumor cell seeding with consequent negative therapeutic and prognostic implications. HPV and Epstein Barr Virus (EBV) testing are suggested for SCC or undifferentiated histology. An HPV-positive test strongly suggests an oropharyngeal occult primary located in the homolateral tonsil or base of tongue. Positive EBV testing hints at a nasopharyngeal tumor.

Computed tomography (CT) and/or magnetic resonance imaging (MRI) with contrast are usually the first line of imaging. In case of negative results, a total body PET-CT scan (preferably before the biopsy) should be performed. Examination under anesthesia with NBI inspection of the entire mucosal sites is a recommended diagnostic step, together with clinical/radiological guided biopsies of primary site.

Transoral diagnostic surgery [lingual or palatine tonsillectomy with Transoral Laser Microsurgery (TLM) and transoral Robotic Surgery (TORS)] have emerged as effective modalities to increase the detection of occult primary [25]. However, the therapeutic benefit of these surgical procedures over radiation treatment is still uncertain.

43.4 Natural History

The vast majority of HNCs arise from the surface epithelium of the aerodigestive track; therefore, their early presentation is usually one of a superficial lesion. Invasion of the underling muscular layer is frequent, allowing for tumor spread along muscular fibers and fascias even further away from the primary site. Advanced lesions usually present bony structure erosions, but sometimes periosteal invasion can be found also in smaller lesion arising from the gum, nasal, and paranasal mucosa. Usually, bony and cartilage structures represent a barrier for tumor spread. On the other hand, cancer cells can grow and migrate along nerves fibers, with histotypes such as SCC or salivary gland cancers (especially adenoid cystic carcinoma) able to recur at distant sites from their origin, such as the skull base. Also, vascular space invasion is associated with a higher metastatic rate.

HNCs, especially SCCs, usually do not cause discomfort and symptoms at early stages, thus leading to frequent diagnosis (about 80% of the cases) in a locoregionally advanced disease stage [6]. Neck lymph nodes enlargement is one of the most common signs that prompts diagnostic workup. Indeed, nodal involvement at diagnosis is quite common, with variable probability according to T stage and relative richness of lymphatic vessels of the district. Metastases are rarely detected at baseline; metastatic spread is more common in cases with higher nodal stage or pathologic lymph nodes below the level of the thyroid notch.

Early diagnosis and timely start of treatment are crucial to improve HNC outcome. Oral cancer occurs in site easily accessible by physical examination. Therefore, prevention in high-risk individuals could be carried out through routine oral mucosa examinations. Screening initiatives have been undertaken worldwide, demonstrating that a primary care strategy reduces the mortality rate of oral cancer in high-risk individuals and increases the proportion of tumors detected in early stages. Whether these strategies are cost-effective is not known and further randomized controlled trials are necessary to assess benefit of a visual examination as part of a population-based screening program [26].

Educational campaigns have been organized worldwide with the aim of raising awareness on HNCs symptoms and subsequently drive earlier presentation, diagnosis, and referral (e.g., *Oral, Head and Neck Cancer Awareness Week* in the US; *Make Sense* campaign in Europe).

43.5 Pathological Features

43.5.1 Histological Type

Almost 90% of epithelial HNCs arise from the surface epithelium and are SCC or one of its several described variants, such as lymphoepithelioma, spindle cell carcinoma, verrucous carcinoma, and undifferentiated carcinoma. Spindle cell carcinoma, usually located in the larynx, consists of a high grade carcinoma with a component of mesenchyimal-like cell [27]. Verrucous carcinoma is more often found in the oral cavity (gum) and is usually a low-grade carcinoma frequently associated with chronic chewing of tobacco. Neuroendocrine neoplasms of the larynx, although rare, are the most common nonsquamous tumors of this organ. Tumor classification is based on its grade of differentiation, with aggressiveness being inversely correlated to differentiation.

43.6 Diagnostic Work-Up

43.6.1 Assessment of HPV Infection

Assessment of HPV infection is indicated in all cases of SCC arising from the oropharynx and from cervical nodes metastasis of unknown primary. No single analysis is considered the *gold standard* for HPV identification. Due to its cheap and reproducible methodology, p16 immunohistochemistry (IHC) is the optimal surrogate for detection of HPV infection and this is the diagnostic test approved for OPC in the latest TNM classification (VIII edition). p16 has high sensitivity, close to 100%, although up to 25% of analyzed cases have discordant results between p16 IHC and HPV in situ *hybridization* (HPV ISH) – which is a more specific but less sensitive test. In those cases, a more sophisticated test, such as mRNA and or DNA qPCR for viral protein E6, is indicated.

Commonly, diagnostic algorithm recommends upfront p16 IHC, given its ability to spare further testing. Human papilloma virus ISH's high specificity allows its use either simultaneously to IHC or as a confirmation test for p16 positive cases. In case of discordant results, it is possible to employ ISH for less common HPV types and perform qPCR (◘ Table 43.2).

◘ **Table 43.2** Methods for HPV detection

Methods	Cost	Sensitivity	Specificity
p16 immunohistochemestry (p16 IHC)	+	+++	+
In situ hybridization for high-risk HPV (HPV ISH)	++	++	+++
Viral E6 mRNA/DNA quantitative polymerase chain reaction (E6 mRNA-DNA qPCR)	+++	++	+++

43.6.2 Imaging

Imaging plays a crucial role in HNC detection, particularly in those tumors not assessable by direct clinical examination or endoscopy. Furthermore, imaging helps to stage the tumor according to the TNM system: delineating lesion size and extension, its invasion of adjacent structures, local lymph nodes involvement, and the presence of distant metastases [28].

Imaging is essential for initial evaluation and guiding biopsies for pathological diagnosis in order to plan proper oncologic treatment; it is also crucial in evaluating tumor response during follow up and therefore plays a pivotal tool to detect early recurrences, which may allow for salvage therapy.

Appropriate imaging modality selection is crucial. Cross-sectional imaging modalities available include: ultrasound (US), CECT, MRI, and positron emission tomography-CT with fluorine-18-deoxy-D-glucose (FDG-PET-CT) [29].

Several factors influence the selection of the imaging techniques, such as the availability of the technology, the primary tumor site and histology, and the presence of contraindications. For example, MRI is contraindicated in patients with pacemakers, metal foreign body, or implants, while CT examination is contraindicated in patients with allergy to iodinated contrast media or renal failure.

Ultrasound is an easy and cheap imaging modality. It has the advantage of sparing ionizing radiation to patients and is ideal for guiding biopsy of superficial lesions. US has the limitation of being operator-dependent and not being able to visualize deeper structures. In fact, US waves are not transmitted through bones and air. In the head and neck area, it is usually reserved for evaluation of *major salivary glands, thyroid gland, and cervical lymph nodes*.

Contrast Enhanced Computer Tomography is a widely available modality with limited execution time. CECT is the best imaging technique to assess bone structures. It has the limitations of using ionizing radiations and showing poor tissue contrast resolution compared to MRI. However, in some cases, its short time of examination resulting in less motion artifacts may make it preferable to MRI. CECT is the preferred technique for the evaluation of *primary laryngeal* or *hypopharyngeal* malignancies and for the detection of adjacent cartilaginous and bony structures involvement. Computed tomography is also crucial in staging malignancies as it allows for detection of distant metastases. It may be used as an alternative to US in guiding biopsies, especially in deeper lesions adjacent to vascular and nervous structures (e.g., parapharyngeal space lesions) [29, 30].

Magnetic Resonance Imaging is the gold standard technique for the assessment of most HNCs based on its superb soft tissue contrast resolution. MRI has the advantage of not using ionizing radiations and is the best modality to assess perineural spread, evident as irregular thickening and post-contrast abnormal enhancement of the affected nerves [30]. MRI also allows for evaluation of blood vessels without injection of contrast media, by means of specific sequences.

More recently, MRI functional techniques, such as diffusion weighted imaging (DWI) or dynamic contrast enhanced (DCE) imaging has been developed. These techniques may help to evaluate response to treatment, to detect early recurrences, to distinguish between residual/recurrence disease and post-treatment changes. The main disadvantages of MRI include its high costs and long acquisition time, with low image's quality due to motion artifacts (e.g., swallowing). Therefore, adequate patient compliance is required.

Flourine-18-Deoxy-Glucose-Positron Emission Tomography/Computer Tomography permits whole body evaluation with a single exam, including the site of primary disease; for this reason, it is used as an alternative modality to computed tomography for staging malignancies. In addition to computed tomography, it has the advantage of evaluating metabolic activity of the tumor, measured by the uptake of a radioactive tracer (FDG, fluoro-deoxy-glucose). Thanks to this peculiarity, FDG-PET is essential during follow up of patient with head and neck malignancies as it helps to detect disease persistence/recurrence [31]. However, since infection and inflammation may also result in FDG uptake, this exam is usually performed at least 12 weeks after the end of treatments to minimize false-positive findings. Compared to CECT, it has superior accuracy for detecting nodal metastases, but may produce false-negative results in cases of nodal disease measuring less than 1 cm. FDG-PET/CT does not adequately assess deep, soft-tissue extension or bone involvement and, therefore, does not provide satisfying anatomical road map for treatment. It has the limitation of using ionizing radiation and requires long acquisition time (total investigation time: 2–3 hours).

43.7 Staging

In order to standardize communication between health professionals, the *American Joint Committee on Cancer Staging System* has been adopted. We invite to refer to the latest edition in order to properly stage your patients. Recently, the VIII edition has been released, introducing major changes [15, 32]. Among them, we want to underline:

A. A distinct staging system adopted for HPV-positive and negative OPC.
B. The introduction of different T-stages in oral cavity carcinomas depending on the depth of tumor invasion. This change acknowledges the different biological behavior of invasive tumors, where deeply invasive cancers (>10 mm) are associated with worse prognosis and are classified with higher T stage (T3).
C. The emphasis on extranodal extension (ENE) for HPV-negative neoplasm. ENE is defined as the presence of carcinoma extension through the fibrous capsule of the lymph node into the surrounding connective tissue. It negatively affects prognosis and it has been classified as N3b.

Neck nodal structures are commonly divided into levels [33], as shown in ▪ Fig. 43.1. Positive nodal involvement is predictive of the site of origin. Indeed, nasal cavity, lip and oral cavity malignancies initially spread to level I-II, while oropharyngeal neoplasm are associated to level II-III. Laryngeal and hypopharyngeal carcinomas spread to level II-III-IV. Level V involvement is typical of nasopharyngeal malignancies.

43.8 General Principles of Curative Treatment

HNCs affect organs vital to a patient's social life (e.g., larynx, oral cavity). Treatments needed to eradicate the malignancy can lead to several physical and functional sequelae with a serious impact on quality of life. Since therapy of locoregional malignancies has a curative intent, therapeutic efforts must not only be focused on cure of the patient but also should aim for minimizing disfigurement outcomes and late side effects. Given the complexity of multimodality treatment, patient's management should be handled from the initial diagnosis by a multidisciplinary team of health care providers with relevant expertise (surgeons, radiation oncologists, medical oncologists, dentists, speech pathologists, physical/occupational therapists, nutritionists, and skilled nurses) [34, 35].

Furthermore, SCCHN patients usually bear several comorbidities, especially metabolic (e.g., diabetes) and cardiovascular (e.g., arterial vasculopathies; hypertension; renal failure). A thorough inquiry on patient's medical history and social environment (i.e., presence of accountable caregiver) is of paramount importance for determining the actual ability to sustain the treatments.

Surgery and RT, alone or combined, are the curative treatments for HNC patients. Although chemotherapy by itself is not considered a curative treatment, it enhances the effects of RT and it is routinely used as part of combined modality treatment (i.e., concomitant chemoradiation), particularly in patients with locally advanced disease. The optimal combination of these treatment modalities depends on the anatomic site of the cancer as well as the disease stage.

43.8.1 Surgical Principles

Surgical treatment is strictly dependent on tumor site, size, and involved structures. Accurate preoperative clinical and radiological evaluations allow to adequately plan surgery according to such specific characteristics. The basic principle of HN oncologic surgery is the achievement of complete tumor resection (with free surgical margins), while maintaining as low as possible the occurrence of postoperative sequelae (attended and unavoidable negative consequences of a given therapeutic act) and complications (unattended and avoidable negative consequences). In this view, whenever feasible, minimally-invasive endoscopic/endoluminal approaches are often favored. These are represented by a number of continuously evolving techniques and approaches, such as TLM, TORS [36], and transnasal endoscopic surgery (TES) [37]. These therapeutic modalities accomplish tumor resection through natural orifices (mouth and nostrils), thus limiting the morbidity due to external scars and traumas to uninvolved surrounding tissues. However, locally advanced tumors may require an extensive resection with more conventional "open" procedures, in which cervicotomy, facial bone osteotomy and/ or craniotomy must be applied in order to access the lesion itself and allow its safe removal. In these scenarios, reconstructive surgical techniques play an essential role in granting an effective esthetic and functional restoration, leading to acceptable results even in case of wide composite resections [38]. In association with surgery of the primary lesion, it is often necessary to remove cervical lymph nodes that may be involved by metastatic (clinically overt or occult) neoplastic localization. This is obtained through different types of lateral and/or central compartment neck dissections. This is a major surgical procedure that has to be well distinguished from the neck node biopsy that is usually used in hematologic diseases for a diagnostic purpose, but not recommended in HNCs. During neck dissections, all involved or potentially involved lymph nodes with the surrounding fat tissue within the neck fascial compartments are removed for prophylactic or therapeutic reasons. While in the first clinical scenario, elective neck dissection will remove only the neck levels at higher risk of harboring metastatic cells according to the site of the primary tumor, in the latter one, therapeutic neck dissection will accomplish removal of all the six neck levels (uni- or bilaterally, according to the tumor relationships with the midline).

43.8.2 Radiotherapy Principles

RT plays a pivotal role in the curative treatment of early and locally advanced SCCHN [39]. Intensity Modulated RT (IMRT) is the standard of care in HNCs. IMRT with or without CT has been established as a radical and effective treatment approach, scoring better than 3D-conformal RT in terms of toxicity and quality of life. However, late radiation-related effects, such as xerostomia or dysgeusia, are important issues that need to be addressed. The advantages of irradiation over surgery may include the following: (1) the avoidance of major postoperative complications, (2) reduction of functional or cosmetic defects since no tissues are removed, (3) elective irradiation of the neck lymph nodes, and (4) irradiation failures could be surgically salvaged.

The treatment intent could be either curative or palliative. Curative IMRT is used for the purpose of permanently eradicating the tumor; in this context, RT could be radical or adjuvant (i.e., postoperative). Palliative RT is designed to ameliorate a specific symptom (e.g., pain, bleeding, etc.) within incurable malignancy.

For early-stage cancer, surgery or RT alone are both effective. RT can be delivered via external beam or interstitial brachytherapy (where radiation sources are inserted into needles placed through the tumor). For intermediate- and advanced-stage cancers, possible alternative strategies are surgery followed by radiation or definitive RT, with or without chemotherapy. Unresectable cancers can be cured by RT alone or chemo-radiation. Nasopharyngeal cancers are treated only by RT or chemoradiation, reserving surgery as salvage treatment in case of failure.

Adjuvant RT is indicated when factors predicting local recurrence after surgery are present: positive resection margins when no further surgery is possible, locally advanced tumors (stage III-IV, nodal extension to level IV or V, extracapsular spread), close resection margins (<5 mm), high-grade tumors and perineural or vascular invasion [40]. In those cases, the addition of concomitant cisplatin 100 mg/m^2 each 3 weeks significantly improves the PFS at least in case of close/positive margins and/or extracapsular spread of disease.

The best evidence for estimating the risk of recurrence in the clinically negative neck comes from historical series of neck node dissections or observational follow-up. If the risk of nodal recurrence is 20% or higher, prophylactic neck treatment is recommended. Selecting the appropriate nodal levels to be treated depends on a thorough knowledge of lymph node drainage pathways of the head and neck areas as well as data from previous series of patients found to have nodal metastases when clinically N0. The choice between surgery or RT to treat the N0 neck usually depends on the treatment of the primary tumor.

When staging exams indicate lymph node involvement, the neck is treated with a neck dissection, RT, or a combination of the two. RT with or without chemotherapy can control neck disease, particularly when involved nodes are smaller than 3 cm at diagnosis. For N2 and N3 disease, particularly where nodes are 3 cm in diameter or larger, a combination of surgery and RT is recommended. Surgery followed by RT presents the advantage of obtaining fast local control of disease, useful for rapidly growing mass or in cases of skin involvement; this approach also provides definitive staging information. Anyway, postoperative RT volumes are more difficult to define with certainty. A selective neck dissection 3 months after radiation should be performed in cases of residual nodal disease. For HPV-positive OPCs, a longer follow up is required to obtain the clearance of the neck nodes after RT or chemoradiotherapy.

After neck dissection, adjuvant RT is recommended in the presence of macroscopic residual disease (e.g., nodes dissected off the carotid artery) or if two or more nodes contain tumor. Adjuvant RT should also be considered if a single involved node exceeds 3 cm in diameter. Chemotherapy can be avoided in the lack of negative pathological prognostic factors listed in ⬛ Table 43.3.

— *Side Effects*

Side effects depend on site, extent, and dose of irradiation to the head and neck areas. They may be divided into acute, when they develop during or soon after treatment, and late, if they appear months (at least >6 months) or years after RT completion. Generally, acute side effects become apparent about 2 weeks after RT start, when dysphagia, dysgeusia, xerostomia, and skin reactions may occur. Dysphagia is the main side effect that makes the course of RT difficult. In fact, when patient's nutritional and fluids oral intake becomes insufficient, causing severe weight loss, feeding tube placement is required. In cases with adequate baseline nutritional status, a reactive approach with temporary naso-gastric tube placement is preferred. On the contrary, when baseline malnutrition or dysphagia are present, or in case of extended field of RT for locally advanced disease (where dysphagia is predictable), a more stable solution, such as gastrostomy, might provide durable support.

Other RT toxicities are changes in voice caused by swelling and scarring, loss of appetite, edema, bone pain, nausea, fatigue, mouth sores. Late side effects may include xerostomia, skin fibrosis, hearing loss, hypothyroidism.

Because RT can cause tooth decay, damaged teeth may need to be removed. Therefore, prior to any RT for HNCs, patients should be examined by a dentist or oral oncologist.

— *Technical Tips*

Before starting RT, the patient undergoes a computed tomography-simulation. It consists of acquiring a computed tomography scan while the patient is positioned and immobilized in the same setting as future treatment. Therefore, the patient must be in a proper position suitable for acquiring CT images and treatment delivery, but at the same time, the patient should also be in a comfortable and reproducible position. The patient is positioned supine on the treatment couch with the head and neck supported by a neck rest, which can be customized as required to find the best position for treatment. A thermoplastic mask constructed from a cast of the patient's head has been regarded as the most accurate method for immobilizing the patient.

Conformal volume-based RT of HNCs requires knowledge of anatomy and patterns of disease spread, which are often specific to each primary tumor site and histology. Cancers in the head and neck region spread in four main ways: (1) direct extension from the primary site to adjacent structures; (2) spread through the lymphatic vessels to lymph nodes; (3) diffusion along nerves (perineural spread) to other HN areas; (4) enter blood vessels and disseminate to distant sites. In SCCHN, a spread to the lymph nodes in the neck is relatively common. When planning treatment volumes, all these dissemination pathways should be taken into account. Furthermore, surrounding critical normal structures and their own radiation sensitivity should also be delineated and may significantly influence treatment planning and/or prescribed dose.

⬛ **Table 43.3** High-risk pathologic features and relative indications for adjuvant treatment (SCC from oral cavity, oro-hypopharynx, and larynx)

Pathologic features	Indications for adjuvant treatment
AJCC Disease stage III-IV	Postoperative RT (PORT)
Level IV-V nodal extension	PORT
Perineural invasion, vascular embolism	PORT
Microscopic marginal resection (R1)	PORT + concurrent CT
Extra nodal extension	PORT + concurrent CT

A radiation therapy regimen (schedule) usually consists of a specific number of treatments given over a set time period. The standard of care in curative RT for SCCHN consists in 2-Gy daily fractions delivered 5 days a week. The standard radical dose to the primary tumor and involved nodes is 70 Gy. In the adjuvant setting, the standard dose is 60 Gy, with 66 Gy delivered on sites of positive resection margins or extranodal spread. 50 Gy prophylactic dose to uninvolved nodal levels is recommended. Improved local control and cure rates can be achieved by using altered fractionation regimens, by combining systemic agents with radiation or possibly by a combination of these approaches.

Altered fractionation regimens comprise accelerated RT, hyperfractionation, and hypofractionation. Accelerated radiation schedules shorten the overall treatment time to reduce tumor repopulation during a course of RT and theoretically increase local control and cure. Hyperfractionation schedules reduce the dose per fraction and use two fractions per day in order to reduce the risk of late effects and allow dose escalation with an improved therapeutic ratio. Hypofractionated regimens give larger doses per fraction in a shorter overall treatment time with the aim of reducing the risk of tumor repopulation at the cost of a theoretical increase in late effects.

— *Brachytherapy*

Brachytherapy is a form of RT where a sealed radiation source is placed inside or next to the neoplastic lesion, thereby concentrating the radiation dose, with a rapid dose fall-off. When expertise is available, it can be used as definitive treatment for small tumors of the lip, oral tongue, floor of mouth, buccal mucosa, and nasal vestibule. It can also be used as retreatment modality in selected cases.

— *Radiotherapic Salvage Treatment*

Despite the advances made in the primary disease setting, still up to 30–50% of all curatively treated SCCHN patients will develop a locoregional recurrence. In addition, the development of a second primary tumor in the HN region represents a constant threat for those who survive. Salvage surgery remains the standard of care for these patients, although it is feasible in only 20% of the cases, with 25% to 45% of patients experiencing long-term disease control.

Potentially curative re-irradiation, with or without concurrent chemotherapy, could be considered whenever the disease is unresectable or the patient is ineligible for surgery. In case of adverse prognostic factors, immediate postoperative (chemo-)re-irradiation after salvage surgery can be administered safely and significantly

improves locoregional control. Re-irradiation for locoregional failure or second primary tumors poses a daunting problem for radiation oncologists. Traditionally, the administration of a second course of RT to tissues within a previous radiation field has been considered unsafe and avoided due to concerns regarding toxicity. Nevertheless, when RT can be safely administered, it provides a reasonable chance of long-term survival (approximately 15–20%). Therefore, patient selection is of utmost importance. Suitable patients should have excellent performance status, no significant medical comorbidities, no severe sequelae from the previous course of radiation. Furthermore, disease-free interval from previous malignancy should be at least 1 year and the target volume as small as possible. Patient should be fully aware of the increased risk of potentially serious acute and late effects. Intensity Modulated RT (IMRT) techniques, Stereotactic Body RT (SBRT), and heavy particle therapy (proton or carbon ion-therapy) can be useful to conform more closely the dose to target volumes, to minimize the high-dose treated volume and the dose to surrounding critical structures.

43.8.3 Systemic Agents as Part of Curative Treatments

Systemic agents might be employed in the curative setting as part of: (1) induction chemotherapy (CT); (2) concomitant CT during radiation treatment; (3) adjuvant CT.

43.8.3.1 Induction Chemotherapy

The role of induction CT is still under discussion. Since the ability of induction CT to increase overall survival in SCCHN patient is not clear, its use is currently reserved only for organ preservation strategy of hypopharyngeal and laryngeal tumors [41–44]. The presently preferred induction chemotherapy regimen (TPF) comprises a combination of three drugs, docetaxel, cisplatin, and 5-fluorouracil (5FU). In previously untreated SCCHN, this combination yields major response rates approximating 70% to 90%, depending on the type of patients treated (resectable vs. unresectable) with clinical complete response rates in the 15–30% range. Induction chemotherapy could be used as part of multimodality treatment in unresectable disease and in organ preservation strategy. It may be employed also in cases of rapid tumor evolution in symptomatic patients – bleeding, reduced airway patency – when other techniques are not promptly available or whenever a tumor shrinkage could avoid a tracheostomy or a gastrostomy.

43.8.3.2 Concomitant Chemotherapy During Radiation Treatment

Several evidences support the use of concurrent CT during RT (CTRT). The meta-analysis of CT in HNC (MACH-NC) showed a 6.5% of 5-year survival benefit and better locoregional control in favor of the combined treatment over RT alone [45]. However, based on calendar age (not biological age) this advantage was shown to be less in older patients and in particular seemingly negligible in those over 70 years of age. Concurrent CTRT treatment could be used as single treatment strategy with a curative aim or as part of the postsurgical, adjuvant treatment. When employed in combination with adjuvant RT, CT indications are restricted to patient at high risk of recurrence, identified through specific pathologic features, reported in ◘ Table 43.3.

Although several drugs have been tested, either as single agent or in combination, concomitant treatments with platinum regimens represent the standard of care being more effective than other types of mono-chemotherapy [45]. Cisplatin 100 mg/m^2 q3weeks is considered the standard of care in association to RT. The 3-weekly cisplatin schedule seems preferable to weekly cisplatin, since it resulted in a significantly better locoregional control (but without overall survival benefit) in a randomized controlled trial comparing the 3-weekly high-dose with a weekly rather low dose of 30 mg/m^2, albeit at the cost of increased toxicitiy [46]. The total cumulative dose of the drug has a significant positive correlation with survival; efforts should be aimed to reach at least a dose of 200 mg/m^2 throughout the course of radiotherapy [47].

In case of absolute contraindications to cisplatin (e.g., impaired renal function, inability to sustain high infusion volume due to cardiac pathology, severe hearing loss, and neuropathy), alternatives are available [48]. Carboplatin is generally tolerated better than cisplatin, but it is also less effective. Cetuximab, a monoclonal antibody targeting EGFR, has proved to increase RT performance (cetuximab+RT OS 49 months vs. RT 29.3 months) [49], although cetuximab added to platinum-based RT was not superior to standard platinum-based RT. [50]

43.8.3.3 Adjuvant Chemotherapy

There is no clear evidence of a benefit from adding adjuvant chemotherapy to locoregional treatment [45]; hence, it should not be used in clinical practice.

43.8.4 Supportive Care During Radiation Treatment

HNC treatment can cause a wide spectrum of disabling toxicities. The addition of cisplatin to RT in CTRT enhances both the therapeutic effect and the toxicities.

In the curative setting, it is of paramount importance to avoid RT breaks and treatment suspensions as they could negatively affect outcomes. For this reason, a supportive care program should be planned before treatment start, helping patient to overcome side effects.

First, patients should be encouraged to quit smoking and to reduce alcohol consumption. In fact, these habits may decrease treatment efficacy and increase treatment-related side effects [51]. Behavioral counseling combined with medications to support smoking cessation could be helpful.

Before treatment start, all patients should perform a thorough assessment of nutritional and dental status. Any dental condition at risk of complications must be managed so as not to create complications that could interrupt RT and to reduce the risk of long-term complications. Dental care after RT requires special attention. Fluoride treatments can help to decrease caries incidence. Long-term maintenance of oral hygiene should be initiated in conjunction with cancer treatment [52].

While most HNC patients are already nutritionally compromised because of their disease and/or their unhealthy life-style habits, RT toxicity, such as mucositis, may cause further difficulties in eating. Thus, patients should receive dietary counseling and be evaluated for nutritional risks before treatment start to select those requiring prophylactic gastric tube placement and those to monitor closely during treatment for the need of temporary nasogastric tube feeding interventions. Prophylactic feeding tube placement should be considered in cases of severe weight loss prior to treatment (i.e., 5% weight loss over prior month; 10% weight loss over 6 months), in patients with ongoing dysphagia, those with severe aspiration, or patients in whom long-term swallowing disorders are expected [53, 54].

Baseline assessment by a speech or language therapist should be undertaken and appropriate interventions organized to maintain functions before treatment starts. This may be beneficial in case of aspiration or risk that the treatment itself induces dysphagia problems or complications, such as aspiration pneumonia. Severe swallowing impairment is hardly rehabilitated. In those patients, gastrostomy should be considered.

Here, we will briefly focus on frequent acute side effects occurring during initial treatment.

Xerostomia is usually a late RT side effect but changes in saliva quantity and composition can occur shortly after RT start (1–2 weeks). The best way to minimize salivary gland toxicity is to use highly conformal RT techniques, avoiding unnecessary RT dose to sensitive targets, such as parotid glands. Patients should drink adequate amounts of fluids, rinse and gargle with a weak salt solution or baking soda several times daily during treatment.

Mucositis occurs in nearly all patients receiving head and neck RT. Multinational Association of Supportive Care (MASCC, ▶ http://www.mascc.org) guidelines suggest the use of oral zinc supplements to prevent mucositis in patients receiving radiation or chemoradiation for oral cancer, while the use of benzydamine mouthwash is recommended only in patients receiving moderate radiation doses (up to 50 Gy) without concomitant chemotherapy. Although there is evidence that low-level laser therapy might be beneficial for the prevention of oral mucositis during RT, this expensive technology requires daily treatment and its use is scarce [55]. Mucositis is managed symptomatically with scrupulous oral hygiene (excluding alcohol-containing mouthwashes), dietary modifications, and pain control. Acidic and spicy foods, sharp foods, caffeine, and alcohol consumption should be avoided. Mucosal superinfections by bacterial, fungal, and viral agents should be treated with appropriate therapy. Pain may be significant during and shortly after the course of RT and therefore it should be treated adequately. 0.2% morphine mouthwash may be effective to treat pain due to oral mucositis during CTRT [55], while transdermal fentanyl is an option for dysphagic patients. In some cases, a nasogastric tube placement is necessary to prevent weight loss.

Radiation dermatitis in the treatment field is common during RT and it occurs within the first 4 weeks of treatment. Patients should be instructed about the harm of exposure to potential chemical irritants or to direct sunlight without adequate protection. Hygienic routine should be carried out with water and mild soap/shampoo gentle washing [56]. Beyond that, there is little evidence to support the use of one topical approach over another [57]. Topical products should not be applied shortly before radiation because they can cause a bolus effect, thereby artificially increasing the radiation dose to the epidermis. Prophylactic topical steroids could be used to reduce discomfort or burning and itching [56].

Dysgeusia is an abnormal or impaired sense of taste and it may contribute to nutritional difficulties and weight loss. Pharmacologic intervention using zinc supplementation or amifostine have not shown consistent benefit; however, dietary counseling may be of value [58].

Cisplatin toxicity. As previously mentioned, cisplatin is the chemotherapeutic drug most frequently used in combination to RT. High cisplatin doses can cause neuropathy, nephrotoxicity, and ototoxicity. Conventional audiometry may be used to detect and monitor hearing impairment. Before using cisplatin, it is important to assess patient's baseline renal function by calculating or measuring urinary creatinine clearance and consider all the potential nephrotoxic comorbidities (e.g., uncontrolled hypertension, diabetes, etc.) and drugs in use.

Electrolytes should be frequently monitored, as hypomagnesemia or other urinary wasting syndromes can occur requiring prompt correction. The administration of intravenous saline with magnesium supplementation is the primary approach for preventing cisplatin-induced nephrotoxicity and must be adopted in all patients treated with cisplatin [59].

Pain is experienced frequently and it could be related to the cancer itself and also to treatment toxicities, such as mucositis, inflammation, superinfection and scarring from surgery, or other treatments. Adequate pain management is mandatory and often requires opioid drugs.

Anxiety and depression are common in patients treated for head and neck cancer, and these symptoms can have a significant negative impact on quality of life. Psychological support and antidepressant drugs should be employed as needed.

43.9 Principle for Curative Treatment of Specific Subsite Tumor

43.9.1 Oral Cavity

Surgery is the first-line treatment for oral SCC. Each surgical procedure, together with adjuvant therapies, should be tailored according to the specific risk profile of every single patient. This is especially true considering tumors involving the mobile tongue/floor of the mouth, with the aim to precisely balance surgical invasiveness, functional results, and oncologic outcomes.

Early tumors, with minimal depth of invasion (less than 4 mm) and no clinical and radiologic evidence of lateral neck metastasis, can be considered as low-risk diseases and should be managed by a unimodal treatment (i.e., surgery alone). Transoral resection can adequately remove the entire disease with wide free surgical margins of at least 1 cm from the visible border of the lesion itself, leaving only minimal or null functional impairment with no impacting on speech and swallowing. Complex reconstructive techniques, such as pedicled or free flaps, are rarely required in these cases even if, in some instances, local mucosal flaps may speed up and help the healing process, thereby improving functional outcomes. In situations where the depth of infiltration is greater than 4 mm, most studies agree on the indication for a prophylactic selective (levels I to III) lateral neck dissection due to the high risk of occult (subclinical) nodal metastases.

Locally advanced tumors characterized by a higher depth of invasion (greater than 1 cm) usually require more aggressive surgical approaches, followed by adjuvant radiotherapy, alone or in combination with chemotherapy. The recently proposed concept of tongue compartmental surgery [60] aims at removing the entire tumor-containing anatomic compartment (i.e., hemi-tongue and ipsilateral floor of the mouth) via a pull-through transoral-transcervical approach, with or without mandibulectomy, in continuity with the T-N tract and the draining lymph nodes (levels I to V). After resection, the separation between oral cavity and the neck is restored using microvascular free flaps or pedi-cled flaps as a second-line option. This approach effectively closes the surgical defect, while granting a sufficient volume to restore function of the resected hemi-tongue. High-risk histopathological features as an advanced local extension or microscopically positive – inadequate surgical margins are the primary indications for adju-vant treatment. Similarly, a significant nodal burden and extranodal extension are associated with an increased risk of regional recurrence that can be adequately man-aged by postoperative (chemo)-radiotherapy.

In summary, while the low-risk disease may be ade-quately managed with a unimodal treatment, high-risk tumors should be handled in a multimodal manner (i.e., surgery + (chemo)-radiotherapy).

43.9.2 Larynx

TLM (or, in some cases, TORS) is the treatment of choice in case of early-intermediate neoplasms, shifting to open partial laryngectomies and total laryngectomy in more advanced tumors. Elective neck dissection is fre-quently considered for supraglottic and advanced glottic carcinoma.

For early laryngeal cancer (T1 and T2), TLM and radiotherapy showed comparable results in terms of survival outcomes. Concerning vocal outcome, while no consistent data are available, radiotherapy seems to induce better results in selected subgroups of patients (T1b). However, TLM has the advantage to be a quick, cost-effective, minimally invasive, and repeatable treat-ment, with a high success rate especially in early neo-plasms (T1 and superficially spreading T2). This is particularly true when it is compared with the lengthy treatment course and the significantly lower chances of organ preservation in case of disease relapse when radio-therapy is the first treatment delivered.

Concerning intermediate tumors (bulky T2 and T3), the choice between possible treatment options is even more extensive. TLM offers good results in terms of functional and oncologic outcomes in T2 and selected T3 tumors when performed in experienced centers. However, open partial laryngectomies represent the most frequently applied surgical approach for these dis-eases. Supraglottic, supracricoid, and supratracheal lar-yngectomies (type I, II, and III according to the

European Laryngological Society classification) can effectively address endolaryngeal tumors (T3) with at least one uninvolved cricoarytenoid unit, and even early T4a with a limited anterior extralaryngeal extension. In these procedures, patient selection is crucial: pulmonary and cardiac functions should be carefully assessed, since unfit patients may not tolerate the resulting degree of chronic subclinical aspiration. Furthermore, non-surgical organ preservation strategies (i.e., induction chemo plus radiation in responding patients) play a piv-otal role in selected T3 (glottic site; mobile vocal cords) and should always be considered before resorting to a total laryngectomy. On the other hand, their use in T4 lesions has been demonstrated to carry to an unfavor-able locoregional control with dismal organ preserva-tion rates [61, 62].

Total laryngectomy followed by adjuvant therapy proved to be the most effective treatment for laryngeal cancers with extensive cartilage infiltration or diffuse extralaryngeal invasion. This procedure consists of the complete removal of the larynx with associated prelar-yngeal strap muscles and results in a permanent trache-ostomy. While swallowing frequently returns to normality after the end of the healing process (10–15 days), speech ability is impaired and voice can be restored with a variety of technical and surgical approaches (e.g., external devices, tracheoesophageal puncture with placement of a voice prosthesis) [63].

43.9.3 Oropharynx

Oropharyngeal cancer has been classically considered as a primarily non-surgical neoplasm due to its remarkable radio- and chemosensitivity and to the invasiveness of conventional (transmandibular) surgical approaches. Therefore, open surgical resection and reconstruction are usually reserved for persistent/recurrent tumors after (chemo)-radiotherapy or locally advanced tumors that need a multimodal treatment to achieve a reasonable chance of cure [i.e., surgery + (chemo)-radiotherapy]. However, recent technical developments such as TLM and TORS led to an expansion of minimally invasive procedures for early-stage neoplasms. This is also related to the recent epidemics of HPV-related tumors, resulting in an increased incidence among young (40- and 50-year-old), healthy subjects with less or no alcoholic/tobacco abuse history if compared to the "classic" 60 and 70-year-old head and neck cancer population. The higher curative rates and longer life-span after treatment of this new type of HNC patients shifted the balance between oncologic outcomes and post-treatment sequelae toward the latter, opening a discussion regard-ing the role of TORS (and transoral surgery in general) as an alternative to (chemo)-radiotherapy, at least in selected cases. While randomized trials comparing minimally invasive surgery with (chemo)-radiotherapy are still ongoing in HPV-positive OPC, there is some limited evidence that surgery may grant better functional outcomes for early disease, still maintaining high chances of cure. However, it is crucial to weight each approach according to a careful pretreatment staging to avoid overtreatment (surgery + chemoradiotherapy) in patients that could have been successfully treated by a less aggressive strategy (chemo-radiotherapy or surgery alone). In this view, evaluation of the primary lesion should take into account its pattern of infiltration in order to avoid unexpected postoperative margins positivity or involvement of functionally essential structures (bilateral lingual vessels or hypoglossal nerves). Lateral neck metastasis should also be carefully assessed to exclude bilateral involvement or extranodal extension before embarking on a primary surgical approach.

43.9.4 Hypopharynx

The surgical principles for treatment of hypopharyngeal cancer are strictly related to its aggressive biologic behavior with frequent laryngeal involvement. Most of these tumors are diagnosed in late stages (III-IV). A diffuse field of cancerization with multiple neoplastic foci and a significant submucosal spread, associated to multiple lymph nodes metastases, represent the typical clinical scenario of hypopharyngeal carcinoma, resulting in the need for extensive resections even in presence of relatively small primary tumors. Therefore, conservative surgical approaches, such as TLM, TORS, or open partial hypopharyngectomies, are only exceptionally employed. Considering early and intermediate tumors, (chemo)-radiotherapy often offers the more favorable balance between adverse effects and oncologic results [64]. In these cases, surgery is generally a salvage option, with minimal chances of organ preservation.

On the other hand, hypopharyngolaryngectomy is a viable option for advanced tumors and those not responding to induction chemotherapy. This is always associated with an elective or therapeutic lateral neck dissection in consideration of the advanced stage of the disease and the high frequency of nodal metastasis. Functional results are comparable with those obtained after total laryngectomy alone, but resection of the hypopharyngeal mucosa results more frequently than not in the need for complex reconstructive techniques (pedicled or free flaps) that significantly increase the operative times and the risk for postoperative complications.

43.10 General Principles for HNC Palliative Treatment

Approximately one third of SCCHN patients are diagnosed with early stage disease (T1-2, N0) with excellent prognosis. On the contrary, overall survival for late stage patients is poor, with 40–50% of them alive after 5 years. Distant metastases usually involve the lung. Recurrent/metastatic SCCHN prognosis is dismal; median OS from standard first-line therapy is about 10 months, with only 20% of patients alive after 2 years [65].

The presence of a locoregional recurrence poses significant challenges that require the ability to anticipate as much as possible the issues correlated with the natural disease evolution. Therefore, foreseeing patient's needs and tailoring therapeutic intervention accordingly is crucial for maintaining adequate quality of life. An example of such process is represented by the regular assessment of airway patency and nutritional status. These areas are of paramount importance and frequent evaluations are mandatory. Risk of bleeding by recurrent lesions close or involving the blood vessels of the neck is another relevant medical issue. Hemorrhage might be lethal and rarely anticipated, although a prior hemorrhagic episode is an important "red flag" signaling the potential risk of major complication. Discussion with the patient over invasive procedures, such as gastrostomy and tracheostomy, are recommended, especially considering residual prognosis.

43.10.1 Radiotherapy: Palliative Treatment

Palliative RT may provide control of local symptoms, such as pain. It is indicated in cases when a curative approach is not feasible due to disease characteristics or patients' comorbidities. Palliative RT to the primary tumor could also be useful when metastases are present at diagnosis, or in locally recurrent disease to ameliorate fungating tumor or reduce bleeding.

43.10.2 Systemic Treatment

First-line treatment for recurrent/metastatic SCCHN is an evolving field. For almost a decade, standard first-line treatment for recurrent/metastatic SCCHN has been a combination of a cisplatin, 5FU, and cetuximab [65]. In clinical trial setting, this regimen registered an overall response rate of 36% with a median OS of 10 months. Nevertheless, suboptimal performance status, frequent cardiovascular conditions and anticipated toxicities reduce the proportion of patients susceptible to such combination. Therefore, alternatives, such as two-drug combination without 5FU or three drug regimens with the introduction of paclitaxel (response rate >50%) in spite of 5FU, could be used [66].

Very recently, data from a phase III trial with pembrolizumab in first-line treatment changed the scenario in this setting. The study evaluated pembrolizumab alone or in combination with platinum and 5FU against the SoC (cetuximab-platinum - 5FU combination). Pembrolizumab combined with chemotherapy showed a benefit over SoC in OS in patients with a programmed cell death ligand 1 (PD-L1) combined positive score (CPS) ≥ 20 (median 14.7 months vs. 11.0 months, HR 0.60, 95% CI, 0.45 to 0.82, $P = 0.0004$), CPS ≥ 1 (median 13.6 months vs. 10.4 months, HR 0.65, 95% CI, 0.53 to 0.80, $P < 0.0001$), and in total population. Furthermore, pembrolizumab alone proved to be superior to SoC in the CPS ≥ 20 and CPS ≥ 1 population [67]. Interestingly, the overall response rate was lower for pembrolizumab alone in comparison to the combination of pembrolizumab and chemotherapy. Overall, these data support the use of pembrolizumab, alone or in combination with chemotherapy, as a new SoC in first-line setting for CPS ≥ 1 recurrent/metastatic SCCHN.

The choice of which first-line treatment to deliver to which patient should be informed by the following factors: (1) CPS score; (2) the urgency of a clinical response. For example, an asymptomatic patient with high CPS could be proposed with a chemo-free scheme. On the other hand, a symptomatic, CPS low patient in need for a rapid clinical benefit should be proposed with a treatment that includes chemotherapy in order to obtain higher chance of response.

Platinum-resistant disease, defined as persistent or recurrent tumor within the 6 months after curative therapy with platinum-based agents, is an aggressive disease with a worse prognosis.

Second-line treatment armamentarium for recurrent/metastatic SCCHN includes immunotherapy as well [68]. A randomized trial compared nivolumab to systemic chemotherapy, showed for the first time a significantly prolonged survival of immunotherapy in this subset of patients (7.5 months vs. 5.1 months, HR 0.70; 97.73% CI, 0.51 to 0.96; $P = 0.01$) [69]. Also pembrolizumab demonstrated a benefit in OS compared to standard chemotherapy (8.4 months vs. 6.9 months; HR: 0.80; 95% CI, 0.65 to 0.98; $P = 0.016$) [70].

However, more than 50% of patients do not receive a second-line treatment, and the expected response rate is low (less than 10% with chemotherapy, 13% immunotherapy). Performance status is the main factor that drives treatment choices. However, more than 50% of patients do not receive a second line treatment and in fact half of them cannot receive this because of a poor general condition [71]. Therefore, a multiprofessional balanced care is mandatory in this disease setting with symptomatic progression.

Case Study Oral Lesion

Man, 68 years old.
- *Family history* negative for malignancy.
- *Comorbidities:* Diabetes mellitus type II, chronic atrial fibrillation, active smoker (20 pack/year), and alcohol consumption (3 drinks per day).
- *Recent history:* Long history of oral leukoplakia, occasional surgical removal with negative histological examination. For nearly 2 months, pain located under dental prosthesis.
- *Objective examination:* painful ulcerated area on the mucosal surface of left mandibular gum. Infracentimetric palpable node at level IIa.
- *Blood tests:* Hb 12,1 g/dl; regular biochemistry.

43

Question

What action should be taken?
(1) Surgery (2) Biopsy (3) Other

Answer

Transoral biopsy under local anesthesia
   Histological examination:
   SCC G1 in a field of high-grade dysplasia.

Question

What radiological exams should be performed?
(1) FDG-PET. (2) Head and neck MRI. (3) EGDS

Answer

FDG-PET and MRI.

   Findings: local lesion at left inferior mandibular mucosa with contrast enhancement and FDG uptake diffuse to left mouth floor, no clear signs of bone invasion. Borderline lymph node at left level IIa.

Question

What action should be taken?
(1) Surgery + adjuvant therapy. (2) Induction chemotherapy + RT. (3) Brachytherapy

Answer

→ Compartmental local surgery with bilateral neck dissection. Tumor pathological stage: pT4a (floor of the mouth invasion) pN3b (1/22 ECS positive lymph node) according to AJCC VIII edition.

→ Adjuvant therapy with IMRT plus three high-dose of cisplatin

- Adequate presurgical staging and postsurgical staging with latest TNM
- The importance of adjuvant therapy
- Importance of multidisciplinary management

Case Study Neck Mass

Man, 56 years old
- *Family history* negative for malignancy
- *Comorbidities*: Negative, smoking history (10 packs/year)
- *Recent history*: Asymptomatic slowly growing left neck mass
- *Blood tests*: No abnormalities
- *Objective examination*: No signs of malignancy in the ENT region, both in transoral and fibroscopic NBI/with light examination. Neck mass at the III level.

Question

What action should be taken?
    (1) Surgery. (2) Biopsy. 3) Staging

Answer

Node biopsy, preferable under US: SCC G3, research of HPV and EBV is mandatory. In this case, p16 IHC/HPV DNA was positive.
    Local MRI and whole body FDG PET: confirm left neck cystic adenopathy, 3.5 cm, without clear primitive lesion. No distant lesion.

General anesthesia with oropharyngeal (bilateral tonsils and base of the tongue) biopsy: negative for malignancy.
    AJCC TNM VIII edition: TxN1M0, stage I

Question

What action should be taken?
    (1) Surgery. (2) Induction chemotherapy. (3) Chemo-radiotherapy

Answer:

Chemoradiation with IMRT delivered with radical intent on oropharynx and bilateral neck combined with 3-weekly cisplatin.

Key Points

- HPV and EBV assessment to guide diagnosis and therapy.
- Supportive care in order to complete curative treatment.

Expert Opinion

Jan B. Vermorken

Faculty of Medicine and Health Sciences, University of Antwerp, Antwerp, and Department of Medical Oncology, Antwerp University Hospital, Edegem, Belgium.

A synthetic and schematic description of head and neck cancers (HNCs), due to their heterogeneity is not simple: primitive sites or origin, stage and presence of comorbidities influence the diagnostic process and the therapeutic course. Otherwise, it has been seen that HNCs share lots of risk factors such as smoking, alcohol consumption, HPV infection, or genetic predisposition. Primary prevention is essential to avoid the onset of HNCs, and as a result smoking should be avoided and so the alcohol consump-

tion which has a well-known synergic action with smoke. As other tumours, early diagnosis is essential to provide a radical and non-invasive treatment. Prognosis is very poor in case of advanced stage or metastases: in this setting of patients palliative cares are crucial in order to guarantee a good quality of life; furthermore is relevant to remember the importance of toxicities during the various treatments which can be used: in these situations a multimodal approach is the best option. Nowadays, hopes rely on immunotherapy as it can determine a better OS and PFS in this setting of patients in case of the need of a second-line therapy, so enrolment in clinical trails is encouraged.

1. Head and neck cancers (HNCs) are a group of heterogeneous neoplasms arising from epithelial tissue of the upper aerodigestive regions. They share almost

the same risk factors such as smoking, alcohol consumption, HPV infection, and previous HNCs.

2. Symptoms can be quite characteristic in dependence of the primary site of origin: it is possible to observe dysphagia, pharyngodynia, dysphagia, dysphonia, enlarged lymph nodes, persistent ulcerations, leukoplakia, or erithroplakia.

3. Clinical history and physical examination are useful approaches in order to understand site and features of HNCs. Obviously lots of imaging investigations can be employed such as US, CT, MRI, PET-FDG/CT or techniques such fibro or video laryngoscopes with the eventual use of the narrow band imaging (NBI). In case of occult neoplasm and lymph nodes enlargement, a FNA can be evaluated to determine the origin site of HNC.

4. The most frequent histologic subtype is the classic squamous carcinoma and its variants; other types are the neuroendocrine neoplasms of the larynx, which are the most common nonsquamous tumors in this region.

5. New therapeutic techniques have changed the clinical approach to HNCs: a multimodal approach must be considered in order to guarantee the best therapeutic options; so surgery and radiotherapy (RT), alone or combined, are regarded as curative treatments; chemotherapy has today the role to improve radiation effects. Obviously, the different approaches depend on the site of origin and the stage of each patient; chemotherapy can be used in three different scenarios: induction, concomitant with RT, or adjuvant approach. Otherwise, an assessment of patient's conditions before and after treatments is essential to avoid or control complications such as swallowing disorders.

6. After curative treatments, follow-up strategies must be adopted; in case of incurable disease, periodic evaluations are generally used to understand the effect of therapy or cancer progression. In this peculiar setting, palliative care should be considered.

Recommendations

ESMO
- ▶ www.esmo.org/Guidelines/Head-and-Neck-Cancers/Squamous-Cell-Carcinoma-of-the-Head-and-Neck

ASCO
- ▶ www.asco.org/practice-guidelines/quality-guidelines/guidelines/head-and-neck-cancer#/34961
- ▶ www.asco.org/practice-guidelines/quality-guidelines/guidelines/head-and-neck-cancer#/32806
- ▶ www.asco.org/practice-guidelines/quality-guidelines/guidelines/head-and-neck-cancer#/28176

AIOM
- ▶ https://www.aiom.it/linee-guida-aiom-tumori-della-testa-e-del-collo/

Hints for a Deeper Insight
- The potential for liquid biopsies in head and neck cancer: ▶ https://www.ncbi.nlm.nih.gov/pubmed/29906408
- Experiences of psychological flow as described by people diagnosed with and treated for head and neck cancer: ▶ https://www.ncbi.nlm.nih.gov/pubmed/31622871
- The emerging use of immune checkpoint blockade in the adjuvant setting for solid tumors: a review: ▶ https://www.ncbi.nlm.nih.gov/pubmed/31621445
- Immunotherapy for head and neck cancer : Highlights of the 2019 ASCO Annual Meeting: ▶ https://www.ncbi.nlm.nih.gov/pubmed/31612261

References

1. Gatta G, van der Zwan JM, Casali PG, et al. Rare cancers are not so rare: the rare cancer burden in Europe. Eur J Cancer. 2011;47(17):2493–511. https://doi.org/10.1016/j.ejca.2011.08.008.
2. Ferlay J, Soerjomataram I, Dikshit R, et al. Cancer incidence and mortality worldwide: sources, methods and major patterns in GLOBOCAN 2012. Int J Cancer. 2015;136(5):E359–86. https://doi.org/10.1002/ijc.29210.
3. Siegel RL, Miller KD, Jemal A. Cancer statistics, 2018. CA Cancer J Clin. 2018;68(1):7–30. https://doi.org/10.3322/caac.21442.
4. Poo DCC. Explicit representation of business policies. In: Proceedings - 1998 Asia Pacific software engineering conference, APSEC 1998. Vol 1998-Decem; 1998. p. 136–43. https://doi.org/10.1200/JCO.2013.50.3870.
5. Chaturvedi AK, D'Souza G, Gillison ML, Katki HA. Burden of HPV-positive oropharynx cancers among ever and never smokers in the U.S. population. Oral Oncol. 2016;60 https://doi.org/10.1016/j.oraloncology.2016.06.006.
6. Gatta G, Botta L, Sánchez MJ, et al. Prognoses and improvement for head and neck cancers diagnosed in Europe in early 2000s: the EUROCARE-5 population-based study. Eur J Cancer. 2015;51(15):2130–43. https://doi.org/10.1016/j.ejca.2015.07.043.

7. Talamini R, Bosetti C, La Vecchia C, et al. Combined effect of tobacco and alcohol on laryngeal cancer risk: a case-control study. Cancer Causes Control. 2002;13(10):957–64. http://www.ncbi.nlm.nih.gov/pubmed/12588092. Accessed 5 June 2018.

8. Boakye EA, Buchanan P, Hinyard L, Osazuwa-Peters N, Schootman M, Piccirillo JF. Incidence and risk of second primary malignant neoplasm after a first head and neck squamous cell carcinoma. JAMA Otolaryngol - Head Neck Surg. 2018; 144(8):727–37. https://doi.org/10.1001/jamaoto.2018.0993.

9. Gillison ML, Koch WM, Capone RB, et al. Evidence for a causal association between human papillomavirus and a subset of head and neck cancers. J Natl Cancer Inst. 2000;92(9):709–20. http://www.ncbi.nlm.nih.gov/pubmed/10793107

10. Gillison MLMLML, Restighini C. Anticipation of the impact of human papillomavirus on clinical decision making for the head and neck cancer patient. Hematol Oncol Clin North Am. 2015;29:1045–60. https://doi.org/10.1016/j.hoc.2015.08.003.

11. El-Mofty SK, Patil S. Human papillomavirus (HPV)-related oropharyngeal nonkeratinizing squamous cell carcinoma: characterization of a distinct phenotype. Oral Surg Oral Med Oral Pathol Oral Radiol Endodontol. 2006;101(3):339–45. https://doi.org/10.1016/j.tripleo.2005.08.001.

12. Huang SH, Perez-Ordonez B, Liu FF, et al. Atypical clinical behavior of p16-confirmed HPV-related oropharyngeal squamous cell carcinoma treated with radical radiotherapy. Int J Radiat Oncol Biol Phys. 2012;82(1):276–83. https://doi.org/10.1016/j.ijrobp.2010.08.031.

13. Guha N, Warnakulasuriya S, Vlaanderen J, Straif K. Betel quid chewing and the risk of oral and oropharyngeal cancers: a meta-analysis with implications for cancer control. Int J Cancer. 2014;135(6):1433–43. https://doi.org/10.1002/ijc.28643.

14. Chuang S-C, Jenab M, Heck JE, et al. Diet and the risk of head and neck cancer: a pooled analysis in the INHANCE consortium. Cancer Causes Control. 2012;23(1):69–88. https://doi.org/10.1007/s10552-011-9857-x.

15. Huang SH, O'Sullivan B. Overview of the 8th edition TNM classification for head and neck cancer. Curr Treat Options in Oncol. 2017;18(7):40. https://doi.org/10.1007/s11864-017-0484-y.

16. Michaels L, Hellquist HB. Malignant neoplasms of surface epithelium. In: Ear, nose and throat histopathology. London: Springer London; 2001. p. 186–91. https://doi.org/10.1007/978-1-4471-0235-9_16.

17. Mascharak S, Baird BJ, Holsinger FC. Detecting oropharyngeal carcinoma using multispectral, narrow-band imaging and machine learning. Laryngoscope. 2018; https://doi.org/10.1002/lary.27159.

18. Piazza C, Cocco D, Del Bon F, et al. Narrow band imaging and high definition television in evaluation of oral and oropharyngeal squamous cell cancer: a prospective study. Oral Oncol. 2010;46(4):307–10. https://doi.org/10.1016/j.oraloncology.2010.01.020.

19. Michaels L, Hellquist HB. Normal anatomy and histology. In: Ear, nose and throat histopathology. London: Springer London; 2001. p. 303–17. https://doi.org/10.1007/978-1-4471-0235-9_28.

20. Iocca O, Sollecito TP, Alawi F, et al. Potentially malignant disorders of the oral cavity and oral dysplasia: a systematic review and meta-analysis of malignant transformation rate by subtype. Head Neck. 2019; https://doi.org/10.1002/hed.26006.

21. Villa A, Villa C, Abati S. Oral cancer and oral erythroplakia: an update and implication for clinicians. Aust Dent J. 2011;56(3):253–6. https://doi.org/10.1111/j.1834-7819.2011.01337.x.

22. Yardimci G. Precancerous lesions of oral mucosa. World J Clin Cases. 2014;2(12):866. https://doi.org/10.12998/wjcc.v2.i12.866.

23. Mello FW, Miguel AFP, Dutra KL, et al. Prevalence of oral potentially malignant disorders: a systematic review and meta-analysis. J Oral Pathol Med. 2018; https://doi.org/10.1111/jop.12726.

24. Fizazi K, Greco FA, Pavlidis N, et al. Cancers of unknown primary site: ESMO clinical practice guidelines for diagnosis, treatment and follow-up. Ann Oncol. 2015;26(suppl 5):v133–8. https://doi.org/10.1093/annonc/mdv305.

25. Fu TS, Foreman A, Goldstein DP, de Almeida JR. The role of transoral robotic surgery, transoral laser microsurgery, and lingual tonsillectomy in the identification of head and neck squamous cell carcinoma of unknown primary origin: a systematic review. J Otolaryngol Head Neck Surg. 2016;45(1):28. https://doi.org/10.1186/s40463-016-0142-6.

26. Brocklehurst P, Kujan O, O'Malley LA, Ogden G, Shepherd S, Glenny A-M. Screening programmes for the early detection and prevention of oral cancer. Cochrane Database Syst Rev. 2013;11:CD004150. https://doi.org/10.1002/14651858.CD004150.pub4.

27. Adel K El-Naggar, John KC Chan, Jennifer R Grandis, Takashi Takata PJS. The 4th edition of the World Health Organization classification of head and neck tumours.; 2017.

28. Lewis-Jones H, Colley S, Gibson D. Imaging in head and neck cancer: United Kingdom National Multidisciplinary Guidelines. J Laryngol Otol. 2016;130(S2):S28–31. https://doi.org/10.1017/S0022215116000396.

29. Tshering Vogel DW, Thoeny HC. Cross-sectional imaging in cancers of the head and neck: how we review and report. Cancer Imaging. 2016;16(1):20. https://doi.org/10.1186/s40644-016-0075-3.

30. Abraham J. Imaging for head and neck cancer. Surg Oncol Clin N Am. 2015;24(3):455–71. https://doi.org/10.1016/j.soc.2015.03.012.

31. Yamazaki Y, Saitoh M, Notani K, et al. Assessment of cervical lymph node metastases using FDG-PET in patients with head and neck cancer. Ann Nucl Med. 2008;22(3):177–84. https://doi.org/10.1007/s12149-007-0097-9.

32. Lydiatt WM, Patel SG, O'Sullivan B, et al. Head and neck cancers-major changes in the American Joint Committee on cancer eighth edition cancer staging manual. CA Cancer J Clin. 2017;67(2):122–37. https://doi.org/10.3322/caac.21389.

33. Robbins KT, Shaha AR, Medina JE, et al. Consensus statement on the classification and terminology of neck dissection. Arch Otolaryngol Neck Surg. 2008;134(5):536. https://doi.org/10.1001/archotol.134.5.536.

34. Licitra L, Keilholz U, Tahara M, et al. Evaluation of the benefit and use of multidisciplinary teams in the treatment of head and neck cancer. Oral Oncol. 2016;59:73–9. https://doi.org/10.1016/j.oraloncology.2016.06.002.

35. Vermorken JB. Multidisciplinary decision making and head and neck tumor boards. In: Critical issues in head and neck oncology. Key concepts from the fifth THNO meeting; 2017. p. 99–108.

36. Gorphe P. A contemporary review of evidence for Transoral robotic surgery in laryngeal cancer. Front Oncol. 2018;8:121. https://doi.org/10.3389/fonc.2018.00121.

37. Castelnuovo P, Battaglia P, Turri-Zanoni M, et al. Endoscopic endonasal surgery for malignancies of the anterior cranial base. World Neurosurg. 2014;82(6):S22–31. https://doi.org/10.1016/j.wneu.2014.07.021.

38. Sakuraba M, Miyamoto S, Kimata Y, et al. Recent advances in reconstructive surgery: head and neck reconstruction. Int J Clin Oncol. 2013;18(4):561–5. https://doi.org/10.1007/s10147-012-0513-6.

39. Lee N, Puri DR, Blanco AI, Chao KSC. Intensity-modulated radiation therapy in head and neck cancers: an update. Head Neck. 2007;29(4):387–400. https://doi.org/10.1002/hed.20332.

40. Bernier J, Cooper JS, Pajak TF, et al. Defining risk levels in locally advanced head and neck cancers: a comparative analysis of concurrent postoperative radiation plus chemotherapy trials of the EORTC (#22931) and RTOG (# 9501). Head Neck. 2005;27(10):843–50. https://doi.org/10.1002/hed.20279.

41. Hitt R, Grau JJ, López-Pousa A, et al. A randomized phase III trial comparing induction chemotherapy followed by chemoradiotherapy versus chemoradiotherapy alone as treatment of unresectable head and neck cancer. Ann Oncol. 2014;25(1):216–25. https://doi.org/10.1093/annonc/mdt461.

42. Haddad R, O'Neill A, Rabinowits G, et al. Induction chemotherapy followed by concurrent chemoradiotherapy (sequential chemoradiotherapy) versus concurrent chemoradiotherapy alone in locally advanced head and neck cancer (PARADIGM): a randomised phase 3 trial. Lancet Oncol. 2013;14(3):257–64. https://doi.org/10.1016/S1470-2045(13)70011-1.

43. Zhong L, Zhang C, Ren G, et al. Randomized phase III trial of induction chemotherapy with docetaxel, cisplatin, and fluorouracil followed by surgery versus up-front surgery in locally advanced resectable oral squamous cell carcinoma. J Clin Oncol. 2013;31(6):744–51. https://doi.org/10.1200/JCO.2012.43.8820.

44. Lefebvre JL, Pointreau Y, Rolland F, et al. Induction chemotherapy followed by either chemoradiotherapy or bioradiotherapy for larynx preservation: the TREMPLIN randomized phase II study. J Clin Oncol. 2013;31(7):853–9. https://doi.org/10.1200/JCO.2012.42.3988.

45. Pignon J-P, le Maître A, Maillard E, Bourhis J, MACH-NC Collaborative Group. Meta-analysis of chemotherapy in head and neck cancer (MACH-NC): an update on 93 randomised trials and 17,346 patients. Radiother Oncol. 2009;92(1):4–14. https://doi.org/10.1016/j.radonc.2009.04.014.

46. Noronha V, Joshi A, Patil VM, et al. Once-a-week versus once-every-3-weeks cisplatin chemoradiation for locally advanced head and neck cancer: a phase III randomized noninferiority trial. J Clin Oncol. 2018;36(11):1064–72. https://doi.org/10.1200/JCO.2017.74.9457.

47. Strojan P, Vermorken JB, Beitler JJ, et al. Cumulative cisplatin dose in concurrent chemoradiotherapy for head and neck cancer: a systematic review. Eisele DW, ed Head Neck. 2016;38(S1):E2151–8. https://doi.org/10.1002/hed.24026.

48. Szturz P, Cristina V, Gómez RGH, Bourhis J, Simon C, Vermorken JB. Cisplatin eligibility issues and alternative regimens in locoregionally advanced head and neck cancer: recommendations for clinical practice. Front Oncol. 2019; https://doi.org/10.3389/fonc.2019.00464.

49. Bonner JA, Harari PM, Giralt J, et al. Radiotherapy plus Cetuximab for squamous-cell carcinoma of the head and neck. N Engl J Med. 2006;354(6):567–78. https://doi.org/10.1056/NEJMoa053422.

50. Ang KK, Zhang Q, Rosenthal DI, et al. Randomized phase III trial of concurrent accelerated radiation plus cisplatin with or without cetuximab for stage III to IV head and neck carcinoma: RTOG 0522. J Clin Oncol. 2014;32(27):2940–50. https://doi.org/10.1200/JCO.2013.53.5633.

51. Chen AM, Chen LM, Vaughan A, et al. Tobacco smoking during radiation therapy for head-and-neck cancer is associated with unfavorable outcome. Int J Radiat Oncol. 2011;79(2):414–9. https://doi.org/10.1016/j.ijrobp.2009.10.050.

52. Devi S, Singh N. Dental care during and after radiotherapy in head and neck cancer. Natl J Maxillofac Surg. 2014;5(2):117. https://doi.org/10.4103/0975-5950.154812.

53. Anderson NJ, Jackson JE, Smith JG, et al. Pretreatment risk stratification of feeding tube use in patients treated with intensity-modulated radiotherapy for head and neck cancer. Head Neck. 2018; https://doi.org/10.1002/hed.25316.

54. Brown T, Banks M, Hughes BGM, Lin C, Kenny LM, Bauer JD. Impact of early prophylactic feeding on long term tube dependency outcomes in patients with head and neck cancer. Oral Oncol. 2017;72:17–25. https://doi.org/10.1016/j.oraloncology.2017.06.025.

55. Lalla RV, Bowen J, Barasch A, et al. MASCC/ISOO clinical practice guidelines for the management of mucositis secondary to cancer therapy. Cancer. 2014;120(10):1453–61. https://doi.org/10.1002/cncr.28592.

56. Wong RKS, Bensadoun R-J, Boers-Doets CB, et al. Clinical practice guidelines for the prevention and treatment of acute and late radiation reactions from the MASCC Skin Toxicity Study Group. Support Care Cancer. 2013;21(10):2933–48. https://doi.org/10.1007/s00520-013-1896-2.

57. Ferreira EB, Vasques CI, Gadia R, et al. Topical interventions to prevent acute radiation dermatitis in head and neck cancer patients: a systematic review. Support Care Cancer. 2017;25(3):1001–11. https://doi.org/10.1007/s00520-016-3521-7.

58. Hovan AJ, Williams PM, Stevenson-Moore P, et al. A systematic review of dysgeusia induced by cancer therapies. Support Care Cancer. 2010;18(8):1081–7. https://doi.org/10.1007/s00520-010-0902-1.

59. Crona DJ, Faso A, Nishijima TF, McGraw KA, Galsky MD, Milowsky MI. A systematic review of strategies to prevent cisplatin-induced nephrotoxicity. Oncologist. 2017;22(5):609–19. https://doi.org/10.1634/theoncologist.2016-0319.

60. Calabrese L, Bruschini R, Giugliano G, et al. Compartmental tongue surgery: long term oncologic results in the treatment of tongue cancer. Oral Oncol. 2011;47(3):174–9. https://doi.org/10.1016/j.oraloncology.2010.12.006.

61. Forastiere AA, Zhang Q, Weber RS, et al. Long-term results of RTOG 91-11: a comparison of three nonsurgical treatment strategies to preserve the larynx in patients with locally advanced larynx cancer. J Clin Oncol. 2013;31(7):845–52. https://doi.org/10.1200/JCO.2012.43.6097.

62. Pointreau Y, Garaud P, Chapet S, et al. Randomized trial of induction chemotherapy with cisplatin and 5-fluorouracil with or without docetaxel for larynx preservation. JNCI J Natl Cancer Inst. 2009;101(7):498–506. https://doi.org/10.1093/jnci/djp007.

63. Lorenz KJ. Rehabilitation after total laryngectomy-A tribute to the pioneers of voice restoration in the last two centuries. Front Med. 2017; https://doi.org/10.3389/fmed.2017.00081.

64. Lefebvre J-L, Andry G, Chevalier D, et al. Laryngeal preservation with induction chemotherapy for hypopharyngeal squamous cell carcinoma: 10-year results of EORTC trial 24891. Ann Oncol. 2012;23(10):2708–14. https://doi.org/10.1093/annonc/mds065.

65. Vermorken JB, Mesia R, Rivera F, et al. Platinum-based chemotherapy plus cetuximab in head and neck cancer. N Engl J Med. 2008;359(11):1116–27. https://doi.org/10.1056/NEJMoa0802656.

66. Bossi P, Miceli R, Locati LD, et al. A randomized, phase 2 study of cetuximab plus cisplatin with or without paclitaxel for the first-line treatment of patients with recurrent and/or metastatic squamous cell carcinoma of the head and neck. Ann Oncol. 2017;28(11):2820–6. https://doi.org/10.1093/annonc/mdx439.

43

67. Rischin P final analysis of the phase 3 K-048 trial of pembro-lizumab (pembro) as first-line therapy for recurrent/metastatic head and neck squamous cell carcinoma (R/M HD), Harrington KJ, Greil R, et al. Protocol-specified final analysis of the phase 3 KEYNOTE-048 trial of pembrolizumab (pembro) as first-line therapy for recurrent/metastatic head and neck squamous cell carcinoma (R/M HNSCC). J Clin Oncol. 2019;37(15_suppl):6000. https://doi.org/10.1200/JCO.2019.37.15_suppl.6000.

68. Cavalieri S, Rivoltini L, Bergamini C, Locati LD, Licitra L, Bossi P. Immuno-oncology in head and neck squamous cell cancers: news from clinical trials, emerging predictive factors and unmet needs. Cancer Treat Rev. 2018;65:78–86. https://doi.org/10.1016/j.ctrv.2018.03.003.

69. Ferris RL, Blumenschein G, Fayette J, et al. Nivolumab for recurrent squamous-cell carcinoma of the head and neck. N Engl J Med. 2016;375(19):1856–67. https://doi.org/10.1056/NEJMoa1602252.

70. Cohen EEW, Soulières D, Le Tourneau C, et al. Pembrolizumab versus methotrexate, docetaxel, or cetuximab for recurrent or metastatic head-and-neck squamous cell carcinoma (KEYNOTE-040): a randomised, open-label, phase 3 study. Lancet. 2019;393(10167):156–67. https://doi.org/10.1016/S0140-6736(18)31999-8.

71. Siano M, Infante G, Resteghini C, et al. Outcome of recurrent and metastatic head and neck squamous cell cancer patients after first line platinum and cetuximab therapy. Oral Oncol. 2017;69:33–7. https://doi.org/10.1016/j.oraloncology.2017.04.002.

Central Nervous System Malignancies

Giuseppe Badalamenti, Massimiliano Cani, Lidia Rita Corsini, Lorena Incorvaia, Alessandro Inno, and Stefania Gori

Central Nervous System Malignancies

Contents

© Springer Nature Switzerland AG 2021
A. Russo et al. (eds.), *Practical Medical Oncology Textbook*, UNIPA Springer Series,
https://doi.org/10.1007/978-3-030-56051-5_44

Learning Objectives

By the end of this chapter, the reader will:

- Have learned the key facts of epidemiology and pathophysiology of CNS malignancies and BMs
- Recognize the clinical presentation of CNS malignancies and BMs
- Be able to plan the appropriate diagnostic work-up
- Be able to manage symptoms
- Have learned the basic concepts of treatment

44.1   Introduction

The most frequent malignancies of the central nervous system (CNS) are not primitive neoplasms, but metastasis originating from other sites, such as lung (small cell lung cancer), breast, and skin (melanoma) are the most frequent intracranial lesions [1]. The primitive neoplasms of the CNS are a rare and heterogeneous group of malignancies with different biological behavior and consequently with different prognosis (☐ Fig. 44.1).

In some cases, CNS malignancies can be part of manifestations of a genetic syndrome, such as von Hippel-Lindau (VHL) or neurofibromatosis. In these rare circumstances, the patients show other neoplasms in different sites (kidney, skin, etc.) with facial abnormalities or peculiar manifestations (café-au-lait macules) [2]. In the following sections, a synthetic view of the most important and frequent CNS neoplasms will be provided with a particular insight to the 2016 WHO classification and, subsequently, the mainly pathophysiologic features of brain metastasis (BMs).

44.2   Primary Brain Tumors

Giuseppe Badalamenti, Massimiliano Cani, Lidia Rita Corsini and Lorena Incorvaia

44.2.1   Classification

The WHO classification provides a good system to categorize this heterogeneous group of CNS neoplasms. The 2007 version was replaced in 2016 with the introduction of new categories and groups of tumors together with a fundamental role of the molecular biology. The integration of genetic and phenotypic aspects is the milestone of the new classification [3] (☐ Fig. 44.1).

44.2.2   Diagnosis

Frequently, in case of asymptomatic lesions like meningiomas, diagnosis could be accidental. However, in presence of signs and symptoms of CNS involvement, a correct diagnostic process must be established. First of all, personal and family history of the patient should be collected in order to focus on the symptoms' onset or to investigate the exposure to risk factors. Then physical and neurological examinations should be performed: focal signs and symptoms can conduct to the correct imaging investigation. Indeed, if the clinical suspect is a neoplasm, the patient should be addressed to a contrast MRI exam. Obviously, other tests, such as CT scan,

☐ **Fig. 44.1** 2016 World Health Organization (WHO) Classification of tumors of the Central Nervous System: A summary

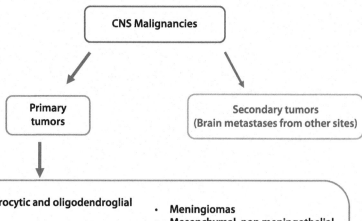

angiography, or PET can be used also as pre-operative investigations [4].

44.2.3 Gliomas

The new 2016 WHO classification has redrawn this group of tumors, which include astrocytomas (II and III grade), oligondendrogliomas (II and III grade), and glioblastomas (IV) together with diffuse gliomas typical of childhood.

The evaluation of the IDH1 status is the first step in the classification system. We can thus identify "IDH mutant gliomas" and "IDH wild type gliomas."

In the context of IDH mutant gliomas, other features must be evaluated to distinguish oligodendrogliomas from astrocitomas, as the co-deletion of 1p/19q and the mutation of ATRX and tp53.

Co-deletion of 1p/19q: diagnosis of oligodendrogliomas (II and III grade).

Mutation of ATRX and tp53: astrocitomas (II and III grade).

Moreover, it is possible to identify different types with different prognosis and molecular features:

— *Diffuse low-grade gliomas*: These include WHO grade II diffuse astrocytomas and oligodendrogliomas, which can be divided into two groups considering the mutation of IDH-1. Early and maximal safe resection is the initial treatment for those patients. Postoperative treatment decisions are based on risk stratification, although the delineation between low-risk and highrisk glioma is highly variable. The wild-type forms are typically diagnosed in elderly patients and the prognosis is poor. Patients with a mutation of IDH-1 are usually younger (≤40 years) and they have best prognosis. In these patients, a watch and wait policy with MRI every 3–6 months is accepted. Patients with highrisk lowgrade gliomas are clinically defined as older than 40 years, have neurological symptoms, large tumor (>5 cm), or subtotal resection. In these cases, current postsurgical standard of care is focal radiotherapy to 50–54Gy followed by six cycles of adjuvant treatment with procarbazine, lomustine, and vincristine (PCV) [5].

— *Diffuse high-grade gliomas*: These include WHO grade III anaplastic astrocytomas and anaplastic oligodendrogliomas. The standard of care for patients with highgrade gliomas is maximal safe surgical resection followed by chemoradiation. Chemoradiation consists of radiotherapy to 60 Gy with either six cycles of adjuvant PCV or concurrent

and adjuvant temozolomide. It is important to notice the role of temozolomide in newly diagnosed anaplastic astrocytomas without 1p/19q co-deletion: in this case temozolomide in the adjuvant setting is linked to a longer overall survival after radiotherapy [6]. Bevacizumab is an option in case of relapse.

44.2.4 Glioblastomas

Glioblastoma is the most lethal of the primary brain tumors in adults.

With the new classification, three different groups of this neoplasm were recognized:

— *IDH1 wild-type glioblastoma*: it is the most frequent form and in general arises in patients older than 55 years old. It can be described as a "the novo" type to easily distinguish it from the other form of glioblastoma, which usually develops after previous gliomas. The milestone of treatment consists in the association of radiotherapy and temozolomide (concurrent and adjuvant), which have improved survival of patients with glioblastoma [7].

Given the important role of temozolomide, the analyses of MGMT promoter methylation in the first steps of the diagnostic process has a prognostic relevance and may inform the treatment, especially in older patients [8]. Another possible treatment is the tumor-treating field, but it is not used today as a first line therapy. In case of progression, nitrosureas, bevacizumab, or temozolomide rechallenge should be considered.

— *IDH1 mutant glioblastoma*: This considers younger patients with a prior diagnosis of lower grade diffuse glioma. The treatment is quite similar to the group of anaplastic astrocytomas [9].

— *NOS glioblastoma*: In this group, all the forms in which a correct evaluation of IDH was not possible are categorized [10].

Recently regorafenib, an oral multikinase inhibitor of angiogenic, stromal, and oncogenic receptor tyrosine kinases, showed an encouraging overall survival benefit in recurrent glioblastoma [11].

44.2.5 Gliomatosis Cerebri

A diffuse clinical involvement defines a clinical condition actually called gliomatosis cerebri, whose treatment differs from other types of malignant forms. In fact, surgery is not the standard of care and some studies have shown an advantage of temozolomide as first line therapy [12].

44.2.6 Ependymomas

Ependymomas are not frequent CNS malignancies. These tumors account for 3.5% of all cases [13] and they usually develop in the IV ventricle, also in children.

Other sites are III ventricle and the vertebral canal. Obviously, signs and symptoms vary according to the site of the tumor, but often they are linked to cranial hypertension. There is also the possibility of spread into the vertebral canal and it depends on the site and grade of the neoplasm.

The risk factors, which can modify the prognosis, are age, the site of the neoplasm, histological grade, and the possibility to perform a curative surgery, although some of them appear controversial even today and there is no solid consensus [14].

In the last 2016 classification, a new variant was introduced: ependymoma RELA fusion-positive, which is actually typical among children. Surgery is the main option in trying to preserve the normal neurologic functions. Post-operative radiotherapy should be considered in case of grade III tumor [15] as some studies have shown an advantage in terms of overall survival. In case of relapse, a medical treatment with cisplatinum or temozolomide should be used [16].

44.2.7 Medulloblastoma

Medulloblastoma is a neoplasm which arises from precursor neuronal cells in the posterior cranial fossa; meanwhile, it is the most frequent tumor of the CNS among children; in adults, it is quite rare. Signs and symptoms are mostly caused by its position and they can be considered a direct consequence of cranial hypertension. The new classification has introduced new molecular entities and actually, they should be integrated with the well-known histologic types, which are as follows:

- Classic
- Desmoplastic/nodular
- Extensive nodularity
- Large cells/anaplastic

The molecular groups are as follows:

- WNT-activated
- SHH-activated
- Group 3
- Group 4

The standard treatment in adults with a standard risk is post-surgery radiotherapy. New studies have shown a better prognosis for patients treated with the combination of both radiotherapy and chemotherapy (cisplatin, etoposide +/− cyclophosphamide) [17].

In case of high risk patients, a combination of radio therapy and chemotherapy is recommended.

During the follow-up, a multidisciplinary approach should be considered for each patient for a correct evaluation of the endocrine, neurologic, and cognitive aspects [18].

44.2.8 Meningiomas

Meningiomas are a group of neoplasms arising from the meninges, which represents the second most frequent tumor in the CNS.

Some well-defined risk factors are: genetic syndromes, such as Neurofibromatosis 2 (NF2), and radiation exposure. Meningiomas are much more frequent in women and a hormonal role in the development of these tumors has been hypothesized [19].

Most frequently, they are diagnosed accidentally, but otherwise, in some cases, they can cause symptoms, such as headache, seizures, nausea, and vomiting as part of a cranial hypertension syndrome.

There are different strategies in case of a diagnosis of meningioma: if it is asymptomatic and characterized by a slow-growth rate, a watchful-wait can be a good approach, while if the neoplasm is associated to symptoms or has a high-growth rate, surgery can be the first approach.

In case of recurrence or unresectable masses, radiotherapy is usually used; chemotherapy is addressed to those patients with a relapse disease who cannot be treated again with surgery or radiotherapy even if solid evidences are lacking [20].

44.2.9 Other Tumors

Other forms of neoplasms which concern the CNS system are as follows:

- Neuromas: This tumor has its origin from the VIII cranial nerve and, even rarely, can be part of a genetic syndrome, such as Neurofibromatosis 2. In most cases, it is localized in the pontocerebellar angle and the most important symptom is tinnitus.
- Pituitary gland neoplasms: Usually they are adenomas and can adopt both secretory and non-secretory forms. Symptoms can depend on both the local compression and the hormones which can be secreted. These neoplasms can be divided into macro and micro adenomas and the standard imaging exam is MRI. In most cases, surgery is the main treatment.

44

Just in case of a prolactinoma, a medical treatment can be used as Dopamine agonists show an inhibitory effect; another option can be gamma-knife treatment.
- Pineal gland tumors: Mainly are germinomas and can be characterized for focal symptoms due to local compression.

44.2.10   Genetic Syndromes

Some genetic syndromes can be characterized for the presence of benign or malign neoplasms in the CNS. Even if they account just for a minority of cases, they should be always taken into consideration in young patients with different lesions also in other sites, such as kidney or skin.

Neurofibromatosis 1 is an autosomal dominant syndrome caused by a mutation in NF1 gene (chromosome 17). It is easy to recognize thanks to peculiar skin lesions called café-au-lait macules, together with neurofibromas and axillary freckling. Regarding the CNS, astrocytomas, meningiomas, gliomas, and ependymomas can appear. Other clinical manifestations can be seizures, mental retardation, and hydrocephalus. *Neurofibromatosis 2* is characterized by a mutation in NF2 gene (chromosome 22). Differently to NF1, café-au-lait macules are less frequent; typically it is possible to find bilateral neuromas which involve the VIII cranial nerve. In addition, in this case, other possible manifestations are meningiomas and gliomas.

In the *von Hippel-Lindau syndrome*, the involvement of CNS is limited to the cerebellum, where the growth of hemangioblastomas is possible; these patients can also suffer from kidney cancer, pheochromocytoma, or liver and pancreatic cysts [21].

> **Key Points**
> - Personal and family histories of the patient, together with a correct physical and neurological examination, are fundamental steps to choose the best imaging test in order to confirm or exclude the diagnosis of a CNS neoplasm.
> - In some rare cases, CNS neoplasms can be part of a genetic syndrome, above all in young patients.
> - The new WHO classification has improved the role of biological features of CNS malignancies, such as IDH mutation or tp53/ATRX. Biological features are very important for diagnosis and prognosis.
> - In most cases, surgery represents the most important treatment. Maximal safe resection improves functional status and reduces mortality in both lowgrade and highgrade glioma. Other

options are radiotherapy and chemotherapy as for glioblastomas (temozolomide with radiotherapy).
- Medulloblastoma is a frequent neoplasm in children, but much less frequent in adults; it is located in the posterior cranial fossa and it can be treated with different approaches.
- Meningiomas are frequent neoplasms; they are usually treated in case of symptomatic conditions.

> **Recommendations**
> - ASCO
>   ▶ https://www.asco.org/research-guidelines/quality-guidelines/guidelines/Neurooncology
> - Hints for a deeper insight
> - The 2016 World Health Organization Classification of Tumors of the Central Nervous System: a summary
>   ▶ https://link.springer.com/article/10.1007/s00401-016-1545-1
> - PD-1/PD-L1 immune-checkpoint inhibitors in glioblastoma: A concise review
>   ▶ https://www.sciencedirect.com/science/article/abs/pii/S1040842818303172?via%3Dihub
> - AIOM
>   ▶ https://www.aiom.it/linee-guida-aiom-neoplasie-cerebrali/

44.3   Brain Metastases

Alessandro Inno and Stefania Gori

Brain metastases (BMs) occur when cancer cells originating in tissues outside the central nervous system (CNS) spread secondarily to the brain. They represent a common complication of many cancers, mainly lung cancer, breast cancer, and melanoma.

The incidence of BMs is thought to be increasing over time due to a combination of factors, including: (1) the improvement in the quality of neuroimaging together with a more frequent use of routine imaging studies of the brain, leading to early detection of clinically silent lesions; (2) effective systemic therapies for the primary cancer resulting into extended survival of cancer patients, thus leading to a larger population of cancer patients at risk for BMs [22].

The occurrence of BMs is generally associated with an adverse impact on survival and quality of life. In fact, despite recent advances in the diagnosis and management of this condition, BMs still carry a dismal prognosis and, therefore, represent an unmet clinical need.

44.3.1 Epidemiology and Risk Factors

BMs are the most frequent intracranial tumor, occurring up to ten times more frequently than primary brain tumors, although their exact incidence is not known. In population studies, the incidence of BMs among cancer patients ranged from 8.5% to 9.6% [23–27]. However, population studies may underestimate the true incidence of BMs. Data from old autopsy studies, in fact, suggest higher frequencies and it is now believed that 20–40% of patients with metastatic cancer will develop BMs during the course of the disease [28, 29].

Virtually, any primary cancer may spread to the brain. The majority of BMs originate from lung cancer (40–50%), breast cancer (15–30%), melanoma (5–20%), kidney cancer (3–10%), colorectal cancer (3–10%) and unknown primary (3–15%) [30, 31]. Therefore, lung cancer, breast cancer, and melanoma account for approximately 80% of BMs overall. However, in more recent cohorts, an increasing prevalence of BMs from colorectal and kidney cancers was reported, possibly due to general improvement in detection, treatment, and prognosis of these two types of cancer [27].

According to the number of brain lesions and the extent of systemic disease, the metastatic involvement of the brain may be defined as follows: solitary BM, in presence of only one brain lesion with a controlled primary tumor and no other metastases; single BM, in presence of only one brain lesion with an active primary tumor and/or systemic metastases; oligo BMs in presence of 2–3 brain lesions; multiple BMs in presence of more than 3 brain lesions [30].

Surgical series and cohort studies reported that among patients with BMs, approximately 40–45% present with one brain lesion, 25–30% with 2–3 lesions, and 20–30% with more than 3 lesions [31, 32]. Breast, colorectal, and kidney cancers have a slightly higher likelihood to be associated with a single BM, whereas lung cancer and melanoma are more likely to develop multiple BMs [30]. The number of patients with a single BM has decreased over time, whereas the proportion of patients with three or more BMs has increased, and this is likely due to the more frequent use of contrast-enhancement brain magnetic resonance imaging (MRI) in the diagnostic work-up.

According to the timing of diagnosis of BMs, they can be classified as: synchronous, if BMs are diagnosed within 2 months from the diagnosis of the primary tumor; metachronous, if BMs are diagnosed more than 2 months after the diagnosis of the primary tumor.

Synchronous BMs are most frequent in lung cancer, while for breast cancer, BMs often represent a late event, with a median time interval of more than 3 years between the diagnosis of primary breast cancer and detection of BMs [31].

The simultaneous diagnosis of BMs and primary cancer has become more common over time, likely because of a more frequent use of neuroimaging in the initial staging assessment [27]. In a recently published descriptive analysis of 2419 patients with BMs, in fact, approximately a quarter of patients presented with synchronous diagnosis of primary tumor and BMs, and 20% of patients received the diagnosis of BMs through routinely performed radiological staging procedures [31].

Several potential risk factors for the development of BMs have been investigated, particularly in breast cancer. Initial studies identified lung metastases as first site of relapse and a negative hormone receptors status as risk factors for the occurrence of BMs in patients with non-brain metastatic breast cancer [33]. Refined knowledge of the molecular classification of breast cancer led to the observation that different intrinsic molecular subtypes are associated with distinctive patterns of metastatic spread, with HER2-positive and triple negative breast cancer having higher the risk of developing BMs, as compared with luminal A subtype [34].

In 2010, Graesslin and colleagues identified age, tumor grade, negative status of hormone receptors and HER2, number of metastatic sites, and short disease-free survival as independent risk factors for subsequent BMs in patients with non-brain metastatic breast cancer. Based on this data, a prediction nomogram for BMs in metastatic breast cancer was developed [35] and, more recently, its validity and exportability were further confirmed by an external validation study [36].

Similarly, nomograms for the prediction of BMs were developed also for patients with non-small-cell lung cancer (NSCLC). Tumor histology, smoking status, pT stage, and the interaction between adenocarcinoma and pN stage were used in a Korean study to build a nomogram for the prediction of BMs as first site of relapse [37], whereas, in a Chinese study, neuron-specific enolase, histology, number of metastatic lymph nodes, and tumor grade were included into a nomogram for predicting BMs in patients with curatively resected NSCLC [38].

Nomograms to predict BMs may represent a helpful tool for identifying high-risk patients in order to personalize follow-up or select candidates for trials specifically designed to evaluate preventive interventions.

44.3.2 Pathophysiology

The propensity to generate BMs differs among different tumor types and also among different cellular clones of the same tumor [39]. Not all cells of a given tumor are able to reach the brain and lead to macroscopic BMs, therefore primary tumors and corresponding BMs may be biologically different [40]. According to the "seed" and "soil" hypothesis, the development of BMs is possibly related to a series of unique characteristics of some tumor cells that allow them to find the brain microenvironment a favorable place for their growth, and that are not necessarily required for successful growth at other organs [41]. Recent investigations are beginning to shed some light into cellular and molecular mechanisms of BMs development. For instance, in metastatic breast cancer, cyclooxygenase-2 (COX2), the epidermal growth factor receptor (EGFR) ligand HB-EGF and a2,6-sialyltransferase ST6GALNAC5 have been identified as mediators of cell passage through the blood–brain barrier (BBB) [42], and the upregulation of SOX2 and OLIG2 genes seems to play a role for the growth of BMs [43].

The metastatic process is a complex series of sequential events governed by a cascade of molecular changes [44]. Metastatic cells that successfully colonize the brain must complete the following steps:

1. Invasion

   Tumor cells dissociate from the primary tumor mass by the loss of the cell-cell adhesion capacity and invade the surrounding stroma through the upregulation of matrix-degrading enzymes and dysregulation of proteins involved in cell motility and migration. In this phase, tumor initiates angiogenesis, which is necessary for tumor growth and also provides a route for detached cells to enter the circulatory system.

2. Intravasation

   Tumor cells interact with more permeable tumor-induced endothelial cells, produce enzymes that degrade the vessel basement membrane, and enter the lumen of capillaries or lymph channels, thus spreading through venous circulation.

3. Transportation

   Once in the bloodstream, tumor cells must avoid detachment-induced apoptosis and escape destruction by the immune system and the mechanical forces to survive.

4. Extravasation

   Through the bloodstream, circulating tumor cells reach the arterial vessels that supply the brain. Access of tumor cells to the brain is governed by the BBB, a physiologic and anatomic structure composed by a monolayer of specialized endothelial cells connected by tight junctions and surrounded by a thick basement membrane without fenestration, and underlying astrocytes that regulate the flow of nutrients, ions, and cells into the brain. The arrest of tumor cells into brain microvessels is favored by specific adhesion molecules to brain endothelials cells, and the process of extravasation and invasion of BBB requires the expression of various cell surface receptors and degradative enzymes.

5. Growth:

   Once in the brain, tumor cells may die or remain quiescent in a dormant state for months or even for years, if the soil is not propitious for tumor growth. Alternatively, the brain may provide a hospitable microenvironment and several growth factors, such as nerve growth factor (NGF) or vascular endothelial growth factor (VEGF), may facilitate the proliferation of tumor cells and the development of macroscopic BMs.

Each step of the metastatic cascade is relatively inefficient and only a small number of primary tumor cells that reach the bloodstream is able to form viable BMs [45].

Although occasionally BMs may occur by direct extension into the CNS from the primary tumor (for instance in case of outer ear, mastoid, rhinopharyngeal, paranasal sinus, or orbital cancer) or from skull metastases, the vast majority of BMs result from hematogenous spread. Therefore, the pattern of distribution of BMs reflects the proportional blood flow to the different anatomical regions of the brain [46], with nearly 80% of BMs involving the cerebral hemispheres, followed by cerebellum (15%) and brainstem (5%).

Within the brain vasculature, single malignant cells or tumor emboli may be entrapped in small size terminal arteries. This might explain the propensity of BMs to develop at the gray/white matter junction and in watershed zones of the cerebral circulation [47].

44.3.3 Clinical Manifestations

Approximately two-thirds of patients with BMs develop neurologic symptoms. Symptoms are extremely variable depending on the location of BMs [48, 49].

Clinical presentation is similar to that of other brain tumors and includes the following:
- Headache
- Seizures
- Nausea and/or vomiting
- Focal neurological dysfunction
- Cognitive dysfunction
- Gait disorders

- Nuchal rigidity
- Photophobia

Headache is the most frequent symptom, occurring in 40–50% of patients with BMs [50]. It may be located on the same side of the tumor mass but can be also diffuse. Patients with multiple BMs or with lesions located in the posterior fossa are at higher risk of headache. Metastasis-related headache is generally a manifestation of intracranial hypertension and it can mainly occur in early morning hours, can be associated with nausea, vomiting, and transient visual impairment, and can be also exacerbated by cough or straining. These typical features, however, are present only in a minority of patients. In most cases, metastasis-related headache is indistinguishable from tension headache or migraine. Therefore, headache characteristics, other than recent worsening, usually fail to predict reliably the presence of BMs, unless focal deficits or papilledema coexist [51].

Seizures occur as the first manifestation of BMs in 20% of patients and a similar percentage of patients may develop symptomatic epilepsy at some point in the course of their disease [52]. Multiple BMs or metastatic melanoma are associated with an increased risk of seizures. Metastasis-related seizures are generally focal with or without secondary generalization.

Focal neurological dysfunction, such as weakness of one limb or hemiparesis, with or without sensory changes, language disorders or visual deficits, is the presenting sign of BMs in 20–40% of patients. Gait disorders characterized by unsteadiness, short steps and widening of lower limbs may develop even in the absence of focal motor deficit and they are typically caused by multiple, bilateral, small size BMs [49].

Patients with BMs can also have cognitive dysfunction, including memory problems and mood or personality changes, especially in case of multiple BMs [53].

Nuchal rigidity or photophobia represent signs of meningeal involvement.

In the majority of cases, the onset of symptoms is subacute due to the gradual growth of the tumor mass and surrounding edema, although some patients can present acutely with seizures or with neurological signs and symptoms resembling stroke or transitory ischemic attack. An acute onset may be due to metastatic hemorrhage, embolization of tumor cells, invasion or compression of cerebral artery by the tumor mass. Melanoma and renal carcinoma are more often associated with hemorrhagic brain metastases [54].

44.3.4 Diagnosis

Neurologic symptoms that are suggestive for BMs require always appropriate investigation, both in patients with and those without a known history of cancer. In fact, neurologic symptoms may represent the first presentation of cancer in about 15% of patients, thus appearing before systemic cancer is diagnosed. On the other hand, up to 10% of brain lesions in cancer patients can be non-metastatic. Differential diagnosis includes primary brain tumors, abscesses, demyelinating diseases, cerebral infarctions or hemorrhages, intracranial hematomas, progressive multifocal leukoencephalopathy, intravascular thrombosis and radiation necrosis [49].

Brain imaging plays a key role for the diagnosis of BMs in cancer patients who develop new neurologic symptoms, but also for the screening of BMs in asymptomatic cancer patients at high-risk of CNS involvement. Computed tomography (CT) scan and MRI represent the key imaging modalities for the diagnosis of BMs (◘ Fig. 44.2) [55].

At imaging, BMs are usually spherical, solid, or cystic, and well-circumscribed lesions of various sizes

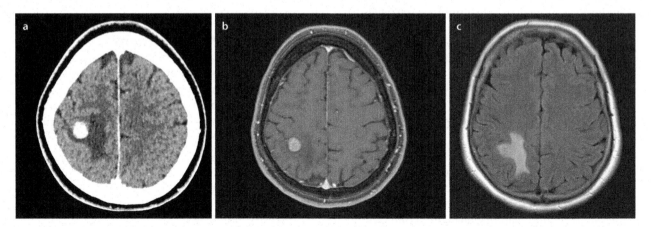

◘ **Fig. 44.2** Right parietal BM from lung adenocarcinoma, with surrounding edema, as showed by: **a** contrast-enhanced CT scan; **b** T1-WI MRI with gadolinium; **c** T2-WI MRI

44

located at the cortico-medullary junction or in watershed areas, with varying amounts of surrounding edema. On non-enhanced CT scan, BMs usually are hypo- or isodense lesions, although hemorrhagic metastases or metastases from melanoma may appear as hyperdense lesions. After iodinate contrast injection, BMs demonstrate enhancement, with surrounding vasogenic edema appearing as hypodense area [56].

Although CT scan is able to detect BMs, MRI represents the gold standard for the diagnosis because of its higher resolution, superior tissue contrast, and no bone artifacts. Standard MRI sequences include T1-weighted imaging (T1-WI) with or without contrast medium, T2-weighted imaging (T2-WI), and fluid-attenuated inversion recovery (FLAIR). On T1-W1, BMs usually generate a low-intermediate intensity signal surrounded by a decreased signal in case of peritumoral edema. When BMs show increased intensity, it can be a sign of intralesional hemorrhage or melanin deposits. After injection of paramagnetic contrast, BMs are often enhanced and may present peripheral ring enhancement with a non-enhancing core corresponding to central necrosis. On T2-WI and FLAIR sequences, both BMs and surrounding edema appear as an area of increased intensity. Metastases from mucinous gastrointestinal adenocarcinomas may appear hypointense in T2-WI, because of high protein content within the lesions. Advanced MRI techniques, such as diffusion-weighted MRI, perfusion MRI, and MRI spectroscopy, represent additional tools for distinguishing BMs from other entities, such as high-grade primary glial tumors, CNS lymphomas, or cerebral abscesses [49, 57].

Fluorodeoxyglucose (FDG) - positron emission tomography (PET)/CT scan is an increasingly used tool in the staging of cancer, particularly lung cancer. However, it is not as sensitive as MRI in the evaluation of BMs [58]. In fact, some BMs may manifest as focal hypermetabolic areas, therefore difficult to detect within the normal cerebral cortex which is FDG avid, or may appear as focal hypometabolic areas indistinguishable from other non-neoplastic conditions, such as brain infarction. Therefore, PET/CT is not routinely indicated for the assessment of BMs. In selected cases, however, FDG-PET/CT or PET/CT with aminoacidic tracers, such as 18F-Tirosine may be helpful to distinguish hypermetabolic local recurrent BMs from hypometabolic post-radiation necrotic lesions [59, 60].

In patients with history of cancer, imaging is generally sufficient to provide diagnosis of BMs, and in most cases, histological confirmation is not required. Stereotactic or open biopsy, or surgical resection of a cerebral lesion should be considered only if at imaging there is some concern regarding diagnosis of BMs, and

in selected patients with BMs as the only site of relapse after successful treatment of the primary tumor and no evidence of extracranial disease.

In patients without known history of cancer, the identification of primary tumor is part of the diagnostic procedure. The diagnostic work-up should consist at least in complete clinical examination, including skin scrutiny, chest and abdomen contrast-enhanced CT and, if CT scan does not show any evidence of primary or systemic cancer, a whole-body FDG-PET/CT. When these examinations are inconclusive, then stereotactic or open biopsy or surgical resection should be performed to establish histological diagnosis and orient to the location of primary tumor [61].

44.3.5 Treatment

(a) *Prognostic Factors*

Despite active treatments, prognosis of patients with BMs remains poor, with a wide heterogeneity of outcomes depending on several prognostic variables. In this regard, a sound prognostic classification is important for both clinical decision-making and design of clinical trials.

In 1997, the Radiation Therapy Oncology Group (RTOG) developed a prognostic index for patients with BMs performing a recursive partitioning analysis (RPA) from a database of 1200 patients treated with whole brain radiotherapy (WBRT) from three RTOG trials conducted between 1979 and 1993 [62]. Based on Karnofsky performance score (KPS), age, control of primary tumor, and extent of extracranial disease, three prognostic classes with different median survival times were identified: class I (patients with KPS $\geq$ 70, age < 65, controlled primary tumor and no extracranial disease), with a median survival of 7.1 months; class II (KPS $\geq$ 70 and one of the following: age $\geq$ 65, uncontrolled primary or extracranial disease), with a median survival of 4.2 months; class III (KPS < 70), with a median survival of 3.4 months.

Since then, several other models have been developed, with the aim to further assess prognostic factors and better predict survival of patients with BMs. Among them, the grading prognostic assessment (GPA), developed in 2008 by Sperduto et al., is considered the least subjective, most quantitative, and based on the most current data from randomized trials [63]. Compared with RPA, GPA excluded the estimation of control of primary tumor, which is subjective and often difficult to evaluate, whereas included the number of BMs, which had proven to represent a relevant prognostic factor.

Table 44.1 Graded prognostic assessment (GPA)

	Score		
	0	0.5	1
Age, years	>60	50–59	<50
KPS	<70	70–80	>80
No. of CNS metastases	>3	2–3	1
Extracranial metastases	Present	–	Absent

CNS central nervous system, *KPS* Karnofsky performance score

According to GPA, a score was assigned for each considered prognostic factor (age, KPS, number of BMs, presence or absence of extracranial metastases), as shown in ◻ Table 44.1.

On the basis of GPA score, four prognostic groups were identified with significantly different median survival times:

- GPA 0–1, 2.6 months
- GPA 1.5–2.5, 3.8 months
- GPA 3, 6.9 months
- GPA 3.5–4, 11.0 months

The original GPA was subsequently refined with diagnosis specific indexes (DS-GPA) which considered different significant prognostic factors for each cancer type (lung, breast, GI, kidney, and melanoma), as summarized in ◻ Table 44.2 [64, 65]. Of note, besides clinical prognostic factors, a relevant prognostic value of molecular characteristics was recognized for breast cancer and NSCLC. Particularly, the status of hormone receptors and HER2 is an integral part of the breast-GPA [66, 67] and, more recently, *EGFR* mutational status and rearrangements of *ALK* have been included into the updated version of DS-GPA for NSCLC, namely, the Lung-molGPA [68].

(b) *Management*

The management of BMs consists of a multimodal approach, including symptomatic treatment, local therapy, such as surgical resection and/or radiation therapy, and systemic therapy [69]. The therapeutic strategy for the individual patient with BMs depends on several factors including the prognosis of the patient, the status of systemic cancer, and the number, size and location of BMs. The appropriate treatment should be discussed within a skilled multidisciplinary team.

For most patients with newly diagnosed BMs, local treatment is the primary approach:

- For patients with newly diagnosed single BM or oligo-BMs, with good performance status (KPS ≥ 70), life expectancy >3 months, controlled systemic disease

and/or available active drugs for systemic disease (RPA class I), upfront treatment options are generally represented by surgical resection or SRS. Surgical resection may be preferred in case of large BMs, BMs surrounded by extensive edema or when histologic diagnosis is needed. The addition of post-operative radiotherapy (WBRT or SRS) or adjuvant WBRT after SRS reduces the risk of intracranial recurrence, without a proven survival benefit.

- For patients with multiple BMs and good prognosis (RPA class I-II), WBRT or SRS represent the primary treatment.
- For patients with BMs and poor performance status (RPA class III) BSC alone is a reasonable option, and alternative options are represented by WBRT or SRS.

Upfront systemic therapy for patients with newly diagnosed BMs can be considered in case of asymptomatic or paucisymptomatic BMs from a chemo-sensitive primary tumor (i.e., germ cell tumor, small-cell lung cancer) or a primary tumor harboring a druggable target (i.e., NSCLC with *EGFR* mutation, *ALK* or *ROS-1* rearrangements, *BRAF*-mutated melanoma or selected cases of *HER2*-positive breast cancer).

A proposal of clinical decision making is summarized in ◻ Table 44.3 [70].

For relapsed or progressive BMs, the treatment should be established considering the local and/or systemic therapies previously done.

Symptomatic treatment should be generally offered to all patients with symptoms related to BMs.

(i) *Symptomatic Treatment*

Symptomatic treatment is often used to reduce the symptoms of BMs. It includes medical decompressive therapy for symptoms associated with increased intracranial pressure, antiepileptic drugs for seizures and analgesic medications for headache.

■ **Medical Decompressive Therapy**

Vasogenic edema associated with BMs plays a major role in the development of neurologic symptoms. By causing an additional mass effect, often exceeding the volume of the BM itself, edema determines an increased intracranial pressure and also leads to neurological disturbances by reducing local blood flow [71].

Corticosteroids are typically used to control cerebral edema in patients with newly diagnosed BMs [72]. The antiedema effects of corticosteroids is attributed to a reduction in the permeability of abnormal tumor capillaries and a stabilization of the disrupted BBB. Dexamethasone is generally considered the drug of choice because of its minimal mineralocorticoid effect and long half-life, although probably any other

⬛ Table 44.2 Disease-specific graded prognostic assessment (DS-GPA)

Primary tumor	Prognostic factor	GPA scoring criteria					Score[a]
Lung cancer							
		0	**0.5**	**1**			
	Age, years	≥70	<70	NA			–
	KPS	<70	80	90–100			–
	ECM	Present	–	Absent			–
	BMs, no	>4	1–4	NA			–
	Gene status	*EGFR* neg/unk and *ALK* neg/unk	NA	*EGFR* pos or *ALK* pos			–
	Total						–
	Adenocarcinoma MS by GPA: 0–1.0, 6.9; 1.5–2.0, 13.7; 2.5–3.0,26.5; 3.5–4.0, 46.8; non-adenocarcinoma MS by GPA: 0–1.0, 5.3; 1.5–2.0, 9.8; 2.5–3.0, 12.8.						
Breast cancer							
		0	**0.5**	**1.0**	**1.5**	**2.0**	
	KPS	≤50	60	70–80	90–100	–	–
	Age, y	≥60	<60	–	–	–	–
	Subtype	Basal like	–	Luminal A	HER2	Luminal B	–
	Total						–
	MS by GPA: 0–1.0 = 3.4; 1.5–2.0 = 7.7; 2.5–3.0 = 15.1; 3.5–4.0 = 25.3						
Melanoma/ RCC							
		0	**1**	**2**			
	KPS	<70	70–80	90–100			–
	BMs, no	>3	2–3	1			–
	Total						–
	Melanoma MS by GPA: 0–1.0 = 3.4; 1.5–2.0 = 4.7; 2.5–3.0 = 8.8; 3.5–4.0 = 13.2; RCC MS by GPA: 0–1.0 = 3.3; 1.5–2.0 = 7.3; 2.5–3.0 = 11.3; 3.5–4.0 = 14.8						
GI cancers							
		0	**1**	**2**	**3**	**4**	
	KPS	<70	70	80	90	100	–
	MS by GPA: 0–1.0 = 3.1; 2.0 = 4.4; 3.0 = 6.9; 4.0 = 13.5						

BMs brain metastases, *ECM* extracranial metastases, *GI* gastrointestinal, *MS* median survival in months, *KPS* Karnofsky Performance Status, *RCC* renal cell carcinoma

[a]Evaluating clinician completes this column

corticosteroid can be effective if given in equipotent doses. Starting doses of 4–8 mg/day of dexamethasone may be considered, unless patients exhibit severe symptoms due to increased intracranial pressure. In these patients, higher doses, such as 16 mg/day or more, should be considered [73]. In view of the definite increase in toxicity with daily doses more than 24 mg and inconclusive dose-response data, daily doses beyond 24 mg are not recommended. The long biological half-life of dexamethasone suggests that the daily dose may be given in two doses, rather than three or four doses. The reported response rates (RRs) in terms of symptom improvements with steroids ranged from 33% to 80% in different studies [74].

Corticosteroids' toxicity includes gastrointestinal adverse events (peptic ulceration, upper gastrointestinal

Table 44.3 Clinical decision-making for BMs

1. Consider systemic therapy when:	BM from highly chemotherapy-sensitive primary tumor BM found on screening MRI with planned systemic treatment BM from primary tumor with identified molecular alteration amenable to targeted therapy Other therapeutic options have been exhausted and there is a reasonable drug available
2. Consider WBRT when:	CNS and systemic progressive disease, with few systemic treatment options and poor PS Multiple (>3) BMs, especially if primary tumor is known to be radiotherapy sensitive Large (>4 cm) BM, not amenable to SRS Postsurgical resection of a dominant BM with multiple (>3) remaining BMs Salvage therapy for recurrent BM after SRS or WBRT failure
3. Consider SRS when:	Oligo-BMs or multiple BMs, especially if primary tumor is known to be radiotherapy resistant Postsurgical resection of a single BM, especially if >3 cm and in the posterior fossa Local relapse after surgical resection of a single BM Salvage therapy for recurrent oligo-BMs after WBRT
4. Consider surgery when:	Uncertain diagnosis of CNS lesion(s) Oligo-BMs, especially when associated with extensive cerebral edema Dominant BM in a critical location
5. BSC alone is reasonable when:	Systemic progressive disease, with few treatment options and poor PS

Modified from Lin and DeAngelis (2015)
BM brain metastasis, *BSC* best supportive care, *CNS* central nervous system, *MRI* magnetic resonance imaging, *PS* performance status, *SRS* stereotactic radiosurgery, *WBRT* whole brain radiotherapy

bleeding or perforation), myopathy, opportunistic infections, cushingoid features, hyperglycemia, behavioral changes (irritability, insomnia, anxiety, depression, and, rarely, florid psychosis), and osteoporosis. Incidence and severity of toxicity are related to higher doses and prolonged treatment duration. Since the majority of responding patients achieve symptoms relief within 48–72 hours, continued use of high starting doses may be neither necessary nor safe. For responding patients, steroid dose has been reduced by 25–50% every fifth day in most studies, although a more rapid tapering every third day may be considered when starting from 16 mg/day, in order to avoid the increased toxicity of steroid use beyond 3 weeks. In patients who worsen on dose reduction, prolonged steroid use may be required. For patients receiving corticosteroids for more than 1 month, prophylaxis of opportunistic infections with trimethoprim/sulfamethoxazole should be considered.

Steroids may be combined with non-steroideal anti-edema agents, such as osmotic cerebral decongestants. Of these agents, only mannitol is currently used in clinical practice. Mannitol is generally reserved for severe neurological manifestations or when a rapid reduction in the intracranial pressure is desirable, such as in impending cerebral herniation [75]. The usual dose is 0.75–1 g/kg given intravenously (usually 125 ml of 18% solution is appropriate for adult patients) every 6 hours. Treatment should be continued for up to 48 hours. Animal experiments suggest that a rapid rate of infusion reduces intracranial pressure more effectively than a slow infusion [76]. Serum electrolytes should be monitored with mannitol use and corrected when required.

Antiepileptic Drugs

Patients with BMs presenting with seizures or those who develop seizures during the course of their disease should be started on antiepileptic drugs.

Among antiepileptic drugs, those inducing P450 cytochromes should be avoided in order to prevent interactions with systemic therapies, as well as those with potential neurotoxic effects in order to not aggravate the neurologic state of the patients with new symptoms that could be wrongly interpreted as progressive disease. For these reasons, phenytoin, phenobarbital, carbamazepine, and oxcarbazepine are not routinely used. Levetiracetam (1000 mg/day–3000 mg/day) has emerged as the preferred treatment because it does not induce the P450 system and does not exhibit any relevant drug interactions. Moreover, levetiracetam is generally well-tolerated, although behavioral irritability has been reported. If necessary, the addition of valproate (20 mg/kg/day) may be considered.

In the absence of seizures, prophylactic antiepileptic drugs should not be routinely started [77]. This recommendation is mostly based on the results of a randomized clinical trial of antiepileptic versus non-antiepileptic prophylaxis in 100 patients with primary brain tumors (n = 40) or BMs (n = 60). In the subgroup of patients with BMs there was no significant difference in terms of seizure incidence between the two arms [78]. Given the lack of benefit and the potential risk of adverse events, published guidelines have recommended against the prophylactic use of antiepileptic drugs for patients with BMs [79, 80]. However, these conclusions are based on data derived from studies with old antiepileptic drugs, including phenytoin and phenobarbital, which are no longer first-choice drugs, whereas newer agents such as levetiracetam, topiramate, lamotrigine, or pregabalin have been not yet systematically investigated in this setting. Therefore, the issue of antiepileptic prophylactic therapy in patients with BMs remains controversial, especially for patients with lesions in highly epileptogenic areas or patients with metastatic melanoma that frequently involves the cerebral cortex.

For patients with BMs undergoing brain surgery, prophylactic antiepileptic drugs may be considered since they reduce the incidence of seizures of 40–50% in the first week after surgery [81]. In patients who do not experience seizures, antiepileptic drugs should be tapered and discontinued after the first post-operative week [80].

(c) *Surgery*

Surgical resection plays a critical role in the treatment of newly diagnosed single BM.

In the 1990s, three randomized clinical trials compared surgery plus WBRT versus WBRT alone for single BM [82–84]. In the first two studies [82, 83], a significant OS benefit for surgery followed by WBRT compared with WBRT alone was reported (approximately 9–10 months vs. 4–6 months) and, in one of these trials [83], the greatest survival advantage was obtained in patients with controlled extracranial disease (12 vs. 7 months; $p = 0.02$). The third trial, which included more patients with an active systemic disease (80% vs. 30–40%) and a lower KPS compared with the first two trials, did not show any survival benefit with the addition of surgery to WBRT [84]. Overall, these data suggest that the survival benefit of surgery is limited to patients with good performance status and controlled systemic disease. There is also some evidence suggesting that in selected patients with 2–3 BMs, complete surgical resection may be beneficial, yielding results that are comparable to those obtained in patients with a single lesion [85].

The goal of surgery is the complete removal of BMs, while protecting functional cortex, subcortical structures, and vascular structures [86]. Although surgical resection is an invasive approach, it is generally well-tolerated in patients with BMs. In fact, a large retrospective review of 208 patients undergoing resection for BMs (191 with single lesions) reported an overall operative mortality of 1.9% [87]. Gross total resection of BMs can be achieved with low morbidity using contemporary image-guided systems, such as preoperative functional MRI, intraoperative neuronavigation, and cortical mapping [88].

Surgical resection allows an immediate relief of symptoms caused by increased intracranial pressure, a reduction of focal neurological deficits, and a rapid steroid tapering in the majority of patients. Furthermore,

surgery helps to establish the histological diagnosis in case of unknown primary or multiple primary tumors, or when imaging is not conclusive.

(i) *SRS*

In the 1980s, SRS was introduced as a minimally invasive option as opposed to surgery for the treatment of oligo-BMs [89].

SRS is a type of external radiation therapy delivered in a single dose to a small target volume (3–4 cm) with high precision. SRS requires precise location of the tumor and head immobilization systems. It can be delivered using either gamma-knife, consisting of multiple collimated cobalt-60 sources, or linear accelerator (Linac). There is no difference in outcome between gamma-knife and Linac. Compared to gamma-knife, however, Linac allows treatment of larger, non-spherical lesions and can deliver treatment both in a single dose and in multiple fractions. In the latter case, the technique is called stereotactic fractionated stereosurgery (SFRT), it represents an alternative to single-dose SRS and may be used for patients with larger lesions or lesions located near critical structures [90]. Studies comparing surgery and SRS suggest similar outcomes, although most of them are not randomized trials [91–93]. SRS for newly diagnosed oligo-BMs achieves symptomatic improvement, a local control of 80–90% at 1 year and median OS of 6–12 months [94]. Patients with single BMs, good performance status (KPS > 70) and controlled extracranial disease have longer survival [95]. Age seems to not affect the outcome, since elderly patients achieve the same benefit as younger patients [96]. BMs from radioresistant primary tumors, such as melanoma or kidney cancer, respond to SRS as well as BMs from radiosensitive tumors [97].

RTOG9508, a randomized phase 3 study in patients with 1–3 BMs, investigated the role of SRS + WBRT compared to WBRT alone, reporting better local control and performance status at six months in the combined therapy group [96]. However, a survival advantage was observed only for patients with a single BM and, in a secondary analysis, for patients with good GPA score (3.5–4.0) regardless of the number of BMs [98], and these observations highlight the need for an appropriate selection of patients for SRS.

In the past 5–10 years, SRS has been increasingly used for patients with higher number of brain metastases, due to improved technology that allows the delivery of SRS with increasing speed while maintaining precision and accuracy [95, 99]. A prospective multicenter Japanese study investigated the use of SRS alone in 1194 patients with 1, 2–4 or 5–10 BMs, and found similar OS and treatment-related toxicity rates between the groups with 2 to 4 and 5 to 10 metastases. Cumulative volume of BMs, rather than the number, was reported as a significant prognostic factor [95].

In recent years, SRS has been used also to treat postsurgical cavities. Several retrospective and one prospective phase 2 trial reported 1-year local control rates ranging from 70% to 90% and a median OS of 10–17 months, suggesting that postoperative SRS may be as effective as WBRT in achieving local control [100]. However, the balance between benefit and risk is currently unknown with unsolved issues (optimal dose and fractionation, impact on survival, quality of life and cognitive function, incidence of complications), therefore randomized trials are needed to clarify the role of postoperative SRS.

Complications of SRS are reported in 10–30% of patients, but severe adverse events are rare. Early complications occur within 2 weeks from treatment and are represented by symptoms related to transient increased intracranial pressure (headache, nausea and vomiting, worsening of preexistent neurological deficits, and seizures) that are generally reversible with steroids. Late adverse events occur months to years after the treatment and include hemorrhage and radionecrosis. The risk of adverse events increases with the increase of lesion size [101].

(ii) *WBRT*

WBRT was historically considered a mainstay in the treatment of BMs and, in the modern era, still plays multiple roles. WBRT is indicated in case of multiple BMs, BMs larger than 4 cm, BMs with poorly controlled systemic disease or BMs in patients with poor performance status. It may be also used as adjuvant therapy with the aim of reducing recurrence after surgery, as salvage therapy after surgery or SRS, or for reirradiation after late WBRT. Standard fractionations are 30 Gy in 10 fractions or 20 Gy in 5 fractions. The addition of radiotherapy sensitizers does not translate into a survival benefit [69, 102].

Different studies in the past reported symptomatic response in up to 60% of patients treated with WBRT, although neurological improvement could be partially attributable to steroids. Median OS reported with WBRT (3–6 months) is longer than that observed in patients not receiving treatment (1–3 months). However, a phase 3 non-inferiority trial on NSCLC patients with BMs that were not candidates to surgery or SRS did not show any survival difference in OS and quality of life between WBRT and BSC [103].

It is still controversial whether, after complete surgical resection or SRS, WBRT should be offered with the aim of destroying microscopic metastatic foci at the original tumor site or at distant intracranial locations. In fact, three large phase 3 trials [104–106] and a meta-analysis [107] demonstrated that omitting WBRT in patients with a limited number of BMs after either complete surgery or SRS results in significantly worse local and distant control in the brain, however, without a significant impact on OS. A recent individual patient data meta-analysis of three randomized studies comparing SRS alone with SRS + WBRT in patients with 1 to 4 BMs suggested a survival advantage for SRS alone and no risk reduction for new BMs with the addition of WBRT in patients aged <50 years, whereas in patients aged ≥50 years the addition of WBRT reduced the risk of recurrence, without improving survival. The reason of these results is not completely clear [108]. WBRT may cause early adverse effects (fatigue, alopecia) and late neurotoxicity. Several studies assessed the impact of adjuvant WBRT on cognitive functions and quality of life, reporting more frequent decline of cognitive functions and more fatigue for SRS + WBRT compared with SRS alone [109–112]. Based on the lack of survival benefit and the increased risk of neurotoxicity, the American Society for Radiation Oncology (ASTRO) has recommended against the routine use of adjuvant WBRT after SRS. The issue of adjuvant WBRT after surgical resection is less well-defined. In a randomized trial on 95 patients with completely resected single BM, the addition of WBRT to surgery compared with surgery alone significantly prevented brain recurrence at site of the original BM (10% vs. 46%, $p < 0.001$) and at other sites in the brain (14% vs. 37%), but, again, without significant difference in survival, that was a secondary endpoint of the study [104].

For patients who do not receive WBRT after surgery or after SRS, close follow up with a brain MRI repeated every 3 months should be performed for early detection and treatment of local or distant brain recurrence. However, it remains unclear whether an active surveillance with salvage local therapy is as effective as immediate adjuvant WBRT. There are no randomized trials in this setting, but case series reported symptom relief in 30–70% patients receiving salvage WBRT [113, 114].

In order to reduce WBRT-associated neurotoxicity, new approaches, including neuroprotective agents and new radiation techniques, have been investigated. In a randomized phase 3 trial, the addition of metamine to WBRT delayed cognitive impairment, but with only 149 patients enrolled, the study was underpowered to achieve significant results [115]. Hippocampus avoidance-WBRT, a novel technique used to reduce the radiation dose to critical hippocampal areas, may be associated with preservation of memory and quality of life without increasing risk of recurrence in the low dose region, as suggested by a phase 2 study [116].

(iii) *Systemic Therapy*

Half of patients with BMs die from progressive systemic cancer, therefore systemic therapy often represents an integral part of the overall treatment strategy. Indeed, the use of systemic therapy as upfront treatment of BMs has been neglected for years, mainly because of the prevailing belief that antitumor drugs do not cross the BBB and also because patients with symptomatic or uncontrolled BMs have been generally excluded from clinical trials of systemic therapies. However, growing evidence suggests that the presence of macroscopic BMs may disrupt the BBB, thus allowing the penetration of therapeutics into the tumor tissue and providing a rationale for clinical investigations of systemic therapy for BMs [117].

For patients with chemo-sensitive primary tumors or tumors harboring a druggable target, systemic therapy may be a reasonable option for upfront treatment, thus delaying the need for local therapy, especially when tumor burden in extracranial sites is prominent and the control of systemic cancer is an urgent issue. Instead, when BMs are symptomatic, large or located in critical areas, or when primary tumor is low chemo-sensitive or not harboring a druggable target, systemic therapy can be postponed after the local treatment of BMs [70].

The choice of systemic therapy in the individual patients depends on multiple factors, including the performance status of the patient, the tumor type and molecular characteristics, and the previous lines of systemic therapy already administered. The following paragraphs are focused on NSCLC and breast cancer, the two cancers that most often metastasize to the brain.

■ NSCLC

NSCLC is a heterogeneous disease composed of several molecular subtypes, some of them associated with specific oncogenic drivers amenable to target therapy.

For patients with metastatic NSCLC, harboring an activating mutation in the *EGFR* gene (10–15% of Caucasian patients and up to 50% of Asian patients), standard first-line systemic therapy is an EGFR tyrosine kinase inhibitor (TKI). EGFR-TKIs are active both against systemic disease and BMs. First-generation (gefitinib, erlotinib, icotinib) and second-generation (afatinib, dacomitinib) agents achieve intracranial RRs of 60–80%, with median PFS in the brain of approximately 7–12 months and median OS of 15–20 months [118]. However, the upfront treatment with EGFR-TKIs may be questionable, since retrospective series with first-generation EGFR-TKIs suggest better OS for patients treated with upfront radiotherapy, especially SRS, compared with patients receiving EGFR-TKIs alone [119]. Moreover, after the initial intracranial response, 26–33% patients eventually experience intracranial progression [120].

About 50% of progressive NSCLC acquire the EGFR T790M mutation, that is a well-known mechanism of resistance to first- and second-generation TKIs [121]. Recently osimertinib, a third-generation EGFR-TKI targeting not only the classic EGFR activating mutations but also T790M mutation, has been approved for metastatic NSCLC. Osimertinib has demonstrated promising activity against BMs. In fact, a pooled analysis of two phase 2 studies on CNS response to osimertinib in patients with T790M-positive metastatic NSCLC reported an encouraging intracranial RR and disease-control rate of 50% and 92%, respectively [122]. These data have been corroborated by the results of a phase 3 randomized trial comparing osimertinib versus platinum-pemetrexed as second-line treatment for patients with T790M-mutated metastatic NSCLC who had progressed during receipt of first-line EGFR-TKI [123]. Among the subgroup of patients with BMs, osimertinib achieved a median PFS significantly longer than chemotherapy (8.5 vs. 4.2 months). Osimertinib seems to be even more effective when administered as first-line treatment as demonstrated by the FLAURA study, a phase 3 study on patients with EGFR-mutant NSCLC randomized to receive osimertinib or a first-generation EGFR-TKI (gefitinib or erlotinib) as first line treatment [124]. Among patients with BMs at trial entry (about 20% of the entire trial population), osimertinib achieved higher intracranial RR compared with standard EGFR-TKI (66% vs. 43%), with longer CNS PFS (not reached vs. 13.9 months), longer duration of response (13.8 vs. 8.5 months) and lower frequency of CNS progression [125].

Although *ALK* rearrangements involve a minority of NSCLC (4–6%), up to 50% of patients with ALK-positive NSCLC eventually develop BMs [126]. Crizotinib was the first ALK inhibitor approved. Pooled analysis of a phase 3 randomized trial (PROFILE 1007) and a single-arm phase 2 trial (PROFILE 1005) with crizotinib reported a 56% of intracranial disease control rate at 3 months, with a RR of 18% in patients with previously untreated BMs and 33% in patients who had previously received brain radiotherapy [127]. Second-generation ALK-TKIs, alectinib, lorlatinib, and brigatinib, have demonstrated efficacy in crizotinib-resistant patients. In a pooled analysis of two studies evaluating CNS response of alectinib in pretreated patients, intracranial RR was 64% [127]. When compared head-to-head as first line treatment in randomized phase 3 trials, alectinib demonstrated an intracranial RR higher than crizotinib (59% vs. 26%) [128, 129].

Based on the high intracranial RRs observed with new-generation TKIs in EGFR-mutant and ALK-positive NSCLC patients, upfront systemic treatment with these agents may be a reasonable option, in order to delay the need for local treatment thus preserving neurocognitive functions [130]. However, as discussed before, some evidence suggests that TKIs given after radiotherapy, particularly SRS, may be a more effective approach than target therapy given upfront, but it should be emphasized that such data derive from non-randomized, retrospective studies with old-generation TKIs [119, 131, 132].

The combination of EGFR-TKIs with radiotherapy is still a controversial approach. In fact, some phase 2 studies investigating the combination of erlotinib plus WBRT or icotinib plus WBRT suggested prolonged survivals [133, 134], but randomized phase 2 and 3 studies on patients unselected for EGFR mutations failed to demonstrate a superiority of the combination of erlotinib with either SRS or WBRT over radiotherapy alone, with higher risk of toxicity [135, 136]. There are only limited data about the safety and tolerability of concomitant ALK-TKIs and radiation therapy [137]. Therefore, a prudential temporary discontinuation of TKIs during radiation therapy may represent an acceptable option. In this regard, SRS has the advantage of few days of temporary systemic therapy discontinuation, as compared to WBRT.

In recent years, immune checkpoint inhibitors have prolonged survival of a subgroup of patients with metastatic NSCLC, and the use of immunotherapy is expected to increase in the near future. Pembrolizumab is approved as first-line treatment for patients with EGFR wild-type, ALK-negative NSCLC with PD-L1 expression ≥50%, and as second-line treatment for patients with PD-L1 expression ≥1%, whereas nivolumab and atezolizumab are approved as second-line treatment, regardless of PD-L1 expression. Although data on immune checkpoint in patients with NSCLC and BMs are limited since most studies excluded untreated BMs and patients requiring a steroid dose ≥10 mg/day of prednisone or equivalent, available evidence suggest activity against BMs. In fact, in a non-randomized, phase 2 study, patients with untreated BMs (18 patients with melanoma and 18 patients with NSCLC) received pembrolizumab, and 33% of patients with NSCLC achieved an intracranial response [138]. Case reports suggest intracranial activity also for nivolumab [139]. Results from larger randomized studies investigating immunotherapy for NSCLC-derived BMs are awaited.

Chemotherapy still represents the mainstay of treatment for many patients with advanced NSCLC who are not candidates to target therapy or immunotherapy. Platinum-based regimens have clinical activity against BMs from NSCLC, with intracranial RR ranging from 23% to 50%, comparable to that expected for the systemic disease. However, the best regimen for BMs has not been identified. In fact, in a randomized phase 3 trial comparing three different chemotherapy regimens (carboplatin plus gemcitabine, paclitaxel plus gemcitabine, or paclitaxel plus carboplatin), in the subgroup of 194 patients with clinically stable BMs, no chemotherapy regimen was proven to be superior to the others in terms of RR, PFS, or OS. In non-squamous histology, the combination of platinum compounds plus pemetrexed has demonstrated interesting activity, with RR of 50% and median OS up to 9 months [140].

- **Breast Cancer**

HER2-positive breast cancer and TNBC have high propensity to metastasize to the brain [141].

The introduction of HER2-targeted agents has dramatically improved the outcome of patients with HER2-positive breast cancer, both in early and in metastatic disease. Despite these improvements, however, approximately 40% of patients with advanced HER2-positive breast cancer relapse in the CNS [142]. Until recently, trastuzumab-based chemotherapy has been the mainstay of treatment for HER2-positive metastatic breast cancer. A survival benefit with trastuzumab was reported also for patients with BMs, but this seems due to the control of systemic disease rather than to an intracranial activity [143]. The addition of pertuzumab to trastuzumab and docetaxel has demonstrated a survival advantage over trastuzumab plus docetaxel, thus becoming the current standard of care as first-line treatment [144]. Unfortunately, patients with BMs were excluded from pivotal trials investigating this combination; therefore, its possible role as upfront treatment of BMs is still unclear. Of note, a secondary analysis of the CLEOPATRA trial reported a longer median time to development of BMs as first site of disease progression for patients in the pertuzumab-trastuzumab-docetaxel arm compared with those in the trastuzumab-docetaxel arm (15.0 versus 11.9 months), suggesting a protective role of the triplet combination against BMs [145]. It is therefore conceivable that for naïve patients, systemic therapy with pertuzumab, trastuzumab, and a taxane following the local treatment of BMs would be a reasonable option to delay disease progression, both in the brain and in extracranial sites.

The dual EGFR/HER2 TKI lapatinib has been extensively investigated in patients with HER2-positive BMs, both as single agent and in combination. As a single agent in pretreated patients, lapatinib has negligible activity with an intracranial RR of less than 3% [146]. Greater activity has been observed in combination with capecitabine, leading to an intracranial RR of 38% in pretreated patients [147], and an intracranial RR of 66% with 1-year survival of 70% in the newly diagnosed setting, as demonstrated by the single-arm phase 2 LANDSCAPE study [148].

Historically, anti-HER2 monoclonal antibodies were thought to be too large to cross the BBB, but there is now evidence from studies utilizing 89Zr-labeled trastuzumab as a PET tracer that there is some penetration of antibodies through BBB disrupted by BMs. This is further supported by accumulating evidence of intracranial activity of T-DM1, with RRs similar to those observed for extracranial disease [149]. Furthermore, an exploratory retrospective analysis of the EMILIA trial showed a survival benefit for patients with brain metastases treated with T-DM1 compared with patients treated with lapatinib and capecitabine (26.8 months versus 12.9 months) [150].

Therefore, for patients with progressive BMs after trastuzumab-based therapy, possible systemic options are T-DM1 or lapatinib plus capecitabine.

Up to 40% of patients with TNBC develop BMs. Unfortunately, no target therapy is available for this subtype, and the only option of systemic therapy is chemotherapy. When treating BMs from breast cancer with chemotherapy, drugs with proven antitumor activity in extracranial sites should be preferred to agents like temozolomide, with known penetration of BBB but limited systemic activity. In fact, temozolomide showed no activity in patients with breast cancer and BMs [151]. Conversely, cisplatin or carboplatin-based combinations achieved objective responses in patients with BMs from breast cancer, particularly TNBC. For instance, a complete brain response of 13% and a partial response of 25% were described with the combination of cisplatin and etoposide in patients with BMs [152]. Data from phase 2 studies also suggest that, in naïve patients with BMs, conventional combination therapies, such as cyclophosphamide/methotrexate/5-fluorouracil (CMF) or 5-fluorouracil/doxorubicin/cyclophosphamide (FAC), may have clinical activity. There is growing investigation of immune checkpoint inhibitors and PARP inhibitors for the treatment of TNBC, but the role of these agents in the treatment of BMs has yet to be elucidated.

(d) *Assessment of Response*

The assessment of response for BMs is still an open issue and there are no standard criteria. Across clinical trials in oncology, dimensional criteria, such as WHO, RECIST, and RECIST 1.1, have been often used to assess the response [153–155]. However, these criteria have many limitations. Particularly, they consider the intracranial and extracranial sites together for the assessment of response, and do not take into account the control of neurologic symptoms, that for patients with BMs represents a crucial goal, as it has an important impact on quality of life. For this reason, Macdonald and colleagues developed response criteria specifically for CNS malignancies [156]. These criteria consider dimensional changes together with neurologic symptoms and need for steroids (◘ Table 44.4).

An important limitation of Macdonald's criteria is that they are derived by WHO criteria which are based on bi-dimensional measurement. Bi-dimensional criteria are more time-consuming and increase the risk of measurement errors compared with uni-dimensional criteria. In order to standardize the response assessment for BMs in clinical trials, the Response Assessment in Neuro-Oncology (RANO) working group has recently proposed new response criteria based on uni-dimensional measurement of lesions, corticosteroids use, and clinical status, but their use in clinical trials is not yet widespread [157].

44.3.6 Conclusion

BMs represent a frequent complication of several solid tumors and their incidence has been rising in the last decades, possibly due to the more widespread use of neuroimaging in asymptomatic patients, but also due to the improved survival of cancer patients obtained by novel anticancer drugs that effectively control systemic disease. Treatment of BMs should be personalized, often requiring a multimodal approach, including both local and systemic treatment.

Although survival of patients with BMs has improved over the last years mainly due to the progress of radiotherapy techniques and the availability of more effective systemic treatments, BMs still have an adverse impact on prognosis and quality of life. The development of more effective treatment for BMs still represents an urgent clinical need.

Table 44.4 Comparison of response criteria

	Image modality	Target lesion	Maximum number of CNS target lesions	Measurement technique	Shrinkage required for partial response	Confirmatory scans	Steroids	Neurological symptoms	Extracranial disease
WHO	Not specified	Minimum size not specified	Not specified	Bi-dimensional	≥50%	Required at least 4 weeks Apart	Not included	Not included	Included
RECIST	CT or MRI	Longest diameter ≥10 mm	5	Uni-dimensional	≥30%	Required in non-randomized trials where response is the primary endpoint	Not included	Not included	Included
RECIST 1.1	CT or MRI	Longest diameter ≥10 mm	2	Uni-dimensional	≥30%	Required in non-randomized trials where response is the primary endpoint	Not included	Not included	Included
Macdonald	CT or MRI	Minimum size not Specified	Not specified	Bi-dimensional	≥50%	Required at least one month Apart	Stable or decreased	Stable to improved	Not applicable

Modified from Lin et al. (2015)

CNS central nervous system, *CT* computed tomography, *MRI* magnetic resonance imaging, *RECIST* Response Evaluation Criteria in Solid Tumors, *WHO* World Health Organization

44

Expert Opinion
Christian Rolfo

- Although any cancer may virtually spread to the brain, the majority of BMs originate from lung cancer, breast cancer, melanoma, kidney cancer, colorectal cancer, and unknown primary.
- In case of neurologic symptoms suggestive for BMs, brain CT scan and/or MRI represent the mainstay of the diagnostic work-up.
- An accurate prognostic assessment through validated prognostic indexes may inform the decision-making process.
- Clinical management is based on a multidisciplinary approach including symptomatic treatment, surgery, radiotherapy (SRS or WBRT), and systemic therapy.
- The goal of symptomatic treatment is to reduce symptoms associated with BMs, particularly symptoms related to cerebral edema through the administration of steroids or mannitol, and seizures through the administration of antiepileptic drugs.
- Surgery represents an option for patients with good performance status and single or oligo-BMs, especially when associated with extensive edema or in case of uncertain diagnosis.
- SRS is a non-invasive approach for patients with good performance status and oligo-BMs, and for selected patients with multiple BMs it can be also delivered as adjuvant treatment after surgical resection of a single BM, or as salvage treatment for recurrence after surgery or WBRT.
- WBRT may be considered for patients with multiple BMs, or as salvage treatment for recurrence after surgery or SRS.
- Systemic treatment is often an integral part of the overall treatment strategy, mainly for the control of systemic disease; some anticancer agents such as *EGFR* or *ALK* inhibitors for oncogene-addicted NSCLC or anti-HER2 drugs for HER2-positive breast cancer have also activity against BMs.

Recommendations
- NICE
  - https://www.nice.org.uk/guidance/ng99/chapter/Recommendations

Hints for a Deeper Insight
- Recent advances in managing brain metastasis: ▸ https://www.ncbi.nlm.nih.gov/pubmed/30473769
- Brain metastases: radiosurgery: ▸ https://www.ncbi.nlm.nih.gov/pubmed/29307350
- Surgery for brain metastases: An analysis of outcomes and factors affecting survival: ▸ https://www.ncbi.nlm.nih.gov/pubmed/29554624
- Management of breast cancer brain metastases: A practical review: ▸ https://www.ncbi.nlm.nih.gov/pubmed/27829201

References

Primary Brain Tumors

1. Lowery FJ, YU D. Brain metastasis: unique challenges and open opportunities. Biochim Biophys Acta Rev Cancer. 2017;1867(1):49–57.
2. Wrensch M, Minn Y, Chew T, Bondy M, Berger MS. Epidemiology of primary brain tumors: current concepts and review of the literature. Neuro-Oncology. 2002;4(4):278–99.
3. Louis DN, Perry A, Reifenberger G, von Deimling A, Figarella-Branger D, Cavenee WK, et al. The 2016 World Health Organization classification of tumors of the central nervous system: a summary. Acta Neuropathol. 2016;131(6):803–20.
4. Perkins A, Liu G. Primary brain tumors in adults: diagnosis and treatment. Am Fam Physician. 2016;93(3):211–7.
5. Weller M, van den Bent M, Tonn JC, Stupp R, Preusser M, et al. European Association for Neuro-Oncology (EANO) guideline on the diagnosis and treatment of adult astrocytic and oligodendroglial gliomas. Lancet Oncol. 2017;18(6):e315–29.
6. van den Bent MJ, Baumert B, Erridge SC, Vogelbaum MA, Nowak AK, Sanson M, et al. Interim results from the CATNON trial (EORTC study 26053-22054) of treatment with concurrent and adjuvant temozolomide for 1p/19q non-co-deleted anaplastic glioma: a phase 3, randomised, open-label intergroup study. Lancet. 2017;390(10103):1645–53.
7. Stupp R, Mason WP, van den Bent MJ, Weller M, Fisher B, Taphoorn MJ, et al. Radiotherapy plus concomitant and adjuvant temozolomide for glioblastoma. N Engl J Med. 2005;352(10):987–96.
8. Weller M, Stupp R, Reifenberger G, Brandes AA, van den Bent MJ, Wick W, et al. MGMT promoter methylation in malignant gliomas: ready for personalized medicine? Nat Rev Neurol. 2010;6(1):39–51.
9. Lu VM, O'Connor KP, Shah AH, Eichberg DG, Luther EM, et al. The prognostic significance of CDKN2A homozygous deletion in IDH-mutant lower-grade glioma and glioblastoma: a systematic review of the contemporary literature. J Neuro-Oncol. 2020;148:221.
10. Davis ME. Glioblastoma: overview of disease and treatment. Clin J Oncol Nurs. 2016;20(5 Suppl):S2–8.
11. Glas M, Kebir S. Regorafenib in glioblastoma recurrence: how to deal with conflicting 'real-life' experiences? Ther Adv Med Oncol. 2019;11:1758835919887667.
12. Sanson M, Cartalat-Carel S, Taillibert S, Napolitano M, Djafari L, Cougnard J, et al. Initial chemotherapy in gliomatosis cerebri. Neurology. 2004;63(2):270–5.
13. Baumert BG, Hegi ME, van den Bent MJ, von Deimling A, Gorlia T, Hoang-Xuan K, et al. Temozolomide chemotherapy versus radiotherapy in high-risk low-grade glioma (EORTC 22033-26033): a randomised, open-label, phase 3 intergroup study. Lancet Oncol. 2016;17(11):1521–32.

14. Metellus P, Guyotat J, Chinot O, Durand A, Barrie M, Giorgi R, et al. Adult intracranial WHO grade II ependymomas: long-term outcome and prognostic factor analysis in a series of 114 patients. Neuro-Oncology. 2010;12(9):976–84.

15. Reni M, Gatta G, Mazza E, Vecht C. Ependymoma. Crit Rev Oncol Hematol. 2007;63(1):81–9.

16. Oya N, Shibamoto Y, Nagata Y, Negoro Y, Hiraoka M. Post-operative radiotherapy for intracranial ependymoma: analysis of prognostic factors and patterns of failure. J Neuro-Oncol. 2002;56(1):87–94.

17. Franceschi E, Bartolotti M, Paccapelo A, Marucci G, Agati R, Volpin L, et al. Adjuvant chemotherapy in adult medulloblastoma: is it an option for average-risk patients? J Neuro-Oncol. 2016;128(2):235–40.

18. Brandes AA, Pasetto LM, Lumachi F, Monfardini S. Endocrine dysfunctions in patients treated for brain tumors: incidence and guidelines for management. J Neuro-Oncol. 2000;47(1):85–92.

19. Wiemels J, Wrensch M, Claus EB. Epidemiology and etiology of meningioma. J Neuro-Oncol. 2010;99(3):307–14.

20. Buerki RA, Horbinski CM, Kruser T, Horowitz PM, James CD, Lukas RV. An overview of meningiomas. Future Oncol. 2018;14(21):2161–77.

21. Melean G, Sestini R, Ammannati F, Papi L. Genetic insights into familial tumors of the nervous system. Am J Med Genet C Semin Med Genet. 2004;129C(1):74–84.

22. Galanti D, Inno A, La Vecchia M, et al. Current treatment options for HER2-positive breast cancer patients with brain metastases. Crit Rev Oncol Hematol. 2021;161:103329. https://doi.org/10.1016/j.critrevonc.2021.103329.

Brain Metastases

23. Walker AE, Robins M, Weinfeld FD. Epidemiology of brain tumors: the national survey of intracranial neoplasms. Neurology. 1985;35:219–26.

24. Counsell CE, Collie DA, Grant R. Incidence of intracranial tumours in the Lothian region of Scotland, 1989-90. J Neurol Neurosurg Psychiatry. 1996;61:143–50.

25. Schouten LJ, Rutten J, Huveneers HA, Twijnstra A. Incidence of brain metastases in a cohort of patients with carcinoma of the breast, colon, kidney, and lung and melanoma. Cancer. 2002;94:2698–705.

26. Barnholtz-Sloan JS, Sloan AE, Davis FG, Vigneau FD, Lai P, Sawaya RE. Incidence proportions of brain metastases in patients diagnosed (1973 to 2001) in the Metropolitan Detroit Cancer Surveillance System. J Clin Oncol. 2004;22:2865–72.

27. Tabouret E, Chinot O, Metellus P, Tallet A, Viens P, Gonçalves A. Recent trends in epidemiology of brain metastases: an overview. Anticancer Res. 2012;32:4655–62.

28. Percy AK. Neoplasms of the central nervous system: epidemiologic considerations. Neurology. 1970;20:398–9.

29. Posner JB, Chernik NL. Intracranial metastases from systemic cancer. Adv Neurol. 1978;19:579–92.

30. Nayak L, Lee EQ, Wen PY. Epidemiology of brain metastases. Curr Oncol Rep. 2012;14:48–54.

31. Berghoff AS, Schur S, Füreder LM, Gatterbauer B, Dieckmann K, Widhalm G, et al. Descriptive statistical analysis of a real life cohort of 2419 patients with brain metastases of solid cancers. ESMO Open. 2016;1:e000024.

32. Stark AM, Stöhring C, Hedderich J, Held-Feindt J, Mehdorn HM. Surgical treatment for brain metastases: prognostic factors and survival in 309 patients with regard to patient age. J Clin Neurosci. 2011;18:34–8.

33. Slimane K, Andre F, Delaloge S, Dunant A, Perez A, Grenier J, et al. Risk factors for brain relapse in patients with metastatic breast cancer. Ann Oncol. 2004;15:1640–4.

34. Kennecke H, Yerushalmi R, Woods R, Cheang MC, Voduc D, Speers CH, et al. Metastatic behavior of breast cancer subtypes. J Clin Oncol. 2010;28:3271–7.

35. Graesslin O, Abdulkarim BS, Coutant C, Huguet F, Gabos Z, Hsu L, et al. Nomogram to predict subsequent brain metastasis in patients with metastatic breast cancer. J Clin Oncol. 2010;28:2032–7.

36. Genre L, Roché H, Varela L, Kanoun D, Ouali M, Filleron T, et al. External validation of a published nomogram for prediction of brain metastasis in patients with extra-cerebral metastatic breast cancer and risk regression analysis. Eur J Cancer. 2017;72:200–9.

37. Won YW, Joo J, Yun T, Lee GK, Han JY, Kim HT, et al. A nomogram to predict brain metastasis as the first relapse in curatively resected non-small cell lung cancer patients. Lung Cancer. 2015;88:201–7.

38. Zhang F, Zheng W, Ying L, Wu J, Wu S, Ma S, et al. A nomogram to predict brain metastases of resected non-small cell lung cancer patients. Ann Surg Oncol. 2016;23:3033–9.

39. Nathoo N, Chahlavi A, Barnett GH, Toms SA. Pathobiology of brain metastases. J Clin Pathol. 2005;58:237–42.

40. Morita R, Fujimoto A, Hatta N, Takehara K, Takata M. Comparison of genetic profiles between primary melanomas and their metastases reveals genetic alterations and clonal evolution during progression. J Invest Dermatol. 1998;111:919–24.

41. Langley RR, Fidler IJ. The seed and soil hypothesis revisited-the role of tumor-stroma interactions in metastasis to different organs. Int J Cancer. 2011;128:2527–35.

42. Bos PD, Zhang XH, Nadal C, Shu W, Gomis RR, Nguyen DX, et al. Genes that mediate breast cancer metastasis to the brain. Nature. 2009;459:1005–9.

43. Lee JY, Park K, Lee E, Ahn T, Jung HH, Lim SH, et al. Gene expression profiling of breast cancer brain metastasis. Sci Rep. 2016;6:28623.

44. Gavrilovic IT, Posner JB. Brain metastases: epidemiology and pathophysiology. J Neuro-Oncol. 2005;75:5–14.

45. Liotta LA, Kohn EC. Cancer's deadly signature. Nat Genet. 2003;33:10–1.

46. Delattre JY, Krol G, Thaler HT, Posner JB. Distribution of brain metastases. Arch Neurol. 1998;45:741–4.

47. Hwang TL, Close TP, Grego JM, Rannon WL, Gonzales F. Predilection of brain metastasis in gray and white matter junction and vascular border zones. Cancer. 1996;77:1551–5.

48. Cairncross JG, Kim JH, Posner JB. Radiation therapy for brain metastases. Ann Neurol. 1980;7:529–41.

49. Gállego Pérez-Larraya J, Hildebrand J. Brain metastases. Handb Clin Neurol. 2014;121:1143–57.

50. Forsyth PA, Posner JB. Headaches in patients with brain tumors: a study of 111 patients. Neurology. 1993;43:1678–83.

51. Argyriou AA, Chroni E, Polychronopoulos P, Argyriou K, Papapetropoulos S, Corcondilas M, et al. Headache characteristics and brain metastases prediction in cancer patients. Eur J Cancer Care. 2006;15:90–5.

52. Lynam LM, Lyons MK, Drazkowski JF, Sirven JI, Noe KH, Zimmerman RS, et al. Frequency of seizures in patients with newly diagnosed brain tumors: a retrospective review. Clin Neurol Neurosurg. 2007;109:634–8.

53. Chang EL, Wefel JS, Maor MH, Hassenbusch SJ 3rd, Mahajan A, Lang FF, et al. A pilot study of neurocognitive function in patients with one to three new brain metastases initially treated with stereotactic radiosurgery alone. Neurosurgery. 2007;60:277–83.

54. Nutt SH, Patchell RA. Intracranial hemorrhage associated with primary and secondary tumors. Neurosurg Clin N Am. 1992;3:591–9.

44

55. Incorvaia L, Madonia G, Corsini LR, et al. Challenges and advances for the treatment of renal cancer patients with brain metastases: From immunological background to upcoming clinical evidence on immune-checkpoint inhibitors. Crit Rev Oncol Hematol. 2021;163:103390.

56. Fink KR, Fink JR. Imaging of brain metastases. Surg Neurol Int. 2013;4(Suppl 4):S209–19.

57. Lee EK, Lee EJ, Kim MS, Park HJ, Park NH, Park S 2nd, et al. Intracranial metastases: spectrum of MR imaging findings. Acta Radiol. 2012;53:1173–85.

58. Rohren EM, Provenzale JM, Barboriak DP, Coleman RE. Screening for cerebralmetastases with FDG PET in patients undergoing whole-body staging of non-central nervous system malignancy. Radiology. 2003;226:181–7.

59. Hustinx R, Pourdehnad M, Kaschten B, Alavi A. PET imaging for differentiating recurrent brain tumor from radiation necrosis. Radiol Clin N Am. 2005;43:35–47.

60. Unterrainer M, Galldiks N, Suchorska B, Kowalew LC, Wenter V, Schmid-Tannwald C, et al. (18)F-FET PET uptake characteristics in patients with newly diagnosed and untreated brain metastasis. J Nucl Med. 2017;58:584–9.

61. Becher MW, Abel TW, Thompson RC, Weaver KD, Davis LE. Immunohistochemical analysis of metastatic neoplasms of the central nervous system. J Neuropathol Exp Neurol. 2006;65:935–44.

62. Gaspar L, Scott C, Rotman M, Asbell S, Phillips T, Wasserman T, et al. Recursive partitioning analysis (RPA) of prognostic factors in three Radiation Therapy Oncology Group (RTOG) brain metastases trials. Int J Radiat Oncol Biol Phys. 1997;37:745–51.

63. Sperduto PW, Berkey B, Gaspar LE, Mehta M, Curran W. A new prognostic index and comparison to three other indices for patients with brain metastases: an analysis of 1,960 patients in the RTOG database. Int J Radiat Oncol Biol Phys. 2008;70:510–4.

64. Sperduto PW, Chao ST, Sneed PK, Luo X, Suh J, Roberge D, et al. Diagnosis-specific prognostic factors, indexes, and treatment outcomes for patients with newly diagnosed brain metastases: a multi-institutional analysis of 4,259 patients. Int J Radiat Oncol Biol Phys. 2010;77:655–61.

65. Sperduto PW, Kased N, Roberge D, Xu Z, Shanley R, Luo X, et al. Summary report on the graded prognostic assessment: an accurate and facile diagnosis-specific tool to estimate survival for patients with brain metastases. J Clin Oncol. 2012a;30:419–25.

66. Sperduto PW, Kased N, Roberge D, Xu Z, Shanley R, Luo X, et al. Effect of tumor subtype on survival and the graded prognostic assessment for patients with breast cancer and brain metastases. Int J Radiat Oncol Biol Phys. 2012b;82:2111–7.

67. Griguolo G, Jacot W, Kantelhardt E, Dieci MV, Bourgier C, Thomssen C, et al. External validation of modified breast graded prognostic assessment for breast cancer patients with brain metastases: a multicentric European experience. Breast. 2018;37:36–41.

68. Sperduto PW, Yang TJ, Beal K, Pan H, Brown PD, Bangdiwala A, et al. Estimating survival in patients with lung cancer and brain metastases: an update of the graded prognostic assessment for lung cancer using molecular markers (lung-molGPA). JAMA Oncol. 2017;3:827–31.

69. Soffietti R, Abacioglu U, Baumert B, Combs SE, Kinhult S, Kros JM, et al. Diagnosis and treatment of brain metastases from solid tumors: guidelines from the European Association of Neuro-Oncology (EANO). Neuro-Oncology. 2017;19:162–74.

70. Lin X, DeAngelis LM. Treatment of brain metastases. J Clin Oncol. 2015;33:3475–84.

71. Stummer W. Mechanisms of tumor-related brain edema. Neurosurg Focus. 2007;22:E8.

72. Ryken TC, McDermott M, Robinson PD, Ammirati M, Andrews DW, Asher AL, et al. The role of steroids in the management of brain metastases: a systematic review and evidence-based clinical practice guideline. J Neuro-Oncol. 2010;96:103–14.

73. Vecht CJ, Hovestadt A, Verbiest HB, van Vliet JJ, van Putten WL, et al. Dose-effect relationship of dexamethasone on Karnofsky performance in metastatic brain tumors: a randomized study of doses of 4, 8, and 16 mg per day. Neurology. 1994;44:675–80.

74. Sarin R, Murthy V. Medical decompressive therapy for primary and metastatic intracranial tumours. Lancet Neurol. 2003;2:357–65.

75. Frank J. Management of intracranial hypertension. Med Clin North Am. 1993;77:61–75.

76. Roberts PA, Pollay M, Engles C, Pendleton B, Reynolds E, Stevens FA. Effect on intracranial pressure of furosemide combined with varying doses and administration rates of mannitol. J Neurosurg. 1987;66:440–6.

77. Mikkelsen T, Paleologos NA, Robinson PD, Ammirati M, Andrews DW, Asher AL, et al. The role of prophylactic anticonvulsants in the management of brain metastases: a systematic review and evidence-based clinical practice guideline. J Neuro-Oncol. 2010;96:97–102.

78. Forsyth PA, Weaver S, Fulton D, Brasher PM, Sutherland G, Stewart D, et al. Prophylactic anticonvulsants in patients with brain tumour. Can J Neurol Sci. 2003;30:106–12.

79. Perry J, Zinman L, Chambers A, Spithoff K, Lloyd N, Laperriere N. The use of prophylactic anticonvulsants in patients with brain tumours—a systematic review. Curr Oncol. 2006;13:222–9.

80. Glantz MJ, Cole BF, Forsyth PA, Recht LD, Wen PY, Chamberlain MC, et al. Practice parameter: anticonvulsant prophylaxis in patients with newly diagnosed brain tumors. Report of the Quality Standards Subcommittee of the American Academy of Neurology. Neurology. 2000;54:1886–93.

81. Temkin NR. Prophylactic anticonvulsants after neurosurgery. Epilepsy Curr. 2002;2:105–7.

82. Patchell RA, Tibbs PA, Walsh JW, Dempsey RJ, Maruyama Y, Kryscio RJ, et al. A randomized trial of surgery in the treatment of single metastases to the brain. N Engl J Med. 1990;322:494–500.

83. Vecht CJ, Haaxma-Reiche H, Noordijk EM, Padberg GW, Voormolen JH, Hoekstra FH, et al. Treatment of single brain metastasis: radiotherapy alone or combined with neurosurgery? Ann Neurol. 1993;33:583–90.

84. Mintz AH, Kestle J, Rathbone MP, Gaspar L, Hugenholtz H, Fisher B, et al. A randomized trial to assess the efficacy of surgery in addition to radiotherapy in patients with a single cerebral metastasis. Cancer. 1996;78:1470–6.

85. Pollock BE, Brown PD, Foote RL, Stafford SL, Schomberg PJ, et al. Properly selected patients with multiple brain metastases may benefit from aggressive treatment of their intracranial disease. J Neuro-Oncol. 2003;61:73–80.

86. Ferguson SD, Wagner KM, Prabhu SS, McAleer MF, McCutcheon IE, Sawaya R. Neurosurgical management of brain metastases. Clin Exp Metastasis. 2017;34:377–89.

87. Paek SH, Audu PB, Sperling MR, Cho J, Andrews DW. Reevaluation of surgery for the treatment of brain metastases: review of 208 patients with single or multiple brain metastases treated at one institution with modern neurosurgical techniques. Neurosurgery. 2005;56:1021–34.

88. Vogelbaum MA, Suh JH. Resectable brain metastases. J Clin Oncol. 2006;24:1289–94.

89. Warnick RE, Darakchiev BJ, Breneman JC. Stereotactic radiosurgery for patients with solid brain metastases: current status. J Neuro-Oncol. 2004;69:125–37.

90. Minniti G, D'Angelillo RM, Scaringi C, Trodella LE, Clarke E, Matteucci P, et al. Fractionated stereotactic radiosurgery for patients with brain metastases. J Neuro-Oncol. 2014;117: 295–301.

91. Auchter RM, Lamond JP, Alexander E, Buatti JM, Chappell R, Friedman WA, et al. A multiinstitutional outcome and prognostic factor analysis of radiosurgery for resectable single brain metastasis. Int J Radiat Oncol Biol Phys. 1996;35:27–35.

92. Muacevic A, Kreth FW, Horstmann GA, Schmid-Elsaesser R, Wowra B, Steiger HJ, et al. Surgery and radiotherapy compared with gamma knife radiosurgery in the treatment of solitary cerebral metastases of small diameter. J Neurosurg. 1999;91:35–43.

93. Muacevic A, Wowra B, Siefert A, Tonn JC, Steiger HJ, Kreth FW. Microsurgery plus whole brain irradiation versus Gamma Knife surgery alone for treatment of single metastases to the brain: a randomized controlled multicentre phase III trial. J Neuro-Oncol. 2008;87:299–307.

94. Lippitz B, Lindquist C, Paddick I, Peterson D, O'Neill K, Beaney R. Stereotactic radiosurgery in the treatment of brain metastases: the current evidence. Cancer Treat Rev. 2014;40:48–59.

95. Yamamoto M, Serizawa T, Shuto T, Akabane A, Higuchi Y, Kawagishi J, et al. Stereotactic radiosurgery for patients with multiple brain metastases (JLGK0901): a multi-institutional prospective observational study. Lancet Oncol. 2014;15: 387–95.

96. Andrews DW, Scott CB, Sperduto PW, Flanders AE, Gaspar LE, Schell MC, et al. Whole brain radiation therapy with or without stereotactic radiosurgery boost for patients with one to three brain metastases: phase III results of the RTOG 9508 randomised trial. Lancet. 2004;363:1665–72.

97. Manon R, O'Neill A, Knisely J, Werner-Wasik M, Lazarus HM, Wagner H, et al. Eastern Cooperative Oncology Group. Phase II trial of radiosurgery for one to three newly diagnosed brain metastases from renal cell carcinoma, melanoma, and sarcoma: an Eastern Cooperative Oncology Group study (E 6397). J Clin Oncol. 2005;23:8870–6.

98. Sperduto PW, Shanley R, Luo X, Andrews D, Werner-Wasik M, Valicenti R, et al. Secondary analysis of RTOG 9508, a phase 3 randomized trial of whole-brain radiation therapy versus WBRT plus stereotactic radiosurgery in patients with 1-3 brain metastases; poststratified by the graded prognostic assessment (GPA). Int J Radiat Oncol Biol Phys. 2014;90:526–31.

99. Bhatnagar AK, Flickinger JC, Kondziolka D, Lunsford LD. Stereotactic radiosurgery for four or more intracranial metastases. Int J Radiat Oncol Biol Phys. 2006;64:898–903.

100. Gans JH, Raper DM, Shah AH, Bregy A, Heros D, Lally BE, et al. The role of radiosurgery to the tumor bed after resection of brain metastases. Neurosurgery. 2013;72:317–25.

101. Maldaun MV, Aguiar PH, Lang F, Suki D, Wildrick D, Sawaya R. Radiosurgery in the treatment of brain metastases: critical review regarding complications. Neurosurg Rev. 2008;31:1–8.

102. Tsao MN, Lloyd N, Wong RK, Chow E, Rakovitch E, Laperriere N, et al. Whole brain radiotherapy for the treatment of newly diagnosed multiple brain metastases. Cochrane Database Syst Rev. 2012a;4:349.55.

103. Langley RE, Stephens RJ, Nankivell M, Pugh C, Moore B, Navani N, et al. Interim data from the Medical Research Council QUARTZ trial: does whole brain radiotherapy affect the survival and quality of life of patients with brain metastases from non-small cell lung cancer? Clin Oncol (R Coll Radiol). 2013;25: 23–30.

104. Patchell RA, Tibbs PA, Regine WF, Dempsey RJ, Mohiuddin M, Kryscio RJ, et al. Postoperative radiotherapy in the treatment of single metastases to the brain: a randomized trial. JAMA. 1998;280:1485–9.

105. Aoyama H, Shirato H, Tago M, Nakagawa K, Toyoda T, Hatano K, et al. Stereotactic radiosurgery plus whole-brain radiation therapy vs stereotactic radiosurgery alone for treatment of brain metastases: a randomized controlled trial. JAMA. 2006;295: 2483–91.

106. Kocher M, Soffietti R, Abacioglu U, Villà S, Fauchon F, Baumert BG, et al. Adjuvant whole-brain radiotherapy versus observation after radiosurgery or surgical resection of one to three cerebral metastases: results of the EORTC 22952-26001 study. J Clin Oncol. 2011;29:134–41.

107. Tsao M, Xu W, Sahgal A. A meta-analysis evaluating stereotactic radiosurgery, whole-brain radiotherapy, or both for patients presenting with a limited number of brain metastases. Cancer. 2012b;118:2486–93.

108. Sahgal A, Aoyama H, Kocher M, Neupane B, Collette S, Tago M, et al. Phase 3 trials of stereotactic radiosurgery with or without whole-brain radiation therapy for 1 to 4 brain metastases: individual patient data meta-analysis. Int J Radiat Oncol Biol Phys. 2015;91:710–7.

109. Aoyama H, Tago M, Kato N, Toyoda T, Kenjyo M, Hirota S, et al. Neurocognitive function of patients with brain metastasis who received either whole brain radiotherapy plus stereotactic radiosurgery or radiosurgery alone. Int J Radiat Oncol Biol Phys. 2007;68:1388–95.

110. Chang EL, Wefel JS, Hess KR, Allen PK, Lang FF, Kornguth DG, et al. Neurocognition in patients with brain metastases treated with radiosurgery or radiosurgery plus whole-brain irradiation: a randomised controlled trial. Lancet Oncol. 2009;10:1037–44.

111. Soffietti R, Kocher M, Abacioglu UM, Villa S, Fauchon F, Baumert BG, et al. A European Organisation for Research and Treatment of Cancer phase III trial of adjuvant wholebrain radiotherapy versus observation in patients with one to three brain metastases from solid tumors after surgical resection or radiosurgery: quality-of-life results. J Clin Oncol. 2013;31: 65–72.

112. Churilla TM, Ballman KV, Brown PD, Twohy EL, Jaeckle K, Farace E, et al. Stereotactic radiosurgery with or without whole-brain radiation therapy for limited brain metastases: a secondary analysis of the North Central Cancer Treatment Group N0574 (Alliance) randomized controlled trial. Int J Radiat Oncol Biol Phys. 2017;99:1173–8.

113. Wong WW, Schild SE, Sawyer TE, Castel H, Laquerriere A, Freger P, et al. Analysis of outcome in patients reirradiated for brain metastases. Int J Radiat Oncol Biol Phys. 1996;34:585–90.

114. Sadikov E, Bezjak A, Yi QL, Wells W, Dawson L, Millar BA, et al. Value of whole brain re-irradiation for brain metastases--single centre experience. Clin Oncol (R Coll Radiol). 2007;19:532–8.

115. Brown PD, Pugh S, Laack NN, Wefel JS, Khuntia D, Meyers C, et al. Memantine for the prevention of cognitive dysfunction in patients receiving whole-brain radiotherapy: a randomized, double blind, placebo-controlled trial. Neuro-Oncology. 2013;15:1429–37.

116. Suh JH. Hippocampal-avoidance whole-brain radiation therapy: a new standard for patients with brain metastases? J Clin Oncol. 2014;32:3789–91.

117. Walbert T, Gilbert MR. The role of chemotherapy in the treatment of patients with brain metastases from solid tumors. Int J Clin Oncol. 2009;14:299–306.

118. Dempke WC, Edvardsen K, Lu S, Reinmuth N, Reck M, Inoue A. Brain metastases in NSCLC - are TKIs changing the treatment strategy? Anticancer Res. 2015;35:5797–806.

119. Magnuson WJ, Lester-Coll NH, Wu AJ, Yang TJ, Lockney NA, Gerber NK, et al. Management of brain metastases in tyrosine kinase inhibitor-Naïve epidermal growth factor receptor-mutant

non-small-cell lung cancer: a retrospective multi-institutional analysis. J Clin Oncol. 2017;35:1070–7.

120. Metro G, Chiari R, Ricciuti B, Rebonato A, Lupattelli M, Gori S, et al. Pharmacotherapeutic options for treating brain metastases in non-small cell lung cancer. Expert Opin Pharmacother. 2016;16:2601–13.

121. Jänne PA, Yang JC, Kim DW, Planchard D, Ohe Y, Ramalingam SS, et al. AZD9291 in EGFR inhibitor-resistant non-small-cell lung cancer. N Engl J Med. 2015;372:1689–99.

122. Goss G, Tsai CM, Shepherd FA, Ahn MJ, Bazhenova L, Crinò L, et al. CNS response to osimertinib in patients with T790M-positive advanced NSCLC: pooled data from two Phase II trials. Ann Oncol. 2017; in press (epub ahead of print).

123. Mok TS, Wu Y-L, Ahn M-J, Garassino MC, Kim HR, Ramalingam SS, et al. Osimertinib or platinum-Pemetrexed in EGFR T790M-positive lung cancer. N Engl J Med. 2017;376:629–40.

124. Soria JC, Ohe Y, Vansteenkiste J, Reungwetwattana T, Chewaskulyong B, Lee KH, et al. Osimertinib in untreated EGFR-mutated advanced non-small-cell lung cancer. N Engl J Med. 2018;378:113–25.

125. Reungwetwattana T, Nakagawa K, Cho BC, Cobo M, Cho EK, Bertolini A, et al. CNS response to Osimertinib versus standard epidermal growth factor receptor tyrosine kinase inhibitors in patients with untreated EGFR-mutated advanced non-small-cell lung cancer. J Clin Oncol 2018 in press.

126. Gainor JF, Ou SH, Logan J, Borges LF, Shaw AT. The central nervous system as a sanctuary site in ALK-positive non-small-cell lung cancer. J Thorac Oncol. 2013;8:1570–3.

127. Costa DB, Shaw AT, Ou SH, Solomon BJ, Riely GJ, Ahn MJ, et al. Clinical experience with Crizotinib in patients with advanced ALK-rearranged non-small-cell lung cancer and brain metastases. J Clin Oncol. 2015;33:1881–8.

128. Gadgeel SM, Shaw AT, Govindan R, Gandhi L, Socinski MA, Camidge DR, et al. Pooled analysis of CNS response to Alectinib in two studies of pretreated patients with ALK-positive non-small-cell lung cancer. J Clin Oncol. 2016;34:4079–85.

129. Peters S, Camidge DR, Shaw AT, Gadgeel S, Ahn JS, Kim DW, et al. Alectinib versus Crizotinib in untreated ALK-positive non-small-cell lung cancer. N Engl J Med. 2017;377:829–38.

130. Hida T, Nokihara H, Kondo M, Kim YH, Azuma K, Seto T, et al. Alectinib versus crizotinib in patients with ALK-positive non-small-cell lung cancer (J-ALEX): an open-label, randomised phase 3 trial. Lancet. 2017;390:29–39.

131. Martínez P, Mak RH, Oxnard GR. Targeted therapy as an alternative to whole-brain radiotherapy in EGFR-mutant or ALK-positive non-small-cell lung cancer with brain metastases. JAMA Oncol. 2017;3:1274–5.

132. Johung KL, Yeh N, Desai NB, Williams TM, Lautenschlaeger T, Arvold ND, et al. Extended survival and prognostic factors for patients with ALK-rearranged non-small-cell lung cancer and brain metastasis. J Clin Oncol. 2016;34:123–9.

133. Zhuang H, Yuan Z, Wang J, Zhao L, Pang Q, Wang P. Phase II study of whole brain radiotherapy with or without erlotinib in patients with multiple brain metastases from lung adenocarcinoma. Drug Des Devel Ther. 2013;7:1179–86.

134. Fan Y, Huang Z, Fang L, Miao L, Gong L, Yu H, et al. A phase II study of icotinib and whole-brain radiotherapy in Chinese patients with brain metastases from non-small cell lung cancer. Cancer Chemother Pharmacol. 2015;76:517–23.

135. Sperduto PW, Wang M, Robins HI, Schell MC, Werner-Wasik M, Komaki R, et al. A phase 3 trial of whole brain radiation therapy and stereotactic radiosurgery alone versus WBRT and SRS with temozolomide or erlotinib for non-small cell lung can-

cer and 1 to 3 brain metastases: Radiation Therapy Oncology Group 0320. Int J Radiat Oncol Biol Phys. 2013;85:1312–8.

136. Lee SM, Lewanski CR, Counsell N, Ottensmeier C, Bates A, Patel N, et al. Randomized trial of erlotinib plus whole-brain radiotherapy for NSCLC patients with multiple brain metastases. J Natl Cancer Inst. 2014;106:177–84.

137. Landi L, Cappuzzo F. Achievements and future developments of ALK-TKIs in the management of CNS metastases from ALK-positive NSCLC. Transl Lung Cancer Res. 2016;5:579–87.

138. Goldberg SB, Gettinger SN, Mahajan A, Chiang AC, Herbst RS, Sznol M, et al. Pembrolizumab for patients with melanoma or non-small-cell lung cancer and untreated brain metastases: early analysis of a non-randomised, open-label, phase 2 trial. Lancet Oncol. 2016;17:976–83.

139. Dudnik E, Yust-Katz S, Nechushtan H, Goldstein DA, Zer A, Flex D, et al. Intracranial response to nivolumab in NSCLC patients with untreated or progressing CNS metastases. Lung Cancer. 2016;98:114–7.

140. Inno A, Di Noia V, D'Argento E, Modena A, Gori S. State of the art of chemotherapy for the treatment of central nervous system metastases from non-small cell lung cancer. Transl Lung Cancer Res. 2016;5:599–609.

141. Galanti D, Inno A, La Vecchia M, et al. Current treatment options for HER2-positive breast cancer patients with brain metastases. Crit Rev Oncol Hematol. 2021;161:103329. https://doi.org/10.1016/j.critrevonc.2021.103329.

142. Brufsky AM, Mayer M, Rugo HS, Kaufman PA, Tan-Chiu E, Tripathy D, et al. Central nervous system metastases in patients with HER2-positive metastatic breast cancer: incidence, treatment, and survival in patients from registHER. Clin Cancer Res. 2011;17:4834–43.

143. Park IH, Ro J, Lee KS, Nam BH, Nam BH, Kwon Y, Shin KH. Trastuzumab treatment beyond brain progression in HER2-positive metastatic breast cancer. Ann Oncol. 2009;20:56–62.

144. Swain SM, Kim SB, Cortés J, Ro J, Semiglazov V, Campone M, et al. Pertuzumab, trastuzumab, and docetaxel for HER2-positive metastatic breast cancer (CLEOPATRA study): overall survival results from a randomised, double-blind, placebo-controlled, phase 3 study. Lancet Oncol. 2013;14:461–71.

145. Swain SM, Baselga J, Miles D, Im YH, Quah C, Lee LF, et al. Incidence of central nervous system metastases in patients with HER2-positive metastatic breast cancer treated with pertuzumab, trastuzumab, and docetaxel: results from the randomized phase III study CLEOPATRA. Ann Oncol. 2014;25:1116–21.

146. Lin NU, Carey LA, Liu MC, Younger J, Come SE, Ewend M, et al. Phase II trial of lapatinib for brain metastases in patients with human epidermal growth factor receptor 2-positive breast cancer. J Clin Oncol. 2008;26:1993–9.

147. Lin NU, Eierman W, Greil R, Campone M, Kaufman B, Steplewski K, et al. Randomized phase II study of lapatinib plus capecitabine or lapatinib plus topotecan for patients with HER2-positive breast cancer brain metastases. J Neuro-Oncol. 2011;105:613–20.

148. Bachelot T, Romieu G, Campone M, Diéras V, Cropet C, Dalenc F, et al. Lapatinib plus capecitabine in patients with previously untreated brain metastases from HER2-positive metastatic breast cancer (LANDSCAPE): a single-group phase 2 study. Lancet Oncol. 2013;14:64–71.

149. Bartsch R, Berghoff AS, Vogl U, Rudas M, Bergen E, Dubsky P, et al. Activity of T-DM1 in Her2-positive breast cancer brain metastases. Clin Exp Metastasis. 2015;32:729–37.

150. Krop IE, Lin NU, Blackwell K, Guardino E, Huober J, Lu M, et al. Trastuzumab emtansine (T-DM1) versus lapatinib plus capecitabine in patients with HER2-positive metastatic breast

cancer and central nervous system metastases: a retrospective, exploratory analysis in EMILIA. Ann Oncol. 2015;26:113–9.

151. Trudeau ME, Crump M, Charpentier D, Yelle L, Bordeleau L, Matthews S, et al. Temozolomide in metastatic breast cancer (MBC): a phase II trial of the National Cancer Institute of Canada—Clinical Trials Group (NCIC-CTG). Ann Oncol. 2006;17:952–6.

152. Franciosi V, Cocconi G, Michiara M, Di Costanzo F, Fosser V, Tonato M, et al. Frontline chemotherapy with cisplatin and etoposide for patients with brain metastases from breast carcinoma, nonsmall cell lung carcinoma, or malignant melanoma: a prospective study. Cancer. 1999;85:1599–605.

153. Miller AB, Hoogstraten B, Staquet M, Winkler A. Reporting results of cancer treatment. Cancer. 1981;47:207–14.

154. Therasse P, Arbuck SG, Eisenhauer EA, Wanders J, Kaplan RS, Rubinstein L, et al. New guidelines to evaluate the response to treatment in solid tumors. J Natl Cancer Inst. 2000;92:20516.

155. Eisenhauer EA, Therasse P, Bogaerts J, Schwartz LH, Sargent D, Ford R, et al. New response evaluation criteria in solid tumours: revised RECIST guideline (version 1.1). Eur J Cancer. 2009;45:228–47.

156. Macdonald DR, Cascino TL, Schold SC Jr, Cairncross JG. Response criteria for phase II studies of supratentorial malignant glioma. J Clin Oncol. 1990;8:1277–80.

157. Lin NU, Lee EQ, Aoyama H, Barani IJ, Barboriak DP, Baumert BG, et al. Response assessment criteria for brain metastases: proposal from the RANO group. Lancet Oncol. 2015;16:e270–8.

Renal Cancer

Lorena Incorvaia, Giuseppe Procopio, and Camillo Porta

Genitourinary Cancers

Contents

© Springer Nature Switzerland AG 2021
A. Russo et al. (eds.), *Practical Medical Oncology Textbook*, UNIPA Springer Series,
https://doi.org/10.1007/978-3-030-56051-5_45

45.1 Introduction

Over the past 10 years, the advances in identification of the molecular mechanisms related to renal cancer tumorigenesis and the understanding of the central role of angiogenesis in cell growth and proliferation allowed in identifying several targets of clinical interest. The development of new drugs, such as tyrosine kinase inhibitors, revolutionized the medical treatment of renal cancer by making possible to target the signaling pathway and the molecular events that are key events for pathogenesis of this malignancy.

Recently, immunoncology, has become a promising frontier for the treatment of renal cancer, improving the organism's competence to direct the immune system against cancer cells. All these findings have resulted in significant improvements in median overall survival (OS) for patients and in a greater number of therapeutic opportunities (◘ Fig. 45.1).

45.2 Epidemiology

— Renal cell carcinoma (RCC), derived from renal tubular epithelial cells, accounts for ~2% of all adult malignancies; it is the seventh most common cancer in men and the tenth most common cancer in women, with a median age of diagnosis of around 60–65 years [1, 2].

— Occurrence in younger ages could be indicative of *hereditary kidney cancer syndrome* (3–5% of all RCCs); the most common is the *Von Hippel Lindau (VHL) disease* [2].

— Over the past two decades, a divergent pattern of increasing incidence and decreasing mortality was observed, especially in the western, industrialized, world [3].

— This is due, probably, to the combined effect of the increasingly incidental detection with abdominal imaging (◘ Fig. 45.2) and the effectiveness of several systemic therapies developed.

45.3 Risk Factors

— Established and well-known risk factors for RCC are *cigarette smoking, hypertension,* and *obesity* [4]. Further clinical conditions that are common in patients with RCC are chronic kidney disease, dialysis, and kidney transplantation [5].

— Furthermore, *genetic factors* also contribute to RCC risk. The *Von Hippel Lindau (VHL) disease* is an autosomal dominant syndrome characterized by mutations affecting the *VHL* tumor suppressor gene [2]. Inactivation of the *VHL gene* leads to accumulation of *HIF (hypoxia inducible factor)*: under normal conditions, HIF is constitutively degraded. HIF promotes transcription of gene involved in the angiogenesis-pathway and tumor progression, including vascular endothelial growth factor (VEGF), PDGF, fibroblast growth factor (FGF), and hepatocyte growth factor (HGF). The aberrant accumulation of HIF results in uncontrolled

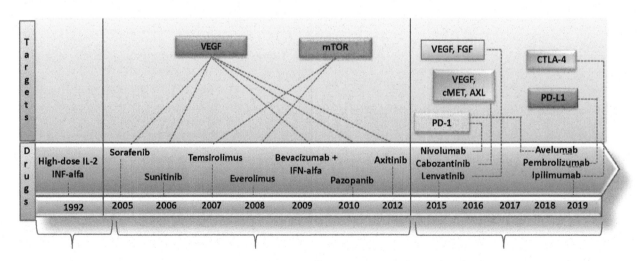

◘ Fig. 45.1 Parallel development of new targets and new drugs for metastatic renal cell carcinoma (RCC)

45

Fig. 45.2 Von Hippel Lindau (VHL) disease. **a** Numerous renal cysts. **b** Renal cell carcinoma, clear cell. (Courtesy of Prof. A. Simonato)

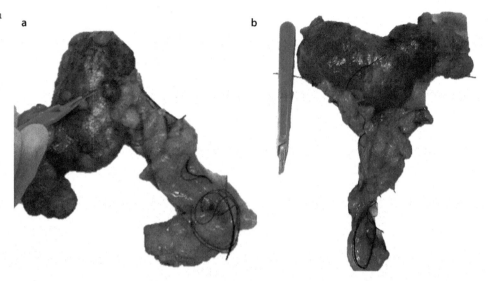

activation of transcription factors and several target genes, predominantly mediators of angiogenesis, that enhance cell survival [6].

- Clinically, suggestive for VHL disease is RCC in young patient, with personal or family history of any other tumor typical of VHL. The most frequent are as follows:
  - Retinal angioma
  - Spinal or cerebellar hemangioblastoma
  - Adrenal or extra-adrenal pheochromocytoma
  - Multiple renal and pancreatic cysts
  - Neuroendocrine tumors of the pancreas. PMID 20301636 (■ Fig. 45.3)

45.4 Histological Subtype and Molecular Profile

Approximately 75% of RCC are *clear cell carcinoma (ccRCC)* (■ Fig. 45.3). The other RCC subtypes are a heterogeneous group of cancer with different morphology, genetic and molecular pathogenesis, and clinical behavior, as a whole known as *non-clear cell RCC (nccRCC)*. In terms of prognosis, the survival of the vast majority of nccRCC patients is significantly inferior compared to ccRCC patients [7].

Today we know that between the histological subtype there are not only histologic difference but also cytogenetic alterations with specific genes mutated (■ Fig. 45.4):

- The *clear cell carcinoma* is a "disease of a chromosome 3p": the *VHL* gene is the most frequently inactivated. This gene resides in the short arm of chromosome 3 (3p), at 3p25, and results mutated, deleted, or hypermethylated. Interestingly, mutations in others tumor suppressor genes located in the 3p, (at 3p21), have also been reported, including Polybromo 1 (*PBRM1*), BRCA associated protein-1 (*BAP1*), and SET Domain Containing1 (*SETD2*). These genes encode chromatin-regulating and histone-regulating proteins. Together with the abnormal expression of kinase of mTOR pathway, these genetic alterations are present in more than 50% of ccRCC patients [8]. According to some authors, ccRCC patients harboring mutations in the mTOR gene should be considered as having a "metabolic" neoplasm, due to the key role of mTOR in the regulation of cell metabolism.
- The *papillary renal cell carcinoma* are ~15% of all renal cancers and are divided into two main subtypes, type 1 and type 2. The type 1 is associated with mutation of gene MET, and type 2 with mutations of CDKN2A, SETD2, and NRF2.
- The *chromophobe renal cell carcinoma* makes up ~5% of kidney tumors. Frequent are mutations of TP53 or PTEN.
- The *oncocytoma*, ~5% of all RCC, is a benign tumor associated with mitochondrial genes alterations (COX1, COX2, MTND4, and MTCYB). Hybrid tumors have been described that present overlapping features of chromophobe RCC and oncocytomas, often observed in Birt–Hogg–Dubé syndrome.

Other minor subtypes include the following:

- *MiT family translocation renal cell carcinoma*, with recurrent translocations, involving Xp11.23 (TFE3), 6p21 (TFEB) and others, that occur typically in young patients.

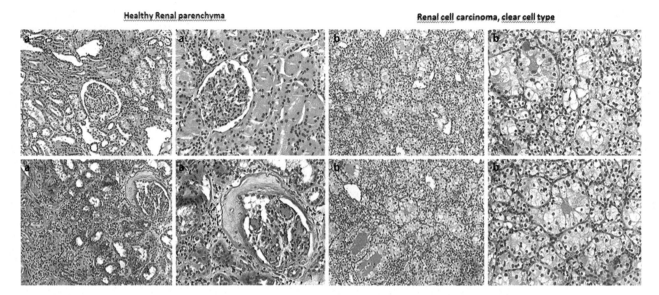

■ **Fig. 45.3** Microscopic picture (H&E 10×, 20× magnification) showing healthy renal parenchima **a** and renal cell carcinoma, clear cell type **b**

■ **Fig. 45.4** Histological subtype and molecular profile of RCC

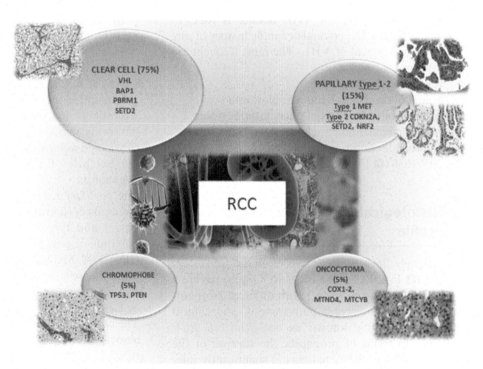

— *Collecting duct carcinoma*, rare and highly aggressive, with unknown gene alterations. Should be considered and treated like urothelial carcinomas of the upper urinary tract, though their prognosis is even worse.

Additional minor subtypes include renal medullary carcinoma, clear cell papillary RCC, hereditary leio-myomatosis, tubulocystic RCC, acquired cystic disease-associated RCC, mucinous tubular and spindle RCC, succinate dehydrogenase-deficient RCC, and RCC-associated RCC [9].

45.5 RCC Pathogenesis and Tumor Evolution

45.5.1 Role of Genes

The genetic and molecular pathogenesis of RCC appears to be much more complex than originally thought. Only 2–3% of ccRCC are accounted for hereditary diseases characterized by a germline mutation of the VHL gene. Conversely, mutations or silencing of the same VHL gene are associated with >80% of sporadic ccRCC.

45

VHL inactivation is the founding event; *BAP1, PBRM1, SETD2, KDM5C* mutations seem to be involved in disease progression and to have effect on clinical outcome [10]. For example, BAP1 is related to larger tumor size, higher Fuhrman nuclear grade, and worse cancer-specific survival [11].

At the same time, VHL loss is early events evident in all ccRCC cell of tumor sampled; driver mutations of BAP1, PBRM1, SET2, MTOR, KDM5C are present heterogeneously (branched mutations) and are mutually exclusive [12]. This leads to hypothesis of molecular subclassification of ccRCC in the future.

Therefore, the *genomic heterogeneity* adds further complexity to RCC pathogenesis: sequential and parallel accumulation of mutations is responsible of subclonal evolution with hypothetical effect on the clinical outcome. How individual genetic alterations and their interactions contribute to the pathogenesis in RCC are largely unknown and no prognostic and predictive biomarkers have been validated to date. But recent report on BAP1, PBRM1, and SETD2 as potential prognostic and predictive biomarkers may foster the possibility of impacting risk profiling.

Genomic heterogeneity translates into *clinical tumor heterogeneity* that has important therapeutic implications. RCC variability, beyond between patients (inter-patient), exists within the same patient (intra-patient) and within a given tumor sample (intra-tumoral). This *spatial* and *temporal biological diversity* changes over time and in response to treatment, and contributes to the development of compensatory mechanisms that result in resistance. The selective pressure first-line antiangiogenic treatments induced on the tumor has been demonstrated to be able to induce further mutations; notably enough, the rate of VHL mutations seems to increase moving from first- to second-line treatment.

45.5.2 Role of Angiogenesis and Tumor Microenvironment

45.5.2.1 Angiogenesis

Due to the above seminal genetic alterations (i.e., those affecting the *VHL* gene), RCCs are *highly vascular*, and *angiogenesis*, the process of new blood vessel formation, is a crucial step in their pathogenesis [13].

The frequent loss of the *VHL* tumor suppressor gene, results in HIF up-regulation. This aberrant accumulation of HIF proteins, translocating into the nucleus, leads to the transcription of several HIF target genes. These genes include angiogenic factors, such as vascular endothelial growth factor (VEGF), platelet-derived growth factor (PDGF), epidermal growth factor (EGF)

and transforming growth factor-α (TGF-α), following the stimulation of angiogenesis (◘ Fig. 45.5).

Furthermore, renal tumor angiogenesis is also stimulated by growth factors through the phosphatidyl-inositol-3 kinase PI3K-AKT-mTOR signal transduction pathway.

Given the highly vascular nature and the central role of angiogenesis in RCCs, several agents targeting the vascular endothelial growth factor (VEGF) pathway have explored this feature. Before 2005, only two drugs were available to treat RCC: High-dose IL-2 (HD IL-2) and interferon α (INF-α), with substantial toxicity and a median survival of ~15 months.

Since 2005, *antiangiogenic drugs*, such as the monoclonal antibody anti-VEGF *bevacizumab*, but especially tyrosine kinase inhibitors (TKI) targeting (mainly, but not exclusively) the VEGF/VEGFRs signaling axis (*sunitinib, pazopanib, axitinib, sorafenib*, and *tivozanib*) and inhibitors of mammalian target of rapamycin (mTOR) pathway (*everolimus, temsirolimus*) revolutionized the treatment of advanced or metastatic RCC, reaching the median overall survival (OS) to ~30 months in 2014.

Sorafenib	The first TKI approved for mRCC treatment. It is a multikinase inhibitor of multiple growth factor receptors as VEGFr, PDGFr, Flt-3 and c-Kit and Raf-1, a member of RAF/MEK/ERK signaling pathway.
Sunitinib, pazopanib	Multitarget oral TKI, with inhibitory activity against VEGF and PDGF receptors.
Axitinib	The next-generation TKI, potent and highly selective for the VEGF receptor 1, 2, and 3.
Everolimus, temsirolimus	The kinase inhibitors of mTOR complex 1 (mTORC1).
Bevacizumab	Unique monoclonal antibody anti-VEGF approved, in combination with immunomodulator interferon α.
Tivozanib	An oral, highly potent, and selective tyrosine kinase inhibitor of VEGF receptors 1, 2, and 3. It has recently been approved by the European Medicines Agency (EMA) for first-line treatment and is at various stages of development in EU countries [14].

However, anti-angiogenic agents have typically *transitory efficacy* because the inhibition of tumor angiogenesis by VEGFR-TKI is reversible. Indeed, clinically durable responses are rare and after an initial period of response, most patients will experience disease progression for the development of treatment resistance.

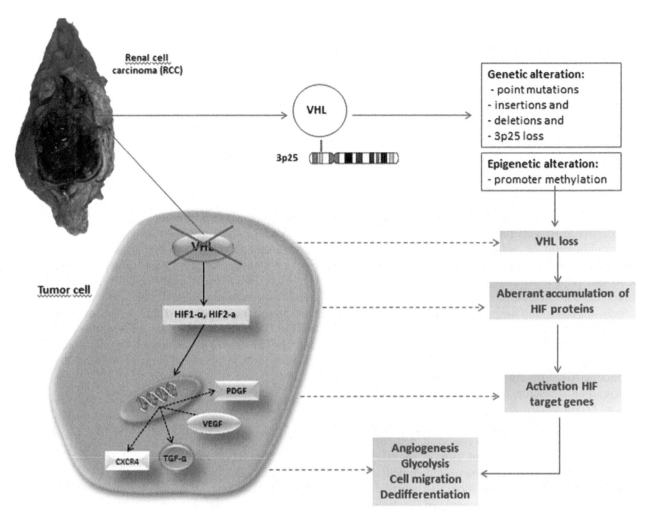

Fig. 45.5 VHL inactivation in clear cell renal cell carcinoma (ccRCC), with accumulation of HIF proteins, activation of HIF target genes and increased angiogenesis

Resistance is mainly caused by adaptive mechanisms of cancer cells with the activation of angiogenesis-related pathways independent of VEGFR and PDGFR.

Furthermore, anti-VEGFR therapies are not definitely precise and "targeted", because VEGF is ubiquitously expressed in solid tumors, although much more in RCC, and anti-VEGFR therapies target endothelial, and not cancer cells.

A strategy to *overcome the resistance* to VEGFR inhibitors is the development of new-generation antiangiogenic drugs targeting multiple distinct pathways, such as *cabozantinib* and *lenvatinib*, characterized by additional targeted mechanism of action.

Inhibiting both VEGFR and accessory pathways simultaneously might avoid the development of resistance to treatment.

| Cabozantinib | A receptor tyrosine kinase inhibitor whose targets include MET (hepatocyte growth factor receptor), VEGFR2, and AXL receptor tyrosine kinase (AXL). |
| Lenvatinib | Third-generation of VEGFR inhibitors. It is a multi-TKI of VEGFR1-3, with inhibitory activity against fibroblast growth factor receptors (FGFR1-4), PDGFRα, glial-cell-line-derived neurotrophic factor receptor (RET) and KIT. |

The Inhibition of MET and AXL with *cabozantinib* has a strong rationale:

- cMET is overexpressed in many ccRCC
- cMET and AXL are induced by VEGF inhibition
- Targeting MET and AXL could to overcome resistance to anti-VEGF [15].

Also the combination of *lenvatinib + everolimus* have an attractive biological rationale of synergistic activity of VEGFR and mTOR pathways inhibition and a randomized phase II trial that show a PFS benefit for this combination, was published recently [16] (◘ Fig. 45.6).

45.5.2.2 Tumor Microenvironment

The observations of high levels of immune infiltrate in the RCC microenvironment and the parallel occurrence of some spontaneous tumor regression of metastases after radical nephrectomy suggested a natural antitumor immunity for metastatic RCC [17].

RCC lesions are often infiltrated by tumor-infiltrating lymphocytes; analyzing T cell infiltration score (TIS) and the corresponding mutation load in 19 cancer types by The Cancer Genome Atlas research program, ccRCC shows the highest TIS. Tumor immune microenvironment characterization in ccRCC identifies prognostic and immunotherapeutically relevant messenger RNA signatures [18].

Despite numerous evidences in solid tumors suggest that increased TILs are associated with good prognosis, several studies showed that high density of CD8+ TILs is associated with poor clinical outcome in RCC: studying the tumor-specific survival in immune infiltration classes, the T cell enriched class has the poorest survival, whereas the non-infiltrated class is associated with better outcomes. Furthermore, the increase in TILs was found to be associated with higher tumor grade and stage [19].

Since the 1990s, before the introduction of TKI for the mRCC treatment, cytokines, such as high-dose IL-2 and interferon-α (IFN-α), were used, alone or in combination, to enhance antitumor immunity in RCC and represented the standards of care, however limited by poor efficacy and severe dose-limiting toxicities. The new generation of *immunotherapy agents*, the immune checkpoint-blocking therapies, are of increasing interest in this disease today.

Immuno-oncology is a promising frontier for RCC and the recent new information relative to the complex role of tumor microenvironment (TME) are resulting in a greater number of therapeutic opportunities [20].

Tumors, indeed, can create an immunosuppressive microenvironment by upregulating inhibitory molecules,

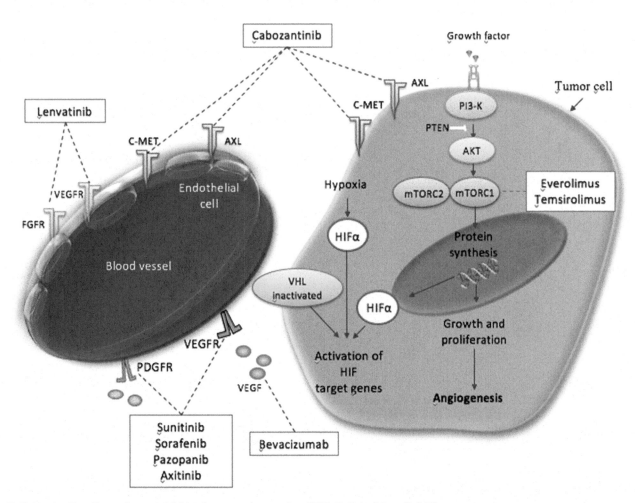

◘ **Fig. 45.6** Signaling pathways inhibition by targeted agents in mRCC. (Adapted from Ref. [6])

such as *programmed cell death protein (PD-1)* on tumor-infiltrating T cells, or its ligand *PD-L1*, on tumors cells [21].

The PD1- PD-L1 pathway downregulates cytotoxic T-cell activity [22].

The blockade of the PD1-PD-L1 interactions with specific antibodies inhibitors, may prevent T-cell suppression: the T-cells remain active and promote the immune killing of the tumor cells.

The *immune checkpoints inhibitors* already developed, or under exploration (alone or within different combinations) in RCC clinical trials are as follows:

- Nivolumab and pembrolizumab, monoclonal antibodies that target PD-1 receptor
- Avelumab and atezolizumab, monoclonal antibodies that target PD-L1-receptor
- Ipilimumab, monoclonal antibody against the cytotoxic T-lymphocyte antigen-4 (CTLA-4), another immune-inhibitory molecule expressed in activated T cells and in suppressor T regulatory cells studied in clinical trials, alone or in combination (◘ Fig. 45.7).

The inhibition of immune checkpoint PD-1 with *nivolumab*, has been demonstrated to be clinically effective on metastatic disease, with significant improvements in median OS for kidney cancer patients treated after the failure of an anti-VEGFR agent [23, 24]. The introduction of these immunotherapy drugs contributed to the revolution in the treatment of mRCC and promise to be translated to a significant number of patients, achieving durable remissions in the near future [25].

45.6 Diagnosis and Staging

The clinical presentation of RCC was, historically, characterized by *flank pain, gross hematuria*, and *a palpable abdominal mass*, depending on the localization and the large size of the tumor.

Currently, the majority of diagnoses (>50%) results from *incidental findings*, suggested by non-invasive radiological techniques, ultrasonography (US), or computed tomography (CT), are often performed for another clinical reason. These RCCs detected incidentally are often early and small tumors, making the classical clinical triad mentioned above less frequent than in the past. Some patients show symptoms related to *paraneoplastic syndromes*, caused by cytokines and hormones production by cancer cells and characterized by hypercalcemia, fever, erythrocytosis, and Stauffer's syn-

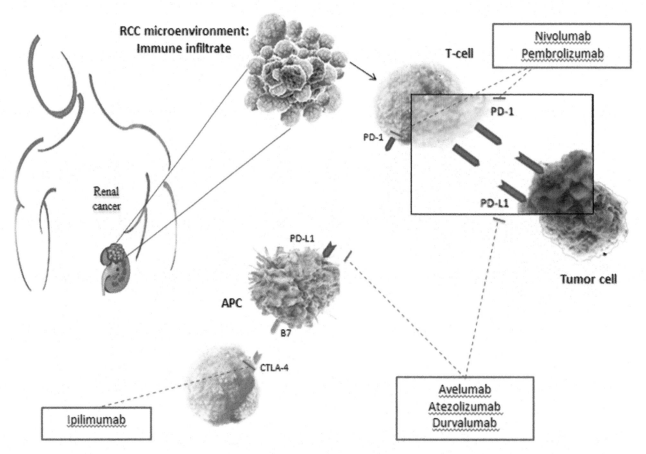

◘ **Fig. 45.7** Immune checkpoints inhibitors approved or available in RCC clinical trials

45

drome (signs of cholestasis unrelated to tumor infiltration of the liver or intrinsic liver disease).

Laboratory examinations could show alterations of several parameters, such as serum creatinine, hemoglobin, leukocyte and platelet counts, lymphocyte to neutrophil ratio, serum calcium and lactate dehydrogenase levels. Some of these tests are used for risk assessment within different prognostic score systems.

Most RCCs are strongly suspected by *imaging studies*, because they have typical radiological features, including intra-tumoral heterogeneity due to necrosis or hemorrhage and exophytic growth, and high uptake of contrast- enhancement agents.

Ultrasonography (US) is usually the first radiological technique that allows the detection of RCC.

Further exams to investigate local invasiveness, lymph node involvement, and distant metastases are contrast-enhanced *chest, abdominal, and pelvic CT scan*, for the study of lung, liver, and lymph nodes metastasis (■ Fig. 45.8).

The use of either bone scan or CT (or MRI) of the brain are usually performed only in symptomatic subject, i.e., when a clinical suspicion of bone or cerebral involvement is present, while 18FDG-PET is not a standard investigation in the diagnosis and staging of ccRCC and should not be used routinely. Abdominal magnetic resonance imaging (MRI) may provide additional information, especially to investigate the venous involvement from the tumors, which frequently causes the vena cava tumor thrombus. *TNM staging* of RCC is based on size, position, and lymph node involvement. The staging system used is the AJCC/UICC TNM classification (American Joint Committee on Cancer -AJCC/Union for International Cancer Control – UICC/tumor–node–metastasis – TNM; 7th edition-2010) (■ Fig. 45.9).

45.7 Management

Approximately 65% of patients with RCC have *localized* tumors, which are treated with *surgery* and can be cured by total nephrectomy or nephron-sparing surgery (e.g., partial nephrectomy). The remaining ~35% of patients present with *metastatic* RCC. Finally, about 20–40% of patients with confined primary tumor at diagnosis will develop metastatic disease after local therapy [26].

45.7.1 Localized Disease

■ Surgery

The standard treatment of localized RCCs is complete surgical excision of the lesion by *partial or radical nephrectomy*, with a curative intent.

The goal of modern surgery is to completely remove the primary tumor, while preserving the largest possible amount of healthy renal parenchyma, limiting invasiveness, iatrogenic renal function impairment, and overtreatment that can increase patients' morbidity.

Radical and partial nephrectomies show similar OS on the basis of a randomized trial (EORTC) and a meta-analysis that included 107 studies with over 180,000 patients [27].

The choice between partial or radical nephrectomy is related to the clinical stage of the disease, predominantly diameter, location, depth, proximity to hilar vessels and the urinary collecting system, and the type of surgical

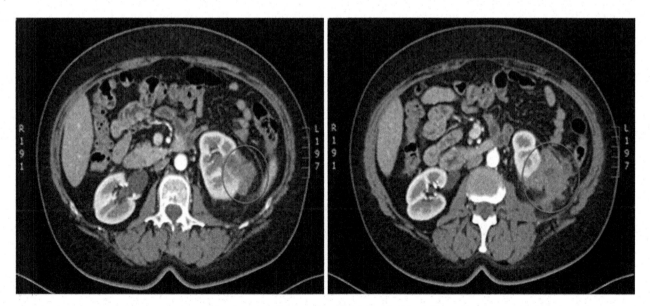

■ **Fig. 45.8** Contrast enhanced CT demonstrates a heterogeneously enhancing mass arising from the lower pole of the left kidney

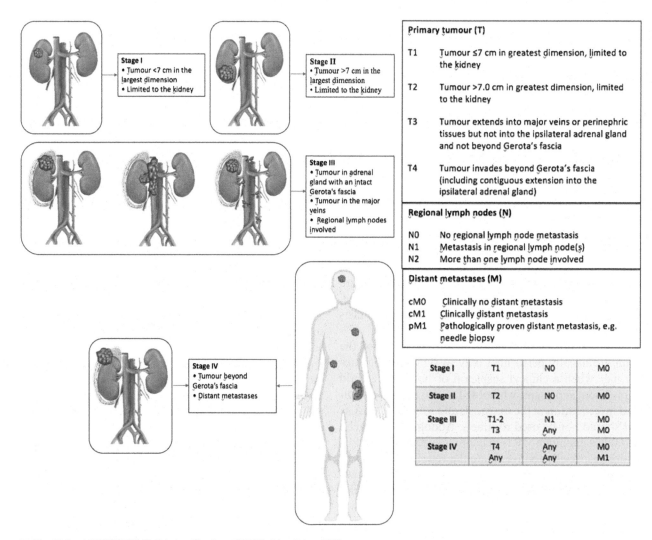

Primary tumour (T)

T1   Tumour ≤7 cm in greatest dimension, limited to the kidney

T2   Tumour >7.0 cm in greatest dimension, limited to the kidney

T3   Tumour extends into major veins or perinephric tissues but not into the ipsilateral adrenal gland and not beyond Gerota's fascia

T4   Tumour invades beyond Gerota's fascia (including contiguous extension into the ipsilateral adrenal gland)

Regional lymph nodes (N)

N0   No regional lymph node metastasis
N1   Metastasis in regional lymph node(s)
N2   More than one lymph node involved

Distant metastases (M)

cM0   Clinically no distant metastasis
cM1   Clinically distant metastasis
pM1   Pathologically proven distant metastasis, e.g. needle biopsy

Stage I
• Tumour <7 cm in the largest dimension
• Limited to the kidney

Stage II
• Tumour >7 cm in the largest dimension
• Limited to the kidney

Stage III
• Tumour in adrenal gland with an intact Gerota's fascia
• Tumour in the major veins
• Regional lymph nodes involved

Stage IV
• Tumour beyond Gerota's fascia
• Distant metastases

Stage I	T1	N0	M0
Stage II	T2	N0	M0
Stage III	T1-2	N1	M0
	T3	Any	M0
Stage IV	T4	Any	M0
	Any	Any	M1

Fig. 45.9 AJCC/UICC TNM classification of RCC, 7th edition-2010

approach (open, laparoscopic, or robotic), and depends, as well as tumor features, also on the surgeon's expertise. Together, these surgical trends highlight the importance of preserved renal function [28] (Fig. 45.10).

■ **Active Surveillance**

Although surgery represents the standard of care for localized RCC, there exists a rationale for active surveillance in well-selected patients. This strategy seems reasonable because of the following:

─ Small renal masses often harbor benign final pathology
─ Some renal tumors have a slow median growth rate with low risk of metastatic progression (2–3 mm/year)
─ A significant proportion of RCC patients with severe comorbidity, particularly the elderly patients, are unfit for surgery, with high risk of surgical complications including death.

A definite protocol for active surveillance, with specifics indications for tumor size and growth rate cut-off, is not yet defined. For these patients, it is commonly suggested imaging every 3 months in the first year, every 6 months during the next 2–3 years, and annually thereafter. Intervention should be proposed for growth >3–4 cm or by >0.4–0.5 cm/year [10].

45.7.1.1 Risk Assessment in Localized Disease

The patient's individual risk of disease recurrence after surgery varies significantly: clinical and pathological variables, such as histology, grading, extent of tumor, have prognostic value in RCC and may be used for the risk assessment. All these features are not perfectly accurate when used alone, but, when combined into integrated systems, have shown to be valuable tools to predict RCC prognosis [29].

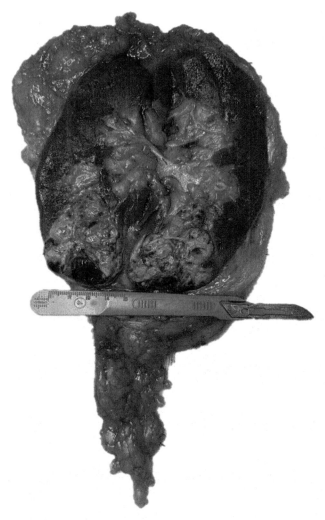

Fig. 45.10 Radical nephrectomy for RCC in the lower pole of the kidney. (Courtesy of Prof. A. Simonato)

The most used and validated systems are as follows:
- The *UCLA Integrated Staging System (UISS)*, that combines TNM stage, Fuhrman grade, and Eastern Cooperative Oncology Group (ECOG) performance status (PS) [30].
- The *SSIGN system (Stage, Size, Grade and Necrosis)*, developed from the Mayo Clinic. It does not consider the performance status or other clinical parameters, and includes tumor necrosis; a limitation of this scoring system is that it is only useful for clear cell renal carcinomas [30].
- The *Karakiewicz nomogram*, similar to the UISS, but tumor size is used as a continuous variable and the ECOG performance status is replaced by a symptom classification that distinguishes asymptomatic, local, and systemic symptoms [31].

- The most recent scoring algorithm developed by *Leibovich et al.* that is a modification of the SSIGN score. It differs from the SSIGN score and from many others because the endpoint is progression to metastatic RCC rather than survival [32].

These risk assessment tools have the potential to allow better risk stratification of patients into low-intermediate- and high-risk groups. To date, no clear preference for a specific prognostic score may be given [33].

■ Adjuvant Therapy

Currently, almost no adjuvant treatment tested, have proved able to improve either disease-free survival (DFS) or OS, within a randomized controlled, phase III trial. A recent study (S-TRAC adjuvant study) reported a DFS benefit of 1 year of sunitinib therapy in comparison with placebo in 615 patients with resected, non-metastatic, high-risk RCC. However, the lack of any OS benefit, together with the suboptimal trade-off of 1 year of toxic therapy in exchange for 1.2 years of DFS benefit, are among the major criticisms regarding this study [34]. Several other trials of adjuvant targeted therapies and immunotherapy are ongoing and the results will be reported in the near future.

45.7.2 Metastatic Disease

One-third of patients with RCC present with distant metastases at diagnosis, and approximately a quarter of patients with localized disease treated with nephrectomy have relapses in distant sites [35]. Distant metastases occur most often in the lymph nodes, lungs, bone, liver, and brain [36] (**■** Fig. 45.11).

45.7.2.1 Risk Assessment in Advanced Disease

Different prognostic models to stratify patients with metastatic RCC for systemic treatment were developed. Key prognostic factors identified include performance status (PS), time from diagnosis to systemic treatment, hemoglobin, calcium, neutrophil and platelet counts in the blood.

The most recent *"International Metastatic RCC Database Consortium (IMDC) score"* is based on six factors. The patients are stratified into three *categories of risk* based on the number of prognostic factors: *favorable* (0 risk factor); *intermediate* (1–2 risk factors); and *poor risk* (3–6 risk factors) (**■** Fig. 45.12).

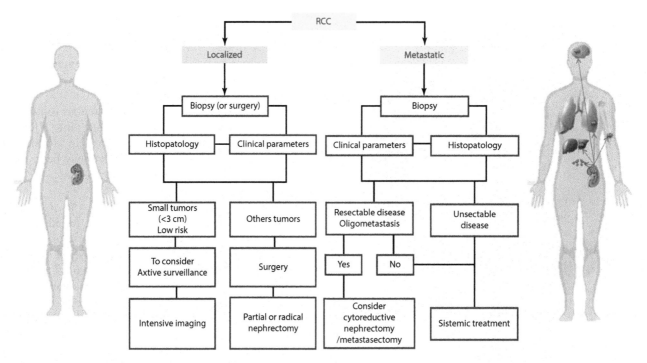

Fig. 45.11 Treatment strategy for renal cell carcinoma; **a** localized disease; **b** metastatic disease and distant sites most frequently involved

Fig. 45.12 Heng criteria (IMDC) and IMDC score. (Heng et al. J Clin Oncol. 2009)

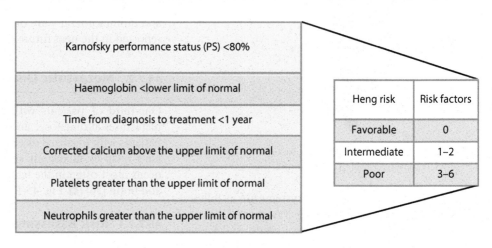

■ **Medical Treatment**

Systemic treatment is indicated for patients with *unresectable* or *metastatic* RCC.

Expanding knowledge of RCC biology and a better understanding of pathways involved in RCC pathophysiology produced in the past 10 years the approval of several novel therapeutic agents tailored to specific molecular drivers described before.

The highly vascular nature of RCCs and the role of "functional hypoxia" and angiogenesis made this tumor an ideal target to exploit this feature with anti-angiogenic drugs.

Tyrosine kinase inhibitors (TKI) targeting *VEGF signaling pathways* have been, in fact, the first drugs that have improved patient outcomes compared with the previous cytokines-based standard of care.

After the approval of Sorafenib in 2005, several targeted agents have been specifically designed and approved, quickly changing the landscape of RCC treatment, targeting VEGF signaling axis (sunitinib, pazopanib, bevacizumab, axitinib) or mTOR pathway (everolimus).

The next paradigm shift occurred in 2015, when three novel agents showed improved outcomes in the post-first-line setting: 2 new-generation antiangiogenic drugs targeting *multiple distinct pathways* (cabozantinib and lenvatinib) and nivolumab, targeting the immune system/tumor microenvironment (■ Fig. 45.13).

Currently, several drugs are available for the treatment of mRCC:

1. Three agents were the first approved for previously untreated mRCC, in *first-line* setting: *sunitinib, pazo-*

Fig. 45.13 Survival outcome and introduction of new therapeutic options for mRCC treatment

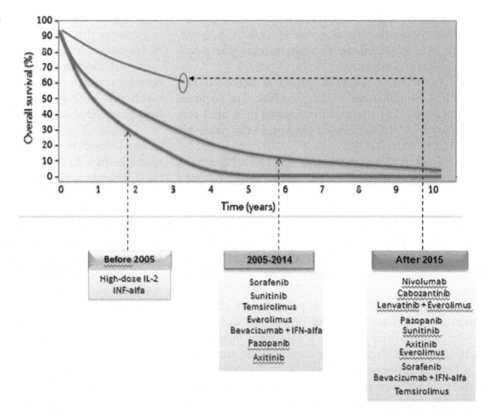

Before 2005
High-dose IL-2
INF-alfa

2005-2014
Sorafenib
Sunitinib
Temsirolimus
Everolimus
Bevacizumab + IFN-alfa
Pazopanib
Axitinib

After 2015
Nivolumab
Cabozantinib
Lenvatinib + Everolimus
Pazopanib
Sunitinib
Axitinib
Everolimus
Sorafenib
Bevacizumab + IFN-alfa
Temsirolimus

panib and the combination of *bevacizumab* and the immunomodulator *interferon-α*.

Sunitinib and pazopanib demonstrated similar median PFS in a randomized trial in first-line setting (COMPARZ), with different safety profile.

Bevacizumab is a monoclonal antibody anti-VEGF approved in 2009, but the TKI sunitinib and pazopanib, showed comparable efficacy, but a distinct safety profile, with the advantage of oral administration compared to the bevacizumab plus interferon regimen.

Afterward, the U.S. Food and Drug Administration (FDA) approved cabozantinib for treatment in the first-line setting, based on data from the CABO-SUN trial. This is a randomized phase II study in patients with intermediate and poor-risk previously untreated RCC. Patients received cabozantinib or sunitinib and cabozantinib treatment significantly prolonged PFS compared with sunitinib [37].

Furthermore, in April 2018, the FDA granted approvals to *nivolumab and ipilimumab* in combination for the treatment of intermediate or poor risk, previously untreated advanced renal cell carcinoma. The approvals were based on the phase 3 CheckMate 214 trial of nivolumab plus ipilimumab versus sunitinib in previously untreated advanced RCC. In this trial, overall survival and objective response rates were significantly higher with nivolumab plus ipilim-

umab than with sunitinib among intermediate- and poor-risk patients [38].

Tivozanib is another option of care when available.

For patients with poor risk, *temsirolimus* is approved, but is associated with modest survival benefits, and requires weekly intravenous administration; thus, sunitinib or pazopanib are usually the preferred options in this setting, not to take into account those unfortunate patients who can receive just best supportive care.

Anti-angiogenic drugs typically have transitory efficacy: they produce more or less durable responses (usually in the range of 8–12 months), followed by disease progression due to the development of resistance to anti-VEGF therapy [39, 40].

2. Current *second-line* therapeutic options for mRCC include *nivolumab*, *cabozantinib*, *lenvatinib + everolimus*, and *axitinib*.

Nivolumab has been compared to everolimus in patients who had failed prior after either one or two TKIs within the CheckMate 025 trial, demonstrating an OS benefit, which led to regulatory approval in both the EU and the USA. However, predicting which patient will benefit from nivolumab still remains an issue, as well as an unmet need. PDL1 is dynamic and the expression in paraffin-embedded tumor from the primary site could not be representative of all metastatic disease.

The subsequent introduction of cabozantinib created more therapeutic options for mRCC patients, but also increased the difficulty in choosing a second-line treatment.

Cabozantinib increased progression-free survival (PFS), overall survival (OS), and objective response rate (ORR) in patients with advanced RCC after previous anti-VEGF targeted therapy, in the phase III METEOR trial [41].

To date, there are no data about direct comparison between nivolumab and cabozantinib and both are effective options after first-line VEGFr-TKI failure. The absence of head-to-head comparisons does not solve the controversy for the choice of treatment at present [42].

Axitinib, everolimus, and lenvatinib + everolimus are considered as alternative options.

Given the increased survival of patients with advanced disease, an increasing number of patients are able to undergo three lines of therapy. Treatment in *third-line* setting depends largely on the choices made previously.

The optimal sequence of agents for the treatment of mRCC is not well defined. Ongoing trials and others recently concluded continue to research new therapies and to elucidate the optimal sequence of the known ones, making the *RCC treatment, a continuously changing scenario.*

Especially, combination therapy with *avelumab + axitinib, pembrolizumab + axitinib,* and *bevacizumab + atezolizumab* are showing promising efficacy in first-line setting.

Given the availability of several promising new drugs with novel mechanisms of action, the immediate challenge is to choose the most effective and specific combination or sequential therapy to prevent resistance in individual patients. The biomarkers can help in the future to formulate personalized treatment, driving the choice of treatment and preventing or overcoming drug resistance.

45.7.2.2 Integrated Management Strategy

Although typically reserved for localized tumors, surgical debulking can also be used with cytoreductive intent in patients with metastatic disease.

Candidates for *cytoreductive nephrectomy* are those patients with good performance status and low systemic disease burden [43]. Although a positive impact of cytoreductive nephrectomy in metastatic ccRCC patients has been demonstrated within two randomized controlled,

phase III trials in the era of cytokines, retrospective data suggest that this paradigm is still valid in the present era of targeted agents.

In addition, surgical resection of metastatic sites remains a treatment option in patients with a solitary metastasis or oligometastatic disease, especially for lung-confined lesions [44].

A subset of patients with advanced tumor, especially having limited sites of metastasis and few adverse prognostic factors, has indolent progression of disease. For these patients, active surveillance can be an initial strategy, that is, observation for a period of time before the start of systemic therapy.

The safety of observation before starting treatment has also been suggested by retrospective and prospective studies, and should be considered in patients with limited tumor burden and in the absence of symptoms [45].

Local treatment strategies of metastases should be discussed in a multidisciplinary team: conventional radiotherapy, whole brain radiotherapy (WBRT), and other type of local radiotherapy, including stereotactic radiosurgery (SRS), stereotactic body radiotherapy (SBRT), CyberKnife radiotherapy, and hypofractionated radiotherapy, can be considered for selected patients after multidisciplinary review [33].

45.8 Emerging Treatment

Recently, immunoncology, represented a new and promising frontier for RCC, with the opportunity of long term survival.

Immune checkpoint inhibitors account for the majority of immunotherapies in use today, but there is a great potential to future developments, including a new generation of immunotherapy agents (◘ Fig. 45.14).

Furthermore, there is a scientific rationale for immunotherapy in combination with VEGF-Inhibitors: angiogenesis, hypoxia, and immunosuppression seem to be strongly related.

The hypothesis of synergistic effect is supported by the observation that antiangiogenic drugs are capable of decreasing immunosuppressive cells and cytokines, such as regulatory T cells, TGF b and IL-10, and inhibitory molecules on T cells, such as immune checkpoint PD-1, enhancing eventually the antitumor immunity. Therefore, targeting the VEGF/VEGFR pathway may attenuate RCC-induced immunosuppression, achieving improved response rates and theoretically can prevent the emergence of escape mechanisms from either agent.

☐ **Fig. 45.14** Immune checkpoint inhibitors and new generation of immunotherapy agents

Novel immunotherapy			
Checkpoint inhibitors	Vaccines	Adoptive T-cell therapy	T-cell agonists
PD-1 inhibitors - Nivolumab - Pembrolizumab PD-L1 inhibitors - Atezolizumab - Avelumab - Durvalumab CTLA-4 inhibitors - Ipilomumab - Tremelimumab	- Dendritic cell - Single peptide - Multipeptide	- CAR T cells - CIK cells	- Agonist antibodies - Cytokines

As mentioned before, several trials with immune checkpoint in combination with VEGF-targeted therapy, or new TKIs, are ongoing to investigate if the bidirectional link between VEGFR- and checkpoint inhibitors is translated into potential clinical benefit for the patients without high toxicity [46–49].

45.9 Follow-Up

No standard recommendation can be given for the follow-up in RCC.

For localized RCC, the time interval of follow-up depends on risk factors. CT scans of thorax and abdomen are routinely carried out; it is recommended to perform CT scans every 3–6 months in high-risk patients for the first 2 years, while yearly on low-risk patients.

During systemic therapy in RCC patients with advanced disease, 2- to 4-month follow-up schemes with CT scan should be advised to determine response and resistance [33].

45.10 Conclusion

Advanced RCC, characterized by a continuously changing treatment scenario.

The introduction of immunotherapy and new generation of oral TKI resulted in a paradigm shift for mRCC, introducing the concept of a possibility of cure.

Sequencing remains, at the moment, the option of choice for treating mRCC, but new available data may change this condition adding an innovative concept of "best patient selection": *predictive biomarkers* are needed to identify patient subgroups for appropriate treatment and to prevent and overcome drug resistance. *Patient selection* will be the key for personalization in the future.

New drugs and new combinations continue to be explored.

Advances in diagnosis, local management, and systemic therapy will help to develop more effective therapeutic strategies and new algorithms for precision therapy (☐ Fig. 45.15).

Summary of Clinical Recommendations
- Linee Guida dell'Associazione Italiana di Oncologia Medica (AIOM)
- Tumori del rene. Edizione 2020.
- Renal cell carcinoma: ESMO Clinical Practice Guidelines for diagnosis, treatment and follow-up. Annals of Oncology 30: 706–720, 2019. ▶ https://doi.org/10.1093/annonc/mdz056. Published online 21 February 2019.
- NCCN (National Comprehensive Cancer Network) GUIDELINES FOR TREATMENT OF CANCER BY SITE: Kidney cancer.

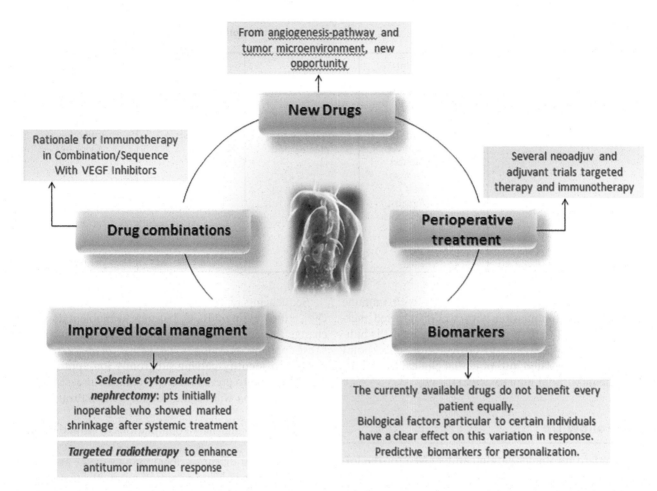

From angiogenesis-pathway and tumor microenvironment, new opportunity

New Drugs

Rationale for Immunotherapy in Combination/Sequence With VEGF Inhibitors

Several neoadjuv and adjuvant trials targeted therapy and immunotherapy

Drug combinations

Perioperative treatment

Improved local managment

Biomarkers

Selective cytoreductive nephrectomy: pts initially inoperable who showed marked shrinkage after systemic treatment

Targeted radiotherapy to enhance antitumor immune response

The currently available drugs do not benefit every patient equally.
Biological factors particular to certain individuals have a clear effect on this variation in response. Predictive biomarkers for personalization.

Fig. 45.15 The near future for the RCC management

45

Case Study

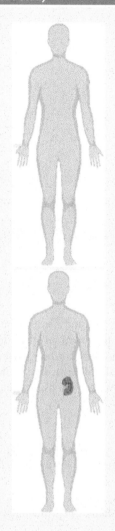

Question

What action should be taken?
1. Surgery
2. neoadjuvant chemotherapy treatment
3. Medical treatment with TKI

Answer

Radical nephrectomy, with a curative intent

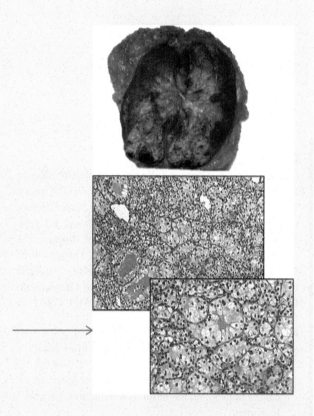

Histological examination: *clear cell carcinoma (ccRCC)*

Question

After surgery?
1. Adjuvant treatment
2. Observation
3. Follow-up

Answer

Follow-up

After 2 years, multiple pulmonary and bone metastases

Man, 65 years old

- *Family history* negative for malignancy
- *APR*: hypertension; cigarette smoking; history of renal lithiasis
- *APP*: in the last 2 months flank pain, then an episode of gross hematuria
- *Objective examination*: Globose abdomen; mild tenderness on deep palpation (quadrant inf.sx); No palpable mass.
- *Blood tests*: Hb 9.2 g/dl; hypercalcemia; platelets and neutrophils greater than the upper limit of normal.
- *Contrast enhanced CT abdomen*: heterogeneously enhancing mass arising from the lower pole of the left kidney.
- *Staging* negative for metastasis.

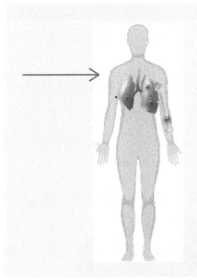

Question

1. Surgery of metastases?
2. Start medical treatment?
3. Follow-up?

Answer

Starts medical treatment

Expert Opinion

(Genitourinary Cancers: Kidney, Antonio Russo, Department of Surgical, Oncological and Oral Sciences, University of Palermo, Palermo, Italy; Marc Peeters, Oncology Department, University of Antwerp, Edegem, Belgium; Lorena Incorvaia, Department of Biomedicine, Neuroscience and Advanced Diagnostics, University of Palermo, Palermo, Italy; Christian Rolfo, Thoracic Medical Oncology, University of Maryl and Greenebaum Comprehensive Cancer Center, Baltimore, MD, USA)

Key Points

- Renal cell carcinoma (RCC), derived from renal tubular epithelial cells, accounts for ~2% of all adult malignancies; it is the seventh most common cancer in men and the tenth most common cancer in women.
- Approximately 75% of RCC are clear cell carcinoma (ccRCC). The other RCC subtypes are a heterogeneous group of cancer with different morphology, genetic and molecular pathogenesis, and clinical behavior, as a whole known as non-clear cell RCC (nccRCC).
- Today we know that between the histological subtypes there are not only histologic difference, but also cytogenetic alterations with specific genes mutated.
- RCC is, indeed, a tumor where new biological knowledge has changed the landscape: antiangiogenic agents and immunotherapy are changing the natural history of the disease.
- Given the availability of several promising new drugs with novel mechanisms of action, the immediate challenge is to choose the most effective and specific combination or sequential therapy to prevent resistance in individual patients. The biomarkers can help in the future to formulate personalized treatment, driving the choice of treatment and preventing or overcoming drug resistance.

Recommendations

- AIOM:
- ▶ https://www.aiom.it/linee-guida-aiom-tumori-del-rene-2019/
- ESMO:
- ▶ https://www.esmo.org/guidelines/genitourinary-cancers/renal-cell-carcinoma

Hints for a Deeper Insight/Suggested Reading

- Kotecha RR, Motzer RJ, Voss MH. Towards individualized therapy for metastatic renal cell carcinoma. Nat Rev Clin Oncol. 2019;16(10):621–33. ▶ https://doi.org/10.1038/s41571-019-0209-1
- Marston Linehan W, Ricketts CJ. The Cancer Genome Atlas of renal cell carcinoma: findings and clinical implications. Nat Rev Urol. 2019;16(9):539–52. ▶ https://doi.org/10.1038/s41585-019-0211-5
- Canino C, Perrone L, Bosco E, Saltalamacchia G, Mosca A, Rizzo M, Porta C. Targeting angiogenesis in metastatic renal cell carcinoma. Expert Rev Anticancer Ther. 2019;19(3):245–57. ▶ https://doi.org/10.1080/14737140.2019.1574574
- Porta C, Rizzo M. Immune-based combination therapy for metastatic kidney cancer. Nat Rev Nephrol. 2019;15(6):324–5.   ▶ https://doi.org/10.1038/s41581-019-0149-0.

References

1. Siegel RL, Miller KD, Jemal A. Cancer statistics, 2016. CA Cancer J Clin. 2016;66(1):7–30.

2. Kaelin WG. Von Hippel-Lindau disease. Annu Rev Pathol. 2007;2:145–73.

3. Levi F, Ferlay J, Galeone C, Lucchini F, Negri E, Boyle P, et al. The changing pattern of kidney cancer incidence and mortality in Europe. BJU Int. 2008;101(8):949–58.

4. Chow WH, Dong LM, Devesa SS. Epidemiology and risk factors for kidney cancer. Nat Rev Urol. 2010;7(5):245–57.

5. McLaughlin JK, Lipworth L, Tarone RE. Epidemiologic aspects of renal cell carcinoma. Semin Oncol. 2006;33(5):527–33.

6. Incorvaia L, Bronte G, Bazan V, Badalamenti G, Rizzo S, Pantuso G, et al. Beyond evidence-based data: scientific rationale and tumor behavior to drive sequential and personalized therapeutic strategies for the treatment of metastatic renal cell carcinoma. Oncotarget. 2016;7(16):21259–71.

7. Ciccarese C, Iacovelli R, Brunelli M, Massari F, Bimbatti D, Fantinel E, et al. Addressing the best treatment for non-clear cell renal cell carcinoma: a meta-analysis of randomised clinical trials comparing VEGFR-TKis versus mTORi-targeted therapies. Eur J Cancer. 2017;83:237–46.

8. Network CGAR. Comprehensive molecular characterization of clear cell renal cell carcinoma. Nature. 2013;499(7456):43–9.

9. Shuch B, Amin A, Armstrong AJ, Eble JN, Ficarra V, Lopez-Beltran A, et al. Understanding pathologic variants of renal cell carcinoma: distilling therapeutic opportunities from biologic complexity. Eur Urol. 2015;67(1):85–97.

10. Hsieh JJ, Purdue MP, Signoretti S, Swanton C, Albiges L, Schmidinger M, et al. Renal cell carcinoma. Nat Rev Dis Primers. 2017;3:17009.

11. Kapur P, Peña-Llopis S, Christie A, Zhrebker L, Pavía-Jiménez A, Rathmell WK, et al. Effects on survival of BAP1 and PBRM1 mutations in sporadic clear-cell renal-cell carcinoma: a retrospective analysis with independent validation. Lancet Oncol. 2013;14(2):159–67.

12. Gerlinger M, Rowan AJ, Horswell S, Math M, Larkin J, Endesfelder D, et al. Intratumor heterogeneity and branched evolution revealed by multiregion sequencing. N Engl J Med. 2012;366(10):883–92.

13. Linehan WM. Molecular targeting of VHL gene pathway in clear cell kidney cancer. J Urol. 2003;170(2 Pt 1):593–4.

14. Kim ES. Tivozanib: first global approval. Drugs. 2017;77(17):1917–23.

15. Zhou L, Liu XD, Sun M, Zhang X, German P, Bai S, et al. Targeting MET and AXL overcomes resistance to sunitinib therapy in renal cell carcinoma. Oncogene. 2016;35(21):2687–97.

16. Rodriguez-Vida A, Hutson TE, Bellmunt J, Strijbos MH. New treatment options for metastatic renal cell carcinoma. ESMO Open. 2017;2(2):e000185.

17. Braren V, Taylor JN, Pace W. Regression of metastatic renal carcinoma following nephrectomy. Urology. 1974;3(6):777–8.

18. Şenbabaoğlu Y, Gejman RS, Winer AG, Liu M, Van Allen EM, de Velasco G, et al. Tumor immune microenvironment characterization in clear cell renal cell carcinoma identifies prognostic and immunotherapeutically relevant messenger RNA signatures. Genome Biol. 2016;17(1):231.

19. Geissler K, Fornara P, Lautenschläger C, Holzhausen HJ, Seliger B, Riemann D. Immune signature of tumor infiltrating immune cells in renal cancer. Onco Targets Ther. 2015;4(1):e985082.

20. Badalamenti G, Fanale D, Incorvaia L, Barraco N, Listì A, Maragliano R, et al. Role of tumor-infiltrating lymphocytes in patients with solid tumors: can a drop dig a stone? Cell Immunol. 2019;343:103753.

21. Incorvaia L, Fanale D, Badalamenti G, et al. Baseline plasma levels of soluble PD-1, PD-L1, and BTN3A1 predict response to nivolumab treatment in patients with metastatic renal cell carcinoma: a step toward a biomarker for therapeutic decisions. Oncoimmunology. 2020;9(1):1832348. Published 2020 Oct 27. https://doi.org/10.1080/2162402X.2020.1832348.

22. Incorvaia L, Fanale D, Badalamenti G, et al. A "Lymphocyte microRNA signature" as predictive biomarker of immunotherapy response and plasma PD-1/PD-L1 expression levels in patients with metastatic renal cell carcinoma: pointing towards epigenetic reprogramming. Cancers (Basel). 2020;12(11):3396. Published 2020 Nov 16. https://doi.org/10.3390/cancers12113396.

23. Motzer RJ, Escudier B, McDermott DF, George S, Hammers HJ, Srinivas S, et al. Nivolumab versus everolimus in advanced renal-cell carcinoma. N Engl J Med. 2015;373(19):1803–13.

24. Motzer RJ, Rini BI, McDermott DF, Redman BG, Kuzel TM, Harrison MR, et al. Nivolumab for metastatic renal cell carcinoma: results of a randomized phase II trial. J Clin Oncol. 2015;33(13):1430–7.

25. Incorvaia L, Madonia G, Corsini LR, Cucinella A, Brando C, Gagliardo C, Santoni M, Fanale D, Inno A, Fazio I, Foti G, Galia M, Badalamenti G, Bazan V, Russo A, Gori S. Challenges and advances for the treatment of renal cancer patients with brain metastases: from immunological background to upcoming clinical evidence on immune-checkpoint inhibitors. Crit Rev Oncol Hematol. 2021 Jun 3:103390. https://doi.org/10.1016/j.critrevonc.2021.103390. Epub ahead of print. PMID: 34090998.

26. Posadas EM, Limvorasak S, Figlin RA. Targeted therapies for renal cell carcinoma. Nat Rev Nephrol. 2017;13(8):496–511.

27. Pierorazio PM, Johnson MH, Patel HD, Sozio SM, Sharma R, Iyoha E, et al. Management of renal masses and localized renal cancer: systematic review and meta-analysis. J Urol. 2016;196(4):989–99.

28. Shingarev R, Jaimes EA. Renal cell carcinoma: new insights and challenges for a clinician scientist. Am J Physiol Renal Physiol. 2017;313(2):F145–F54.

29. Volpe A, Patard JJ. Prognostic factors in renal cell carcinoma. World J Urol. 2010;28(3):319–2.

30. Zisman A, Pantuck AJ, Wieder J, Chao DH, Dorey F, Said JW, et al. Risk group assessment and clinical outcome algorithm to predict the natural history of patients with surgically resected renal cell carcinoma. J Clin Oncol. 2002;20(23):4559–66.

31. Karakiewicz PI, Briganti A, Chun FK, Trinh QD, Perrotte P, Ficarra V, et al. Multi-institutional validation of a new renal cancer-specific survival nomogram. J Clin Oncol. 2007;25(11):1316–22.

32. Leibovich BC, Blute ML, Cheville JC, Lohse CM, Frank I, Kwon ED, et al. Prediction of progression after radical nephrectomy for patients with clear cell renal cell carcinoma: a stratification tool for prospective clinical trials. Cancer. 2003;97(7):1663–71.

33. Escudier B, Porta C, Schmidinger M, Rioux-Leclercq N, Bex A, Khoo V, et al. Renal cell carcinoma: ESMO Clinical Practice Guidelines for diagnosis, treatment and follow-up. Ann Oncol. 2016;27(suppl 5):v58–68.

34. Ravaud A, Motzer RJ, Pandha HS, George DJ, Pantuck AJ, Patel A, et al. Adjuvant sunitinib in high-risk renal-cell carcinoma after nephrectomy. N Engl J Med. 2016;375(23):2246–54.

35. Dabestani S, Thorstenson A, Lindblad P, Harmenberg U, Ljungberg B, Lundstam S. Renal cell carcinoma recurrences and metastases in primary non-metastatic patients: a population-based study. World J Urol. 2016;34(8):1081–6.

36. McKay RR, Kroeger N, Xie W, Lee JL, Knox JJ, Bjarnason GA, et al. Impact of bone and liver metastases on patients with renal cell carcinoma treated with targeted therapy. Eur Urol. 2014;65(3):577–84.

37. Choueiri TK, Hessel C, Halabi S, Sanford B, Michaelson MD, Hahn O, et al. Cabozantinib versus sunitinib as initial therapy for metastatic renal cell carcinoma of intermediate or poor risk (Alliance A031203 CABOSUN randomised trial): progression-free survival by independent review and overall survival update. Eur J Cancer. 2018;94:115–25.

38. Motzer RJ, Tannir NM, McDermott DF, Arén Frontera O, Melichar B, Choueiri TK, et al. Nivolumab plus ipilimumab versus sunitinib in advanced renal-cell carcinoma. N Engl J Med. 2018;378(14):1277–90.

39. Rini BI. Vascular endothelial growth factor-targeted therapy in metastatic renal cell carcinoma. Cancer. 2009;115(10 Suppl):2306–12.

40. Rini BI, Atkins MB. Resistance to targeted therapy in renal-cell carcinoma. Lancet Oncol. 2009;10(10):992–1000.

41. Santoni M, Massari F, Grande E, et al. Cabozantinib in pretreated patients with metastatic renal cell carcinoma with sarcomatoid differentiation: a real-world study [published online ahead of print, 2021 Aug 2]. Target Oncol. 2021. https://doi.org/10.1007/s11523-021-00828-z.

42. Santoni M, Massari F, Bracarda S, et al. Body mass index in patients treated with cabozantinib for advanced renal cell carcinoma: a new prognostic factor?. Diagnostics (Basel). 2021;11(1):138. Published 2021 Jan 18. https://doi.org/10.3390/diagnostics11010138.

43. Heng DY, Wells JC, Rini BI, Beuselinck B, Lee JL, Knox JJ, et al. Cytoreductive nephrectomy in patients with synchronous metastases from renal cell carcinoma: results from the International Metastatic Renal Cell Carcinoma Database Consortium. Eur Urol. 2014;66(4):704–10.

44. Kavolius JP, Mastorakos DP, Pavlovich C, Russo P, Burt ME, Brady MS. Resection of metastatic renal cell carcinoma. J Clin Oncol. 1998;16(6):2261–6.

45. Rini BI, Dorff TB, Elson P, Rodriguez CS, Shepard D, Wood L, et al. Active surveillance in metastatic renal-cell carcinoma: a prospective, phase 2 trial. Lancet Oncol. 2016;17(9):1317–24.

46. Kuusk T, Albiges L, Escudier B, Grivas N, Haanen J, Powles T, et al. Antiangiogenic therapy combined with immune checkpoint blockade in renal cancer. Angiogenesis. 2017;20(2):205–15.

47. Motzer RJ, Penkov K, Haanen J, Rini B, Albiges L, Campbell MT, et al. Avelumab plus axitinib versus sunitinib for advanced renal-cell carcinoma. N Engl J Med. 2019;380(12):1103–15. https://doi.org/10.1056/NEJMoa1816047. Epub 2019 Feb 16.

48. Rini BI, Plimack ER, Stus V, Gafanov R, Hawkins R, Nosov D, et al. Pembrolizumab plus axitinib versus sunitinib for advanced renal-cell carcinoma. N Engl J Med. 2019;380(12):1116–27. https://doi.org/10.1056/NEJMoa1816714. Epub 2019 Feb 16.

49. Santoni M, Heng DY, Bracarda S, Procopio G, Milella M, Porta C, et al. Real-world data on cabozantinib in previously treated patients with metastatic renal cell carcinoma: focus on sequences and prognostic factors. Cancers (Basel). 2019;12(1):pii: E84. https://doi.org/10.3390/cancers12010084. PMID: 31905816.

Bladder Cancer

Hector Josè Soto Parra, Fiorenza Latteri, Laura Noto,
and Marco Maria Aiello

Genitourinary Cancers

Contents

© Springer Nature Switzerland AG 2021
A. Russo et al. (eds.), *Practical Medical Oncology Textbook*, UNIPA Springer Series,
https://doi.org/10.1007/978-3-030-56051-5_46

46.1 Introduction

Bladder cancer is one of the most common urologic cancers with the highest recurrence rate of any malignant disease. In North and South America, Europe, and Asia, the most common histologic subtype is transitional cell carcinoma. Other histotypes include squamous cell carcinoma and adenocarcinomas.

46.2 Epidemiology

Bladder cancer represents the ninth tumor by incidence in the World with an incidence rate of 9 per 100,000 in men and 2.2 per 100,000 in women, turning out to be the fourth tumor by incidence in men (9% of all diagnoses of cancer), and the 11th tumor in women (2.7% of all diagnoses of cancer). In terms of mortality, it represents 4.5% of total cancer deaths in males and 1.7% in women. These data indicate that survival of bladder cancer, considering all the stages, is averagely long, with a statistically declining trend of mortality rate in men (−1.5% per year) and a stable mortality trend in women (+0.3% per year):
- Incidence of bladder cancer increases with age, with a median of diagnosis around 72 years.
- Bladder cancer is rarely diagnosed before age 40 years.
- Bladder cancer is about three times more common in men than in women.
- In the past two decades, the incidence of bladder cancer has been stable in men, but has increased in women (+0.2% per year).

46.3 Etiology

Factors that may increase bladder cancer risk include the following:
- Cigarette Smoke: it is the main risk factor; it causes 50–60% of bladder cancers in men and 20–30% in women. The correlation between bladder cancer's incidence, number of cigarettes and years of smoking is statistically relevant.
- Occupational exposure: exposure to paint components, PAHs, aromatic amines, and diesel exhaust are the second risk factor.
- Diet: consumption of fruits and vegetables reduces bladder cancer incidence.
- Chronic infections: according to numerous scientific works a correlation was found between chronic urinary infections and infiltrating tumor forms and squamous histological subtype (e.g., Schistosoma, Haematobium, and Bilharzia).
- Previous chemotherapy exposures: cyclophosphamide is associated with an increased risk of approximately nine times; radiotherapy of the abdomen and/or pelvis increases the risk of bladder cancer even many years later.
- Genetics: Although some polymorphisms seem to increase susceptibility to bladder cancer in persons with work exposure to substances associated with increased risk, no strong evidence have been observed for hereditary factors in the development of bladder cancer even if familial clusters of bladder cancer have been described.

There is currently no evidence that non-invasive screening investigations could reduce risk of mortality of bladder cancer.

46.4 Clinical Features

Bladder cancer could be asymptomatic for a long time. Symptoms may also vary depending on the location and extension of the tumor. Bladder cancer located at the urethral level could cause acute urinary retention, while superficial forms may be asymptomatic or give irritative symptoms (e.g., increased frequency of urination, increased urgency of urination, urge incontinence, excessive passage of urine at night). Bladder tumors at the ureteral openings could cause hydroureteronephrosis. In advanced stages, the symptomatology may be characterized by asthenia, loss of appetite, weight loss, pain in the sites of metastasis, or organ failure.

46.5 Pathological Features

Ninety percent of bladder cancer derives from the urothelial epithelium so it's called urothelial cell carcinoma. Other uncommon forms are squamous cell carcinoma, mixed forms, sarcomatoid tumors, and small cell carcinomas. Bladder cancer is distinct into invasive and non-invasive carcinoma based on the infiltration of the basal membrane.

46.5.1 Non-Invasive Bladder Cancer

It includes 70% of urothelial cell carcinomas, it is characterized by papillary architecture and subdivided on the basis of cytological nucleus differentiation grade (WHO 2016) in three forms:
- Non-invasive urothelial cell carcinoma of low malignant potential (50% of recurrence risk)
- Non-invasive urothelial cell carcinoma of low grade: >50% of recurrence risk and 10% of metastatic risk
- Non-invasive urothelial cell carcinoma of high grade: >60% of recurrence risk and 30% of metastatic risk.

46.5.2 Invasive Bladder Cancer

It includes all bladder cancers which infiltrate the basal membrane, which are usually high-grade neoplasia with a high recurrence and metastatic risk.

46.6 Molecular Biology

Somatic mutations in fibroblast growth receptor 3 (FGFR-3) and tumor protein p53 (TP53) in tumor cells seem to be crucial molecular events in the non-invasive and invasive pathways, respectively.

FGFR-3, Ras, and PIK3CA mutations occur more frequently in non-invasive bladder cancer, upregulating the AKT and mitogen-activated protein kinase (MAPK) pathway. Loss of heterozygosity (LOH) on chromosome 9 is among the most frequent genetic alterations in bladder cancers and is considered an initial event.

The TP53 gene is found to be altered in approximately 60–65% of invasive bladder cancers and its mutation is significantly related with a short Progression-Free Survival (PFS). The TP53 gene mutation is also considered an independent predictive factor of death in patients with muscle-invasive bladder cancer.

Usually, high-grade invasive cancers also present alterations in PTEN and retinoblastoma (Rb) genes.

In addition to specific cancer cell genetic alterations, the tumor microenvironment may influence the tumor growth and cell proliferation by production of vascular endothelial growth factor (VEGF) and abnormal E-cadherin expression.

46.7 Diagnosis

In case of clinical suspicion of bladder cancer, it is mandatory to proceed with clinical examination, blood tests, urinalysis (to evaluate the presence of anemia from hematuria, acute renal failure from hydronephrosis, and exclude the presence of urinary tract infections). If a bladder cancer is suspected, it is convenient to perform cytological analysis of urinary sediment to eventually identify tumor cells. Eco-ultrasound has a diagnostic sensibility of 80–95% and high diagnostic specificity, with some limitations, such as the inability to diagnose flat bladder neoplasms and to study the upper urinary tract and the fact that it is an operator-dependent exam. Due to these limitations, in case of neoplasm found with the echography or strong clinical suspicion, it is mandatory to perform an endoscopic evaluation. The local staging could be performed both with computerized tomography (CT) and with magnetic resonance imaging (MRI); however, the MRI is more detailed to define the local staging. Once a radiological description of the lesion is obtained it is necessary to complete the diagnostic work-flow with an endoscopic evaluation with flexible cystoscopy in order to evaluate both the number and morphological features (papillary or solid) of the lesions and to describe mucosal anomalies. The transurethral resection of bladder tumor (TURBT) is a diagnostic-staging procedure, also, in the case of small lesions (smaller than a centimeter), allows to perform the radical removal of its implant base and the surrounding margins, to identify a possible involvement of the muscular tunic. These data are essential for the subsequent therapeutic strategy.

46.8 Staging and Prognosis

Bladder tumors could be subdivided into non-muscle invasive (T1, Ta, Tis) and muscle-invasive (T2–T4 – ◘ Table 46.1). The prognosis of non-invasive muscle neoplasms is significantly influenced by the grading of differentiation, by the size, by the number of diagnosed neoplasms, by the number of recurrences, by submucosal invasion, and by the presence of in situ carcinoma, a high-grade flat neoplasm with high risk of invasion. Related to these characteristics, 5 years progression risk ranges from 1% to 45%. In muscle-invasive cancers, recurrence risk and 5-year survival are, respectively, 68% and 66%.

46.9 Treatment

The treatment of bladder cancer is multidisciplinary and should involve urologist, oncologist, and radiotherapist. Treatment algorithm for management of bladder cancer includes non-muscle-invasive bladder cancer, localized muscle-invasive bladder cancer, and metastatic disease (◘ Fig. 46.1).

■ **Table 46.1**   TNM staging system

Primary tumor (T)		Stage	T	N	M
TX	Primary tumor cannot be assessed	Stage 0a	Ta	N0	M0
T0	No evidence of primary tumor	Stage 0is	Tis	N0	M0
Ta	Noninvasive papillary carcinoma	Stage I	T1	N0	M0
Tis	Carcinoma in situ: "flat tumor"	Stage II	T2a	N0	M0
T1	Tumor invades lamina propria (subepithelial connective tissue)		T2b	N0	M0
T2	Tumor invades muscularis propria	Stage IIIA	T3a	N0	M0
pT2a	Tumor invades superficial muscularis propria (inner half)		T3b	N0	M0
pT2b	Tumor invades deep muscularis propria (outer half)		T4a	N0	M0
T3	Tumor invades perivesical tissue		T1–T4a	N1	M0
pT3a	Microscopically	Stage IIIB	T1–T4a	N2, N3	M0
pT3b	Macroscopically (extravesical mass)	Stage IVA	T4b	Any N	M0
T4	Tumor invades any of the following: prostatic stroma, seminal vesicles, uterus, vagina, pelvic wall, abdominal wall		Any T	Any N	M1a
T4a	Tumor invades prostatic stroma, uterus, vagina	Stage IVB	Any T	Any N	M1b
T4b	Tumor invades pelvic wall, abdominal wall				
Regional lymph nodes (N)					
Regional lymph nodes include both primary and secondary drainage regions. All other nodes above the aortic bifurcation are considered distant lymph nodes.					
NX	Lymph nodes cannot be assessed				
N0	No lymph node metastasis				
N1	Single regional lymph node metastasis in the true pelvis (perivesical, obturator, internal and external iliac, or sacral lymph node)				
N2	Multiple regional lymph node metastasis in the true pelvis (perivesical, obturator, internal and external iliac, or sacral lymph node metastasis)				
N3	Lymph node metastasis to the common iliac lymph nodes				
Distant metastasis (M)					
M0	No distant metastasis				
M1	Distant metastasis				
M1a	Distant metastasis limited to lymph nodes beyond the common iliacs				
M1b	Non–lymph node distant metastases				

■ Fig. 46.1 Treatment algorithm for management of blabber cancer

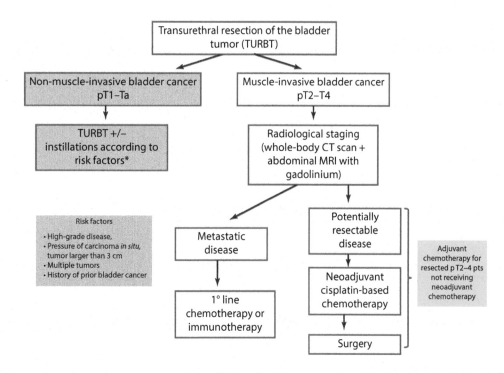

```
                    ┌─────────────────────────────┐
                    │ Transurethral resection of  │
                    │   the bladder tumor (TURBT) │
                    └─────────────────────────────┘
            ┌──────────────────┴────────────────────┐
┌───────────────────────────┐         ┌───────────────────────────┐
│ Non-muscle-invasive        │         │ Muscle-invasive bladder   │
│ bladder cancer pT1–Ta      │         │ cancer pT2–T4             │
└───────────────────────────┘         └───────────────────────────┘
            │                                      │
┌───────────────────────────┐         ┌───────────────────────────┐
│ TURBT +/– instillations    │         │ Radiological staging      │
│ according to risk factors* │         │ (whole-body CT scan +     │
└───────────────────────────┘         │ abdominal MRI with        │
                                       │ gadolinium)               │
                                       └───────────────────────────┘
```

Risk factors
- High-grade disease,
- Pressure of carcinoma *in situ*, tumor larger than 3 cm
- Multiple tumors
- History of prior bladder cancer

Metastatic disease → 1° line chemotherapy or immunotherapy

Potentially resectable disease → Neoadjuvant cisplatin-based chemotherapy → Surgery

Adjuvant chemotherapy for resected p T2–4 pts not receiving neoadjuvant chemotherapy

46.9.1 Treatment of Non-Muscle-Invasive Bladder Cancer

Complete TURBT is the treatment of choice for any initial bladder tumor, followed by instillations according to risk. Risk factors for recurrence and progression include high-grade disease, presence of carcinoma in situ, tumor larger than 3 cm, multiple tumors, and history of prior bladder cancer. Intravesical BCG is the treatment of choice for reducing the risk of cancer progression and is mainly used for cancers with an intermediate or high risk of progressing. It is associated with a risk of significant toxicity, including rare deaths from BCG sepsis, local toxicity, and systemic side effects. Because of concerns about side effects, BCG is not generally used for patients with a low risk of progression. Intravesical therapy with thiotepa, mitomycin C, or doxorubicin is also often used for treatment of patients with multiple tumors or recurrent tumors or as a prophylactic measure. Segmental cystectomy or radical cystectomy is used in highly selected patients at high risk of progression with extensive or refractory superficial high-grade tumors based on reports that up to 20% of patients are at risk of death.

46.9.2 Treatment of Muscle-Invasive Bladder Cancer

Radical cystectomy is the standard treatment option of muscle-invasive bladder cancer and its effectiveness at prolonging survival increases if it is preceded by cisplatin-based multiagent chemotherapy. Radical cystectomy is a major operation with a perioperative mortality rate of 2–3% that is accompanied by pelvic lymph node dissection and includes removal of the bladder, perivesical tissues, prostate, and seminal vesicles in men and removal of the uterus, fallopian tubes, ovaries, anterior vaginal wall, and urethra in women. Postoperative complications may include erectile dysfunction in men and sexual dysfunction in women. After radical cystectomy, approximate 30–40% risk of recurrence still exists for patients with muscle-invasive disease and overall survival has generally been reported to be in the range of 50–60%. Combined treatments with the highest level of evidence supporting their effectiveness are radical cystectomy preceded by multiagent cisplatin-based chemotherapy and radiation therapy with concomitant chemotherapy.

46.9.2.1 Neoadjuvant and Adjuvant Chemotherapy

Because bladder cancer commonly recurs with distant metastases, systemic chemotherapy administered before cystectomy may be preferable to postoperative treatment in order to enhance tumor resectability and treat occult metastatic disease. Additionally, neoadjuvant chemotherapy is better tolerated. The use of cisplatin-based neoadjuvant chemotherapy for bladder cancer is supported by a 5% absolute increase in 5-year OS and a 9% absolute increase in 5-year disease-free survival compared with radical cystectomy alone. This demonstrated survival benefit encourages the use of this approach in patients with good performance status (ECOG 0–1) and renal function (GFR > 60 ml/min) with clinical stage T2–T4, N0. While there is still insufficient evidence for

Fig. 46.2 Treatment algorithm for metastatic disease

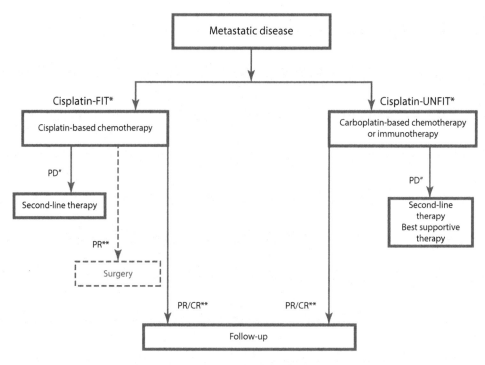

*Cisplatin-FIT: ECOG P5 O-1, Creatinine clearance >60 ml/min, no serious comorbid conditions
** PD: Progressive disease, PR: Partial response, CR: Complete response

the routine use of adjuvant chemotherapy in clinical practice, it is likely that high-risk patients that have not received neoadjuvant chemotherapy, such as those with pT2–T4 and/or node-positive disease, will benefit most from adjuvant cisplatin-based chemotherapy.

46.9.2.2 Radiotherapy With or Without Concomitant Chemotherapy

The approach of organ preservation therapy is a reasonable option for patients seeking an alternative to cystectomy and a palliative option for those who are medically unfit for surgery. In these cases, definitive radiation therapy is a treatment option that yields a 5-year survival of approximately 30–40%, and best results are seen in patients with solitary lesions and without carcinoma in situ or hydronephrosis. The addition of chemotherapy to radiation therapy has been shown to reduce local relapse rates, although it has not been shown to result in increased survival or improved quality of life.

46.9.3 Metastatic Disease

Metastatic disease can arise at the time of diagnosis (about 10% of cases) or, more often, occur after primary surgical treatment in about half of all patients. Distant metastases are more common than local recurrences and they can involve lymph nodes, bones, lungs, or other organs. Patients with metastatic disease are treated with systemic therapy, even if metastasectomy

could be taken into consideration in selected cases with oligometastatic disease, especially located in lung or lymph nodes, and good response to pharmacological treatments (■ Fig. 46.2).

46.9.3.1 First-Line Therapy

Since the 1980s, cisplatin-containing chemotherapy is the gold standard treatment for advanced bladder cancer. In particular, GC (Gemcitabine plus Cisplatin) and HD-MVAC (High Dose of Methotrexate, Vinblastine, Doxorubicin and Cisplatin with growth factor support) regimens represent the recommended first-line treatment options for cisplatin eligible patients thanks to the results of two large phase III trials (Von Der Maase et al., 2000; Sternberg et al., 2001). Cisplatin-based chemotherapy is associated with a median overall survival of 14 months with better efficacy in patients with only lymph node disease and good performance status. For cisplatin ineligible patients (due to compromised renal or liver status, poor performance status, or serious comorbid conditions), representing about one-third of all patients, regimens with lower toxicity profiles are recommended. For example, the use of carboplatin may be a substitute for cisplatin and non-platin-containing regimens, including taxanes and gemcitabine, may be considered in some cases. For selected patients with only lymph node subdiaphragmatic disease who present a partial response after first-line chemotherapy, a surgical approach on residual disease can be considered as part of a multidisciplinary choice. Results of ongoing phase III clinical

□ Table 46.2 Clinical trials of immune-checkpoint inhibitors plus chemotherapy for first-line urothelial cancer

Study	Agent	Phase and type	Primary endpoint
MK347536/ KEYNOTE-361	Pembrolizumab ± chemotherapy vs chemotherapy	Randomised. controlled	PFS, OS
IMvigor130	Alezolizumab ± chemotherapy vs chemotherapy	Randomised, controlled	PFS, OS, % with AEs
DANUBE	Durvalumab ± tremelmimab vs SOC chemotherapy	Randomised, open label	PFS, OS
CheckMate901	Nivolumab ± ipilimmab vs chemotherapy	Randomised, open label	PFS, OS

trials investigating immune-checkpoint inhibitors in combination with chemotherapy for the treatment of first-line urothelial cancer are awaited (□ Table 46.2). Early data from KEYNOTE-361 (pembrolizumab ± chemotherapy versus chemotherapy) and IMvigor130 (atezolizumab ± chemotherapy versus chemotherapy) showed a detrimental effect in terms of overall survival of immunotherapy alone compared to chemotherapy for those patients with a negative PD-L1 expression. For this reason, on May 2018, FDA restricted first-line use of atezolizumab and pembrolizumab for patients who are not eligible for cisplatin and whose tumors express PD-L1 (PD-L1 expression ≥5% and ≥10%, respectively) or in patients who are not eligible for any platinum-containing chemotherapy regardless of PD-L1 expression (NCCN Guidelines Bladder Cancer Version 05.2018).

46.9.3.2 Second-Line Therapy

In patients progressing after first-line therapy, prognosis is very poor with a median overall survival of 5–7 months. Treatment options for subsequent line of therapies include several chemotherapeutic agents (docetaxel, paclitaxel, gemcitabine, pemetrexed), many of which tested in phase II trials with a modest antitumor activity (overall response rate – ORR from 0% to 30%). Vinflunine, a third-generation member of the vinca alkaloid family, is the only drug that showed a survival benefit in this setting. Based on a 2.6-month median survival gain compared with best supportive care in a randomized phase III clinical trial (Bellmunt et al., 2009), it was approved as second-line treatment option in metastatic transitional cell carcinoma of the urothelium by the European Medicines Agency (EMA), but not by the US Food and Drug Administration (FDA).

46.9.3.3 New Agents

Given the high rate of somatic mutations reported in bladder cancer, immunotherapy has shown a significant impact as a treatment option for this pathology. □ Table 46.3

summarizes recent data of immunotherapy in metastatic urothelial cancer both in the first and second lines. Based on these results, the PD-1 inhibitors nivolumab and pembrolizumab as well as the PD-L1 inhibitor atezolizumab are approved by FDA and EMA for the treatment of locally advanced or metastatic urothelial cell carcinoma that has progressed during or after platinum-based chemotherapy or within 12 months of neoadjuvant or adjuvant platinum-containing chemotherapy. In addition, durvalumab and avelumab (PD-L1 inhibitors) are approved for the same indication only by FDA.

Although immune checkpoint inhibitors have improved outcomes in some patients with platinum-resistant metastatic or unresectable urothelial carcinoma, many others may not benefit from this kind of approach. A part of immune-refractory patients are carriers of FGFR (fibroblast growth factor receptor) alterations, which are found in 10–20% of metastatic urothelial carcinoma and are typical of the immunologically "cold" luminal 1 molecular subtype. Erdafitinib, a pan-FGFR inhibitor, demonstrated promising activity among patients with FGFR alterations in the recently presented open-label phase 2 study BLC2001: 42% confirmed ORR (3% CR, 39% PR) and 80% disease control rate (CR + PR + SD), data through which FDA granted Breakthrough Therapy Designation for erdafitinib in the treatment of urothelial cancer (Siefker-Radkte et al., ASCO-GU abstract #411, ASCO Annual Meeting 2018 abstract 4503). A phase III trial is ongoing.

46.10 Follow-Up

Timing, plan, and follow-up duration may vary based on risk categories. In general, for non-muscle invasive disease, the first cystoscopy performed after 3 months since the diagnosis represents an important prognostic factor. In the following tables, useful follow-up algorithms are shown.

Table 46.3 Trials with immunotherapy in metastatic urothelial cancer both in the first and second lines (Jiang et al., 2018)

Setting	ICI	Phase	n	ORR (%)	PFS (mo)	OS (mo)	PD-L1 biomarker analysis			SAEs	HrQOL
							Assay	Cells	Cut-off		
Metastatic second line therapy	Alezolizumab vs. chemotherapy[a]	III	931	22	2.1	11.1 vs 10.6	VentanaSP142	IC	5%	20	Improved fatigue and physical function
	Prembroliziamab vs. chemotherapy[a]	III	542	210	2.1	10.3 vs 7.4	Dako IIIC22C3	TC and IC	10%	15	–
	Nivolumab	II	270	20	2.0	8.74	Ventana SP142	TC and IC	1%, 5%	18	Stable or improved
	Avelumab	I	249	17	1.58	6.5	Dako IHC73-10	TC	5%	8	–
	Durvalumab	I/II	191	17.8	1.5	18.2	Ventana SP263	TC or IC	25%	4.9	–
Metastatic firstline[b]	Atezolizumab	II	119	23	2.7	15.9	Ventana SP142	TC	<1%, 1–4%, ≥5%	16	–
	Pembrolizumab	III	370	29	2.0	11.0	Dako IHC22C3	TC and IC	<1%, 1–9%, ≥10%	16	–

ICI immune checkpoint inhibitor, *ORR* objective response rate, *PFS* progression free survival, *OS* overall survival, *SAEs* severe adverse events, *HrQOL* health-related quality of life, *IC* immune cells, *TC* tumor cells

[a]Chemotherapy was physician's choice of docetauel (74 mg/m^2), paclitaxel (175 mg/m^2), or vinflunine (320 mg/m^2) every 3 weeks

[b]Cisplatin-ineligible patient

46

46.10.1 Non-Muscle Invasive Bladder Cancer

Low risk	*Cystoscopy*: after 3 and 12 months; then annually up to 5 years *Imaging*: upper tract and abdominal-pelvic imaging baseline
Intermediate risk	*Cystoscopy and urine cytology*: after 3 and 6 months, then every 6 months up to 2 years, then annually up to 5 years *Imaging*: upper tract and abdominal-pelvic imaging baseline
High risk	*Cystoscopy and urine cytology*: every 3 months up to 2 years, every 6 months up to 5 years, then annually up to 10 years *Imaging*: upper tract and abdominal-pelvic imaging baseline, upper tract imaging every 1–2 years up to 5 years

46.10.2 Muscle Invasive Bladder Cancer

Post-bladder sparing (partial cystectomy or chemoradiation)	*Cystoscopy*: every 3 months up to 2 years; every 6 months up to 4 years, then annually up to 10 years *Urine cytology*: every 6–12 months up to 2 years *Blood tests*: every 3–6 months up to 2 years *Imaging*: chest, upper tract, and abdominal-pelvic imaging every 3–6 months up to 2 years, then annually up to 5 years
Post-cystectomy pT2 N0	*Urine cytology*: every 6–12 months up to 2 years *Blood tests*: every 3–6 months up to 2 years, then every 9–12 months up to 5 years *Imaging*: chest and abdominal-pelvic imaging (CT scan) every 6 months up to 2 years, then annually up to 5 years
Post-cystectomy pT3–4 and/or pN+	*Urine cytology*: every 6–12 months up to 2 years *Blood tests*: every 3–6 months up to 2 years, then every 9–12 months up to 5 years *Imaging*: chest and abdominal-pelvic imaging (CT scan) every 4 months up to 2 years, then every 6 months up to 5 years *Blood tests*: CBC (cell blood count), renal, and liver function testing

Man, 67 years old. Smoker of 20 cigarettes die
- *Family history* negative for malignancy
- *APR*: Hypertension
- *APP*: Hematuria and dysuria for nearly 4 months
- *Objective examination*: Globose abdomen; mild pain during deep palpation on right flank with palpable mass
- *Blood tests*: Anemia (Hb 9.1 g/dl)
- *Urine cytology*: Positive for malignant tumor cells
- *CT abdomen mdc*: Lesion in the right renal pelvis
  - No lymphadenopathies
  - No distant metastases

Question

What action should be taken?
   (1) Surgery. (2) Biopsy. (3) Other

Answer

Surgery: right nefro-ureterectomy + TURBT
   Histological examination:
(a) Kidney, paracaval lymph node, and ureter: high-grade papillary and solid urothelial carcinoma infiltrating the pelvis wall at full thickness and the peripielic fat. Free the renal parenchyma. Multiple foci of high-grade urothelial neoplasia along the ureter mucosa. pT3N0
(b) Bladder: high-grade solid urothelial carcinoma infiltrating the muscularis propria. pT2

Conclusion:

Resected renal pelvis urothelial carcinoma pT3N0 + endoscopically resected bladder urothelial carcinoma pT2

Question

What action should be taken?
   (1) Surgery. (2) Medical therapy. (3) Radiotherapy

Answer

Surgery: radical cystectomy + bilateral pelvic lymphadenectomy

   Histological examination: high-grade urothelial carcinoma of the bladder infiltrating the bladder wall and the perivesical fat. Metastasis in 1/6 right iliac lymph nodes. pT3a N1

   Staging of disease with CT thorax-abdomen and PET-FDG: right lung metastasis in the medium lobe + right external iliac lymphadenopathies and metastasis on the abdominal wall in hypogastrium

Question

What action should be taken?
   (1) Surgery. (2) Medical therapy. (3) Radiotherapy

Answer

Medical therapy: the patient begins first-line chemotherapy with Cisplatin + Gemcitabine

   Response evaluation after 6 months of therapy with Cisplatin + Gemcitabine: Partial response to CT; partial metabolic response to PET-FDG (reduction in extension and intensity of metastatic lesions)

Lung Metastasis
Basal

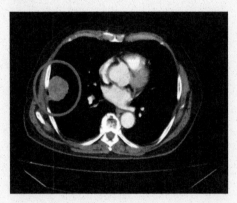

After 6 months of chemotherapy

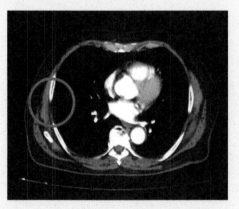

CT

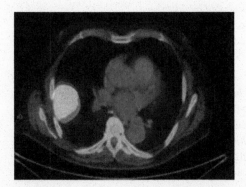

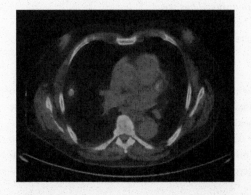

PET-FDG

**Hypogastric Abdominal Wall Metastasis
Basal**

After 6 months of chemotherapy

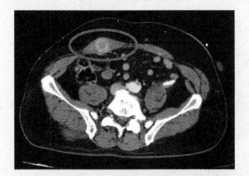

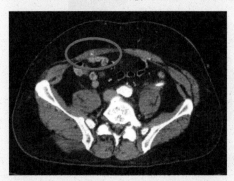

CT

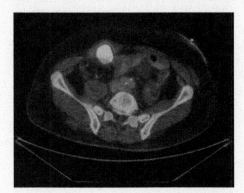

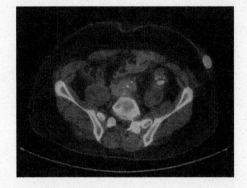

PET-FDG

Question

What action should be taken?

(1) Metastasectomy. (2) Follow-up. (3) Continues chemotherapy

Answer

Surgical evaluation: metastasectomy not indicated due to initial disease extension and tumor aggressiveness → the patient begins *follow-up*

After 6 months of follow-up, progression disease (lung right lesion 40 versus 14 mm and appearance of new nodules + increase of the right external iliac lymphadenopathy)

Before treatment

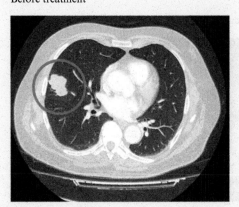

Key Points

- The importance of a correct disease staging to avoid unnecessary surgery
- The importance of a multidisciplinary approach

Question

What action should be taken?

(1) Second-line chemotherapy. (2) Cisplatin-gemcitabine re-challenge. (3) Immunotherapy

Answer

The patient begins second-line chemotherapy with Vinflunine (immunotherapy not available)

- *Response evaluation after 3 months of therapy with Vinflunine*: Partial pulmonary response, lymph nodal stable disease to CT, he continues chemotherapy until progression or unacceptable toxicity

After 3 months of Vinflunine

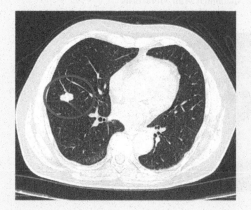

- Correct management of medical treatment side effects
- Choice of best therapeutic option for the patient

Case Study: Platin-Unfit Patient

Man, 77 years old
- *Family history* negative for malignancy
- *APR*: severe ischemic cardiopathy, hypertension, renal failure
- *APP*: after the appearance of hematuria TURBT with diagnosis of high-grade urothelial papillary carcinoma infiltrating the prostate (pT4)
- *CT Thorax-Abdomen mdc*: thickening of the bladder wall that involves the ureteral meatus causing hydroureteronephrosis, iliac lymphadenopathies, and lung metastasis (metastatic disease)
- *Blood tests*: serum creatinine 1.7 mg/dl (renal failure due to hydroureteronephrosis)

Question

What action should be taken?

(1) Surgery. (2) Nephrostomy. (3) Immediate first-line chemotherapy

Answer

Nephrostomy: the patient underwent bilateral nephrostomy placement with only partial renal function recovery

Question

What action should be taken?

(1) Platin-based poli-chemotherapy. (2) Mono-chemotherapy. (3) Immunotherapy

Answer

Mono-chemotherapy: patient begins first-line mono-chemotherapy with gemcitabine due to persistent moderate renal failure and concomitant cardiopathy (immunotherapy not available)

After 3 months of Gemcitabine: SD, after 6 months: local progression of the bladder lesion with urinary symptoms, pulmonary stability

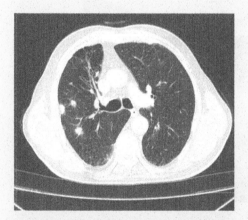
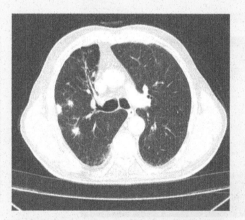

Pulmonary stability after 3 and 6 months of gemcitabine

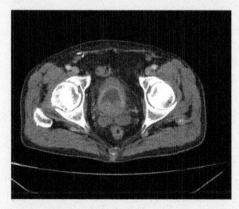
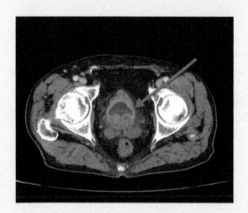

Local PD after 6 months

Question

What action should be taken?

   (1) Second-line chemotherapy. (2) Immunotherapy. (3) Best supportive care

Answer

Second-line chemotherapy: the patient begins second-line chemotherapy with weekly paclitaxel

   After 6 months of paclitaxel: stable disease, he continues with the same therapy until progression or unacceptable toxicity

Before paclitaxel

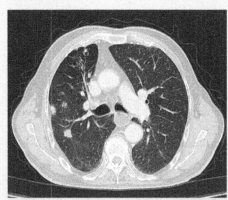

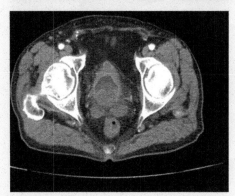

After 6 months of paclitaxel

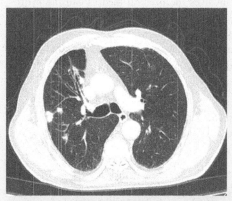

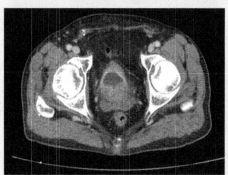

Key Points

- Importance of comorbidity evaluation in order to decide the best medical treatment
- It could be useful to consider immunotherapy for platin-unfit patients when possible
- The duration of therapy is based on tolerability and efficacy
- Importance of symptoms management in the context of simultaneous care

Expert Opinion
Giuseppe Procopio

Key Points

1. Bladder cancer is a common neoplasm that affects frequently men with a median age at the diagnosis of 72 years old. The most important risk factors are cigarette smoke, professional exposure to paint components or aromatic amines, chronic infections (i.e., Schistosoma Haemotobium, and Bilharzia), previous chemotherapies, and gene predisposition.

2. Symptoms vary from hematuria, increased frequency or urgency of urination, hydroureteronephrosis, and acute urinary retention, and they actually depend on the primitive site of cancer. Systemic symptoms are asthenia and weight loss, while others can depend on the sites of metastases.

3. There are different histological types, but the most frequent is the transitional cell carcinoma. Other types are squamous cell carcinoma, mixed forms, sarcomatoid tumors, and small cell carcinomas. Moreover, they can be divided in non-invasive and invasive subtypes considering the basal membrane infiltration. It is crucial to understand this aspect in order to administer the correct treatment.

4. Clinical examination, blood test, and urine analyses are the first steps in the diagnostic approach. US is quite useful but flexible cystoscopy is essential to study both the number and morphological features of the lesions. It is possible to investigate the local involvement thanks to MRI or CT which can be implied also for a complete staging. The transurethral resection of bladder tumor (TURBT) is the most important step, which can have also a therapeutic intent, and it allows to study the basal membrane invasion.

5. Treatments are different considering the infiltration of the basal membrane: in non-invasive cancers, TURBT is the treatment of choice followed by instillations according to the risk. In invasive forms, radical cystectomy is recommended preferable if preceded by cisplatin-based multitarget chemotherapy.

6. Radiation therapy can be used to prevent cystectomy or for those who are unfit for surgery. In case of metastatic disease, a platinum-based chemotherapy is recommended together with gemcitabine or high dose of Methotrexate, Vinblastine, Doxorubicin with growth factor support. In case of second-line therapy, Vinflunine is the only drug that showed a survival benefit.

7. PD-1 inhibitors Nivolumab and Pembrolizumab and the PD-L1 inhibitor Atezolizumab are approved for the treatment of locally advanced or metastatic urothelial cell carcinoma that has progressed during or after platinum-based chemotherapy or within 12 months of neoadjuvant or adjuvant platinum-containing chemotherapy.

8. Timing, plan, and follow-up duration may vary based on risk categories and can consist in cystoscopy, urine cytology, blood test, or imaging such as CT scan.

Recommendations

- ESMO
- ▶ https://www.esmo.org/Guidelines/Genitourinary-Cancers/Bladder-Cancer
- ASCO
- ▶ www.asco.org/practice-guidelines/quality-guidelines/guidelines/genitourinary-cancer#/25246
- ▶ www.asco.org/practice-guidelines/quality-guidelines/guidelines/genitourinary-cancer#/10691
- AIOM
- ▶ www.aiom.it/linee-guida-aiom-2020-tumori-urotelio/

Hints for a Deeper Insight

- Update on the Guideline of Guidelines: Non-Muscle Invasive Bladder Cancer: ▶ https://www.ncbi.nlm.nih.gov/pubmed/31597003
- Epidemiology of Bladder Cancer: A Systematic Review and Contemporary Update of Risk Factors in 2018: ▶ https://www.ncbi.nlm.nih.gov/pubmed/30268659
- Bladder cancer: Present and future: ▶ https://www.ncbi.nlm.nih.gov/pubmed/28736063

Suggested Reading

Jiang DM, Sridhar SS. Prime time for immunotherapy in advavnced urothelial cancer. Asia Pac J Clin Oncol. 2018;14:24–32.

Bibliography

Advanced Bladder Cancer (ABC) Meta-analysis Collaboration. Adjuvant chemotherapy for invasive bladder cancer (individual patient data). Cochrane Database Syst Rev. 2006;2:CD006018.

Babjuk M, Burger M, Zigeuner R, et al. EAU guidelines on non-muscleinvasive urothelial carcinoma of the bladder: update 2013. Eur Urol. 2013;64:639–53.

Brierley JD, Gospodarowicz MK, Wittekin CH. TNM classification of malignant tumours. 8th ed. Chichester: Wiley-Blackwell; 2017.

Cancer Stat Facts: Bladder Cancer. National Cancer Institute. Available at https://seer.cancer.gov/statfacts/html/urinb.html. Accessed 16 August 2018.

Chan KS, Espinosa I, Chao M, Wong D, Ailles L, Diehn M, et al. Identification, molecular characterization, clinical prognosis, and therapeutic targeting of human bladder tumor-initiating cells. Proc Natl Acad Sci U S A. 2009;106(33):14016–21.

Dawson C, Whitfield H. ABC of urology. Urological malignancy – II: Urothelial tumours. BMJ. 1996;312(7038):1090–4.

James ND, Hussain SA, Hall E, et al. Radiotherapy with or without chemotherapy in muscle-invasive bladder cancer. N Engl J Med. 2012;366:1477–88.

Leow JJ, Martin-Doyle W, Rajagopal PS, et al. Adjuvant chemotherapy for invasive bladder cancer: a 2013 updated systematic review and meta-analysis of randomized trials. Eur Urol. 2014;66:42–54.

Milosevic M, Gospodarowicz M, Zietman A, et al. Radiotherapy for bladder cancer. Urology. 2007;69:80–92.

Rödel C, Weiss C, Sauer R. Trimodality treatment and selective organ preservation for bladder cancer. J Clin Oncol. 2006;24:5536–44.

Siegel RL, Miller KD, Jemal A. Cancer statistics, 2018. CA Cancer J Clin. 2018;68(1):7–30.

Stimson CJ, Chang SS, Barocas DA, et al. Early and late perioperative outcomes following radical cystectomy: 90-day readmissions, morbidity and mortality in a contemporary series. J Urol. 2010;184:1296–300.

Prostate Cancer: Locoregional Disease

Roberto Iacovelli, Claudia Mosillo, Chiara Ciccarese, Renzo Mazzarotto, and Maria Angela Cerruto

Genitourinary Cancers

Contents

© Springer Nature Switzerland AG 2021
A. Russo et al. (eds.), *Practical Medical Oncology Textbook*, UNIPA Springer Series,
https://doi.org/10.1007/978-3-030-56051-5_47

47.1 Epidemiologic Evidence and Risk Factors of Prostate Cancer

47.1.1 Epidemiology

Prostate cancer (PCa) is the most frequently diagnosed non-skin cancer among Western men aged >50 years with an estimated incidence of 161,360 new cases in 2017 in the United States. More than 80% of PCa diagnoses are represented by localized disease [1].

Incidence rates in the United States fluctuated during the last decade with a peak of 240,000 new cases in the 1993. The great increase in incidence between the late 1980s and the mid-1990s were due to the large number of cases detected once PSA became available and widely utilized. Since 1992, incidence rates declined as a result of changing of PCa screening [2].

With regard to mortality rates in Western countries, PCa is the third leading cause of cancer death behind lung and colorectal cancer. In 2017, in the United States, 26,730 people died of PCa. A steady decline in mortality has been noted during the last decade due to the screening and numerous new treatments. Currently, the 5-year survival is approximately 91% [1].

47.1.2 Risk Factors

PCa is a multifactorial disease. The different role of constitutional and environmental risk factors in tumor carcinogenesis has yet to be elucidated [2].

The established constitutional risk factors are advancing age, positive family history, and the race. PCa develops mainly in older men; about six cases in ten are diagnosed in men aged 65 or older. A study of age-specific incidence reveals that PCa risk begins to rise after age 55 years and peaks at age 70–74, declining slightly thereafter [2].

Heredity plays a significant role in PCa. Men who have a family history of PCa are more likely to develop it themselves. Pathogenic variants in genes of high and moderate penetrance (e.g., BRCA1, BRCA2, the mismatch repair genes, and HOXB13) confer lifetime risk of PCa. However, these alterations probably explain no more than 10% of all cases [3].

Regarding race, PCa is more common among men of African descent than in Caucasian and Asiatic ethnicity. These men seem to develop a more aggressive disease and at a younger age than others racial groups [4]. The exact reasons for these differences are not known and may involve socioeconomic causes or other factors. Observation of Asian migrants provides the most compelling argument for environmental influences linked to Western lifestyle as causal factors [5].

The environmental risk factors potentially associated with PCa development include obesity, physical activity, sexual activity, smoking, and occupational exposures [5, 6].

47.2 Initial Prostate Cancer Diagnosis and Disease Staging

47.2.1 Prostate Cancer Screening

Secondary prevention is the most appropriate instrument to influence the natural history of a disease and to reduce its lethality. For a long time, the periodic dosage of prostate specific antigen (PSA) was considered the more useful screening test for early detection of PCa with a consequent dramatic increase in the incidence rate between the 1980s and the 1990s [2].

PSA evaluation and digital rectal examination (DRE) are the two components of the modern PCa screening program. The ERSPC (European Randomized Study of Screening for Prostate Cancer) and PLCO (Prostate, Lung, Colorectal, and Ovarian Cancer Screening Trial) trials were designed to define the effects of screening on prostate cancer-related mortality [7, 8]. Both trials showed that PSA screening, with or without the support of DRE, was associated with an increased of diagnosis rate. However, only the European study showed a reduction in PCa mortality in the screening arm compared to the control arm (RR 0.8; 95% CI, 0.65–0.98) after a median follow-up of 9 years [7–9]. In other words, to prevent one death from prostate cancer, 1410 (95% CI, 1132–1721) men need to be screened and 48 men treated [7].

Therefore, there are convincing evidence that the screening is associated with over-diagnosis and over-treatment [9]. Consequently, the decision to undergo PSA testing should be discussed between the patient and his physician, balancing advantages and disadvantages (opportunistic screening). Currently, the principal international guidelines do not recommend population-based PSA screening for prostate cancer annually. Individual screening may be considered for high-risk populations: from the age of 50 years (or from the age of 45 years for African American men and family history of PCa) for men who have at least a 10-year life expectancy, with positive family history [10, 11].

47.2.2 Laboratory Test and Imaging for Diagnosis of Prostate Cancer

The main diagnostic tools to identify a prostate tumor include serum concentration of PSA, DRE, and prostate imaging. However, the only test that can confirm the diagnosis of PCa is tumor biopsy.

The PSA is a protein produced within the prostate gland and secreted into seminal fluid. Circulating PSA level can be elevated not only in the presence of cancer, but also in physiological conditions (recent ejaculation or intense physical activity), in case of benign pathologies (prostatic hypertrophy, prostatitis, prostatic infarction, urinary retention) and after diagnostic investigations (digital rectal examination, transrectal ultrasound, endorectal coil prostate magnetic resonance) [12]. There are two types of PSA: free PSA that moves freely in the blood, and complex PSA attached to other proteins. PCa cells produce more complex PSA than other physiological and pathological situations. Consequently, the higher the amount of free PSA, the less likely prostate cancer will be diagnosed. Therefore, several controversies exist regarding PSA level cutoffs and reference ranges [13].

DRE is a simple procedure to examine the peripheral zone of prostate gland where most often PCa is found. Any lumps, hard or irregular areas encountered during this procedure may indicate the presence of cancer. A prospective clinical trial, conducted by Catalona et al., compared DRE and serum PSA in the early detection of PCa. The study enrolled 6630 males, 50 years or older, who underwent PSA determination and/or DRE. The biopsies were performed if the PSA level was greater than 4 mcg/l and/or the DRE was suspicious. Of 1167 biopsies performed, cancer was detected in 264 cases. PSA identified significantly more tumors (82%, 216 of 264 cancers) than DRE (55%, 146 of 264 cancers, $p = 0.001$). The cancer detection rate was 3.2% for DRE, 4.6% for PSA and 5.8% for the two methods combined. The author concluded that the use of PSA in conjunction with DRE enhanced early PCa diagnosis; prostatic biopsy should be considered if either the PSA level was greater than 4 mcg/l or DRE was suspicious for cancer [14].

Transrectal ultrasound (TRUS) and multiparametric magnetic resonance imaging (mpMRI) are the two main imaging methods used for localized PCa detection [15]. TRUS could identify hypoechoic areas that are commonly associated with cancer. Currently, this technique plays an essential role in guiding prostate biopsy. mpMRI has better soft tissue resolution than TRUS. It uses more sequence in addition to the anatomic T2-weighted images, such as diffusion-weighted MRI, derived apparent-diffusion coefficient from diffusion-weighted MRI, and dynamic contrast-enhanced MRI [16]. mpMRI can be helpful in the characterization of suspicious lesions and in the staging of PCa to accurately define the capsular infiltration and assist the physician for surgical planning. Moreover, it is suggested for low-risk localized PCa in the active surveillance program [17, 18]. The use of mpMRI prior to starting active surveillance could identify missed lesions or, conversely, support this option for patients with minimal disease. Preliminary results speculate on the role of mpMRI in selecting patients for active surveillance [17, 18]. Less certain is the role of mpMRI in monitoring patients on active surveillance because larger validation studies are still necessary.

On the basis of the PSA level and/or a suspicious DRE, the TRUS-guided transperineal prostate core biopsy has become the standard way to obtain material for an accurate histopathologic diagnosis [19].

47.2.3 Histology and Grading Score

Prostatic adenocarcinoma is the most commonly diagnosed form of PCa (more than 90% of cases). One of the major characteristics of prostate adenocarcinoma is its heterogenic structure, with variably differentiated glandular structures formed by tumor cells that express PSA and androgen receptors [20].

Prostatic adenocarcinoma is subject to Gleason scoring to give an overall evaluation of the tumor differentiation and heterogeneity. The grading system consists of five different histologic patterns (from 1 to 5) based on the differentiation of tumor growth pattern compared to normal glandular structure. Two different scores are assigned at each prostate tumor, the first one refers to the most common pattern (which represents more than 50% of the tumor tissue) and the second one is the non-dominant cell pattern with the highest grade; the final Gleason score (GS) is the sum of these two scores [21]. The Gleason grading system remains one of the most powerful prognostic predictors in prostate cancer. However, this system has undergone significant revisions. The last revision was made during the 2014 International Society of Urological Pathology (ISUP) Consensus Conference on Gleason Grading of Prostatic Carcinoma [22]. The new grading system includes five distinct Grade Groups based on the Gleason score groups (Grade group 1 = GS 6, Grade group 2 = GS 7 3 + 4, Grade group 3 = GS 7 4 + 3, Grade group 4 = GS 8, Grade group 5 = GS 9–10). Gleason score groups, initially described in 2013 in a study from Johns Hopkins

Hospital and then validated in a multi-institutional study on 20,845 radical prostatectomies, were shown to be more accurate in predicting tumor progression than the Gleason risk stratification groups (GS ≤ 6, GS 7, GS 8–10) [23, 24]. Moreover, even though the GS can range from 2 to 10, the last ISUP revision identified GS 6 as the lowest score that can be assigned.

47.2.4 Staging of Localized Prostate Cancer

The decision to proceed with further staging workup is guided by clinical and pathological features that define the risk of systemic spread: the number and the site of positive biopsy cores (Table 47.1), the tumor grade, and the level of serum PSA [25].

The most common sites of PCa spread are bone and lymph nodes. Abdominal-pelvic CT scan and bone scan are useful for defining the cancer dissemination [26].

Patients with clinical stage T2 or less, PSA < 10 ng/ml, Gleason score ≤7% and <50% positive biopsy cores have <10% likelihood of having node metastases and can be spared nodal evaluation with CT scan [23]. In addition, the bone scan may be avoided in asymptomatic cT1 patients, if the serum PSA level is <20 ng/ml and in asymptomatic cT2 patients with PSA level <10 ng/ml, but only for well-differentiated or moderately differentiated tumors (Gleason score ≤7) [27].

The international guidelines recommend the use of thoraco-abdominal computed tomography (CT) scan, abdominal Magnetic Resonance Imaging (MRI), and bone scan to complete PCa staging in intermediate- and

---

Table 47.1 TNM staging for prostate cancer

Clinical (c) primary tumor (T)	Pathologic (p) primary tumor (T)
cTx Primary tumor cannot be assessed	
cT0 No evidence of primary tumor	
cT1 Clinically inapparent tumor neither palpable nor visible by imaging cT1a Tumor incidental histologic finding in 5% or less of tissue resected cT1b Tumor incidental histologic finding in more than 5% of tissue resected cT1c Tumor identified by needle biopsy (e.g., because of elevated PSA)	
cT2 Tumor confined within prostate cT2a Tumor involves one-half of one lobe or less cT2b Tumor involves more than one-half of one lobe but not both lobes cT2c Tumor involves both lobes	pT2 Organ confined pT2a Unilateral, involving one-half of one side or less pT2b Unilateral, involving more than one-half of one side but not both sides pT2c Bilateral disease
cT3 Tumor extends through the prostatic capsule cT3a Extracapsular extension cT3b Tumor invades the seminal vesicle	pT3 Extraprostatic extension pT3a Extraprostatic extension or microscopic invasion of the bladder neck pT3b Seminal vesicle invasion
cT4 Tumor is fixed or invades adjacent structures other than seminal vesicles: bladder, levator muscles, and/or pelvic wall	pT4 Invasion of bladder, rectum
Clinical (c) regional lymph nodes (N)	Pathological (p) regional lymph nodes (N)
cNx Regional lymph nodes were not assessed	pNx Regional nodes not sampled
cN0 No regional lymph node metastasis	pN0 No positive regional nodes
cN1 Metastasis in regional lymph node(s)	pN1 Metastasis in regional nodes(s)
Clinical (c) distant metastasis (M)	
cM0 No distant metastasis	
cM1 Distant metastasis cM1a Non-regional lymph node(s) cM1b Bone(s) cM1c Other site(s) with or without bone disease	

high-risk disease or in symptomatic patients [28]. Choline positron emission tomography/CT (PET/CT) is not considered standard for PCa staging.

47.3 Treatment Options for Localized Prostate Cancer

According to clinical risk groups for recurrence of localized and locally advanced PCa (□ Table 47.2), several treatments can be proposed [25]. The international guidelines consider radiotherapy (RT) and radical prostatectomy (RP) the standard treatments with curative intent for localized PCa. However, which of these approaches offers survival benefit over the other remains controversial. Therefore, choosing between RP and RT is based on the different toxicity profile. In addition, in particular conditions observational strategies can be adopted.

47.3.1 Observational Strategies: Active Surveillance and Watchful-Waiting

The active surveillance (AS) is an observational strategy that consists in a periodic monitoring of disease course, reserving surgery or radiation therapy in case of disease progression. The AS offers to selected men with PCa the chance to delay or avoid an invasive treatment and its associated side effects. Currently, this approach includes the PSA blood test and the DRE every 6 months, and prostate biopsies every year.

The ProtecT is the only prospective randomized clinical trial comparing the AS with an immediate curative treatment. Of the 82,429 patients who were screened,

□ **Table 47.2** Clinical risk groups for recurrence of localized and locally advanced prostate cancer

Risk group	Low	Intermediate	High
Localized PCa	PSA < 10 ng/ml and GS < 7 (ISUP grade 1) and cT1–2a	PSA 10–20 ng/ml or GS7 (ISUP grade 2/3) or cT2b	PSA > 20 ng/ml or GS > 7 (ISUP grade 4/5) or cT2c
Locally advanced PCa			Any PSA; any GS; cT3–4 or cN+; any ISUP grade

PCa prostate cancer, *PSA* prostatic specific antigen, *GS* gleason score, *ISUP* International Society of Urological Pathology

1643 men were randomized in three arms: AS (n = 545), RP (n = 533), and 74 Gy of 3D conformal external beam RT (EBRT) (n = 545). In the AS group, the trigger for intervention included PSA kinetics (PSA doubling time less than 12 months), appearance of symptoms, changes in DRE, and patient anxiety. The patients had a median age of 62 years, median PSA of 4.6 ng/ml (90% of patients have PSA < 10 ng/ml) and not palpable disease (T1c). Moreover, 75% of the entire population had a Gleason Score 6. The primary aim was 10-year disease-specific survival. The secondary endpoints were all-cause mortality, the incidence of clinical progression, and the incidence of metastasis. Approximately, 80% of patients assigned to the surveillance arm did not demonstrate any clinical progression. However, almost 50% of men enrolled in this arm opted for treatment intervention. There was no statistical difference in OS among the three study arms (98.8% in the AS group; 99% in the surgery group; 99.8% in the radiant therapy group at 10 years; p = 0.48). However, the prostatectomy and the radiant therapy were associated with lower rates of disease progression, including metastasis, than active monitoring (112 patients in the AS group; 46 patients in the surgery group; 46 patients in the radiotherapy group; p < 0.001 for the overall comparison) [29].

According to the international guidelines, the AS strategy can be offered to patients with a life expectancy of 10 years or less with low-risk disease (T1–2a, Gleason score ≤6 and the PSA level <10 ng/ml), but also to patients with low-risk disease and a life expectancy greater than 10 years to avoid side effects related to surgery or radiant treatments.

The watchful-waiting is another option for men with early-stage prostate cancer. It consists in a less intensive follow-up with specific attention to the cancer-related symptoms to decide if a treatment is needed.

The Scandinavian Prostate Cancer Group Study number 4 (SPCG-4) is a prospective, randomized trial to compare the surgical treatment with watchful-waiting in men with localized PCa. After randomization, 348 patients were assigned to watchful-waiting arm and 347 men to RP. The study enrolled patients with localized PCa (cT1–2), age <75 years and PSA values <50 ng/ml. Moreover, approximately 50% of patients were classified as intermediate or high risk. The endpoints of this trial were all-cause mortality, specific survival and the incidence of metastasis. After a follow-up of 18 years, the data revealed that the risk of death from PCa was significantly lower in the RP arm than in the watchful-waiting group (17.7% vs. 28.7%, HR: 0.56; p = 0.001). Similarly, the risk of death from all causes was 56.1% in the RP arm and 68.9% in the watchful-waiting group (HR: 0.71; p < 0.001). Moreover, the risk of spreading was significantly lower for patients treated with RP (26.1% vs. 38.3%, RR 0.56; p < 0.001). Moreover, the subgroup analysis showed a greater survival benefit of immediate treatment for younger patients (<65 years) and for high-risk disease [30].

By contrast, the Prostate Cancer Intervention versus Observation Trial (PIVOT) showed that RP did not significantly reduce PCa specific and overall mortality after a follow-up of 12 years. The PIVOT study enrolled 731 patients with a localized PCa (cT1–2) and PSA values <50 ng/ml who were younger than 75 years and had a life expectancy <10 years [31]. Although the inclusion criteria were similar, the two studies did not enroll a homogeneous population (cT1c: 12% in the SPCG-4 trial and 50% in the PIVOT; intermediate and high risk: 50% in the SPCG-4 trial vs. 35% in the PIVOT). The differences between study populations and the historic period (before or during the era of PSA testing in the SPCG-4 and PIVOT, respectively) make the results of these trials not fully comparable. In conclusion, watchful-waiting could be recommended for patients with cT1c prostate tumor and a life expectancy <10 years.

47.3.2 Surgical Approaches

RP represents the most common and effective treatment for localized PCa. RP can be performed by open, laparoscopic, or robot-assisted (RARP) approaches. The goal of each approach must be complete eradication of disease, while preserving continence and, whenever possible, potency [32]. In a randomized phase III trial, RARP showed to reduce admission times and blood loss but not early (12 weeks) functional or oncological outcomes [33, 34].

Actually many men with localized PCa will not benefit from definitive treatment, and 45% of men with PSA-detected PCa may be candidates for deferred management. In men with co-morbidity and a limited life expectancy, treatment of localized PCa may be deferred to avoid loss of quality of life (QoL).

47.3.2.1 Radical Prostatectomy and Prostate Cancer Risk Groups

RP has to be offered to patients with low- and intermediate-risk PCa and a life expectancy >10 years.

In low-risk PCa, a lymph node dissection (LND) is not recommended. In intermediate-risk PCa, a nerve-sparing surgery is recommended in patients with a low-risk of extracapsular disease (referring to specific nomograms). In order to select patients for nerve sparing procedures it is possible to use mpMRI.

An extended LND (eLND) has to be performed if the estimated risk for positive lymph nodes exceeds 5%. A limited LND is not recommended.

RP can be offered in patients with high-risk localized PCa and a life expectancy of >10 years only as a part of multimodal strategy. In high-risk PCa, a neoadjuvant hormonal therapy before RP is not recommended. In high-risk PCa an eLND is mandatory.

It is possible to offer RP also in selected patients with locally advanced (cT3a) disease and a life expectancy >10 years, but only as a part of multi-modal therapy. A nerve-sparing surgery can be offered to patients with a low risk of extracapsular disease (referring to specific nomograms). In high-risk disease the use of mpMRI is recommended as a decision-making tool to select patients for nerve-paring procedures. In highly selected patients with high-risk locally advanced PCa (cT3b-T4 N0 or any T N1), an RP can be offered only as a part of multimodal therapy.

47.3.2.2 Radical Prostatectomy in Senior Adult Patients (>70 Years of Age)

In senior adults with PCa it is recommended to perform a systematic health status evaluation using a geriatric screening with G8 and mini-COGTM.

Treatment options for senior adults according to their health status are as follows:

- Standard treatment to fit or healthy older men
- Standard treatment to frail patients with reversible impairment after the resolution of geriatric problems
- Adapted treatment to disabled patients
- Only symptomatic palliative treatment to patients who are too sick with terminal illness

47.3.2.3 After Radical Prostatectomy for Curative Intent

After RP, PSA should be undetectable (<0.1 ng/ml). A PSA of >0.1 ng/ml after RP is a signal of residual prostate tissue. Palpable nodules and increasing serum PSA are often signs of local recurrence. After an undetectable PSA is obtained following RP, a PSA >0.2 ng/ml and rising is associated with recurrent disease. In patients with pT3N0M0 PCa and an undetectable PSA, it is recommended to discuss with the patients about the possibility of adjuvant external beam radiotherapy (EBRT) because it at least improves biochemical-free survival. It is recommended to inform patients with pT3N0M0 PCa and an undetectable PSA the possibility to use a salvage irradiation as an alternative to adjuvant EBRT when PSA increases. An adjuvant hormonal therapy for pN0 disease is not recommended.

The role of adjuvant ADT after RP is controversial. The only prospective randomized trial, designed to evaluate the efficacy of immediate ADT compared to ADT deferred at disease progression in node-positive PCa patients after radical prostatectomy and pelvic lymphadenectomy, showed significant OS and PFS improvements with immediate ADT [35]. However, the positive results might be affected by the gross lymph node disease involvement and the high percentage of positive margins and seminal vesicle invasion (more than 60%). Therefore, in PCa patients with microscopic lymph node metastases, adjuvant ADT cannot be recommended.

A routine follow-up of asymptomatic patients should be obtained by a disease-specific history and PSA measurement supplemented by DRE. This kind of follow-up should be performed at 3, 6, and 12 months after treatment, then every 6 months until 3 years, and then annually. Imaging to detect local recurrence is only recommended if it affects treatment planning. Biopsy is usually not necessary before second-line therapy. Bone scans and other imaging modalities are not routinely recommended for asymptomatic patients if there are no signs of biochemical relapse. In case of bone pain or other symptoms of progression, a re-staging should be considered irrespective of serum PSA level.

47.3.2.4 Oncological Outcomes

It is very difficult to compare open RP with the laparoscopic (LRP) and RARP approaches because the available clinical studies have several limitations. Almost all of the available data derive from prospective non-randomized trials, or retrospective studies, which provide a low level of evidence [36].

Positive surgical margins (PSMs) are the most used and collected data for oncological RP analysis. This is mainly because of the lack of long-term biochemical recurrence and disease-free survival rate data. Analysing the overall PSM rates and pT2 PSM rates among comparative studies, similar PSM rates have been found for RRP and LRP (22.45% and 22.04%, respectively, $p = 0.000$), whereas RARP was only slightly better compared with the other techniques (21.14%). These differences become significant considering only the pT2 stage with similar rates for the RRP and LRP series (16.64% and 17.44% pT2 PSM rates, respectively, $p = 0.045$) and lower rates for RARP (10.53% pT2 PSM rates). Randomized trials are necessary, however, to draw definitive conclusions.

47.3.2.5 Functional Outcomes

A critical point in the evaluation of the RP outcomes is whether patients who obtain good cancer control also obtain a good functional result. This is a relevant issue considering that urinary incontinence (UI) and erectile dysfunction can have a significant negative impact on patients' health-related quality of life.

Thus, in the last decade, the desire to reduce the invasiveness of traditional open and laparoscopic surgery and, above all, the attempt of achieving better functional results, produced the increased interest in and the popularity of robotic techniques both in Europe and the USA.

Although recent systematic reviews and meta-analysis found that RARP had higher postoperative continence rates than retropubic or laparoscopic radical prostatectomy, UI and sexual dysfunction remain the most bothersome postoperative complications even after RARP [36, 37].

The evaluation of UI rates between different studies published in the literature is difficult. This is due mainly to the lack of standard data collection methods (the use of non-validated questionnaires or simple interviews) and the use of different definitions. Furthermore, follow-up is often insufficient or only partial.

The weighted mean continence rates at 6 months for the RRP, LRP, and RARP series are 73.71%, 63.82%, and 89.12%, respectively ($p = 0.000$). After a 12-month follow-up, the continence rates for the RRP, LRP, and RARP series are 83.22%, 70.77%, and 92.78%, respectively ($p = 0.001$). Evaluation at 24 months of follow-up is not possible because few papers conducted follow-up using this interval. These data support the statement that the continence rates after RRP and LRP are similar, with RRP performing slightly better than LRP. Randomized prospective studies are necessary, however, to accurately compare the continence rates between the three surgical approaches.

Regarding erectile dysfunction rates, the data are too limited for definitive conclusions. Data from the available comparative studies suggest an advantage in terms of urinary continence and erectile function for patients who underwent RARP compared with those patients subjected to the RRP and LRP techniques, but future studies are needed to confirm this trend.

47.3.2.6 RP as Second-Line Treatment

RP as salvage treatment can be offered to treat highly selected patients with localized PCa and a histologically proven local recurrence. Due to the increased rate of side effects, a salvage RP should be performed only in experienced centers.

47.3.3 Radiotherapy

RT for PCa was first introduced during the second decade of the twentieth century, by positioning radium applicators in hollow organs adjacent to the prostate, like urethra, bladder, or rectum. Unfortunately, this type of treatment, a form of endocavitary brachytherapy, was associated with high-dose to the organ's mucosa that caused significant morbidity. During the 1920s–1940s,

EBRT was introduced, but due to the availability of machines generating low-energy x-ray beams, it had palliative intent with significant side effects. The role of EBRT in the management of prostate carcinoma became clearer with the introduction of technological advancements that allowed the use of megavoltage radiation (energy >1000 kV) that penetrated more deeply in the body, and that were associated with less skin and subcutaneous morbidity. During the 1950s and 1960s, megavoltage radiation was more commonly available from the decay of radioactive isotopes (Cobalt-60 units, 1.25 MeV), while in the following decades, high-energy X-rays, produced by linear accelerators, became increasingly popular and are now the most common form of EBRT [38]. Furthermore, linear accelerators provide beams with more sharply delineated borders, thus allowing to escalate tumor dose and to minimize acute and late toxicity to normal tissues. Improved technology, including 3-dimensional conformal radiotherapy (3D-CRT), intensity-modulated radiotherapy (IMRT), and image-guided radiotherapy (IGRT), associated with improvement in treatment planning and dosimetry, made RT, together with RP, one of the primary treatment options for patients with both localized and locally advanced non-metastatic PCa, and a treatment option for patients with persistent disease or who relapse after surgery. RT may be administered using EBRT alone, EBRT combined with a brachytherapy (BT) boost, or BT alone.

47.3.3.1 External Beam Radiation Therapy

A large body of medical literature on radiotherapy in the management of PCa regards the use of conventional EBRT, which was typically delivered using a 4-field technique (anteroposterior, posteroanterior, left lateral, right lateral) usually designed to include the prostate, seminal vesicles, and regional lymphatics, for a cumulative dose of 45–50 Gy delivered over 5–5.5 weeks. Subsequently, an additional dose of approximately 20 Gy to a boost field was administered to the prostate and periprostatic tissues to a total dose of 66.6–70 Gy. The results of this treatment in patients with T1–2 disease were similar to those achieved after RP, with 10-year survival rates for both treatments in excess of 60% [39, 40]. More modern techniques, 3D-CRT and IMRT, allow delivering of higher doses of at least 72–80 Gy with an improvement of local and regional control [41, 42].

Clinical trials involving 3D-CRT, demonstrated relevant advantages of this technique over conventional RT: less morbidity associated to 3D-CRT, make possible dose escalation to the target organs with improvement of biochemical outcome, as well documented in a trial by MD Anderson CC, in which the outcomes following 70 and 78 Gy were compared, and by MGH with dose comparisons of 70 and 79 Gy [41–43]. 3D-CRT tech-

niques are now considered the minimum standard EBRT approach in patients with prostate cancer.

During the last decades, IMRT has rapidly become a highly precise method of delivering increasing doses of radiotherapy to the prostate and immediate periprostatic tissues, by achieving tightly conformal dose distributions with the use of non-uniform radiation beams. Complex treatment-planning software algorithms allow exceedingly high doses of radiation to be delivered to the target, while significantly smaller doses are delivered to the adjacent normal tissue. Data from the Memorial Sloan Kettering Cancer Center have demonstrated the safe delivery of doses of more than 80 Gy using IMRT [44].

The treatment of prostate cancer with IMRT techniques need the reproducible identification of the target and surrounding organs on daily treatments. IGRT, which refers to the use of verification tools in an attempt to ensure proper target localization during the course of radiotherapy, is of paramount importance to assure daily reproducibility if high conformal techniques are used [45, 46]. IGRT thus further minimizes the margin of normal tissue that would otherwise need to be irradiated. The term IGRT has been used to identify wide range imaging techniques as simple as daily port films, to those as complex as computer-assisted patient repositioning devices. Intraprostatic implantable fiducial markers, and daily three-dimensional imaging IGRT, are frequently utilized for accurate target localization if IMRT is the modality of choice; without such specificity, the logic of using IMRT is questionable.

Furthermore, many efforts have been recently attempted to address the importance of organ movement during the daily treatment fraction [47]. This issue is particularly important because many intensity-modulated radiation treatments can require 20–30 minutes or longer to be performed. In the attempt to manage intrafraction movement, new forms of target tracking have become clinically available, such as the use of small radio transponder devices implanted into the prostate [48].

Conventional EBRT is usually delivered using photon beams. Charged particle therapy, i.e., proton beam therapy, has been successfully used in the management of PCa. Early work from the cyclotron center at Harvard formed an important basis for current clinical trials. A unique feature of proton beam therapy is the way in which it deposits its most concentrated radiation dose. Proton beams have a characteristic Bragg peak; beyond this point, where energy deposit in target tissues is at a maximum, radiation rapidly falls off, which is important in the management of normal tissue toxicity.

Data from Loma Linda and Harvard suggest that prostate cancer can be effectively managed with conformal proton beam therapy [49, 50]. Although proton beam therapy is being more widely used in men with prostate cancer, as new treatment facilities become available, there is currently no evidence that this approach offers any advantages over IMRT.

Radiation therapy is also widely used in an adjuvant setting after radical prostatectomy. Selection of candidates for this approach is difficult. Multi-institutional data from the American Society of Therapeutic Radiation Oncology (ASTRO) consensus conference suggest that in patients treated for rising PSA levels, postoperative radiotherapy (dose range of 60–65 Gy) offers a PSA remission rate of 70% with a durability of the response ranging from 25 to 67 months.

47.3.3.2 Brachytherapy

In brachytherapy (BT), radioactive sources are directly implanted within the prostate, thus providing the highest of radiation over a very limited distance, allowing to maximize irradiation to the tumor, while minimizing the dose to normal structures [51]. BT can be used as a single modality, or as a boost in association to EBRT. BT implants may be permanent or temporary; in both cases radiation sources are inserted into the prostate using a transperineal approach, under transrectal ultrasound guidance. BT requires only one or limited number of treatments, rather than the daily therapy required by EBRT.

Permanent implants are characteristic of low dose-rate BT (LDR), which is delivered by permanently implanting numerous radioactive seed, typically either Iodine-125 or Palladium-103. The recommended prescribed doses for LDR monotherapy are 145 Gy for Iodine-125 and 125 Gy for Palladium-103. The corresponding boost dose after 40–50 Gy EBRT are 110 Gy and 90–100 Gy, respectively. LDR BT is usually completed in a single outpatient procedure [52].

Temporary implants are used in High Dose-Rate BT (HDR). This type of BT uses a single radiation source (Iridium-192) which is inserted into the prostate, by a computer-driven after-loading machine, through hollow catheters or needles, that have been previously positioned under transrectal ultrasound, and then removed at the end of the treatment. HDR BT can be used alone or in combination with EBRT (40–50 Gy). A commonly used regimen for HDR treatment alone includes 13.5 Gy × 2 fractions, while commonly used boost regimens include 9.5–11.5 Gy × 2 fractions, 5.5–7.5 Gy × 3 fractions, and 4.0–6.0 Gy × 4 fractions. HDR BT typically requires a 48-hour hospitalization for each session, and can be completed in one or few procedures [53].

Indication of BT for individual patients is based upon technical feasibility, the absence of coexistent urinary conditions and the ability to adequately irradiate all disease. A large prostate gland (usually more than 60 g) is associated with a higher rate of treatment-related complications and represents a relative contraindication to BT. In these cases, a course of androgen deprivation therapy prior to BT may help to reduce the organ volume. BT alone is considered an appropriate option in men with low or intermediate-risk disease, but its interest for high-risk patients, particularly as a boost in association with EBRT, is increasing [54].

47.3.3.3 Complications of RT

The morbidity of both EBRT and BT when performed with advanced techniques and in high experience Centers are very low. Acute radiation proctitis of moderate severity is reported in less than 20% of patients treated with EBRT, depending on radiation dose and treatment volume [55]. If pelvic lymph nodes are included in the target volume, radiation enteritis may also be observed. After RT completion, acute symptoms usually disappeared within 1–2 months. A small percentage of patients require a procedure, such as colonoscopy, following EBRT due to the persistence of diarrhea, rectal urgency, or hematochezia [56]. Less than 50% of patients experience urinary symptoms, including urinary frequency, dysuria, or urgency due to cystitis or urethritis during RT. Symptoms completely disappear after the completion of therapy. With modern techniques, late side effects are extremely uncommon.

After RT, erectile dysfunction increases over time and its frequency is associated to other factors, including older age, concurrent comorbidities, such as hypertension, cardiovascular disease, and diabetes [55]. The use of anti-androgen deprivation therapy is also an important factor.

47.3.3.4 Results of RT

For man with low-risk clinically localized prostate cancer, EBRT, BT, and radical prostatectomy all provide an extremely high degree of freedom from local or distal recurrence in series with long follow-up. For selected patients with a low or very low-risk of recurrence, active surveillance with delayed definitive treatment if necessary, represent an appropriate option [57, 58]. If disease control is similar, different treatment approaches show important differences in the pattern of associated toxicity that may address patients' choice. For man with regionally localized intermediate, high, and very high-risk prostate cancer, RT administered using EBRT alone or combined with a BT boost and associated with ADT, or radical prostatectomy with pelvic lymph node dissection, in patients without tumor fixation to adjacent structure, are both treatment options. In patients managed with radical prostatectomy and with more extensive local disease, positive surgical margins, or lymph nodes involvement at histologic examination, adjuvant RT should be recommended. The choice of treatment,

47

surgery versus RT, depends upon a detailed, informed, patient decision, taking into consideration the potential advantages and disadvantages associated with each approach, balanced with the specific side effects associated with each different treatment technique. For men treated with RT, therapy should be administered using high conformal techniques, such as image guided IMRT, with the aim to ensure the delivery of high curative doses to the target, while minimizing the dose to surrounding normal tissues [44]. The association of EBRT plus BT may be helpful in attempting dose escalation [59–63].

47.3.4 Neoadjuvant and Adjuvant ADT After RT

The role of neoadjuvant ADT has been evaluated in several randomized trials. The Trans-Tasman Radiation Oncology Group (TROG) 96-01 trial demonstrated a significant OS advantage [HR 0.63 (0.48–0.83)] with RT plus 6 months neoadjuvant and concurrent combined androgen blockade (CAB) compared to RT alone in 818 locally advanced PCa patients [64]. Similarly, the Radiation Therapy Oncology Group (RTOG) trial 8610 showed an improvement in 10-year prostate cancer-specific mortality (23% vs. 36%; $p = 0.01$) with the addition of 4 months neoadjuvant and concurrent ADT to RT in 456 PCa patients with T2–4 disease [65].

Therefore, neoadjuvant and concurrent ADT for 4–6 months are recommended for high-risk PCa patients receiving radical RT, and can be considered for men with intermediate-risk disease.

Adjuvant ADT has been investigated in several trials, showing an OS improvement among patients with locally advanced PCa treated with EBRT combined with androgen suppression as compared with the use of EBRT alone and deferral of hormonal treatment until relapse. An EORTC randomized phase III trial comparing EBRT alone and EBRT combined with an ADT for 3 years for T1–2 PCa tumors of WHO grade 3 or T3–4 N0–1 M0 tumors, revealed a significant improvement in disease-free (5-year DFS 40% vs. 74%; $p = 0.0001$) and overall survival (5-year OS 62% vs. 78%; $p = 0.0002$) in favor of the combined therapy [66].

As concerns the optimal duration of adjuvant ADT, two randomized trials support the role of long-term ADT. In particular, the RTOG 92-02 trial demonstrated significant improvement with long-term ADT (28 months) compared to short-term ADT (4 months) in addition to RT in term of disease-free survival, disease-specific survival, local progression, distant metastasis, and biochemical failure. An OS advantage was limited to the subgroup of patients with a Gleason score of 8–10 (81.0% vs. 70.7%, $p = 0.044$) [67]. Analogously, the EORTC-22961 trial showed a 4.7% advantage in 5-year OS in favor of long-term adjuvant ADT (36 months, 6 months concurrent to RT and 2.5 years of further treatment) compared to short-term hormonal therapy (6 months, concurrent to RT) in locally advanced PCa patients treated with external-beam radiotherapy [68].

Therefore, concomitant (with or without neoadjuvant) and adjuvant ADT, for 2–3 years, is recommended for high-risk locally advanced PCa patients treated with radical EBRT.

Updates:
- Prostate-specific membrane antigen (PSMA) positron-emission tomography (PET)/computed tomography (CT) scanning could be more sensitive than conventional imaging to detect occult lesions in prostate cancer patients.
- A novel magnetic resonance imaging (MRI)-guided ultrasound procedure for localized prostate cancer (TULSA) is able to spare healthy nerve tissue enveloping prostate gland. The TACT trial results showed 80% of patients without clinically relevant prostate cancer and 65% with negative biopsy at 12 months.
- Data from the RADICALS-RT trials suggested the role of radiotherapy as salvage strategy rather than as adjuvant treatment of men with prostate cancer.

Expert Opinion
Giuseppe Procopio

Key Points
- Prostate cancer is the most frequent solid tumor diagnosed in male people and due to its high incidence and prevalence, screening programs have been adopted among population such as the valuation of PSA; otherwise, for the frequent over-diagnosis and over-treatments, nowadays, the screening program should be carefully discussed with the patient.

- After diagnosis of PCa, the decision to proceed with systemic staging workup is guided by the risk of disease systemic spread. Curative treatments or observational strategies may be proposed according to the risk of recurrence, life expectancy, and patients' preferences.
- RP or radiotherapy (external beam or brachytherapy) are two options for low- or intermediate-risk disease.
- RP plus pelvic lymphadenectomy or external beam RT plus hormone treatment are two alternative options for high-risk or locally advanced PCa.

- Long-term adjuvant ADT is recommended for high-risk PCa patients treated with radical EBRT.
- ADT represents the cornerstone of treatment for metastatic prostate cancer.
- The early addiction of docetaxel or abiraterone acetate to ADT improves the overall survival of mHSPC, mainly in the subpopulation of high-volume and in high-risk patients.
- Several therapeutic options have demonstrated to improve patients' outcomes in the mCRPC setting, including docetaxel, cabazitaxel, abiraterone and enzalutamide, and Radium-223.

Summary of Clinical Recommendations

- The annual PSA-based screening program should be discussed with the patient for the risk of over-diagnosis and over-treatment.
- After diagnosis of PCa, the decision to proceed with systemic staging workup is guided by the risk of disease systemic spread.
- Curative treatments or observational strategies may be proposed according to the risk of recurrence, life expectancy, and patients' preferences.
- RP or radiotherapy (external beam or brachytherapy) are two options for low- or intermediate-risk disease.
- RP plus pelvic lymphadenectomy or external beam RT plus hormone treatment are two alternative options for high-risk or locally advanced PCa.
- Long-term adjuvant ADT is recommended for high-risk PCa patients treated with radical EBRT.

Recommendations

- ESMO
  - ▶ www.esmo.org/Guidelines/Genitourinary-Cancers/ESMO-Consensus-Guidelines-Prostate-cancer
- NCCN
  - ▶ jnccn.org/view/journals/jnccn/17/5/article-p479.xml
- ASCO
  - ▶ www.asco.org/practice-guidelines/quality-guidelines/guidelines/genitourinary-cancer#/32796
  - ▶ www.asco.org/practice-guidelines/quality-guidelines/guidelines/genitourinary-cancer#/33301
  - ▶ www.asco.org/practice-guidelines/quality-guidelines/guidelines/genitourinary-cancer#/25251
  - ▶ www.asco.org/practice-guidelines/quality-guidelines/guidelines/genitourinary-cancer#/24836

Hints for a Deeper Insight

- Phase II study of pembrolizumab (MK-3475) in patients with metastatic castration-resistant prostate cancer (KEYNOTE-199)-study AP 93/16 of the AUO:
  - ▶ https://www.ncbi.nlm.nih.gov/pubmed/28980011
- Prostate cancer between prognosis and adequate/proper therapy: ▶ https://www.ncbi.nlm.nih.gov/pubmed/28255369
- Prostate Cancer Genetics: Variation by Race, Ethnicity, and Geography: ▶ https://www.ncbi.nlm.nih.gov/pubmed/27986209

References

1. SEER Cancer Statistics Review (1975–2014). National Cancer Institute, Bethesda, November 2016. http://seer.cancer.gov/csr/1975_2014/. Posted to the SEER web site April 2017.
2. Montie JE. Observations on the epidemiology and natural history of prostate cancer. Urology. 1994;44:2–8.
3. Hemminki K. Familial risk and familial survival in prostate cancer. World J Urol. 2012;30(2):143–8.
4. Kheirandish P. Ethnic differences in prostate cancer. Br J Cancer. 2011;105(4):481–5.
5. Leitzmann MF. Risk factors for the onset of prostatic cancer: age, location, and behavioral correlates. Clin Epidemiol. 2012;4:1–11.
6. Laurence N. Dietary fat and prostate cancer: current status. J Natl Cancer Inst. 1999;91:414–28.
7. Wolters T. The effect of study arm on prostate cancer treatment in the large screening trial ERSPC. Int J Cancer. 2010;126:2387.
8. Shoag JE, Reevaluating PSA. Testing rates in the PLCO trial. N Engl J Med. 2016;374:1795.
9. Ilic D. Screening for prostate cancer: an updated cochrane systematic review. BJU Int. 2011;107:882.
10. Mottet N. EAU-ESTRO-SIOG guidelines on prostate cancer. Part 1: Screening, diagnosis, and local treatment with curative intent. Eur Urol. 2017;71(4):618–29.
11. Wolf AM. American Cancer Society guideline for the early detection of prostate cancer: update 2010. CA Cancer J Clin. 2010;60(2):70–98.
12. Tchetgen MB. The effect of prostatitis, urinary retention, ejaculation, and ambulation on the serum prostate-specific antigen concentration. Urol Clin North Am. 1997;24:283.
13. Punglia RS. Effect of verification bias on screening for prostate cancer by measurement of prostate-specific antigen. N Engl J Med. 2003;349:335.
14. Catalona WJ. Comparison of digital rectal examination and serum prostate specific antigen in the early detection of prostate cancer: results of a multicenter clinical trial of 6,630 men. J Urol. 1994;151:1283.
15. Ahmed HU. Diagnostic accuracy of multi-parametric MRI and TRUS biopsy in prostate cancer (PROMIS): a paired validating confirmatory study. Lancet. 2017;389:815.
16. Panebianco V. Multiparametric magnetic resonance imaging vs. standard care in men being evaluated for prostate cancer: a randomized study. Urol Oncol. 2015;33:17e1.

17. Somford DM. The predictive value of endorectal 3 Tesla multiparametric magnetic resonance imaging for extraprostatic extension in patients with low, intermediate and high risk prostate cancer. J Urol. 2013;190:1728.

18. Gordon LG. Cost-effectiveness analysis of multiparametric MRI with increased active surveillance for low-risk prostate cancer in Australia. J Magn Reson Imaging. 2017;45:1304.

19. Eichler K. Diagnostic value of systematic biopsy methods in the investigation of prostate cancer: a systematic review. J Urol. 2006;175:1605–12.

20. Humphrey PA. Histological variants of prostatic carcinoma and their significance. Histopathology. 2012;60:59–74.

21. Gleason DF. Prediction of prognosis for prostatic adenocarcinoma by combined histological grading and clinical staging. J Urol. 1974;111(1):58–64.

22. Epstein JI. The 2014 International Society of Urological Pathology (ISUP) consensus conference on Gleason grading of prostatic carcinoma: definition of grading patterns and proposal for a new grading system. Am J Surg Pathol. 2016;40(2):244–52.

23. Pierorazio PM. Prognostic Gleason grade grouping: data based on the modified Gleason scoring system. BJU Int. 2013;111(5):753–60.

24. Epstein JI. A contemporary prostate cancer grading system: a validated alternative to the Gleason score. Eur Urol. 2016;69(3):428–35.

25. D'Amico AV, Whittington R, Malkowicz SB, et al. Biochemical outcome after radical prostatectomy, external beam radiation therapy, or interstitial radiation therapy for clinically localized prostate cancer. JAMA. 1998;280:969–74.

26. Hoivels AM. The diagnostic accuracy of CT and MRI in the staging of pelvic lymph nodes in patients with prostate cancer: a meta-analysis. Clin Radiol. 2008;63:387–95.

27. Briganti A. When to perform bone scan in patients with newly diagnosed prostate cancer: external validation of the currently available guidelines and proposal of a novel risk stratification tool. Eur Urol. 2010;57:551–8.

28. Prostate Cancer Clinical Guideline Update Panel. Clinically localized prostate cancer: AUA/ASTRO/SUO guideline. American Urological Association, 2017. Available at: https://www.auanet.org/guidelines/clinically-localized-proste-cancer-new-(aua/astro/suo-guideline-2017). Accessed 22 July 2017.

29. Hamdy FC. 10-year outcomes after monitoring, surgery, or radiotherapy for localized prostate cancer. N Engl J Med. 2016;375:1415–24.

30. Bill-Axelson A. Radical prostatectomy or watchful waiting in early prostate cancer. N Engl J Med. 2014;370:932–42.

31. Wilt TJ. Radical prostatectomy versus observation for localized prostate cancer. N Engl J Med. 2012;367:203–13.

32. Bianco FJ. Radical prostatectomy: long-term cancer control and recovery of sexual and urinary function ("trifecta"). Urology. 2005;66:83.

33. Yaxley JW. Robot-assisted laparoscopic prostatectomy versus open radical retropubic prostatectomy: early outcomes from a randomised controlled phase 3 study. Lancet. 2016;388:1057.

34. Allan C. Laparoscopic versus robotic-assisted radical prostatectomy for the treatment of localised prostate cancer: a systematic review. Urol Int. 2016;96:373.

35. Messing EM, Eastern Cooperative Oncology Group Study EST 3886. Immediate versus deferred androgen deprivation treatment in patients with node-positive prostate cancer after radical prostatectomy and pelvic lymphadenectomy. Lancet Oncol. 2006;7(6):472–9.

36. De Carlo F. Retropubic, laparoscopic, and robot-assisted radical prostatectomy: surgical, oncological, and functional outcomes: a systematic review. Urol Int. 2014;93:373–83.

37. Ficarra V. Systematic review and meta-analysis of studies reporting urinary continence recovery after robot-assisted radical prostatectomy. Eur Urol. 2012;62(3):405–17.

38. Brame RS. Regarding the focal treatment of PCa: inference of the Gleason grade from MRI. Int J Radiat Oncol Biol Phys. 2009;74(1):110–4.

39. Bagshaw MA. Radiation therapy for localized prostate cancer. Justification by long-term follow-up. Urol Clin North Am. 1990;17(4):787–802.

40. Perez CA. Clinical assessment of outcome of prostate cancer (TCP, NTCP). Rays. 2005;30(2):109–20.

41. Pollack A. Preliminary results of a randomized radiotherapy dose-escalation study comparing 70 Gy with 78 Gy for prostate cancer. J Clin Oncol. 2000;18(23):3904–11.

42. Zietman AL. Comparison of conventional-dose vs high-dose conformal radiation therapy in clinically localized adenocarcinoma of the prostate: a randomized controlled trial. JAMA. 2005;294(10):1233–9.

43. Roach M. Phase III trial comparing whole-pelvic versus prostate-only radiotherapy and neoadjuvant versus adjuvant combined androgen suppression: Radiation Therapy Oncology Group 9413. J Clin Oncol. 2003;21(10):1904–11.

44. Zelefsky MJ. Long-term results of conformal radiotherapy for prostate cancer: impact of dose escalation on biochemical tumor control and distant metastases-free survival outcomes. Int J Radiat Oncol Biol Phys. 2008;71(4):1028.

45. Zelefsky MJ. Clinical experience with intensity modulated radiation therapy (IMRT) in prostate cancer. Radiother Oncol. 2000;55:241.

46. Zelefsky MJ. Improved clinical outcomes with high-dose image guided radiotherapy compared with non-IGRT for the treatment of clinically localized prostate cancer. Int J Radiat Oncol Biol Phys. 2012;84(1):125.

47. Pinkawa M. Image-guided radiotherapy for prostate cancer. Implementation of ultrasound-based prostate localization for the analysis of inter- and intrafraction organ motion. Strahlenther Onkol. 2008;184(12):679–85.

48. Noel C. Prediction of intrafraction prostate motion: accuracy of pre- and post-treatment imaging and intermittent imaging. Int J Radiat Oncol Biol Phys. 2009;73(3):692–8.

49. Slater JD. Proton therapy for prostate cancer: the initial Loma Linda University experience. Int J Radiat Oncol Biol Phys. 2004;59(2):348–52.

50. Gardner BG. Late normal tissue sequelae in the second decade after high dose radiation therapy with combined photons and conformal protons for locally advanced prostate cancer. J Urol. 2002;167(1):123–6.

51. Nag S. American Brachytherapy Society (ABS) recommendations for transperineal permanent brachytherapy of prostate cancer. Int J Radiat Oncol Biol Phys. 1999;44:789.

52. Davis BJ. American Brachytherapy Society consensus guidelines for transrectal ultrasound-guided permanent prostate brachytherapy. Brachytherapy. 2012;11(1):6.

53. Wojcieszek P. Prostate cancer brachytherapy: guidelines overview. J Contemp Brachytherapy. 2012;4(2):116.

54. Davis BJ. ACR appropriateness criteria: permanent source brachytherapy for prostate cancer. Brachytherapy. 2017;16:266.

55. Sanda MG. Quality of life and satisfaction with outcome among prostate cancer survivors. N Engl J Med. 2008;358:1250.

56. Sheets NC. Intensity modulated radiation therapy, proton therapy, or conformal radiation therapy and morbidity and disease control in localized prostate cancer. JAMA. 2012;307:1611.

57. Hamdy FC. 10-year outcomes after monitoring, surgery, or radiotherapy for prostate cancer. N Engl J Med. 2016;375:1415.

58. Donovan JL. Patient-reported outcomes after monitoring, surgery, or radiotherapy for prostate cancer. N Engl J Med. 2016; 375:1425.

59. Stone NN. Multicenter analysis of effect of high biologic effective dose on biochemical failure and survival outcomes in patients with Gleason score 7-10 prostate cancer treated with permanent prostate brachytherapy. Int J Radiat Oncol Biol Phys. 2009;73: 341.

60. Koonz BF. Morbidity and prostate-specific antigen control of external beam radiation therapy plus low-dose-rate brachytherapy boost for low, intermediate and high-risk prostate cancer. Brachytherapy. 2009;8:191.

61. Morris WJ. Androgen suppression combined with elective nodal and dose escalated radiation therapy (the ASCENDE-RT trial): an analysis of survival endpoints for a randomized trial comparing a low-dose-rate brachytherapy boost to a dose-escalated esternal beam boost for high and intermediate risk prostate cancer. Int J Radiat Oncol Biol Phys. 2017;98:275.

62. Hsu IC. Phase II trial of combined high-dose-rate brachytherapy and external beam radiotherapy for adenocarcinoma of the prostate: preliminary results of RTOG 0321. Int J Radiat Oncol Biol Phys. 2010;78:751.

63. Hoskin PJ. Randomized trial of external beam radiotherapy alone or combined with high-dose-rate brachytherapy boost for localized prostate cancer. Radiother Oncol. 2012;103:217.

64. Denham JW. Short-term neoadjuvant androgen deprivation and radiotherapy for locally advanced prostate cancer: 10-year data from the TROG 96.01 randomised trial. Lancet Oncol. 2011; 12(5):451–9.

65. Roach M. Short-term neoadjuvant androgen deprivation therapy and external-beam radiotherapy for locally advanced prostate cancer: long-term results of RTOG 8610. J Clin Oncol. 2008;26:585–91.

66. Bolla M. Long-term results with immediate androgen suppression and external irradiation in patients with locally advanced prostate cancer (an EORTC study): a phase III randomised trial. Lancet. 2002;360(9327):103–6.

67. Hanks GE. Phase III trial of long-term adjuvant androgen deprivation after neoadjuvant hormonal cytoreduction and radiotherapy in locally advanced carcinoma of the prostate: the Radiation Therapy Oncology Group Protocol 92-02. J Clin Oncol. 2003;21:3972–8.

68. Bolla M. Duration of androgen suppression in the treatment of prostate cancer. N Engl J Med. 2009;360(24):2516–27.

Prostate Cancer: Advanced and Metastatic Disease

Roberto Iacovelli, Raffaele Ratta, Chiara Ciccarese, Emanuela Fantinel, Davide Bimbatti, Elena Verzoni, and Giuseppe Procopio

Genitourinary Cancers

Contents

© Springer Nature Switzerland AG 2021
A. Russo et al. (eds.), *Practical Medical Oncology Textbook*, UNIPA Springer Series,
https://doi.org/10.1007/978-3-030-56051-5_48

🔄 **Learning Objectives**

By the end of the chapter, the reader will:

- Be able to distinguish between hormone-sensitive and castration-resistant prostate cancer
- Have learned the basic concepts of metastatic prostate cancer therapeutic algorithm
- Have reached in-depth knowledge of prostate cancer hormonal therapy, chemotherapy, and particle-emitting radionuclides (efficacy and safety profile)
- Be able to put acquired knowledge into clinical practice for the evaluation of metastatic prostate cancer patients' prognosis and the management of different treatment options

48.1 Introduction

Advanced or metastatic prostate cancer includes two main clinical patterns: patients that develop metachronous locoregional or distant metastases (after a variable interval from the diagnosis, and the treatment, of the primary tumor) and patients that present with metastasis at the time of diagnosis.

Although the spread of prostate cancer screening has resulted in an apparent migration of the diagnosis in earlier stages, with consequent improvement in long-term survival and decrease in the rate of patients with metastatic cancer, however, it is estimated that currently up to 3–6% of patients have metastatic prostate cancer at the time of diagnosis in the United States [1] and in Europe [2], with an incidence of 6.7 per 100,000 cases per year [3]. De novo metastatic prostate cancer usually affects younger subjects, with a mean age at diagnosis of 62 years, and a proportion of diagnoses in men aged 35–50, 51–55, and 56–60 of 4.4%, 8.5%, and 12.5%, respectively [3].

According to tumor sensibility to hormonal therapy, which constitutes the fundamental treatment of advanced prostate cancer as will be clarified later, it is possible to distinguish two different metastatic prostate cancer stages: hormone-sensitive disease (metastatic hormone-sensitive prostate cancer (mHSPC)) and castration-resistant disease (metastatic castration-resistant prostate cancer (mCRPC)).

48.2 Metastatic Hormone-Sensitive Prostate Cancer

48.2.1 Prognosis

Compared to patients that develop metachronous metastases, the worst prognosis of patients with newly diagnosed metastatic prostate cancer reflects the peculiar aggressiveness of this condition [4]. The median survival of patients with de novo metastatic prostate cancer is about 42 months [5, 6]. However, it must be underlined that this population is extremely heterogeneous and differs in terms of clinical presentation, tumor biology, and prognosis. In fact, alongside very aggressive forms (symptomatic patients, undifferentiated tumors, visceral metastases, large bone involvement), there are considerably more indolent clinical patterns (asymptomatic, oligo-metastatic patients).

The heterogeneity of prostate carcinoma makes it difficult to correctly predict its clinical evolution since the diagnosis; therefore, the debate on the prognostic evaluation of the single men affected by this pathology is still open.

In contrast to CRPC, there is little evidence regarding the main factors influencing prognosis in the hormone-sensitive disease setting. Several clinical features have been recognized as potential prognostic factors, including the number and the site of bone metastases, the presence of visceral metastases, the Gleason score of the primary tumor, the performance status and the patient's age, and the initial values of PSA and alkaline phosphatase [7]. Of note, no prognostic factor has been validated prospectively.

- *Gleason score*: As reported by Crawford, well-differentiated tumors (Gleason 2–4) at the time of diagnosis are associated with lower rates of progression and mortality and, vice versa, prostate cancer presenting a low degree of differentiation (Gleason 7–10) progresses faster toward metastatic disease [8].
- *PSA*: The prognostic role of PSA at the time of the diagnosis is still a matter of debate, as it is not always correlated with the biological behavior of the tumor. For example, tumors with high Gleason score and low PSA levels at the diagnosis have been associated with worse prognosis than those with higher PSA [9]. However, it should be noted that high-grade tumors could produce less PSA per gram of tumor, reducing the reliability of this marker. Therefore PSA is more reliable in the diagnostic phase and as a parameter to monitor responses to treatments.

The potential prognostic role of the absolute value of PSA was prospectively evaluated after 7 months from the beginning of androgen deprivation therapy in the cohort of patients enrolled in the SWOG-9346 study. Three different prognostic groups were distinguished: PSA <0.2 ng/mL with median overall survival (mOS) of 75 months, PSA <4 ng/mL with mOS of 44 months, and PSA > 4 ng/mL with mOS of only 13 months [10]. However, this stratification requires further confirmation.

- *Alkaline phosphatase*: A recent sub-analysis of the GETUG-AFU-15 study reported the role of alkaline phosphatase (ALP) – an indicator of disease bone involvement – as a potentially useful factor for assessing patients with high bone metastases who might benefit from more aggressive treatments. ALP was in fact the strongest prognostic factor in the discrimination of patients with good or poor prognosis, with mOS of 69.1 months in patients with normal ALP compared to 33.6 months of patients with high ALP values and 5-year survival rates of 62.1% and 23.2%, respectively [11].

— *Site of metastases and tumor burden*: Bone and lymph nodes are the most common sites of distant metastases. It has been estimated, through autopsy studies, that the prevalence of skeletal involvement in patients who die of prostate cancer is more than 90%. The presence of clinically evident bone metastases and the appearance of skeletal events represent a negative prognostic factor [12]. Up to 15% of patients with metastatic prostate cancer at diagnosis have visceral metastases [13, 14]. The visceral metastatic involvement and the presence of multiple sites affected represent two unfavorable prognostic factors, so that any new metastatic site involved is associated with an increase of about 20% of the mortality risk. However, we should note that the negative impact of visceral metastases on mortality is maintained even when focusing exclusively on patients with only one metastatic site involved [13].

Although there is a consensus in considering the disease volume as one of the main factors influencing the prognosis of mHSPC patients and therefore in guiding the therapeutic choices, the correct definition of high volume (or low volume) still remains to be stated unequivocally. Several classifications have in fact been used over the years in many studies, many of which agree to consider the visceral metastatic involvement and/or the involvement of the appendicular skeleton as the main factors correlated to poor prognosis.

Of interest, Glass defined a prognostic model based on the outcome of patients enrolled in the prospective SWOG-8894 study, identifying three different prognostic groups on the basis of four risk factors: bone metastases (appendicular or axial skeleton involvement), performance status (PS) of the patient according to ECOG classification, PSA value, and tumor Gleason score [7]. Patients at good prognosis include those without appendicular disease and without visceral metastases or with appendicular and/or visceral involvement but with ECOG-PS of 0 and Gleason <8; patients at intermediate prognosis are those with appendicular and/or visceral involvement and ECOG-PS of 0 with Gleason ≥8, or with ECOG-PS ≥1 and PSA <65 ng/ml; and finally poor prognosis patients are those with appendicular skeletal and/or visceral metastases and PS-ECOG ≥1 and PSA ≥65 ng/ml.

Good, intermediate, and poor prognosis risk groups were associated with 5-year survival rates of 42%, 21%, and 9%, respectively [7]. However, this model was based on data from patients treated more than 20 years ago (in the period between 1989 and 1994). To limit this bias, Gravis et al. re-tested Glass's prognostic system in a more updated patient cohort, the GETUG-15 study population, highlighting the persistence of a significant difference in OS between good and intermediate and between good and poor prognostic groups, while the difference was not confirmed among patients belonging to the intermediate group and to poor prognosis. However, the small sample size of the poor prognosis group (83 patients) may have affected these results [11].

48.2.2 Therapy

Prostate cancer treatment has different objectives, depending on the extent and aggressiveness of the disease but also on the patient's life expectancy and the presence of comorbidities that may represent a risk of death higher than that represented by the same prostatic cancer. In contrast to the treatment of localized and locally advanced disease, in which surgery and radiotherapy play a central role, the therapeutic approach for metastatic prostate cancer is systemic. Radiotherapy is a palliative option for controlling cancer-related pain.

48.2.2.1 Androgen Deprivation Therapy for mHSPC

Prostate cancer is an androgen-dependent tumor; therefore, androgen deprivation therapy (ADT) represents the fundamental treatment of mHSPC since the 1940s when Huggins and Hodges demonstrated for the first time the responsiveness of prostate cancer to androgen deprivation [15].

Survival and proliferation of tumor cells, as the normal ones, depend on the binding of androgens (testosterone and dihydrotestosterone) to the androgen receptor (AR). AR is a member of the superfamily of nuclear steroid receptors that, in the absence of its ligand, is kept confined in the cytoplasm by the chaperone protein HSP90. The binding of androgenic hormones with AR, instead, causes the dissociation of AR from HSP90 and its migration into the nucleus, where it dimers and subsequently binds the promoter regions of target genes, inducing their transcription. If prostate cells (or neoplastic cells) are deprived of androgen stimulation, resulting from the reduction of testosterone to castration levels, they undergo apoptosis. Any treatment aimed at suppressing androgen activity (reduction of circulating testosterone levels) is called ADT. The purpose of ADT is therefore to lower serum testosterone to castration levels (<50 ng/dl, or more recently <20 ng/dl), thus limiting the survival of tumor cells and inducing tumor regression. DT can be achieved by surgery (orchiectomy) or with medical castration drugs.

Surgical Castration

Surgical castration, which permanently reduces circulating testosterone levels to less than 50 ng/dl, is still the most rapid and economical method to achieve this goal. Bilateral orchiectomy is a simple and low-cost surgical procedure; however, it has fallen into disuse due to the negative psychological impact on patients. Since orchiectomy induces a rapid fall of testosterone levels (95% within 3 hours), it can still be reserved for patients with bone metastases at high risk of bone marrow compression.

Medical Castration

The medical approach remains the most used therapeutic modality for castration. Several classes of drugs, with different mechanisms of action, are able to induce a reduction of serum testosterone up to castration levels. Medical castration is, at least in part, reversible.

- LHRH analogs: Medical therapy with analogs of hypothalamic LHRH has provided results, in the short and long term, comparable to those of bilateral orchiectomy [16]. LHRH is normally secreted by the hypothalamus in a pulsatile way and stimulates the pituitary gland to secrete LH and FSH, which in turn promote testicular testosterone synthesis. Exposure to stable concentrations of LHRH inhibits the production of pituitary hormones. The chemical castration is nowadays mostly carried out by LHRH analog molecules that lead to a saturation of the pituitary receptors for Gn-RH and therefore inhibition of the increase in LH. This inhibition is however preceded by a transient phase of stimulation of the pituitary LHRH receptors and consequently of increased testosterone levels. This phenomenon is called flare-up and starts about 2–3 days after the first injection of LHRH analogs and persists for at least a week. Chronic exposure to LHRH analogs results in a downregulation of LHRH receptors; this suppresses the pituitary secretion of FSH and LH and therefore the production of testosterone, whose levels fall to castration values generally within 2–4 weeks.

Flare-up may be responsible for a worsening of symptoms due to an initial transient increase in testosterone levels that, by stimulating tumor growth, may precipitate bone marrow compression or urinary tract obstruction, or lead to a worsening of the bone-metastases pain. Flare-up can be avoided by the concomitant use of anti-androgens, which antagonize the action of androgens at the peripheral (receptor) level, thus neutralizing the proliferative effects of testosterone on the target tissues, including the primary prostate tumor.

- LHRH antagonists: These drugs compete with the LHRH for binding to the pituitary receptors, therefore blocking the secretion of LH and FSH as well as of testosterone. The LHRH antagonists, by definition, have no agonist effect and therefore are responsible for a more rapid reduction of testosterone with an optimal safety profile, avoiding the flare-up phenomenon [17]. The efficacy of this class of drugs is comparable to LHRH analogs in reducing testosterone to castration levels [18].

- Anti-androgens: Anti-androgens compete with testosterone and DHT for binding to the prostatic nuclear receptor, promoting apoptosis and inhibiting tumor growth.

According to their chemical structure, anti-androgens are classified into steroidal (synthetic hydroxyprogesterone derivatives) and non-steroidal anti-androgens. Both classes compete with androgens at the receptor level. This is the only non-steroidal anti-androgen action. In addition steroidal anti-androgens have progestogenic properties due to central pituitary inhibition (they inhibit the release of gonadotropins, LH, and FSH). As a consequence, non-steroidal anti-androgens, not suppressing testosterone secretion, are associated with preservation of libido, physical potency, and bone mass.

The use of anti-androgens as monotherapy can only be considered in M0 patients, but not in metastatic disease. In fact, a meta-analysis assessing the efficacy of different steroidal (cyproterone acetate) and non-steroidal (flutamide, nilutamide, bicalutamide) anti-androgens showed the inferiority of anti-androgen monotherapy compared to other methods of surgical or pharmacological castration in metastatic patients [19].

- Total androgenic blockade (BAT): One of the strategies still under debate is the total androgenic blockade (BAT), obtained by associating to the medical or surgical castration the anti-androgens not only for the short period of time necessary to counteract the flare effect. Numerous studies have been conducted to confirm the superiority of BAT compared to monotherapy with LHRH analogs, with conflicting results [20–22].

A meta-analysis of the Prostate Cancer Trialists' Collaborative Group, published in 2000 on *The Lancet*, examined the results of 27 randomized trials (8275 patients) comparing LHRH analog monotherapy to BAT. The 5-year survival rate was 25.4% in patients undergoing BAT compared to 23.6% in patients treated with ADT alone ($p = 0.11$). However, the subgroup analysis showed that BAT induced a 3% increase in

5-year survival in patients treated with non-steroidal anti-androgens (27.6% BAT vs. 24.7% with LHRH analogs, $p = 0.005$); on the contrary, in patients treated with cyproterone acetate, the combination therapy reduced survival compared to LHRH analog monotherapy (15.4% BAT vs. 18.1% LHRH analogs, $p = 0.04$). This difference is due to the increase in non-cancer-related mortality in patients treated with cyproterone acetate in combination with LHRH analogs [23]. A Cochrane review, which excluded studies with cyproterone acetate, confirmed a statistically significant benefit in terms of 5-year survival in favor of BAT (risk difference, 0.048; 95% CI, 0.02–0.077) [24].

Therefore, BAT determines a small but statistically significant advantage in terms of survival compared to monotherapy, accompanied however by a further deterioration of the quality of life in several areas: sexuality, cognitive functions, and thermoregulation. For this reason, BAT is an option to be considered only in selected patients.

ADT is generally well tolerated, but this therapy is not free from side effects such as hot flashes, loss of power and libido, fatigue, muscle mass reduction, osteoporosis, dysmetabolic syndrome, and increased cardiovascular risk.

In order to overcome ADT side effects, intermittent androgen deprivation (IAD) has been evaluated as a potential therapeutic strategy. IAD consists in alternating periods of treatment with LHRH analogs to periods of therapy interruption. The rationale of the IAD is based on the fact that an intermittent therapy would allow a cyclic recovery of the gonadal function with consequent reduction of the collateral side effects and improvement of the quality of life; moreover the reestablishment of the testosterone blood concentration would delay the selection of androgen-independent cellular clones, procrastinating disease progression and increasing overall survival.

A non-inferiority phase 3 study that compared IAD to continuous ADT treatment enrolled 3040 patients with metastatic disease and PSA >5 ng/ml. Patients treated with goserelin and bicalutamide for 7 months whose PSA values reached <4 ng/ml were randomized to continue the current therapy or to interrupt it with the reserve or take it back in case of clinical or biochemical disease progression. Although some indicators of quality of life have improved among patients undergoing IAD, overall survival was not non-inferior compared to continuous therapy (5.1 years vs. 5.8 years, HR 1.10, 90% CI 0.99–1.23) [25]. Therefore, IAD should not be considered an alternative to continuous ADT in metastatic prostate cancer patients, out of highly personalized strategies.

48.2.2.2 Chemotherapy for mHSPC

Historically, the role of chemotherapy in prostate cancer was reserved to castration-resistant disease. Recently the research has focused on HSPC, significantly modifying the whole therapeutic paradigm. In recent years, in fact, several studies have been carried out to evaluate the possibility of associating to ADT other therapeutic agents in order to enhance the antitumor activity, delay the development of resistance, and improve the patients' prognosis. A relevant question is whether the administration of chemotherapy to mHSPC patients may improve the efficacy and tolerability of docetaxel. Docetaxel, indeed, exerts its cytotoxic activity through androgen-mediated effects that target androgen-dependent cells before they can adapt to become androgen-independent. Taxanes have a direct effect on the androgen signaling pathway. In fact, docetaxel stabilizes microtubules and maintains the AR in the cytoplasm, inhibiting its translocation into the nucleus in response to androgens or via ligand-independent pathways. In addition, taxanes act through the FOXO1 transcriptional repressor to prevent gene expression responsive to androgens. The inhibition of AR signal, rather than antimitotic activity, may indeed be the reason that explains the antitumor activity of taxanes in prostate cancer [26, 27]. Therefore, the early combination of docetaxel with ADT could delay the development of resistance to ADT (delay the CRPC phase) and maximize the efficacy of docetaxel.

The efficacy of first-line therapy with the association of ADT and docetaxel in mHSPC patients has been shown in three randomized phase 3 trials:

- GETUG-AFU15 study: It is a small phase 3 study conducted in France and published in November 2015 [28]. It randomized a total of 385 patients to receive ADT monotherapy (orchiectomy or LHRH analogs, with or without non-steroidal anti-androgens) or the association of ADT with docetaxel for nine cycles. The majority of patients had metastatic disease at the time of diagnosis (71%, 272/385), while only a minority of them became metastatic after treatment for localized disease. The study failed to demonstrate a survival advantage with chemotherapy in the overall population: median survival was 58.9 months (95% CI 50.8–69.1) in the docetaxel plus ADT arm compared to 54.2 months (42.2–not achieved) in the ADT arm (HR 1.01, 95% CI 0.75–1.36). Combination therapy had been shown to significantly prolong the biochemical PFS (22.9 vs. 12.9 months, HR 0.72, 0.57–0.91, $p = 0.005$) and the radiological PFS (23.5 vs. 15.4 months, HR 0.75, 0.59–0.94, $p = 0.015$) [28]. One of the major limits of this study was the enrollment of patients mainly with low disease burden. A subsequent retrospective analysis, in fact, has reclassified patients according to the disease volume using the CHAARTED study criteria. In the high-volume subgroup of patients (47% of total), there was a trend in favor of the combination therapy of ADT plus docetaxel, with a 22% reduction in the risk of death and an improvement of 4.7 months in overall survival (mOS 39.8 vs. 35.1 months, HR 0.78, 95% CI 0.56–1.09, $p = 0.14$) [29].

- CHAARTED study: It is a randomized phase 3 study, published in August 2015 in the *New England Journal of Medicine*, involving a total of 790 patients with mHSPC randomized to receive ADT alone or the association of ADT with docetaxel for six cycles within 4 months from the beginning of the ADT. The study included mainly metastatic patients at diagnosis (75%), compared to patients who developed metachronous metastases. At a median follow-up of 28.9 months, there was a statistically significant and clinically relevant overall survival advantage (about 13.6 months) for patients treated with docetaxel plus ADT (mOS 57.6 vs. 44 months, HR 0.61, 95% CI 0.47–0.80, $p < 0.001$), which translates into a reduction in the risk of death by 39%. The survival benefit was more evident in patients with high-volume disease (65% of cases), defined by the presence of visceral metastases or four or more bone lesions, of which at least one is located outside the axial skeleton and pelvis (mOS 49.2 vs. 32.2 months, HR 0.60, 95% CI 0.45–0.81, $p < 0.001$) [30].

- The STAMPEDE study: It is a multi-factorial study that enrolled 2962 patients, with metastatic disease at diagnosis (M1, 1817 subjects), with localized high-risk disease (N0, 697), or with lymph node involvement (N+, 448), but all candidates received long-term hormone therapy. Patients were randomized to ADT alone ($n = 1184$), ADT in association with docetaxel for six cycles ($n = 592$), the combination of ADT and zoledronic acid for 2 years ($n = 593$), or ADT in combination with docetaxel and zoledronic acid ($n = 592$). The main objective of the study was to evaluate the efficacy of combined treatment with ADT and docetaxel compared to ADT monotherapy and to evaluate the possible benefit of the addition of zoledronic acid in the population of hormone-sensitive patients. At a median follow-up of 43 months, patients who received docetaxel (with or without zoledronic acid) associated with ADT showed a significant advantage in overall survival of about 10 months (mOS 81 vs. 71 months, HR 0.78, $p = 0.006$). This advantage was even more significant in the subgroup of metastatic patients (mOS 60 vs. 45 months, $p = 0.0005$) compared to those with only biochemical disease recurrence. However, the limited number of patients with non-metastatic disease, along with the small number of deaths in this subgroup, underestimated the power of all survival analyses. Early docetaxel was also associated with a PFS advantage, while no benefit in terms of DFS and OS was observed by the addition of zoledronic acid [31].

The results suggest a paradigmatic shift in the therapeutic algorithm of mHSPC, providing a solid rationale about the possibility of improving patients' survival by starting docetaxel in a hormone-sensitive stage, rather than procrastinating chemotherapy in the castration-resistant phase.

The results of GETUG-AFU15, CHAARTED, and STAMPEDE trials were included in two meta-analyses, which analyzed the role of docetaxel addition to ADT in the treatment of hormone-naïve metastatic patients, confirming the statistically significant advantage in favor of early combination therapy [32, 33]. In particular, the meta-analysis of Vale and co-authors showed an increase in overall survival with the early use of docetaxel together with ADT in patients with metastatic disease at diagnosis estimated at around 9% at 4 years (from 40% to 49%), with a hazard ratio of 0.77 (95% CI 0.68–0.87, $p < 0.0001$). Furthermore, chemotherapy in combination with ADT improved the failure-free survival, with an HR of 0.64 (0.58–0.70, $p < 0.0001$), which translated into an absolute reduction in the rate of therapeutic failure of 16% at 4 years (95% CI 12–19) [32]. For this reason, the combination of ADT and docetaxel is a viable option for those hormone-naïve patients who have metastases at diagnosis, are with "high-volume" disease, and are in good clinical condition.

The adequate selection of mHSPC patients destined to achieve a significant benefit from this therapeutic strategy still represents a matter of debate. It should also be emphasized that chemotherapy with docetaxel is a treatment associated with remarkable toxicity, especially hematologic; in the CHAARTED study, the grade 3–4 neutropenia rate was about 12%, with febrile neutropenia in about 6% and severe infections associated with neutropenia in 2% of cases. Obviously it is important to remember that in patients with multiple bone metastases, of advanced age, and with comorbidities, the expected toxicity is even higher. The results of the CHAARTED study showed a major advantage of docetaxel restricted to the subgroup of "high-volume" disease compared to patients with "low-volume" disease. Robust data are not available to recommend the routine use of the early combination of docetaxel and ADT in patients with low-volume, oligo-metastatic, and slowly evolving hormone-sensitive disease. In this subgroup ADT remains the therapeutic standard of care.

48.2.2.3 Second-Generation Hormonal Therapy for mHSPC

Similarly to what has been described for chemotherapy, the efficacy of early use of the combination of ADT with second-generation anti-androgen in mHSPC disease has recently been investigated. Abiraterone acetate, pro-drug of the corresponding active form abiraterone, is a selective and irreversible inhibitor of cytochrome P-450c17 (17α-hydroxylase/C17,20-lyase), a crucial enzyme in the biosensitization of androgen hormones in testicular and adrenal tissues and in neoplastic prostate tissues. Blocking CYP17 inhibits the testicular, adrenal, and neoplastic biosynthesis of androgens.

The LATITUDE trial evaluated the use of abiraterone acetate and prednisone in association with ADT in 1199 patients with mHSPC. All patients included in the study had a high-risk disease, defined by the presence of at least two of the following criteria: Gleason score equal to or greater than 8, a minimum number of bone lesions equal to 3, and evidence of measurable visceral metastases. The main objective of the study was to demonstrate an advantage in terms of overall survival and radiological PFS resulting from the early addition of abiraterone to standard hormone therapy. At a median follow-up of 30.4 months, the addition of abiraterone to ADT resulted in a statistically significant prolongation of survival (mOS not reached vs. 34.7 months, HR 0.62, 95% CI 0.51–0.76, $p < 0.001$), with a 38% reduction in the risk of death compared to the placebo group. Abiraterone also prolonged PFS (33.0 vs. 14.8 months, HR 0.47, 95% CI 0.39–0.55, $p < 0.001$), time to pain worsening, time to the beginning of subsequent therapies, and time to biochemical progression [34]. It is important to underline that, given the significant benefit in OS observed at the interim analysis, crossover to abiraterone was allowed for patients in the placebo treatment arm. Grade 3 and 4 toxicities were reported in 63% of patients in the abiraterone treatment arm (mainly mineralocorticoid toxicity, with hypertension and hypokalemia) and in 48% of those in the placebo group [34]. Therefore, the data support the hypothesis that a more effective inhibition of the AR-mediated signal pathway as initial systemic therapy in mHSPC patients at higher risk, albeit with a greater incidence of side effects related to the use of abiraterone compared to ADT alone, leads to better results than ADT alone.

The role of abiraterone plus ADT for mHSPC was confirmed in the STAMPEDE study. The *New England Journal of Medicine* published the results of the STAMPEDE study relative to the comparison between abiraterone acetate and prednisolone in addition to ADT compared to ADT alone in a cohort of 1917 mHSPC patients (52% with newly diagnosed metastatic prostate cancer, 20% with lymph node metastasis, and 28% with a locally advanced disease or a disease previously treated with surgery or radiotherapy and relapse with high-risk characteristics). At a median follow-up of 40 months, the combination of abiraterone/prednisone and ADT showed significantly longer survival compared to ADT alone, with a 3-year survival rate of 83% versus 76% (HR 0.63, 95% CI 0.52–0.76, $p < 0.001$). The survival advantage in favor of abiraterone was even more significant in the subgroup of patients with metastatic disease (HR 0.61, 95% CI 0.49–0.75). Grade 3–5 adverse events occurred in 47% of patients in the abiraterone treatment arm and in 33% of patients treated with ADT and were primarily hypertension, transaminase increase, and respiratory disorders [35]. It is important to underline that a randomized phase 3 study comparing the combination of ADT and enzalutamide to ADT plus placebo in patients with mHSPC is currently ongoing (NCT02677896).

Of interest, at the 2017 ESMO Congress, the results of an analysis about the direct comparison between the two treatment cohorts evaluated in the STAMPEDE trial (the combination of abiraterone acetate and ADT vs. the combination of docetaxel and ADT) were presented. There was no difference in survival between the two different combinations (HR for the OS of 1.16), while a statistically significant advantage in terms of biochemical relapse and disease progression in favor of abiraterone compared to docetaxel was noticed [36]. However, these preliminary data do not allow to draw definitive recommendations.

48.3 Metastatic Castration-Resistant Prostate Cancer

48.3.1 Introduction

All men with metastatic prostate cancer will progress to castration-resistant disease with a mortality rate of over 50% [37]. Castrate-resistant prostate cancer (CRPC) is defined by disease progression despite androgen deprivation therapy (ADT) and may present as one or any combination of castrate serum testosterone <50 ng/dL or 1.7 nmol/L plus either biochemical progression (defined as three consecutive rises in PSA 1 week apart resulting in two 50% increases over the nadir and a PSA > 2 ng/mL) or radiological progression (defined by the appearance of two or more new bone lesions on bone scan or a soft tissue lesion using RECIST (Response Evaluation Criteria in Solid Tumours)) [38]. Symptomatic progression alone is not sufficient to diagnose CRPC.

There are currently six systemic therapies approved by the Food and Drug Administration (FDA) and the European Agency for the Evaluation of Medicinal

◘ Table 48.1 Phase 3 trials of single agents leading to regulatory approval in castration-resistant prostate cancer

Trial: therapy (approved date)	N	Disease state	Comparator	HR	OS (months)	P value
TAX327: docetaxel (2004) [11]	1.006	First-line	Mitoxantrone Prednisone	0.76	18.9 vs. 16.5	0.009
TROPIC: cabazitaxel (2010) [13]	755	Post-chemotherapy	Mitoxantrone Prednisone	0.70	15.1 vs. 12.7	<0.0001
COU-AA-301: abiraterone acetate (2011) [24]	1195	Post-docetaxel	Placebo Prednisone	0.74	15.8 vs. 11.2	<0.0001
COU-AA-302: abiraterone acetate (2013) [26]	1.088	Pre-chemotherapy	Placebo Prednisone	0.81	34.7 vs. 30.3	0.0033
AFFIRM: enzalutamide (2012) [34]	1199	Post-docetaxel	Placebo	0.63	18.4 vs. 13.6	<0.0001
PREVAIL: enzalutamide (2014) [35]	1717	Pre-chemotherapy	Placebo	0.71	32.4 vs. 30.2	p < 0.001
ALSYMPCA: radium-223 (2013) [22]	922	Pre- and post-docetaxel Symptomatic	Placebo	0.695	14.0 vs. 11.2	0.00085

Products (EMEA) that offer a survival benefit for the treatment of metastatic castration-resistant prostate cancer (mCRPC). These include docetaxel, cabazitaxel, enzalutamide, abiraterone acetate, sipuleucel-T (approved only in the United States), and radium-223 (◘ Table 48.1).

48.3.2 Therapy

48.3.2.1 Chemotherapy for mCRPC

The first available chemotherapeutic options for patients with mCRPC, mitoxantrone and estramustine, had a limited clinical benefit because these agents did not show to prolong overall survival (OS) [39–41]. Estramustine was approved for the treatment of mCRPC in 1981 on the basis of small non-randomized studies, which showed improved rates of disease control over comparators [42, 43]. Estramustine was associated with a high rate of toxicity when given in combination, and while it may improve PSA response, it did not consistently improve OS [44, 45]. A meta-analysis of 742 patients demonstrated better PSA response and OS with the addition of estramustine to chemotherapy, but at the cost of significant adverse events (AEs) [46]. Mitoxantrone was associated with significant palliative benefits and improved PSA response rates, which led to its approval in 1996 and subsequent establishment as standard of care [40–43].
▬ *Docetaxel*

In 2004 the taxane chemotherapy, docetaxel, replaced mitoxantrone as the standard of care following two phase 3 studies (TAX327 and SWOG-9916) in which docetaxel prolonged OS in patients with mCRPC [47, 48].

TAX327 was a randomized, non-blinded, phase 3 study in which 1006 patients with mCRPC received 5 mg of prednisone twice daily and were randomly assigned to receive 12 mg of mitoxantrone per square meter of body-surface area every 3 weeks, 75 mg of docetaxel per square meter every 3 weeks, or 30 mg of docetaxel per square meter weekly for 5 of every 6 weeks.

The primary end point of the study was overall survival; secondary end points were predefined reductions in pain, an improvement in the quality of life, a reduction in serum PSA levels of at least 50%, and objective tumor responses.

Patients treated with docetaxel every 3 weeks had a significantly higher survival rate compared with the mitoxantrone group ($p = 0.009$); on the contrary, patients treated with weekly docetaxel did not show any survival superiority ($p = 0.36$). The median duration of survival was 18.9 months (95% confidence interval [CI], 17.0–21.2) in the group given docetaxel every 3 weeks, 17.4 months (95% CI, 15.7–19.0) in the group given weekly docetaxel, and 16.5 months (95% CI, 14.4–18.6) in the mitoxantrone group. The hazard ratio for death in the group treated with docetaxel every 3 weeks, as compared with the mitoxantrone group, was 0.76. Visceral involvement, high baseline alkaline phosphatase level, and low hemoglobin level were negative prognostic factors in the multivariate models, whereas rising serum PSA as the sole indicator of progression was a favorable factor. Post hoc analysis indicated that high Gleason score (8, 9, or 10) was an adverse prognostic factor for survival.

A reduction in pain was more frequent among patients receiving docetaxel every 3 weeks than among those treated with mitoxantrone (35% vs. 22%, $p = 0.01$), but the percentage of patients with reduced pain in the weekly docetaxel group (31%) did not differ significantly from that of the mitoxantrone group.

Rates of PSA response were significantly higher in the docetaxel groups (45% in the group treated with docetaxel every 3 weeks and 48% in the group of weekly docetaxel, $p < 0.001$ for both comparisons) than in the mitoxantrone group (32%). Patients with measurable soft-tissue lesions who received docetaxel every 3 weeks had a higher rate of tumor response than patients who received mitoxantrone every 3 weeks (12% vs. 7%, $p = 0.11$), but this difference was not significant.

As to the AEs, the incidence of grade 3 and 4 neutropenia was relatively low, and febrile neutropenia was rare. There was a higher incidence of cardiac events among patients who received mitoxantrone. Most other types of AEs were more frequent among patients treated with docetaxel, and there was no trend toward a lower frequency with weekly docetaxel than with docetaxel given every 3 weeks. Low-grade AEs that occurred in at least 15% of patients in one of the groups included fatigue, nausea or vomiting or both, alopecia, diarrhea, nail changes, sensory neuropathy, anorexia, changes in taste, stomatitis, dyspnea, tearing, peripheral edema, and epistaxis. More patients in the docetaxel groups than in the mitoxantrone group had at least one serious adverse event, with rates of 26% among those in the group given docetaxel every 3 weeks, 29% among those given weekly docetaxel, and 20% among those given mitoxantrone. AEs leading to discontinuation of treatment included fatigue, musculoskeletal or nail changes, sensory neuropathy, and infection in the docetaxel groups and cardiac dysfunction in the mitoxantrone group.

The percentage of patients who had an improvement in the quality of life was similar in the two docetaxel groups (22% in the group given docetaxel every 3 weeks and 23% in the group given weekly docetaxel) and significantly higher than that in the mitoxantrone group (13%, $p = 0.009$ and $p = 0.005$, respectively).

SWOG-9916 was also a randomized, phase 3 trial in which 770 men were randomly assigned to one of two treatments, each given in 21-day cycles: 280 mg of estramustine three times daily on days 1 through 5, 60 mg of docetaxel per square meter of body-surface area on day 2, and 60 mg of dexamethasone in three divided doses before docetaxel, or 12 mg of mitoxantrone per square meter on day 1 plus 5 mg of prednisone twice daily. The primary end point was overall survival; secondary end points were progression-free survival, objective response rates, and post-treatment declines of at least 50 percent in PSA levels.

In an intention-to-treat analysis, the median overall survival was longer in the group of patients treated with docetaxel and estramustine than in the group who received mitoxantrone and prednisone (17.5 months vs. 15.6 months, $p = 0.02$), and the corresponding hazard

ratio for death was 0.80 (95% CI, 0.67–0.97). The median time to progression was 6.3 months in the group given docetaxel and estramustine and 3.2 months in the group given mitoxantrone and prednisone ($p < 0.001$). PSA declines of at least 50 percent occurred in 50% and 27% of patients, respectively ($p < 0.001$), and objective tumor responses were observed in 17% and 11% of patients with bidimensionally measurable disease, respectively ($p = 0.30$). Grade 3 or 4 neutropenic fevers ($p = 0.01$), nausea and vomiting ($p < 0.001$), and cardiovascular events ($p = 0.001$) were more common among patients receiving docetaxel and estramustine than among those receiving mitoxantrone and prednisone.

The TAX327 and the SWOG-9916 trials have provided support for the treatment with docetaxel in men with mCRPC.

Cabazitaxel

Cabazitaxel, a second-generation taxane, was developed to overcome resistance to docetaxel. Its efficacy was evaluated in the TROPIC phase 3 trial [49]. This was a randomized trial in which 755 mCRPC patients received oral prednisone 10 mg daily and were randomly assigned to receive cabazitaxel 25 mg per square meter intravenously or mitoxantrone 12 mg per square meter intravenously on day 1 of each 21-day cycle and were stratified for disease measurability (measurable vs. non-measurable) and ECOG performance status (0–1 vs. 2). 50% of patients had measurable soft-tissue disease and 25% had visceral (poor prognosis) disease. One dose reduction (cabazitaxel 20 mg per square meter or mitoxantrone 10 mg per square meter) per patient was allowed in this study.

Median overall survival was 15.1 months for patients in the cabazitaxel arm (95% CI, 14.1–16.3) versus 12.7 months for the mitoxantrone arm (95% CI, 11.6–13.7). This result corresponds to a 30% reduction in relative risk of death (HR 0.70; 95% CI, 0.59–0.83; $p < 0.0001$). Median progression-free survival was 2.8 months (95% CI, 2.4–3.0) in the cabazitaxel group and 1.4 months (95% CI, 1.4–1.7) in the mitoxantrone group (HR 0.74; 95% CI, 0.64–0.86; $p < 0.0001$). Patients treated with cabazitaxel had significantly higher rates of tumor response and PSA response than did those who received mitoxantrone, as well as significant improvements in time to tumor progression and time to PSA progression.

The most common toxic effects of cabazitaxel were hematological; the most frequent hematological grade 3 or higher AEs were neutropenia, leukopenia, and anemia. The most common non-hematological grade 3 or higher adverse event was diarrhea. Grade 3 peripheral neuropathy was uncommon.

On the basis of these results, cabazitaxel was approved in 2010 for the treatment of patients with mCRPC who have previously received docetaxel-based regimens [42].

The PROSELICA study, which compared the two allowed doses of cabazitaxel (20 and 25 mg per square meter) as second-line therapy in patients with mCRPC, concluded that the 20 mg per square meter dose maintains at least 50% of the survival benefit observed in the TROPIC study [49, 50]. This study reported lower toxicity for 20 mg per square meter than for 25 mg per square meter cabazitaxel dose with similar OS, suggesting that the dose may be reduced in patients who require the reduction [50].

More recently, cabazitaxel 25 and 20 mg per square meter (every 3 weeks) were compared with docetaxel in terms of OS in patients with chemotherapy-naïve mCRPC (FIRSTANA) [51]. No statistically significant differences between the three treatment groups were observed for OS or PFS; the study did not demonstrate the superiority of cabazitaxel over docetaxel. Treatment with cabazitaxel at the lower dose resulted in a similar OS and less hematological toxicity than the higher dose.

48.3.2.2 Radiopharmaceutical
Radium-223

Radium-223, a bone-seeking calcium mimetic, forms hydroxyapatite complexes during bone mineralization in areas of high osteoblast activity and increased bone turnover around prostate cancer metastatic lesions [52–54]. Radium-223 decays to emit predominantly high-energy alpha particles over a short range (<1 mm), leading to cytotoxicity through the production of predominantly unrepairable DNA double-strand breaks in nearby tumor and cells forming the cancer microenvironment. The short path of the alpha particles also means that toxic effects on adjacent healthy tissue and particularly the bone marrow may be minimized.

In phase 1 and 2 clinical trials of patients with bone metastases, radium-223 was associated with a favorable safety profile, with minimal myelotoxicity [55, 56]. Phase 2 studies have shown that radium-223 reduces pain and improves disease-related biomarkers (e.g., bone alkaline phosphatase and PSA) [57, 58], suggesting a survival benefit in patients with CRPC and bone metastases. To evaluate the effect of radium-223 on survival, a phase 3, randomized, double-blind, multinational study has been conducted (the Alpharadin in Symptomatic Prostate Cancer Patients (ALSYMPCA) study), which has compared the efficacy and safety of radium-223 versus placebo in patients with CRPC and bone metastases [59]. A total of 921 patients have been enrolled in the ALSYMPCA study (614 in the radium-223 group and 307 in the placebo group). The median number of injections was six in the radium-223 group and five in the placebo group.

At the interim analysis, the median overall survival was 14.0 months in the radium-223 group and 11.2 months in the placebo group; radium-223 was asso-

ciated with a 30% reduction in the risk of death (HR 0.70; 95% CI, 0.55–0.88; two-sided $p = 0.002$). The advantage of radium-223 over placebo was confirmed also in the updated analysis, where median overall survival was 14.9 months in the radium-223 group and 11.3 months in the placebo group; the updated analysis confirmed the 30% reduction in the risk of death among patients in the radium-223 group as compared with the placebo group (HR 0.70; 95% CI, 0.58–0.83; $p < 0.001$). Radium-223, as compared with placebo, significantly prolonged the time to the first symptomatic skeletal event (median, 15.6 months vs. 9.8 months; HR 0.66; 95% CI, 0.52–0.83; $p < 0.001$), the time to an increase in the total alkaline phosphatase level (HR 0.17; 95% CI, 0.13–0.22; $p < 0.001$), and the time to an increase in the PSA level (HR, 0.64; 95% CI, 0.54–0.77; $p < 0.001$).

The associated toxicity was mild and, apart from slightly more hematologic toxicity and diarrhea with radium-223, this did not differ significantly from that in the placebo arm. Grade 3 febrile neutropenia was reported in one patient (<1%) in each group. A significantly higher percentage of patients who received radium-223, as compared with those who received placebo, had a meaningful improvement in the quality of life during the period of study-drug administration (25% vs. 16%, $p = 0.02$).

Therefore, although radium-223 is most often used as a second- or third-line therapy for mCRPC, it is reasonable to use it in bone-predominant, symptomatic disease even in the pre-docetaxel setting.

48.3.2.3 Novel Androgen-Directed Agents
Abiraterone Acetate

Abiraterone acetate is a selective inhibitor of androgen biosynthesis that potently blocks cytochrome P450 c17 (CYP17), a critical enzyme in testosterone synthesis, thereby blocking androgen synthesis by the adrenal glands and testes and within the prostate tumor. The efficacy of abiraterone acetate, in combination with prednisone, has been evaluated in two pivotal phase 3 studies in both men with mCRPC after chemotherapy with docetaxel (COU-AA-301 trial) [60, 61] and in men who were chemotherapy-naïve (COU-AA-302 trial) [62–64].

In the two phase 3 trials, patients received oral abiraterone acetate 1000 mg or placebo once daily in combination with oral prednisone 5 mg twice daily.

In the COU-AA-301 trial, 1195 patients were randomly assigned to receive abiraterone acetate plus prednisone (797 patients) or placebo plus prednisone (398 patients) [60]. At the time of the preplanned interim analysis, treatment with abiraterone acetate plus prednisone resulted in a 35.4% reduction in the risk of death as compared with placebo plus prednisone (HR 0.65; 95% CI, 0.54–0.77; $p < 0.001$). The mOS was

14.8 months in the abiraterone acetate group and 10.9 months in the placebo group. The effect of abiraterone acetate and prednisone on OS was consistent across all subgroups, and the significance of the treatment effect on OS was robust after adjustment for stratification factors in a multivariate analysis (HR for death, 0.66; 95% CI, 0.55–0.78; $p < 0.001$). Abiraterone acetate demonstrated its superiority over placebo for all the secondary end points analyzed, including the confirmed PSA response rate (29% vs. 6%, $p < 0.001$), the objective response rate on the basis of RECIST among patients with measurable disease at baseline (14% vs. 3%, $p < 0.001$), time to PSA progression (10.2 months vs. 6.6 months), and median PFS on the basis of radiographic evidence (5.6 vs. 3.6 months). At a median follow-up of 20.2 months, median OS was 15.8 months (95% CI, 14.8–17.0) in the abiraterone group compared with 11.2 months (10.4–13.1) in the placebo group (HR 0.74, 95% CI 0.64–0.86, $p < 0.0001$) [61]. The most common adverse event was fatigue, which occurred at a similar frequency in the two treatment groups [60]. Other common AEs in both groups were back pain (30% in the abiraterone acetate group and 33% in the placebo group), nausea (30% and 32%, respectively), constipation (26% and 31%), bone pain (25% and 28%), and arthralgia (27% and 23%). Most of these events were grade 1 or 2. AEs associated with elevated mineralocorticoid levels due to CYP17 blockade (fluid retention and edema, hypokalemia, and hypertension), as well as cardiac disorders and liver-function test abnormalities, were more common in the abiraterone acetate group than in the placebo group (55% vs. 43%, $p < 0.001$). The incidence of fluid retention and edema was higher in the abiraterone acetate group (31%, vs. 22% in the placebo group, $p = 0.04$). Grade 1 or 2 peripheral edema accounted for most of these events. Hypokalemia also occurred in a higher proportion of patients in the abiraterone acetate group (17%, vs. 8% in the placebo group, $p < 0.001$). Cardiac events (primarily grade 1 or 2) occurred at a higher rate in the abiraterone acetate group than in the placebo group (13% vs. 11%, $p = 0.14$), but the difference was not significant. The most frequently reported cardiac events were tachycardia (3% in the abiraterone acetate group and 2% in the placebo group, $p = 0.22$) and atrial fibrillation (2% and 1%, respectively, $p = 0.29$). Abiraterone acetate treatment has been associated with an elevation in aminotransferase levels. A grade 4 elevation in an aminotransferase level early in the study led to a protocol amendment specifying more frequent monitoring with liver-function tests during the first 12 weeks of treatment. Overall, however, abnormalities in liver-function tests occurred at a similar frequency in the abiraterone acetate and placebo groups, including changes of any grade in liver-function tests (10% and 8%, respectively), grade 3 or 4 changes in liver-function tests (3.5% and 3.0%), grade 3 or 4 elevations in aspartate aminotransferase levels (1.4% and 1.6%), grade 3 or 4 elevations in alanine aminotransferase levels (1.0% and 1.1%), and grade 4 elevations in aminotransferase levels (0.3% and 0.5%).

In the COU-AA-302 trial, co-primary end points were radiographic progression-free survival (rPFS) and OS defined as the time from randomization to death from any cause [62–64]. The median follow-up duration for all patients was 22.2 months. At the time of the first interim analysis, treatment with abiraterone plus prednisone, as compared with placebo plus prednisone, resulted in a 57% reduction in the risk of radiographic progression or death (median not reached vs. median of 8.3 months; HR for abiraterone-prednisone vs. prednisone alone, 0.43; 95% CI, 0.35–0.52; $p < 0.001$). At the time of the second interim analysis, the median time to rPFS was 16.5 months in the abiraterone-prednisone group and 8.3 months in the prednisone-alone group (HR 0.53; 95% CI, 0.45–0.62; $p < 0.001$).

The planned interim analysis of overall survival was performed after 333 deaths (43% of 773 events) were observed. Median OS was not reached for the abiraterone-prednisone group and was 27.2 months (95% CI, 26.0 to not reached) in the prednisone alone group. A 25% decrease in the risk of death in the abiraterone-prednisone group was observed (HR, 0.75; 95% CI, 0.61–0.93; $p = 0.01$), indicating a strong trend toward improved survival with abiraterone-prednisone. The effect of abiraterone on OS was consistently favorable across all prespecified subgroups.

The final analysis showed that there was a significant decrease in the risk of death in the abiraterone acetate group compared with the placebo group (HR 0.81, 95% CI 0.70–0.93, $p = 0.0033$) [63]. At a median follow-up of 49.2 months, mOS was significantly longer in the abiraterone acetate group than in the placebo group (34.7 months [95% CI 32.7–36.8] vs. 30.3 months [28.7–33.3], HR 0.81 [95% CI 0.70–0.93], $p = 0.0033$) [63].

In a multivariate analysis baseline PSA, lactate dehydrogenase, alkaline phosphatase, hemoglobin, bone metastases, and age were all significant prognostic factors for overall survival but ECOG performance status score was not. Abiraterone acetate plus prednisone decreased the risk of time to opiate use for prostate cancer-related pain compared with placebo plus prednisone at this final analysis (HR 0.72, 95% CI 0.61–0.85, $p < 0.0001$). Median time to opiate use for prostate cancer-related pain was 33.4 months (95% CI 30.2–39.8) in the abiraterone acetate group versus 23.4 months (95% CI 20.3–27.5) in the placebo group [63].

As to the safety profile, AEs of special interest, including events related to mineralocorticoid excess, were more common in the abiraterone acetate group than in the placebo group. Most of them were of grade 1 or grade 2 in severity. The most common AEs in the final analysis resulting in death in the abiraterone acetate group were disease progression and general physical health deterioration as a sign of clinical progression in three (1%) and three (1%) patients, respectively. No treatment-related deaths occurred. Abiraterone acetate therapy was also associated with significant ($p < 0.05$) improvements in health-related quality of life (HR-QOL) compared with placebo plus prednisone in terms of patient-reported fatigue (assessed by Brief Fatigue Inventory questionnaire) [65] and functional status (assessed by Functional Assessment of Cancer Therapy-Prostate total score (FACT-P)) [66].

On the basis of the results of the COU-AA-301 and COU-AA-302 trials, abiraterone acetate has been approved by the national agencies for drug regulation and is now part of clinical practice in mCRPC treatment algorithm.

Enzalutamide

Enzalutamide is an androgen-receptor-signaling inhibitor chosen for clinical development on the basis of activity in prostate-cancer models with overexpression of the androgen receptor. Enzalutamide inhibits nuclear translocation of the androgen receptor, DNA binding, and coactivator recruitment. It also has a greater affinity for the receptor, induces tumor shrinkage in xenograft models (in which conventional anti-androgen agents only retard growth), and has no known agonistic effects [67, 68].

In a phase 1–2 trial enrolling men with CRPC (some of whom had undergone previous chemotherapy) conducted by the Prostate Cancer Clinical Trials Consortium [69], enzalutamide had shown significant antitumor activity regardless of previous chemotherapy status. On the basis of these findings, a dose of enzalutamide was identified for further study [70].

The efficacy of enzalutamide has been evaluated in two pivotal phase 3 studies in both men with mCRPC after chemotherapy with docetaxel (AFFIRM trial) [71] and in men who were chemotherapy-naïve (PREVAIL trial) [72].

In the AFFIRM trial, 1199 patients were randomly assigned to receive either enzalutamide (800 patients) or placebo (399 patients) [71]. The primary end point was OS, defined as the time from randomization to death from any cause. Secondary end points included measures of response (in the PSA level, in soft tissue, and in the quality-of-life score) and measures of progression (time to PSA progression, radiographic PFS, and time to the first skeletal-related event).

The mOS was 18.4 months (95% CI, 17.3 to not yet reached) for patients receiving enzalutamide and 13.6 months (95% CI, 11.3–15.8) among patients who received placebo. The use of enzalutamide resulted in a 37% reduction in the risk of death, as compared with placebo (HR for death 0.63; 95% CI, 0.53–0.75; $p < 0.001$). The survival benefit was consistent across all subgroups, including age, baseline pain intensity, geographic region, and type of disease progression at entry. The superiority of enzalutamide over placebo was shown for all secondary end points, including PSA-level response rate (54% vs. 2%, $p < 0.001$), soft-tissue response rate (29% vs. 4%, $p < 0.001$), FACT-P quality-of-life response (43% vs. 18%, $p < 0.001$), the time to PSA progression (8.3 vs. 3.0 months; HR, 0.25; $p < 0.001$), radiographic PFS (8.3 vs. 2.9 months; HR, 0.40; $p < 0.001$), and the time to the first skeletal-related event (16.7 vs. 13.3 months, HR 0.69, $p < 0.001$).

In terms of safety, the enzalutamide group had a lower incidence of AEs of grade 3 or above (45.3%, vs. 53.1% in the placebo group). The median time to the first adverse event was 12.6 months in the enzalutamide group, as compared with 4.2 months in the placebo group. A higher incidence of all grades of fatigue, diarrhea, hot flashes, musculoskeletal pain, and headache was observed in the enzalutamide group than in the placebo group. Cardiac disorders were noted in 6% of patients receiving enzalutamide and in 8% of patients receiving placebo (with cardiac disorders of grade 3 in 1% and 2%, respectively). Hypertension or increased blood pressure was observed in 6.6% of patients in the enzalutamide group and 3.3% of those in the placebo group. Liver-function abnormalities were reported as AEs in 1% of patients receiving enzalutamide and in 2% of those receiving placebo. Five of the 800 patients in the enzalutamide group (0.6%) were reported by the investigators to have had a seizure; no seizures were reported in the placebo group. One case of status epilepticus (confusion associated with partial complex status epilepticus) required medical intervention; the four other seizures were self-limited and did not recur after study-drug discontinuation. However, potentially predisposing factors were present in several patients. Caution should be used in administering enzalutamide to patients with a history of seizure or who have other predisposing factors, including underlying brain injury, stroke, brain metastases, or alcoholism, or to patients receiving concomitant medication that may lower the seizure threshold.

In the PREVAIL trial, a total of 1717 patients were enrolled randomly assigned to enzalutamide ($n = 872$) and placebo ($n = 845$) [72]. At 12 months of follow-up, the rate of radiographic PFS was 65% in the enzalutamide group and 14% in the placebo group. Treatment with enzalutamide, as compared with placebo, resulted in an 81% reduction in the risk of radiographic progression or death (HR in the enzalutamide group, 0.19; 95% CI, 0.15–0.23; $p < 0.001$). Fewer patients in the enzalutamide group than in the placebo group had radiographic progression or died (118 of 832 patients [14%] vs. 321 of 801 patients [40%]). The median radiographic PFS was not reached in the enzalutamide group, as compared with 3.9 months in the placebo group. The treatment effect of enzalutamide on radiographic PFS was consistent across all prespecified subgroups.

As to the OS, at the planned interim analysis, the median duration of follow-up for survival was approximately 22 months. Fewer deaths occurred in the enzalutamide group than in the placebo group (241 of 872 patients [28%] vs. 299 of 845 patients [35%]). Treatment with enzalutamide, as compared with placebo, resulted in a 29% decrease in the risk of death (HR, 0.71; 95% CI, 0.60–0.84; $p < 0.001$). The mOS was estimated at 32.4 months in the enzalutamide group and 30.2 months in the placebo group. The treatment effect of enzalutamide on overall survival was consistent across all prespecified subgroups.

Enzalutamide has showed superiority over placebo with respect to all secondary end points. The median time to the initiation of cytotoxic chemotherapy was 28.0 months in the enzalutamide group, as compared with 10.8 months in the placebo group (HR, 0.35; $p < 0.001$). Treatment with enzalutamide also resulted in a reduction in the risk of a first skeletal-related event, which occurred in 278 patients (32%) in the enzalutamide group and 309 patients (37%) in the placebo group (HR, 0.72; $p < 0.001$) at a median of approximately 31 months in each of the two groups. Among patients with measurable soft-tissue disease at baseline, 59% of the patients in the enzalutamide group, as compared with 5% in the placebo group, had an objective response ($p < 0.001$): complete and partial responses were observed in 20% and 39% of the patients, respectively, in the enzalutamide group, as compared with 1% and 4%, respectively, in the placebo group. Enzalutamide was also superior to placebo with respect to reductions of at least 50% and 90% in the PSA level, the time until PSA progression, and the time until a decline in the quality of life. The median time until a quality-of-life deterioration, as measured on the FACT-P scale, was 11.3 months in the enzalutamide

group and 5.6 months in the placebo group (HR, 0.63; $p < 0.001$).

As to the safety profile, a grade 3 or higher adverse event was reported in 43% of the patients in the enzalutamide group, as compared with 37% in the placebo group; however, the median time until the first event of grade 3 or higher was 22.3 months in the enzalutamide group and 13.3 months in the placebo group. The most common adverse events leading to death were disease progression and a general deterioration in physical health, with similar incidences in the two groups. Adverse events that occurred in 20% or more of patients receiving enzalutamide at a rate that was at least 2 percentage points higher than that in the placebo group were fatigue, back pain, constipation, and arthralgia. The most common event of grade 3 or higher in the enzalutamide group was hypertension, which was reported in 7% of the patients. The most common cardiac event was atrial fibrillation, which was reported in 2% of the patients in the enzalutamide group and in 1% of those in the placebo group. One patient in each study group had a seizure. No evidence of hepatotoxicity was observed in the enzalutamide group.

On the basis of the results of the AFFIRM and PREVAIL trials, enzalutamide has been approved by the national agencies for drug regulation and is now part of clinical practice in mCRPC treatment algorithm.

Updates:

— The phase 3 PROfound trial results suggested a role for olaparib, an inhibitor of PARP enzyme, for castration-resistant prostate cancer patients who carry genetic -alteration in BRCA1, BRCA2, or ATM genes and other genes involved in the homologous recombination mechanism.

— TITAN phase 3 randomized trial results showed a significant delay in second progression-free survival for castration-sensitive metastatic prostate cancer patients who received apalutamide in association with standard androgen deprivation therapy (ADT) versus standard ADT.

— Immunotherapy could have a significant role in advanced prostate cancer management. In particular, preliminary results from the phase 2 KEYNOTE-199 underlined a role for the addition of anti-PD1 pembrolizumab to standard enzalutamide in a cohort of chemo-naïve metastatic castration-resistant prostate cancer patients.

Case Study Metastatic Prostate Cancer

Man, 50 years old
- *Family history:* Negative for malignancy
- *APR:* Negative
- *APP:* April 2018, lower back pain on the right, VAS 9. Prostate adenocarcinoma Gleason score 9 (4 + 5)
- Right femoral metastasis and treated since 2016 with ADT
- *Blood tests:* PSA 6 ng/dl (vs. 2.5 ng/dl vs. 11.8 ng/dl), testosterone <0.04 ng/dl
- *PET with choline:* Hypermetabolic areas in the right femur (SUV max 6 vs. 4) + right iliac wing (SUV max 5 vs. 3.8) + left iliac wing (SUV max 6 vs. 3.4) + L3-L4-L5 (SUV max 3.2). Evidence of hypermetabolic area at L1 (SUV max 5.0) and left femur (SUV max 6)

Questions

What is the disease setting?
1. mCRPC
2. mCSPC
3. Locally advanced prostate cancer

Answer

mCRPC

Question

What is the preferred therapy option in this setting?
1. Abiraterone acetate
2. Enzalutamide
3. Chemotherapy

Answer

Abiraterone acetate + corticosteroid if there are no important cardiovascular comorbidities, otherwise enzalutamide. Chemotherapy could be preferred if high disease volume or visceral metastatic sites are involved.

Key Points

- The importance of the correct disease setting
- The importance of new-generation hormonal therapies

Expert Opinion
Giuseppe Procopio

Key Points
- Prostate cancer is the most frequent solid tumor diagnosed in male people and due to its high incidence and prevalence, screening programs have been adopted among population such as the valuation of PSA; otherwise, for the frequent over-diagnosis and over-treatments, nowadays, the screening program should be carefully discussed with the patient.
- After diagnosis of PCa, the decision to proceed with systemic staging workup is guided by the risk of disease systemic spread. Curative treatments or observational strategies may be proposed according to the risk of recurrence, life expectancy, and patients' preferences.
- RP or radiotherapy (external beam or brachytherapy) are two options for low- or intermediate-risk disease.
- RP plus pelvic lymphadenectomy or external beam RT plus hormone treatment are two alternative options for high-risk or locally advanced PCa.
- Long-term adjuvant ADT is recommended for high-risk PCa patients treated with radical EBRT.

- ADT represents the cornerstone of treatment for metastatic prostate cancer.
- The early addiction of docetaxel or abiraterone acetate to ADT improves the overall survival of mHSPC, mainly in the subpopulation of high-volume and in high-risk patients.
- Several therapeutic options have demonstrated to improve patients' outcomes in the mCRPC setting, including docetaxel, cabazitaxel, abiraterone and enzalutamide, and Radium-223.

Recommendations
- ESMO
  ▶ www.esmo.org/Guidelines/Genitourinary-Cancers/ESMO-Consensus-Guidelines-Prostate-cancer
- NCCN
  ▶ jnccn.org/view/journals/jnccn/17/5/article-p479.xml
- ASCO
  ▶ www.asco.org/practice-guidelines/quality-guidelines/guidelines/genitourinary-cancer#/32796
  ▶ www.asco.org/practice-guidelines/quality-guidelines/guidelines/genitourinary-cancer#/33301

▶ www.asco.org/practice-guidelines/quality-guide-lines/guidelines/genitourinary-cancer#/25251

▶ www.asco.org/practice-guidelines/quality-guide-lines/guidelines/genitourinary-cancer#/24836

Hints for a Deeper Insight

- Phase II study of pembrolizumab (MK-3475) in patients with metastatic castration-resistant prostate cancer (KEYNOTE-199)-study AP 93/16 of the AUO: ▶ https://www.ncbi.nlm.nih.gov/pubmed/28980011
- Prostate cancer between prognosis and adequate/proper therapy: ▶ https://www.ncbi.nlm.nih.gov/pubmed/28255369
- Prostate Cancer Genetics: Variation by Race, Ethnicity, and Geography: ▶ https://www.ncbi.nlm.nih.gov/pubmed/27986209

References

1. Weiner AB, Matulewicz RS, Eggener SE, Schaeffer EM. Increasing incidence of metastatic prostate cancer in the United States (2004–2013). Prostate Cancer Prostatic Dis. 2016;19:395–7.
2. Buzzoni C, Auvinen A, Roobol MJ, et al. Metastatic Prostate Cancer incidence and prostate-specific antigen testing: new insights from the European Randomized Study of Screening for Prostate Cancer. Eur Urol. 2015;68(5):885–90. https://doi.org/10.1016/j.eururo.2015.02.042.
3. Cetin K, Beebe-Dimmer JL, Fryzek JP, Markus R, Carducci MA. Recent time trends in the epidemiology of stage IV prostate cancer in the United States: analysis of data from the surveillance, epidemiology, and end results program. Urology. 2010;75(6):1396–404.
4. Finianos A, Gupta K, Clark B, Simmens SJ, Aragon-Ching JB. Characterization of differences between prostate cancer patients presenting with De Novo versus primary progressive metastatic disease. Clin Genitourin Cancer. 2017. pii: S1558-7673(17)30247-1. https://doi.org/10.1016/j.clgc.2017.08.006. [Epub ahead of print].
5. James ND, Spears MR, Clarke NW, Dearnaley DP, De Bono JS, Gale J, Hetherington J, Hoskin PJ, Jones RJ, Laing R, Lester JF, McLaren D, Parker CC, Parmar MKB, Ritchie AWS, Russell JM, Strebel RT, Thalmann GN, Mason MD, Sydes MR. Survival with newly diagnosed metastatic prostate cancer in the "Docetaxel Era": data from 917 patients in the control arm of the STAMPEDE Trial (MRC PR08, CRUK/06/019). Eur Urol. 2015;67(6):1028–38.
6. Berg KD, Thomsen FB, Mikkelsen MK, Ingimarsdóttir IJ, Hansen RB, Kejs AM, Brasso K. Improved survival for patients with de novo metastatic prostate cancer in the last 20 years. Eur J Cancer. 2017;72:20–7.
7. Glass TR, Tangen CM, Crawford ED, Thompson I. Metastatic carcinoma of the prostate: identifying prognostic groups using recursive partitioning. J Urol. 2003;169(1):164–9.
8. Crawford ED. Understanding the epidemiology, natural history, and key pathways involved in prostate cancer. Urology. 2009;73(5 Suppl):S4–10.
9. McGuire BB, Helfand BT, Loeb S, Hu Q, O'Brien D, Cooper P, Yang X, Catalona WJ. Outcomes in patients with Gleason score 8-10 prostate cancer: relation to preoperative PSA level. BJU Int. 2012;109(12):1764–9.
10. Hussain M, Tangen CM, Higano C, Schelhammer PF, Faulkner J, Crawford ED, Wilding G, Akdas A, Small EJ, Donnelly B, MacVicar G, Raghavan D, Southwest Oncology Group Trial 9346 (INT-0162). Absolute prostate-specific antigen value after androgen deprivation is a strong independent predictor of survival in new metastatic prostate cancer: data from Southwest Oncology Group Trial 9346 (INT-0162). J Clin Oncol. 2006;24(24):3984–90.
11. Gravis G, Boher JM, Fizazi K, Joly F, Priou F, Marino P, Latorzeff I, Delva R, Krakowski I, Laguerre B, Walz J, Rolland F, Théodore C, Deplanque G, Ferrero JM, Pouessel D, Mourey L, Beuzeboc P, Zanetta S, Habibian M, Berdah JF, Dauba J, Baciuchka M, Platini C, Linassier C, Labourey JL, Machiels JP, El Kouri C, Ravaud A, Suc E, Eymard JC, Hasbini A, Bousquet G, Soulie M, Oudard S. Prognostic factors for survival in noncastrate metastatic prostate cancer: validation of the glass model and development of a novel simplified prognostic model. Eur Urol. 2015;68(2):196–204.
12. Nørgaard M, Jensen AØ, Jacobsen JB, Cetin K, Fryzek JP, Sørensen HT. Skeletal related events, bone metastasis and survival of prostate cancer: a population based cohort study in Denmark (1999 to 2007). Mk J Urol. 2010;184(1):162–7.
13. Gandaglia G, Karakiewicz PI, Briganti A, Passoni NM, Schiffmann J, Trudeau V, Graefen M, Montorsi F, Sun M. Impact of the site of metastases on survival in patients with metastatic prostate cancer. Eur Urol. 2015;68(2):325–34.
14. Vinjamoori AH, Jagannathan JP, Shinagare AB, Taplin ME, Oh WK, Van den Abbeele AD, Ramaiya NH. Atypical metastases from prostate cancer: 10-year experience at a single institution. Hu AJR Am J Roentgenol. 2012;199(2):367–72.
15. Huggins C, Stephens RE, Hodges CV. Studies on prostate cancer II. The effects of castration on advanced carcinoma of the prostate. Arch Surg. 1941;43:209–23.
16. Pagliarulo V, Bracarda S, Eisenberger MA, Mottet N, Schröder FH, Sternberg CN, Studer UE. Contemporary role of androgen deprivation therapy for prostate cancer. Eur Urol. 2012;61(1):11–25.
17. Crawford ED, Hou AH. The role of LHRH antagonists in the treatment of prostate cancer. Oncology. 2009;23(7):626–30.
18. Weckermann D, Harzmann R. Hormone therapy in prostate cancer: LHRH antagonists versus LHRH analogues. Eur Urol. 2004;46:279–83.
19. Seidenfeld J, Samson DJ, Hasselblad V, Aronson N, Albertsen PC, Bennett CL, Wilt TJ. Single-therapy androgen suppression in men with advanced prostate cancer: a systematic review and meta-analysis. Ann Intern Med. 2000;132(7):566–77.
20. Eisenberger MA, Blumenstein BA, Crawford ED, Miller G, McLeod DG, Loehrer PJ, Wilding G, Sears K, Culkin DJ, Thompson IM Jr, Bueschen AJ, Lowe BA. Bilateral orchiectomy with or without flutamide for metastatic prostate cancer. N Engl J Med. 1998;339:1036–42.

21. Crawford ED, Eisenberger MA, McLeod DG, Spaulding JT, Benson R, Dorr FA, Blumenstein BA, Davis MA, Goodman PJ. A controlled trial of leuprolide with and without flutamide in prostatic carcinoma. N Engl J Med. 1989;321:419–24.

22. Akaza H, Hinotsu S, Usami M, Arai Y, Kanetake H, Naito S, Hirao Y. Combined androgen blockade with bicalutamide for advanced prostate cancer: long-term follow-up of a phase 3, double-blind, randomized study for survival. Cancer. 2009;115: 3437–45.

23. Prostate Cancer Trialists' Collaborative Group. Maximum androgen blockade in advanced prostate cancer: an overview of the randomised trials. Lancet. 2000;355:1491–8.

24. Samson DJ, Seidenfeld J, Schmitt B, et al. Systematic review and meta-analysis of monotherapy compared with combined androgen blockade for patients with advanced prostate carcinoma. Cancer. 2002;95:361–76.

25. Hussain M, Tangen CM, Berry DL, Higano CS, Crawford ED, Liu G, Wilding G, Prescott S, Kanaga Sundaram S, Small EJ, Dawson NA, Donnelly BJ, Venner PM, et al. Intermittent versus continuous androgen deprivation in prostate cancer. N Engl J Med. 2013;368:1314–25.

26. Fitzpatrick JM, de Wit R. Taxane mechanisms of action: potential implications for treatment sequencing in metastatic castration-resistant prostate cancer. Eur Urol. 2014;65(6): 1198–204.

27. Gan L, Chen S, Wang Y, Watahiki A, Bohrer L, Sun Z, Wang Y, Huang H. Inhibition of the androgen receptor as a novel mechanism of taxol chemotherapy in prostate cancer. Cancer Res. 2009;69(21):8386–94.

28. Gravis G, Fizazi K, Joly F, Oudard S, Priou F, Esterni B, Latorzeff I, Delva R, Krakowski I, Laguerre B, Rolland F, Théodore C, Deplanque G, Ferrero JM, Pouessel D, Mourey L, Beuzeboc P, Zanetta S, Habibian M, Berdah JF, Dauba J, Baciuchka M, Platini C, Linassier C, Labourey JL, Machiels JP, El Kouri C, Ravaud A, Suc E, Eymard JC, Hasbini A, Bousquet G, Soulie M. Androgen-deprivation therapy alone or with docetaxel in non-castrate metastatic prostate cancer (GETUG-AFU 15): a randomised, open-label, phase 3 trial. Lancet Oncol. 2013;14(2):149–58.

29. Gravis G, Boher JM, Joly F, Soulié M, Albiges L, Priou F, Latorzeff I, Delva R, Krakowski I, Laguerre B, Rolland F, Théodore C, Deplanque G, Ferrero JM, Culine S, Mourey L, Beuzeboc P, Habibian M, Oudard S, Fizazi K, GETUG. Androgen deprivation therapy (ADT) plus docetaxel versus ADT alone in metastatic non castrate prostate Cancer: impact of metastatic burden and long-term survival analysis of the randomized phase 3 GETUG-AFU15 trial. Eur Urol. 2016;70(2):256–62.

30. Sweeney CJ, Chen YH, Carducci M, Liu G, Jarrard DF, Eisenberger M, Wong YN, Hahn N, Kohli M, Cooney MM, Dreicer R, Vogelzang NJ, Picus J, Shevrin D, Hussain M, Garcia JA, DiPaola RS. Chemohormonal therapy in metastatic hormone-sensitive prostate cancer. N Engl J Med. 2015;373(8):737–46.

31. James ND, Sydes MR, Clarke NW, Mason MD, Dearnaley DP, Spears MR, Ritchie AW, Parker CC, Russell JM, Attard G, de Bono J, Cross W, Jones RJ, Thalmann G, Amos C, Matheson D, Millman R, Alzouebi M, Beesley S, Birtle AJ, Brock S, Cathomas R, Chakraborti P, Chowdhury S, Cook A, Elliott T, Gale J, Gibbs S, Graham JD, Hetherington J, Hughes R, Laing R, McKinna F, McLaren DB, O'Sullivan JM, Parikh O, Peedell C, Protheroe A, Robinson AJ, Srihari N, Srinivasan R, Staffurth J, Sundar S, Tolan S, Tsang D, Wagstaff J, Parmar MK, STAMPEDE investigators. Addition of docetaxel, zoledronic acid, or both to first-line long-term hormone therapy in prostate cancer (STAMPEDE): survival results from an adaptive, multi-arm, multistage, platform randomised controlled trial. Lancet. 2016;387(10024):1163–77.

32. Vale CL, Burdett S, Rydzewska LHM, Albiges L, Clarke NW, Fisher D, Fizazi K, Gravis G, James ND, Mason MD, Parmar MKB, Sweeney CJ, Sydes MR, Tombal B, Tierney JF, STOpCaP Steering Group. Addition of docetaxel or bisphosphonates to standard of care in men with localised or metastatic, hormone-sensitive prostate cancer: a systematic review and meta-analyses of aggregate data. Lancet Oncol. 2016;17(2):243–56.

33. Tucci M, Bertaglia V, Vignani F, Buttigliero C, Fiori C, Porpiglia F, Scagliotti GV, Di Maio M. Addition of docetaxel to androgen deprivation therapy for patients with hormone-sensitive metastatic prostate cancer: a systematic review and meta-analysis. Eur Urol. 2016;69(4):563–73.

34. Fizazi K, Tran N, Fein L, Matsubara N, Rodriguez-Antolin A, Alekseev BY, Özgüroğlu M, Ye D, Feyerabend S, Protheroe A, De Porre P, Kheoh T, Park YC, Todd MB, Chi KN, LATITUDE Investigators. Abiraterone plus prednisone in metastatic, castration-sensitive prostate cancer. N Engl J Med. 2017;377(4): 352–60.

35. James ND, de Bono JS, Spears MR, Clarke NW, Mason MD, Dearnaley DP, AWS R, Amos CL, Gilson C, Jones RJ, Matheson D, Millman R, Attard G, Chowdhury S, Cross WR, Gillessen S, Parker CC, Russell JM, Berthold DR, Brawley C, Adab F, Aung S, Birtle AJ, Bowen J, Brock S, Chakraborti P, Ferguson C, Gale J, Gray E, Hingorani M, Hoskin PJ, Lester JF, Malik ZI, McKinna F, McPhail N, Money-Kyrle J, O'Sullivan J, Parikh O, Protheroe A, Robinson A, Srihari NN, Thomas C, Wagstaff J, Wylie J, Zarkar A, MKB P, Sydes MR, STAMPEDE Investigators. Abiraterone for prostate cancer not previously treated with hormone therapy. N Engl J Med. 2017;377(4):338–51.

36. Sydes MR, Mason MD, Spears MR, et al. Adding abiraterone acetate plus prednisolone (AAP) or docetaxel for patients (pts) with high-risk prostate cancer (PCa) starting long-term androgen deprivation therapy (ADT): directly randomised data from STAMPEDE (NCT00268476), Abstract LBA31_PR, ESMO 2017.

37. Scher HI, Solo K, Valant J, et al. Prevalence of prostate cancer clinical states and mortality in the United States: estimates using a dynamic progression model. PLoS One. 2015;10:e0139440.

38. Mottet N, Bellmunt J, Briers E et al. EAU-ESTRO-SIOG guidelines on prostate cancer; 2016.

39. Eisenberger MA, Simon R, O'Dwyer PJ, et al. A reevaluation of nonhormonal cytotoxic chemotherapy in the treatment of prostatic carcinoma. J Clin Oncol. 1985;3:827–41.

40. Tannock IF, Osoba D, Stockler MR, et al. Chemotherapy with mitoxantrone plus prednisone or prednisone alone for symptomatic hormone resistant prostate cancer: a Canadian randomized trial with palliative end points. J Clin Oncol. 1996;14: 1756–64.

41. Berry W, Dakhil S, Modiano M, et al. Phase III study of mitoxantrone plus low dose prednisone versus low dose prednisone alone in patients with asymptomatic hormone refractory prostate cancer. J Urol. 2002;168:2439–43.

42. D'Amico AV. US Food and Drug Administration approval of drugs for the treatment of prostate cancer: a new era has begun. J Clin Oncol. 2014;32:362–4.

43. Figg W, Chau CH, Small EJ, editors. Drug management of prostate cancer. New York NY: Springer; 2010.

44. Albrecht W, Van Poppel H, Horenblas S, et al. Randomized phase II trial assessing estramustine and vinblastine combination chemotherapy vs. estramustine alone in patients with progressive hormone-escaped metastatic prostate cancer. Br J Cancer. 2004;90:100–5.

48

45. Eymard JC, Priou F, Zannetti A, et al. Randomized phase II study of docetaxel plus estramustine and single-agent docetaxel in patients with metastatic hormone-refractory prostate cancer. Ann Oncol. 2007;18:1064–70.

46. Fizazi K, Le Maitre A, Hudes G, et al. Addition of estramustine to chemotherapy and survival of patients with castration-refractory prostate cancer: a meta-analysis of individual patient data. Lancet Oncol. 2007;8:994–1000.

47. Tannock IF, de Wit R, Berry WR, et al. Docetaxel plus prednisone or mitoxantrone plus prednisone for advanced prostate cancer. N Engl J Med. 2004;351:1502–12.

48. Petrylak DP, Tangen CM, Hussain MH, et al. Docetaxel and estramustine compared with mitoxantrone and prednisone for advanced refractory prostate cancer. N Engl J Med. 2004;351: 1513–20.

49. de Bono JS, Oudard S, Ozguroglu M, et al. Prednisone plus cabazitaxel or mitoxantrone for metastatic castration-resistant prostate cancer progressing after docetaxel treatment: a randomised open-label trial. Lancet. 2010;376:1147–54.

50. de Bono JS, Hardy-Bessard AC, Kim CS, et al. Phase III noninferiority study of cabazitaxel (C) 20 mg/m2 (C20) versus 25 mg/m2 (C25) in patients (pts) with metastatic castration-resistant prostate cancer (mCRPC) previously treated with docetaxel (D). J Clin Oncol. 2016;34(Abstr 5008)

51. Sartor O, Oudard S, Sengelov L, et al. Cabazitaxel vs. docetaxel in chemotherapy-naïve patients with metastatic castration-resistant prostate cancer: a three-arm phase III study (FIRSTANA). J Clin Oncol. 2016;34(Abstr 5006)

52. Henriksen G, Breistol K, Bruland OS, et al. Significant antitumor effect from bone-seeking, alpha-particle-emitting (223)Ra demonstrated in an experimental skeletal metastases model. Cancer Res. 2002;62:3120–5.

53. Bruland OS, Nilsson S, Fisher DR, et al. High-linear energy transfer irradiation targeted to skeletal metastases by the alpha-emitter 223Ra: adjuvant or alternative to conventional modalities? Clin Cancer Res. 2006;12:6250s–7s.

54. Suominen MI, Fagerlund KM, Rissanen JP, et al. Radium-223 inhibits osseous prostate cancer growth by dual targeting of cancer cells and bone microenvironment in mouse models. Clin Cancer Res. 2017;23:4335–46.

55. Nilsson S, Larsen RH, Foss SD, et al. First clinical experience with alpha-emitting radium-223 in the treatment of skeletal metastases. Clin Cancer Res. 2005;11:4451–9.

56. Nilsson S, Franzén L, Parker C, et al. Bone-targeted radium-223 in symptomatic, hormone-refractory prostate cancer: a randomised, multicentre, placebo-controlled phase II study. Lancet Oncol. 2007;8:587–94.

57. Parker CC, Pascoe S, Chodacki A, et al. A randomized, double-blind, dose-finding, multicenter, phase 2 study of radium chloride (Ra-223) in patients with bone metastases and castration-resistant prostate cancer. Eur Urol. 2013;63:189–97.

58. Nilsson S, Strang P, Aksnes AK, et al. A randomized, dose-response, multicenter phase II study of radium-223 chloride for the palliation of painful bone metastases in patients with castration-resistant prostate cancer. Eur J Cancer. 2012;48:678–86.

59. Parker C, Nilsson S, Heinrich D, et al. Alpha emitter radium-223 and survival in metastatic prostate cancer. N Engl J Med. 2013;369:213–23.

60. de Bono JS, Logothetis CJ, Molina A, et al. Abiraterone and prednisone increased survival in metastatic prostate cancer. N Engl J Med. 2011;364(21):1995–2005.

61. Fizazi K, Scher HI, Molina A, et al. Abiraterone acetate for treatment of metastatic castration-resistant prostate cancer: final overall survival analysis of the COU-AA-301 randomised, double-blind, placebo-controlled phase 3 study. Lancet Oncol. 2012;13(10):983–92.

62. Ryan CJ, Smith MR, de Bono JS, et al. Abiraterone in metastatic prostate cancer without previous chemotherapy. N Engl J Med. 2013;368(2):138–48.

63. Ryan CJ, Smith MR, Fizazi K, et al. Abiraterone acetate plus prednisone versus placebo plus prednisone in chemotherapy-naive men with metastatic castration-resistant prostate cancer (COU-AA-302): final overall survival analysis of a randomised, double-blind, placebo-controlled phase 3 study. Lancet Oncol. 2015;16(2):152–60.

64. Rathkopf DE, Smith MR, de Bono JS, et al. Updated interim efficacy analysis and long-term safety of abiraterone acetate in metastatic castration-resistant prostate cancer patients without prior chemotherapy (COU-AA-302). Eur Urol. 2014;66(5):815–25.

65. Sternberg CN, Molina A, North S, et al. Effect of abiraterone acetate on fatigue in patients with metastatic castration-resistant prostate cancer after docetaxel chemotherapy. Ann Oncol. 2013;24(4):1017–25.

66. Harland S, Staffurth J, Molina A, et al. Effect of abiraterone acetate treatment on the quality of life of patients with metastatic castration-resistant prostate cancer after failure of docetaxel chemotherapy. Eur J Cancer. 2013;49(17):3648–57.

67. Jung ME, Ouk S, Yoo D, et al. Structure-activity relationship for thiohydantoin androgen receptor antagonists for castration-resistant prostate cancer (CRPC). J Med Chem. 2010;53:2779–96.

68. Tran C, Ouk S, Clegg NJ, et al. Development of a second-generation antiandrogen for treatment of advanced prostate cancer. Science. 2009;324:787–90.

69. Morris MJ, Basch EM, Wilding G, et al. Department of Defense prostate cancer clinical trials consortium: a new instrument for prostate cancer clinical research. Clin Genitourin Cancer. 2009;7:51–7.

70. Scher HI, Beer TM, Higano CS, et al. Antitumour activity of MDV3100 in castration-resistant prostate cancer: a phase 1-2 study. Lancet. 2010;375:1437–46.

71. Scher HI, Fizazi K, Saad F, et al. Increased survival with enzalutamide in prostate cancer after chemotherapy. N Engl J Med. 2012;367(13):1187–97.

72. Beer TM, Armstrong AJ, Rathkopf DE, et al. Enzalutamide in metastatic prostate cancer before chemotherapy. N Engl J Med. 2014;371(5):424–33.

Testicular Cancer

Andreia Coelho, Patricia Gago, Miguel Barbosa, and Antonio Teira

Genitourinary Cancers

Contents

© Springer Nature Switzerland AG 2021
A. Russo et al. (eds.), *Practical Medical Oncology Textbook*, UNIPA Springer Series,
https://doi.org/10.1007/978-3-030-56051-5_49

Learning Objectives

By the end of the chapter, the reader will:

- Be able to detect a possible patient with testicular cancer
- Have learned how to manage the work-up and diagnosis of testicular cancer
- Have reached in-depth knowledge of treatment of this pathology
- Be able to put acquired knowledge into clinical practice
- Be able to follow-up these patients both to detect relapse and late toxicity

49.1 Introduction

Testicular cancer is the most common malignant solid tumor in young men between the second and fourth decade of life, and it accounts for approximately 1% of all cancers in men [1].

The classification of testicular cancer includes several types of testicular cancers but the germ-cell tumor (GCT) is the most frequent (about 95%). Approximately 50% are pure seminoma and the other 50% are non-seminoma [2].

The 5-year survival for localized testicular cancer is 99.2%, while for metastatic testicular cancer it is 73.2% [3]; therefore, a careful staging at diagnosis, adequate early treatment based on a multidisciplinary approach, and strict follow-up and salvage therapies are very important approaches for the delivery of the best treatment.

49.2 Epidemiology

Nearly 8.850 men are diagnosed with testicular cancer yearly in the United States, but only around 410 will die of their disease [1]. In Europe the rate of incidence is 5.8% (21.532/100.000) and the mortality rate is 0.4% (1612/100.000) [4].

There are some known risk factors such as:
- Cryptorchidism [5]
- Personal or family history of testicular cancer [6–8]
- Infertility or subfertility [9]

49.3 Clinical Features

Testicular cancer usually presents as a nodule or a painless swelling in one testicle.

When there are metastases, symptoms can vary from neck mass (supraclavicular adenopathy), cough or dyspnea (lung metastases), abdominal or lumbar back pain (retroperitoneal disease), bone pain (bone metastases), central nervous system (CNS) symptoms (CNS metastases), or lower extremities swelling (obstruction or thrombosis).

In about 5% of the GCT patients, they can be presented with gynecomastia, which is a systemic endocrine manifestation associated with production of human chorionic gonadotropin (hCG) by foci of choriocarcinoma or trophoblastic cells in the tumor [10].

49.4 Diagnosis

49.4.1 Clinical Examination

In the case of a suspected testicular nodule or swelling, the physical examination should include scrotum palpation to evaluate the nodule or swelling. A complete physical examination should be performed to search for any other findings such as gynecomastia, abdominal palpable mass, or supraclavicular mass.

49.4.2 Imaging

Testicular ultrasound is useful to confirm the presence of a testicular mass and explore the contralateral testis [2]. It is a very sensitive diagnostic method and it is important to evaluate whether the mass is intra- or extra-testicular.

If a patient is diagnosed with a retroperitoneal mass or has elevated serum tumor marker suggesting extragonadal GCT, a testicular ultrasound should be performed even in the absence of palpable testicular mass [11] (EAU guidelines).

The imaging studies should also include a chest radiography.

49.4.3 Serum Tumor Markers

The serum tumor markers assume a crucial role in testicular cancer. Alpha-fetoprotein (AFP), lactate dehydrogenase (LDH), and beta-hCG are essential in the diagnosis, staging, prognosis, and assessment of treatment outcome. They should be measured before and after treatment and throughout the follow-up period [11].

AFP is produced by non-seminomatous cells and it has a half-life of 5–7 days; therefore, a non-seminoma is associated with elevated AFP. If a pure seminoma has an elevated AFP, then an undetected focus of non-seminoma is present [12]. Beta-hCG can be elevated in both seminoma and non-seminoma tumors and it has a half-life of about 1–3 days.

49.4.4 Screening

There are no recommendations for screening for testicular cancer. However, individuals with risk factors and especially in patients with a family history of testicular cancer, family members and the patient should be informed about the importance of physical self-examination [11].

49.5 Differential Diagnosis

The differential diagnoses are:
- Epididymitis
- Orchitis
- Hydrocele
- Abdominal hernias
- Varicocele
- Lymphoma
- Trauma
- Metastases from other tumors
- Testicular torsion

49.5.1 Pathology

The natural evolution of the disease depends of the histological subtype [13, 14] (▶ Box 49.1):

Box 49.1 Classification of testicular cancer according to the World Health Organization Classification of Tumors 2016

Germ-cell tumors
Seminoma
Non-seminoma
- Embryonal carcinoma
- Choriocarcinoma
- Yolk sac tumor
- Teratoma
- Teratoma with malignant/somatic transformation
- Mixed germ-cell tumor

Spermatocytic tumor
Sex cord-stromal tumors
- Sertoli cell tumor
- Leydig cell tumor
- Granulosa cell tumor
- Mixed types
- Unclassified

Mixed germ-cell and stromal tumors
- Gonadoblastoma

Adnexal and paratesticular tumors
- Adenocarcinoma of rete testis
- Adenocarcinoma of the epididymis
- Mesothelioma
  - Malignant mesothelioma
  - Adenomatoid tumor

Miscellaneous tumors
- Carcinoid
- Lymphoma
- Metastatic tumors

- Seminoma: It represents approximately 45% of testicular tumors. At diagnosis 25% of the patients presented lymphatic and up to 5% visceral metastases (lung and bone mainly).
- Spermatocytic seminoma represents 4% of seminomas and usually appears in older patients with germ-cell tumor and more frequent in patients older than 70 years. They are most often bilateral and its metastatic potential is minimal.
- Pure choriocarcinoma: It is rare (0.3%). It is the most aggressive and metastasizes quickly through hematogenous spread. It has elevated HCG and normal alpha-fetoprotein concentrations.
- Yolk sac tumor: It produces AFP; it has worse prognosis in adults compared to children.
- Embryonal carcinoma: In pure form it represents 3% of the cases and in the mixed form it is present in more than 40% of adult testicular tumors. It is a tumor consisting of undifferentiated cells. 33% of elevation of AFP is associated.
- Teratoma: You can see the three germ layers' (ectoderm, mesoderm, and endoderm) fabrics; it may undergo a malignant transformation and this produces metastasis. The most common is the mesodermal differentiation.

Other tumors with less constraints:
- Leydig cell tumor, Sertoli cell tumor, and granulosa cell tumor: They do not present serious elevations of AFP or hCG. They can produce metastases. Sertoli cell tumors are chemo-resistant. Granulosa cell tumors have juvenile and adult forms and usually have a benign behavior [15–17].
- Rhabdomyosarcoma: It is more frequent in those younger than 20 years old. Metastatic potential is fundamentally to lymph nodes and lungs.

49

49.6 Staging

Physical examination; history; determination of serum level of AFP, beta-hCG, and LDH; pathology; and imaging studies define the extension of disease and appropriate treatment [13].

The recommended staging system is based on the classification of the International Union Against Cancer (UICC), with the TNMS system (tumor, node, metastasis, and serum markers) including the anatomical extension (T), the invasion of regional nodes (N), and the presence of metastasis (M) with local characterization (■ Tables 49.1 and 49.2). Serum concentrations of tumor markers, AFP, beta-hCG, and LDH and the nadir value post-orchiectomy are incorporated into the S category [18].

49.6.1 Imaging Studies

Computed tomography (CT): It is used to identify metastatic involvement above and below the diaphragm. Oral and intravenous contrast is the best for identifying retroperitoneal lymphadenopathy [19].

Positron emission tomography (PET): It yields no improvement in clinical staging and no value in post-chemotherapy management [20].

Magnetic resonance imaging (MRI): It occasionally provides valuable information regarding vascular anatomy or liver disease [13].

49.6.2 Risk Classification for Advanced Disease

For the advanced disease, the International Germ Cell Cancer Collaborative Group (IGCCCG) defined a prognostic classification system based on the extent of disease and levels of serum tumor markers post-orchiectomy and divides seminomas and non-seminomas in good-, intermediate-, and poor-risk groups (■ Table 49.3) [2].

49.7 Treatment

49.7.1 Fertility Issues

Patients with testicular cancer frequently present sperm alterations, and the chemotherapy and radiotherapy contribute to fertility impairment. It is important to assess their fertility pretreatment and they should be informed of their options, e.g., cryopreservation [11].

■ **Table 49.1** Staging system of testicular cancer according to the TNMS system

TNM category	Description
Primary tumor (T)	
TX	Primary tumor cannot be assessed
T0	No evidence of primary tumor
Tis	Intratubular germ-cell neoplasia
T1	Tumor limited to the testis and epididymis or tumor invasion into the tunica albuginea only
T2	Tumor extending through the tunica albuginea with involvement of the tunica vaginalis
T3	Tumor invades the spermatic cord
T4	Tumor invades the scrotum
Regional lymph nodes – Clinical (N) or pathologic (pN) staging	
NX	Regional lymph nodes cannot be assessed
N0	No regional lymph node metastasis
N1	Metastases to single or multiple lymph nodes, each <2 cm in size
N2	Metastases to single or multiple lymph nodes, >2 cm but <5 cm in size
N3	Metastases to lymph node, >5 cm in greatest dimension
Distant metastasis (M)	
MX	Distant metastasis cannot be assessed
M0	No distant metastasis
M1	Distant metastasis
M1a	Nonregional nodal or pulmonary metastasis
M1b	Distant metastasis other than to nonregional lymph nodes and lungs
Serum tumor markers	
SX	Unavailable or not performed
S0	Within normal limits
S1	Lactate dehydrogenase (LDH) level <1.5 times normal, human chorionic gonadotropin (HCG) level <5000 IU/L, alpha-fetoprotein (AFP) level <1000 ng/mL
S2	LDH 1.5–10 times normal; HCG level, 5000–50,000 IU/L; AFP level, 1000–10,000 ng/mL
S3	LDH >10 times normal; HCG level >50,000 IU/L; AFP level >10,000 ng/mL

Table 49.2 Anatomical staging and prognostic groups

Stage	T	N	M	S
0	pTis	N0	M0	S0, Sx
I	pT1 – pT4	N0	M0	Sx
IA	pT1	N0	M0	S0
IB	pT2-pT4	N0	M0	S0
IS	Any pT	N0	M0	S1 – 3
II	Any pT	N1 – N3	M0	Sx
IIA	Any pT	N1	M0	S0
		N1	M0	S1
IIB	Any pT	N2	M0	S0
	Any pT	N2	M0	S1
IIC	Any pT	N3	M0	S0
	Any pT	N3	M0	S1
III	Any pT	Any N	M1	Sx
IIIA	Any pT	Any N	M1a	S0
	Any pT	Any N	M1a	S1
IIIB	Any pT	N1-N3	M0	S2
	Any pT	Any N	M1a	S2
IIIC	Any pT	N1-N3	M0	S3
	Any pT	Any N	M1a	S3
	Any pT	Any N	M1b	Any S

Table 49.3 Risk classification for advanced disease

Risk status	Non-seminoma	Seminoma
Good risk	Testicular or retroperitoneal primary tumor	Any primary site
	No nonpulmonary visceral metastases	No nonpulmonary visceral metastases
	AFP <1000 ng/mL hCG <5000 IU/L LDH <1.5 × upper limit of normal	Normal AFP Any hCG Any LDH
Intermediate risk	Testicular or retroperitoneal primary tumor	Any primary site
	No nonpulmonary visceral metastases	Nonpulmonary visceral metastases
	Post-orchiectomy markers – Any of the following: hCG 5000–50,000 IU/L LDH 1.5–10 × upper limit of normal	Normal AFP Any hCG Any LDH
Poor risk	Mediastinal primary tumor	No patients classified as poor Prognosis
	Nonpulmonary visceral metastases	
	Post-orchiectomy markers – any of the following: AFP >10,000 ng/mL hCG >50,000 IU/L LDH >10 × upper limit of normal	

49.7.2 Management of Testicular Cancer

The treatment of seminoma and NSGCT involves surgery, radiotherapy, and chemotherapy and depends on the disease stage [2, 11, 18].

49.7.2.1 Primary Treatment
The primary treatment for the majority of testis tumors is radical inguinal orchiectomy. A testicular prosthesis should be offered to every patient.

Seminoma germ-cell tumor first-line treatment (⬛ Algorithm 49.1)

49.7.2.2 Stage I Seminoma
In this stage, most of the patients are cured after surgery and the rate of relapse is small, so the toxicity should be minimized. Surveillance is the preferred option for this stage.

In alternative, one course of adjuvant carboplatin therapy AUC 7 can be used or adjuvant radiotherapy as seminoma cells are extremely radiosensitive.

The risk factors that divide seminoma stage I into low- and high-risk groups for occult metastatic disease are tumor size >4 cm and rete testis invasion.

49.7.2.3 Stage IS Seminoma
Stage IS is a very rare type of seminoma with persistent elevation of serum tumor markers after surgery, which can be evidence of metastatic disease. The extent of disease should be determined by imaging studies. The chemotherapy is similar to the non-seminoma tumors.

49.7.2.4 Stage IIA Seminoma
In this stage, adjuvant radiotherapy of the para-aortic region and ipsilateral iliac nodes reaches an overall survival of almost 100%. In case of multiple node involvement, chemotherapy with EP (etoposide and cisplatin) × 4 or BEP (bleomycin, etoposide, and cisplatin) × 3 is an option.

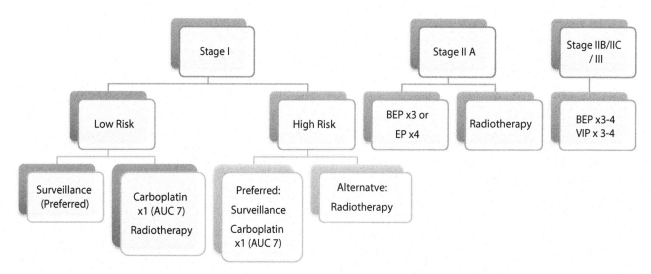

☐ **Algorithm 49.1**   Seminoma germ-cell tumor first-line treatment

49.7.2.5   Stage IIB Seminoma

Adjuvant radiotherapy can be an option for stage IIB seminoma (non-bulky disease). For cases with adenopathy greater than 3 cm, adjuvant chemotherapy with EP × 4 or BEP × 3 is an option.

49.7.2.6   Stage IIC Seminoma

Adjuvant chemotherapy with BEP × 3 or EP × 4 is recommended.

49.7.2.7   Stage III Seminoma

Stage III patients are divided into good or intermediate risk (nonpulmonary visceral metastases).

In the good-risk group, adjuvant chemotherapy with BEP × 3 or EP × 4 is recommended.

In the intermediate group, chemotherapy with BEP × 4 or VIP (etoposide, mesna, ifosfamide, and cisplatin) × 4 is recommended.

49.7.2.8   Post-chemotherapy Management of Seminoma Stages II–III

Serum tumor markers and CT scan are used to evaluate the presence of residual mass. In case of normal serum tumor markers and no residual mass or mass less than 3 cm, no more treatment is needed and the patient should be on surveillance.

In case of residual tumor, a PET scan should be performed 6 weeks after chemotherapy. If the PET scan is negative, the patient should go under follow-up. If the PET scan is positive, biopsy of the mass or resection should be considered, and if the results show seminoma, chemotherapy with EP × 2 or TIP (paclitaxel, ifosfamide, and cisplatin) × 2 is recommended. In case of incomplete resection, TIP × 4 or

VeIP (vinblastine, ifosfamide, and cisplatin) × 4 is recommended.

Non-seminoma germ-cell tumor first-line treatment

49.7.2.9   Stage I Non-seminoma

This stage has high survival rates. It can be divided into low or high risk based on absence or presence of vascular invasion, respectively.

In the low-risk group, surveillance is standard, but if it is not possible, adjuvant chemotherapy with one or two cycles of BEP is recommended. If the patient is not fit for chemotherapy, open nerve-sparing retroperitoneal lymph node dissection (RPLND) is an option.

In the high-risk group, surveillance and chemotherapy (one or two cycles of BEP) are options. Open nerve-sparing RPLND can be an option.

49.7.2.10   Stage IS Non-seminoma

Chemotherapy with EP ×4 or BEP ×3 is recommended. Hepatobiliary disease, use of marijuana, and hypogonadism may be the reason for elevated serum tumor markers post-orchiectomy, so results should be interpreted with caution.

49.7.2.11   Stage IIA Non-seminoma

The treatment for these patients depends on the serum tumor marker levels:

— In case of normal serum tumor markers post-orchiectomy, RPLND or chemotherapy with four cycles of EP or three cycles of BEP is recommended.
  — If the disease is multifocal, chemotherapy is the best option.
— In case of persistent elevation of serum tumor markers, the risk of relapse is elevated, so induction chemotherapy is recommended.

49.7.2.12 Management of Non-seminoma Stage IIA After Primary Treatment

After primary chemotherapy, AFP and beta-hCG levels should be assessed and an abdominal and pelvic CT with contrast should be done and a chest CT or X-rays may be considered.

In case of negative serum tumor markers or residual mass <1 cm, surveillance is an option. In case of residual mass >1 cm, RPLND must be considered. This procedure must be done in high-volume centers.

After primary RPLND:
- Surveillance for pN0 and pN1
- Chemotherapy for selected pN1, pN2, and pN3

For pN1 and pN2, the regimen is BEP or EP for two cycles. For pN3 disease, four cycles of EP or three cycles of BEP are recommended.

49.7.2.13 Stage IIB Non-seminoma

The patient's treatment also depends on both post-orchiectomy tumor marker levels and radiographic findings:
- If normal tumor markers and imagological findings of retroperitoneum disease:
  - Nerve-sparing RPLND followed for adjuvant treatment
  - Primary chemotherapy and nerve-sparing RPLND or surveillance
- In presence of imagological findings of metastatic disease:
  - Chemotherapy, followed by RPLND or surveillance
- In case of persistent elevation of tumor markers, the primary treatment should be chemotherapy and RPLND is not recommended.

49.7.2.14 Advanced Metastatic Non-seminoma

The choice of the chemotherapy regimen depends on the risk classification:
Good-risk group:
- There are two regimens recommended for this group: BEP ×3 or EP ×4.

Intermediate-risk group:
- There are two regimens recommended for this group: BEP ×4 or VIP ×4 (patients with bleomycin intolerance).

Poor-risk group:
- The regimen recommended is BEP ×4 and VIP ×4 (patients with bleomycin intolerance) (◘ Algorithm 49.2).

Post-chemotherapy management:
- In the end of chemotherapy, the patient should undergo a CT scan and evaluation of serum tumor markers.

In case of negative tumor markers and imagological complete response, the following are recommended:
- Surveillance in case of initial stage IS
- Surveillance or RPLND in case of IIA, S1, IIB, S1, IIC, or IIIA

In case of residual mass, the recommended treatment is surgery followed by chemotherapy.

Second-Line Therapy for Metastatic Germ-Cell Tumors

Patients who present recurrence or do not have a durable complete response to first-line therapy can be divided in two groups: favorable or unfavorable prognosis based on prognostic factors.

In the favorable prognosis group (complete response to first-line therapy, low levels of post-orchiectomy serum tumor markers, and low-volume disease), the use of conventional chemotherapy or high-dose chemotherapy is recommended. Participation in clinical trials is encouraged.

In the unfavorable prognosis group (incomplete response to first-line treatment, high levels of serum markers, high-volume disease, and presence of extragonadal primary tumor), participation in a clinical trial is the preferred option, or conventional chemotherapy or high-dose chemotherapy.

49.8 Follow-Up

The main objective of follow-up visits is to allow an early detection and treatment of relapse. The follow-up plan must be adapted to the individual patients and the schedules published should only provide a general guidance.

Late relapses after 5 years are a rare event occurring in nearly 0.5% of patients. Therefore, beyond 5 years of follow-up, its aim shifts toward detection of late side effects of treatment [11].

49.9 Survivorship

Although testicular cancer represents the most curable solid tumor, there is considerable long-term morbidity related to the treatment and extensive follow-up. Neurotoxicity, nephrotoxicity, cardiovascular disease,

◻ Algorithm 49.2
Non-seminoma germ-cell
tumor first-line treatment

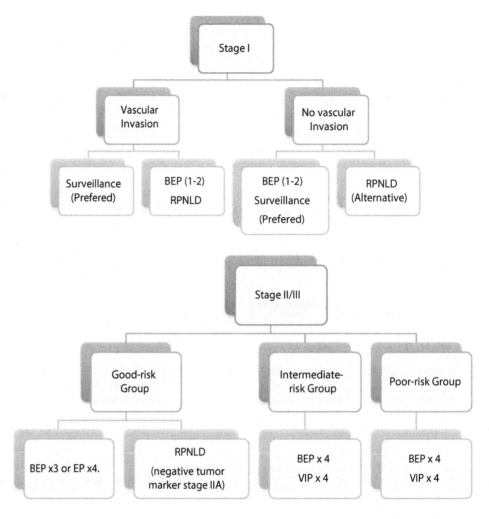

pulmonary toxicity, hypogonadism, decreased fertility, psychosocial problems, and even the development of second malignant neoplasms are all possible outcomes late in life for testicular cancer patients. In this regard, the institution of lifelong follow-up of testicular cancer survivors should be considered [21].

Case study

Male, 36 years old, healthy
- *Family history:* Negative for malignancy
- *APP:* For nearly 4 months, left lower back pain. Recently with irradiation to the abdomen and palpable abdominal mass
- *Objective examination:* Palpable mass of stony consistency in the upper left abdominal quadrant with 60 × 100 mm
- *Blood tests:* Elevated LDH (1668 U/L)
- *Abdominal ultrasound:* Well-defined and lobulated bulky mass (retroperitoneal?) of 108 × 134 mm, solid, heterogeneous, with cystic areas
- *Abdominal and pelvic CT:* Bulky left retroperitoneal mass (139 × 109, 7 mm) as described by the ultrasound. Suggesting MRI

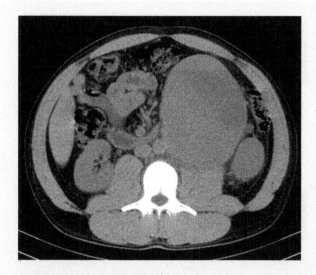

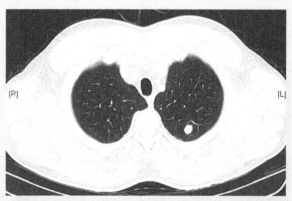

— *Thoracic CT:* Multiple lung metastasis

— *Abdominal and pelvic* MRI: Bulky expansive left retroperitoneal mass, with 11/12 cm, heterogeneous, cystic areas and hemorrhagic areas. Probably a sarcoma or extragonadal germ-cell tumor

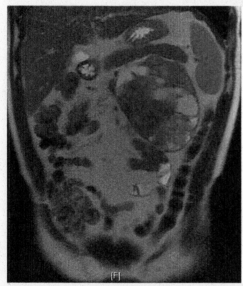

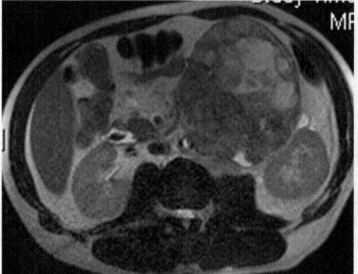

Question

What should we do?

1. Serum tumor markers
2. Surgery
3. Biopsy

Answer

Serum tumor markers and biopsy
    Beta-hCG was elevated (1804 mlU/mL)
    Histology: Carcinoma extensively necrotic

Question

What should we do next?

1. Surgery
2. Chemotherapy
3. Testicular ultrasound

Answer

Testicular ultrasound
    Multifocal tumor in the left testis

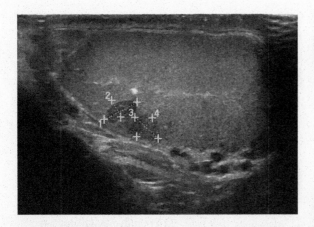

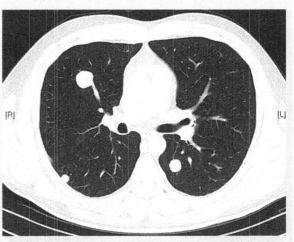

Question

What should we do next?

1. Biopsy
2. Chemotherapy
3. Other

Answer

Chemotherapy

Four cycles of BEP (bleomycin, etoposide, and cisplatin)

Response Assessment

Thoracic, abdominal, and pelvic CT: Significant reduction of retroperitoneal mass dimension as well as lung metastasis

The patient was sent to the IPO (Portuguese Oncology Institute) of Lisbon where they performed surgery: radical left orchiectomy + appendectomy + excision of the retroperitoneal residual mass.

- Histology: Germ-cell intratubular tumor with 2 mm in the left testis and a metastasis of a non-seminomatous germ-cell tumor, with tumor in the surgical margins
- Serum tumor markers: AFP and beta-hCG normal

Two months later, the patient had an increase of AFP and the CT shows disease progression (lung and retroperitoneal).

Question

What should we do next?

1. Chemotherapy
2. Surgery
3. Others

Answer

Chemotherapy

The patient started chemotherapy with TIP (paclitaxel, ifosfamide, and cisplatin) followed by autologous bone marrow transplantation.

Response Assessment

Thoracic, abdominal, and pelvic CT: No evidence of oncological disease

Key Points

- Importance of serum tumor markers and biopsy: Differential diagnosis with other neoplasia.
- Do not forget to look for a testicular mass even in the extragonadal germ-cell tumors.
- When appropriately treated, testicular cancer can have high survival rates even in the metastatic setting.

Case study

Man, 33 years old, healthy

- *Family history:* Negative for malignancy
- *APP:* Palpable nodule in the right testis after a trauma that increased its dimensions
- *Objective examination:* Palpable suspicious mass in the right testis

- *Blood tests:* AFP and LDH normal, beta-hCG elevated (5.7 U/L)
- *Scrotum ultrasound:* Increased volume of the right testis with cystic suspicious testicular cancer

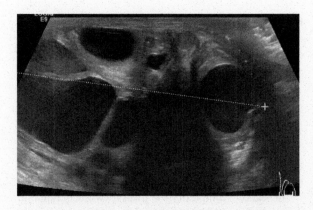

- *Thoracic, abdominal, and pelvic CT:* Increased volume of right testis with multiple cystic formations, no evidence of other disease sites

Question

What should we do next?
1. Biopsy
2. Surgery
3. Others

Answer

Surgery

The patient underwent a right radical orchiectomy with prosthetic implantation.

Histology: Cystic teratoma with foci of embryonal carcinoma and foci of seminoma.

Question

What should we do next?
1. Chemotherapy
2. Serum tumor markers
3. Radiotherapy

Answer

Serum tumor markers

Post-orchiectomy tumor marker levels are used for risk stratification and are incorporated into the American Joint Committee on Cancer TNM Staging System for Testis Cancer.

- LDH, AFP, and beta-hCG normal
- Stage IA, low risk

Question

What should we do next?
1. Chemotherapy
2. Active surveillance
3. Radiotherapy

Answer

Active surveillance

Key Points

- Importance of serum tumor markers before and after the surgery.
- Early diagnosis leads to high rates of survival.
- Active surveillance is the preferred treatment option in low-risk patients.

Expert Opinion
Antonio Russo

Key Points
1. Testicular cancer is the most common cancer in 20-40 years old men; its incidence in Europe is around 5.8%, with a mortality rate of 0.4%.
2. Clinically it usually appears as a nodule or a painless swelling in one testicle; sometimes symptoms are linked to the metastatic diffusion (i.e., dyspnea or cough can appear in case of lung metastases). Some testicular cancers can produce human chorionic gonadotropin (hCG) which causes gynecomastia.
3. It is possible to identify different histological subtypes according to the latest WHO classification: seminoma (the most frequent form), spermatocytic seminoma, choriocarcinoma, yolk sac tumor, embryonal carcinoma, teratoma, Leydig cell tumor, Sertoli tumor, granulosa cell tumor, and rhabdomyosarcoma.
4. When a testicular cancer is suspected, a physical examination should be performed followed by US and blood test with the evaluation of beta-hCG, alpha-fetoprotein (AFP), and lactate dehydrogenase (LDH). They can give useful information about the type of testicular cancer and they are also implied during the follow-up. For a correct and complete staging, CT is recommended.
5. Treatment differs from each patient; the primary one in most cases consist in a radical inguinal orchiectomy. The subsequent approaches depend on the his-

tological subtype and stage; they can comprise just follow-up (stage I seminoma), radiotherapy, or even chemotherapy with different schedules.

6. At the end of the treatment, the patient should undergo follow-up periodic evaluations which must be adapted to the single patient.

Reccomendetions
- ESMO
- ▸ www.esmo.org/Guidelines/Genitourinary-Cancers/Testicular-germ-cell-cancer
- ▸ www.esmo.org/Guidelines/Genitourinary-Cancers/Testicular-Seminoma-and-Non-Seminoma American Urological Association
- ▸ www.auanet.org/guidelines/testicular-cancer-guideline

Hints for a Deeper Insight
- Epidemiology and Diagnosis of Testis Cancer: ▸ www.ncbi.nlm.nih.gov/pubmed/26216814
- Clinical presentation, management and follow-up of 83 patients with Leydig cell tumors of the testis: a prospective case-cohort study: ▸ https://www.ncbi.nlm.nih.gov/pubmed/31532522
- Relapse surveillance of patients with testicular germ cell tumor: ▸ https://www.ncbi.nlm.nih.gov/pubmed/31495441
- Cancer-testis antigens and immunotherapy in the light of cancer complexity: ▸ https://www.ncbi.nlm.nih.gov/pubmed/25901859
- Testicular Cancer Biomarkers: A Role for Precision Medicine in Testicular Cancer: ▸ https://www.ncbi.nlm.nih.gov/pubmed/30497810

References

1. Siegel RB, Miller KD, Jemal A. Cancer statistics, 2017. CA Cancer J Clin. 2017;67:7–30. https://doi.org/10.3322/caac.21387.
2. Oldenburg J, Fosså SD, Nuvei J, Heidenreich A, Schmoll H-J, Bokemeyer C, Horwich A, Beyer J, Kataja V, on behalf of the ESMO Guidelines Working Group. Testicular seminoma and non-seminoma: ESMO Clinical Practice Guidelines for diagnosis, treatment and follow-up. Ann Oncol. 2013;24 Suppl 6:vi125–32. https://doi.org/10.1093/annonc/mdt304.
3. Surveillance, Epidemiology, and End Results (SEER) Program of the National Cancer Institute. https://seer.cancer.gov/. Accessed 18 Nov 2017.
4. EUCAN International Agency for Research on Cancer. http://eco.iarc.fr/EUCAN/Default.aspx. Accessed 18 Nov 2017.
5. Lip SZ, Murchison LE, Cullis PS, Govan L, Carachi R. A meta-analysis of the risk of boys with isolated cryptorchidism developing testicular cancer in later life. Arch Dis Child. 2013;98:20–6.
6. Schaapveld M, van den Belt-Dusebout AW, Gietema JA, de Wit R, Horenblas S, Witjes JA, Hoekrtra HJ, Kiemeney LALM, Louwman WJ, Ouwens GM, Aleman BMP, van Leeuwen FE. Risk and prognostic significance of metachronous contralateral testicular germ cell tumors. Br J Cancer. 2012;107:1637–43. https://doi.org/10.1038/bjc.2012.448.
7. Green MH, Kratz CP, Mai PL, Mueller C, Peters JA, Bratslavsky G, Ling A, Choyke PM, Premkumar A, Bracci J, Watkins R, McMaster ML, Korde LA. Familial testicular germ cell tumors in adults: 2010 summary of genetic risk factors and clinical phenotype. Endoc Relat Cancer. 2010;17:109–21. https://doi.org/10.1677/ERC-09-0254.
8. Holzik MFL, Rapley EA, Hoekstra HJ, Sleijfer DT, Nolte IM, Sijmons RH. Genetic predisposition to testicular germ-cell tumours. Lancet Oncol. 2004;5:363–71. https://doi.org/10.1016/S1470-2045(04)01493-7.
9. Peng X, Zeng X, Peng S, Deng D, Zhang J. The association risk of male subfertility and testicular cancer: a systematic review. PLoS One. 2009;4:5591. https://doi.org/10.1371/journal.pone.0005591.
10. Tseng A, Horning S, Freiha F, Resser K, Hannigan J, Torti F. Gynecomastia in testicular cancer patients: prognostic and therapeutic implications. Cancer. 1985;56:2534–8.
11. Albers P, Albrecht W, Algaba F, Bokemeyer C, Cohn-Cedermark G, Fizazi K, Horwich A, Laguna MP, Nicolai N, Oldenburg JEAU. Guidelines on Testicular. Cancer. 2017. https://uroweb.org/guideline/testicular-cancer/. Accessed 18 Nov 2017.
12. Nazeer T, Ro JY, Amato RJ, Park YW, Ordonez NG, Ayala AG. Histologically pure seminoma with elevated alpha-fetoprotein: a clinicopathologic study of ten cases. Oncol Rep. 1998;5:1425–34. https://doi.org/10.3892/or.5.6.1425.
13. Casciato DA, Territo MC, Einhorn LH, et al. Text book of medical oncology. 6th ed: Wolters Kluwer Health/Lipincott Williams &Wikins.
14. Devita, Hellman and Rosemberg's. Cancer principles & practice of oncology. 9th ed: Wolters Kluwer Health/Lipincott Williams &Wikins.
15. CosentinoM AF, Saldaña L, Bujons A, Caffaratti J, Garat JM, et al. Juvenile granulose cell tumor of the testis. Urology. 2014;84:694–6.
16. Hemley JD, Young RH, Ulbright TM. Malignant Sertoli cell tumors of the testis. Am J Surg Patthol. 2002;26:541–50.
17. Grem JL, Robins HI, Wilson KS, Gilchrist K, et al. Metastatic Leydig cell tumor of the testis. Cancer. 1986;58:2116–9.
18. National Comprehensive Cancer Network. NCCN clinical practice guidelines in oncology.
19. Leibovitch L, RS F, Kopeky K, et al. Improved accuracy of computerized tomography based clinical staging. J Urol. 1995;157:1759.
20. Oechsle K, Hartmman M, Brenner W, et al. The German multi-center positron emission tomography study group. J Clin Oncol. 2004;22:1034.
21. Travis L, Beard C, Allan J, et al. Testicular Cancer survivorship: research strategies and recommendations. J Natl Cancer Inst. 2010;102(15):1114–30.

Cancer of the Penis

Alchiede Simonato, Cristina Scalici Gesolfo, and Alberto Abrate

Genitourinary Cancers

Contents

© Springer Nature Switzerland AG 2021
A. Russo et al. (eds.), *Practical Medical Oncology Textbook*, UNIPA Springer Series,
https://doi.org/10.1007/978-3-030-56051-5_50

Learning Objectives

By the end of the chapter, the reader will:
- Be able to identify patients/lesions at risk for penile cancer
- Have learned the basic investigation method for a good staging of penile cancer
- Be able to apply the acquired knowledge in clinical practice in order to make an early diagnosis and choose the best treatment for the patient

50.1 Epidemiology and Cancer Prevention

Penile carcinoma, though a rare neoplasm in developed countries, is an aggressive disease with devastating effect in affected patients. In developing countries such as South America, Africa, and Asia, where its incidence is higher, early detection is a goal that urologists try to achieve, in order to limit the damage and the mortality related to the progression of this tumor.

Squamous cell carcinoma (SCC) represents the commonest histological type followed by basaloid carcinoma, warty carcinoma, and papillary carcinoma as shown in Table 50.1. It arises from the prepuce or glans and its natural history and pathology are similar to other locations of SCC such as the oropharynx, female genitalia, and anus. The incidence of penile SCC is related to age, with a peak in the sixth decade, and changes dramatically from the Western countries to the Third World.

In fact, while in Europe and the USA it is a rare disease, with an incidence <1/100,000 males, in some parts of Africa, South America, and Asia, it can represent the 1–2% of malignant disease in men [1].

Furthermore, distribution around the world in terms of incidence is related to the prevalence of HPV. The higher the prevalence of HPV in a certain country, the higher the incidence of penile carcinoma [1]. According to this evidence, HPV infection (especially sustained by subtypes HPV-16 and HPV-18) is one of the major risk factors, as it probably acts as a cofactor in the carcinogenesis through an interaction with oncogenes and oncosuppressor genes such as p53 and Rb [2]. Supporting this hypothesis, HPV DNA is present in the histological samples of the 70–100% intraepithelial neoplasms and in the 30–40% of invasive penile cancers.

However, HPV infection is not the only cause of penile carcinoma. It is probable that chronic infection/inflammation in general could promote this oncogenesis. This fact could explain the association between phimosis and penile carcinoma [3]. The mechanical micro-trauma and the poor hygienic conditions linked to phimosis could promote infections and inflammations and sustain their chronicity. In this sense, it is not surprising that the lowest incidence of penile carcinoma is recorded in those cultures or countries where neonatal circumcision is routinely performed, as this not only improves hygiene and reduces the risk of chronic infection/inflammation but also removes the majority of the tissue that could develop a penile carcinoma.

Table 50.1 Prevalence and prognosis according to histological type of penile carcinoma

Prevalence and prognosis according to histological type of penile carcinoma			
Histological type	% of cases	Prognosis	Metastasis
Common squamous cell carcinoma (SCC)	48–65	Depends on location, stage, and grade	Early inguinal nodal metastasis could be present
Basaloid carcinoma	4–10	Poor prognosis	Early inguinal nodal metastasis
Warty carcinoma	7–10	Good prognosis	Rare
Verrucous carcinoma	3–8	Good prognosis	None
Papillary carcinoma	5–15	Good prognosis	Rare
Sarcomatoid carcinoma	1–3	Very poor prognosis	Early vascular metastasis
Mixed carcinoma	9–10	Heterogeneous group	Depending on histological types
Pseudohyperplastic carcinoma	<1	Good prognosis	Not reported
Carcinoma cuniculatum	<1	Good prognosis	Not reported
Pseudoglandular carcinoma	<1	Poor prognosis	Early metastasis
Warty-basaloid carcinoma	9–14	Poor prognosis	High metastatic potential
Adenosquamous carcinoma	<1	Low mortality	High metastatic potential
Mucoepidermoid carcinoma	<1	Poor prognosis	Not reported
Clear cell variant of penile carcinoma	1–2	Poor prognosis	Early metastasis, frequent lymphatic metastasis

Despite this encouraging data, the incidence of carcinoma in situ (CIS) seems not to be affected by neonatal circumcision [3]; furthermore, no significant changes in incidence have been recorded in adults having undergone circumcision. Another important risk factor for penile carcinoma is cigarette smoking, which increases three- to fivefold the risk of penile carcinoma, which in its turn has been found to be dose dependent [3].

50.2 Genetic Aspects of Hereditary Cancer

Currently, cancer of the penis has not been correlated to a hereditary disorder or a hereditary genetic mutation.

50.3 Differential Diagnosis

Squamous cell carcinoma represents the commonest histological type of penile carcinoma (up to 95%), with smaller percentages also of melanoma, basal cell carcinoma, and Paget disease. Furthermore, the incidence of penile Kaposi's disease increased following the incidence of HIV.

SCC is often preceded by a premalignant lesion [4]. Recognizing and treating the premalignant lesion is important to prevent the evolution to penile cancer. ◘ Table 50.2 summarizes the most common premalignant lesions and their characteristics.

◘ **Table 50.2** Types of premalignant lesions

Types of premalignant lesions		
Premalignant lesion	Risk factor	Appearance
Leukoplakia	Diabetes	White, hard, may ulcerate
Balanitis xerotica obliterans (BXO)	Chronic phimosis, chronic infections, poor hygiene, vigorous sexual activity, lichen sclerosus, paraphimosis	Penile skin fusion to the head of the penis, indurated and narrowed
Giant condyloma acuminata	HPV infection	Bulky exophytic growth and tumor size that often exceeds 10 cm in greatest diameter
Bowen disease		Sharply defined plaques of scaly erythema, may ulcerate and crusted

50.4 Typical Signs and Symptoms

The primitive tumor is localized on the glans in the 48% of cases, on the prepuce in the 21% of cases, on both in the 9% of cases, and on the coronal line and on the penile rod in the 6% and 2% of cases, respectively [5]. At physical examination, penile carcinoma presents as a small, hard, and erythematous area, sometimes ulcerated, or as a small endophytic or exophytic node. The commonest symptoms are pain, discomfort, and burning sensations.

50.5 Diagnostic Strategies and Staging

Physical examination is the first important step for the diagnosis of penile carcinoma. Lesions could be hidden by a phimosis; in this case circumcision should be performed before choosing local treatment of the lesion in order to avoid under- or over-treatment.

During physical examination, attention must be paid to the inguinal lymph nodes. The physical examination should be reported as complete as possible with indication of side, number, and mobility of enlarged nodes. The absence of palpable lymph nodes in the presence of penile cancer deposes for an early lymphadenectomy without need for further imaging investigation; in fact 20% of patients with absence of palpable lymph nodes have nodal micrometastases [6]. At diagnosis enlarged palpable inguinal lymph nodes are present in about 58% of patients, of which 17–45% are positive for metastasis [7], while in the other cases the enlargement is due to inflammation. In order to distinguish the inflammatory enlarged nodes from the metastatic ones, patient should be reexamined after at least a week of antibiotics. Bilateral involvement of lymph nodes is possible due to the presence of a high number of lymphatic vessels that cross in the subcutaneous tissue of the penis. Patients with positive lymph nodes should be assessed for distant metastasis through a CT scan of the abdomen and pelvis and chest X-rays [8].

Histological examination is crucial for the diagnosis and treatment of penile carcinoma.

Based on the clinical presentation of the primitive lesion, a total excision or a biopsy should be considered. When the lesion appears deep and invasiveness is suspected, a penile US or MRI must be performed in order to exclude involvement of the corpora cavernosa [9].

In any case a biopsy should be performed.

Aggressiveness criteria are used to choose the timing for demolitive treatment. One of these criteria is the differentiation grading that varies from 0 to 4, from more differentiated to more undifferentiated and aggressive disease. The staging of penile carcinoma follows the

Jackson classification and the TNM classification as reported in Tables 50.3 and 50.4. Negative prognostic factors for metastatic spread are tumors with vertical growths and with vascular and lymphatic invasion.

50.6 Treatment Options

The treatment of penile carcinoma tries to achieve two ideal goals:
- Complete eradication of the tumor
- Organ preservation

For small, superficial, and localized lesions, organ preservation is generally an achievable goal as complete eradication can be performed with excisional surgery, laser ablation, brachytherapy, or external beam radiotherapy.

First-line treatment of carcinoma in situ (CIS) can consist of topical chemotherapy with imiquimod or 5-FU, though a strict follow-up is required in consideration of the high risk of failure of the treatment or recurrence both in the short and long term. Total or partial glans resurfacing can be performed both in the first or second line of treatment.

Table 50.3 Jackson classification of penile carcinoma

Jackson classification	
Stage	Description
I	Confined to the glans or prepuce
II	Invasion into shaft or corpora
III	Operable inguinal lymph node metastasis
IV	Tumor invades adjacent structures, inoperable inguinal lymph node metastasis

Table 50.4 2016 TNM clinical and pathological classification of penile carcinoma

2016 TNM clinical classification of penile carcinoma	
T – Primary tumor	
TX	Primary tumor cannot be assessed
T0	No evidence of primary tumor
Tis	Carcinoma in situ
Ta	Non-invasive verrucous carcinoma
T1	Tumor invades subepithelial connective tissue
	T1a without lymphovascular invasion and is not poorly differentiated
	T1b with lymphovascular invasion or is poorly differentiated
T2	Tumor invades corpus spongiosum with or without invasion of the urethra
T3	Tumor invades corpus cavernosum with or without invasion of the urethra
T4	Tumor invades other adjacent structures
N – Regional lymph nodes	
NX	Regional lymph nodes cannot be assessed
N0	No palpable or visibly enlarged inguinal lymph node
N1	Palpable mobile unilateral inguinal lymph node
N2	Palpable multiple unilateral or bilateral inguinal lymph nodes
N3	Fixed inguinal nodal mass or pelvic lymphadenopathy, unilateral or bilateral

Table 50.4 (continued)

M – Distant metastasis	
M0	No distant metastasis
M1	Distant metastasis
2016 TNM pathological classification of penile carcinoma	
pT – Categories that correspond to the clinical T categories	
pN – Regional lymph nodes (from biopsy or surgical excision)	
pNX	Regional lymph nodes cannot be assessed
pN0	No regional lymph node metastasis
pN1	Metastasis in one or two inguinal lymph nodes
pN2	Metastasis in more than two unilateral inguinal nodes or bilateral inguinal lymph nodes
pN3	Metastasis in pelvic lymph node(s), unilateral or bilateral extranodal or extension of regional lymph node metastasis
pM – Distant metastasis	
pM1	Distant metastasis microscopically confirmed
G – Histopathological grading	
GX	Grade of differentiation cannot be assessed
G1	Well differentiated
G2	Moderately differentiated
G3	Poorly differentiated
G4	Undifferentiated

In patients with small, localized, invasive lesions, a conservative approach is recommended with an extemporary analysis of the margins. To consider the reliability of the negativity of a margin, it should be at least 5 mm from the lesion.

Possible conservative treatments for T1/T2 diseases are:
- Laser therapy
- Mohs micrographic surgery
- Glans resurfacing
- Glansectomy
- Partial penectomy

There is not enough evidence to prefer one organ-conserving strategy over another in terms of outcome and conservative surgery could improve the patient's quality of life.

In patients with T1 and T2 disease with a diameter <4 cm, radiotherapy could be a valid conservative treatment with local control rate ranging from 70% to 90%; however, recurrence rates after radiotherapy are higher than after partial penectomy. Common complications of radiant treatments are urethral stenosis, meatal stenosis, glans necrosis, and late fibrosis of corpora cavernosa.

Treatment of T2/T3 disease consists of partial amputation with at least 5 mm of free margin. Surgery must be followed by a strict follow-up. Radiotherapy could be considered as treatment.

In patients with locally advanced disease (T3/T4), a total penectomy with perineal urethrostomy must be performed. In patients with T4 penile cancer, neoadjuvant chemotherapy should be performed and followed by surgery in responders. In non-responders, adjuvant chemotherapy and palliative radiotherapy are options.

50.6.1 Nodal Anatomy, Drainage, and Treatment

It is important to devote a paragraph to the treatment of the inguinal nodes. In fact, nodal involvement could be considered the major prognostic factor for survival in patients affected by penile SCC. As discussed above, survival is related to the absence or presence of nodal metastases.

The lymphatic drainage of the penis is entrusted to superficial and deep inguinal nodes and is characterized by a well-known anatomy crossover between those two groups, both ipsilateral and bilateral. The sentinel node of the prepuce is located on the upper-medial zone and drains from this to the superficial inguinal nodes (8–25 nodes), while glans and corpora cavernosa could drain into superficial inguinal node or directly into the deep inguinal nodes and into the external iliac nodes. For this reason, in patients undergoing lymphadenectomy, both the superficial and deep inguinal nodes are removed according to the ilioinguinal lymph node dissection (IILND). In fact, contralateral metastases could be found in more than 50% of patients treated with a bilateral inguinal lymphadenectomy, despite the absence of palpable lymph nodes.

Several studies demonstrated the importance of an early lymphadenectomy, considering that micrometastases were found in the 25% of patients with non-palpable lymph nodes who underwent surgery. An improvement of survival has been found in patients undergoing early nodal dissection while delayed nodal dissection could only rarely save recurring patients.

Surveillance in case of non-palpable lymph nodes should be offered only to Ta, T1, and CIS patients with high compliance and after a complete information about the risk of worst survival in case of lymphadenectomy of lateral regional recurrence. In this case survival decreases from 90% to 40% at 5 years comparing early lymphadenectomy with lymphadenectomy for later regional recurrence. Whenever surveillance is indicated, it is important to schedule a strict follow-up schedule in order to intervene immediately, should there appear to be a change in nodal stage.

The choice of timing and extension of lymphadenectomy should follow the algorithm shown in ▢ Fig. 50.1. Approaching inguinal nodal dissection, it is important to establish the correct balance between therapeutic goals and minimal morbidity for the patient. In fact the IILND often causes important complications such as severe lymphedema and necrosis of the skin flap (30–50%), wound infection, phlebitis, and pulmonary embolism. In order to decrease this rate of complications in patients with clinically negative inguinal lymph nodes, different procedures have been tested:
- Fine-needle aspiration cytology (FNAC): In both ultrasonography and lymphangiography guidance, the FNAC did not show sufficient sensitivity to be considered as a staging procedure [10].
- Sentinel lymph node biopsy: This procedure is no longer recommended due to unreliability in identifying microscopic metastasis.
- Dynamic sentinel node biopsy: This procedure uses the injection of radiant and colored substances that produce gamma emissions near the lesion. These substances are absorbed from the lymphatic system and collected to regional lymph nodes that can be detected, identified, and dissected during surgery. However, this technique currently shows good results in terms of sensitivity only in high-volume centers with trained surgeons and nuclear medicine specialists [11].
- Superficial node dissection: This consists of the removal of those nodes which are superficial to the

Fig. 50.1 Algorithm of timing and extension of lymphadenectomy

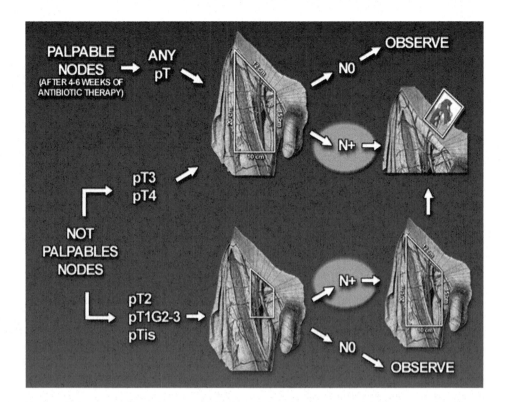

fascia lata. If no metastatic nodes are found, a complete IILND is not performed due to evidence of absence of recurrence in up to 3 years of follow-up in cohort studies [12].

- Complete modified inguinal dissection: This technique was proposed by Catalona in 1988 [13] and allows the performance of a small cutaneous incision, preserving the saphenous vein. No muscle transposition is needed in order to protect the femoral vessel, and furthermore this technique allows the dissection of both superficial and deep nodes. The Catalona modified inguinal dissection is shown in ◘ Fig. 50.2. With the modified IILND by Catalona, though still present, comorbidities are less frequent and less severe as demonstrated by different studies [14–16].
- Laparoscopic and robotic minimally invasive inguinal lymphadenectomy: At present, the results obtained with minimally invasive approaches are comparable to open surgery [17].
- Pelvic lymphadenectomy: It should be performed in case of positivity of the inguinal node due to the uncommon presence of pelvic lymph node metastasis with negative inguinal nodes. Suspicion of nodal pelvic involvement in absence of inguinal node metastasis should be evaluated through pelvic CT scan.

50.6.2 Non-surgical Treatments

Neoadjuvant chemotherapy (four cycles of cisplatin- and taxane-based regimen) should precede radical surgery in patients with non-resectable or recurrent lymph nodes (LE 2a GR B) [18].

Adjuvant chemotherapy should be offered to patients with pN2/pN3 or systemic disease and a limited metastatic load (LE 2b-3 GR C). Second-line therapy with anti-EGFR monoclonal antibodies and tyrosine-kinase inhibitor has been investigated but further studies are necessary (LE 4) [19, 20].

50.7 Conclusions

Penile carcinoma is a malignant disease which benefits from early diagnosis and treatment. After a complete staging, a multidisciplinary approach is mandatory to ensure the best therapy for the patients. However, timing plays a crucial role; whatever the chosen treatment, it must be performed as early as possible to increase the chances of success.

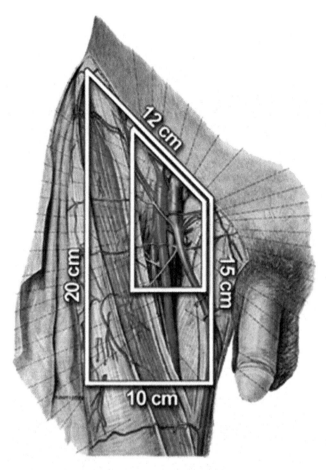

Fig. 50.2 IILND resection area: **a** Classic IILND involves lymph node both superficial and deep to the fascia lata contained within the femoral triangle. **b** Completed modified inguinal dissection according to Catalona that excludes the area lateral to the femoral artery and caudal to the fossa ovalis and saphenous vein preservation, with no need for sartorius muscle transposition

Summary of Clinical Recommendation

Diagnosis and Staging:

- Perform a physical examination, and record morphology, extent, and invasion of penile structures. Perform a physical examination of both groins, and record the number, laterality, and characteristics of inguinal lymph nodes and:
  - Non-palpable nodes → offer invasive lymph node staging in high-risk patients (≥T1b).
  - Palpable nodes → abdominopelvic computed tomography (CT) or positron emission tomography (PET)/CT and chest X-ray for staging.
- In patients with systemic disease or with relevant symptoms, obtain a bone scan.

Treatment:

- For localized penile cancer (from Tis to T2 confined to the glans) → offer local treatment like laser, glans resurfacing, radiotherapy, and glansectomy.

- For T2 with invasion of the corpora cavernosa → offer partial amputation and reconstruction/radiotherapy/brachytherapy.
- For T3 with invasion of the urethra → offer partial/total penectomy with perineal urethrostomy.
- T4 → offer neoadjuvant chemotherapy followed by surgery in responders or palliative external beam radiation.

Management of Nodal Metastases:

- Non-palpable inguinal nodes (cN0):
  - Tis, Ta G1, T1a → surveillance
  - ≥ T1b → invasive staging by bilateral modified inguinal lymphadenectomy/dynamic sentinel node biopsy
- Palpable inguinal nodes (cN1/cN2) → radical inguinal lymphadenectomy
- Fixed inguinal lymph nodes(cN3) → neoadjuvant chemotherapy followed by radical inguinal lymphadenectomy in responders
- Pelvic lymphadenopathy → ipsilateral pelvic lymphadenectomy if two or more inguinal nodes are involved on one side (pN2) and if extracapsular nodal metastasis (pN3) is confirmed
- pN2/pN3 patients after radical lymphadenectomy → adjuvant chemotherapy

Follow-Up:

- Minimum length of 5 years, with an interval of 3 months for the first 2 years for any categories of patients.
- Penile-preserving treatment: Interval of 6 months after the first 2 years with regular physician/self-examination. If positive, repeat biopsy after topical or laser treatment for carcinoma in situ.
- Amputation: Interval of 1 year after the first 2 years with regular physician/self-examination.
- Inguinal lymph nodes under surveillance: Interval of 6 months after the first 2 years with regular physician/self-examination.
- Inguinal lymph nodes pN0 at initial treatment: Interval of 1 year after the second year of follow-up with regular physician/self-examination. Ultrasound with fine-needle aspiration biopsy optional.
- Inguinal lymph nodes pN+ at initial treatment: Interval of 6 months after 2 years of follow-up with regular physician/self-examination. Ultrasound with fine-needle aspiration cytology optional, CT/MRI optional.

[a]According to the most recent guidelines available [e.g., ASCO, EAU, AUA]

Expert Opinion
Lorena Incorvaia

Key Points

- In case of suspected penile cancer, early diagnosis and treatment are mandatory.
- Treatment of penile carcinoma aims to completely eradicate the tumor, while preserving the organ integrity when possible.
- Nodal involvement is the major prognostic factor.

Hints for Deeper Insight

- Pathological subtype, perineural invasion, lymphovascular invasion, depth of invasion, and grade in the primary tumor are strong predictors of poor prognosis and high cancer-specific mortality.
- In doubtful cases, before definitive surgical treatment, confirmatory frozen section excisional biopsy can be done.

- In case of clinically normal inguinal regions (cN0), imaging studies are not helpful (except in obese patients) for N-staging.

Suggested Reading

- Hakenberg, O.W., et al. EAU Guidelines on Penile Cancer. ▶ https://uroweb.org/guideline/penile-cancer/
- Engelsgjerd, J.S., et al. Cancer, Penile. StatPearls [Internet]. Treasure Island (FL): StatPearls Publishing; 2019. ▶ https://www.ncbi.nlm.nih.gov/books/NBK499930/
- Azizi, M., et al. Current controversies and developments on the role of lymphadenectomy for penile cancer. UrolOncol, 2019. 37:201.
- Ficarra, V., et al. Prognostic factors in penile cancer. Urology. 2010. 76(2 Suppl 1): S66.

References

1. Backes DM, et al. Systematic review of human papillomavirus prevalence in invasive penile cancer. Cancer Causes Control. 2009;20:449.
2. Gunia S, et al. p16(INK4a) is a marker of good prognosis for primary invasive penile squamous cell carcinoma: a multi-institutional study. J Urol. 2012;187:899.
3. Maden C, et al. History of circumcision, medical conditions, and sexual activity and risk of penile cancer. J Natl Cancer Inst. 1993;85:19.
4. Teichman JM, et al. Non-infectious penile lesions. Am Fam Physician. 2010;81:167.
5. Sufrin G, Huben R. Benign and malignant lesion of the penis. In: Jy G, editor. Adult and pediatric urology. 2nd ed. Chicago, IL: Year Book Medical Publisher; 1991. p. 1643.
6. Hakenberg OW, et al. EAU guidelines Penile. Cancer. 2015;
7. Ornellas AA, et al. Surgical treatment of invasive squamous cell carcinoma of the penis: retrospective analysis of 350 cases. J Urol. 1994;151:1244–9.
8. Schlenker B, et al. Detection of inguinal lymph node involvement in penile squamous cell carcinoma by 18F-fluorodeoxyglucose PET/CT: a prospective single-center study. Urol Oncol. 2012; 30:55.
9. Bertolotto M, et al. Primary and secondary malignancies of the penis: ultrasound features. Abdom Imaging. 2005;30:108.
10. Colecchia M, et al. pT1 penile squamous cell carcinoma: a clinicopathologic study of 56 cases treated by CO2 laser therapy. Anal Quant Cytol Histol. 2009;31:153.
11. Zou ZJ, et al. Radiocolloid-based dynamic sentinel lymph node biopsy in penile cancer with clinically negative inguinal lymph node: an updated systematic review and meta-analysis. Int Urol Nephrol. 2016;48(12):2001–13. Epub 2016 Aug 30.
12. Spiess PE, et al. Preoperative lymphoscintigraphy and dynamic sentinel node biopsy for staging penile cancer: results with pathological correlations. J Urol. 2007;177:2157–61.
13. Catalona WJ. Modified inguinal lymphadenectomy for carcinoma of the penis with preservation of saphenous veins: technique and preliminary results. J Urol. 1988;140(2):306–10.
14. Yao K, et al. Modified technique of radical inguinal lymphadenectomy for penile carcinoma: morbidity and outcome. J Urol. 2010;184(2):546–52. https://doi.org/10.1016/j.juro.2010.03.140. Epub 2010 Jun 17.
15. Parra RO, et al. Accurate staging of carcinoma of the penis in men with nonpalpable inguinal lymph nodes by modified inguinal lymphadenectomy. J Urol. 1996;155(2):560–3.
16. Bouchot O, et al. Morbidity of inguinal lymphadenectomy for invasive penile carcinoma. Eur Urol. 2004;45(6):761–5; discussion 765–6.
17. Russell CM, et al. Minimally invasive inguinal lymphadenectomy in the management of penile carcinoma. Urology. 2017;106:113–8. https://doi.org/10.1016/j.urology.2017.04.022. Epub 2017 Apr 24.
18. Pond GR, et al. Prognostic risk stratification derived from individual patient level data for men with advanced penile squamous cell carcinoma receiving first-line systemic therapy. Urol Oncol. 2014;32:501.
19. Gou HF, et al. Epidermal growth factor receptor (EGFR)-RAS signaling pathway in penile squamous cell carcinoma. PLoS One. 2013;8:e62175.
20. Zhu Y, et al. Feasibility and activity of sorafenib and sunitinib in advanced penile cancer: a preliminary report. UrolInt. 2010;85:334.

Ovarian Cancer, Early Primary Disease

Domenica Lorusso, Giuseppa Maltese, Ilaria Sabatucci, and Elisa Tripodi

Gynecological Cancers

Contents

© Springer Nature Switzerland AG 2021
A. Russo et al. (eds.), *Practical Medical Oncology Textbook*, UNIPA Springer Series,
https://doi.org/10.1007/978-3-030-56051-5_51

Learning Objectives

By the end of the chapter, the reader will:

- Be able to apply diagnostic and staging procedures in the management of early ovarian cancer
- Have learned the basic concepts of surgical management of disease
- Have reached in-depth knowledge of indications to adjuvant treatments
- Be able to put acquired knowledge into clinical practice for the management of early stage particularly by referring patients to tertiary centers where multidisciplinary management can be performed

51.1 Introduction

Ovarian cancer represents the seventh most common cause of cancer among women worldwide, and the vast majority of malignant ovarian cancers (about 90%) are epithelial tumors (EOC) [1, 2].

Ovarian cancer is staged according to FIGO staging system (International Federation of Gynecology and Obstetrics) and, less commonly, to AJCC-TNM staging system.

FIGO stage I disease describes a neoplasm exclusively limited to ovaries, while in FIGO stage II the tumor is confined to the pelvis, as shown in ◘ Fig. 51.1. Both conditions are defined as "early-stage ovarian cancers"[3]. Early-stage ovarian cancers are usually asymptomatic and have a relatively good prognosis with a 5-year survival rate of about 90%. Unfortunately, only 20–30% of all ovarian cancer cases are diagnosed at early stage [4].

51.2 Epidemiology

The incidence of ovarian cancer differs among geographic areas, with the higher rates in industrialized countries, especially Europe and North America, with approximately 22,200 new cases diagnosed during 2016 in the USA resulting in 14,240 deaths [5].

The incidence increases with age and is prevalent in postmenopause, with a median age at presentation of 60 years. The age at diagnosis is earlier in patients with genetic or familial predisposition, generally in the fifth decade of life [6].

Over the past 30 years, the 5-year survival rate of women with ovarian cancer has increased to about 10%, ranging from 30% to 40%, depending primarily on the stage of disease at diagnosis. The improvement of surgical techniques [6], surgical expertise, and the decrease of the use of postmenopausal hormonal therapy [7] have possibly contributed to the survival amelioration.

Approximately 25% of women with ovarian cancer are diagnosed at FIGO stages I and II, generally due to an accidental finding, for example, during sonography, computerized tomography (CT) scanning, or laparoscopy performed for other reasons.

51.3 Ovarian Cancer Staging

All the most important international scientific guidelines underline the importance of staging on treatment and prognosis of ovarian cancer.

Ovarian cancer is classified according to size, extent, and localization of the disease, using two different staging systems: the FIGO (International Federation of

---

◘ **Fig. 51.1** FIGO staging of early stage ovarian cancer (2014) (IIC has recently been eliminated in 2014 FIGO Staging)

FIGO Stage I

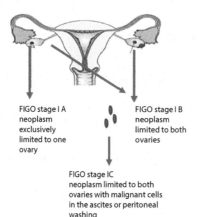

FIGO stage I A neoplasm exclusively limited to one ovary

FIGO stage I B neoplasm limited to both ovaries

FIGO stage IC neoplasm limited to both ovaries with malignant cells in the ascites or peritoneal washing

FIGO Stage II

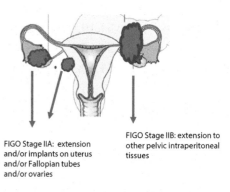

FIGO Stage IIA: extension and/or implants on uterus and/or Fallopian tubes and/or ovaries

FIGO Stage IIB: extension to other pelvic intraperitoneal tissues

◘ Table 51.1 FIGO and AJCC-TNM staging classification of ovarian, fallopian tube, and peritoneal cancer

Stage FIGO	Classification	TNM	Incidence (%)	Year survival (%)
I	*Tumor limited to ovaries or fallopian tube(s)* *Stage IA*: Tumor is limited to one ovary or fallopian tube; the capsule is intact, no tumor on ovarian surface. No malignant cells on the ovarian surface or in peritoneal washings or ascites. *Stage IB*: Tumor is limited to both ovaries or fallopian tube; the capsule is intact, no tumor on ovarian surface. No malignant cells on the ovarian surface or in peritoneal washings or ascites *Stage IC:* Tumor is limited to one or both ovaries or fallopian tubes, with any the following: surgical spill (*IC1*), capsule rupture before surgery or tumor on surface (*IC2*), or malignant cell in the ascites or peritoneal washings (*IC3*) *Capsule rupture and positive cytological washings are considered as independent predictors of poor disease-free survival [9]	T1 T1a T1b T1c1 T1c2 T1c3	20%	92
II	*Tumor involves one or both ovaries with pelvic extension* *IIA:* Extension and/or implants on uterus and/or fallopian tubes and/or ovaries *IIB:* Extension to other pelvic intraperitoneal tissues *IIC is recently eliminated in 2014 FIGO stage	T2 T2a T2b	5%	73–78

Gynecology and Obstetrics) [3] and the AJCC-TNM staging systems [8]. Both staging systems are also applied to fallopian tube carcinoma and primary peritoneal adenocarcinoma. In ◘ Table 51.1 incidence and survival rates by stage are shown.

Objectives of staging are:
- To describe prognosis
- To plan appropriate treatment

The FIGO staging system is exclusively pathological and based on the findings at surgical intervention. A preoperative instrumental evaluation is necessary to evaluate neoplasm extension and to exclude the presence of extraperitoneal metastases. Surgical exploration and adequate staging are necessary to determine postoperative treatment.

51.4 Risk Factors

51.4.1 Non-genetic

Most part of epithelial ovarian tumors is sporadic. Nulliparity, older age (>40 years), obesity, long-term postmenopausal estrogen therapy use, and infertility increase the risk for ovarian cancer. On the contrary, multiparity, oral contraceptive use, younger age at first pregnancy, and breastfeeding are protective factors (◘ Table 51.2) [10].

A recent meta-analysis demonstrated that a long-term oral contraceptive use reduces the risk of ovarian cancer in general population, especially in patients with BRCA mutation [11].

◘ Table 51.2 Risk factors for ovarian cancer

Patient characteristics	Increasing age Personal history of breast cancer Familial history of breast and ovarian cancer
Reproductive factors	Nulliparity Early menarche and late menopause Infertility Hormonal replacement therapy
Environmental factors	Obesity Talc exposure
Genetic factors	BRCA1/2 mutations Lynch syndrome Other genetic syndromes

The role of smoking, talc exposure, diet, and nonsteroidal anti-inflammatory drugs is still controversial [12, 13].

51.4.2 Genetic Syndromes

Familial genetic syndromes are diagnosed in approximately 10–12% of women with EOC [14, 15]. Hereditary breast-ovarian cancer syndrome and hereditary nonpolyposis colorectal cancer (Lynch syndrome) are the most frequent; other syndromes, although less frequent, have been associated with an increased risk of ovarian cancer (◘ Table 51.3).

■ *BRCA-associated ovarian cancer*

An important risk factor for ovarian cancer is the BRCA1 or BRCA2 gene mutation, which is the cause of hereditary breast-ovarian cancer syndrome. In families with a history of breast or ovarian cancer, BRCA germ-line mutations are responsible for approximately 90% of cases of ovarian cancer [16].

Both BRCA genes are tumor suppressor genes that produce proteins involved in DNA damage repair; BRCA mutation carriers are unable to repair double-strand DNA damage, which ultimately leads to the accumulation of genetic alterations and to cancer development (■ Fig. 51.2).

Characteristics of BRCA-mutated ovarian cancer patients:

- BRCA mutations are prevalent in the Jewish population [17].
- BRCA1 mutations are more common than BRCA2 mutations (incidence: 20–40% vs. 10–20%, respectively) [18].
- The predicted lifetime risk of ovarian cancer is greater in patient with BRCA1 than BRCA2 mutation (40–60% vs. 10–30%, respectively).
- BRCA-mutated tumors are associated with improved progression-free survival (PFS) and overall survival (OS), with a better prognosis compared to sporadic ovarian cancers [19, 20].
- BRCA mutations are generally associated with high-grade serous ovarian cancer and less frequently with other histological subtypes (e.g., high-grade endometrioid tumors and clear cells).
- BRCA1/2-mutated tumors are particularly sensitive to PARP inhibitors.
- BRCA status is associated with greater chemosensitivity, mainly to platinum [18, 20] but also to other chemotherapies, for example, pegylated liposomal doxorubicin [21, 22] or trabectedin [23].

■ **Table 51.3** Genetic syndromes associated with an increased risk of ovaria cancer

Syndrome	Gene mutation	Pathologies
Hereditary breast and ovarian cancer	BRCA1 and BRCA2 mutation, HRD positive	Breast, ovarian, fallopian tube, peritoneal, and pancreatic cancer
Hereditary non-polyposis colorectal cancer (Lynch syndrome)	MLH1, MLH3, MSH2, MSH6, tgfbr2, pms1, pms2	Colorectal, endometrial, and ovarian cancer
Peutz-Jeghers syndrome	STH11	Colorectal, stomach, esophageal, small intestine, and ovarian cancer
PTEN hamartoma tumor syndrome (Cowden syndrome)	PTEN	Thyroid, breast, and ovarian cancer
MUTYH-associated polyposis	MUTYH	Colorectal, small intestine, bladder, and ovarian cancer

■ **Fig. 51.2** Role of BRCA 1–2 genes

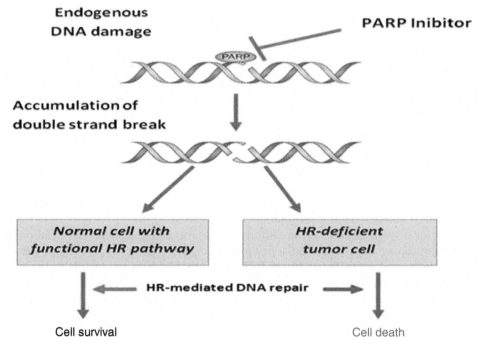

Endogenous DNA damage

PARP Inibitor

Accumulation of double strand break

Normal cell with functional HR pathway

HR-deficient tumor cell

HR-mediated DNA repair

Cell survival

Cell death

Other genetic syndromes:

Hereditary non-polyposis colorectal cancer (Lynch syndrome) is an autosomal-dominant inherited disorder, associated with several cancers mainly with colorectal and less frequently with gastric, small intestine, endometrial, ovarian and hepatobiliary malignancies [24].

The typical germline mutations are in DNA mismatch repair (MMR) genes MLH1, MLH2, MSH2, MSH6, and PMS2 [25] and only 2–3% of ovarian cancers are attributable to this syndrome [24, 26].

The lifetime risk of ovarian cancer is approximately 10% in patients with MMR gene mutations [25].

A small proportion of ovarian cancer, generally early stage at diagnosis, is diagnosed in women with Li-Fraumeni syndrome, a cancer predisposition characterized by germline mutations in p53 gene.

51.5 Screening

Several studies have been conducted to verify the feasibility of ovarian cancer screening, evaluating both the benefits and the costs of a needless surgery. Systematic pelvic examination, transvaginal ultrasonography, and biomarker levels have been evaluated, but at present, there is no valid screening program for ovarian cancer, because simply there is no test able to anticipate the diagnosis at an earlier stage [27, 28]. The most important screening studies are as follows:

1. PLCO study (USA) compared annual transvaginal ultrasound and 4-month CA125 blood tests for 4 years versus no screening. After a median follow-up of 12 years, no decrease in mortality was reported; in addition, false-positive results led to serious complications after surgery in 15% of women.

2. UKCTOCS study (UK) compared transvaginal ultrasound plus CA-125 (annual multimodality screening) versus ultrasound alone versus no screening. Preliminary results suggested that the multimodality screening is more effective in detecting early-stage tumors; however, after a median follow-up of 11 years, a significant mortality reduction was not observed.

3. Birmingham School of Medicine (USA) randomized 32,000 women to receive transvaginal ultrasound or CA125 evaluation annually versus no screening, without benefit in cancer-related mortality.

Ultrasound and biochemical monitoring are however suggested for patients with familiarity and with BRCA mutations, even though, also in these cases, no benefit in survival was reported.

51.6 Histological Subtypes

Epithelial ovarian tumors are classified according to the WHO histological classification (◻ Fig. 51.3). Recent classification of these tumors considers cell type, degree of malignancy, and infiltration, distinguishing benign lesions from low malignant potential lesions and from malignant invasive carcinomas. Borderline tumors (low malignant potential) do not exhibit stromal invasion and therefore have a good prognosis, while invasive carcinomas, which have a worse prognosis, have a papillary structure, stromal invasion, and high mitotic activity [29].

Epithelial ovarian cancer comprises five main histological subtypes, including high-grade serous carcinoma (HGSC), low-grade serous carcinoma (LGSC), endometrioid carcinoma (EC), clear-cell carcinoma (CCC),

◻ **Fig. 51.3** WHO histological classification (2014)

Serous tumors
- Serous cystadenoma
- Serous adenofibroma
- Serous surface papilloma
- Serous borderline tumor/atypical proliferative serous tumor
- Serous borderline tumor-micropapillary variant/non-invasive low-grade serous carcinoma
- Low-grade serous
- High-grade serous

Mucinous tumors
- Mucinous cystadenoma
- Mucinous adenofibroma
- Mucinous borderline tumor/atypical proliferative mucinous tumor
- Mucinous carcinoma

Endometrioid tumors
- Endometriotic cyst
- Endometriotic cystadenoma
- Endometriotic adenofibroma
- Endometrioid borderline tumor/atypical proliferative endometrioid tumor
- Endometrioid carcinoma

Clear cell tumors
- Clear cell cystadenoma
- Clear cell adenofibroma
- Clear cell borderline tumor/atypical proliferative clear cell tumor
- Clear cell carcinoma

□ Table 51.4 Tumor histotypes, incidence, and involved genetic pathway

Subtypes	Incidence	Genetic pathway correlated	Microscopic features
High-grade serous carcinoma (HGSC)	70%	TP53: Encodes a protein that regulates the cell cycle BRCA1/2: Encodes proteins that are involved in DNA repair mechanism	
Low-grade serous carcinoma (LGSC)	5%	BRAF KRAS	
Endometrioid carcinoma (EC)	15%	PTEN TP53/BRCA1/2	
Clear-cell carcinoma (CCC)	5%	PTEN ARID1A PIK3CA	
Mucinous carcinoma (MC)	2%	KRAS	

and mucinous carcinoma (MC) [30]. These tumor types really represent different diseases because they are associated with different risk factors (epidemiologic and genetic factors); different incidences, prognosis, and outcomes; different types of response to chemotherapy; and finally different abnormal biomolecular pathways. About 70% of patients have high-grade serous histology, while mucinous and clear-cell carcinomas are extremely rare [31, 32]. Recent histological review distinguished low-grade (grade 1) from high-grade (grade 2 or 3) serous carcinomas recognizing them as different tumor entities (□ Table 51.4) [33, 34].

51.7 Patterns of Spread of Epithelial Ovarian Cancer

- Lymphatic dissemination to pelvic and para-aortic lymph nodes is common in epithelial ovarian cancer. Retroperitoneal lymphatic dissemination in stage I and II tumors has been reported in 5–20% of cases depending on grade and histology [35]. Spread through the retroperitoneal and diaphragmatic lymphatics can result in metastasis to the supraclavicular lymph nodes; in rare cases, retro-

grade invasion of inguinal/femoral lymph nodes is reported.
- Direct extension to adjoining organs, like adhesions to the intestine, is frequent, while the involvement of the lumen of the intestine is uncommon.
- Exfoliation of clonogenic cells that directly implant on peritoneal surfaces (pelvis, paracolic gutters, intestinal mesenteries, right hemidiaphragm) is the principal pattern of spread; tumor cells tend to follow the path of circulation of peritoneal fluid from the right pericolic gutter cephalic to the right hemidiaphragm.
- Hematogenous spread is uncommon, with involvement of the liver, lung, CNS, and bone.

Patterns of spread and dissemination of epithelial ovarian cancer are shown in □ Fig. 51.4.

Various genetic and molecular factors responsible for ovarian carcinoma cell dissemination, able to impact either on peritoneal dissemination or vascular metastasization, have been identified.

The passive dissemination, which impacts on peritoneal involvement, interests numerous enzymes with proteolytic activity (integrin, spheroids, transglutaminases, various interleukins, vascular endothelial growth factor)

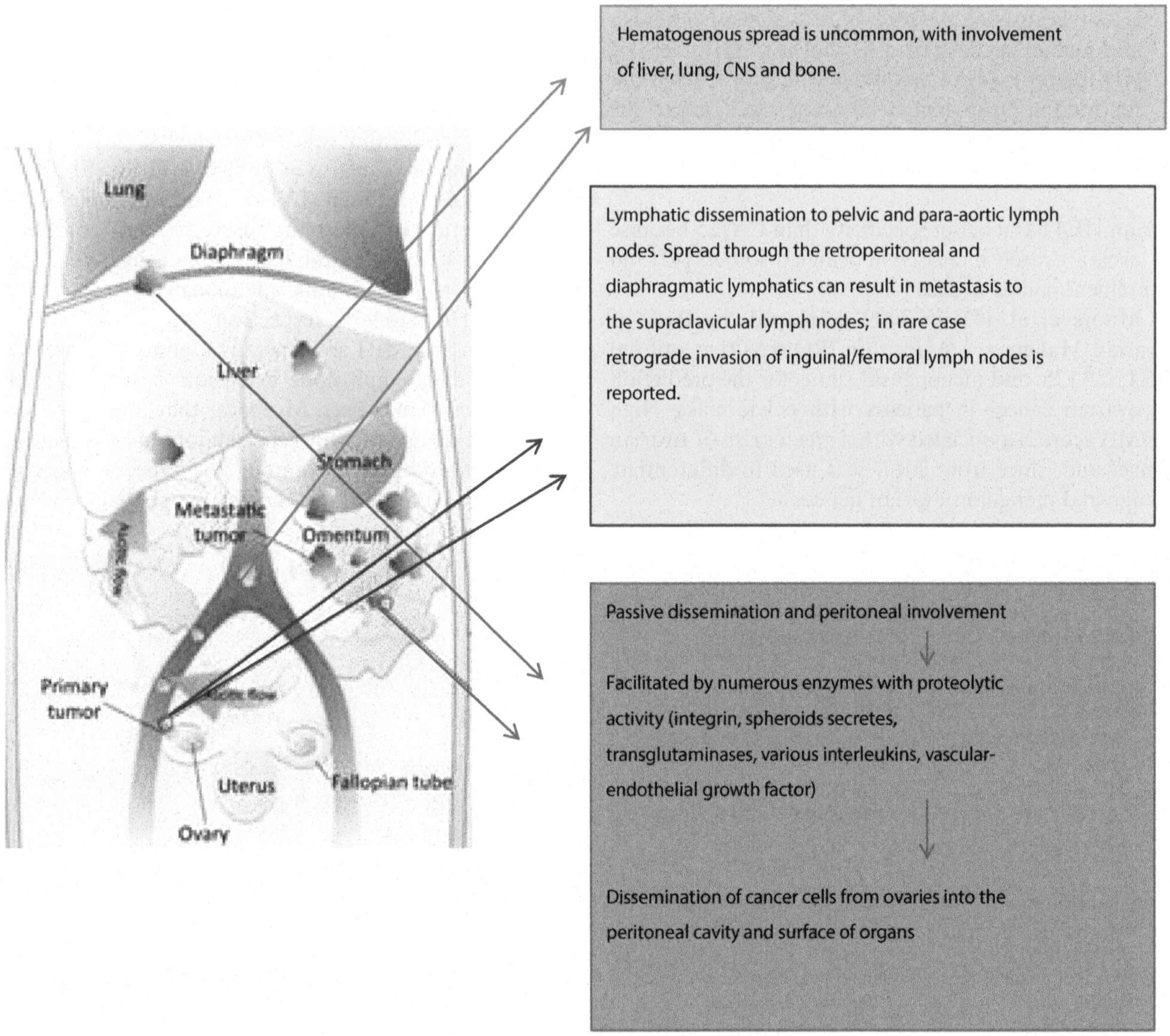
Hematogenous spread is uncommon, with involvement of liver, lung, CNS and bone.
Lymphatic dissemination to pelvic and para-aortic lymph nodes. Spread through the retroperitoneal and diaphragmatic lymphatics can result in metastasis to the supraclavicular lymph nodes; in rare case retrograde invasion of inguinal/femoral lymph nodes is reported.
Passive dissemination and peritoneal involvement
Facilitated by numerous enzymes with proteolytic activity (integrin, spheroids secretes, transglutaminases, various interleukins, vascular-endothelial growth factor)
Dissemination of cancer cells from ovaries into the peritoneal cavity and surface of organs
Lung
Diaphragm
Liver
Stomach
Metastatic tumor
Omentum
Primary tumor
Uterus
Fallopian tube
Ovary

Fig. 51.4 Patterns of spread and dissemination of epithelial ovarian cancer

responsible for dissemination and adhesion of cancer cells into the peritoneal surface [36, 37].

Thereafter, peritoneal implants produce enzymes necessary for new vessel creation. A group of vascular endothelial growth factors (VEGFs) activate vascular and lymphatic endothelium receptors to form new blood and lymphatic vessels with high permeability.

51.8 Diagnosis

Approximately 70% of women with ovarian cancers are diagnosed with advanced disease.

The most common symptoms associated with ovarian cancer are vague and non-specific and include pelvic or abdominal pain, abdominal discomfort, bloating, change in bowel habits, increased abdominal size, dyspepsia and nausea, difficulty eating, early satiety, weight loss, vomiting, and acute abdomen [38].

Rarely ovarian cancer may appear with paraneoplastic syndromes, such as hypercalcemia, thrombophlebitis, Cushing syndrome, and neurologic syndrome with cerebellar ataxia and peripheral neuropathy [39].

The diagnostic evaluation of ovarian cancer is based on:

- Pelvic examination: Gynecologic evaluation with rectovaginal examination is indicated to assess suspicious pelvic or abdominal masses.
- Physical examination: It is indicated, in advanced stage, to assess ascites, superficial lymphadenopathy (generally in supraclavicular and inguinal areas), and pleural effusion.
- Laboratory testing: Cancer biomarkers suggestive of ovarian cancer are CA125 (cancer antigen 125) and HE4 (human epididymis protein 4). CA125 level is elevated in approximately 80% of advanced epithelial ovarian tumors and in 50–60% of patients with early-stage disease [40]. The sensitivity of CA125 in ovarian cancer correlates to tumor stage; specificity

is low because the marker is increased in other benign and malignant disorders, as shown in ▣ Table 51.5 [41]. Better positive predictive values of CA125 are reported in postmenopausal women, because of the higher probability of cancer and the lower prevalence of benign lesions after menopause.

Serum HE4 has a better specificity than CA125 because its levels are rarely increased in benign disorders [42] and in premenopausal women [40].

Moore et al. [43] in 2009 developed the Risk of Ovarian Malignancy Algorithm (ROMA) that utilized HE4, CA125, and menopausal status for the prediction of ovarian cancer in patients with pelvic mass. High ROMA score is associated with a greater risk of ovarian cancer and, since from 2012, it is used to differentiate benign and malignant ovarian masses.

Imaging techniques: Transvaginal ultrasound (TVU) is an important diagnostic tool in the evaluation of patients with a pelvic mass. The typical sonographic finding of malignancy is a "complex" cyst, defined as containing cystic and solid components; presence of septa and papillae can also be observed (▣ Fig. 51.5 and ▣ Table 51.6). Although, TVU is able to evaluate ovarian architecture and mass vascularization and to detect ascites, the sensitivity and specificity in distinguishing benign from malignant adnexal lesions varies from 86% to 94% and 94% to 96%, respectively [44].

CT scan and MRI are generally used to evaluate the peritoneal and lymph node extension in women with suspected ovarian cancer. Moreover they are useful for differential diagnosis with other abdominal neoplasms and are important for planning the type of surgery. Chest study, with X-ray or CT scan, is essential for identifying a pleural effusion.

▣ Table 51.5 Disorders associated to elevated CA125 levels

Benign disorders	Malignant disorders
Pelvic mass correlated Ovarian hyperstimulation syndrome Meigs syndrome	Primary pelvic tumor Ovarian cancer Uterine cancer (advanced stage) Fallopian-tube cancer (advanced stage) Rectal or bladder cancer (advanced stage)
Non-pelvic mass associated Pancreatitis Nephrotic syndrome Liver failure Peritonitis	Secondary pelvic association Peritoneal metastasis in breast cancer Pancreatic carcinoma Peritoneal metastasis in gastric cancer (Krukenberg) Lymphoma

▣ Table 51.6 Typical sonographic finding of benign and malignant masses

Benign mass	Malignant mass
Unilocular cysts	Irregular solid tumor
Presence of solid components <7 mm	Presence of ascites
Presence of acoustic shadowing	At least four papillary structures
Smooth multilocular mass with largest diameter <100 mm	Irregular multilocular solid tumor with largest diameter >100 mm
No blood flow (color score 1)	Very strong blood flow (color score 4)

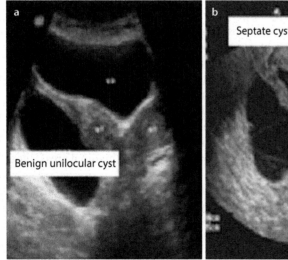
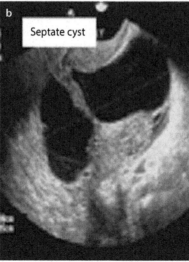
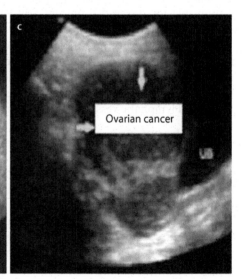

▣ Fig. 51.5 **a** Benign unilocular cyst. **b** Septate cyst. **c** Ovarian cancer

The value of positron emission tomography (PET) has been recently studied. Hypermetabolic lesions are often associated with adnexal malignancies, but several false-positives (follicular cysts or benign cystadenomas) have been identified in pre-menopausal women. PET positivity in postmenopausal patients is always suspicious and must be investigated. However, several studies have documented a sensitivity and specificity inferior to other techniques such as CT scan or MRI (58% and 78%, respectively) and in consequence PET scan is not routinely used [45].

More recently, the role of 18-F-FDG-PET-CT (positron emission tomography CT scan) has been investigated as a more accurate method to characterize adnexal masses. The studies appear very encouraging, demonstrating a superior sensitivity with respect to other techniques (93% and 77% vs. 96% and 38% for PET-CT scan and CT scan alone, respectively) [46]. Unfortunately, a significant percentage of false-negative (borderline tumors, low-grade serous carcinomas, mucinous and clear-cell carcinomas) and false-positive (myomas or corpus luteum) does not advice a routine use of this method.

51.9 Prognostic Factors

Prognostic factors in ovarian cancer are:
- *Ethnicity and race*: At the same stage of diagnosis, Afro-American patients have a 30% greater risk to die when compared to Caucasian women [47].
- *Age:* Younger patents have a survival rate higher than older population across all stages (75% vs. 40%, respectively) [48].
- *Performance status* is an independent prognostic factor: Patients with good PS have a better tolerance to treatments (both surgery and chemotherapy) [49, 50].
- *FIGO stage:* Most powerful predictor of prognosis and most important factor influencing survival (as shown in ▣ Table 51.7) [51]. Careful surgical staging is crucial to address appropriate treatment and assure better survival.
- *In early stage* the most important factors correlating with poor prognosis are histopathological subtype

▣ **Table 51.7** Correlation between FIGO stage and 5-year overall survival

Stage FIGO	5-year overall survival
I	70–90%
II	50–60%
III	20–40%
IV	10%

(serous vs. other histotypes), grade of differentiation (G1-G2-G3), and cyst rupture (spontaneous before surgery or during surgery) [52, 53].
- *Grading* is particularly important for stage I disease and distinguishes three subcategories [54]:
  1. Low risk (good prognosis) → FIGO stage IA, grade 1 with 5-year overall survival >90%
  2. Intermediate risk(FIGO stage IA G2, or IB and IC G1)
  3. High risk (poor prognosis) → (FIGO stage IA grade 3, IB or IC grade 2–3, FIGO stage II, any clear-cell carcinoma) with 5-year overall survival of 50–60%
- *Genetic factors:* Genetic predisposition linked to BRCA1/2 mutation genes is associated with a better prognosis [55]. In several studies, BRCA mutations have been correlated with younger age and improved response to antitumoral treatment, mainly PARP inhibitor [56] and platinum-based chemotherapy [18, 20] but also pegylated liposomal doxorubicin (PLD) [21, 57] or trabectedin [23, 58].
- *Immunologic factors*: Presence of tumor-infiltrating lymphocytes and higher expression of immune signature are considered as good prognostic factors. Immunohistochemical studies demonstrated that the elevated expression of PD-1 and PD-L1 and the elevated concentration of CD3+ and CD8+ TILs, mostly in HR-deficient tumors, were independent positive prognostic factors [59].

51.10 Treatment

The treatment of ovarian cancer is based on the stage of disease which is the reflection of the extent and spread of the cancer. There are generally three approaches for the treatment of ovarian cancer: surgery, chemotherapy, and, only in selected cases, radiation treatment.

51.10.1 Surgery

Surgery is the primary treatment for ovarian cancer. It is used for diagnosis, staging (according to FIGO system), and treatment with the intent of maximal cytoreduction [60]. A small rate of patients with early-stage disease is treated with surgery alone. In all other cases, systemic chemotherapy is added. The standard surgical management of early-stage invasive ovarian cancer consists of:
- Peritoneal washings
- Intact tumor removal
- Total abdominal hysterectomy and bilateral salpingo-oophorectomy (TAH/BSO), only unilateral salpingo-oophorectomy (USO) in selected cases
- Infracolic omentectomy
- Random peritoneal biopsies

— Biopsy of all adhesions and suspicious lesions
— Bilateral pelvic and para-aortic lymph node sampling

A midline vertical incision is critical for an adequate exploration of abdomen. The pelvis and upper abdomen and specifically all peritoneal surfaces (liver, stomach, spleen, large and small bowel, and diaphragms) are carefully explored to identify metastatic implants.

Any ascites is collected for cytology. If no ascites, peritoneal washings should be obtained.

Laparoscopy Several studies have investigated the safety of minimally invasive laparoscopic approach (with the same intra-abdominal procedures) for staging and treatment of early-stage ovarian cancer, mainly to reduce hospital stay and postoperative complications (reduced blood loss, fewer infections) [61, 62]. A systematic review [63] demonstrated that laparoscopy is associated with several disadvantages such as a higher rate of intraoperative cyst rupture and port-site metastasis [64, 65, 66] so it is only considered in experienced centers.

Conservative management of patients desiring to preserve fertility (fertility-sparing surgery) This approach can be considered for young and nulliparous woman with unilateral, low-risk tumors (stage IA or stage IC with grade 1 or 2 and favorable histology [67]. Fertility- sparing surgery includes unilateral salpingo-oophorectomy (preserving the uterus and contralateral ovary) after careful exploration and biopsies of abdominal cavity to exclude metastatic disease, lymphadenectomy, and curettage of the uterine cavity to exclude a synchronous endometrial tumor [60].

The rate of microscopic disease (including positive node, cytology, peritoneal and omental metastases), in apparently EOC, is up to 25% [68]. A recent GOG review on early- stage high-risk ovarian cancer established a 5-year recurrence and overall survival of 75.5% and 81.7%, respectively [12]. Thus surgical restaging in apparent stage I tumors may help in identifying patients requiring adjuvant treatment and is an independent prognostic factor.

51.10.2 Adjuvant Chemotherapy

Systemic adjuvant chemotherapy for early-stage disease is recommended in all patients with high-risk tumors stage IA and IB grade 3 or IC any grade serous, endometrioid, and mucinous and for all stages of clear-cell carcinomas.

The optimal adjuvant therapy for intermediate-risk group (FIGO stage IA G2, IB and IC G1) and high-risk group (FIGO stage IAG3, IB G2-G3, IC G2-G3, and clear cell) had not yet been established until 2003 when solid scientific proof of the clinical effectiveness of adjuvant chemotherapy was provided.

■ **Adjuvant Trials**

In 2003 two large prospective randomized trials (ICON1 and ACTION) [69, 70, 71] and two relevant meta-analyses [72] demonstrated that women who received adjuvant platinum-based chemotherapy had better overall survival and progression-free survival than those who did not.

ICON1: In this trial patients with FIGO stage I–II ovarian cancers requiring adjuvant chemotherapy were randomized to receive platinum-based chemotherapy or observation. Carboplatin (AUC5) for six cycles was administered in most patients (87%). The trial reported a significant benefit in OS (72% vs. 64%) and PFS (70% vs. 60%) for chemotherapy-treated patients versus the observation arm [73]. Subgroup post hoc analysis suggested that high-risk patients (IA G3, IB or IC G2 or G3, clear cell) benefit more from adjuvant chemotherapy.

ACTION: Patients with stage IA and IB G2-G3, all stage IC, and stage IIA, after intensive surgical staging, were randomized to receive platinum-based chemotherapy (47% cisplatin plus cyclophosphamide and 33% single-agent carboplatin) for at least four cycles versus no treatment. The final results reported a significant benefit for chemotherapy-treated patients in terms of PFS (HR 0.63) and OS (HR 0.69). In a subgroup analysis, significant advantages in terms of OS and PFS were identified in sub-optimally staged patients, whereas, among optimally staged patients, there was no significant difference in survival outcomes.

The analysis of the combined trials [70, 71], a Cochrane review [54], and a relevant meta-analysis [74] confirmed the amelioration of survival and PFS for patients receiving adjuvant chemotherapy despite the non-uniformity of data on the type of surgery, the number of cycles, and the type of chemotherapy.

■ **Type of Chemotherapy**

The standard treatment for early-stage disease is carboplatin-based chemotherapy. Single agent or combination is a controversial issue. Literature data present several limitations (different chemotherapy regimens, retrospective data, small number of patients, different surgical approaches, and different postoperative residuals). Specifically, three retrospective trials have compared platinum monotherapy versus platinum-paclitaxel combination in early-stage ovarian cancer [75, 76] suggesting no significant advantage in terms of recurrence and deaths for the combined treatment at the price of a higher toxicity. Despite controversial data, according to published guidelines of the 4th Ovarian Cancer Consensus Conference [2], carboplatin-paclitaxel remains the standard treatment for early-stage disease. Carboplatin alone is a reasonable alternative for patients with poor performance status and comorbidity and, probably, for intermediate-risk disease.

■ **Duration of Treatment**

The optimal number of cycles of adjuvant chemotherapy in early-stage ovarian cancer is not defined. ACTION and ICON trials have demonstrated identical benefit when using four or six courses of platinum-based chemotherapy. The GOG 157 trial [77], comparing three versus six cycles of platinum-paclitaxel chemotherapy, has demonstrated no significant difference in recurrence rate (25% and 20%, respectively) with a higher risk of toxicity in the six-cycle arm. The authors concluded that three cycles of carboplatin-paclitaxel chemotherapy could be considered a sufficient number of cycles in early stage. A subgroup analysis of the same study [78] showed a significant reduction of the risk of recurrence with six cycles of chemotherapy for serous histotypes, while no benefit was reported for other histotypes with a longer treatment.

■ **Viewpoint**

The objective of future research should be to identify possible prognostic and predictive factors able to identify which patients with EOC can benefit from adjuvant chemotherapy. Several studies [79, 80, 81] have shown that DNA ploidy is an independent prognostic factor in early-stage disease distinguishing poor from good prognosis patients and able to separate patients who do not require adjuvant chemotherapy. Other ongoing studies attempt to identify molecular markers, serum protein patterns, gene expression, and microarray profiles with prognostic and predictive roles [82, 83, 84].

51.10.3 Radiotherapy

Radiotherapy is not generally used in the management of patients with early-stage ovarian cancer. Two randomized phase II studies [85, 86] have investigated the role of pelvic radiotherapy in stage I epithelial ovarian cancer, comparing radiotherapy with no postoperative treatment. The trials suggested that pelvic irradiation presents severe toxicity and could reduce the rate of pelvic relapses but does increase OS, because relapses occurred generally in the peritoneal cavity. Otherwise, for clear-cell carcinomas, a mono-institutional study [87] reported a significantly higher 5-year OS and PFS in women with stage I to III OCCC when treated with adjuvant whole abdominal radiation (WAR) probably because the majority of cases are confined to the pelvis and because the disease is generally chemoresistant. On the contrary a recent study [88] has not reported a survival benefit for patients with stage I and II ovarian clear-cell carcinoma treated with adjuvant RT.

Summary of Clinical Recommendations

Chemotherapy recommendations based on risk group:

— Low-risk group: FIGO stage IA and IB grade 1 → chemotherapy is not recommended; patients in this stage have an excellent prognosis without adjuvant treatment.

— Intermediate-risk group: FIGO IA G2, IB G1–G2, IC G1 → the advantage of chemotherapy (carboplatin AUC5-7.5 g1 q 21 single agent or carboplatin plus paclitaxel 175 mg/mq g1 q 21 for three to six cycles) is minimal and this option is to be discussed with patients.

— High-risk group: FIGO stage IA G3, IB G3, IC G2–G3, FIGO stage II, any clear-cell carcinoma: Adjuvant chemotherapy is recommended with carboplatin AUC5-7.5 g1 q 21 plus paclitaxel 175 mg/mq g1 q 21 for three to six cycles; single-agent carboplatin AUC5 is considered for patients with contraindication for doublets.

Case Study 1: Management of Solid Ovarian Masses

36-year-old female, G2P2.

— Family history: Mother (deceased) for endometrial cancer.

— *APR:* No prior history of pelvic infections or abnormal Pap tests.

— *APP:* In the last 3 months, pelvic pain, worsening with defecation.

— Pelvic examination revealed a solid pelvic mass.

Question

What action should be taken?

(1) Surgery. (2) Pelvis transvaginal ultrasound. (3) PET-FDG

Answer

Pelvic ultrasound showed an enlarged right ovary containing a 2.8 × 2.8 cm heterogeneous mass (hypoechoic cystic with a solid component). The image demonstrates increased vascularity within the solid component of the right ovarian mass (suspicion for malignancy).

Question

What action should be taken?

(1) MRI. (2) Surgery. (3) Follow-up

Answer

MRI showed an enlarged right ovary plus peripheral follicles with heterogeneous enhancement. Pelvic free fluid is also apparent.

- CT scan: No evidence of distant metastasis.
- CA125 level was normal.

Question

What action should be taken?
(1) Surgery. (2) Chemotherapy. (3) Radiotherapy

Answer

Monolateral right oophorectomy was performed with frozen section: The histologic report was a serous high-grade ovarian cancer. Immediately contralateral salpingo-oophorectomy, total abdominal hysterectomy, omentectomy, peritoneal washings, random peritoneal biopsies, and bilateral pelvic and para-aortic lymph node sampling were performed → The final pathologic report:

tumor is limited to one ovary; the capsule is intact, no tumor on ovarian surface. No malignant cells are present in peritoneal washings in the peritoneum or lymph nodes (FIGO stage IA grade 1).

Question

What action should be taken?
(1) Follow-up. (2) Chemotherapy. (3) Radiotherapy

Answer

Follow-up
Low-risk group: FIGO stage IA and IB grade 1 → Chemotherapy is not recommended; patients in this stage have an excellent prognosis without other treatments.

Key Points

- Multidisciplinary consultation in the primary management of EOC
- Role of surgery for adequate diagnosis and staging

Case Study 2: Management of Solid Ovarian Masses

46-year-old female
- *APR and APP:* No prior history of gynecologic disorders
- During routine gynecological examination, the gynecologist revealed a pelvic mass with complex characteristics by transvaginal ultrasound

Question

What action should be taken?
(1) Surgery. (2) Follow up. (3) Consultation at a reference center

Answer

The patient was referred to a gynecological center where she received accurate work-up by:
- Transvaginal ultrasound (TVU) → Irregular solid mass with papillary structures and high-density vascularization
- Laboratory testing → CA125 and HE4 at normal levels
- CT scan: Negative for secondary lesions
- Pelvic MRI: Suspicious implants on the uterus and homolateral fallopian tube

Question

What action should be taken?
(1) Surgery. (2) Chemotherapy. (3) Radiotherapy
- The patient underwent surgery → Mass removal with frozen section intraoperative examination was per-

formed. The histology report was suggestive for an epithelial ovarian tumor. The patient underwent complete surgical staging with bilateral salpingo-oophorectomy, total abdominal hysterectomy, omentectomy, peritoneal washings, random peritoneal biopsies, and homolateral pelvic and para-aortic lymphadenectomy → The final pathologic report was ovarian endometrioid carcinoma G3 with implants on the uterus (FIGO stage IIB).

Question

What action should be taken?
(1) Chemotherapy. (2) Follow-up. (3) Radiotherapy

Answer

- In patients with FIGO stage II, classified as high risk, adjuvant chemotherapy is recommended with carboplatin AUC5-7.5 g1 q 21 plus paclitaxel 175 mg/mq g1 q 21 for six cycles.

Key Points

- Surgery has a key role in early-stage tumors for diagnosis and adequate staging.
- High-risk patients should receive adjuvant chemotherapy.
- Suspicious mass should be referred to referral centers for ovarian cancer treatment where adequate preoperative work-up and surgical procedures can be performed.

Expert Opinion
Peter van Dam

Unit of Gynecologic Oncology, Department of Obstetrics & Gynecology, Antwerp University Hospital, Antwerp, Belgium.

Key Points

1. Ovarian cancer is a neoplasm affecting female people with a median age of 60 years old; incidence has increased in the last years, but on the contrary mortality has decreased. The main risk factors are age, genetic predisposition, obesity, and long-term postmenopausal oestrogen therapy. Some genetic syndromes have been associated with the onset of ovarian cancer such as Lynch syndrome and hereditary breast and ovarian syndrome (BRCA1/2).

2. Almost 70% of women are diagnosed with an advanced disease; symptoms are vague and nonspecific, such as abdominal pain, bloating, weight loss, nausea, vomiting, or acute abdomen. The diagnostic assessment is based on pelvic and physical examination, evaluation of Ca125 and HE4 (ROMA Index), US, CT, MRI, and 18F-FDG-PET. Up to date, no screening programs are useful for an early diagnosis, even if ultrasound (US) and biochemical monitoring is suggested for patients with familiarity and BRCA mutations.

3. The main classification schemes are the FIGO and the AJCC staging systems. There are several histological subtypes, such as high-grade serous carcinoma (70% of types), low-grade serous carcinoma, endometroid carcinoma, clear-cell carcinoma, and mucinous carcinoma. Each subtype has different features, and prognosis varies according to the histological group.

4. Ovarian cancer can spread to other organs thanks to different mechanisms: lymphatic dissemination, direct extension to adjoining organs, exfoliation of clonogenic cells that directly implant on peritoneal surfaces and hematogenous spread, which is actually uncommon.

5. Treatment is based on the stage of the neoplasm and it can consist in surgery, chemotherapy, and in selected cases, radiotherapy. Surgery has a diagnostic, staging, and therapeutic intent. A small percentage of patients with early stage are treated with surgery alone; otherwise, chemotherapy is usually added. Carboplatin-paclitaxel remains the standard for early stage disease. Carboplatin alone can be used in patients with comorbidity, poor performance status, and maybe intermediate risk disease.

Recommendations

- ESMO
  - ▸ https://www.esmo.org/Guidelines/Gynaecological-Cancers/ESMO-ESGO-Consensus-Conference-Recommendations-on-Ovarian-Cancer
- AIOM

Hints for a Deeper Insight

- Laparoscopy versus laparotomy for FIGO stage I ovarian cancer: ▸ https://www.ncbi.nlm.nih.gov/pubmed/27737492
- Newly Diagnosed and Relapsed Epithelial Ovarian Carcinoma: ESMO Clinical Practice Guidelines: ▸ https://www.esmo.org/Guidelines/Gynaecological-Cancers/Newly-Diagnosed-and-Relapsed-Epithelial-Ovarian-Carcinoma
- Staging classification for cancer of the ovary, fallopian tube, and peritoneum: ▸ https://www.ncbi.nlm.nih.gov/pubmed/24219974
- 2010 Gynecologic Cancer InterGroup (GCIG) consensus statement on clinical trials in ovarian cancer: report from the Fourth Ovarian Cancer Consensus Conference: ▸ https://www.ncbi.nlm.nih.gov/pubmed/21543936
- Adjuvant (post-surgery) chemotherapy for early stage epithelial ovarian cancer: ▸ https://www.ncbi.nlm.nih.gov/pubmed/22419298

Surgery for Ovarian Cancer

- Surgery is the corner stone of treatment of ovarian cancer. It enables the clinician to confirm the diagnosis histologically, to assess the extent and spread of the disease, and to attempt resect all visible tumor if possible. The concept of cytoreduction was introduced by Griffiths in 1975 and has been validated in several subsequent studies. In patients with advanced epithelial ovarian cancer, surgery is used in conjunction with chemotherapy consisting of a taxane and platinum compound. In most cases, six cycles of paclitaxel and carboplatin are given. Patients with early ovarian cancer often do not require adjuvant chemotherapy. The optimal type of surgical access to the abdomen depends upon the clinical presentation. In young patients who want to preserve their fertility with a tumor of less than 10 cm diameter, which seems to be limited to the ovary(ies), a laparoscopic approach can be considered. In patients with larger tumors and disseminated disease, a (midline) laparotomy is preferred. For patients with no apparent extra-ovarian disease, adequate surgical staging is mandatory as microscopic metastasis can be found in up to 25% of cases, which is an indication for additional chemotherapy. The staging procedure should include inspection of the entire peritoneal cavity, multiple peritoneal biopsies, an (infracolic) omentectomy, a pelvic and paraaortic-lymph node sampling. In patients who do not want to become pregnant anymore and in patients with advanced disease the ovaries, fallopian tubes and uterus are removed. An appendectomy is performed in case of a mucinous tumor. If extra-ovarian disease is visualized, the surgeon should aim to remove all macroscopic tumor. This may require extensive surgery including resection of large- and/or small bowel, excision of implants of peritoneal or liver surface, a splenectomy, etc. Organ resections are performed in about 30% of patients in order to remove all macroscopic disease. Complete surgical resection rates of epithelial ovarian cancer are higher if the surgery is performed by a specialized gynecological oncologist or in high-volume hospitals, but also depend on the biology of the disease (e.g., higher for endometrioid carcinoma). Survival of patients is clearly better after a complete (optimal) debulking. In expert centers, this can be achieved in 70–85% of patients with advanced disease.

- If peri-operative assessment shows that not all macroscopic disease can be removed surgically, interval debulking surgery should be considered. This may be particularly the case in patients with a high upper abdominal tumor load and extensive peritoneal carcinomatosis with a lot of ascites. These patients should receive three to four cycles of chemotherapy after their initial diagnostic and/or staging procedure. Approximately 60% of these patients can have a successful optimal interval cytoreductive operation. Postoperatively these patients are treated with three cycles of additional chemotherapy. A prospective randomized trial showed that the survival of these patients was significantly improved by the second attempt to remove disease. A meta-analysis found no survival benefit of interval debulking surgery compared to primary surgery, but noted a better survival in patients whose primary surgery was not performed by gynecologic oncologists or who had primary suboptimal surgery. The current consensus is that patients should have at least one surgical attempt to remove all visible disease by an experienced team. If possible this should be performed as primary procedure but if not feasible an interval debulking operation should be performed.

- The role of hyperthermic intraperitoneal chemotherapy (HIPEC) in conjunction with cytoreductive surgery remains controversial for patients with ovarian cancer. HIPEC is a highly concentrated, heated chemotherapy treatment that is delivered directly to the abdomen during surgery. A recent Dutch and Korean randomized study gave contradictory results, so the final word remains to be said about this indication. Secondary cytoreductive surgery in patients with recurrent ovarian cancer is safe and effective in selected cases. Preferentially the patients should have platinum-sensitive disease, a disease-free interval of more than 24 months after primary treatment and optimal cytoreduction.

References

1. Eisenhauer EA, Vermorken JB, Van Glabbeke M. Predictors of response to subsequent chemotherapy in platinum pretreated ovarian cancer: a multivariate analysis of 704 patients. Ann Oncol. 1997;8(10):963–8. https://doi.org/10.1023/A:1008240421028.

2. Stuart GCE, Kitchener H, Bacon M, duBois A, Friedlander M, Ledermann J, et al. 2010 Gynecologic Cancer InterGroup (GCIG) consensus statement on clinical trials in ovarian cancer. Int J Gynecol Cancer. 2011;21(4):750–5. https://doi.org/10.1097/IGC.0b013e31821b2568.

3. Prat J, Committee F. International Journal of Gynecology and Obstetrics Staging classi fi cation for cancer of the ovary , fallopian tube , and peritoneum ☆. Int J Gynecol Obstet. 2013;124:1), 1–5. https://doi.org/10.1016/j.ijgo.2013.10.001.

4. Maringe C, Walters S, Butler J, Coleman MP, Hacker N, Hanna L, et al. Stage at diagnosis and ovarian cancer survival: evidence from the international cancer benchmarking partnership. Gynecol Oncol. 2012;127(1):75–82. https://doi.org/10.1016/j.ygyno.2012.06.033.

5. Siegel RL, Miller KD, Jemal A. Cancer statistics, 2016. CA Cancer J Clin. 2016;66(1):7–30. https://doi.org/10.3322/caac.21332.

6. Siegel R, Naishadham D, Jemal A. Cancer statistics, 2013. CA Cancer J Clin. 2013;63(1):11–30. https://doi.org/10.3322/caac.21166.

7. Mosher WD, Jones J. Use of contraception in the United States: 1982-2008. Vital Health Stat. Series 23, Data from the National Survey of Family Growth. 2010;(29):1–44. Retrieved from http://www.ncbi.nlm.nih.gov/pubmed/20939159.

8. Edge SB, Compton CC. The american joint committee on cancer: the 7th edition of the AJCC cancer staging manual and the future of TNM. Ann Surg Oncol. 2010; https://doi.org/10.1245/s10434-010-0985-4.

9. Seidman JD, Yemelyanova AV, Khedmati F, Bidus MA, Dainty L, et al. Prognostic factors for stage I ovarian carcinoma. Int J Gynecol Pathol. 2010;29(1):1–7. https://doi.org/10.1097/PGP.0b013e3181af2372.

10. Morch LS, Lokkegaard E, Andreasen AH, Kjaer SK, Lidegaard O. Hormone therapy and different ovarian cancers: a National Cohort Study. Am J Epidemiol. 2012;175(12):1234–42. https://doi.org/10.1093/aje/kwr446.

51

11. Moorman PG, Havrilesky LJ, Gierisch JM, Coeytaux RR, Lowery WJ, Urrutia RP, et al. Oral contraceptives and risk of ovarian cancer and breast cancer among high-risk women: a systematic review and meta-analysis. J Clin Oncol. 2013;31(33):4188–98. https://doi.org/10.1200/JCO.2013.48.9021.

12. Chan JK, Tian C, Monk BJ, Herzog T, Kapp DS, Bell J, et al. Prognostic factors for high-risk early-stage epithelial ovarian cancer. Cancer. 2008;112(10):2202–10. 10.1002/cncr.23390

13. Modugno F. Ovarian cancer and high-risk women—implications for prevention, screening, and early detection. Gynecol Oncol. 2003;91(1):15–31. https://doi.org/10.1016/S0090-8258(03)00254-3.

14. Pruthi S, Gostout BS, Lindor NM. Identification and management of women with BRCA mutations or hereditary predisposition for breast and ovarian cancer. Mayo Clin Proc. 2010; https://doi.org/10.4065/mcp.2010.0414.

15. Jelovac D, Armstrong DK. Recent progress in the diagnosis and treatment of ovarian cancer. CA Cancer J Clin. 2011;61(3):183–203. https://doi.org/10.3322/caac.20113.

16. Gori S, Barberis M, Bella MA, et al. Recommendations for the implementation of BRCA testing in ovarian cancer patients and their relatives. Crit Rev Oncol Hematol. 2019;140:67–72. https://doi.org/10.1016/j.critrevonc.2019.05.012.

17. Metcalfe KA, Poll A, Royer R, Nanda S, Llacuachaqui M, Sun P, Narod SA. A comparison of the detection of BRCA mutation carriers through the provision of Jewish population-based genetic testing compared with clinic-based genetic testing. Br J Cancer. 2013;109(3):777–9. https://doi.org/10.1038/bjc.2013.309.

18. Alsop K, Fereday S, Meldrum C, DeFazio A, Emmanuel C, George J, et al. BRCA mutation frequency and patterns of treatment response in BRCA mutation-positive women with ovarian cancer: a report from the Australian ovarian cancer study group. J Clin Oncol. 2012;30(21):2654–63. https://doi.org/10.1200/JCO.2011.39.8545.

19. Hennessy BTJ, Timms KM, Carey MS, Gutin A, Meyer LA, Flake DD, et al. Somatic mutations in BRCA1 and BRCA2 could expand the number of patients that benefit from poly (ADP ribose) polymerase inhibitors in ovarian cancer. J Clin Oncol. 2010;28(22):3570–6. https://doi.org/10.1200/JCO.2009.27.2997.

20. Tan DSP, Rothermundt C, Thomas K, Bancroft E, Eeles R, Shanley S, et al. "BRCAness" syndrome in ovarian cancer: a case-control study describing the clinical features and outcome of patients with epithelial ovarian cancer associated with BRCA1 and BRCA2 mutations. J Clin Oncol. 2008;26(34):5530–6. https://doi.org/10.1200/JCO.2008.16.1703.

21. Kaye SB, Lubinski J, Matulonis U, Ang JE, Gourley C, Karlan BY, et al. Phase II, open-label, randomized, multicenter study comparing the efficacy and safety of olaparib, a poly (ADP-ribose) polymerase inhibitor, and pegylated liposomal doxorubicin in patients with BRCA1 or BRCA2 mutations and recurrent ovarian cancer. J Clin Oncol. 2012;30(4):372–9. https://doi.org/10.1200/JCO.2011.36.9215.

22. Safra T, Borgato L, Nicoletto MO, Rolnitzky L, Pelles-Avraham S, Geva R, et al. BRCA mutation status and determinant of outcome in women with recurrent epithelial ovarian cancer treated with pegylated liposomal doxorubicin. Mol Cancer Ther. 2011;10(10):2000–7. https://doi.org/10.1158/1535-7163.MCT-11-0272.

23. Lorusso D, Scambia G, Pignata S, Sorio R, Amadio G, Lepori S, et al. Prospective phase II trial of trabectedin in BRCA-mutated and/or BRCAness phenotype recurrent ovarian cancer patients: the MITO 15 trial. Ann Oncol. 2016;27(3):487–93. https://doi.org/10.1093/annonc/mdv608.

24. Hunn J, Rodriguez GC. Ovarian cancer: etiology, risk factors, and epidemiology. Clin Obstet Gynecol. 2012;55(1):3–23. https://doi.org/10.1097/GRF.0b013e31824b4611.

25. Bonadona V, Bonati B, Olschwang S, Grandjouan S, Huiart L, Longy M, et al. Cancer risks associated with germline mutations in MLH1, MSH2, and MSH6 genes in lynch syndrome. JAMA. 2011;305(22):2304–10. https://doi.org/10.1001/jama.2011.743.

26. Ferlay J, Shin HR, Bray F, Forman D, Mathers C, Parkin DM. Estimates of worldwide burden of cancer in 2008: GLOBOCAN 2008. Int J Cancer. 2010;127(12):2893–917. https://doi.org/10.1002/ijc.25516.

27. Buys SS. Effect of screening on ovarian cancer mortality. JAMA. 2011;305(22):2295. https://doi.org/10.1001/jama.2011.766.

28. Moyer VA. Screening for ovarian cancer: U.S. preventive services task force reaffirmation recommendation statement. Ann Intern Med. 2012; https://doi.org/10.7326/0003-4819-157-11-201212040-00539.

29. Meinhold-Heerlein I, Fotopoulou C, Harter P, Kurzeder C, Mustea A, Wimberger P, et al. The new WHO classification of ovarian, fallopian tube, and primary peritoneal cancer and its clinical implications. Arch Gynecol Obstet. 2016;293(4):695–700. https://doi.org/10.1007/s00404-016-4035-8.

30. Lee KR, Young RH. The distinction between primary and metastatic mucinous carcinomas of the ovary: gross and histologic findings in 50 cases. Am J Surg Pathol. 2003;27(3):281–92. https://doi.org/10.1097/00000478-200303000-00001.

31. Gilks CB, Prat J. Ovarian carcinoma pathology and genetics: recent advances. Hum Pathol. 2009;40(9):1213–23. https://doi.org/10.1016/j.humpath.2009.04.017.

32. Prat J. Ovarian carcinomas: five distinct diseases with different origins, genetic alterations, and clinicopathological features. Virchows Arch. 2012; https://doi.org/10.1007/s00428-012-1203-5.

33. Gourley C, Farley J, Provencher DM, Pignata S, Mileshkin L, Harter P, et al. Gynecologic Cancer InterGroup (GCIG) consensus review for ovarian and primary peritoneal low-grade serous carcinomas. Int J Gynecol Cancer. 2014;24(9 Suppl 3):S9–S13. https://doi.org/10.1097/IGC.0000000000000257.

34. McCluggage WG. Morphological subtypes of ovarian carcinoma: a review with emphasis on new developments and pathogenesis. Pathology. 2011; https://doi.org/10.1097/PAT.0b013e328348a6e7.

35. Berek JS, Bertelsen K, du Bois A, Brady MF, Carmichael J, Eisenhauer EA, et al. Epithelial ovarian cancer (advanced stage): consensus conference (1998). Gynecol Obstet Fertil. 2000;28(7–8):576–83. Retrieved from http://www.ncbi.nlm.nih.gov/pubmed/10996969.

36. Hwang JY, Mangala LS, Fok JY, Lin YG, Merritt WM, Spannuth WA, et al. Clinical and biological significance of tissue transglutaminase in ovarian carcinoma. Cancer Res. 2008;68(14):5849–58. https://doi.org/10.1158/0008-5472.CAN-07-6130.

37. Moser TL, Pizzo SV, Bafetti LM, Fishman DA, Stack MS. Evidence for preferential adhesion of ovarian epithelial carcinoma cells to type I collagen mediated by the alpha2beta1 integrin. Int J Cancer. 1996;67(5):695–701. https://doi.org/10.1002/(SICI)1097-0215(19960904)67:5<695::AID-IJC18>3.0.CO;2-4.

38. Goff BA, Mandel LS, Melancon CH, Muntz HG. Frequency of symptoms of ovarian cancer in women presenting to primary care clinics. J Am Med Assoc. 2004;291(22):2705–12. https://doi.org/10.1001/jama.291.22.2705.

39. Cannistra SA. Cancer of the ovary. N Engl J Med. 2004;351(24):2519–29. https://doi.org/10.1056/NEJMra041842.

40. Wu L, Dai Z-Y, Qian Y-H, Shi Y, Liu F-J, Yang C. Diagnostic value of serum human epididymis protein 4 (HE4) in ovarian carcinoma: a systematic review and meta-analysis. Int J Gynecol Cancer. 2012;22(7):1106–12. https://doi.org/10.1097/IGC.0b013e318263efa2.

41. Escudero JM, Auge JM, Filella X, Torne A, Pahisa J, Molina R. Comparison of serum human epididymis protein 4 with can-

cer antigen 125 as a tumor marker in patients with malignant and nonmalignant diseases. Clin Chem. 2011;57(11):1534–44. https://doi.org/10.1373/clinchem.2010.157073.

42. Moore RG, Miller MC, Steinhoff MM, Skates SJ, Lu KH, Lambert-Messerlian G, Bast RC. Serum HE4 levels are less frequently elevated than CA125 in women with benign gynecologic disorders. Am J Obstet Gynecol. 2012;206(4):351.e1–8. https://doi.org/10.1016/j.ajog.2011.12.029.

43. Moore RG, McMeekin DS, Brown AK, DiSilvestro P, Miller MC, et al. A novel multiple marker bioassay utilizing HE4 and CA125 for the prediction of ovarian cancer in patients with a pelvic mass. Gynecol Oncol. 2009;112(1):40–6. https://doi.org/10.1016/j.ygyno.2008.08.031.

44. Timmerman D, Testa AC, Bourne T, Ameye L, Jurkovic D, Van Holsbeke C, et al. Simple ultrasound-based rules for the diagnosis of ovarian cancer. Ultrasound Obstet Gynecol. 2008;31(6):681–90. https://doi.org/10.1002/uog.5365.

45. Rieber A, Nüssle K, Stöhr I, Grab D, Fenchel S, Kreienberg R, et al. Preoperative diagnosis of ovarian tumors with MR imaging. Am J Roentgenol. 2001;177(1):123–9. https://doi.org/10.2214/ajr.177.1.1770123.

46. Dauwen H, Van Calster B, Deroose CM, Op De Beeck K, Amant F, Neven P, et al. PET/CT in the staging of patients with a pelvic mass suspicious for ovarian cancer. Gynecol Oncol. 2013;131(3):694–700. https://doi.org/10.1016/j.ygyno.2013.08.020.

47. Zeng C, Wen W, Morgans AK, Pao W, Shu XO, Zheng W. Disparities by race, age, and sex in the improvement of survival for major cancers: results from the National Cancer Institute Surveillance, Epidemiology, and End Results (SEER) program in the United States, 1990 to 2010. JAMA Oncol. 2015;1(1):88–96. https://doi.org/10.1001/jamaoncol.2014.161.

48. Lee C, Pires de Miranda M, Ledermann J, Ruiz de Elvira M-C, Nelstrop A, Lambert H, et al. Outcome of epithelial ovarian cancer in women under 40 years of age treated with platinum-based chemotherapy. Eur J Cancer. 1999;35(5):727–32. https://doi.org/10.1016/S0959-8049(99)00011-8.

49. Akahira JI, Yoshikawa H, Shimizu Y, Tsunematsu R, Hirakawa T, Kuramoto H, et al. Prognostic factors of stage IV epithelial ovarian cancer: a multicenter retrospective study. Gynecol Oncol. 2001;81(3):398–403. https://doi.org/10.1006/gyno.2001.6172.

50. Chan JK, Zhang M, Kaleb V, Loizzi V, Benjamin J, Vasilev S, et al. Prognostic factors responsible for survival in sex cord stromal tumors of the ovary - a multivariate analysis. Gynecol Oncol. 2005;96(1):204–9. https://doi.org/10.1016/j.ygyno.2004.09.019.

51. Jemal A, Siegel R, Ward E, Murray T, Xu J, Thun MJ. Cancer statistics, 2007. CA Cancer J Clin. n.d.;57(1):43–66. Retrieved from http://www.ncbi.nlm.nih.gov/pubmed/17237035.

52. Malkasian GD, Melton LJ, O'Brien PC, Greene MH. Prognostic significance of histologic classification and grading of epithelial malignancies of the ovary. Am J Obstet Gynecol. 1984;149(3):274–84. https://doi.org/10.1016/0002-9378(84)90227-8.

53. Vergote I, Trimbos BJ. Treatment of patients with early epithelial ovarian cancer. Curr Opin Oncol. 2003;15(6):452–5.

54. Winter-Roach BA, Kitchener HC, Lawrie TA. Adjuvant (post-surgery) chemotherapy for early stage epithelial ovarian cancer. In: Winter-Roach BA, editor. Cochrane database of systematic reviews. Chichester, UK: Wiley; 2012. p. CD004706. https://doi.org/10.1002/14651858.CD004706.pub4.

55. Bolton KL. Association between BRCA1 and BRCA2 mutations and survival in women with invasive epithelial ovarian cancer. JAMA. 2012;307(4):382. https://doi.org/10.1001/jama.2012.20.

56. McLachlan J, George A, Banerjee S. The current status of PARP inhibitors in ovarian cancer. Tumori. 2016; https://doi.org/10.5301/tj.5000558.

57. Adams SF, Marsh EB, Elmasri W, Halberstadt S, Vandecker S, Sammel MD, et al. A high response rate to liposomal doxorubicin

is seen among women with BRCA mutations treated for recurrent epithelial ovarian cancer. Gynecol Oncol. 2011;123(3):486–91. https://doi.org/10.1016/j.ygyno.2011.08.032.

58. Russo A, Incorvaia L, Malapelle U, et al. The tumor-agnostic treatment for patients with solid tumors: a position paper on behalf of the AIOM-SIAPEC/IAP-SIBIOC-SIF italian scientific societies [published online ahead of print, 2021 Aug 6]. Crit Rev Oncol Hematol. 2021;103436. https://doi.org/10.1016/j.critrevonc.2021.103436.

59. Strickland KC, Howitt BE, Shukla SA, Rodig S, Ritterhouse LL, Liu JF, et al. Association and prognostic significance of BRCA1/2-mutation status with neoantigen load, number of tumor-infiltrating lymphocytes and expression of PD-1/PD-L1 in high grade serous ovarian cancer. Oncotarget. 2016;7(12):13587–98. https://doi.org/10.18632/oncotarget.7277.

60. Liu JH, Zanotti KM. Manejo de la Masa Anexial. Obstet Gynecol. 2011;117(6):1413–28. https://doi.org/10.1097/AOG.0b013e31821c62b6.

61. Ghezzi F, Cromi A, Uccella S, Bergamini V, Tomera S, Franchi M, Bolis P. Laparoscopy versus laparotomy for the surgical management of apparent early stage ovarian cancer. Gynecol Oncol. 2007;105(2):409–13. https://doi.org/10.1016/j.ygyno.2006.12.025.

62. Qureshi ZP, Norris L, Sartor O, McKoy JM, Armstrong J, Raisch DW, et al. Caveat oncologist: clinical findings and consequences of distributing counterfeit erythropoietin in the United States. J Oncol Pract/Am Soc Clin Oncol. 2012;8(2):84–90. https://doi.org/10.1200/JOP.2011.000325.

63. Falcetta FS, Lawrie TA, Medeiros LR, da Rosa MI, Edelweiss MI, Stein AT, et al. Laparoscopy versus laparotomy for FIGO stage I ovarian cancer. In: Rosa DD, editor. Cochrane database of systematic reviews. Chichester, UK: Wiley; 2016. https://doi.org/10.1002/14651858.CD005344.pub4.

64. Muzii L, Angioli R, Zullo M, Panici PB. The unexpected ovarian malignancy found during operative laparoscopy: incidence, management, and implications for prognosis. J Minim Invasive Gynecol. 2005;12(1):81–9. https://doi.org/10.1016/j.jmig.2004.12.019.

65. Spirtos NM, Eisekop SM, Boike G, Schlaerth JB, Cappellari JO, Mackey D. Laparoscopic staging in patients with incompletely staged cancers of the uterus, ovary, fallopian tube, and primary peritoneum: a Gynecologic Oncology Group (GOG) study. Am J Obstet Gynecol. 2005;193(5):1645–9. https://doi.org/10.1016/j.ajog.2005.05.004.

66. Vaisbuch E, Dgani R, Ben-Arie A, Hagay Z. The role of laparoscopy in ovarian tumors of low malignant potential and early-stage ovarian cancer. Obstet Gynecol Surv. 2005; https://doi.org/10.1097/01.ogx.0000161373.94922.33.

67. Ledermann JA, Raja FA, Fotopoulou C, Gonzalez-Martin A, Colombo N, Sessa C. Newly diagnosed and relapsed epithelial ovarian carcinoma: ESMO clinical practice guidelines for diagnosis, treatment and follow-up. Ann Oncol. 2013;24(SUPPL.6):vi24–32. https://doi.org/10.1093/annonc/mdt333.

68. Young RC, Decker DG, Wharton JT, Piver MS, Sindelar WF, Edwards BK, Smith JP. Staging laparotomy in early ovarian cancer. JAMA. 1983;250(22):3072–6. https://doi.org/10.1001/jama.1983.03340220040030.

69. Colombo N, Guthrie D, Chiari S, Parmar M, Qian W, Swart AM, et al. International Collaborative Ovarian Neoplasm trial 1: a randomized trial of adjuvant chemotherapy in women with early-stage ovarian cancer. J Natl Cancer Inst. 2003;95(2):125–32. https://doi.org/10.1093/jnci/95.2.125.

70. Trimbos JB, Parmar M, Vergote I, Guthrie D, Bolis G, Colombo N, et al. International Collaborative Ovarian Neoplasm trial 1 and Adjuvant ChemoTherapy In Ovarian Neoplasm trial: two parallel randomized phase III trials of adjuvant chemotherapy in patients with early-stage ovarian carcinoma. J Natl Cancer Inst. 2003;95(2):105–12. https://doi.org/10.1093/jnci/95.2.105.

71. Trimbos JB, Vergote I, Bolis G, Vermorken JB, Mangioni C, Madronal C, et al. Impact of adjuvant chemotherapy and surgical staging in early-stage ovarian carcinoma: European Organisation for Research and Treatment of Cancer-Adjuvant ChemoTherapy in Ovarian Neoplasm trial. J Natl Cancer Inst. 2003;95(2):113–25. https://doi.org/10.1093/jnci/95.2.113.

72. Winter-Roach BA, Kitchener HC, Lawrie TA. Adjuvant (post-surgery) chemotherapy for early stage epithelial ovarian cancer. Cochrane Database Syst Rev. 2009;(3) https://doi.org/10.1002/14651858.CD004706.pub3.

73. Tropé C, Kaern J. Adjuvant chemotherapy for early-stage ovarian cancer: review of the literature. J Clin Oncol. 2007; https://doi.org/10.1200/JCO.2007.11.1013.

74. Winter-Roach B, Hooper L, Kitchener H. Systematic review of adjuvant therapy for early stage (epithelial) ovarian cancer. Int J Gynecol Cancer. 2003;13(4):395–404. Retrieved from http://www.ncbi.nlm.nih.gov/pubmed/12911714.

75. Adams G, Zekri J, Wong H, Walking J, Green JA. Platinum-based adjuvant chemotherapy for early-stage epithelial ovarian cancer: single or combination chemotherapy? BJOG. 2010;117(12):1459–67. https://doi.org/10.1111/j.1471-0528.2010.02635.x.

76. Skírnisdóttir I, Lindborg K, Sorbe B. Adjuvant chemotherapy with carboplatin and taxane compared with single drug carboplatin in early stage epithelial ovarian carcinoma. Oncol Rep. 2007;18(5):1249–56. Retrieved from http://www.ncbi.nlm.nih.gov/pubmed/17914581.

77. Bell J, Brady MF, Young RC, Lage J, Walker JL, Look KY, et al. Randomized phase III trial of three versus six cycles of adjuvant carboplatin and paclitaxel in early stage epithelial ovarian carcinoma: a Gynecologic Oncology Group study. Gynecol Oncol. 2006;102(3):432–9. https://doi.org/10.1016/j.ygyno.2006.06.013.

78. Chan JK, Tian C, Fleming GF, Monk BJ, Herzog TJ, Kapp DS, Bell J. The potential benefit of 6 vs. 3 cycles of chemotherapy in subsets of women with early-stage high-risk epithelial ovarian cancer: an exploratory analysis of a Gynecologic Oncology Group study. Gynecol Oncol. 2010;116(3):301–6. https://doi.org/10.1016/j.ygyno.2009.10.073.

79. But I, Gorisek B. DNA-ploidy as an independent prognostic factor in patients with serous ovarian carcinoma. Int J Gynaecol Obstet. 2000;71(3):259–62. https://doi.org/10.1016/S0020-7292(00)00277-0.

80. Kristensen GB, Kildal W, Abeler VM, Kaern J, Vergote I, Tropé CG, Danielsen HE. Large-scale genomic instability predicts long-term outcome for women with invasive stage I ovarian cancer. Ann Oncol. 2003;14(10):1494–500. https://doi.org/10.1093/annonc/mdg403.

81. Schueler JA, Trimbos JB, vd Burg M, Cornelisse CJ, Hermans J, Fleuren GJ. DNA index reflects the biological behavior of ovarian carcinoma stage I-IIa. Gynecol Oncol. 1996;62(1):59–66. Retrieved from http://www.ncbi.nlm.nih.gov/pubmed/8690293.

82. De Cecco L, Berardi M, Sommariva M, Cataldo A, Canevari S, Mezzanzanica D, et al. Increased sensitivity to chemotherapy induced by CpG-ODN treatment is mediated by microRNA modulation. PLoS One. 2013;8(3):e58849. https://doi.org/10.1371/journal.pone.0058849.

83. Mok SC, Chao J, Skates S, Wong K, Yiu GK, Muto MG, et al. Prostasin, a potential serum marker for ovarian cancer: identification through microarray technology. J Natl Cancer Inst. 2001;93(19):1458–64. https://doi.org/10.1093/jnci/93.19.1458.

84. Trope C, Kaern J, Tropé C. Adjuvant chemotherapy for early-stage ovarian cancer: review of the literature. J Clin Oncol. 2007; 25(20):2909–20. https://doi.org/10.1200/JCO.2007.11.1013.

85. Dembo AJ. Epithelial ovarian cancer: the role of radiotherapy. Int J Radiat Oncol Biol Phys. 1992;22(5):835–45. Retrieved from http://www.ncbi.nlm.nih.gov/pubmed/1555974.

86. Engelen MJA, Snel BJ, Schaapveld M, Pras E, de Vries EGE, Gietema JA, et al. Long-term morbidity of adjuvant whole abdominal radiotherapy (WART) or chemotherapy for early stage ovarian cancer. Eur J Cancer. 2009;45(7):1193–200. https://doi.org/10.1016/j.ejca.2009.01.006.

87. Nagai Y, Inamine M, Hirakawa M, Kamiyama K, Ogawa K, Toita T, et al. Postoperative whole abdominal radiotherapy in clear cell adenocarcinoma of the ovary. Gynecol Oncol. 2007;107(3):469–73. https://doi.org/10.1016/j.ygyno.2007.07.079.

88. Hogen L, Thomas G, Bernardini M, Bassiouny D, Brar H, Gien LT, et al. The effect of adjuvant radiation on survival in early stage clear cell ovarian carcinoma. Gynecol Oncol. 2016;143(2):258–63. https://doi.org/10.1016/j.ygyno.2016.09.006.

Ovarian Cancer: Primary Advanced and Recurrent Disease

Domenica Lorusso, Giuseppa Maltese, Lorena Incorvaia, Ilaria Sabatucci, and Stefano Lepori

Gynecological Cancers

Contents

© Springer Nature Switzerland AG 2021
A. Russo et al. (eds.), *Practical Medical Oncology Textbook*, UNIPA Springer Series,
https://doi.org/10.1007/978-3-030-56051-5_52

52

By the end of the chapter, the reader will:
 - Be able to apply medical and surgical procedures in the management of primary advanced and recurrent EOC
 - Have learned the basic concepts and the clinical indications to primary and secondary cytoreductive surgery
 - Have reached in-depth knowledge of recurrence treatment strategy in order to build an algorithm that allow patients to receive all the available treatment options, possibly in the more appropriate temporary order
 - Be able to apply acquired knowledge about molecular and genetic characteristics of ovarian cancer to ameliorate treatment options and targeted therapy approaches

52.1 Introduction

About 70% of patients with epithelial ovarian cancer (EOC) are diagnosed at advanced International Federation of Gynecology and Obstetrics (FIGO) stage III or IV disease, with a 5-year survival that ranges from 39% to 17% [1].

Generally, more than 70% of women with advanced disease obtain a complete clinical and instrumental remission at the completion of primary treatment, but unfortunately 50–70% of them will develop a recurrence after a median PFS of approximately 18 months [2].

In the last years, the survival rate of patients with advanced and recurrent ovarian cancer has increased thanks to the improvement of surgery and the utilization of novel antitumoral agents. Moreover, a significant increase in the knowledge of molecular and genetic characteristics of ovarian cancer has led to the improvement of treatment options including targeted therapies.

52.2 Epidemiology, Diagnosis, Pathogenesis, and Prognosis

Ovarian cancer typically spreads to peritoneal surfaces and the omentum and can diffuse by local extension, lymphatic invasion, intraperitoneal implantation, hematogenous dissemination, and transdiaphragmatic passage. Intraperitoneal dissemination is the most common: malignant cells can spread anywhere in the peritoneal cavity but are more likely to implant in sites of stasis along the peritoneal fluid circulation (e.g., pelvis, paracolic gutters, intestinal mesenteries, right hemidiaphragm).

When disease spreads beyond the ovaries, determining an advanced stage, patients experience persistent but not specific symptoms such as abdominal bloating, constipation, digestive difficulties, nausea, loss of appetite, sense of pelvic weight, or lower back pain. Patients with advanced disease are instrumentally evaluated with CT scan, PET-FDG, or MRI in order to assess site, size, and distribution of metastases particularly for preoperative appraisal of resectability.

Preoperative serum Ca125 level is elevated in 75% of cases; it frequently reflects the burden of disease and does not appear to be predictive of survival. The postoperative and during chemotherapy reduction of Ca125 value is associated with a more favorable outcome.

Recently, Zeng et al. reported that normalization of Ca125 levels after three cycles of neoadjuvant chemotherapy is associated with more favorable outcomes, as well as achievement of a Ca125 nadir equal or less than 10 U/L after completion of treatment [3].

Other prognostic and predictive factors are [4]:
 - FIGO tumor stage
 - Age
 - Histology (mucinous and clear cell histotypes are associated with poor prognosis than other histotypes)
 - Grade of differentiation
 - Performance status
 - BRCA mutational status
 - Residual tumor after cytoreductive surgery
 - Markers of proliferation and growth factors receptors (Bcl-2, EGFR, GST, LRP, p16, p21, P-pg, and TNF-α)
 - Expression of genes associated with metastasization

52.3 Staging of Ovarian Cancer

Ovarian cancer is staged according to the International Federation of Gynecology and Obstetrics (FIGO) surgical staging system (🔲 Table 52.1) [5].

52.4 Primary Treatment of Advanced Disease

Management of primary advanced disease includes:
 - Primary cytoreductive surgery or neoadjuvant chemotherapy (NACT) followed by interval debulking surgery (IDS)
 - Chemotherapy (intravenous chemotherapy or intraperitoneal chemotherapy)
 - Maintenance therapy

◻ Table 52.1 FIGO staging of advanced ovarian cancer (2014)

Stage III	Tumor involves one or both ovaries with cytologically or histologically confirmed spread to the peritoneum outside the pelvis and/or metastasis to the retroperitoneal lymph nodes
IIIA	Positive retroperitoneal lymph nodes and/or microscopic metastasis beyond the pelvis IIIA1 positive retroperitoneal lymph nodes only IIIA1(i) metastasis ≤10 mm IIIA1(ii) metastasis >10 mm
IIIA2	Microscopic, extrapelvic (above the brim) Peritoneal involvement ± positive Retroperitoneal lymph nodes
IIIB	Macroscopic, extrapelvic, peritoneal Metastasis ≤2 cm ± positive Retroperitoneal lymph nodes. Includes Extension to capsule of the liver/spleen
IIIC	Macroscopic, extrapelvic, peritoneal Metastasis >2 cm ± positive Retroperitoneal lymph nodes. Includes Extension to capsule of the liver/spleen
Stage IV	Distant metastasis excluding peritoneal metastasis
IVA	IVA pleural effusion with positive cytology
IVB	Hepatic and/or splenic parenchymal Metastasis, metastasis to extra-abdominal organs (including inguinal lymph nodes and lymph nodes outside of the abdominal cavity)

52.4.1 Primary Debulking

The standard treatment of patients with advanced EOC is radical cytoreductive surgery followed by platinum-based chemotherapy for six to eight cycles [6]. The role of primary surgery is to provide histological diagnosis, stage the disease, and provide, when possible, a complete tumor debulking [7, 8].

The primary debulking surgery (PDS) involves:
- Total abdominal hysterectomy (TAH)
- Bilateral salpingo-oophorectomy (BSO)
- Peritoneal washing
- Omentectomy
- Biopsies of peritoneal surfaces
- Pelvic and para-aortic lymphadenectomy of bulky nodes
- Removal of all visible lesions and biopsies of any suspected areas

Furthermore, other more invasive procedures, such as splenectomy, bowel resection, partial hepatectomy/gastrectomy, or cystectomy, are frequently required to adequately and radically debulk all visible disease [9, 10].

Primary optimal cytoreductive surgery is considered an essential step in the management of advanced ovarian cancer because it confers better outcome and prognosis to patients [11]. Another important role of primary surgery is to remove large necrotic lesions promoting drug failure and chemoresistance; furthermore, removing bulky intra-abdominal lesions ameliorates patient symptoms decreasing the risk of bowel obstruction or perforation [12].

The success of debulking surgery depends on various aspects, such as patient performance status, extension of disease, and, probably the most important one, surgeon expertise [13].

The objective of debulking surgery is to achieve maximal cytoreduction by removing all visible disease; in general, cytoreductive surgery is defined as optimal when all macroscopic disease is resected and is defined optimal when the largest residual tumor after procedure is less than 1 cm in maximum diameter [14]. Residual disease at primary surgery and outcome are strictly related; in this context, all studies report a statistical survival advantage in patients with ≤1 cm residual disease compared to patients with residual disease >1 cm [11, 15].

▪ Systematic Lymphadenectomy

Actually, the standard management of stage IIIC–IV ovarian cancer involves removal of pelvic and para-aortic lymph nodes only if clinically suspicious. Systematic lymphadenectomy of non-suspicious nodes during primary surgery has recently been discouraged because of the lack of evidence for therapeutic role [16].

An Italian perspective randomized trial evaluated FIGO stage IIIB–IIIC and IV EOC patients to receive systematic pelvic and para-aortic lymphadenectomy at primary debulking surgery versus removal of only bulky nodes. The final results showed an improvement in progression-free but not in overall survival in patients who had undergone systematic lymphadenectomy [17].

The recently published results of a prospective randomized AGO trial (LION), which investigated the role of systematic pelvic and para-aortic lymphadenectomy versus no lymphadenectomy in FIGO stage IIB–IV epithelial ovarian cancer patients achieving complete intraperitoneal debulking during primary surgery, showed no improvement in overall and progression-free survival in patients subjected to systematic lymphadenectomy.

Recent international guidelines do not recommend systematic lymphadenectomy other than the removal of suspicious and/or enlarged nodes in patients with advanced EOC [18, 19].

▪ Ultra-radical Surgery

The criteria of "extension of debulking" evolved in the last years since postoperative residual tumor is considered the most important survival prognostic factor.

Unanimously recent international guidelines recommend the maximum surgical effort at primary cytoreduction, with the goal of no macroscopic residual disease [20].

Ultra-radical surgery is defined as an aggressive approach aiming to obtain the complete macroscopic resection of all visible disease. The ultra-radical debulking is comprehensive of the already described surgical procedures with eventually bowel resection, splenectomy, cholecystectomy, caudal pancreatectomy, large stripping of the peritoneum, and diaphragm or hepatic resection, if involvement is demonstrated. Retrospective data suggest that patients receiving aggressive surgical debulking have a significant improved survival when compared to those with suboptimal cytoreduction at the price of increased complications [9, 10, 21].

- ■ Neoadjuvant Chemotherapy (NACT)

Neoadjuvant chemotherapy is defined as a treatment given before surgery (defined as interval debulking surgery or IDS) to reduce tumor dimensions and increasing surgical radicality. The objective of NACT is to increase the complete resection rate at interval debulking surgery and decrease perioperative morbidity and mortality. This approach is typically considered an option for patients with stage IIIC and IV EOC who are not good candidates to upfront surgery for several reasons (comorbidities, poor performance status, high perioperative risk, low possibility of optimal cytoreduction,

or non-removable sites of metastasis) [22]. Generally patients receive three cycles of carboplatin-paclitaxel chemotherapy, and subsequently, if there is evidence of response, they undergo interval debulking surgery followed by additional three cycles of the same chemotherapy.

Actually, information about the therapeutic role of NACT followed by interval debulking surgery is controversial. The approach is supported by two phase III international randomized trials, EORTC 55971 and CHORUS studies, which compared NACT followed by interval debulking surgery to primary debulking surgery followed by adjuvant chemotherapy in stage IIIC–IV patients with potentially resectable disease. The final results showed no difference in PFS and OS in both arms with less morbidity in patients receiving NACT [23, 24]. Both studies have been criticized because of the scanty median OS, the slow mean operative time, and the rates of optimal cytoreduction in the primary surgery arm (■ Fig. 52.1).

A recently published meta-analysis showed that neoadjuvant chemotherapy helps the gynecologic surgeons to achieve an increased rate of optimal cytoreduction, while a meta-analysis by Bristow et al. showed a negative survival effect in patients undergoing interval debulking surgery compared with those receiving primary surgery [25].

Therefore, the choice between primary cytoreductive surgery and NACT remains unclear. A position

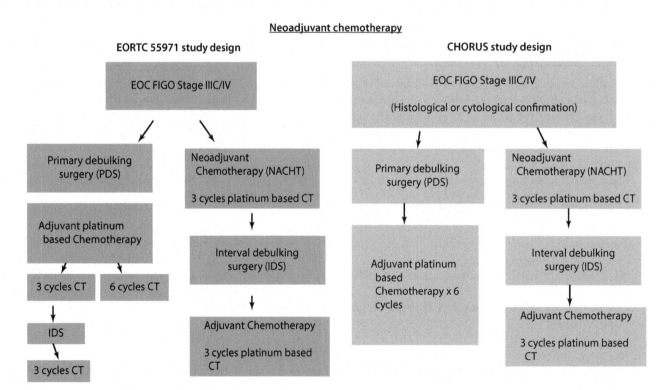

■ **Fig. 52.1** EORTC 55971 and CHORUS study design

paper concerning the appropriate use of NACT in advanced ovarian cancer has recently been published by the American Society of Clinical Oncology and the Society of Gynecologic Oncology [26]. The consensus panel concluded that PDS is recommended in patients fit for surgery and with a good chance of achieving optimal cytoreduction while NACT followed by IDS is the preferred approach for patients with advanced-stage disease less fit for surgery and with low possibility of achieving upfront radical cytoreduction. Both conditions have to be assessed by a gynecologic oncologist.

The number of NACT cycles (ranging from three to six) and consequently the optimal surgery timing are still controversial. Colombo et al. retrospectively evaluated patients with stages IIIC–IV EOC according to the number of neoadjuvant chemotherapy cycles (<4 = group B1; >4 = group B2) and compared them with patients receiving PDS (group A) [27]. Final results showed an inverse relationship between prognosis and number of NACT cycles; patients receiving late IDS had a worse survival compared to patients treated with early IDS or PDS. Similar results are reported in the Bristow meta-analysis, which demonstrated an inverse relationship between survival and the number of NACT cycles with each additional chemotherapy cycle beyond the third associated with a 4-month decrease in overall survival. In conclusion, IDS should be attempted as soon as possible, preferably no later than three or four cycles of NACT.

52.5 Systemic Treatment

Intravenous platinum-paclitaxel chemotherapy is the standard of care in patients with stage III and IV ovarian cancer. A complete clinical remission is achieved in approximately 70% of treated patients, but up to 80% of them will experience disease recurrence after a median PFS of approximately 18 months [28]. At current time, platinum-taxane combination is the gold standard of treatment, showing improved survival compared to platinum single agent or to platinum-non-taxane combinations [29].

As reported by several studies, the addition of a third non-cross-resistant agent (e.g., liposomal doxorubicin, gemcitabine, or topotecan) does not improve survival compared to platinum-paclitaxel doublet [30, 31, 32, 33, 34, 35].

There is no evidence that continuing first-line platinum-paclitaxel chemotherapy beyond six cycles confers additional benefit to patients with advanced ovarian cancer; similarly there is no evidence that maintenance treatment with a different chemotherapy agent increases OS in advanced disease.

■ **Schedules of Intravenous Chemotherapy**

The established doses of chemotherapy are carboplatin AUC 5–6 and paclitaxel 175 mg/m^2 every 3 weeks. The JGOG 3016 study compared platinum-taxane doublet every 3 weeks with the "dose-dense" paclitaxel schedule (carboplatin AUC 6 administered every 3 weeks plus weekly paclitaxel 80 mg/m^2) for six cycles, in women with stages III–IV EOC. The final results showed that dose-dense schedule was associated with improved PFS (median 28 vs. 17.5 months) and OS (100.5 vs. 62 months) and a better toxicity profile with respect to the standard approach [36, 37].

In the Western populations, the same advantages have not been documented. The GOG 262 trial [38], the MITO 7 trial [39], and the ICON8 trial [40] did not report any difference in PFS or OS between the schedules at the price of notable differences in the toxicity profile and quality of life (QOL).

■ **Bevacizumab in First-Line Treatment**

Bevacizumab, a potent inhibitor of vascular endothelial growth factor receptor (VEGFR), blocks the growth of new tumor blood vessels, starving the cancer of the nutrition and oxygen it needs to survive; moreover it increases the effects of chemotherapy by improving drug delivery to the tumor. In ovarian cancer, bevacizumab has been explored as a single agent and in combination and maintenance after chemotherapy. GOG 218 and ICON7 are the two phase III trials investigating bevacizumab in combination with carboplatin-paclitaxel in the adjuvant setting.

■ **GOG 218**

Patients with FIGO stage IIIB–C and IV epithelial ovarian cancer who had undergone optimal debulking surgery were randomized to receive three different treatments, as shown in ◘ Fig. 52.2:

A. Standard chemotherapy with 3-weekly intravenous paclitaxel plus carboplatin for 6 cycles plus 3-weekly placebo for 22 cycles

B. Standard chemotherapy with 3-weekly intravenous paclitaxel plus carboplatin for 6 cycles plus bevacizumab 15 mg/kg during chemotherapy followed by 3-weekly placebo for 22 cycles

C. Standard chemotherapy with 3-weekly intravenous paclitaxel plus carboplatin for 6 cycles plus bevacizumab 15 mg/kg during chemotherapy followed by bevacizumab for a total of 15 months

Final results showed a prolongation of PFS in arm C with respect to control arm A (10.3 vs. 14.1 months, respectively). Progression was assessed by biochemical progression based on Ca125 levels (GCIG criteria) and radiological progression with imaging RECIST criteria. When an analysis of treatment efficacy was done only

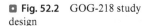

Fig. 52.2 GOG-218 study design

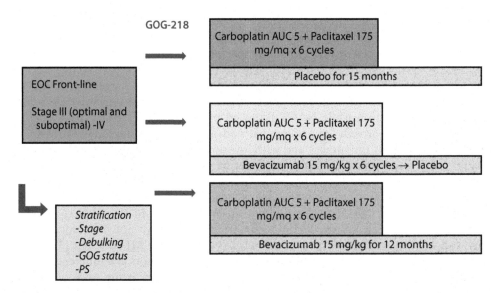

Fig. 52.3 ICON-7 study design

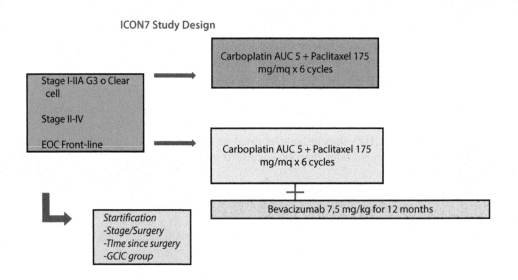

with radiological method, patients in arm C had a 6.2-month improvement in PFS compared to the control group and a 36% reduction in the risk of cancer progression or death [41].

ICON 7

Patients with high-risk stage I or II and stage III and IV epithelial ovarian cancer that had undergone debulking surgery (optimal and suboptimal) were randomized to receive:

A. Standard chemotherapy with 3-weekly intravenous paclitaxel plus carboplatin for six cycles

B. Six cycles of three weekly carboplatin-paclitaxel plus bevacizumab (7.5 mg/kg) for six cycles followed by bevacizumab in maintenance for 12 months (Fig. 52.3)

In the intention-to-treat population, a 1.7-month improvement in PFS was reported in the bevacizumab arm. In high-risk patients (stage III with >1.0 cm residual disease or stage IV), a median PFS improvement from 10.5 to 15.9 months in the bevacizumab arm was registered [42]. A recently published final analysis of survival data showed a statistically significant advantage in OS in patients with high-risk disease (39.3 vs. 34.9 months, in bevacizumab- and non-bevacizumab-treated patients, respectively).

Results from these two studies supported the European Commission (EMA) approval of bevacizumab in combination with carboplatin and paclitaxel in front-line treatment of patients with advanced FIGO stage IIIB–C and IV ovarian cancer (Table 52.2).

■ **Intraperitoneal Chemotherapy**

This procedure provides direct delivery of chemotherapy (cisplatin and/or paclitaxel) into the peritoneal cavity through a catheter, in addition to administering intravenous chemotherapy (■ Fig. 52.4) [43].

The rationale of this approach is based on the following:

– The most common route of ovarian cancer spread is within the peritoneal cavity.
– The ability to reduce tumor volume with debulking is essential to favor drug penetration.
– The residual peritoneal tumor is exposed to increased concentration of drug for a prolonged time period compared to intravenous (IV) treatment.

Patients eligible for this treatment should present:

– Good performance status
– Stage III–IV EOC with optimally cytoreduced disease (residual <1 cm after surgery) because penetration of IP chemotherapy into tumors is limited to 1–2 mm

■ **Table 52.2** PFS and OS results in ICON7 and GOG 218 studies

Trial	Arms	PFS	OS (HR, *p* value)
ICON7 *N* = 1528 Beva: 7.5 mg/kg	A: CP B: CP + Beva → Beva 12 cycles	17.4 months 19.8 months	44.6 months 44.5 months
GOG 218 *N* = 1873 Beva: 15 mg/kg	CP CP + Beva CP + Beva → Beva 22 cycles	10.3 months 11.2 months 14.1 months	39.3 months 38.7 months 39.7 months

Abbreviations: *CP* carboplatin-paclitaxel, *Beva* bevacizumab

Side effects: Abdominal pain, nausea, and vomiting.

Complications: Bowel obstructions, infections (peritonitis, abdominal wall or catheter infections), and intestinal perforations.

A Cochrane meta-analysis [44] showed that IV/IP therapy improved median progression-free survival and overall survival and decreased the risk of recurrence and death, compared to IV therapy; unfortunately a relevant rate of patients is unable to complete IP cycles for related treatment-related toxicities (neurotoxicity and abdominal discomfort impacting on self-reported QOL) or catheter-related complications [45, 46]. In the GOG 172 trial, only 42% of patients completed treatment, 8% never started, and 34% received only one or two cycles.

For these reasons, despite the interesting data, this approach is difficult to apply in clinical practice to the majority of patients.

■ **Treatment of Recurrent Disease**

In advanced-stage EOC, the relapse rate is approximately 70–80%, even after complete response to systemic first-line treatment [47].

At recurrence the treatment options are:

1. Systemic therapy (standard and novel chemotherapeutic agents and biological agents)
2. Surgery: Secondary cytoreductive surgery (SCS) followed by chemotherapy

The choice depends on different factors such as previous treatments, the BRCA mutational status, the performance status, the number and sites of metastases, and finally the interval time between the last cycle of first-line chemotherapy and recurrence (platinum-free interval: PFI) (■ Figs. 52.5 and 52.6).

■ **Platinum Agents**

Platinum compounds remain the most active agents currently used in the treatment of recurrent platinum-sensitive epithelial ovarian cancer (PFI >6 months). As

■ **Fig. 52.4** Intraperitioneal chemotherapy procedures and mechanism of action

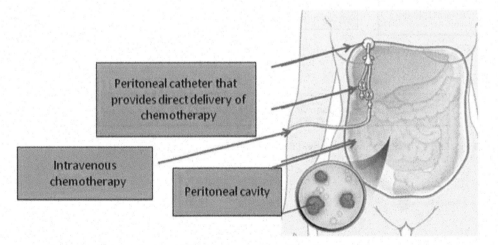

Peritoneal catheter that provides direct delivery of chemotherapy

Intravenous chemotherapy

Peritoneal cavity

52

Fig. 52.5 Treatment algorithm of recurrent ovarian cancer

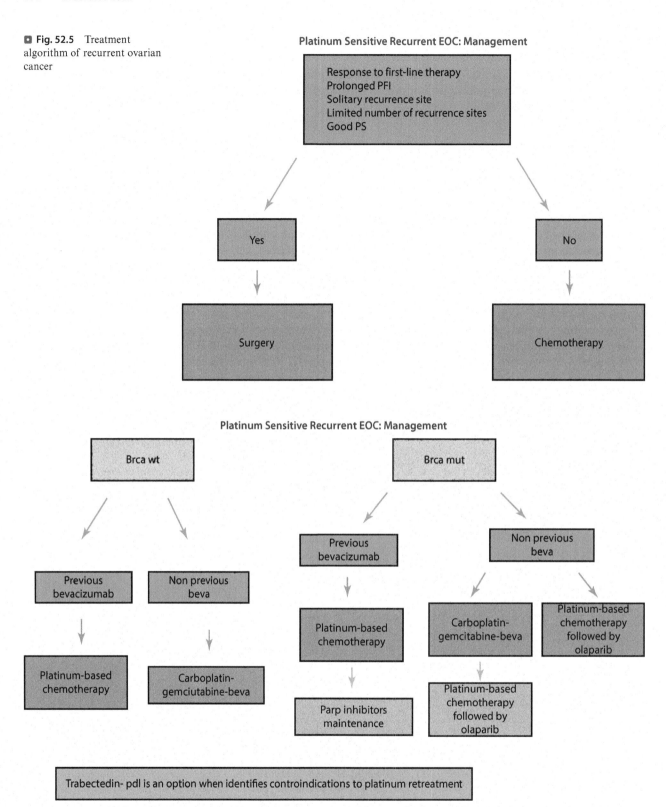

Platinum Sensitive Recurrent EOC: Management

Response to first-line therapy
Prolonged PFI
Solitary recurrence site
Limited number of recurrence sites
Good PS

Yes

No

Surgery

Chemotherapy

Platinum Sensitive Recurrent EOC: Management

Brca wt

Brca mut

Previous bevacizumab

Non previous beva

Previous bevacizumab

Non previous beva

Platinum-based chemotherapy

Carboplatin-gemciutabine-beva

Platinum-based chemotherapy

Carboplatin-gemcitabine-beva

Platinum-based chemotherapy followed by olaparib

Parp inhibitors maintenance

Platinum-based chemotherapy followed by olaparib

Trabectedin- pdl is an option when identifies controindications to platinum retreatment

Fig. 52.6 Platinum sensitive recurrent EOC management

for the adjuvant setting, extending administration beyond six cycles has not improved long-term outcomes but increased the risk of hematologic and non-hematologic cumulative toxicity [48]. In patients with platinum-sensitive recurrence, platinum-based treatment, generally given as a doublet, is recommended. Usually carboplatin (AUC 4–5) is given in association with pegylated liposomal doxorubicin (PLD, 30 mg/m^2) every 4 weeks or with paclitaxel (175 mg/m^2) every 3 weeks or with gemcitabine (1000 mg/m^2 days 1 and 8) every 3 weeks. Overlapping oncologic outcome with different hematologic and non-hematologic toxicities has been reported with the different regimens, so that the choice is mainly based on previous toxicity and patient's preference.

Cisplatin has a comparable efficacy to carboplatin and could be associated with the same drugs (gemcitabine, paclitaxel, and PLD) but is usually considered a second choice because of the worse toxicity profile. Moreover it is generally used in case of hypersensitivity reactions to carboplatin [49].

Carboplatin-PLD combination: The efficacy of this association was established by the CALYPSO study which compared, in platinum-sensitive recurrent EOC, carboplatin-paclitaxel to carboplatin-PLD. The final results showed an improvement in median PFS in the PLD regimen compared to the paclitaxel regimen (11.3 vs. 9.4 months, respectively) and equivalent OS. As for the toxicity profile, carboplatin-PLD was characterized by less neuropathy (5% vs. 27%), myalgia (4% vs. 19%), and carboplatin-hypersensitivity reactions (16% vs. 33%), but higher percentages of mucositis (14% vs. 7%) and hand-foot syndrome (HFS) (12% vs. 2%) compared to paclitaxel regimen were reported [50, 51].

Carboplatin-paclitaxel combination: The efficacy of this association was evaluated in ICON4 and AGO-OVAR-2.2 trials [52, 53] which compared single-agent platinum to platinum-paclitaxel combination in platinum-sensitive recurrent ovarian cancer. Final data showed a significant OS benefit (29 vs. 24 months) in the experimental arm with a higher percentage of neurotoxicity and alopecia, compared to carboplatin alone.

Carboplatin-gemcitabine combination: An AGO-GCIG study, comparing carboplatin-gemcitabine to carboplatin alone, has reported an advantage in response rate (47% vs. 31%) and PFS (8.6 vs. 5.8 months) for the combination arm without a significant OS advantage. The doublet is associated with a significant myelosuppression, mainly thrombocytopenia [54].

In platinum-sensitive patients not able to receive platinum for residual neurotoxicity or for anaphylactic reaction, a non-platinum doublet is available. The combination of trabectedin-PLD has reported increased PFS (9.2 vs. 7.5, respectively) and increased OS (23.0 vs. 17.1, respectively) with respect to PLD single agent in partially platinum-sensitive recurrent EOC [55, 56].

■ **Non-platinum agents**

Generally, recurrence in platinum-resistant patients (platinum-free interval <6 months) is treated with single-agent non-platinum chemotherapy. Among available agents, the most used are:

Paclitaxel: Generally the weekly schedule (60–80 mg/m^2 continuously or the 3 weeks on and 1 week off schedule) is a well-tolerated regimen and it is recommended in patients without residual neuropathy. The response rate is approximately 13–25%. Neuropathy is the most frequent toxicity [57].

PLD: Single-agent PLD is administered once every 4 weeks at the dose of 40 mg/m^2. This schedule is well tolerated and hand-foot syndrome and stomatitis are the main toxicities. Approximately, the ORR is about 12–15%, the time to progression 9–12 weeks, and the median OS 35–40 weeks [58].

Gemcitabine: Single agent is administered at the dose of 1000 mg/m^{2}d1 and d8 every 21 days. The objective response rate is 9–11% with 55% of stabilizations of disease. Median PFS and OS are 3 and 13 months, respectively. Gemcitabine is associated with considerable myelosuppression, mostly thrombocytopenia [59].

Topotecan: Single-agent administration considers two different schedules: daily (1.5 mg/mq/day on days 1–5 of a 21-day cycle) or weekly (4 mg/mq on days 1, 8, and 15 of a 28-day cycle). High-grade hematological toxicity was reported in 27.9% and 4.8% of patients in the 3-weekly and weekly schedule, respectively, without difference in objective response rate (9–19%), PFS, and OS [60].

Other drugs used as single agent in this setting are etoposide (50 mg/m^2 daily for 21 days every 4 weeks) and pemetrexed (900 mg/m^2 every 21 days) with response rate of 27% [61] and 10–20%, respectively [62].

■ **Antiangiogenic Agents:**

Bevacizumab: The OCEANS study is a phase III randomized trial evaluating the role of bevacizumab in combination with chemotherapy in platinum-sensitive recurrent ovarian cancer. Patients received gemcitabine and carboplatin for six cycles plus placebo or bevacizumab in combination and maintenance until disease progression. The final results reported a median 4-month PFS advantage in patients receiving bevacizumab compared with placebo (12.4 months vs. 8.4 months, respectively), without difference in overall survival [63]. Moreover the bevacizumab arm registered an increased response rate compared to placebo arm (78.5% vs. 57.4%, respectively).

The phase III randomized AURELIA trial [64] evaluated the efficacy of bevacizumab in combination with standard chemotherapy versus chemotherapy alone in patients with platinum-resistant recurrent ovarian cancer. Enrolled patients received either single-agent chemotherapy (at investigator's choice between weekly paclitaxel, pegylated liposomal doxorubicin (PLD), or topotecan) or chemotherapy in combination and maintenance with bevacizumab until disease progression or unacceptable toxicity. Patients enrolled in the bevacizumab arm experienced a 3.3-month improvement in median PFS and a significant amelioration in quality of life [65] with respect to chemotherapy alone-treated patients. Final results did not show a significant improvement in OS, probably due to crossover of 40% of patients receiving bevacizumab therapy after progression.

Actually, the prescription of bevacizumab has different indications across the world. In fact, despite evidence of activity in different treatment settings, there is no international consensus about the most appropriate setting of disease in which to use the antiangiogenic agent [66].

Multitargeted TKIs: Various agents are being investigated in several phase II–III studies demonstrating single-agent activity in EOC:

(a) *Pazopanib*: It is an oral tyrosine kinase inhibitor targeting VEGF receptor 1, 2, and 3, platelet-derived growth factor receptor α and β, and c-kit and inhibiting angiogenesis and tumor proliferation. When used as maintenance treatment after first-line carboplatin-paclitaxel chemotherapy in advanced ovarian cancer (AGO-OVAR 16), the drug demonstrated a 6-month PFS benefit [67]). The MITO 11 trial [68] is a phase II trial, evaluating the efficacy of pazopanib in combination with weekly paclitaxel in patients with platinum-resistant recurrent ovarian cancer versus chemotherapy alone. The study showed a significant 2.9-month improvement in PFS for the pazopanib arm (median 6.3 vs. 3.4 months for experimental arm vs. standard arm, respectively).

(b) *Cediranib:* It is a VEGFR 1, 2, and 3 oral tyrosine kinase inhibitor demonstrating a particular activity in recurrent ovarian cancer [69]. In ICON6 trial [70, 71], a randomized controlled phase III trial, the efficacy of cediranib given concurrently with platinum-based chemotherapy and as maintenance in women with platinum-sensitive relapsed ovarian cancer was assessed. Final results showed a significant improvement in terms of PFS and OS for the experimental arm. Recently, data on the association to olaparib plus cediranib versus olaparib alone in patients with relapsed platinum-sensitive ovarian cancer were reported and documented. Improvements in objective response rate (80% vs. 48%), disease stabilization (17.7 vs. 9 months), and PFS for the combination arm were reported regardless of BRCA status [72].

(c) *Nintedanib* is an oral triple angiokinase inhibitor that blocks VEGFR 1, 2, and 3, platelet-derived growth factor receptors (PDGFR), and fibroblast growth factor receptors (FGFR) 1, 2, and 3. When used as maintenance treatment in first-line setting after chemotherapy (AGO-OVAR 12), nintedanib showed a 1.2-month increase in PFS versus placebo. This advantage was considered insufficient for promoting further development of the drug [73].

■ **PARP Inhibitors**

Approximately 50% of patients with high-grade EOC are deficient in the DNA homologous recombination repair pathway.

In about 25% of cases, this defect is related to mutations (germline or somatic) of BRCA 1/2 genes or epigenetic inactivation of the same genes. In the remaining 25% of cases, patients present mutations in a series of minor genes, involved in the homologous recombination deficiency (HRD) [74], as shown in ◘ Fig. 52.7.

Poly(ADP-ribose) polymerase (PARP) plays an integral role in single-strand DNA break repair via the base excision pathway. Normal cells can repair DNA damage using alternative pathways, for example, homologous recombination pathway (HR), sufficient to maintain genomic integrity; in cells with deficient homologous recombination (as are BRCA-mutated cells), DNA damage accumulates and consequently leads to cell death (apoptosis).

Based on this mechanism, PARP inhibitors selectively kill tumor cells compared with normal cells, a concept recognized as "synthetic lethality." HRD increases sensitivity also to platinum-based chemotherapy because the deficiency impairs the ability of cancer cells to repair the direct platinum-induced double-strand DNA breaks. For these reasons, platinum sensitivity is often associated with an HRD tumor phenotype (◘ Fig. 52.8).

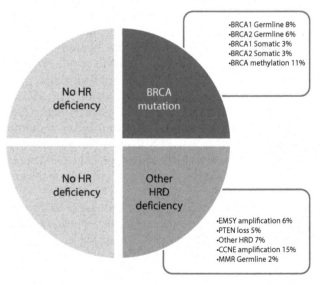

◘ **Fig. 52.7** Genes and intracellular proteins involved in homologous recombination deficiency

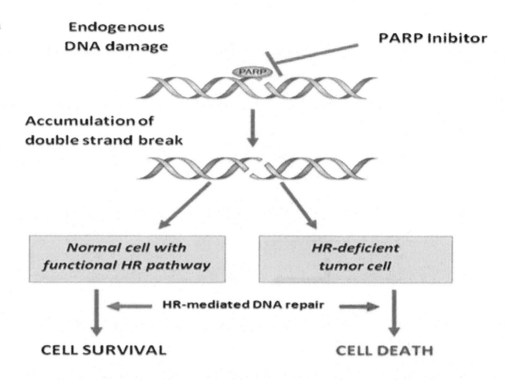

Fig. 52.8 PARP inhibition and tumor-selective synthetic lethality

PARP inhibition is a novel approach to target tumors with deficiencies in DNA repair mechanisms. BRCA mutation is the first and currently the unique predictive biomarker for targeted therapy in ovarian cancer. The availability of PARP inhibitors as a treatment option in EOC opened the door for routine testing of BRCA mutations in blood (germline test) and in the tumor specimen (somatic test) [75]. Information about BRCA status, according to the most recent guidelines, should be obtained at the time of diagnosis, in order to create a suitable therapeutic algorithm. Robust data support the role of PARP inhibitors in the treatment of patients with *BRCA*-associated ovarian cancer. Moreover responses are also described in non-*BRCA*-mutated patients (particularly in platinum-sensitive) suggesting that the clinical utility of PARP inhibitors can be extended to a larger patient population [76].

Common features of PARP inhibitors:
- Inhibition of PARP-associated DNA repair pathway.
- Particularly effective in presence of BRCA mutation.
- Oral drug.
- Well tolerated.
- Common side effects are nausea, fatigue, vomiting, diarrhea, and bone marrow suppression (increased risk infection, bleeding, anemia).
- Rare serious toxicity such as leukemia and lung inflammation (interstitial pneumonia).

Olaparib:

Olaparib (AZD2281, KU-0059436) is a potent PARP inhibitor (PARP 1, 2, and 3) that is being developed as an oral therapy, both as single agent (including maintenance) and in combination with chemotherapy and other antineoplastic agents. Actually, olaparib indications are different in the United States and European Union.

In the United States olaparib is approved in monotherapy for patients with BRCA-mutated ovarian cancer who received three or more previous chemotherapy treatments and as maintenance in platinum-sensitive, platinum-responding ovarian cancer, regardless of BRCA mutational status. In Europe olaparib is approved for the maintenance treatment of patients with relapsed platinum-sensitive, BRCA-mutated (germline or somatic), high-grade serous epithelial ovarian cancer who are responding (partial or complete) to platinum-based chemotherapy. In both cases, the recommended dose is 400 mg twice daily, until disease progression or unacceptable toxicity.

Study 19 is an international, double-blind, pivotal, randomized, phase II trial showing antitumor activity of olaparib in maintenance treatment of patients with platinum-sensitive high-grade serous relapsed EOC (Fig. 52.9).

The study reported a significant 3.6-month increase in median PFS for olaparib maintenance therapy compared with placebo (8.4 months vs. 4.8 months, respectively) in the overall population; moreover, in a subgroup analysis, the benefit was greater in patients with germline or somatic BRCA mutation, with a significant 6.9-month increase in median PFS and a 82% risk reduction of disease progression or death in olaparib arm without detrimental impact on global health-related quality of life (HRQoL).

Fig. 52.9 STUDY-19 study design

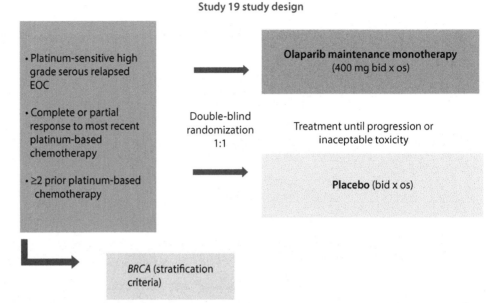

Study 19 study design

- Platinum-sensitive high grade serous relapsed EOC
- Complete or partial response to most recent platinum-based chemotherapy
- ≥2 prior platinum-based chemotherapy

Double-blind randomization 1:1

Olaparib maintenance monotherapy (400 mg bid x os)

Treatment until progression or inaceptable toxicity

Placebo (bid x os)

BRCA (stratification criteria)

On November 2016, the Lancet Oncology reported overall survival data of Study 19 demonstrating that patients with platinum-sensitive recurrent EOC receiving olaparib maintenance treatment have longer overall survival with respect to patients receiving placebo (median survival was 29.8 months vs. 27.8 months in olaparib and placebo arm, respectively). Moreover, in BRCA-mutated patients, the median survival was 34.9 months versus 30.2 months for olaparib and placebo, respectively [70, 71].

Rucaparib

Rucaparib is a small-molecule PARP 1 and PARP 2 inhibitor which is administered at the dose of 600 mg twice daily. This drug is being developed as maintenance treatment for recurrent platinum-sensitive EOC in ARIEL3 study, in which rucaparib was administered to prespecified groups of patients, categorized according to homologous recombination deficiency (HRD) status (BRCA-mutated, BRCA-like/high loss of heterozygosity (LOH), and the intention-to-treat population), as maintenance treatment after platinum-based chemotherapy in comparison to placebo.

Final results showed a statistically significant improvement in progression-free survival (PFS) in each of the three populations: median progression-free survival in patients with BRCA mutation was 16.6 months in the rucaparib arm versus 5.4 months in the placebo arm. In patients with a homologous recombination deficiency, median PFS was 13.6 months versus 5.4 months in the rucaparib and placebo arm, respectively. In the intention-to-treat population, median PFS was 10.8 months versus 5.4 months for rucaparib and placebo, respectively.

Rucaparib is already approved by the FDA as single agent for the treatment of BRCA-mutated (either germline or somatic) recurrent EOC patients who had received at least two previous CHT lines based on a pooled analysis of two phase II trials (ARIEL2 and Study 10) reporting 54% response rate and 10-month median PFS when rucaparib was used a single agent for the treatment of active disease [77].

The ARIEL4 trial is a phase III ongoing multicenter randomized study evaluating rucaparib versus clinician choice chemotherapy in relapsed ovarian cancer patients with BRCA mutations who failed two prior lines of therapy.

Niraparib

Niraparib is a small-molecule PARP 1 and PARP 2 inhibitor administered at the dose of 300 mg daily. In the phase III NOVA trial, niraparib was given as maintenance treatment in patients with recurrent epithelial ovarian cancer who are in complete or partial response to platinum-based chemotherapy in comparison to placebo. Two parallel and independent cohorts of patients were enrolled: germline BRCA-mutated patients and platinum-sensitive patients without germline mutation. Final results reported a decrease in risk of progression or death compared with placebo for the BRCA-mutated patients.

Median PFS was 21 months in patients with germline *BRCA* mutations, 12.9 months in germline BRCA wild-type patients who carry a homologous recombination deficiency (HRD), and 9.3 months in BRCA wild-type patients without HRD deficiency. The corresponding figures for the placebo arm were 5.5 months, 3.7 months, and 3.8 months, respectively. Based on these data, the FDA has approved niraparib as maintenance treatment for patients with recurrent epithelial ovarian, fallopian tube, or primary peritoneal cancer in complete or partial response to platinum-based chemotherapy, regardless of BRCA mutational status (Fig. 52.10).

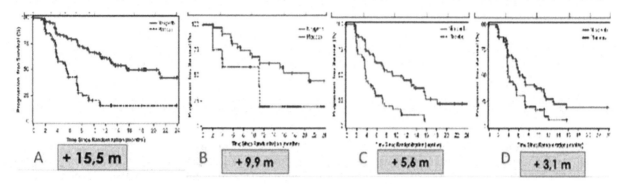

	Germline BRCA mut	**Somatic BRCA mut HRD +**	**BRCAwt HRD +**	**BRCAwt HRD neg**
Niraparib	21.0 months	20.9 months	9.3 months	6.9 months
Placebo	5.5 months	11.0 months	3.7 months	3.8 months

Fig. 52.10 The Kaplan-Meier curves of PFS for the 2 treatments arms in the different population: A: gBRCA mutated cohort; B: sBRCA mutated cohort; C: HRD positive-BRCA WT patients; D: HRD Negative patients

Alpha-Folate Receptor

The folate receptors (FR) constitute a group of proteins that mediate accumulation of folate into cells and regulate folate homeostasis and consequently synthesis, methylation, and DNA repair [78].

Alpha-folate receptor (aFR), an isoform of this family, can be over-expressed by several epithelial-derived tumors, including ovarian cancer, where it is present in approximately 75% of cases [79]. The over-expression of aFR is considered a negative prognostic factor and associated with poorer overall survival (OS) [80].

Recently, aFR is receiving more interest in gynecologic cancers as an excellent target for new targeted therapies [81]. aFR is expressed on cancer cell surface and has the ability to connect through folic acid several ligand molecules (e.g., antineoplastic agents) that can selectively penetrate into cancer cells minimizing systemic toxic side effects. This family of molecules, also called immunoconjugates, includes:

- Farletuzumab (MORAb-003), a humanized monoclonal antibody that targets glycoprotein 3 (GP-3) and triggers a host immune response against GP-3-expressing cells resulting in apoptosis [82]. This drug has shown activity against advanced epithelial ovarian cancer, mainly in platinum-sensitive disease (MORAB study).
- Mirvetuximab soravtansine (IMGN853), an alpha-folate receptor-targeting antibody-drug conjugate that combines an alpha-folate receptor-binding antibody and a novel antitumoral agent (tubulin-disrupting maytansinoid DM4). This drug has shown activity against advanced epithelial ovarian cancer, mainly in platinum-resistant disease (FORWARD 1 study) [83].

- Vintafolide (EC145), an alpha-folate receptor ligand conjugated with vinca alkaloid-derived drug that targets FR-expressing cells, explored in a randomized phase II trial in "platinum-resistant" ovarian cancer versus PLD with deluding results (PRECEDENT study) [84].

52.6 Secondary Cytoreductive Surgery

Chemotherapy is the standard treatment of recurrent epithelial ovarian cancer, but surgery can also be performed in selected patients.

The role of secondary cytoreductive surgery (SCS) in the standard management of recurrence remains poorly defined. Generally, the eligibility criteria for secondary cytoreduction are:

1. Response to first-line therapy and prolonged platinum-free interval (PFI) [12, 85, 86]
2. Solitary recurrence site or limited number of recurrence sites [86, 87]
3. Good PS

The DESKTOP OVAR I retrospective trial and the DESKTOP OVAR II prospective trial have identified and validated a panel of selection criteria for SCS and a predictive score to identify patients who could have a complete resection during secondary cytoreductive surgery (AGO score: ECOG PS 0, no residual tumor after first surgery, and ascites less than 500 ml) [88].

DESKTOP IIII and GOG 213 are two prospective randomized controlled phase III trials investigating the role of secondary cytoreductive surgery for recurrent EOC.

Final results of DESKTOP III trial showed that secondary cytoreductive surgery translates in 6-month improvement in PFS with respect to chemotherapy alone; the benefit was exclusively seen in patients with complete resection (CR) indicating the importance of selecting patients and centers in which the surgical procedure is performed.

■ **Treatment Algorithms for Recurrent Ovarian Cancer**

The option of second-line chemotherapy for recurrent disease is based on platinum-free interval (PFI), defined as the time interval between the last dose of platinum to the progression of disease [89].

Patients are generally divided into four groups:

A. Platinum-refractory: Patients who progressed during platinum-based chemotherapy or within 4 weeks after last dose
B. Platinum-resistant: Patients with a disease progressing within 6 months from last platinum dose
C. Partially platinum-sensitive: Patients who progressed between 6 and 12 months from last platinum dose
D. Fully platinum-sensitive: Patients who progressed with an interval of more than 12 months from last platinum dose

PFI is considered the most important criterion for predicting the response to chemotherapy in recurrent ovarian cancer and is also the main factor leading the choice of therapeutic strategy. PFI is not only expression of the biology of the disease but is highly influenced by several factors, such as the type of surgery (primary debulking surgery or neoadjuvant chemotherapy) and the type of chemotherapy (with or without bevacizumab in first line). Moreover, the PFI value has recently been criticized for arbitrary definition and categorizations of recurrences particularly because the date of disease progression is somewhat variable according to the method used to evaluate progression (either radiological assessment, Ca125 level increase, or clinical progression) [90].

Recently, the Fifth Word Consensus Conference on Ovarian Cancer reported that the PFI should not be considered more as the only parameter to take into account in choosing treatment at recurrence of disease particularly in the era of targeted therapies and biological characterization of ovarian tumors.

Other important tools for the decision-making are platinum-free-interval, BRCA mutational status, previous treatments, and toxicity. The ultimate goal of treatment strategy is to build an algorithm which allows patients to receive all the available treatment options, possibly in the more appropriate temporary order.

■ **When Platinum Is an Option**

In patients with platinum-sensitive recurrent epithelial ovarian cancer who do not present contraindication to platinum retreatment, platinum-based combinations with paclitaxel, gemcitabine, or pegylated liposomal doxorubicin are recommended.

Some other considerations are mandatory before starting with second-line chemotherapy such as ECOG performance status, mutational status of BRCA 1 and 2 genes, and previous received treatments.

A. BRCA 1/2 wild-type patients never exposed to bevacizumab

Recommended choice is represented by the combination of carboplatin AUC 4 on day 1 plus gemcitabine 1000 mg/m^2 on days 1 and 8 associated with bevacizumab 15 mg/kg on day 1 every 21 days until progression of disease or unacceptable toxicity.

B. BRCA 1/2 wild-type patients previously exposed to bevacizumab

Recommended choice, according to physician's judgment, is platinum-based combinations with paclitaxel, gemcitabine, or pegylated liposomal doxorubicin chosen according to the toxicity profile and patient's preference. The recommended schedules are:

- Carboplatin AUC 4 on day 1 plus gemcitabine 1000 mg/m^2 on days 1 and 8 every 21 days [54]
- Carboplatin AUC 5 plus pegylated liposomal doxorubicin (PLD) 30 mg/m^2 on day 1 every 28 days [50, 51]
- Carboplatin AUC 5 plus paclitaxel 175 mg/m^2 on day 1 every 21 days [53]

C. BRCA 1/2 mutation carrier patients previously exposed to bevacizumab

Recommended choice is a platinum-based chemotherapy (for four to six cycles) followed by maintenance treatment with the licensed PARP inhibitor until progression of disease or unacceptable toxicity.

D. BRCA 1/2 mutation carriers never exposed to bevacizumab

Available choices are:

Combination of carboplatin AUC 4 on day 1 plus gemcitabine 1000 mg/m^2 on days 1 and 8 associated with bevacizumab 15 mg/kg on day 1 every 21 days until progression of disease or unacceptable toxicity

Platinum-based chemotherapy (for four to six cycles) followed by maintenance treatment with the licensed

PARP inhibitor until progression of disease or unacceptable toxicity

The choice between two regimens should be based on patient's preference and disease characteristics and discussed with patients.

■ **When Platinum Is Not an Option**

When the physician identifies contraindications to platinum retreatment, despite the patient being platinum-sensitive, such as in the case of previous anaphylactic reactions to platinum [91] which occurs in up to 40% of cases, residual neurotoxicity, or intermediate sensitivity to platinum (patients who progressed between 6 and 12 months from last platinum dose), a platinum-free strategy with the combination of trabectedin 1.1 mg/m² plus PLD 30 mg/m² on day 1 every 21 days can be offered [55].

OVA-301 trial is a randomized phase III trial comparing the efficacy and the safety of trabectedin 1.1 mg/m² associated with PLD 30 mg/m² on day 1 every 21 days versus PLD 50 mg/m² alone on day 1 every 28 days. The study reported a benefit in PFS in the combination arm, especially in the platinum-partially sensitive cohort (median PFS was 9.2 months vs. 7.5 months and median OS was 23.0 months vs. 17.1 months, respectively) [92].

Moreover a post hoc analysis suggests that this combination is particularly active in terms of response rate, PFS, and OS in BRCA-mutated patients [93]. Preclinical and clinical data suggest a benefit in the trabectedin → platinum sequence suggesting that trabectedin administered before carboplatin is able to select cellular clones more sensitive to subsequent carboplatin treatment. This hypothesis will be tested in the ongoing prospective randomized INOVATYON trial.

In patients with platinum-resistant disease, the objective of treatment is symptoms palliation and maintenance of QoL. Sequential single-agent non-platinum therapies are recommended and, as reported in a recent Cochrane systematic review, paclitaxel, PLD, and topotecan have similar efficacy (ORR 10–15% and median PFS 3–4 months) but different toxicity profile, which should be discussed with the patient [94].

Summary of Clinical Recommendations
Management of primary advanced disease includes:
- Primary cytoreductive surgery or NACT followed by interval cytoreductive surgery
- Intravenous chemotherapy
- Intraperitoneal chemotherapy
- Dose-dense chemotherapy
- Maintenance treatment

Intravenous chemotherapy → carboplatin AUC 5–6 + paclitaxel 175 mg/m² every 3 weeks plus bevacizumab in combination with chemotherapy and in maintenance for 15 months
Management of recurrent disease includes:
1. Systemic therapy (standard and novel chemotherapeutic agents and biological agents)
2. Surgery: Secondary cytoreductive surgery (SCS)

The choice depends on many factors such as the previous received treatments, the BRCA mutational status, the performance status, the site and number of recurrences, and finally the time interval between the last cycle of first-line chemotherapy and recurrence.
When Platinum Is an Option
BRCA 1/2 wild-type patients never exposed to bevacizumab → carboplatin AUC 4 on day 1 plus gemcitabine 1000 mg/m² on days 1 and 8 associated with bevacizumab 15 mg/kg on day 1 every 21 days until progression of disease or unacceptable toxicity
BRCA 1/2 wild-type previously exposed to bevacizumab → platinum-based combinations with paclitaxel, gemcitabine, or pegylated liposomal doxorubicin
BRCA 1/2 mutation carriers previously exposed to bevacizumab → platinum-based chemotherapy (for four to six cycles) followed by maintenance treatment with the licensed PARP inhibitor until progression of disease or unacceptable toxicity.
BRCA 1/2 mutation carriers never exposed to bevacizumab → (a) Combination of carboplatin AUC 4 on day 1 plus gemcitabine 1000 mg/m² on days 1 and 8 associated with bevacizumab 15 mg/kg on day 1 every 21 days until progression of disease or unacceptable toxicity. (b) Platinum-based chemotherapy (for four to six cycles) followed by maintenance treatment with the licensed PARP inhibitor until progression of disease or unacceptable toxicity.
When Platinum Is Not an Option
In patients with platinum-partially sensitive disease → trabectedin 1.1 mg/m² plus PLD 30 mg/m² on day 1 every 21 days
In patients with platinum-resistant disease → sequential single non-platinum agents (paclitaxel, PLD, and topotecan)

Woman, 64 years old, ECOG PS0
- *Family history:* Negative for malignancy
- *APR:* Hypercholesterolemia treated with statin, well-controlled hypertension treated with spironolactone

- *APP:* Nausea, asthenia, and diffuse abdominal pain
- *CT scan chest-abdomen* (20/09/2002): Presence of pelvic mass, ascites, carcinomatosis, and clinically suspected pelvic lymph nodes, Ca125 level of 622 U/ml

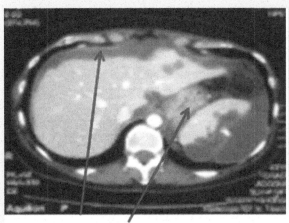

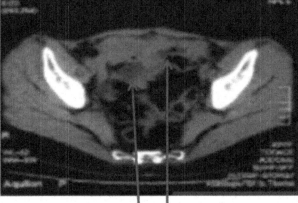

ascitis

pelvic mass and carcinomatosis

- *Surgery* (02/10/2002): Laparotomy with total abdominal hysterectomy, bilateral salpingo-oophorectomy (BSO), peritoneal washing, total peritonectomy and omentectomy, removal of bulky pelvic and para-aortic lymph nodes, and removal of peritoneal nodules. Postoperative residual tumor = absent (RT0)

- *Pathologic assessment* showed stage IIIC high-grade serous ovarian cancer.
- From 22/11/2002 to 4/04/2003, the patient received six cycles of chemotherapy treatment with carboplatin AUC 5 plus paclitaxel 175 mg/mq g1 q 21.
- Follow-up labs showed normalization of Ca125 to less than 10 U/ml and CT scan was NED (non-evidential disease upon completion of chemotherapy).
- In 2016 the patients developed abdominal pain. Physical examination was normal but laboratory analyses showed a Ca125 level of 190 U/ml.
- *CT scan* (30/06/2016) revealed enlarged retroperitoneal para-aortic lymph nodes suspected to be metastatic. This data were confirmed by PET-FGD performed on 11/07/2016.

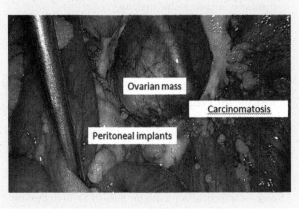

Ovarian mass

Carcinomatosis

Peritoneal implants

52

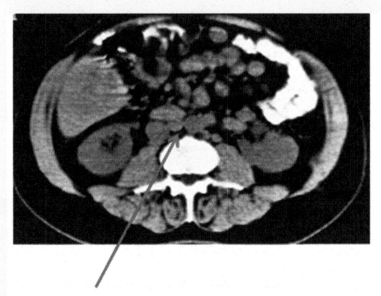

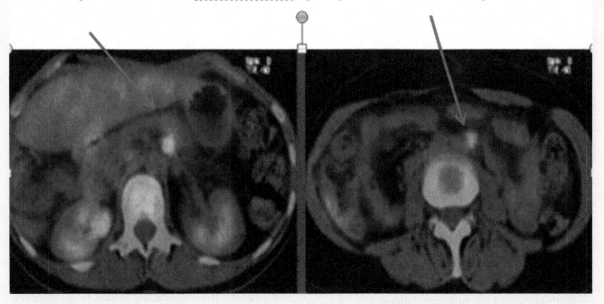

retroperitoneal paraortic lymph nodes suspected

Question

What action should be taken?
1. Secondary cytoreductive surgery
2. Systemic chemotherapy
3. Wait and see strategy

Answer

Considering the good PS, the prolonged PFI, and the limited number of recurrent sites of disease, the choice was for secondary cytoreduction surgery.

22/07/2016: Patient underwent secondary cytoreductive surgery (removal of para-aortic lymph nodes through laparotomy).

20/06/2016: Although she had no family history of ovarian and breast malignancies, she was offered BRCA testing for hereditary risk assessment. The test showed a pathogenic BRCA 2 mutation.

What action should be taken?
1. Carboplatin-gemcitabine followed by licensed PARP inhibitor maintenance
2. Carboplatin -gemcitabine-bevacizumab followed by bevacizumab as maintenance
3. Non-platinum combination

Answer

Considering the platinum-free interval (>12 months) and the prior received treatments (only platinum-based chemotherapy without bevacizumab), despite the BRCA mutation, given the limitation in bevacizumab reimbursement which is labelled only in the first platinum-sensitive recurrence, after discussing with the patient the treatment strategy, our choice was carboplatin-gemcitabine in combination and maintenance with bevacizumab.

- From 22/08/2016 to 14/12/2016, patient received six cycles of carboplatin AUC 4 g1 plus gemcitabine 1000 mg/mq g1, 8 q21 plus bevacizumab 15 mg/kg.
- Since 8/01/2017, maintenance therapy with bevacizumab 15 mg/kg is ongoing.

52

Case study 2: Management of patient with stage IV ovarian cancer and BRCA germline mutation

Woman, 60 years old, ECOG PS1
- *APR:* Severe obesity, well-controlled hypertension and diabetes mellitus treated with oral hypoglycemic drug
- *BRCA 1 germline mutation carrier*

- *APP:* In December2016, she referred abdominal pain, increased abdominal size, and anorexia. Patient has undergone CT scan and PET-FDG showing multiple liver metastasis, peritoneal nodules, and multiple para-aortic bulky lymph nodes.

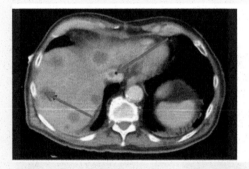 multiple liver metastasis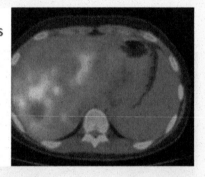

Question

What action should be taken?
A. Cytoreductive surgery and subsequently adjuvant platinum-based chemotherapy
B. Laparoscopic-TC-guided biopsy and subsequently neoadjuvant platinum-based chemotherapy
C. Platinum-based chemotherapy alone

Answer

- Considered the comorbidities, the poor performance status, the low possibility of optimal cytoreduction, and the non-resectable sites of metastasis, the choice was option B.
- On 09/01/2017, during laparoscopy, unilateral salpingo-oophorectomy and biopsy of liver metastasis were performed. The histologic examination showed a high-grade serous carcinoma FIGO stage IV.
- From 20/01/2017 to 10/03/2017, the patient received three cycles of chemotherapy treatment with carboplatin AUC 5 plus paclitaxel 175 mg/mq g1 q 21.

- After the third CHT cycle, the Ca125 level was within the range of normality; radiologic imaging showed a partial response in lymph nodes and a complete response in liver metastasis (with only a residual small subglissonian metastases).
- On 10/04/2017, the patient underwent interval debulking surgery (total abdominal hysterectomy, unilateral salpingo-oophorectomy, peritoneal washing, total omentectomy, biopsy of suspected peritoneal surfaces, and removal of pelvic and para-aortic bulky lymph nodes). Residual disease at the end of the procedure was absent.

What action should be taken?
(a) Other three cycles of carboplatin-paclitaxel
(b) Other three cycles of carboplatin-paclitaxel plus bevacizumab followed by bevacizumab maintenance
(c) Other three cycles of carboplatin-paclitaxel followed by PARP inhibitor maintenance

Considering the excellent response to chemotherapy, the known BRCA mutational status, and the possibility of subsequently administering bevacizumab (at first recurrence), our choice was option C. In fact, the patient was enrolled in PRIMA trial, a phase III randomized, double-blind multicenter study, evaluating the efficacy of niraparib versus placebo as maintenance treatment in patients with stage III or IV ovarian cancer responding to front-line platinum-based chemotherapy.

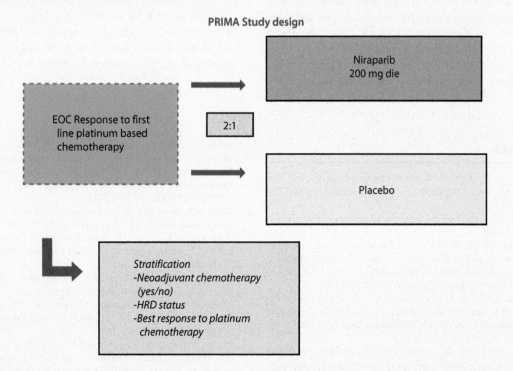

PRIMA Study design

Key Points

— Multidisciplinary consultation in the primary management of EOC.
— Patient selection for neoadjuvant systemic treatment.

— Personalization of treatment according to BRCA mutation is important (also considering patients as possible candidates for clinical trials).

Expert Opinion
Domenica Lorusso

Key Points
1. Management of primary advanced disease includes the following:
   — Primary cytoreductive surgery or NACT followed by interval cytoreductive surgery
   — Intravenous chemotherapy
   — Intraperitoneal chemotherapy
   — Dose-dense chemotherapy
   — Maintenance treatment
2. Management of recurrent disease includes the following:

   — Systemic therapy (standard and novel chemotherapeutic agents and biological agents)
   — Surgery: secondary cytoreductive surgery (SCS)
     The choice depends on many factors such as the previous received treatments, the BRCA mutational status, the performance status, the site and numbers of recurrences, and finally the time interval between the last cycle of first-line chemotherapy and recurrence.

Recommendations
ESMO
— ▶ https://www.esmo.org/Guidelines/Gynaecological-Cancers/ESMO-ESGO-Consensus-Conference-Recommendations-on-Ovarian-Cancer
AIOM

52

References

1. Jemal A, Siegel R, Xu J, Ward E. Cancer statistics, 2010. CA Cancer J Clin. 2010;60(5):277–300. https://doi.org/10.3322/caac.20073.
2. Ozols RF. Update on the management of ovarian cancer. Cancer J. 2002;8 Suppl 1:S22–30.
3. Zeng J, Huang H, Shan Y, Li Y, Jin Y, Pan L. The effect of CA125 nadir level on survival of advanced-stage epithelial ovarian carcinoma after interval debulking surgery. J Cancer. 2017;8(17):3410–5. https://doi.org/10.7150/jca.21362.
4. Ezzati M, Abdullah A, Shariftabrizi A, Hou J, Kopf M, Stedman JK, et al. Recent advancements in prognostic factors of epithelial ovarian carcinoma. Int Scholar Res Not. 2014;2014:1–10. https://doi.org/10.1155/2014/953509.
5. Prat J, Committee F. International Journal of Gynecology and Obstetrics Staging classification for cancer of the ovary, fallopian tube, and peritoneum ☆. Int J Gynecol Obstet. 2013;124(1):1–5. https://doi.org/10.1016/j.ijgo.2013.10.001.
6. Marchetti C, Pisano C, Facchini G, Bruni GS, Magazzino FP, Losito S, Pignata S. First-line treatment of advanced ovarian cancer: current research and perspectives. Expert Rev Anticancer Ther. 2010; https://doi.org/10.1586/ERA.09.167.
7. Bristow RE, Chang J, Ziogas A, Anton-Culver H. Adherence to treatment guidelines for ovarian cancer as a measure of quality care. Obstet Gynecol. 2013;121(6):1226–34. https://doi.org/10.1097/AOG.0b013e3182922a17.
8. du Bois A, Quinn M, Thigpen T, Vermorken J, Avall-Lundqvist E, Bookman M, et al. 2004 consensus statements on the management of ovarian cancer: final document of the 3rd International Gynecologic Cancer Intergroup Ovarian Cancer Consensus Conference (GCIG OCCC 2004). Ann Oncol. 2005;16(SUPPL. 8):7–12. https://doi.org/10.1093/annonc/mdi961.
9. Eisenhauer EL, Abu-Rustum NR, Sonoda Y, Levine DA, Poynor EA, Aghajanian C, et al. The addition of extensive upper abdominal surgery to achieve optimal cytoreduction improves survival in patients with stages IIIC-IV epithelial ovarian cancer. Gynecol Oncol. 2006;103(3):1083–90. https://doi.org/10.1016/j.ygyno.2006.06.028.
10. Wimberger P, Lehmann N, Kimmig R, Burges A, Meier W, Du Bois A. Prognostic factors for complete debulking in advanced ovarian cancer and its impact on survival. An exploratory analysis of a prospectively randomized phase III study of the Arbeitsgemeinschaft Gynaekologische Onkologie Ovarian Cancer Study Group (AGO-OVA). Gynecol Oncol. 2007;106(1):69–74. https://doi.org/10.1016/j.ygyno.2007.02.026.
11. Bristow RE, Tomacruz RS, Armstrong DK, Trimble EL, Montz FJ. Survival effect of maximal cytoreductive surgery for advanced ovarian carcinoma during the platinum era: a meta-analysis. J Clin Oncol. 2002;20(5):1248–59. https://doi.org/10.1200/JCO.2002.20.5.1248.
12. Fader AN, Rose PG. Role of surgery in ovarian carcinoma. J Clin Oncol. 2007; https://doi.org/10.1200/JCO.2007.11.0932.
13. Schorge JO, Garrett LA, Goodman A. Cytoreductive surgery for advanced ovarian cancer: quo vadis? Oncology (Williston Park, N.Y.). 2011;25(10):928–34.
14. Bristow BRE, Tomacruz RS, Armstrong DK, Trimble EL, Montz FJ. Effect maximal cytoreductive surgery for advanced ovarian carcinoma during the platinum era. J Clin Oncol. 2008;20(5):1248–59. https://doi.org/10.1200/JCO.2002.20.5.1248.
15. Elattar A, Bryant A, Winter-Roach BA, Hatem M, Naik R. Optimal primary surgical treatment for advanced epithelial ovarian cancer. In: Elattar A, editor. Cochrane database of systematic reviews. Chichester, UK: Wiley; 2011. p. CD007565. https://doi.org/10.1002/14651858.CD007565.pub2.
16. Aletti GD, Powless C, Bakkum-Gamez J, Wilson TO, Podratz KC, Cliby WA. Pattern of retroperitoneal dissemination of primary peritoneum cancer: basis for rational use of lymphadenectomy. Gynecol Oncol. 2009;114(1):32–6. https://doi.org/10.1016/j.ygyno.2009.03.020.
17. Panici PB, Maggioni A, Hacker N, Landoni F, Ackermann S, Campagnutta E, et al. Systematic aortic and pelvic lymphadenectomy versus resection of bulky nodes only in optimally debulked advanced ovarian cancer: a randomized clinical trial. J Natl Cancer Inst. 2005;97(8):560–6. https://doi.org/10.1093/jnci/dji102.
18. Chan JK, Urban R, Hu JM, Shin JY, Husain A, Teng NN, et al. The potential therapeutic role of lymph node resection in epithelial ovarian cancer: a study of 13,918 patients. Br J Cancer. 2007;96(12):1817–22. https://doi.org/10.1038/sj.bjc.6603803.
19. Takeshima N, Hirai Y, Umayahara K, Fujiwara K, Takizawa K, Hasumi K. Lymph node metastasis in ovarian cancer: difference between serous and non-serous primary tumors. Gynecol Oncol. 2005;99(2):427–31. https://doi.org/10.1016/j.ygyno.2005.06.051.
20. Karam A, Ledermann JA, Kim J-W, Sehouli J, Lu K, Gourley C, et al. Fifth ovarian cancer consensus conference of the gynecologic cancer intergroup: first-line interventions. Ann Oncol. 2017;28(4):711–7. https://doi.org/10.1093/annonc/mdx011.
21. Chi DS, Eisenhauer EL, Zivanovic O, Sonoda Y, Abu-Rustum NR, Levine DA, et al. Improved progression-free and overall survival in advanced ovarian cancer as a result of a change in

surgical paradigm. Gynecol Oncol. 2009;114(1):26–31. https://doi.org/10.1016/j.ygyno.2009.03.018.

22. Morrison J, Haldar K, Kehoe S, Lawrie TA. Chemotherapy versus surgery for initial treatment in advanced ovarian epithelial cancer. Cochrane Database Syst Rev. 2012;8:CD005343. https://doi.org/10.1002/14651858.CD005343.pub3.

23. Kehoe S, Hook J, Nankivell M, Jayson GC, Kitchener H, Lopes T, et al. Primary chemotherapy versus primary surgery for newly diagnosed advanced ovarian cancer (CHORUS): an open-label, randomised, controlled, non-inferiority trial. Lancet. 2015;386(9990):249–57. https://doi.org/10.1016/S0140-6736(14)62223-6.

24. Vergote I, Tropé CG, Amant F, Kristensen GB, Ehlen T, Johnson N, et al. Neoadjuvant chemotherapy or primary surgery in stage IIIC or IV ovarian cancer. N Engl J Med. 2010;363(10):943–53. https://doi.org/10.1056/NEJMoa0908806.

25. Bristow RE, Chi DS. Platinum-based neoadjuvant chemotherapy and interval surgical cytoreduction for advanced ovarian cancer: a meta-analysis. Gynecol Oncol. 2006;103(3):1070–6. https://doi.org/10.1016/j.ygyno.2006.06.025.

26. Wright AA, Bohlke K, Armstrong DK, Bookman MA, Cliby WA, Coleman RL, et al. Neoadjuvant chemotherapy for newly diagnosed, advanced ovarian cancer: Society of Gynecologic Oncology and American Society of Clinical Oncology Clinical Practice Guideline. J Clin Oncol. 2016;34(28):3460–73. https://doi.org/10.1200/JCO.2016.68.6907.

27. Colombo PE, Labaki M, Fabbro M, Bertrand M, Mourregot A, Gutowski M, et al. Impact of neoadjuvant chemotherapy cycles prior to interval surgery in patients with advanced epithelial ovarian cancer. Gynecol Oncol. 2014;135(2):223–30. https://doi.org/10.1016/j.ygyno.2014.09.002.

28. Stuart GCE, Kitchener H, Bacon M, duBois A, Friedlander M, Ledermann J, et al. 2010 Gynecologic Cancer InterGroup (GCIG) consensus statement on clinical trials in ovarian cancer. Int J Gynecol Cancer. 2011;21(4):750–5. https://doi.org/10.1097/IGC.0b013e31821b2568.

29. Kyrgiou M, Salanti G, Pavlidis N, Paraskevaidis E, Ioannidis JPA. Survival benefits with diverse chemotherapy regimens for ovarian cancer: meta-analysis of multiple treatments. J Natl Cancer Inst. 2006;98(22):1655–63. https://doi.org/10.1093/jnci/djj443.

30. Aravantinos G, Fountzilas G, Bamias A, Grimani I, Rizos S, Kalofonos HP, et al. Carboplatin and paclitaxel versus cisplatin, paclitaxel and doxorubicin for first-line chemotherapy of advanced ovarian cancer: a Hellenic cooperative oncology group (HeCOG) study. Eur J Cancer. 2008;44(15):2169–77. https://doi.org/10.1016/j.ejca.2008.06.035.

31. Bolis G, Scarfone G, Raspagliesi F, Mangili G, Danese S, Scollo P, et al. Paclitaxel/carboplatin versus topotecan/paclitaxel/carboplatin in patients with FIGO suboptimally resected stage III-IV epithelial ovarian cancer a multicenter, randomized study. Eur J Cancer. 2010;46(16):2905–12. https://doi.org/10.1016/j.ejca.2010.06.124.

32. Bookman MA, Brady MF, McGuire WP, Harper PG, Alberts DS, Friedlander M, et al. Evaluation of new platinum-based treatment regimens in advanced-stage ovarian cancer: a phase III trial of the gynecologic cancer intergroup. J Clin Oncol. 2009;27(9):1419–25. https://doi.org/10.1200/JCO.2008.19.1684.

33. du Bois A, Herrstedt J, Hardy-Bessard A-C, Müller H-H, Harter P, Kristensen G, et al. Phase III trial of carboplatin plus paclitaxel with or without gemcitabine in first-line treatment of epithelial ovarian cancer. J Clin Oncol. 2010;28(27):4162–9. https://doi.org/10.1200/JCO.2009.27.4696.

34. Du Bois A, Weber B, Rochon J, Meier W, Goupil A, Olbricht S, et al. Addition of epirubicin as a third drug to carboplatin-paclitaxel in first-line treatment of advanced ovarian cancer: a

prospectively randomized Gynecologic Cancer Intergroup trial by the Arbeitsgemeinschaft Gynaekologische Onkologie Ovarian Cancer Study G. J Clin Oncol. 2006;24(7):1127–35. https://doi.org/10.1200/JCO.2005.03.2938.

35. Hoskins P, Vergote I, Cervantes A, Tu D, Stuart G, Zola P, et al. Advanced ovarian cancer: phase III randomized study of sequential cisplatin-topotecan and carboplatin-paclitaxel vs carboplatin-paclitaxel. J Natl Cancer Inst. 2010;102(20):1547–56. https://doi.org/10.1093/jnci/djq362.

36. Katsumata N, Yasuda M, Isonishi S, Takahashi F, Michimae H, Kimura E, et al. Long-term results of dose-dense paclitaxel and carboplatin versus conventional paclitaxel and carboplatin for treatment of advanced epithelial ovarian, fallopian tube, or primary peritoneal cancer (JGOG 3016): a randomised, controlled, open-label trial. Lancet Oncol. 2013;14(10):1020–6. https://doi.org/10.1016/S1470-2045(13)70363-2.

37. Katsumata N, Yasuda M, Takahashi F, Isonishi S, Jobo T, Aoki D, et al. Dose-dense paclitaxel once a week in combination with carboplatin every 3 weeks for advanced ovarian cancer: a phase 3, open-label, randomised controlled trial. Lancet. 2009;374(9698):1331–8. https://doi.org/10.1016/S0140-6736(09)61157-0.

38. Seagle B-LL, Shahabi S. Cost-effectiveness analysis of dose-dense versus standard intravenous chemotherapy for ovarian cancer: an economic analysis of results from the Gynecologic Oncology Group protocol 262 randomized controlled trial. Gynecol Oncol. 2017;145(1):9–14. https://doi.org/10.1016/j.ygyno.2017.02.014.

39. Pignata S, Scambia G, Katsaros D, Gallo C, Pujade-Lauraine E, De Placido S, et al. Carboplatin plus paclitaxel once a week versus every 3 weeks in patients with advanced ovarian cancer (MITO-7): a randomised, multicentre, open-label, phase 3 trial. Lancet Oncol. 2014;15(4):396–405. https://doi.org/10.1016/S1470-2045(14)70049-X.

40. Milani A, Kristeleit R, McCormack M, Raja F, Luvero D, Widschwendter M, et al. Switching from standard to dose-dense chemotherapy in front-line treatment of advanced ovarian cancer: a retrospective study of feasibility and efficacy. ESMO Open. 2016;1(6):e000117. https://doi.org/10.1136/esmoopen-2016-000117.

41. Burger RA, Brady MF, Bookman MA, Fleming GF, Monk BJ, Huang H, et al. Incorporation of bevacizumab in the primary treatment of ovarian cancer. N Engl J Med. 2011;365(26):2473–83. https://doi.org/10.1056/NEJMoa1104390.

42. Perren, T. J., Swart, A. M., Pfisterer, J., Ledermann, J. A., Pujade-Lauraine, E., Kristensen, G., … ICON7 Investigators. (2011). A phase 3 trial of bevacizumab in ovarian cancer. N Engl J Med, 365(26), 2484–2496. https://doi.org/10.1056/NEJMoa1103799.

43. Armstrong DK, Bundy B, Wenzel L, Huang HQ, Baergen R, Lele S, et al.; Gynecologic Oncology Group. Intraperitoneal cisplatin and paclitaxel in ovarian cancer. N Engl J Med, 2006:354(1);34–43. https://doi.org/10.1056/NEJMoa052985.

44. Jaaback K, Johnson N, Lawrie TA. Intraperitoneal chemotherapy for the initial management of primary epithelial ovarian cancer. In: Jaaback K, editor. Cochrane database of systematic reviews. Chichester, UK: Wiley; 2016. https://doi.org/10.1002/14651858.CD005340.pub4.

45. Davidson SA, Rubin SC, Markman M, Jones WB, Hakes TB, Reichman B, et al. Intraperitoneal chemotherapy: analysis of complications with an implanted subcutaneous port and catheter system. Gynecol Oncol. 1991;41(2):101–6.

46. Walker JL, Armstrong DK, Huang HQ, Fowler J, Webster K, Burger RA, Clarke-Pearson D. Intraperitoneal catheter outcomes in a phase III trial of intravenous versus intraperitoneal chemotherapy in optimal stage III ovarian and primary peritoneal cancer: a Gynecologic Oncology Group study. Gynecol Oncol. 2006;100(1):27–32. https://doi.org/10.1016/j.ygyno.2005.11.013.

47. Bhoola S, Hoskins WJ. Diagnosis and management of epithelial ovarian cancer. Obstet Gynecol. 2006; https://doi.org/10.1097/01.AOG.0000220516.34053.48.

48. Jakobsen A, Bertelsen K, Andersen JE, Havsteen H, Jakobsen P, Moeller KA, et al. Dose-effect study of carboplatin in ovarian cancer: a Danish Ovarian Cancer Group study. J Clin Oncol. 1997;15(1):193–8. https://doi.org/10.1200/JCO.1997.15.1.193.

49. Bergamini A, Pisano C, Di Napoli M, Arenare L, Della Pepa C, Tambaro R, et al. Cisplatin can be safely administered to ovarian cancer patients with hypersensitivity to carboplatin. Gynecol Oncol. 2017;144(1):72–6. https://doi.org/10.1016/j.ygyno.2016.10.023.

50. du Bois A, Pfisterer J, Burchardi N, Loibl S, Huober J, Wimberger P, et al. Combination therapy with pegylated liposomal doxorubicin and carboplatin in gynecologic malignancies: a prospective phase II study of the Arbeitsgemeinschaft Gynäekologische Onkologie Studiengruppe Ovarialkarzinom (AGO-OVAR) and Kommission Uterus (AGO-K-U). Gynecol Oncol. 2007;107(3):518–25. https://doi.org/10.1016/j.ygyno.2007.08.008.

51. Pujade-Lauraine E, Wagner U, Aavall-Lundqvist E, Gebski V, Heywood M, Vasey PA, et al. Pegylated liposomal doxorubicin and carboplatin compared with paclitaxel and carboplatin for patients with platinum-sensitive ovarian cancer in late relapse. J Clin Oncol. 2010;28(20):3323–9. https://doi.org/10.1200/JCO.2009.25.7519.

52. Parmar, M. K. B., Ledermann, J. A., Colombo, N., du Bois, A., Delaloye, J.-F., Kristensen, G. B., ... ICON and AGO Collaborators. (2003). Paclitaxel plus platinum-based chemotherapy versus conventional platinum-based chemotherapy in women with relapsed ovarian cancer: the ICON4/AGO-OVAR-2.2 trial. Lancet (London, England), 361(9375), 2099–2106.

53. Wagner U, Marth C, Largillier R, Kaern J, Brown C, Heywood M, et al. Final overall survival results of phase III GCIG CALYPSO trial of pegylated liposomal doxorubicin and carboplatin vs paclitaxel and carboplatin in platinum-sensitive ovarian cancer patients. Br J Cancer. 2012;107(4):588–91. https://doi.org/10.1038/bjc.2012.307.

54. Pfisterer J, Plante M, Vergote I, Du Bois A, Hirte H, Lacave AJ, et al. Gemcitabine plus carboplatin compared with carboplatin in patients with platinum-sensitive recurrent ovarian cancer: an intergroup trial of the AGO-OVAR, the NCIC CTG, and the EORTC GCG. J Clin Oncol. 2006;24(29):4699–707. https://doi.org/10.1200/JCO.2006.06.0913.

55. Monk BJ, Herzog TJ, Kaye SB, Krasner CN, Vermorken JB, Muggia FM, et al. Trabectedin plus pegylated liposomal doxorubicin in recurrent ovarian cancer. J Clin Oncol. 2010;28(19):3107–14. https://doi.org/10.1200/JCO.2009.25.4037.

56. Monk BJ, Sill MW, McMeekin DS, Cohn DE, Ramondetta LM, Boardman CH, et al. Phase III trial of four cisplatin-containing doublet combinations in stage IVB, recurrent, or persistent cervical carcinoma: a Gynecologic Oncology Group study. J Clin Oncol. 2009;27(28):4649–55. https://doi.org/10.1200/JCO.2009.21.8909.

57. Gore ME, Levy V, Rustin G, Perren T, Calvert AH, Earl H, Thompson JM. Paclitaxel (Taxol) in relapsed and refractory ovarian cancer: the UK and Eire experience. Br J Cancer. 1995;72(4):1016–9. https://doi.org/10.1038/bjc.1995.453.

58. Gordon AN, Fleagle JT, Guthrie D, Parkin DE, Gore ME, Lacave AJ. Recurrent epithelial ovarian carcinoma: a randomized phase III study of pegylated liposomal doxorubicin versus topotecan. J Clin Oncol. 2001;19(14):3312–22. https://doi.org/10.1200/JCO.2001.19.14.3312.

59. Ferrandina G, Ludovisi M, Lorusso D, Pignata S, Breda E, Savarese A, et al. Phase III trial of gemcitabine compared with pegylated liposomal doxorubicin in progressive or recurrent ovarian cancer. J Clin Oncol. 2008;26(6):890–6. https://doi.org/10.1200/JCO.2007.13.6606.

60. Bruchim I, Ben-Harim Z, Piura E, Haran G, Fishman A. Analysis of two topotecan treatment schedules in patients with recurrent ovarian cancer. J Chemother. 2016;28(2):129–34. https://doi.org/10.1080/1120009X.2015.1115195.

61. Rose PG, Blessing JA, Mayer AR, Homesley HD. Prolonged oral etoposide as second-line therapy for platinum-resistant and platinum-sensitive ovarian carcinoma: a gynecologic oncology group study. J Clin Oncol. 1998;16(2):405–10. https://doi.org/10.1200/JCO.1998.16.2.405.

62. Miller DS, Blessing JA, Krasner CN, Mannel RS, Hanjani P, Pearl ML, et al. Phase II evaluation of pemetrexed in the treatment of recurrent or persistent platinum-resistant ovarian or primary peritoneal carcinoma: a study of the gynecologic oncology group. J Clin Oncol. 2009;27(16):2686–91. https://doi.org/10.1200/JCO.2008.19.2963.

63. Aghajanian C, Blank SV, Goff BA, Judson PL, Teneriello MG, Husain A, et al. OCEANS: a randomized, double-blind, placebo-controlled phase III trial of chemotherapy with or without bevacizumab in patients with platinum-sensitive recurrent epithelial ovarian, primary peritoneal, or fallopian tube cancer. J Clin Oncol. 2012;30(17):2039–45. https://doi.org/10.1200/JCO.2012.42.0505.

64. Pujade-Lauraine E, Hilpert F, Weber B, Reuss A, Poveda A, Kristensen G, et al. Bevacizumab combined with chemotherapy for platinum-resistant recurrent ovarian cancer: the AURELIA open-label randomized phase III trial. J Clin Oncol. 2014;32(13):1302–8. https://doi.org/10.1200/JCO.2013.51.4489.

65. Stockler MR, Hilpert F, Friedlander M, King MT, Wenzel L, Lee CK, et al. Patient-reported outcome results from the open-label phase III AURELIA trial evaluating bevacizumab-containing therapy for platinum-resistant ovarian cancer. J Clin Oncol. 2014;32(13):1309–16. https://doi.org/10.1200/JCO.2013.51.4240.

66. Grunewald T, Ledermann JA. Targeted therapies for ovarian cancer. Best Pract Res Clin Obstet Gynaecol. 2016; https://doi.org/10.1016/j.bpobgyn.2016.12.001.

67. Du Bois A, Floquet A, Kim JW, Rau J, Del Campo JM, Friedlander M, et al. Incorporation of pazopanib in maintenance therapy of ovarian cancer. J Clin Oncol. 2014;32(30):3374–81. https://doi.org/10.1200/JCO.2014.55.7348.

68. Pignata S, Lorusso D, Scambia G, Sambataro D, Tamberi S, Cinieri S, et al. Pazopanib plus weekly paclitaxel versus weekly paclitaxel alone for platinum-resistant or platinum-refractory advanced ovarian cancer (MITO 11): a randomised, open-label, phase 2 trial. Lancet Oncol. 2015;16(5):561–8. https://doi.org/10.1016/S1470-2045(15)70115-4.

69. Matulonis UA, Berlin S, Ivy P, Tyburski K, Krasner C, Zarwan C, et al. Cediranib, an oral inhibitor of vascular endothelial growth factor receptor kinases, is an active drug in recurrent epithelial ovarian, fallopian tube, and peritoneal cancer. J Clin Oncol. 2009;27(33):5601–6. https://doi.org/10.1200/JCO.2009.23.2777.

70. Ledermann JA, Embleton AC, Raja F, Perren TJ, Jayson GC, Rustin GJS, et al. Cediranib in patients with relapsed platinum-sensitive ovarian cancer (ICON6): a randomised, double-blind, placebo-controlled phase 3 trial. Lancet. 2016a;387(10023):1066–74. https://doi.org/10.1016/S0140-6736(15)01167-8.

71. Ledermann JA, Harter P, Gourley C, Friedlander M, Vergote I, Rustin GJS, et al. Overall survival (OS) in patients (pts) with platinum-sensitive relapsed serous ovarian cancer (PSR SOC) receiving olaparib maintenance monotherapy: an interim analysis. ASCO Ann Meet. 2016b;17(11)., Abstract number 5501. https://doi.org/10.1016/S1470-2045(16)30376-X.

72. Liu JF, Barry WT, Birrer M, Lee JM, Buckanovich RJ, Fleming GF, et al. Combination cediranib and olaparib versus olaparib

alone for women with recurrent platinum-sensitive ovarian cancer: a randomised phase 2 study. Lancet Oncol. 2014;15(11):1207–14. https://doi.org/10.1016/S1470-2045(14)70391-2.

73. du Bois A, Kristensen G, Ray-Coquard I, Reuss A, Pignata S, Colombo N, et al. Standard first-line chemotherapy with or without nintedanib for advanced ovarian cancer (AGO-OVAR 12): a randomised, double-blind, placebo-controlled phase 3 trial. Lancet Oncol. 2016;17(1):78–89. https://doi.org/10.1016/S1470-2045(15)00366-6.

74. Bono M, Fanale D, Incorvaia L, et al. Impact of deleterious variants in other genes beyond BRCA1/2 detected in breast/ovarian and pancreatic cancer patients by NGS-based multigene panel testing: looking over the hedge [published online ahead of print, 2021 Aug 6]. ESMO Open. 2021;6(4):100235. https://doi.org/10.1016/j.esmoop.2021.100235.

75. Gori S, Barberis M, Bella MA, et al. Recommendations for the implementation of BRCA testing in ovarian cancer patients and their relatives. Crit Rev Oncol Hematol. 2019;140:67–72. https://doi.org/10.1016/j.critrevonc.2019.05.012.

76. Russo A, Incorvaia L, Malapelle U, et al. The tumor-agnostic treatment for patients with solid tumors: a position paper on behalf of the AIOM-SIAPEC/IAP-SIBIOC-SIF italian scientific societies [published online ahead of print, 2021 Aug 6]. Crit Rev Oncol Hematol. 2021;103436. https://doi.org/10.1016/j.critrevonc.2021.103436.

77. Jenner ZB, Sood AK, Coleman RL. Evaluation of rucaparib and companion diagnostics in the PARP inhibitor landscape for recurrent ovarian cancer therapy. Future Oncol. 2016;12(12):1439–56. https://doi.org/10.2217/fon-2016-0002.

78. Ledermann JA, Canevari S, Thigpen T. Targeting the folate receptor: diagnostic and therapeutic approaches to personalize cancer treatments. Ann Oncol. 2015; https://doi.org/10.1093/annonc/mdv250.

79. Bueno R, Appasani K, Mercer H, Lester S, Sugarbaker D. The α folate receptor is highly activated in malignant pleural mesothelioma. J Thorac Cardiovasc Surg. 2001;121(2):225–33. https://doi.org/10.1067/mtc.2001.111176.

80. Kalli KR, Oberg AL, Keeney GL, Christianson TJH, Low PS, Knutson KL, Hartmann LC. Folate receptor alpha as a tumor target in epithelial ovarian cancer. Gynecol Oncol. 2008;108(3):619–26. https://doi.org/10.1016/j.ygyno.2007.11.020.

81. Ponte JF, Ab O, Lanieri L, Lee J, Coccia J, Bartle LM, et al. Mirvetuximab soravtansine (IMGN853), a folate receptor alpha–targeting antibody-drug conjugate, potentiates the activity of standard of care therapeutics in ovarian cancer models. Neoplasia (United States). 2016;18(12):775–84. https://doi.org/10.1016/j.neo.2016.11.002.

82. Jelovac D, Armstrong K. Role of farletuzumab in epithelial ovarian carcinoma. Curr Pharm Des. 2012;18(25):3812–5. https://doi.org/10.2174/138161212802002698.

83. Moore KN, Martin LP, O'Malley DM, Matulonis UA, Konner JA, Vergote I, et al. A review of mirvetuximab soravtansine in the treatment of platinum-resistant ovarian cancer. Fut Oncol (London, England). 2017;14(2):123–36. https://doi.org/10.2217/fon-2017-0379.

84. Naumann RW, Coleman RL, Burger RA, Sausville EA, Kutarska E, Ghamande SA, et al. PRECEDENT: a randomized phase II trial comparing vintafolide (EC145) and pegylated liposomal doxorubicin (PLD) in combination versus PLD alone in patients with platinum-resistant ovarian cancer. J Clin Oncol. 2013;31(35):4400–6. https://doi.org/10.1200/JCO.2013.49.7685.

85. Eisenkop SM, Friedman RL, Spirtos NM. The role of secondary cytoreductive surgery in the treatment of patients with recurrent epithelial ovarian carcinoma. Cancer. 2000;88(1):144–53.

86. Salani R, Santillan A, Zahurak ML, Giuntoli RL, Gardner GJ, Armstrong DK, Bristow RE. Secondary cytoreductive surgery for localized, recurrent epithelial ovarian cancer: analysis of prognostic factors and survival outcome. Cancer. 2007;109(4):685–91. https://doi.org/10.1002/cncr.22447.

87. Scarabelli C, Gallo A, Visentin MC, Canzonieri V, Carbone A, Zarrelli A. Systematic pelvic and Para-aortic lymphadenectomy in advanced ovarian cancer patients with no residual intraperitoneal disease. Int J Gynecol Cancer. 1997;7(1):18–26.

88. Harter P, Du Bois A, Hahmann M, Hasenburg A, Burges A, Loibl S, et al. Surgery in recurrent ovarian cancer: the Arbeitsgemeinschaft Gynaekologische Onkologie (AGO) DESKTOP OVAR trial. Ann Surg Oncol. 2006;13(12):1702–10. https://doi.org/10.1245/s10434-006-9058-0.

89. Ushijima K. Treatment for recurrent ovarian cancer—at first relapse. J Oncol. 2010;2010:1–7. https://doi.org/10.1155/2010/497429.

90. Pujade-Lauraine E, Combe P. Recurrent ovarian cancer. Ann Oncol. 2016;27(suppl 1):i63–5. https://doi.org/10.1093/annonc/mdw079.

91. Makrilia N, Syrigou E, Kaklamanos I, Manolopoulos L, Saif MW. Hypersensitivity reactions associated with platinum antineoplastic agents: a systematic review. Metal-Based Drugs. 2010; https://doi.org/10.1155/2010/207084.

92. Poveda A, Vergote I, Tjulandin S, Kong B, Roy M, Chan S, et al. Trabectedin plus pegylated liposomal doxorubicin in relapsed ovarian cancer: outcomes in the partially platinum-sensitive (platinum-free interval 6–12 months) subpopulation of OVA-301 phase III randomized trial. Ann Oncol. 2011;22(1):39–48. https://doi.org/10.1093/annonc/mdq352.

93. Monk BJ, Ghatage P, Parekh T, Henitz E, Knoblauch R, et al. Effect of BRCA1 and XPG mutations on treatment response to trabectedin and pegylated liposomal doxorubicin in patients with advanced ovarian cancer: exploratory analysis of the phase 3 OVA-301 study. Ann Oncol. 2015;26(5):914–20. https://doi.org/10.1093/annonc/mdv071.

94. Edwards SJ, Barton S, Thurgar E, Trevor N. Topotecan, pegylated liposomal doxorubicin hydrochloride, paclitaxel, trabectedin and gemcitabine for advanced recurrent or refractory ovarian cancer: a systematic review and economic evaluation. Health Technol Assess. 2015;19(7):1–524. https://doi.org/10.3310/hta19070.

Endometrial and Cervical Cancers

Lorena Incorvaia, Luisa Castellana, Lavinia Insalaco, Giuseppa Maltese, and Domenica Lorusso

Gynecological Cancers

Contents

Lorena Incorvaia and Luisa Castellana should be considered equally co-first authors.

© Springer Nature Switzerland AG 2021
A. Russo et al. (eds.), *Practical Medical Oncology Textbook*, UNIPA Springer Series,
https://doi.org/10.1007/978-3-030-56051-5_53

Learning Objectives

By the end of the chapter, the reader will:

- Have learned the most important knowledge of uterine and cervical cancers
- Be able to define the diagnostic and therapeutic procedures relative to uterine cancers and apply them into clinical practice
- Have understood the most innovative therapeutic strategies of uterine cancers
- Have known the potential future therapeutic perspectives of both uterine and cervical cancers

53.1 Introduction

The uterus can be essentially divided into two distinct anatomic regions (Fig. 53.1):

- Corpus
- Cervix

Uterine corpus and cervical cancers represent two malignancies very different from each other in terms of epidemiology, risk and etiological factors, histopathology/molecular biology, and therapeutic approaches. Thus, we will deal with these two arguments as separated topics in this chapter.

53.2 Uterine Corpus Cancers

Uterine corpus cancers are the fourth most common malignancy and the sixth leading cause of cancer-related death in female sex in the United States, with estimated incidence and mortality rates of 7% (61,880

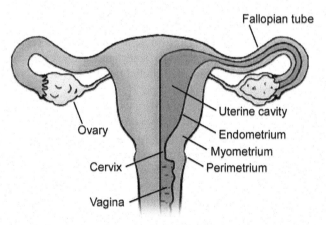

Fig. 53.1 In the cranio-caudal direction, we can distinguish the *fundus* (the uppermost rounded part), *uterine corpus* and *uterine cavity*, *internal uterine orifice*, *cervix* (known also as "uterine neck" and protruding into the vagina) and *cervical canal*, and *external uterine orifice*. The uterine wall is composed of three layers: *endometrium* (the innermost), *myometrium*, and *perimetrium* (the outermost)

Breast (30 %)
Lung and bronchus (13 %)
Colon and rectum (8 %)
Uterine corpus (7 %)
Melanoma of the skin (4 %)
Thyroid (4 %)
Non-Hodgkin lymphoma (4 %)
Kidney and renal pelvis (3 %)
Pancreas (3 %)
Leuka emia (3 %)

Fig. 53.2 Estimated incidence rate by cancer types in female sex, United States, 2019

Lung and bronchus (23 %)
Breast (15 %)
Colon and rectum (8 %)
Pancreas (8 %)
Ovary (5 %)
Uterine corpus (4 %)
Liver and intrahepatic bile ducts (4 %)
Leuka emia (3 %)
Non-Hodgkin lymphoma (3 %)
Brain and other nervous system (3 %)

Fig. 53.3 Estimated mortality rate by cancer types in female sex, United States, 2019

new cases) and 4% (12,160 deaths), respectively, in 2019 [1] (Figs. 53.2 and 53.3).

These numbers are in line with epidemiological data emerged from Europe in 2018: incidence rate 6.6% (121,600 new cases) and mortality rate 3.5% (29,600 deaths). Particularly, corpus cancers were found to be at the fourth and seventh places, respectively, in terms of incidence and mortality [2] (Figs. 53.4 and 53.5).

53.3 Endometrial Cancer

53.3.1 Epidemiology

Endometrial cancer (EC) is the sixth most common cancer in women with over 382,000 new cases and 90,000

Breast (28,2 %)

Colon and rectum (12,3 %)

Lung and bronchus (3,5 %)

Uterine corpus (6,6 %)

Melanoma of the skin (3,9 %)

Ovary (3,7 %)

Pancreas (3,5 %)

Cervix (3,3%)

Thyroid (3 ,3 %)

Non-Hodgkin lymphoma (2,8 %)

Fig. 53.4 Incidence rate by cancer types in female sex, Europe, 2018

Breast (6,2 %)

Lung and bronchus (14,2 %)

Colon and rectum (13,2 %)

Pancreas (7,4 %)

Ovary (5,2 %)

Stomach (4, 7 %)

Uterine corpus (3,5 %)

Leukaemia (3,2 %)

Liver and intrahepatic bile ducts (3,2 %)

Cervix (3 %)

Fig. 53.5 Mortality rate by cancer types in female sex, Europe, 2018

deaths found in 2018 worldwide. The countries with the highest incidence rate in 2018 are represented in the Fig. 53.6 [3]. EC is at the first place in terms of frequency among uterine corpus cancers and the most representative gynecological tumor in developed countries (likely due to environmental and dietetic factors); there, over the last decades, a gradual increase both in the incidence and mortality rate has been registered, related to prolonged life expectancy, bad lifestyle habits, rise of advanced-stage cases, and poor-risk histologies [4]. EC is typically diagnosed in post-menopausal women (>90% in the 50–70 age group, median age 63 years) and at an early stage ($\simeq$67% at stage I) [5] (Fig. 53.7). Five-year survival rate varies according to the stage at the diagnosis [6] (Fig. 53.8).

53.3.2 Etiological, Risk, and Protective Factors

Increased estrogen levels, especially not enough to be counterbalanced by adequate progesterone levels, are the most important predisposing factor to the endometrial cancer onset. We can divide the *risk factors* as shown in Table 53.1.

Contrariwise, we can recognize as *protective factors*:

- Active lifestyle, maintaining of a normal weight, consumption of dietary fibers, and coffee consumption [24]
- Use of combined estrogen-progestin contraceptives (CCs) [25–27]
- Use of combined estrogen-progestin HRT in menopause [28]

53.3.3 Prevention and Screening

Any validated screening test for EC is designed for the general population; certainly, it is recommended to adopt primary and/or secondary prevention measures for those women who present with increased or high risk to develop an endometrial cancer.

Primary prevention may carry out correcting some risk factors: adoption of healthy dietary habits and active lifestyle.

Women who have an *increased risk* of EC onset (for the presence of concomitant risk factors) should undergo a careful surveillance if any endometrial thickness ($\geq$3 mm) is detected on ultrasonography or if any unexpected vaginal bleeding has recently appeared, especially when in treatment with unopposed estrogen or tamoxifen. Likewise, the same can be even more so applied to *high-risk* groups: women who underwent a fertility-sparing treatment for adult granulosa cell tumor (AGCT), epithelial estrogen-secreting ovarian tumor, endometrioid EC (EEC), and well-differentiated (G1), premalignant lesions (atypical endometrial hyperplasia (AEH), endometrial intraepithelial neoplasia (EIN)).

Lynch syndrome (LS) type II deserves a separate discussion. Mutations relative to genes involved in the mismatch repair (MMR) system (MLH1, MSH2, MSH6, PMS2) can occur up to 5% of EC cases, thus typically presenting with microsatellite instability (MSI) on immunohistochemistry (IHC) [29, 30].

Genetic counselling and testing should be proposed to all those patients who had an EC and colorectal cancer, especially when younger than 50 years and/or with a significant related family history [31–35].

Patients with known germline LS mutations should respect at least a close surveillance program from the age of 35 years that includes annual clinical gynecological examination, trans-vaginal ultrasonography (TVUS), and endometrial biopsy [33–36].

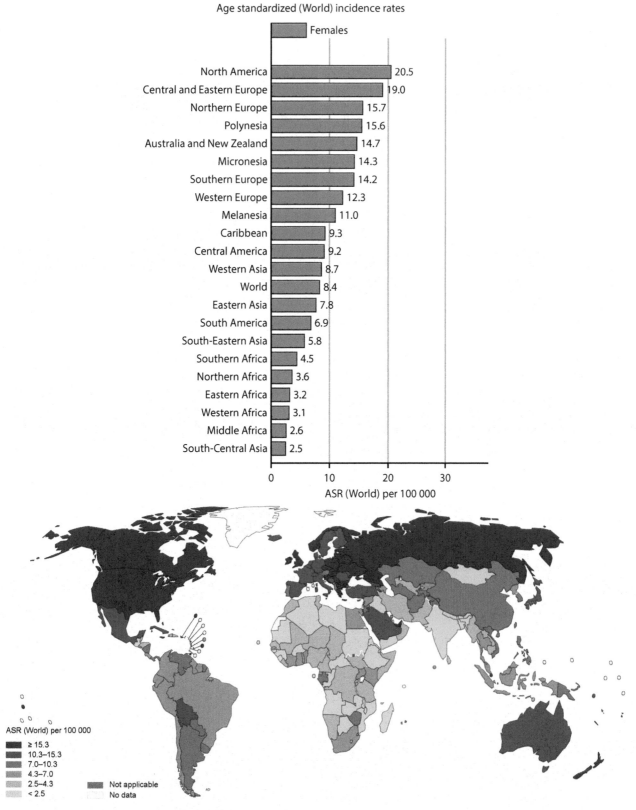

Fig. 53.6 Age-standardized incidence rates of EC in the world

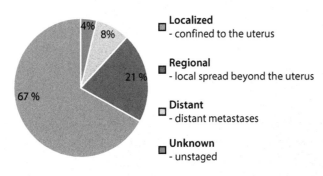

Fig. 53.7 Percent of cases by stage at the diagnosis

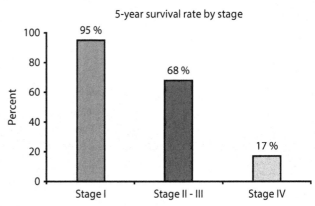

Fig. 53.8 5-year survival rate according to the stage

53

■ **Table 53.1** Principal *risk factors* for endometrial cancer

Enviromental factors	Hormonal factors	Hereditary/familial factors

Overweight (BMI 25–29,9 kg/m²)/obesity (BMI ≥ 30 kg/m²):
  Higher BMI associated with higher relative risk (RR) [7–10]
  Chronic hyperinsulinemia leads to:
    (a) Higher levels of free insulin-like growth factor (IGF) with mitogenic/anti-apoptotic effect
    (b) Higher estrogen levels secondary to sex hormone-binding globulin (SHBG) lowering [11]
  Medical history of metabolic syndrome, type II diabetes mellitus (T2DM), hypertension, chronic hepatopathy, and sedentary habits may be observed [12]
  Correlation with good prognostic factors: low grade, endometrioid histology, and presentation at early stage
	Early menarche (<12 years)
	Late menopause (>55 years) [15]
		Lynch syndrome (LS)/hereditary Non-polyposis colorectal cancer Syndrome (HNPCC):
		  Lifetime risk for EC and colorectal cancer 40–60% [23]
		  Lifetime risk for ovarian cancer 9–12%
		  Correlation with poor prognosis

Eating habits:
  High consumption of red meat (100 g/die) [13]
  High consumption of saturated fat [14]
	Nulliparity/infertility	

	Polycistic ovarian syndrome (PCOS) [16]	
	Estrogen-producing tumors *Ovarian granulosa tumors* *Theca cell tumors* [17]	
	Use of uncombined menopausal hormone replacement therapy (HRT) [18]	

	Use of tamoxifen for breast cancer treatment:
	  Estrogenic/proliferative activity on endometrium [19–21]
	  Increased risk in post-menopausal women [22]
	  Increased risk correlated to dose and time of treatment	

53.3.4 Histopathology and Molecular Biology

An old and outdated dualistic model divided ECs into two pathogenic entities, as shown in ▫ Table 53.2 [39]. Recently, The Cancer Genome Atlas (TCAG) Research Network, innovatively, identified four different EC subgroups on the basis of molecular profiles [40] (▫ Table 53.3).

POLE ultramutated and MSI hypermutated subgroups appear to be related to a better prognosis [41]; thus, the preliminary molecular characterization of an endometrial carcinoma could help clinicians to make more tailored therapeutic decisions, mostly in those apparent high-risk cases which could benefit or not from such a treatment on the basis of their molecular profiles.

▫ Table 53.4 shows the main EC histological subtypes and their relative frequencies. The ECC is typically composed of glands, recalling those of normal endometrium, well/moderately differentiated with respective solid component <5% (G1) and 6–50% (G2). Atypical endometrial hyperplasia (AEH) and endometrial intraepithelial neoplasia (EIN) are considered precursor lesions. Likewise, the serous endometrial intraepithelial

carcinoma (SEIC) would seem the premalignant lesion of serous ECs.

All the other special histotypes represent high-grade and more aggressive epithelial variants of ECs. Serous-papillary and clear cell ECs usually involve more elderly women [42]. The first is frequently related to pelvic irradiation and tamoxifen-based hormone treatment; the second, indeed, embraces a heterogeneous group of typical and less typical (serous-like) clear cell carcinoma. Mucinous and squamous ECs must be carefully distinguished from respective cervical cancer histotypes. The carcinosarcoma, also known as malignant-mixed Müllerian tumor (MMMT), is considered a metaplastic epithelial tumor [43, 44]. The undifferentiated ECs are very rare clinical entities, microscopically composed of undifferentiated cells organized in solid mass. They included both small cell neuroendocrine (chromogranin, synaptophysin-positive) and de-differentiated carcinomas [45]. The latter is commonly found in LS and is characterized by the concomitant presence of G1/G2 adeno- and undifferentiated components.

53.3.5 Clinical Presentation and Diagnosis

Almost all patients with EC present with abnormal (post-menopausal or intermenstrual) vaginal bleeding. Leukorrhea, pelvic and low back pain, leg edema consequent to intra-abdominal lymph node involvement, bowel obstruction, bone pain related to the presence of metastases, and dyspnea could be other possible symptoms complained by patients usually with advanced EC.

When an EC is suspected, the common clinical practice provides, first of all, the execution of a TVUS (+/− color Doppler) to detect any eventual focal or diffuse endometrial thickening [46, 47]. A post-menopausal endometrial thickness >3 mm or an inappropriate pre-menopausal endometrial thickening, associated with a vaginal bleeding, must be seen as a "wake-up call," and further investigations are necessary. Particularly, endometrial sampling through US-/hysteroscopy-guided biopsy or dilatation and curettage (D & C) is usually the next step. Conventional D & C is associated with lower accuracy and discomfort for patients, whereas highly sensitive devices, like Pipelle, Vabra aspirator or Tao brush, and SAP-1, are increasingly established and better-tolerated endometrial samplers]. Obviously, the visually direct endometrial biopsy by hysteroscopy guide implies a higher accuracy [48]. Besides, saline infusion sonography enables to differentiate focal from diffuse endometrial involvement. Histological examination is based on morphological features, supported by IHC stains and, sometimes, by the research for specific molecular alterations. The differential diagnosis between benign and malignant lesions is allowed by

▫ **Table 53.2** *Dualistic model*

Principal characteristics	Type I	Type II
Histology	Endometrioid	Serous, clear cell
Relation to estrogen	Yes	No
Differentiation grade	G1/G2	G3
Prognosis	Good	Poor
Molecular alterations	PI3K, PTEN silencing, defects on repair system genes, MSI, KRAS, CTNNB1	Serous → TP53, p16 inactivation, E-cadherin lowering, HER-2 overexpression Clear cell → ARID1A

G1 well differentiated, *G2* moderately differentiated, G3 poorly differentiated, PI3K phosphatidylinositol 3-kinase, *PTEN* phosphatase and tensin homolog, *HER-2* human epidermal growth factor receptor 2, *CTNNB1* catenin-β 1 gene, *ARID1A* AT-rich interactive domain-containing protein 1A

□ Table 53.3 *New model* by TCGA

POLE ultramutated	MSI hypermutated	Copy number (CN) low	Copy number (CN) high
High mutagenicity	High mutagenicity	Low mutagenicity	Low mutagenicity
Mutations on POLE 58 exonucleasic domain	MSI consequent to dysfunction of MMR proteins (above all, MLH1 promoter hypermethylation)	Microsatellite stability (MSS)	MSS
Infrequent copy number aberration	Infrequent copy number aberration	Low copy number aberration	High copy number aberration
Mutations on PI3KCA, PI3KR1, PTEN, KRAS, and FBXW7	Mutations on PTEN, KRAS, and RPL22	Mutations on CTNNB1	Mutations on TP53, FBXW7, and PPP2R1A
Mostly high-grade (G3) EECs	Mostly EECs	Mostly EECs with positive estrogen and progesterone receptors (ER/PR)	Mostly serous ECs
Good prognosis (5-yr RFS = 93%)	Good prognosis (5-yr RFS = 95%)	Poor prognosis (5-yr RFS = 52%)	Poor prognosis (5-yr RFS = 42%)

POLE 58 DNA polymerase subunit ε, *RFS* relapse-free survival, *PI3KCA* PI3K catalytic subunit α, *PI3KR1* PI3K regulatory subunit α, *FBXW7* F-box/WD repeat-containing protein 7, *yr* year, *RPL22* ribosomal protein L22, *PPP2R1A* protein phosphatase 2 scaffold subunit α

□ Table 53.4 *EC histotypes*

Histotype	Frequency (%)
Endometrioid	≃80%
Serous-papillary	<10%
Clear cell	≃4%
Mucinous	≃1%
Squamous	<1%
Mixed[a]	<1%
Carcinosarcoma	<1%
Undifferentiated	<1%

[a]All tumors whose non-predominant component exceeds 10%

all these analyses. For example, AEH/EIN is typically characterized by loss of PTEN and PAX-2 (paired box gene-2) expression compared to benign lesions; or the loss of p53 commonly identifies a SEIC, in contrast to its benign mimics. Wilms tumor gene (WT-1) is searched for serous EC. Moreover, to distinguish an endocervical EC from a cervical cancer, searching for ER/PR, vimentin, carcinoembryonic antigen (CEA), and p16 is recommended. Histotype and grade differentiation are the most important features to be taken into account when a malignant endometrial sample is analyzed, as these will influence the therapeutic choice.

53.3.6 Pre-operative Work-Up, Staging, and Risk Groups

The pre-operative work-up may be schematized as shown in □ Fig. 53.9.

The current staging system for EC is based on the last FIGO (*Fédération Internationale de Gynécologie et d'Obstétrique*) classification, revised and published in the year 2009 [49] (□ Table 53.5).

Unfavorable prognostic factors associated with high risk of recurrence not reported by the FIGO staging but to be taken into consideration are myometrial invasion ≥50%; special histotypes; high-grade differentiation; lymphovascular space invasion (LVSI); tumor size >2 cm; nodal, lower uterine segment and extrauterine involvement; young age; and molecular LS profile [50–52]. Indeed, based on these clinico-pathological factors, a risk-group classification can help clinicians to make therapeutic decisions in adjuvant setting (□ Table 53.6).

53.3.7 Surgical Treatment, Lymphadenectomy, and SLND

In the figure below (□ Fig. 53.10), we report the surgical management algorithm of EC.

As regards stage I, the gold standard for surgery consists of extrafascial simple total hysterectomy without vaginal cuff [55]. Minimally (laparoscopic, robotic) invasive surgery would not seem to negatively affect the overall survival (OS) and progression-free survival

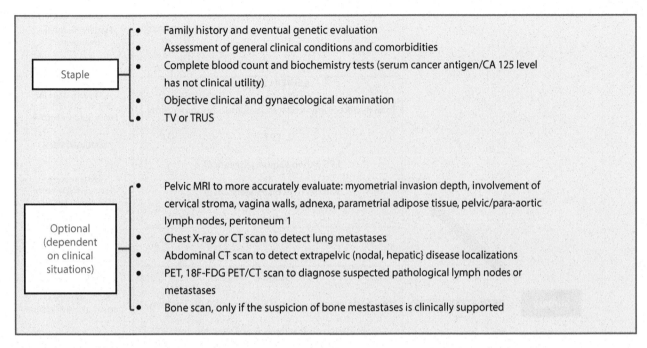

Fig. 53.9 Pre-operative work-up. TRUS trans-rectal ultrasonography, MRI magnetic resonance imaging, CT computed tomography, PET positron emission tomography, FDG fluorodeoxyglucose

Table 53.5 EC staging according to the FIGO classification (2009)

Stage I	Tumor confined to the uterine corpus
IA	<50% myometrial invasion
IB	≥50% myometrial invasion
Stage II	Tumor confined to the uterus, but with cervical stromal involvement
Stage III	Local and/or regional extension of the tumor
IIIA	Uterine corpus serosa and/or adnexa
IIIB	Vagina and/or parametrium
IIIC	Pelvic or para-aortic lymph nodes
IIIC1	Pelvic lymph nodes
IIIC2	Para-aortic lymph nodes (+/− pelvic lymph nodes)
Stage IV	Tumor involves bladder and/or bowel mucosa and/or distant metastases
IVA	Bladder and/or bowel mucosa
IVB	Distant metastases[a] (including also intra-abdominal and inguinal lymph nodes)

[a]Most frequent metastasizing sites are the lymph nodes, liver, lung, brain, and bone (vertebrae)

Table 53.6 Risk groups

Risk group	Prognostic factors
Low	Stage IA, endometrioid, G1/2, LVSI negative
Low/ intermediate	Stage IB, endometrioid, G1/2, LVSI negative
High/ intermediate	Stage IA, endometrioid, G3, LVSI negative/ positive
	Stage IA/IB, endometrioid, G1/2, LVSI positive
High	Stage IB, endometrioid, G3, LVSI negative/ positive
	Stage II
	Stage III without residual disease (R0)
	All stage special histotypes (serous-papillary, clear cell, mucinous, squamous, carcinosarcoma, small cell neuroendocrine carcinoma, de-differentiated carcinoma)

53

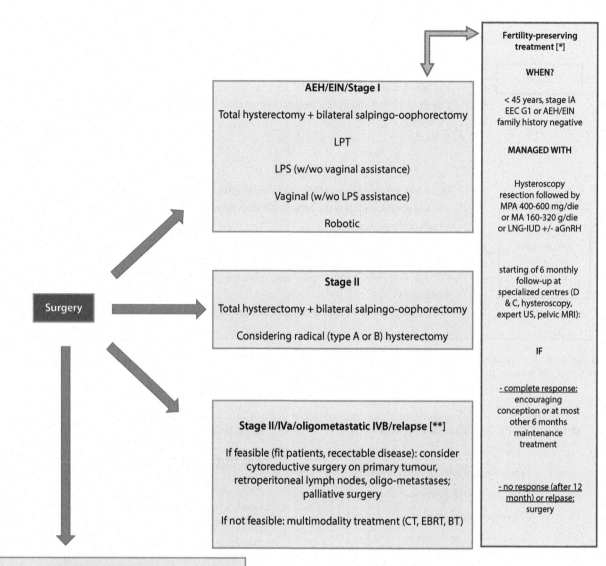

Surgery

AEH/EIN/Stage I

Total hysterectomy + bilateral salpingo-oophorectomy

LPT

LPS (w/wo vaginal assistance)

Vaginal (w/wo LPS assistance)

Robotic

Stage II

Total hysterectomy + bilateral salpingo-oophorectomy

Considering radical (type A or B) hysterectomy

Stage II/IVa/oligometastatic IVB/relapse [**]

If feasible (fit patients, recectable disease): consider cytoreductive surgery on primary tumour, retroperitoneal lymph nodes, oligo-metastases; palliative surgery

If not feasible: multimodality treatment (CT, EBRT, BT)

Unfit patients (all stages)

Vaginal hysterectomy +/- bilateral salpingo-oophorectomy if low risk patients

In alternative:

-hormone treatment

-radiotherapy

- multimodality treatment

Fertility-preserving treatment [*]

WHEN?

< 45 years, stage IA EEC G1 or AEH/EIN family history negative

MANAGED WITH

Hysteroscopy resection followed by MPA 400-600 mg/die or MA 160-320 g/die or LNG-IUD +/- aGnRH

starting of 6 monthly follow-up at specialized centres (D & C, hysteroscopy, expert US, pelvic MRI):

IF

- complete response: encouraging conception or at most other 6 months maintenance treatment

- no response (after 12 month) or relpase: surgery

◻ **Fig. 53.10** Surgical management algorithm. LPT laparotomy, LPS laparoscopy, w/wo with or without, MPA medroxyprogesterone acetate, MA megestrol acetate, LNG-IUD levonorgestrel intrauter-ine device, aGnRH gonadotropin-releasing hormone analogue, CT chemotherapy, EBRT external beam radiotherapy, BT intracavitary brachytherapy, * [53], ** [54]

(PFS), as demonstrated by Gynecologic Oncology Group/GOG-LAP2 and LACE studies; besides, it is associated, particularly the robotic approach, with shorter hospitalization, less intra- and post-operative complications, and better quality of life versus laparotomy [56–59]. Thus, it may be recommended in low- and intermediate-risk patients and could be considered for high-risk ones. The vaginal approach is contemplated for low-risk or unfit patients [60].

A radical hysterectomy, with the lateral extension of resection on parametrium (type A or modified-type B depending on the lateral level of resection), is the surgical procedure carried out from stage II with clear peritoneum involvement, to ensure the highest possibility of free margins. Exenteration (removal of the uterus, bladder, and rectum and permanent uro- and colostomy) is an option in extensively locally advanced stage III/IV cases or in central recurrence (after RT), when the possibility to obtain no residual macroscopic disease is high.

The standard surgical approach remains the same for special histotypes, but in addition a staging omentectomy should be executed for serous-papillary histotype.

The role of systematic lymphadenectomy (pelvic and para-aortic up to the level of renal veins) is crucial to reduce the lymphatic spread, for staging purposes, and to guide adjuvant therapies (◘ Fig. 53.11). As demonstrated by the SEPAL study results, the removal of para-aortic lymph nodes increases the OS in high-risk population, and the number of excised lymph nodes has an important impact [61].

Intermediate-risk patients would not seem to benefit from systematic lymphadenectomy in terms of OS and PFS, but it should be considered for staging intent and, therefore, to choose the proper adjuvant treatment [62, 63]. Also stage III/IV cases do not gain advantages

in OS and PFS from a systematic lymphadenectomy, but it represents an integral part of the comprehensive staging.

The technique of SLND (sentinel lymph node dissection) has been studied over the last few years for the uterine cancers and to date is to be considered experimental. The cervical tracer injection, like fluorescent indocyanine green, enables to individuate bilaterally sentinel lymph nodes (SLNs) with high sensitivity, identifying even micrometastases or isolated tumor cells (ITC). This could allow to avoid an improper and not free from morbidity lymphadenectomy in those clinico-pathological high-risk cases with SLN negative or, conversely, to ensure a more radical surgery in low-risk patients with SLN positive, for which initially there was no planning for a lymph node systematic removal [64, 65].

53.3.8 Adjuvant Treatment

In the figures below (◘ Figs. 53.12, 53.13, 53.14, and 53.15), we report different flowcharts relative to adjuvant treatment algorithms by disease stage and risk groups, based on more recent clinical trial results.

■ Stage I – *low, intermediate, and high risk*
BT has the role to reduce vaginal recurrence, while EBRT has been associated with a lower risk of pelvic recurrence and major local toxic effects versus BT. BT does not seem to increase neither the local control of disease nor the OS in low-risk patients. As demonstrated from several studies, the intermediate-risk patients do not gain advantages in terms of OS from EBRT, though this increases the local control of disease, mostly in the presence of high-risk factors. Therefore, BT is consid-

◘ **Fig. 53.11** Role of systematic lymphadenectomy. SLND sentinel lymph node dissection

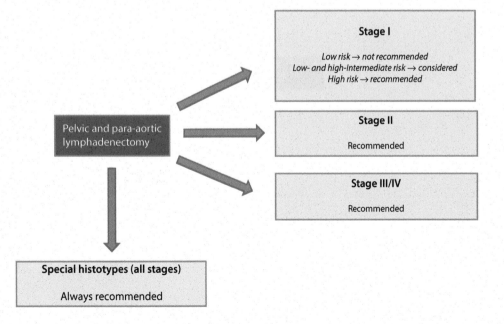

53

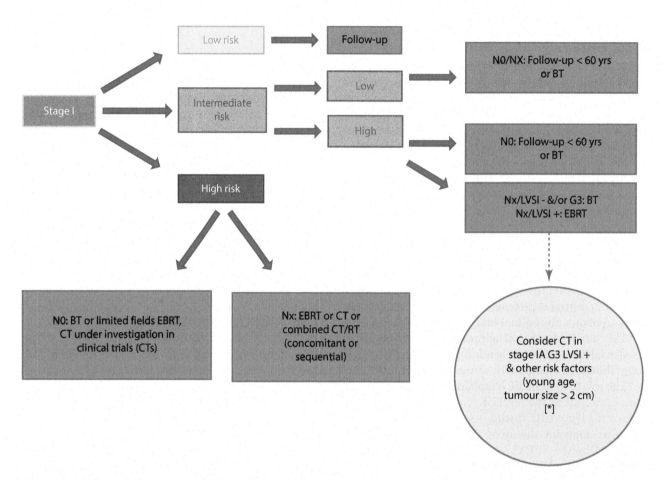

Fig. 53.12 Adjuvant treatment in stage I. N0 no regional lymph nodes involved, Nx regional lymph nodes not assessable, * [66]

Fig. 53.13 Adjuvant treatment in stage II. N+ regional lymph nodes involved

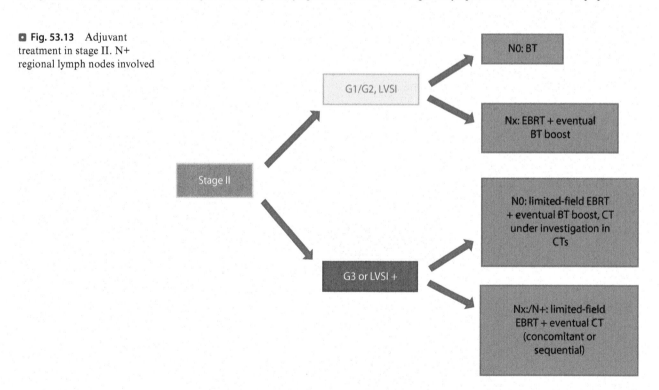

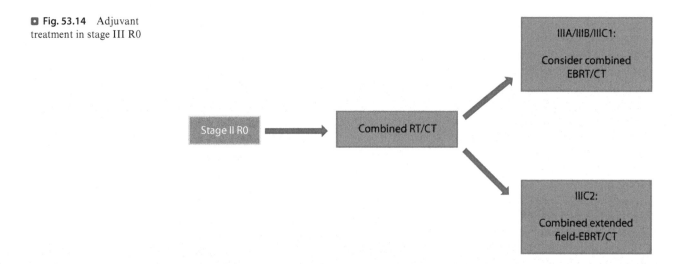

■ **Fig. 53.14** Adjuvant treatment in stage III R0

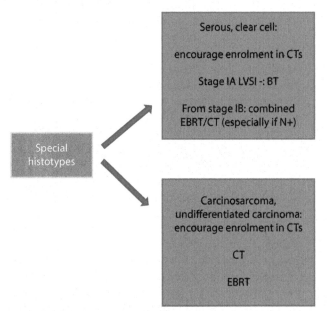

■ **Fig. 53.15** Adjuvant treatment for special histotypes

ered sufficient to reduce vaginal recurrence in this group, except in those cases with several high-risk factors which likely deserve an EBRT [67].

- **Stage II – *high risk***

- **Stage III without Residual Disease – *high risk***

- **Special Histotypes – *high risk***

The PORTEC-3 trial, after a median follow-up of 6 years, has recently revealed that combined platinum-based CT/RT (concomitant cisplatin/RT followed by four carboplatin-paclitaxel cycles) increases both relapse-free survival (RFS) and OS in all high-risk groups (from stage I-high risk, without nodal status assessment, to stage III and special histotypes) [68, 69].

Interestingly, the impact of adjuvant CT was also investigated for each of the four molecular subgroups (see ■ Table 53.3), using tissue samples from PORTEC-3 trial patients, and the results of this research were presented at the European Society for Medical Oncology (ESMO) 2019 meeting. The aim was to assign to specific molecular alterations the proper predictive value in terms of response to adjuvant CT/RT, to better identify patients who could benefit more from concomitant therapies. It was found that CN-high and POLE ultra-mutated subgroups report improved RFS if treated with the combination, unlike the MSI hypermutated population, who seems to not benefit from CT [70].

53.3.9 Advanced and Recurrent Disease

Locally advanced disease (stage IIIA/IIIB/IIIC with residual disease, IVA) typically benefits from multimodality treatments.

The role of surgery, as discussed above, has to be considered when the maximum cytoreductive effort (on primary tumor, pelvic and para-aortic and/or other enlarged lymph nodes, oligo-metastases in stage IVB) could likely ensure the absence of post-operative residual disease, though there are few evidence about its efficacy in such cases as distant metastatic diseases. Alternatively, the surgical approach may have a palliative purpose.

When surgery is not feasible (unfit patients, medical contraindications, unresectable tumors), radical frontline RT (EBRT and BT) plays an incisive role. Likewise, as surgery, also radiotherapy may exercise a palliative role, both on regional complications (bleeding, local pain, etc.) and distant lesions (painful bone metastases).

Sometimes, a multimodality approach is associated with a better outcome, such as reported for bulky diseases, in which carrying out systemic therapy (chemo- or hormone) or surgery before RT could provide a more radical result.

A doublet chemotherapy, generally 3-weekly carboplatin-paclitaxel administered for six cycles, represents the standard of first-line medical care in unresectable patients [71]. Recently, as revealed by a phase II single-arm study (KCOGG1303), a dose-dense paclitaxel (days 1, 8, 15) plus carboplatin (day 1 every 3 weeks) regimen, in advanced or recurrent uterine corpus cancers, was assessed alike as safe and effective [72]. The triplet cisplatin-paclitaxel-adriamycin has been demonstrated to increase the response rate (RR), PFS, and OS versus the doublet cisplatin-adriamycin, at the price of increased toxic effects especially in fragile patients [73]. Interestingly, mono-platinum, anthracyclines, and taxane-based therapy have been associated with objective response rate (ORR) > 20%.

To date, there is not a standard second-line chemotherapy validated for patients who progressed on first-line platinum-based treatment. A recent meta-analysis has reported ifosfamide, oxaliplatin, pegylated liposomal doxorubicin (PLD), topotecan, and docetaxel as the most active chemotherapeutics in this setting [74, 75].

In selected cases, including either ER/PR-positive G1/G2 not rapidly progressive EEC or unfit patients, a progestin-based front-line treatment (MPA 200 mg/die, MA 160 mg/die), resulting in ORR 15–30% and OS 7–11 months, has to be taken into consideration [76]. After disease progression, tamoxifen, fulvestrant, and aromatase inhibitors (AIs) w/wo aGnRH could be considered as second-line hormone therapy [77]. The results of a phase II trial, based on the use of ribociclib (400 mg/die) and letrozole (2.5 mg/die) in patients with relapsed ER-positive EC, were recently presented at the American Society of Clinical Oncology (ASCO) 2019 meeting. After a median of two previous chemo-regimens, a PFS12 (PFS at 12 weeks) rate of 55% was achieved, thus encouraging efforts in revisiting old standard hormone treatment in specific subsets of EC patients [78].

Local relapse disease, similarly to locally advanced tumors, could take advantages from combined treatments. Patients who previously received RT and present with pelvic recurrence could undergo where feasible to prompt surgery (even exenteration) or chemo-/hormone therapy with neoadjuvant intent followed by surgery. Conversely, when never received, RT could be curative in a high percent of central-vaginal recurrence thanks to combined EBRT/BT [79]; besides, in regional or high-risk relapsed disease, patients could benefit from the RT/CT combination. The ongoing trial GOG-0238 will evaluate if the concomitant RT/cisplatin-based CT is also valid for vaginal relapse versus the only RT treatment [80].

53.3.10 New and Potential Future Therapeutic Perspectives

The treatment of metastatic endometrial cancer still represents an unmet clinical need; in fact, the median OS (mOS) is no longer than 12–15 months in advanced and recurrent disease. That is why a lot of efforts are moving toward the search and development of innovative tailored therapeutic opportunities, mainly considering patients' genetic and molecular characteristics and incorporating them as eligibility and stratification factors into CTs.

Several targeted therapies, relying on molecular pathways typically altered in EC, are being studied into phase II/III clinical trials; however, to date, none has been extended to clinical practice.

— *Mammalian Target of Rapamycin (mTOR) Inhibitors*
Discouraging results come from phase II CTs, evaluating the use of mTOR inhibitors (temsirolimus, ridaforolimus) in chemo-naïve or pretreated patients and reporting alterations on PTEN-PIK3CA-AKT-mTOR signaling proliferative pathway [81]. A more recent phase II study reported an increased OS for ridaforolimus versus hormone and chemotherapy [82]. Other altered pathways as object of study include RAS-RAF-MEK-ERK-MAPK and FGFR-2 [83].

— *Anti-angiogenic Agents*
It has been hypothesized that patients overexpressing vascular endothelial growth factor (VEGF), which is known to play an immunosuppressive action, could benefit from the use of anti-angiogenic agents, as resulted from preliminary clinical data [84–86]. Unfortunately, some randomized CTs (GOG-86P, MITO (Multicenter Italian Trials in Ovarian Cancer and Gynecologic Malignancies), END-2) have recently reported that the addition of the anti-angiogenic bevacizumab to standard CT does not significantly improve PFS nor in never-treated patients [87, 88].

The ongoing NICCC study is recruiting patients with ovarian or endometrial recurrent clear cell carcinoma, randomizing them to receive standard CT or the multi-kinase anti-angiogenic inhibitor nintedanib, to evaluate if the experimental arm is associated or not to a longer PFS as primary endpoint [89].

— *Immune Checkpoint Inhibitors (iCKPi)*
Encouraging results are emerging from the possible use of iCKPi particularly in those endometrial cancers associated with high genomic instability and mutational and neoantigen load, like POLE ultra-mutated and MSI hypermutated subgroups, usually presenting increase in tumor-infiltrating lymphocytes (TILs) and PD-1/PD-L1 protein expression

[90]. Preliminary positive clinical data moved the research toward the design of prospective randomized CTs, to compare immunotherapy (alone or combined with CT) to standard of care.

Recently, the Food and Drug Administration (FDA) approved the use of the anti-PD-1 monoclonal antibody pembrolizumab for PD-L1-positive pretreated EC patients, after the phase II KEYNOTE-158 study results, showing durable disease control rate (DCR) (73%) in heavily pretreated MSI-H (high) advanced EC [91].

The phase II PHAEDRA trial, discussed at the ASCO 2019 meeting, showed the activity of the anti-PD-L1 monoclonal antibody durvalumab in patients with advanced EC who received ≤3 prior CT. In detail, the d-MMR (deficient mismatch repair) cohort obtained higher objective tumor response rate (OTRR) and DCR compared to pMMR (proficient mismatch repair) cohort [92].

The phase I/II GARNET trial reported the efficacy of dostarlimab/TSR-042 (anti-PD-1 monoclonal antibody) in treating advanced/recurrent EC, obtaining significant RR regardless of MMR status [93].

The ongoing phase II randomized MITO END-3 trial will confront the experimental combination of carboplatin-paclitaxel with the anti-PD-L1 monoclonal antibody avelumab versus carboplatin-paclitaxel in first or subsequent lines of therapy. Analogously, the phase III randomized AtTEnd/ENGOT-en 7 (European Network for Gynaecological Oncological Trial groups) study is recruiting patients with advanced or recurrent EC to evaluate if the addition of the anti-PD-L1 monoclonal antibody atezolizumab to carboplatin-paclitaxel would improve PFS and OS compared to CT alone. An ongoing phase II trial by Oaknin et al. is investigating the role of the combination pembrolizumab-doxorubicin in advanced EC patients, treated with at least one previous platinum-based CT [94].

 — *Combined Anti-angiogenic-iCKPi Therapy*
At the ESMO 2019 meeting, Mekker et al. presented the results of a phase Ib/II trial comprising a cohort of patients with metastatic EC, pretreated with no more than two CT lines and enrolled to receive the combination of the multi-kinase anti-angiogenic inhibitor lenvatinib with pembrolizumab. The synergistic combination showed a promising antitumor activity with an ORR at 24 weeks of 40% in overall population and significant efficacy also in not MSI-H/d-MMR subgroup. This leads to the combination approval by FDA as second-line treatment or for patients not candidate to definitively curative surgery or RT or, finally, in not MSI-H/d-MMR subgroups [95]. However, a high percent of severe adverse events (AEs) was recorded (grade 3–4 AEs

almost in 70% of population, discontinuation rate 20%). The respective prospective randomized phase III trial (lenvatinib-pembrolizumab versus CT) is still recruiting [96].

 — *Poly(ADP-Ribose) Polymerase (PARP) Inhibitors*
Also poly(ADP-ribose) polymerase (PARP) inhibitors – alone or combined with anti-angiogenic agents – could have a role in the treatment of advanced EC showing mutations in homologous recombination repair (HRR) genes (PTEN loss, ARID1A, etc.), as already shown from preclinical data. The rationale of a PARPi-anti-angiogenic combination therapy arises from the observation, into preclinical studies, of an HRR gene suppression and a major sensitivity to PARPi, in hypoxic states, with consequent synergistic effect [97, 98]. The randomized phase II three-arm NRG GY012 study is investigating if single-agent olaparib, single-agent cediranib, or the combination would prolong the PFS in recurrent, persistent, or metastatic EC [99]. Also the synergistic association of PARPi and iCKPi in more immunogenic EC subtypes (POLE and MSI positive) would seem promising, leading physicians to test this combination into CTs [100]; the phase II DOMEC study was designed to evaluate the efficacy of olaparib + durvalumab in advanced, persistent, or metastatic EC [101].

53.3.11 Follow-Up

The surveillance program after a radical and curative treatment for EC may be schematized as in ▣ Table 53.7.

Besides the clinical and physical examination, further investigation would not seem to impact on OS and should be performed only when the clinical suspicion of relapsed disease is high [103]. Certainly, these decisions must be entrusted to the clinical judgment depending on the individual and primary tumor risk group. The ongoing Italian multicenter randomized TOTEM trial could provide more indications regarding the best surveillance attitude, as it is evaluating different follow-up strategies, depending on relative patient risk [104].

▣ **Table 53.7** Follow-up for EC after curative therapy

Clinical and physical (gynecological/pelvic) examination	Every 3–4 months for the first 2 years and then 6-monthly until the 5th year from primary treatment [102]
Not ordinarily recommended exams	Tumor markers: CEA, CA 125, CA 19.9, and AFP, chest X-ray, abdominal US, CT scan, pelvic MRI, 18F-FDG PET/CT scan, whole-body bone scan

53.4 Cervical Cancer

53.4.1 Epidemiology

Cervical cancer (CC) is the most common gynecological tumor in developing countries, where it is even reported as a leading cause of cancer-related death, as consequence of a higher human papillomavirus (HPV) infection prevalence and a less availability of effective screening tools. Contrariwise, industrialized countries are experiencing a progressive decrease in the incidence and mortality rate, thanks to the implementation of efficacious primary and secondary prevention measures against HPV infection, and this is contributing also to the steady decline of global CC incidence and mortality. It has been calculated that the global prevalence of HPV infection exceeds 80%.

Worldwide, CC represents the fourth most frequent tumor in female sex with 570,000 new cases and 310,000 deaths registered in 2018, predominantly concentrated in Africa, Latin America, and Asia (these countries contributing to almost 90% of global deaths) [105] (◼ Fig. 53.16). The estimated new cases and deaths in the United States in 2019 are 13,170 and 4250, respectively, whereas the not insignificant numbers in Europe in 2018 were 61,100 and 25,800, respectively, with an incidence rate of 3.3% and a mortality rate of 3% [1, 2].

Most cases of cervical carcinoma in situ (CIS) are diagnosed in younger age (25–35 years), whereas the peak incidence of invasive CC concerns the 40–65 age group, with a 5-year survival rate variable according to the stage (90%, 66%, and 40% for early, locally advanced, and metastatic disease, respectively) [106].

53.4.2 Pathogenesis and Molecular Biology

The primary cause of CC is represented by a persistent HPV infection, most commonly involving the basal cells of the transformation zone (TZ), which is a transitional area between the endocervical columnar epithelium and the squamous epithelium of the vagina; indeed, the HPV DNA is detected in almost all cases of cervical cancer (99.7%) [107]. Most ($\simeq$ 80%) carriers naturally eliminate HPV within 1–2 years, but the contemporary intervention of other risk factors predisposes to a chronic infection, spreading locally without systemic viremic phase, tough to overcome, initially leading to the development of precancerous lesions and secondarily of cervical cancer [108, 109] (◼ Fig. 53.17).

Precancerous lesions refer to dysplastic conditions characterized by abnormal cervical cell growth and are known as cervical intraepithelial neoplasia (CIN) 1, 2, or 3, on the basis of dysplasia grade (see ▶ Sect. 53.3.4).

The human papillomavirus is a double-stranded DNA virus, with a capsid consisting of 72 capsomeres (◼ Fig. 53.18). Its genome codifies for six early proteins (E1, E2, E4, E5, E6, and E7), which are responsible for the viral replication, and for two late structural proteins (L1 and L2), then assembled into capsomeres in different percentages (80 and 20%, respectively). When HPV integrates its DNA with that of the host cell, E2 stops inhibiting E6/E7 with consequent p53-retinoblastoma protein (pRb) suppression and morphological/functional cellular alterations. When persistently repeated, this process leads to a neoplastic transformation and progression within about 15 years or less.

Two-thirds of invasive CC cases are related to HPV 16 and 18 oncogenic genotypes, which predominantly affect the 30–39 age group [112] (◼ Table 53.8). Less frequent oncogenic subtypes are responsible for the other 30% of cervical carcinomas, with HPV 31, 33, 35, 45, 52, and 58 being the most common after HPV 16 and 18.

As we can observe from ◼ Table 53.8, the prevalence of HPV 16 and 18 varies according to the histotype, with HPV 16 more related to squamous histology and HPV 18 to adenocarcinomas [113]. Other subtypes (6, 11) are frequently related to benign conditions, being responsible for 90% of genital warts [114].

As for ECs, the efforts of physicians are moving toward the attempt of characterizing CCs on the basis of their molecular profiles. At last ESMO 2019, some authors present the molecular characterization of 37 patients with advanced cervical carcinoma, finding 34 different pathogenic mutations (PI3KCA and KRAS being the most frequent) in about the 70% of the population. They individuated a correlation between KRAS mutations and adeno-/adenosquamous histologies, associated with a worse prognosis. Instead, PIK3CA mutations seem to be related to a better prognosis of mixed histology tumors. Knowing the biological profile could help clinicians to direct patients to increasing tailored therapies (see ▶ Sect. 53.3.12).

53.4.3 Primary and Secondary Prevention

For several decades, the Papanicolaou test (PAP test/smear) has represented the only validated screening tool to anticipate the diagnosis and the treatment of cervical precancerous/cancerous lesions. It works in identifying cytological alterations on a small scratched TZ cell sample, resulting in a low-sensitivity (50%) and strongly operator-dependent procedure (both on the execution and the interpretation of results). Lately, it has been outdone by the more sensitive and effective HPV test, which works in detecting the higher-risk genotype DNA on cervical cells [115, 116]. However, the PAP test maintains its usefulness in the 21–29 age group, whereas the HPV test alone or combined with the PAP test (co-test) is recommended from 30 years [117] (◼ Fig. 53.19).

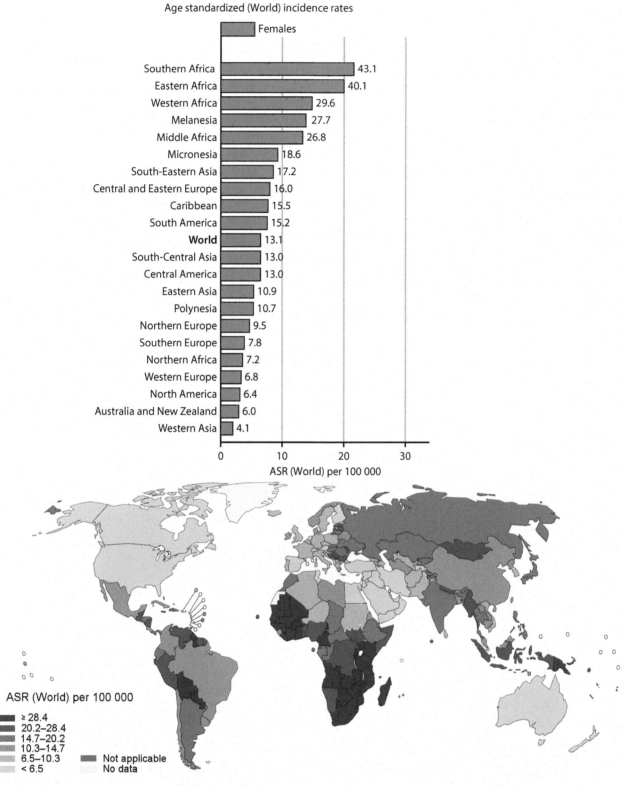

Fig. 53.16 Age-standardized incidence rates of cervical cancer in the world

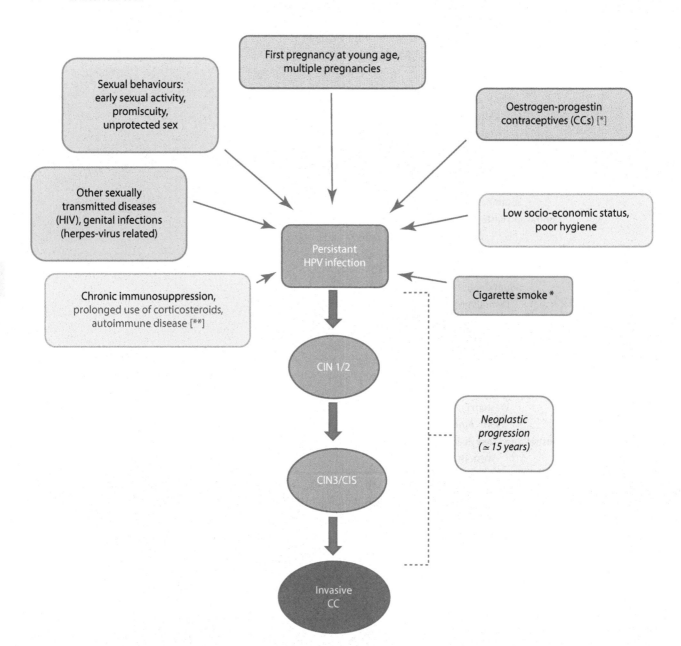

Fig. 53.17 Risk factors intervening on chronic HPV infection. HIV human immunodeficiency virus. *The correlation smoke-CC is strong for squamous histotype and, depending on lower immune local defense, consequent to a smoke-induced reduction of cervical Langerhans cells, * [110],** [111]

– Vaccines

Almost 90% of the general population comes, at least once in life, into contact with HPV and the peak incidence of the infection regards the 16–25 age group. Accordingly, the pharmaceutical industry has developed, in recent years, efficacious vaccines directed against the higher-risk HPV genotypes and to be administered at an early age. Currently, three vaccines are available for the primary prevention of HPV infection and its related pathologies (■ Table 53.9).

These three vaccines, in addition to offering a type-specific protection, would seem to have some cross-protective activity against other oncogenic viruses.

The duration of vaccine-induced protection, differentiated according to the number of doses received, will be better defined by longer follow-up of CTs. From observational studies till now conducted, it has emerged that vaccines reach almost 100% of protection efficacy against persistent infection and precancerous lesions up to 9 years (Cervarix®) [119, 120]. Furthermore, early findings from some clinical trials would support the

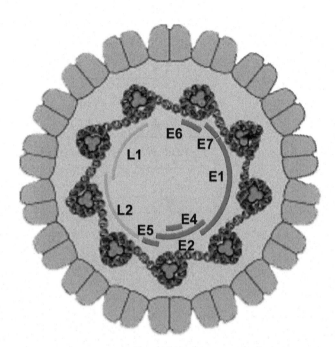

◨ **Table 53.8** Prevalence of HPV genotypes by most frequent histotypes (squamous and adenocarcinoma)

Genotypes	Squamous carcinoma	Adenocarcinoma
16	59%	36%
18	13%	37%
31, 33,35, 39, 45, 52, 58, 59, 67, 68, 70, 85	≃ 28%	≃ 27%

comparable effect in long-term protection of one single vaccine dose versus two or three dose schedules. This could lead, in the future, to the introduction of one single dose schedule, facilitating the adhesion to screening program from low-income countries [121, 122].

A large randomized trial revealed that the nine-valent vaccine immunizes almost 100% of the population against all nine HPV genotypes, preventing effectively precancerous lesions, carcinomas in situ, and invasive cancers and showing 96% of efficacy against 6-month persistent infection, sustained by HPV 31, 33, 45, 52, and 58 genotypes. Thus, Gardasil 9® adds a cover against the genotypes responsible for 15% of cervical cancer and 4% of HPV-related pathologies in men (penile, anal, oropharyngeal cancers, genital warts) [123–125].

The immunization of young population will produce a drastic reduction in the prevalence of HPV infection and relative benign/malignant pathologies. Some CTs

confirmed the efficacy, although lower, of vaccines even when administered to adult population (24–45 years) [126, 127]. Consequently, current screening programs need to be extended to older women and men. In women aged 20–29 with 80% vaccine coverage, a reduction in the invasive CC incidence rate of 63% within 2025 is expected.

Obviously, proper lifestyle (quitting smoking) and sexual habits (avoiding promiscuity and unprotected sex) have to be considered as useful primary prevention tools in reducing the risk of CC onset.

53.4.4 Histopathology

The World Health Organization (WHO) recognizes three categories of cervical epithelial tumors (◨ Table 53.10).
- — *Squamous Tumors*
  All squamous tumors and their precursors are related to HPV infections, mostly sustained by HPV 16 genotype, which is also associated with poorer prognosis (see ◨ Table 53.8).

  The *squamous cell carcinoma*, based on the growth pattern and morphological features, could microscopically present as one of the following variants: *keratinizing*, characterized by rare mitosis and the presence of keratin pearls, *non-keratinizing*, and *special histotypes* (*basaloid, verrucous, warty, papillary, lymphoepithelioma-like, squamo-transitional*).
- — *Squamous intraepithelial neoplasia* refers to *CIN3/CIS*. Cervical intraepithelial neoplasia is generally considered as a precancerous lesion limited to the cervical epithelium (usually the TZ epithelium), which may present with various grades of dysplasia extension:
  - – CIN1, mild dysplasia, involves the lower third of the epithelial thickness.
  - – CIN2, moderate dysplasia, involves from one-third to two-thirds of the epithelial thickness.
  - – CIN3, severe dysplasia, involves ≥ two-thirds of the epithelial thickness and practically coinciding with CIS, without going beyond the basement membrane.
- — *Glandular Tumors*
  Most *adenocarcinomas* (80%) are endocervical and microscopically presenting architecturally well-differentiated (cytologically G2/G3) and eosinophilic cytoplasm. Variants include *mucinous,* the most common, with mucin-rich cells, usually G1 and associated with good prognosis and including, in turn, *endocervical, intestinal, signet-ring cell, minimal deviation,* and *villoglandular* subtypes; *endometrioid, clear cell, serous,* and *mesonephric* are all other rare variants.

  Glandular tumors and their precursors present a heterogeneous correlation with HPV, with the usual-type endocervical adenocarcinomas and AIS being

53

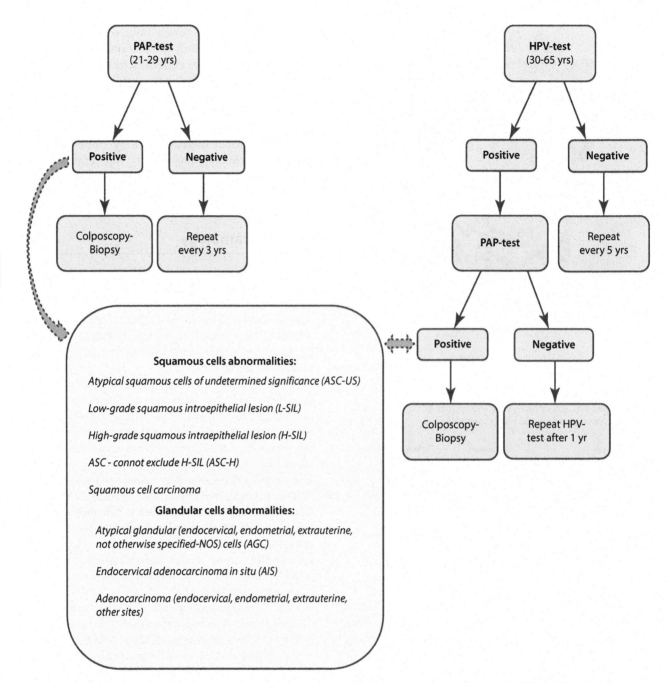

Squamous cells abnormalities:

Atypical squamous cells of undetermined significance (ASC-US)

Low-grade squamous introepithelial lesion (L-SIL)

High-grade squamous intraepithelial lesion (H-SIL)

ASC - connot exclude H-SIL (ASC-H)

Squamous cell carcinoma

Glandular cells abnormalities:

Atypical glandular (endocervical, endometrial, extrauterine, not otherwise specified-NOS) cells (AGC)

Endocervical adenocarcinoma in situ (AIS)

Adenocarcinoma (endocervical, endometrial, extrauterine, other sites)

◘ **Fig. 53.19** PAP and HPV tests execution flowchart. The cytological alterations detected on PAP test are reported according to the *Bethesda system* (2001) [118]. L-SIL corresponds to mild dysplasia/CIN1 and H-SIL to moderate-severe dysplasia/CIN2 and CIN3/ CIS. Women with known risk factors (HIV positivity, immunosuppression, previous cervical precancerous/cancerous lesions) and beyond 65 years old should undergo more frequent screening tests

highly related to HPV (90 and 100%, respectively), especially with HPV 18 genotype; conversely rarer variants appear unrelated to viral etiology. Although AIS occurs rarely, its incidence rate seems to be rising up; it is typically difficult to detect at colposcopy and to manage, being multifocal and extending inside the cervical canal [128].

■ *Other Epithelial Tumors*

Also *adenosquamous carcinomas* show a correlation with HPV 18. *Neuroendocrine tumors* (carcinoid, atypical carcinoid, small cell carcinoma, large cell carcinoma) are diagnosed on histology and usually present with higher neuroendocrine marker distant spread.

◨ **Table 53.9** Principal characteristics of the three licensed HPV vaccines

Characteristics	Bivalent (Cervarix®)	Quadrivalent (Gardasil®)	Nine-valent (Gardasil 9®)
Genotype protection	16, 18	6, 11 16, 18	6, 11 16, 18 31, 33, 45, 52, 58
Indications	*Prevention of:*	*Prevention of:*	*Prevention of:*
	Cervical, vaginal, vulvar precancerous lesions	Cervical, vaginal, vulvar precancerous lesions	Cervical, vaginal, vulvar precancerous lesions
	Cervical cancer	Cervical cancer	Cervical cancer
		Anal precancerous lesions, anal cancer	Anal precancerous lesions, anal cancer
		Genital warts	Genital warts
Indications by age, sex, and relative schedule	Females	Females	Females
		Males	Males
	9–14 years old: Two doses (0–6 months)	9–13 years old: Two doses (0-6 months)	9–14 years old: Two doses (0–6 months)
	≥15 years old: Three doses (0–1–6 months)	≥14 years old: Three doses (0–2–6 months)	≥15 years old: Three doses (0–2–6 months)

53.4.5 Clinical Presentation and Diagnosis

CC is often asymptomatic, especially at an early stage; instead, when locally advanced, patients could complain spontaneous or after coitus abnormal vaginal bleeding and discharge, dyspareunia, and pelvic pain. Patients with metastatic small cell neuroendocrine cervical carcinoma may clearly present with paraneoplastic syndromes and relative symptoms: syndrome of inappropriate antidiuretic hormone secretion (SIADH), Cushing syndrome, hypercalcemia, neurological disorders, and weight loss.

Ordinarily, the suspicion of a cervical carcinoma arises from an abnormal PAP test or a positive HPV test. As shown in ◨ Fig. 53.19, the second-level procedure to further investigate the presence of a CC is represented by the colposcopy w/wo biopsy. Particularly, this exam allows to obtain a magnified view of the cervix, thanks to the use of a binocular microscope equipped with a light source, called colposcope. During the observation, the cervix will be first cleansed with saline solution to detect eventual abnormal vascularization; then, an acetic acid 3–5% wash will show up as whitish areas possible dysplastic lesions; and, finally, the *Schiller test*, which consists of the application of an iodine solution (*Lugol's solution*) on the cervical surface, will individuate as negative-iodine (clearer) eventual pathological areas. Therefore, colposcopy enhances the possibility to individuate suspected lesions and to achieve more addressed biopsies and histological characterization.

Macroscopically, a cervical cancer could appear as exophytic with outward-growing or endophytic with predominant stromal infiltration.

53.4.6 Pre-operative Work-Up, Staging, and Risk Assessment

After histological diagnosis, a pre-operative work-up to better define the cervical carcinoma extension is mandatory; it should include clinical examination and radiological imaging as schematized in ◨ Fig. 53.20.

Until recently, the staging system for CC was based on the 8th FIGO and Union for International Cancer Control (UICC)-Tumor-Node-Metastasis (TNM) classification [131] (◨ Table 53.11).

A new revisited FIGO classification, published in 2018, reported some changes in cervical cancer staging, shown in green in ◨ Table 53.11 [132].The tumor risk assessment is based on the evaluation of some clinico-pathological factors: tumor size, stromal invasion depth, and LVSI, which help physicians to define the relative risk class (low, intermediate, high) and to choose the proper adjuvant treatment (◨ Table 53.12). Greater tumor size (>2 cm), deeper stromal invasion, and the presence of LVSI (correlating with a higher risk of lymph node metastasis) are associated with a worse prognosis. Other prognostic factors include lymph node status/number of lymph nodes involved and stage, which appear directly related to each other, differentiation

Table 53.10 WHO histological classification of cervical tumors

Histotype		Frequency (%)
Epithelial		*95%*
Squamous tumors and precursors	Squamous cell carcinoma, NOS: Keratinizing Non-keratinizing Special histotypes	85%
	Early invasive/microinvasive squamous cell carcinoma	
	Squamous intraepithelial neoplasia (CIN3/CIS)	
	Benign squamous cell lesions (condyloma acuminatum, squamous papilloma, fibroepithelial polyp)	
Glandular tumors and precursors	Adenocarcinoma: Mucinous Endometrioid Clear cell Serous Mesonephric	10–12%
	Early invasive adenocarcinoma	
	Adenocarcinoma in situ (AIS)	
	Glandular dysplasia	
	Benign glandular lesions (Müllerian papilloma, endocervical polyp)	
Other epithelial tumors	Adenosquamous carcinoma (glassy cell carcinoma variant)	3–5%
	Neuroendocrine tumors	
	Undifferentiated carcinoma	
	Adenoid cystic carcinoma	
	Adenoid basal carcinoma	
Not epithelial		*<5%*
Mesenchymal tumors		
Mixed epithelial and mesenchymal tumors		
Melanocytic tumors		
Miscellaneous tumors		
Lymphoid and hematopoietic tumors		
Secondary tumors		

grade, histological subtype (adenocarcinoma – worse than squamous carcinoma), margin status, parametria and vaginal cuff status, and levels of squamous cell carcinoma antigen (SCC) and hemoglobin at the moment of diagnosis [133, 134].

53.4.7 Treatment of Pre-invasive Tumors

Usually, CIN1 lesions spontaneously regress; hence, no excisional treatment is routinely recommended in these cases [135]. Patients presenting with a CIN1 at colposcopy will have to repeat, after 1 year, co-test (≥30 years) or only PAP smear (<30 years) and eventually a new colposcopy. If CIN1 persists, an excision will be preferred, primarily when H-SIL or ASC-H has been cytologically detected.

Conversely, CIN2 and CIN3/CIS should always deserve an excisional treatment, even if CIN2 could regress without intervening, certainly more easily than CIN3. Thus, young patients presenting with a CIN2 could be alternatively addressed to a surveillance strategy, repeating PAP test and colposcopy every 6 months for 1 year and undergoing an excisional procedure if CIN2 persists.

The excisional treatment consists of the removal of a cervical cone (conization), trying to obtain clear margins and to allow the re-establishment of a new TZ. Possible procedures include LEEP (loop electrosurgical excision procedure), cold knife conization, and laser conization. Besides, ablative techniques, such as cryosurgery or laser ablation (CO2 laser), are admitted when the entire borders of the lesion are visible, the endocervical sampling is negative, and there are no glandular abnormalities at cytological test; generally, ablation seems to be associated with higher recurrence rate than excision [136, 137].

Total hysterectomy represents the gold standard for women who satisfied the offspring desire and presenting with an AIS, with the risk of post-conization persistent disease being high (multifocal, endocervical growth). Alternatively, a conservative fertility-sparing excisional treatment may be preferred for fertile women.

53.4.8 Treatment of Early Invasive Tumors (FIGO 2018 - IA1/2, IB1/2, IIA1)

In the figure below (◘ Fig. 53.21), we report the treatment algorithms for early cervical carcinomas.

The standard primary treatment for early invasive CC is represented by simple or radical hysterectomy, depending on the substage and class risk, and bilateral

Fig. 53.20 Pre-operative work-up, * [129],** [130]

> **Gynaecological examination** (if difficult or unclear vaginal/parametrial involvement, <u>examination under anaesthesia</u> w/wo cervical and vaginal mapping has to prefer)
>
> **Cystoscopy/rectoscopy +/- biopsies** (if infiltration is suspected)
>
> **Abdominal/pelvic MRI w/wo contrast** to evaluate with high sensitivity and specifity: tumour size, distance between tumour and internal uterine orifice, cervical length, involvement of cervical stroma/parametrial tissue and infiltration depth, involvement of corpus uteri, vagina, bladder, rectum, pelvic/para-aortic lymph nodes, peritoneum, presence of hydronephrosis [*]
>
> **Abdominal CT scan w/wo contrast** to study eventual pathological lymph nodes and abdominal metastases; to evaluate the response to neoadjuvant treatments
>
> **CT scan w/wo contrast** to detect possible lung metastases
>
> **18F-FDG PET/CT scan** to diagnose with high sensitivity and specificity suspected pathological lymph nodes or metastases, mostly in advanced disease rather than early tumours [**]

Table 53.11 CC staging according to the 8th edition of FIGO (2014) and UICC-TNM classification

TNM	FIGO	Definition
T – primary tumor		
Tx		**Primary tumor cannot be assessed**
T0		**No evidence of primary tumor**
Tis		**Carcinoma in situ**
T1	**I**	**Tumor confined to the cervix**
T1a	**IA**	Microinvasive carcinoma (diagnosed only by microscopy) Stromal invasion[a] <5 mm and horizontal spread ≤7 mm
T1a1	IA1	Stromal invasion <3 mm, horizontal spread ≤7 mm
T1a2	IA2	Stromal invasion ≥3 mm and <5 mm, horizontal spread ≤7 mm
T1b	**IB**	Clinically visible carcinoma or microscopic carcinoma greater than IA
T1b1	IB1	≤4 cm
	IB1 *(FIGO 2018)*	Stromal invasion ≥5 mm and tumor size <2 cm
T1b2	IB2	>4 cm
	IB2 *(FIGO 2018)*	Tumor size ≥2 cm and <4 cm
	IB3 *(FIGO 2018)*	Tumor size ≥4 cm
T2	**II**	**Tumor extends beyond the uterus but not to the lower third vagina/pelvic wall**
T2a	IIA	No parametrial invasion
T2a1	IIA1	<4 cm
T2a2	IIA2	≥4 cm
T2b	IIB	Parametrial invasion

Table 53.11 (continued)

TNM	FIGO	Definition
T3	**III**	**Tumor extends to the lower third vagina/pelvic wall or causes hydronephrosis/ non-functioning kidney**
T3a	IIIA	Tumor extends to the lower third vagina
T3b	IIIB	Tumor extends to the pelvic wall or causes hydronephrosis/non-functioning kidney
	IIIC1r/p (*FIGO 2018*)	Pelvic lymph node metastasis
	IIIC2r/p (*FIGO 2018*)	Para-aortic lymph node metastasis
T4	**IVA**	**Tumor involves bladder/rectum mucosa or extends beyond true pelvis**
N – regional lymph nodes		
Nx		**Regional lymph nodes cannot be assessed**
N0		**No regional nodal metastasis**
N1		**Regional nodal metastasis**
M – distant metastasis		
M0		**No distant metastasis**
M1	**IVB**	**Distant metastasis**

[a]Stromal invasion is calculated from the base of epithelium to the deepest point of infiltration. In green, changes in staging system reported by FIGO 2018 classification. r radiological, p pathological. M1 includes inguinal lymph nodes and peritoneal disease; the extension of tumor to the vagina, adnexa, and pelvic serosa is not to be defined as M1

Table 53.12 Risk groups

Risk group	Prognostic factors		
	Tumor size	Stromal invasion depth	LVSI
Low	<2 cm	Superficial 1/3	Negative
Intermediate	<2 cm	Any	Positive
	≥2 cm	Any	Negative
High	≥2 cm	Any	Positive

PLND (except for squamous IA1 LVSI-negative carcinomas), w/wo PALND [138]. Some ongoing randomized CTs will better establish which is more appropriate between a simple and a radical procedure [139]. Bilateral annessiectomy is also usually executed, in addition to hysterectomy, especially in post-menopause or patients who satisfied the offspring desire.

The sentinel lymph node mapping, through the intra-operative injection on the cervix of a tracer (fluorescent indocyanine green, the most favorite), would allow to avoid an inappropriate and not completely free from morbidity PLND or, conversely, to support a lymphadenectomy (if SLNs are negative or positive, respectively), above all in stages from IA1 with LVSI positivity to IB1,

for which high detection rate and sensitivity have been reported in literature [140, 141].

However, considering the not widely standardized procedure, often physicians prefer to remove PLNs, regardless of SLN mapping results [142].

The PALN involvement appears to be more related to the presence of pelvic lymph node metastases and tumors larger than 2 cm; hence, PALND should ensure a better prognosis from stage IB1.

Minimally invasive (laparoscopic, robotic) surgery, in the past years, had been thought to offer similar outcomes than laparotomy in early invasive CC and to be advantageous in terms of less intra- and post-operative complications. Nevertheless, some recent CTs have dem-

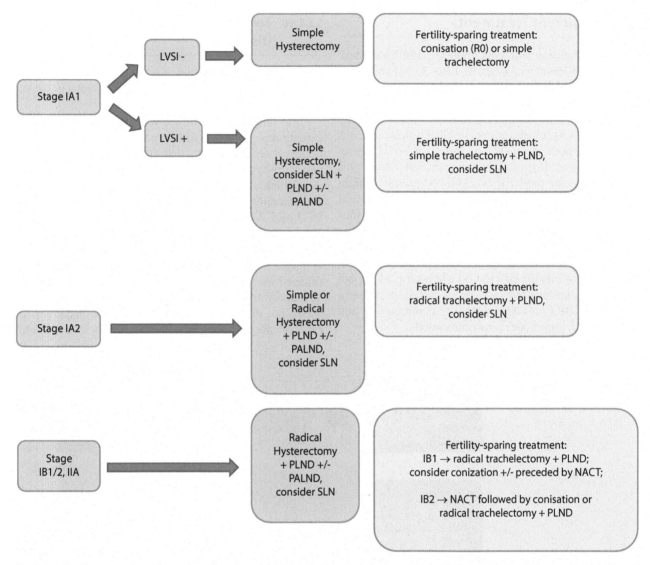

Fig. 53.21 Surgical algorithms for early invasive cervical tumors. PLND pelvic lymph nodes dissection, PALND para-aortic lymph node dissection, NACT neoadjuvant chemotherapy

onstrated that laparoscopic and robotic approaches failed in improving PFS and OS and reducing recurrence rate, compared to open surgery, moreover for tumors >2 cm.

Almost half of early tumors concern women of childbearing age; thus, it is fundamental to define fertility-sparing approaches. Trachelectomy consists of the removal of the cervix (via the abdomen or vagina) and nearby tissue (paracervix/parametrial tissue), upper part of the vagina, and pelvic lymph nodes [143]. Depending on the lateral extension level of resection, trachelectomy may be defined as simple (resection at cervical border) or radical (resection at ureter bed), with the latter preferred for tumors >2 cm as they are associated with higher risk of parametrial involvement, LVSI, lymph node metastases, and recurrence [144].

NACT can be exploited to downstage IB1/2 disease, before fertility-sparing treatments (both conization and trachelectomy), and, although under experimental validation, also IB3 stage (FIGO 2018) [145].

– Exclusive Radiotherapy
Exclusive RT approach, consisting of simultaneous EBRT and intravaginal-cervical BT (80–85 Gy overall dose), could be also applied, as valid primary treatment and alternatively to surgery, in IB1–IIA1 stages [146]. In fact, RT seems to ensure comparable outcomes in terms of local control of disease, PFS and OS, and safety profile [147]. Surgery could be preferred in adeno-histologies, younger age, and low-risk groups who would not necessitate further adjuvant treatments (CT or RT), in relation to favorable prognostic factors and considering the increased toxicity arising from combined approaches. Otherwise, RT should be considered as the treatment of choice.

53.4.9 Adjuvant Treatment

Patients presenting with concomitant pathological risk factors (see ▶ Sect. 53.3.6 and ◻ Table 53.12) are candidates to receive further adjuvant therapies, after surgery (◻ Fig. 53.22).

Particularly, it seems that intermediate-risk group could benefit from adjuvant pelvic EBRT alone in terms of PFS, without improving of overall survival; therefore, the option of no further treatment after surgery is equally valid for these patients [148]. Conversely, high-risk patients should undergo concomitant adjuvant RT (45–50, 4 Gy total dose) and at least three to four cycles of cisplatin-based CT (weekly radio-sensitizing dose of 40 mg/mq), resulting in increased PFS and OS when the combined strategy is used [149]. In addition, there is also a role for BT (10 Gy) when surgical vaginal margin resulted positive or close at pathology. Finally, large-field EBRT on eventual positive common iliac and para-aortic lymph nodes is recommended.

53.4.10 Treatment of Locally Advanced Disease

The treatment algorithm for locally advanced disease may be schematized as in the flowchart below (◻ Fig. 53.23).

The standard of care for locally advanced cervical carcinomas (w/wo positive pelvic/para-aortic lymph nodes) is represented by definitive concomitant EBRT/platinum-based CT, with the addition of endocavitary/interstitial vaginal-cervical brachytherapy. In fact, this multimodality approach allows to gain better both local and distant control of disease and also absolute improvement in OS and PFS, compared to any monotherapy; however, these advantages mostly concern I/II stages than III/IVA ones [150]. Normally, EBRT is directed on the uterus, upper third vagina, parametria, and obturator/pre-sacral lymph nodes (45–50 Gy total dose), but an extended-field RT could be necessary in case of positive iliac/para-aortic lymph nodes (until

◻ **Fig. 53.22** Algorithm for adjuvant treatment according to Sedlis (on the top) and Peters (on the bottom) criteria

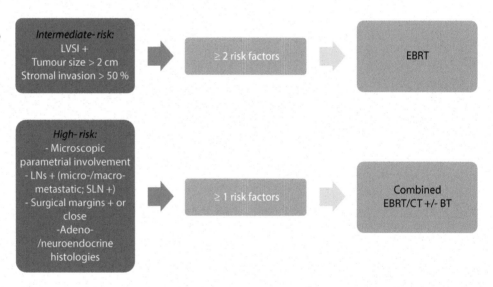

◻ **Fig. 53.23** Flowchart on locally advanced CC treatment

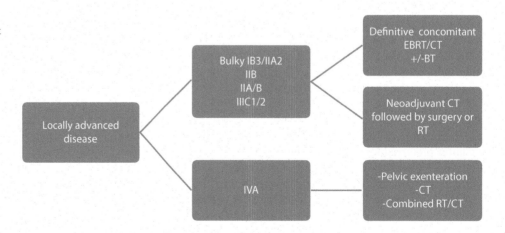

55–60 Gy of overall dose for macroscopic metastases) and of inguinal lymph nodes in stage IIIA (extension to lower third of vagina). In IIIB stage, protective endoureteral stent or nephrostomy placement is required to ensure both kidney function and nephrotoxic cisplatin administration.

The addition of BT (25–30 Gy) is crucial to increase the local disease-free survival (DFS) in IIB/IIIB stages, although its effect on OS is unknown; besides, the interstitial approach could be associated with the traditional endocavitary BT for high paracervical tumoral residue, after EBRT/CT, with probable benefits on survival [151]. Therefore, an optimal RT treatment has to reach elevated overall dose (90–95 Gy) and, furthermore, should be administered within 7–8 weeks [152].

The concomitant CT consists of the administration of weekly 40 mg/mq cisplatin for the whole time of RT, generally for six cycles. Alternatively, a concomitant doublet cisplatin-gemcitabine, followed by two further adjuvant cycles of the same CT regimen, has shown to improve OS and PFS. Noteworthy, the worse safety profile of this combination makes difficult the routine application in clinical practice [153].

Some authors are trying to establish the potential role on survival of salvage hysterectomy after definitive radiotherapy/concurrent chemoradiotherapy in case of residual cervical disease [154].

As alternative to concomitant RT/CT, high-dose neoadjuvant CT followed by radical surgery (type C hysterectomy) may be also carried out. Generally, doublet cisplatin-paclitaxel is the most preferred regimen, considering the higher hematological toxicity occurring with use of triplets, such as cisplatin-paclitaxel-ifosfamide.

Recently, the phase III randomized EORTC trial results have been presented at ASCO 2019. This study has compared outcomes arising from platinum-based NACT followed within 6 weeks by radical surgery versus concomitant RT/CT in IB2 (FIGO 2014) and IIA/B stages. It was found that sequential NACT-radical surgery approach does not improve DFS and OS compared to concomitant treatment [155]. A similar phase III clinical trial found that concomitant RT/CT produces advantages in terms of PFS but not OS versus sequential NACT-radical surgery, with a mildly worse toxicity profile for concomitant treatment [156]. Thus, the choice of the most appropriate therapy should individually rely on safety and quality of life.

The role of sequential RT or concomitant CT/RT following NACT is still controversial. An ongoing phase III trial (INTERLACE) will provide insights on the better treatment between induction dose-dense CT (carboplatin AUC2-paclitaxel for six cycles) followed by concomitant RT/CT and standard RT/CT alone [157]. Besides, a phase III randomized study (OUTBACK) is testing the role of additional four cycles of adjuvant carboplatin-paclitaxel-based CT, after definitive concurrent RT/CT in locally advanced disease [158].

Finally, efforts are moving toward the definition of a molecular prediction model of response to chemoradiation, so as to improve clinical outcome in cervical cancer patients [151].

53.4.11 Recurrent and Metastatic Disease

Generally, most relapses occur within 2 years from first diagnosis of CC and may present as locoregional, extrapelvic, and metastatic distant disease (lungs, bones, etc.).

CC local relapses may occur at vaginal cuff (central relapse) or at pelvic wall (lateral relapse). Managing of recurrence depends on previous received treatment. Particularly, pelvic recurrences after surgery or outside the previous field of radiation may be treated with radical concurrent RT/platinum-based mono-CT (or combined with 5-fluorouracil) w/wo BT. Alternatively, post-radiated patients may undergo pelvic exenteration w/wo intraoperative RT (IORT) and subsequent reconstructive surgery. Besides, patients with small (<2 cm) isolated central pelvic relapse could be treated with a more conservative surgery (radical hysterectomy) or endocavitary/interstitial BT. Lateral relapses could benefit too from both concurrent EBRT/CT and surgery w/wo IORT [159].

The standard first-line chemotherapy regimen for patients presenting with distant metastases (stage IVB) is represented by 3-weekly cisplatin-paclitaxel doublet associated with bevacizumab, since the GOG-240 trial reported improvement of response rate, PFS, and OS (gain of 4 months) with the addition of the anti-angiogenic agent [160]. Alternatively, for patients not candidate to receive cisplatin (renal dysfunction, early relapse after previous cisplatin-based treatment), carboplatin-based doublet CT could be applied [161]. Other active platinum-based doublets include agents such as topotecan, gemcitabine, vinorelbine, ifosfamide, and 5-fluorouracil which result in higher response rate compared to monotherapies [162].

Any standardized regimen is expected for patients who progress following a first-line CT, but, usually, one of the most active abovementioned agents is used, if not previously administered. Other possible chemotherapeutics, which are in any way not associated with impressive improving in OS, are pegylated liposomal doxorubicin, docetaxel, and irinotecan.

Also in metastatic setting, there is a role for high-dose RT, especially in controlling oligo-metastatic disease and lymph node metastases (pelvic, para-aortic, mediastinal, supraclavicular), whereas short-course RT could be applied for treating symptomatic distant metastases (e.g., painful bone metastases) [163].

53.4.12 New and Potential Future Perspectives

As for ECs, the treatment of recurrent and metastatic cervical cancers is still considered an unmet clinical need, considering the short survival related to this disease setting (<17 months after first-line therapy) [164]. Therefore, it is not surprising that clinical efforts are moving toward the identification of innovative and targeted therapies, which could affect selected altered molecular pathways.

– *Anti-angiogenic Agents*
   The viral oncogenic E5 and E7 proteins are known to act inducing VEGF overexpression; in fact, in addition to bevacizumab, some CTs have tested multikinase inhibitors with anti-angiogenic activity (sunitinib, pazopanib, apatinib), finding a mild prolongation in terms of PFS associated with the use of pazopanib [165, 166].

– *Anti-EGFR Agents*
   Although the EGFR (epidermal growth factor receptor) overexpression is reported in more than 50% of CCs, studies on the administration of anti-EGFR molecules (erlotinib, gefitinib, cetuximab) have reported uncertain and discouraging results [167].

– *iCKPi*
   Promising results are coming from CTs testing iCKPi, such as nivolumab (monoclonal anti-PD-1 antibody), ipilimumab (monoclonal anti-CTLA4), and pembrolizumab, which have shown to increase ORR in recurrent or metastatic CCs [168].

   Particularly, the phase II KEYNOTE-158 trial resulted in the FDA approval of pembrolizumab for PD-L1 positive patients, pretreated with chemotherapy (from second-line) [169]. An ongoing phase III randomized trial (GOG-3016) is testing the activity of a new anti-PD-1 antibody (cemiplimab) versus standard of care in advanced setting [170]. Recently, at ESMO 2019, the interim analysis results of the CheckMate 358 trial have been presented, showing the safety of combination nivolumab + ipilimumab in recurrent/metastatic CC pretreated or not with CT, regardless of PD-L1 expression.

   Probably, the most satisfying results will come from the synergistic effect of combined iCKPi-based treatment with chemotherapy and anti-angiogenic agents. The phase III randomized KEYNOTE-826 trial is enrolling patients with persistent, recurrent, or metastatic cervical cancer to receive pembrolizumab plus CT versus CT alone. Interestingly, BEATcc is an ongoing randomized phase III study on the use of standard cisplatin-paclitaxel-bevacizumab with or without atezolizumab as first-line treatment for advanced disease. Besides, iCKPi-CT is being evalu-

ated also in locally advanced setting, such as in the phase III CALLA trial; particularly it is randomizing patients to receive durvalumab with and following concurrent RT/CT versus RT/CT alone.

– *Therapeutic Vaccines*
   Encouraging activities are emerging from the use of therapeutic vaccines, consisting of the infusion of E6/E7-activated T lymphocytes or autologous tumor-infiltrating lymphocytes (LN-145) after in vitro clonal expansion, in combination with interleukin 2 (IL-2) and/or CT.

53.4.13 Follow-Up

The surveillance program after a definitive treatment for CC may be schematized as in ◘ Table 53.13 [171, 172]. Effect on survival of follow-up strategies should be defined within prospective studies.

53.5 Conclusions

Endometrial and cervical cancers are showing, over the last decades, increasing incidence and mortality in developed and low-income countries, respectively. Regarding EC, this is essentially related to prolonged life expectancy and bad lifestyle habits, whereas, for CC, it depends on low availability of effective screening programs and tests in poor countries. On the other hand, innovative therapeutic strategies are emerging for the management of advanced gynecological malignancies. In fact, efforts of clinicians are increasingly moving toward the experimentation of targeted therapies, trying to ensure to patients more proper and tailored solutions, on the basis of predictive molecular profiles of response to specific and selected agents or combination of them. Thus, in the next years, this could lead to prolonging

◘ **Table 53.13** Follow-up for CC after radical treatment

Clinical and physical (gynecological/pelvic/rectal) examination	Every 3–6 months for the first 2 years and then 6-monthly until the 5th year from primary treatment
PAP test if feasible +/− HPV test	Annually
Not ordinarily recommended exams *Admitted for symptomatic or high-risk patients when physical examination appears difficult*	Tumor markers: CEA, CA 125, CA 19.9, and AFP, chest X-ray, abdominal US, CT scan, pelvic MRI, 18F-FDG PET/CT scan, whole-body bone scan

overall survival and progression-free survival of more advanced settings, whose management is still considered an unmet clinical need. Furthermore, thanks to the wide implementation of clinical trials on the definition of risk factors and predisposing conditions, prevention, through lifestyle correction and/or validated screening tests, represents an efficacious tool to diagnose earlier and reduce mortality of uterine cancers.

Case Study: Management of a Patient Affected by Locally Advanced Endometrial Cancer

63 years old
- *Family history:* negative for malignancies
- *PMH:* Obese (BMI = 32 kg/m^2), Systemic Arterial Hypertension
- *RMH:* Complain of abnormal vaginal bleeding and pelvic pain
- *Objective examination*: painful lower abdominal regions
- *Blood tests*: lower hemoglobin (10.1 mg/dL)

Question

What action should be taken in the first instance?
1. Abdominal Ultrasound
2. Gynaecological examination and Trans-Vaginal Ultrasound
3. Pelvic MRI w/wo contrast

Answer

Gynaecological examination and Trans-Vaginal Ultrasound (for searching eventual origin of bleeding from uterus)

Question

A diffuse (9 mm) endometrial thickness is detected on TVUS. What should be the next step?
1. Hysteroscopy-guided biopsy
2. Pelvic MRI w/wo contrast
3. Planning of hysterectomy

Answer

Hysteroscopy-guided biopsy

Although the presence of an abnormal vaginal bleeding associated to pelvic pain and endometrial thickness at US is highly suggestive for an endometrial cancer, a histological characterization should be recommended before considering other staging exams and/or surgery.

Question

Pathology concludes for a serous-papillary EC. *What should be the next step?*
1. Combined RT/CT
2. Complete staging (Pelvic MRI, Abdominal CT scan, Chest CT scan) and planning of surgery
3. Hysteroscopy surveillance

Answer

Complete staging (Pelvic MRI, Abdominal CT scan, Chest CT scan) and planning of surgery

The patient is affected by a high-risk histology EC. A pre-operative work-up should be recommended in all patients with pathological confirmed endometrial tumours, considering as optional some radiological exams. In this case, because of the more aggressive and prognostically unfavorable histology, a depth pre-operative evaluation should be highly taken into account to better establish the disease loco-regional and distant spread.

Question

The pre-operative work-up has detected a suspected pelvic lymph nodes involvement (stage IIIC), without distant localizations. Which surgical strategy should be preferred?
1. Extrafascial simple total hysterectomy without vaginal cuff + bilateral salpingo-oophorectomy
2. Radical hysterectomy + bilateral salpingo-oophorectomy + pelvic and para-aortic lymphadenectomy + staging omentectomy
3. Radical hysterectomy + pelvic lymphadenectomy

Answer

Radical hysterectomy + bilateral salpingo-oophorectomy + pelvic and para-aortic lymphadenectomy + staging omentectomy

Simple hysterectomy is considered the gold standard for stage I EC. Instead, starting from stage II a radical hysterectomy associated to systematic lymphadenectomy is recommended, independently from the macroscopic lymph nodes involvement. Our patient was clinically staged as a IIIC, thus even more so deserving a systematic lymph nodes removal to reduce lymphatic spread risk, but also for staging purposes and better guiding adjuvant treatment. Moreover, a staging omentectomy is strongly recommended, because of the high peritoneal spread risk by serous EC.

Question

Pathology confirms a IIIC1 stage for pelvic and no para-aortic lymph nodes involvement. Should the patient undergo to further treatments?

1. No, but she must follow a surveillance program
2. Yes: 3-weekly carboplatin-paclitaxel administered for 6 cycles
3. Yes: combined platinum-based CT/RT

Answer

Yes: combined platinum-based CT/RT

A multimodality approach is strongly suggested for special histotypes, especially in presence of a N-positive disease, as several clinical studies have found longer PFS and/or OS linked to combined treatments.

Key Points

- Start with medical history, physical examination and histological definition
- A proper pre-operative work-up should be always proposed, especially in presence of high-risk disease
- A radical hysterectomy should be accompanied by an optimal surgical staging (omentectomy), when a serous-papillary histology is diagnosed
- Adjuvant combined RT/CT is basically the preferred approach after EC surgery, especially in high-risk clinico-pathological conditions.

53

Case Study: Management of a Patient Affected by Metastatic Cervical Cancer

49 years old
- *Family history:* negative for malignancies
- *PMH:* tobacco smoker for 30 years; 3 years ago → positive HPV-test for 16 genotype; positive PAP-TEST for L-SIL; colposcopy-guided biopsy conclusive for CIN1
- *RMH:* 6-months history of vaginal discharge, dyspareunia, pelvic discomfort, lumbar pain, legs lymphedema
- *Physical examination:* painful hypogastric region, pain on pressing lumbar region, vaginal discharge on gynaecological examination
- *Laboratory tests:* no abnormalities
- *New HPV and PAP-tests:* positivity for 16 genotype HPV and the presence of squamous carcinoma cells, respectively.

Question

Which investigations should be performed?
1. 18F-FDG PET/CT scan
2. Colposcopy-guided biopsy and a complete radiological staging
3. Hysteroscopy

Answer

Colposcopy-guided biopsy and a complete radiological staging

Considering the presence of squamous carcinoma cells on PAP-TEST, past and recent medical history and objective findings on physical examination, the suspicion for an advanced cervical cancer is very high. Thus, a colposcopy-guided biopsy and a complete staging of the disease are mandatory.

Pathology confirms the presence of a squamous cell carcinoma and the radiological staging the extension to pelvic lymph nodes with right hydronephrosis, two suspected left lung and one L3 metastases.

Question

What action should be taken?
1. First-line CT
2. Radical hysterectomy + bilateral salpingo-oophorectomy + systematic lymphadenectomy
3. First-line CT and consider high-dose and/or short-course RT

Answer

First-line CT and consider high-dose and/or short-course RT

Although the patient is affected by a metastatic cervical cancer and a first-line chemotherapy is tightly required, a multimodality approach should be considered. Indeed, the role of high-dose RT in controlling oligometastatic disease and lymph nodes metastases is quite recognized. Moreover, a short-course RT could be applied for treating symptomatic distant metastases, for example painful bone metastases like in this case (L3 lesion).

Question

Which CT regimen should be preferred?
1. 3 weekly cisplatin-paclitaxel doublet associated to Bevacizumab
2. 3 weekly cisplatin-paclitaxel doublet
3. 3 weekly carboplatin-paclitaxel doublet +/- Bevacizumab

Answer

3 weekly carboplatin-paclitaxel doublet associated +/- Bevacizumab

The standard first-line CT regimen for metastatic patients consists in the combination of the 3 weekly cisplatin-paclitaxel doublet and the anti-angiogenic Bevacizumab. But, considering the right hydronephrosis detected on radiological exams, our patient should be candidate to receive carboplatin, instead of cisplatin, to reduce the renal dysfunction risk. In fact, in similar cases, a protection nephrostomy placement should be recommended, primarily in those patients could benefit from a high-dose RT on abdominal lymph nodes.

Question

After 12-months treatment, the radiological revaluation shows a disease progression on lungs and mediastinal lymph nodes. What should be the next step?

1. Pegylated liposomal doxorubicin administration
2. Gemcitabine administration
3. Refer the patient to a specialized center for the eventual enrolling into clinical trials

Answer

All the options are valid therapeutic strategies.

To date, any standardized regimen is recommended for patients who progress to a first-line platinum-based doublet; in fact, a series of several chemotherapy agents could be used in this setting: pegylated liposomal doxorubicin, gemcitabine, topotecan, vinorelbine, ifosfamide, 5-fluo-rouracil docetaxel, irinotecan. Besides that, the phase II KEYNOTE 158 trial resulted in the FDA approval of pembrolizumab for PD-L1 positive patients, pretreated with chemotherapy (from second-line); thus, also in this case, the possibility to evaluate the PD-L1 expression by tumoural cells and, consequently, to administer iCKPi should be taken into account. Certainly, referring the patient to a center that handles ongoing clinical trials could represent an optimal therapeutic strategy and opportunity.

Key Points

– Start with medical history, physical examination and histological definition
– Proper pre-operative work-up and imagine techniques are crucial to establish the effective extension of the disease
– Multimodality treatment could find its usefulness even in metastatic setting
– The choice of the most effective and tailored treatment should be discussed or realized in high volume gynaecologic oncology centers handling clinical trials on targeted therapies

Expert Opinion

Peter van Dam

Unit of Gynecologic Oncology, Department of Obstetrics & Gynecology, Antwerp University Hospital, Antwerp, Belgium.

Key Points

Endometrial cancer is the most common gynecological cancer affecting about 320000 women worldwide. As most cases are diagnosed in an early stage due to the occurrence of vaginal bleeding, the overall survival rate is high. However, nearly one-fifth of women have aggressive endometrial cancer with a survival of about 1 year. There are two different types of endometrial carcinoma, named as type I and type II. Type I endometrioid endometrial cancer represents most sporadic cases, is driven by estrogens, often is well differentiated, and has a good prognosis. Type II endometrial cancer consists of clear cell, serous, mucinous, adenosquamous, and mixed carcinomas and typically presents with advanced stage disease and is associated with a high mortality. About 10% of endometrial carcinomas are triggered by germline alterations in DNA mismatch repair genes (MMR). Those patients often develop endometrial cancer at a young age. Standard management of endometrial cancer at diagnosis involves surgery consisting of a hysterectomy, bilateral salpingo-oophorectomy, and in high-risk cases pelvic- and paraaortic lymphadenectomy and staging. A 2012 review found that for early-stage primary endometrioid adenocarcinoma of the endometrium, laparoscopy and laparotomy are associated with similar rates of disease-free and overall survival and that laparoscopy is associated with reduced operative morbidity and shorter hospital stays. In patients with advanced disease, adjuvant chemotherapy and/or radiotherapy should be considered. The Cancer Genome Atlas (TCGA) group used whole genome sequencing to characterize genetic aberrations in endometrial cancers. Recurrent translocations of gene were found in important cancer pathways, such as WNT-EGFR-MAPK-RAS, PI3K, and RB1. Frequent translocations were discovered in the BCL family and novel POLE hotspot mutations were identified. PTEN, PIK3R1, PIK3CA, FBXW7, and KRAS were found to be frequently mutated. These genomic alterations are crucial for the development of genome-driven precision care, pharmacogenomics, and the development of targeted drugs. Next-generation sequencing assays looking at MMR genes are currently already actively used for the identification of individuals at risk for developing endometrial cancer.

Cancer of the uterine cervix (CC) reflects the disparities in access to healthcare across the world. Although being highly preventable, this disease is still a major public health problem in less developed regions. Globally it is the second most prevalent cancer in women, with most cases diagnosed in an advanced stage. Inoperable CC will continue to be highly prevalent during the next decades as screening programs and vaccination campaigns are still unavailable in most countries while not being entirely effective. Currently, locally advanced disease is treated with (chemo)radiotherapy and metastatic disease with platinum-based chemotherapy (+/- bevacizumab). First- and second-line systemic treatments are not very effective, and early clinical trials with targeted therapy have not yet identified new targeted drugs with superior response rates. Up to now, the scientific society and pharmaceutical industry have shown little interest in developing new (targeted) treatment modalities to improve the outcome of patients with advanced and recurrent CC. In fact, CC is often not included in phase I-II basket trials assessing experimental drugs. Traditionally, testing novel systemic treatments in advanced CC requires large and expensive randomized clinical trials involving hundreds of patients, with follow-up extending several years before results emerge. Neoadjuvant experimental therapy (NET) provides a unique opportunity for faster and cheaper studies assessing the responsiveness to targeted drugs and/or immunotherapy. CC is easily and safely accessible for repeated tumor biopsies allowing intra-patient comparisons. NET can be performed in a concept of proof setting as short (2-4 weeks) treatment courses before standard treatment, using biomarkers as endpoints. It can also be tested with randomized trials comparing standard chemotherapy versus a combination of experimental treatment using operability and/or pathological response as endpoints, jointly with biomarkers for response, thereby gaining insight into molecular changes associated with tumor response. While immunotherapy is emerging as a potential treatment modality of CC, NET may offer a unique opportunity to assess the immune response in vivo. Patients with recurrent metastatic disease are often immunocompromised, and it is therefore important to assess immunotherapy in earlier stage patients. We therefore advocate the use of NET as a tool to accelerate translational and clinical research into better treatment of CC. Performing this research in parts of the world with a high incidence of the disease is mandatory to achieve this goal. Such an approach is only ethically defendable if strategies are developed to reduce costs and access to new active drugs in these countries.

References

1. Siegel RL, Miller KD, Jemal A. Cancer statistics, 2019. CA Cancer J Clin. 2019;69:7–34.
2. Ferlay J, Colombet M, Soerjomataram I, Dyba T, Randi G, Bettio M, Gavin A, Visser O, Bray F. Cancer incidence and mortality patterns in Europe: estimates for 40 countries and 25 major cancers in 2018. Eur J Cancer. 2018;103:356–87.
3. Endometrial cancer statistics Available online.: https://www.wcrf.org/dietandcancer/cancer-trends/endometrial-cancer-statistics.
4. Cook LS, Weiss NS, Doherty JA, Chen C. Endometrial Cancer: Oxford University Press; 2006. ISBN 978-0-19-986506-2.
5. Siegel RL, Miller KD, Jemal A. Cancer statistics, 2017. CA Cancer J Clin. 2017;67:7–30.
6. Endometrial Cancer Treatment (PDQ®)–Health Professional Version Available online.: https://www.cancer.gov/types/uterine/hp/endometrial-treatment-pdq.
7. Renehan AG, Tyson M, Egger M, Heller RF, Zwahlen M. Body-mass index and incidence of cancer: a systematic review and meta-analysis of prospective observational studies. Lancet. 2008;371:569–78.
8. Crosbie EJ, Zwahlen M, Kitchener HC, Egger M, Renehan AG. Body mass index, hormone replacement therapy, and endometrial cancer risk: a meta-analysis. Cancer Epidemiol Biomark Prev. 2010;19:3119–30.
9. Esposito K, Chiodini P, Capuano A, Bellastella G, Maiorino MI, Giugliano D. Metabolic syndrome and endometrial cancer: a meta-analysis. Endocrine. 2014;45:28–36.
10. Zhang Y, Liu H, Yang S, Zhang J, Qian L, Chen X. Overweight, obesity and endometrial cancer risk: results from a systematic review and meta-analysis. Int J Biol Markers. 2014;29:e21–9.
11. Calle EE, Kaaks R. Overweight, obesity and cancer: epidemiological evidence and proposed mechanisms. Nat Rev Cancer. 2004;4:579–91.
12. Rosato V, Zucchetto A, Bosetti C, Dal Maso L, Montella M, Pelucchi C, Negri E, Franceschi S, La Vecchia C. Metabolic syndrome and endometrial cancer risk. Ann Oncol. 2011;22:884–9.
13. Bandera EV, Kushi LH, Moore DF, Gifkins DM, McCullough ML. Consumption of animal foods and endometrial cancer risk: a systematic literature review and meta-analysis. Cancer Causes Control. 2007;18:967–88.
14. Zhao J, Lyu C, Gao J, Du L, Shan B, Zhang H, Wang H-Y, Gao Y. Dietary fat intake and endometrial cancer risk. Medicine (Baltimore). 2016;95:e4121.
15. Zucchetto A, Serraino D, Polesel J, Negri E, De Paoli A, Dal Maso L, Montella M, La Vecchia C, Franceschi S, Talamini R. Hormone-related factors and gynecological conditions in relation to endometrial cancer risk. Eur J Cancer Prev. 2009;18:316–21.
16. Barry JA, Azizia MM, Hardiman PJ. Risk of endometrial, ovarian and breast cancer in women with polycystic ovary syndrome: a systematic review and meta-analysis. Hum Reprod Update. 2014;20:748–58.
17. Peiretti M, Colombo N. Sex cord-stromal tumors of the ovary. In: Ayhan A, Reed N, Gultekin M, Dursun P, editors. Textbook of gynaecological oncology: Gunes Publishing; 2012. ISBN 978-975-277-387-5.

18. Humans, I.W.G. on the E. of C.R. to Hormonal contraception and post-menopausal hormonal therapy; International Agency for Research on Cancer, 1999.

19. Hu R, Hilakivi-Clarke L, Clarke R. Molecular mechanisms of tamoxifen-associated endometrial cancer (review). Oncol Lett. 2015;9:1495–501.

20. Assikis VJ, Neven P, Jordan VC, Vergote I. A realistic clinical perspective of tamoxifen and endometrial carcinogenesis. Eur J Cancer. 1996;32A:1464–76.

21. Kim HS, Jeon YT, Kim YB. The effect of adjuvant hormonal therapy on the endometrium and ovary of breast cancer patients. J Gynecol Oncol. 2008;19:256–60.

22. Fisher B, Costantino JP, Wickerham DL, Redmond CK, Kavanah M, Cronin WM, Vogel V, Robidoux A, Dimitrov N, Atkins J, et al. Tamoxifen for prevention of breast cancer: report of the National Surgical Adjuvant Breast and Bowel Project P-1 Study. J Natl Cancer Inst. 1998;90:1371–88.

23. Lancaster JM, Powell CB, Chen L-M, Richardson DL. SGO Clinical Practice Committee Society of Gynecologic Oncology statement on risk assessment for inherited gynecologic cancer predispositions. Gynecol Oncol. 2015;136:3–7.

24. Friberg E, Orsini N, Mantzoros CS, Wolk A. Coffee drinking and risk of endometrial cancer – a population-based cohort study. Int J Cancer. 2009;125:2413–7.

25. Mueck AO, Seeger H, Rabe T. Hormonal contraception and risk of endometrial cancer: a systematic review. Endocr Relat Cancer. 2010;17:R263–71.

26. Chin J, Konje JC, Hickey M. Levonorgestrel intrauterine system for endometrial protection in women with breast cancer on adjuvant tamoxifen. Cochrane Database Syst Rev. 2009:CD007245.

27. Luo L, Luo B, Zheng Y, Zhang H, Li J, Sidell N. Oral and intrauterine progestogens for atypical endometrial hyperplasia. Cochrane Database Syst Rev. 2018;12:CD009458.

28. Brinton LA, Felix AS. Menopausal hormone therapy and risk of endometrial cancer. J Steroid Biochem Mol Biol. 2014;142:83–9.

29. Resnick KE, Hampel H, Fishel R, Cohn DE. Current and emerging trends in Lynch syndrome identification in women with endometrial cancer. Gynecol Oncol. 2009;114:128–34.

30. Russo A, Incorvaia L, Malapelle U, et al. The tumor-agnostic treatment for patients with solid tumors: a position paper on behalf of the AIOM-SIAPEC/IAP-SIBIOC-SIF italian scientific societies [published online ahead of print, 2021 Aug 6]. Crit Rev Oncol Hematol. 2021;103436. https://doi.org/10.1016/j.critrevonc.2021.103436.

31. Obermair A, Youlden DR, Young JP, Lindor NM, Baron JA, Newcomb P, Parry S, Hopper JL, Haile R, Jenkins MA. Risk of endometrial cancer for women diagnosed with HNPCC-related colorectal carcinoma. Int J Cancer. 2010;127:2678–84.

32. Win AK, Lindor NM, Winship I, Tucker KM, Buchanan DD, Young JP, Rosty C, Leggett B, Giles GG, Goldblatt J, et al. Risks of colorectal and other cancers after endometrial cancer for women with Lynch syndrome. J Natl Cancer Inst. 2013;105:274–9.

33. Meyer LA, Broaddus RR, Lu KH. Endometrial cancer and Lynch syndrome: clinical and pathologic considerations. Cancer Control. 2009;16:14–22.

34. Lancaster JM, Powell CB, Kauff ND, Cass I, Chen L-M, Lu KH, Mutch DG, Berchuck A, Karlan BY, Herzog TJ, et al. Society of Gynecologic Oncologists Education Committee statement on risk assessment for inherited gynecologic cancer predispositions. Gynecol Oncol. 2007;107:159–62.

35. Bonnet D, Selves J, Toulas C, Danjoux M, Duffas JP, Portier G, Kirzin S, Ghouti L, Carrère N, Suc B, et al. Simplified identification of Lynch syndrome: a prospective, multicenter study. Dig Liver Dis. 2012;44:515–22.

36. Manchanda R, Saridogan E, Abdelraheim A, Johnson M, Rosenthal AN, Benjamin E, Brunell C, Side L, Gessler S, Jacobs I, et al. Annual outpatient hysteroscopy and endometrial sampling (OHES) in HNPCC/Lynch syndrome (LS). Arch Gynecol Obstet. 2012;286:1555–62.

37. Smith RA, Cokkinides V, Brawley OW. Cancer screening in the United States, 2012: a review of current American Cancer Society guidelines and current issues in cancer screening. CA Cancer J Clin. 2012;62:129–42.

38. Kwon JS, Scott JL, Gilks CB, Daniels MS, Sun CC, Lu KH. Testing women with endometrial cancer to detect Lynch syndrome. J Clin Oncol. 2011;29:2247–52.

39. Bokhman JV. Two pathogenetic types of endometrial carcinoma. Gynecol Oncol. 1983;15:10–7.

40. Cancer Genome Atlas Research Network, Kandoth C, Schultz N, Cherniack AD, Akbani R, Liu Y, Shen H, Robertson AG, Pashtan I, Shen R, et al. Integrated genomic characterization of endometrial carcinoma. Nature. 2013;497:67–73.

41. Stelloo E, Nout RA, Osse EM, Jürgenliemk-Schulz IJ, Jobsen JJ, Lutgens LC, van der Steen-Banasik EM, Nijman HW, Putter H, Bosse T, et al. Improved risk assessment by integrating molecular and clinicopathological factors in early-stage endometrial cancer-combined analysis of the PORTEC cohorts. Clin Cancer Res. 2016;22:4215–24.

42. Soslow RA, Bissonnette JP, Wilton A, Ferguson SE, Alektiar KM, Duska LR, Oliva E. Clinicopathologic analysis of 187 high-grade endometrial carcinomas of different histologic subtypes: similar outcomes belie distinctive biologic differences. Am J Surg Pathol. 2007;31:979–87.

43. D'Angelo E, Prat J. Pathology of mixed Müllerian tumours. Best Pract Res Clin Obstet Gynaecol. 2011;25:705–18.

44. Kernochan LE, Garcia RL. Carcinosarcomas (malignant mixed Müllerian tumor) of the uterus: advances in elucidation of biologic and clinical characteristics. J Natl Compr Canc Netw. 2009;7:550–6.

45. Tafe LJ, Garg K, Chew I, Tornos C, Soslow RA. Endometrial and ovarian carcinomas with undifferentiated components: clinically aggressive and frequently underrecognized neoplasms. Mod Pathol. 2010;23:781–9.

46. Epstein E, Van Holsbeke C, Mascilini F, Måsbäck A, Kannisto P, Ameye L, Fischerova D, Zannoni G, Vellone V, Timmerman D, et al. Gray-scale and color Doppler ultrasound characteristics of endometrial cancer in relation to stage, grade and tumor size. Ultrasound Obstet Gynecol. 2011;38:586–93.

47. Timmermans A, Opmeer BC, Khan KS, Bachmann LM, Epstein E, Clark TJ, Gupta JK, Bakour SH, van den Bosch T, van Doorn HC, et al. Endometrial thickness measurement for detecting endometrial cancer in women with postmenopausal bleeding: a systematic review and meta-analysis. Obstet Gynecol. 2010;116:160–7.

48. Clark TJ, Voit D, Gupta JK, Hyde C, Song F, Khan KS. Accuracy of hysteroscopy in the diagnosis of endometrial cancer and hyperplasia: a systematic quantitative review. JAMA. 2002;288:1610–21.

49. Pecorelli S. Revised FIGO staging for carcinoma of the vulva, cervix, and endometrium. Int J Gynaecol Obstet. 2009;105:103–4.

50. Doll KM, Tseng J, Denslow SA, Fader AN, Gehrig PA. High-grade endometrial cancer: revisiting the impact of tumor size and location on outcomes. Gynecol Oncol. 2014;132:44–9.

51. Schink JC, Lurain JR, Wallemark CB, Chmiel JS. Tumor size in endometrial cancer: a prognostic factor for lymph node metastasis. Obstet Gynecol. 1987;70:216–9.

52. Benedetti Panici P, Basile S, Salerno MG, Di Donato V, Marchetti C, Perniola G, Palagiano A, Perutelli A, Maneschi F, Lissoni AA, et al. Secondary analyses from a randomized clinical trial: age as the key prognostic factor in endometrial carcinoma. Am J Obstet Gynecol. 2014;210:363.e1–363.e10.

53. Falcone F, Laurelli G, Losito S, Di Napoli M, Granata V, Greggi S. Fertility preserving treatment with hysteroscopic resection followed by progestin therapy in young women with early endometrial cancer. J Gynecol Oncol. 2017;28:e2.

54. Barlin JN, Puri I, Bristow RE. Cytoreductive surgery for advanced or recurrent endometrial cancer: a meta-analysis. Gynecol Oncol. 2010;118:14–8.

55. Querleu D, Morrow CP. Classification of radical hysterectomy. Lancet Oncol. 2008;9:297–303.

56. Eddib A, Danakas A, Hughes S, Erk M, Michalik C, Narayanan MS, Krovi V, Singhal P. Influence of morbid obesity on surgical outcomes in robotic-assisted gynecologic surgery. J Gynecol Surg. 2014;30:81–6.

57. Shah CA, Beck T, Liao JB, Giannakopoulos NV, Veljovich D, Paley P. Surgical and oncologic outcomes after robotic radical hysterectomy as compared to open radical hysterectomy in the treatment of early cervical cancer. J Gynecol Oncol. 2017;28:e82.

58. Janda M, Gebski V, Davies LC, Forder P, Brand A, Hogg R, Jobling TW, Land R, Manolitsas T, Nascimento M, et al. Effect of total laparoscopic hysterectomy vs total abdominal hysterectomy on disease-free survival among women with stage I endometrial cancer: a randomized clinical trial. JAMA. 2017;317:1224–33.

59. Walker JL, Piedmonte MR, Spirtos NM, Eisenkop SM, Schlaerth JB, Mannel RS, Barakat R, Pearl ML, Sharma SK. Recurrence and survival after random assignment to laparoscopy versus laparotomy for comprehensive surgical staging of uterine cancer: gynecologic oncology group LAP2 study. J Clin Oncol. 2012;30:695–700114.

60. Susini T, Massi G, Amunni G, Carriero C, Marchionni M, Taddei G, Scarselli G. Vaginal hysterectomy and abdominal hysterectomy for treatment of endometrial cancer in the elderly. Gynecol Oncol. 2005;96:362–7.

61. Todo Y, Kato H, Kaneuchi M, Watari H, Takeda M, Sakuragi N. Survival effect of para-aortic lymphadenectomy in endometrial cancer (SEPAL study): a retrospective cohort analysis. Lancet. 2010;375:1165–72.

62. ASTEC study group, Kitchener H, Swart AMC, Qian Q, Amos C, Parmar MKB. Efficacy of systematic pelvic lymphadenectomy in endometrial cancer (MRC ASTEC trial): a randomised study. Lancet. 2009;373:125–36.

63. Benedetti Panici P, Basile S, Maneschi F, Alberto Lissoni A, Signorelli M, Scambia G, Angioli R, Tateo S, Mangili G, Katsaros D, et al. Systematic pelvic lymphadenectomy vs. no lymphadenectomy in early-stage endometrial carcinoma: randomized clinical trial. J Natl Cancer Inst. 2008;100:1707–16.

64. Geppert B, Lönnerfors C, Bollino M, Persson J. Sentinel lymph node biopsy in endometrial cancer-feasibility, safety and lymphatic complications. Gynecol Oncol. 2018;148:491–8.

65. Ballester M, Dubernard G, Lécuru F, Heitz D, Mathevet P, Marret H, Querleu D, Golfier F, Leblanc E, Rouzier R, et al. Detection rate and diagnostic accuracy of sentinel-node biopsy in early stage endometrial cancer: a prospective multicentre study (SENTI-ENDO). Lancet Oncol. 2011;12:469–76.

66. Bendifallah S, Canlorbe G, Raimond E, Hudry D, Coutant C, Graesslin O, Touboul C, Huguet F, Cortez A, Daraï E, et al. A clue towards improving the European Society for Medical Oncology risk group classification in apparent early stage endometrial cancer? Impact of lymphovascular space invasion. Br J Cancer. 2014;110:2640–6.

67. Creutzberg CL, Nout RA, Lybeert MLM, Warlam-Rodenhuis CC, Jobsen JJ, Mens J-WM, Lutgens LCHW, Pras E, van de Poll-Franse LV, van Putten WLJ, et al. Fifteen-year radiotherapy outcomes of the randomized PORTEC-1 trial for endometrial carcinoma. Int J Radiat Oncol Biol Phys. 2011;81:E631–8.

68. de Boer SM, Powell ME, Mileshkin L, Katsaros D, Bessette P, Haie-Meder C, Ottevanger PB, Ledermann JA, Khaw P, D'Amico R, et al. Adjuvant chemoradiotherapy versus radiotherapy alone in women with high-risk endometrial cancer (PORTEC-3): patterns of recurrence and post-hoc survival analysis of a randomised phase 3 trial. Lancet Oncol. 2019;20:1273–85.

69. de Boer SM, Powell ME, Mileshkin L, Katsaros D, Bessette P, Haie-Meder C, Ottevanger PB, Ledermann JA, Khaw P, Colombo A, et al. Adjuvant chemoradiotherapy versus radiotherapy alone for women with high-risk endometrial cancer (PORTEC-3): final results of an international, open-label, multicentre, randomised, phase 3 trial. Lancet Oncol. 2018;19:295–309.

70. Creutzberg CL, Leon-Castillo A, de Boer SM, Powell ME, Mileshkin LR, Mackay HJ, Leary A, Nijman HW, Singh N, Pollock P, et al. Molecular classification of the PORTEC-3 trial for high-risk endometrial cancer: impact on adjuvant therapy. In: Proceedings of the annals of oncology, vol. 30: Oxford University Press; 2019. p. 899–900.

71. DeLeon MC, Ammakkanavar NR, Matei D. Adjuvant therapy for endometrial cancer. J Gynecol Oncol. 2014;25:136–47.

72. Hori K, Nishio S, Ushijima K, Kasamatsu Y, Kondo E, Takehara K, Kakubari R, Ito K. A phase II, open labeled, single-arm study of dose-dense paclitaxel plus carboplatin in advanced or recurrent uterine corpus cancer: KCOGG1303 study. JCO. 2019;37:5584.

73. Fleming GF, Brunetto VL, Cella D, Look KY, Reid GC, Munkarah AR, Kline R, Burger RA, Goodman A, Burks RT. Phase III trial of doxorubicin plus cisplatin with or without paclitaxel plus filgrastim in advanced endometrial carcinoma: a Gynecologic Oncology Group Study. J Clin Oncol. 2004;22:2159–66.

74. Humber CE, Tierney JF, Symonds RP, Collingwood M, Kirwan J, Williams C, Green JA. Chemotherapy for advanced, recurrent or metastatic endometrial cancer: a systematic review of Cochrane collaboration. Ann Oncol. 2007;18:409–20.

75. Makker V, Hensley ML, Zhou Q, Iasonos A, Aghajanian CA. Treatment of advanced or recurrent endometrial carcinoma with doxorubicin in patients progressing after paclitaxel/carboplatin: Memorial Sloan-Kettering Cancer Center experience from 1995 to 2009. Int J Gynecol Cancer. 2013;23:929–34.

76. Fiorica JV, Brunetto VL, Hanjani P, Lentz SS, Mannel R, Andersen W. Gynecologic Oncology Group study Phase II trial of alternating courses of megestrol acetate and tamoxifen in advanced endometrial carcinoma: a Gynecologic Oncology Group study. Gynecol Oncol. 2004;92:10–4.

77. Mileshkin L, Edmondson R, O'Connell RL, Sjoquist KM, Andrews J, Jyothirmayi R, Beale P, Bonaventura T, Goh J, Hall M, et al. Phase 2 study of anastrozole in recurrent estrogen (ER)/progesterone (PR) positive endometrial cancer: the PARAGON trial - ANZGOG 0903. Gynecol Oncol. 2019;154:29–37.

78. Colon-Otero G, Weroha SJ, Zanfagnin V, Foster NR, Asmus E, Wahner Hendrickson AE, Jatoi A, Block MS, Langstraat CL, Glaser GE, et al. Results of a phase 2 trial of ribociclib and letrozole in patients with either relapsed estrogen receptor (ER)-positive ovarian cancers or relapsed ER-positive endometrial cancers. JCO. 2019;37:5510.

79. Huh WK, Straughn JM, Mariani A, Podratz KC, Havrilesky LJ, Alvarez-Secord A, Gold MA, McMeekin DS, Modesitt S, Cooper AL, et al. Salvage of isolated vaginal recurrences in women with surgical stage I endometrial cancer: a multiinstitutional experience. Int J Gynecol Cancer. 2007;17:886–9.

80. Radiation Therapy With or Without Cisplatin in Treating Patients With Recurrent Endometrial Cancer - Full Text View - ClinicalTrials.gov Available online: https://clinicaltrials.gov/ct2/show/NCT00492778. Accessed on 20 Jan 2020.

53

81. Oza AM, Elit L, Tsao M-S, Kamel-Reid S, Biagi J, Provencher DM, Gotlieb WH, Hoskins PJ, Ghatage P, Tonkin KS, et al. Phase II study of temsirolimus in women with recurrent or metastatic endometrial cancer: a trial of the NCIC Clinical Trials Group. J Clin Oncol. 2011;29:3278–85.

82. Oza AM, Pignata S, Poveda A, McCormack M, Clamp A, Schwartz B, Cheng J, Li X, Campbell K, Dodion P, et al. Randomized phase II trial of Ridaforolimus in advanced endometrial carcinoma. J Clin Oncol. 2015;33:3576–82.

83. Yeramian A, Moreno-Bueno G, Dolcet X, Catasus L, Abal M, Colas E, Reventos J, Palacios J, Prat J, Matias-Guiu X. Endometrial carcinoma: molecular alterations involved in tumor development and progression. Oncogene. 2013;32:403–41354.

84. Gavalas NG, Tsiatas M, Tsitsilonis O, Politi E, Ioannou K, Ziogas AC, Rodolakis A, Vlahos G, Thomakos N, Haidopoulos D, et al. VEGF directly suppresses activation of T cells from ascites secondary to ovarian cancer via VEGF receptor type 2. Br J Cancer. 2012;107:1869–75.

85. Terme M, Pernot S, Marcheteau E, Sandoval F, Benhamouda N, Colussi O, Dubreuil O, Carpentier AF, Tartour E, Taieb J. VEGFA-VEGFR pathway blockade inhibits tumor-induced regulatory T-cell proliferation in colorectal cancer. Cancer Res. 2013;73:539–49.

86. Shrimali RK, Yu Z, Theoret MR, Chinnasamy D, Restifo NP, Rosenberg SA. Antiangiogenic agents can increase lymphocyte infiltration into tumor and enhance the effectiveness of adoptive immunotherapy of cancer. Cancer Res. 2010;70:6171–80.

87. Aghajanian C, Filiaci V, Dizon DS, Carlson JW, Powell MA, Secord AA, Tewari KS, Bender DP, O'Malley DM, Stuckey A, et al. A phase II study of frontline paclitaxel/carboplatin/bevacizumab, paclitaxel/carboplatin/temsirolimus, or ixabepilone/carboplatin/bevacizumab in advanced/recurrent endometrial cancer. Gynecol Oncol. 2018;150:274–81.

88. Lorusso D, Ferrandina G, Colombo N, Pignata S, Pietragalla A, Sonetto C, Pisano C, Lapresa MT, Savarese A, Tagliaferri P, et al. Carboplatin-paclitaxel compared to Carboplatin-Paclitaxel-Bevacizumab in advanced or recurrent endometrial cancer: MITO END-2 - a randomized phase II trial. Gynecol Oncol. 2019;155:406–12.

89. Study Of Nintedanib compared to chemotherapy in patients with recurrent clear cell carcinoma of the ovary or endometrium - full text view - ClinicalTrials.gov Available online: https://clinicaltrials.gov/ct2/show/NCT02866370.

90. Howitt BE, Shukla SA, Sholl LM, Ritterhouse LL, Watkins JC, Rodig S, Stover E, Strickland KC, D'Andrea AD, Wu CJ, et al. Association of Polymerase e-mutated and microsatellite-instable endometrial cancers with neoantigen load, number of tumor-infiltrating lymphocytes, and expression of PD-1 and PD-L1. JAMA Oncol. 2015;1:1319–23.

91. Chung HC, Ros W, Delord J-P, Perets R, Italiano A, Shapira-Frommer R, Manzuk L, Piha-Paul SA, Xu L, Zeigenfuss S, et al. Efficacy and safety of Pembrolizumab in previously treated advanced cervical cancer: results from the phase II KEYNOTE-158 study. J Clin Oncol. 2019;37:1470–8.

92. Antill YC, Kok PS, Robledo K, Barnes E, Friedlander M, Baron-Hay SE, Shannon CM, Coward J, Beale PJ, Goss G, et al. Activity of durvalumab in advanced endometrial cancer (AEC) according to mismatch repair (MMR) status: the phase II PHAEDRA trial (ANZGOG1601). JCO. 2019;37:5501.

93. A phase 1 dose escalation and cohort expansion study of TSR-042, an anti-PD-1 monoclonal antibody, in patients with advanced solid tumors - full text view - ClinicalTrials.gov Available online: https://clinicaltrials.gov/ct2/show/NCT02715284

94. Pembrolizumab in combination with doxorubicin in advanced, recurrent or metastatic endometrial cancer - full text view - ClinicalTrials.gov Available online: https://clinicaltrials.gov/ct2/show/NCT03276013.

95. Makker V, Rasco D, Vogelzang NJ, Brose MS, Cohn AL, Mier J, Di Simone C, Hyman DM, Stepan DE, Dutcus CE, et al. Lenvatinib plus pembrolizumab in patients with advanced endometrial cancer: an interim analysis of a multicentre, open-label, single-arm, phase 2 trial. Lancet Oncol. 2019;20: 711–8.

96. Lenvatinib in Combination With Pembrolizumab Versus Treatment of Physician's Choice in Participants With Advanced Endometrial Cancer (MK-3475-775/E7080-G000–309 Per Merck Standard Convention [KEYNOTE-775]) - Full Text View - ClinicalTrials.gov Available online: https://clinicaltrials.gov/ct2/show/NCT03517449.

97. Bindra RS, Gibson SL, Meng A, Westermark U, Jasin M, Pierce AJ, Bristow RG, Classon MK, Glazer PM. Hypoxia-induced down-regulation of BRCA1 expression by E2Fs. Cancer Res. 2005;65:11597–604.

98. Chan N, Bristow RG. "Contextual" synthetic lethality and/or loss of heterozygosity: tumor hypoxia and modification of DNA repair. Clin Cancer Res. 2010;16:4553–60.

99. Mackay H, Rimel B, Bender D. NRG GY012: a randomized phase II study comparing single-agent olaparib, single agent cediranib, and the combination of cediranib/olaparib in women with recurrent, persistent or metastatic endometrial cancer. JCO. 2019;37:TPS5609–TPS5609.

100. Higuchi T, Flies DB, Marjon NA, Mantia-Smaldone G, Ronner L, Gimotty PA, Adams SF. CTLA-4 blockade synergizes therapeutically with PARP inhibition in BRCA1-deficient ovarian cancer. Cancer Immunol Res. 2015;3:1257–68.

101. Durvalumab and Olaparib in Metastatic or Recurrent Endometrial Cancer - Full Text View - ClinicalTrials.gov Available online: https://clinicaltrials.gov/ct2/show/NCT03951415.

102. Salani R, Backes FJ, Fung MFK, Holschneider CH, Parker LP, Bristow RE, Goff BA. Posttreatment surveillance and diagnosis of recurrence in women with gynecologic malignancies: Society of Gynecologic Oncologists recommendations. Am J Obstet Gynecol. 2011;204:466–78.

103. Lajer H, Jensen MB, Kilsmark J, Albæk J, Svane D, Mirza MR, Geertsen PF, Reerman D, Hansen K, Milter MC, et al. The value of gynecologic cancer follow-up: evidence-based ignorance? Int J Gynecol Cancer. 2010;20:1307–20.

104. Trial between two follow up regimens with different test intensity in endometrial cancer treated patients - full text view - ClinicalTrials.gov Available online: https://clinicaltrials.gov/ct2/show/NCT00916708.

105. Bray F, Ferlay J, Soerjomataram I, Siegel RL, Torre LA, Jemal A. Global cancer statistics 2018: GLOBOCAN estimates of incidence and mortality worldwide for 36 cancers in 185 countries. CA Cancer J Clin. 2018;68:394–424.

106. Sant M, Chirlaque Lopez MD, Agresti R, Sánchez Pérez MJ, Holleczek B, Bielska-Lasota M, Dimitrova N, Innos K, Katalinic A, Langseth H, et al. Survival of women with cancers of breast and genital organs in Europe 1999-2007: results of the EUROCARE-5 study. Eur J Cancer. 2015;51:2191–205.

107. Marth C, Landoni F, Mahner S, McCormack M, Gonzalez-Martin A, Colombo N. ESMO guidelines committee cervical cancer: ESMO clinical practice guidelines for diagnosis, treatment and follow-up. Ann Oncol. 2017;28:iv72–83.

108. Shanmugasundaram S, You J. Targeting persistent human papillomavirus infection. Viruses. 2017;9:229.

109. Berrington de González A, Green J. International Collaboration of Epidemiological Studies of Cervical Cancer Comparison of risk factors for invasive squamous cell carcinoma and adenocarcinoma of the cervix: collaborative reanalysis of individual data on 8,097 women with squamous cell carcinoma and 1,374 women with adenocarcinoma from 12 epidemiological studies. Int J Cancer. 2007;120:885–91.

110. International Collaboration of Epidemiological Studies of Cervical Cancer, Appleby P, Beral V, Berrington de González A, Colin D, Franceschi S, Goodhill A, Green J, Peto J, Plummer M, et al. Cervical cancer and hormonal contraceptives: collaborative reanalysis of individual data for 16,573 women with cervical cancer and 35,509 women without cervical cancer from 24 epidemiological studies. Lancet. 2007;370: 1609–21.

111. Dugué P-A, Rebolj M, Garred P, Lynge E. Immunosuppression and risk of cervical cancer. Expert Rev Anticancer Ther. 2013;13:29–42.

112. Hammer A, Rositch A, Qeadan F, Gravitt PE, Blaakaer J. Age-specific prevalence of HPV16/18 genotypes in cervical cancer: a systematic review and meta-analysis. Int J Cancer. 2016;138:2795–803.

113. Li N, Franceschi S, Howell-Jones R, Snijders PJF, Clifford GM. Human papillomavirus type distribution in 30,848 invasive cervical cancers worldwide: variation by geographical region, histological type and year of publication. Int J Cancer. 2011;128:927–35.

114. Psyrri A, DiMaio D. Human papillomavirus in cervical and head-and-neck cancer. Nat Clin Pract Oncol. 2008;5:24–31.

115. Wright TC, Stoler MH, Behrens CM, Sharma A, Zhang G, Wright TL. Primary cervical cancer screening with human papillomavirus: end of study results from the ATHENA study using HPV as the first-line screening test. Gynecol Oncol. 2015;136:189–97.

116. Ronco G, Dillner J, Elfström KM, Tunesi S, Snijders PJF, Arbyn M, Kitchener H, Segnan N, Gilham C, Giorgi-Rossi P, et al. Efficacy of HPV-based screening for prevention of invasive cervical cancer: follow-up of four European randomised controlled trials. Lancet. 2014;383:524–32.

117. US Preventive Services Task Force, Curry SJ, Krist AH, Owens DK, Barry MJ, Caughey AB, Davidson KW, Doubeni CA, Epling JW, Kemper AR, et al. Screening for cervical cancer: US preventive services task force recommendation statement. JAMA. 2018;320:674–86.

118. Solomon D, Davey D, Kurman R, Moriarty A, O'Connor D, Prey M, Raab S, Sherman M, Wilbur D, Wright T, et al. The 2001 Bethesda system: terminology for reporting results of cervical cytology. JAMA. 2002;287:2114–9.

119. Apter D, Wheeler CM, Paavonen J, Castellsagué X, Garland SM, Skinner SR, Naud P, Salmerón J, Chow S-N, Kitchener HC, et al. Efficacy of human papillomavirus 16 and 18 (HPV-16/18) AS04-adjuvanted vaccine against cervical infection and precancer in young women: final event-driven analysis of the randomized, double-blind PATRICIA trial. Clin Vaccine Immunol. 2015;22:361–73.

120. FUTURE II Study Group. Quadrivalent vaccine against human papillomavirus to prevent high-grade cervical lesions. N Engl J Med. 2007;356:1915–27.

121. Sankaranarayanan R, Joshi S, Muwonge R, Esmy PO, Basu P, Prabhu P, Bhatla N, Nene BM, Shaw J, Poli URR, et al. Can a single dose of human papillomavirus (HPV) vaccine prevent cervical cancer? Early findings from an Indian study. Vaccine. 2018;36:4783–91.

122. Safaeian M, Sampson JN, Pan Y, Porras C, Kemp TJ, Herrero R, Quint W, van Doorn LJ, Schussler J, Lowy DR, et al. Durability of protection afforded by fewer doses of the HPV16/18 vaccine: the CVT trial. J Natl Cancer Inst. 2018;110:205.

123. Petrosky E, Bocchini JA, Hariri S, Chesson H, Curtis CR, Saraiya M, Unger ER, Markowitz LE. Centers for Disease Control and Prevention (CDC) use of 9-valent human papillomavirus (HPV) vaccine: updated HPV vaccination recommendations of the advisory committee on immunization practices. MMWR Morb Mortal Wkly Rep. 2015;64:300–4.

124. Joura EA, Giuliano AR, Iversen O-E, Bouchard C, Mao C, Mehlsen J, Moreira ED, Ngan Y, Petersen LK, Lazcano-Ponce E, et al. A 9-valent HPV vaccine against infection and intraepithelial neoplasia in women. N Engl J Med. 2015;372:711–23.

125. Alemany L, Cubilla A, Halec G, Kasamatsu E, Quirós B, Masferrer E, Tous S, Lloveras B, Hernández-Suarez G, Lonsdale R, et al. Role of human papillomavirus in penile carcinomas worldwide. Eur Urol. 2016;69:953–61.

126. Castellsagué X, Muñoz N, Pitisuttithum P, Ferris D, Monsonego J, Ault K, Luna J, Myers E, Mallary S, Bautista OM, et al. End-of-study safety, immunogenicity, and efficacy of quadrivalent HPV (types 6, 11, 16, 18) recombinant vaccine in adult women 24-45 years of age. Br J Cancer. 2011;105:28–37.

127. Skinner SR, Szarewski A, Romanowski B, Garland SM, Lazcano-Ponce E, Salmerón J, Del Rosario-Raymundo MR, Verheijen RHM, Quek SC, da Silva DP, et al. Efficacy, safety, and immunogenicity of the human papillomavirus 16/18 AS04-adjuvanted vaccine in women older than 25 years: 4-year interim follow-up of the phase 3, double-blind, randomised controlled VIVIANE study. Lancet. 2014;384:2213–27.

128. Sherman ME, Wang SS, Carreon J, Devesa SS. Mortality trends for cervical squamous and adenocarcinoma in the United States. Relation to incidence and survival. Cancer. 2005;103:1258–64.

129. Wagenaar HC, Trimbos JB, Postema S, Anastasopoulou A, van der Geest RJ, Reiber JH, Kenter GG, Peters AA, Pattynama PM. Tumor diameter and volume assessed by magnetic resonance imaging in the prediction of outcome for invasive cervical cancer. Gynecol Oncol. 2001;82:474–82.

130. Patel CN, Nazir SA, Khan Z, Gleeson FV, Bradley KM. 18F-FDG PET/CT of cervical carcinoma. AJR Am J Roentgenol. 2011;196:1225–33.

131. TNM classification of malignant tumours. 8th ed: Wiley. Available online: https://www.wiley.com/en-us/TNM+Classification+of+Malignant+Tumours%2C+8th+Edition-p-9781119263579. Accessed on 20 Jan 2020.

132. Bhatla N, Aoki D, Sharma DN, Sankaranarayanan R. Cancer of the cervix uteri. Int J Gynaecol Obstet. 2018;143(Suppl 2):22–36.

133. Mabuchi S, Okazawa M, Matsuo K, Kawano M, Suzuki O, Miyatake T, Enomoto T, Kamiura S, Ogawa K, Kimura T. Impact of histological subtype on survival of patients with surgically-treated stage IA2-IIB cervical cancer: adenocarcinoma versus squamous cell carcinoma. Gynecol Oncol. 2012;127:114–20.

134. Kim SM, Choi HS, Byun JS. Overall 5-year survival rate and prognostic factors in patients with stage IB and IIA cervical cancer treated by radical hysterectomy and pelvic lymph node dissection. Int J Gynecol Cancer. 2000;10:305–12.

135. Moscicki A-B, Shiboski S, Hills NK, Powell KJ, Jay N, Hanson EN, Miller S, Canjura-Clayton KL, Farhat S, Broering JM, et al. Regression of low-grade squamous intra-epithelial lesions in young women. Lancet. 2004;364:1678–83.

53

136. Mello V, Sundstrom RK. Cancer, cervical intraepithelial neoplasia (CIN). In: StatPearls. Treasure Island: StatPearls Publishing; 2019.

137. Massad LS, Einstein MH, Huh WK, Katki HA, Kinney WK, Schiffman M, Solomon D, Wentzensen N, Lawson HW. 2012 ASCCP consensus guidelines conference 2012 updated consensus guidelines for the management of abnormal cervical cancer screening tests and cancer precursors. J Low Genit Tract Dis. 2013;17:S1–S27.

138. Querleu D, Cibula D, Abu-Rustum NR. 2017 update on the Querleu–Morrow classification of radical hysterectomy. Ann Surg Oncol. 2017;24:3406–12.

139. Radical versus simple hysterectomy and pelvic node dissection in patients with low-risk early stage cervical cancer (SHAPE) - full text view - ClinicalTrials.gov Available online: https://clinicaltrials.gov/ct2/show/NCT01658930.

140. Lécuru F, Mathevet P, Querleu D, Leblanc E, Morice P, Daraï E, Marret H, Magaud L, Gillaizeau F, Chatellier G, et al. Bilateral negative sentinel nodes accurately predict absence of lymph node metastasis in early cervical cancer: results of the SENTICOL study. J Clin Oncol. 2011;29:1686–91.

141. Diab Y. Sentinel lymph nodes mapping in cervical cancer a comprehensive review. Int J Gynecol Cancer. 2017;27:154–8.

142. Cormier B, Diaz JP, Shih K, Sampson RM, Sonoda Y, Park KJ, Alektiar K, Chi DS, Barakat RR, Abu-Rustum NR. Establishing a sentinel lymph node mapping algorithm for the treatment of early cervical cancer. Gynecol Oncol. 2011;122:275–80.

143. Yoneda JY, Braganca JF, Sarian LO, Borba PP, Conceição JCJ, Zeferino LC. Surgical treatment of microinvasive cervical cancer: analysis of pathologic features with implications on radicality. Int J Gynecol Cancer. 2015;25:694–8.

144. Lanowska M, Mangler M, Spek A, Grittner U, Hasenbein K, Chiantera V, Hertel H, Schneider A, Köhler C, Speiser D. Radical vaginal trachelectomy (RVT) combined with laparoscopic lymphadenectomy: prospective study of 225 patients with early-stage cervical cancer. Int J Gynecol Cancer. 2011;21:1458–64.

145. Fanfani F, Landoni F, Gagliardi ML, Fagotti A, Preti E, Moruzzi MC, Monterossi G, Scambia G. Sexual and reproductive outcomes in early stage cervical cancer patients after excisional cone as a fertility-sparing surgery: an Italian experience. J Reprod Infertil. 2014;15:29–34.

146. Baalbergen A, Veenstra Y, Stalpers L. Primary surgery versus primary radiotherapy with or without chemotherapy for early adenocarcinoma of the uterine cervix. Cochrane Database Syst Rev. 2013:CD006248.

147. Landoni F, Colombo A, Milani R, Placa F, Zanagnolo V, Mangioni C. Randomized study between radical surgery and radiotherapy for the treatment of stage IB-IIA cervical cancer: 20-year update. J Gynecol Oncol. 2017;28:e34.

148. Rotman M, Sedlis A, Piedmonte MR, Bundy B, Lentz SS, Muderspach LI, Zaino RJ. A phase III randomized trial of postoperative pelvic irradiation in stage IB cervical carcinoma with poor prognostic features: follow-up of a gynecologic oncology group study. Int J Radiat Oncol Biol Phys. 2006;65:169–76.

149. Peters WA, Liu PY, Barrett RJ, Stock RJ, Monk BJ, Berek JS, Souhami L, Grigsby P, Gordon W, Alberts DS. Concurrent chemotherapy and pelvic radiation therapy compared with pelvic radiation therapy alone as adjuvant therapy after radical surgery in high-risk early-stage cancer of the cervix. J Clin Oncol. 2000;18:1606–13.

150. Chemoradiotherapy for Cervical Cancer Meta-analysis Collaboration (CCCMAC). Reducing uncertainties about the effects of chemoradiotherapy for cervical cancer: individual patient data meta-analysis. Cochrane Database Syst Rev. 2010:CD008285.

151. Marth C, Vulsteke C, Rubio MJ, Makker V, Braicu EI, McNeish IA, Radoslaw M, Ayhan A, Hasegawa K, Wu X, et al. 1063TiPENGOT-EN9/LEAP-001: a phase III, randomized, open-label study of pembrolizumab plus lenvatinib versus chemotherapy for first-line treatment of advanced or recurrent endometrial cancer. Ann Oncol. 2019;30

152. Pötter R, Haie-Meder C, Van Limbergen E, Barillot I, De Brabandere M, Dimopoulos J, Dumas I, Erickson B, Lang S, Nulens A, et al. Recommendations from gynaecological (GYN) GEC ESTRO working group (II): concepts and terms in 3D image-based treatment planning in cervix cancer brachytherapy-3D dose volume parameters and aspects of 3D image-based anatomy, radiation physics, radiobiology. Radiother Oncol. 2006;78:67–77.

153. Dueñas-González A, Zarbá JJ, Patel F, Alcedo JC, Beslija S, Casanova L, Pattaranutaporn P, Hameed S, Blair JM, Barraclough H, et al. Phase III, open-label, randomized study comparing concurrent gemcitabine plus cisplatin and radiation followed by adjuvant gemcitabine and cisplatin versus concurrent cisplatin and radiation in patients with stage IIB to IVA carcinoma of the cervix. J Clin Oncol. 2011;29:1678–85.

154. Takekuma M, Takahashi F, Arimoto T, Ishikawa M, Ota Y, Kagabu M, Kasamatsu T, Kanao H, Kawamura N, Kitagawa R, et al. Determination of eligibility criteria for salvage hysterectomy after definitive radiotherapy/concurrent chemoradiotherapy for residual cervical disease. JCO. 2019;37:5524.

155. Kenter G, Greggi S, Vergote I, Katsaros D, Kobierski J, Massuger L, van Doorn HC, Landoni F, Van Der Velden J, Reed NS, et al. Results from neoadjuvant chemotherapy followed by surgery compared to chemoradiation for stage Ib2-IIb cervical cancer, EORTC 55994. JCO. 2019;37:5503.

156. Gupta S, Maheshwari A, Parab P, Mahantshetty U, Hawaldar R, Sastri Chopra S, Kerkar R, Engineer R, Tongaonkar H, Ghosh J, et al. Neoadjuvant chemotherapy followed by radical surgery versus concomitant chemotherapy and radiotherapy in patients with stage IB2, IIA, or IIB squamous cervical cancer: a randomized controlled trial. J Clin Oncol. 2018;36:1548–55.

157. Induction Chemotherapy Plus Chemoradiation as First Line Treatment for Locally Advanced Cervical Cancer - Full Text View - ClinicalTrials.gov Available online: https://clinicaltrials.gov/ct2/show/NCT01566240. Accessed on 20 2020.

158. Mileshkin LR, Narayan K, Moore KN, Rischin D, King M, Kolodziej I, Martyn J, Friedlander M, Quinn M, Small W, et al. A phase III trial of adjuvant chemotherapy following chemoradiation as primary treatment for locally advanced cervical cancer compared to chemoradiation alone: Outback (ANZGOG0902/GOG0274/RTOG1174). JCO. 2014;32:TPS5632–TPS5632.

159. Friedlander M, Grogan M. U.S. Preventative Services Task Force Guidelines for the treatment of recurrent and metastatic cervical cancer. Oncologist. 2002;7:342–7.

160. Tewari KS, Sill MW, Penson RT, Huang H, Ramondetta LM, Landrum LM, Oaknin A, Reid TJ, Leitao MM, Michael HE, et al. Bevacizumab for advanced cervical cancer: final overall survival and adverse event analysis of a randomised, controlled, open-label, phase 3 trial (Gynecologic Oncology Group 240). Lancet. 2017;390:1654–63.

161. Kitagawa R, Katsumata N, Shibata T, Kamura T, Kasamatsu T, Nakanishi T, Nishimura S, Ushijima K, Takano M, Satoh T, et al. Paclitaxel plus carboplatin versus paclitaxel plus cisplatin in metastatic or recurrent cervical cancer: the open-label randomized phase III trial JCOG0505. J Clin Oncol. 2015;33:2129–35.

162. Monk BJ, Sill MW, McMeekin DS, Cohn DE, Ramondetta LM, Boardman CH, Benda J, Cella D. Phase III trial of four cisplatin-containing doublet combinations in stage IVB, recur-

rent, or persistent cervical carcinoma: a Gynecologic Oncology Group study. J Clin Oncol. 2009;27:4649–55.

163. Smith SC, Koh WJ. Palliative radiation therapy for gynaeco-logical malignancies. Best Pract Res Clin Obstet Gynaecol. 2001;15:265–78.

164. Cohen PA, Jhingran A, Oaknin A, Denny L. Cervical cancer. Lancet. 2019;393:169–82.

165. Mackay HJ, Tinker A, Winquist E, Thomas G, Swenerton K, Oza A, Sederias J, Ivy P, Eisenhauer EA. A phase II study of sunitinib in patients with locally advanced or metastatic cer-vical carcinoma: NCIC CTG trial IND.184. Gynecol Oncol. 2010;116:163–7.

166. Monk BJ, Mas Lopez L, Zarba JJ, Oaknin A, Tarpin C, Termrungruanglert W, Alber JA, Ding J, Stutts MW, Pan-dite LN. Phase II, open-label study of pazopanib or lapatinib monotherapy compared with pazopanib plus lapatinib combi-nation therapy in patients with advanced and recurrent cervical cancer. J Clin Oncol. 2010;28:3562–9.

167. Pignata S, Scambia G, Lorusso D, De Giorgi U, Nicoletto MO, Lauria R, Mosconi AM, Sacco C, Omarini C, Tagliaferri P, et al. The MITO CERV-2 trial: a randomized phase II study of cetuximab plus carboplatin and paclitaxel, in advanced or recurrent cervical cancer. Gynecol Oncol. 2019;153:535–40.

168. Naumann RW, Hollebecque A, Meyer T, Devlin M-J, Oaknin A, Kerger J, López-Picazo JM, Machiels J-P, Delord J-P, Evans TRJ, et al. Safety and efficacy of Nivolumab monotherapy in recurrent or metastatic cervical, vaginal, or vulvar carcinoma: results from the phase I/II CheckMate 358 trial. J Clin Oncol. 2019;37:2825–34.

169. Chung HC, Ros W, Delord J-P, Perets R, Italiano A, Shapira-Frommer R, Manzuk L, Piha-Paul SA, Xu L, Zeigenfuss S, et al. Efficacy and safety of Pembrolizumab in previously treated advanced cervical cancer: results from the phase II KEYNOTE-158 study. J Clin Oncol. 2019;37:1470–8.

170. Minion LE, Tewari KS. Cervical cancer - state of the science: from angiogenesis blockade to checkpoint inhibition. Gynecol Oncol. 2018;148:609–21.

171. Elit L, Fyles AW, Devries MC, Oliver TK, Fung-Kee-Fung M. Gynecology Cancer Disease Site Group follow-up for women after treatment for cervical cancer: a systematic review. Gynecol Oncol. 2009;114:528–35.

172. Salani R, Backes FJ, Fung MFK, Holschneider CH, Parker LP, Bristow RE, Goff BA. Posttreatment surveillance and diag-nosis of recurrence in women with gynecologic malignancies: Society of Gynecologic Oncologists recommendations. Am J Obstet Gynecol. 2011;204:466–78.

53

Vulvar and Vaginal Cancers

Nicla La Verde, Aurelia Ada Guarini, Lavinia Insalaco, and Domenica Lorusso

Gynecological Cancers

Contents

© Springer Nature Switzerland AG 2021
A. Russo et al. (eds.), *Practical Medical Oncology Textbook*, UNIPA Springer Series,
https://doi.org/10.1007/978-3-030-56051-5_54

Learning Objectives

By the end of the chapter, the reader will:

- Have learned the basic concepts of epidemiology, histological subtype, and clinical manifestation of vulvar and vaginal cancer
- Be able to define staging strategies and diagnostic and therapeutic procedures
- Be able to put acquired knowledge into clinical practice
- Be able to realize future perspectives of vulvar and vaginal cancer

54.1 Vulvar Cancer

54.1.1 Overview

Vulvar cancer is considered as a rare tumor and it accounts for 4 % of gynecologic malignancies; the median age of diagnosis is 68 years. The 5-year survival rates range from 86 % of localized disease (stage I and II) to 53 % of locally advanced disease (stage III) and 19 % for patients with metastatic disease (stage IV). The most common histologic path is the squamous cell carcinoma (SCC). There are also many other rarer histologies: melanoma, Bartholin gland adenocarcinoma, verrucous carcinoma, extramammary Paget disease, and sarcoma.

Risk factors are represented by human papillomavirus (HPV) infection, cigarette smoking, inflammatory conditions of the vulva, aging, and immunodeficiency.

Ninety percent of vulvar cancer is of SCC histology. The noninvasive vulvar intraepithelial neoplasias (VINs) are correlated in approximately 52–100 % of cases to human papillomavirus (HPV). VINs can be divided into "usual" VIN (uVIN), normally caused by HPV infection, and "differentiated" VIN (dVIN), not caused by infection but correlated to inflammatory lesions, like lichen sclerosus.

The International Society for the Study of Vulvovaginal Disease defined a new classification in low-grade squamous intraepithelial lesion (LSIL), including condyloma and HPV effect, and high-grade squamous intraepithelial lesion (HSIL), which corresponds to uVIN of the previous classification and dVIN. There is another variant called Bowenoid papulosis (BP) that can appear similar to uVIN or HSIL but it disappears spontaneously (World Health Organization Classification of Tumours of Female Reproductive Organs, 4th edn., IARC).

There are many benign conditions that may develop into vulvar carcinoma; *lichen sclerosus* is the most common inflammatory, noninfectious disorder of the vulva, and it can be associated with VIN and vulvar carcinoma in 15% to 40% of cases. Lichen planus is a dermatosis but, as well as lichen sclerosis, it can evolve into erosive vulvar disease, which has been associated with invasive vulvar squamous cell carcinoma.

Extramammary Paget disease of the vulva is an eczematous lesion that appears on the vulva and, rarely, it may be associated with underlying cutaneous adenocarcinoma [1].

54.1.2 Clinical Presentation, Diagnosis, and Work-Up

Currently the guidelines used are the International Federation of Gynecology and Obstetrics (FIGO) and American Joint Committee on Cancer (AJCC) TNM staging systems. There are a few updates on these available guidelines that include the revision of stage III that now includes the positivity of the groin lymph nodes, while patients with positive pelvic lymph nodes are considered stage IVB.

The clinical presentation of vulvar cancer can be varied. The most common presentation is within the labia majora; other possible sites are the clitoris, mons, or perineum. Patients with HPV-positive tumors can have multifocal lesions and concurrent cervical neoplasia can be present. Many cases may be asymptomatic while itchiness, bleeding, pain, and irritation can occur as the most common symptoms.

Diagnosis is made through biopsy of the suspicious areas. Once the diagnosis of vulvar cancer is confirmed, the work-up includes history and physical examination, while the imaging techniques used are CT, PET-CT, and MRI that may be helpful to stage the disease and to delineate the extent of the tumor. CT scan is a useful tool to do a clinical staging of the disease and to detect distant metastases. MRI is performed to understand the real extension of the disease; in the TNM system staging, the parameters T and N can be studied through this abovementioned technique. PET-CT scan is performed when the disease is locally advanced to better understand if the first approach should be surgical or medical. HPV testing is always recommended while HIV testing is suggested in younger patients.

54.1.3 Prognostic Factors and Surgical Staging

AJCC and FIGO TNM staging systems are both used to delineate the disease. The clinical staging alone is not useful to define the lymph node involvement; the node (N) parameter is a fundamental prognostic factor to establish the vulvar cancer survival [2].

A complete lymph node staging requires a full inguinofemoral lymphadenectomy. However, common practice has included the use of the sentinel lymph node (SLN) biopsy in order to obtain a proper disease staging in the early disease, where lymphadenectomy could be avoided because of its morbidity.

Other prognostic factors in vulvar cancer represent the tumor site, tumor size, number of tumor foci, histologic type and grade, depth of stromal invasion, surgical margin status, and presence of lymphovascular invasion. Additionally, tumor involvement of tissues/organs such as vagina, urethra, anus, and rectal mucosa is an important prognostic factor [3, 4].

■ **Primary Tumor Resection**

The surgical technique used can be local excision or vulvectomy: it depends on tumor extent. However, the surgical techniques mentioned involve resection of approximately 1- to 2-cm radial margin of grossly normal tissue and a minimum of 1-cm-deep margin of deep fascia.

Vulvar cancer has a high recurrence rate and the goal of primary resection is the complete removal with 1- to 2-cm margins; moreover, in a recent study of Arvas et al., tumor-free margins of at least 2 mm have been associated to a decreased local recurrence risk [5].

■ **Lymph Node Evaluation**

Lymph node dissection in patients can be omitted in patients with stage IA, since the lymph node involvement at this stage is less than 1%. The SLN and inguinofemoral lymphadenectomy is recommended starting from the stage IB, because the risk of lymph node involvement is greater than 8% and it grows for stages beyond the IB [6].

The *SLN assessment* has the role to avoid a unilateral or bilateral inguinofemoral lymphadenectomy that can have many side effects like lymphedema. The safety and accuracy of SLN assessment has been examined in a multicenter observational study (GROINSS-VI). 403 women with vulvar tumors<4 cm did not undergo lymphadenectomy if SLN was negative. The median follow-up period was 35 months and recurrence was observed in only 6 of 259 patients with a unifocal primary tumor and negative SLN. The study demonstrated that in early-stage vulvar cancer, the groin recurrence was low when the SLN assessment was performed [7].

54.1.4 Management

■ **Early-Stage Disease**

In the early-stage disease, the better treatment is represented by radical local incision or vulvectomy; the right approach is still debated and remains a surgical decision.

Stehman et al. have compared groin dissection versus groin irradiation and they noted that the surgical removal of lymph nodes had a better outcome and disease control and lower recurrence rates than radiation therapy.

T1 tumors should undergo local resection or radical local resection and the SLN is recommended. Surgery of T1b or smaller T2 is led by tumor location. Lateralized lesions at >2 cm from the vulvar midline should undergo radical resection or modified radical vulvectomy and ipsilateral groin node evaluation.

Patients with midline vulvar lesions should undergo radical local resection or modified radical vulvectomy [8].

■ **Adjuvant Treatment**

There are limited prospective randomized trials on the adjuvant treatment of vulvar cancer due to the rarity of the disease.

Node involvement is an important prognostic factor and adjuvant treatment should be addressed to these patients.

The GOG 37 enrolled 114 patients with groin node-positive vulvar cancer after radical vulvectomy and bilateral inguinofemoral lymphadenectomy. Patients were randomly assigned to receive pelvic node dissection or adjuvant radiotherapy to the groin/pelvis. A long-term follow-up demonstrated that the higher rates of disease-related death were registered in the group that received pelvic node dissection compared with pelvic/groin RT [9].

A more recent study showed that, among 444 elderly patients (median age of 78) with node-positive vulvar cancer, the better outcomes were reached from the patients that underwent adjuvant radiotherapy.

External beam irradiation should be performed as adjuvant treatment in patients with close margins or with positive sentinel lymph node or with one or more lymph nodes positive for metastases at inguinofemoral lymphadenectomy (see ▫ Table 54.1).

■ **Locally Advanced Disease**

In the past, the locally advanced disease was primarily treated with radical surgery such as en bloc radical vulvectomy with bilateral inguinofemoral lymphadenectomy; however, these surgeries had significant postoperative complications.

Nowadays, a multimodality treatment has been explored and implemented. Preoperative radiotherapy is demonstrated to have a debulking role and to reduce the surgical treatment morbidity. Additionally, chemotherapy is demonstrated to sensitize the disease to radiations [10].

■ **Chemoradiation**

Patients with stage III/IV disease may benefit from a concurrent chemo- and radiation therapy treatment: this choice results in a longer survival rate and recurrence rate [11].

Table 54.1 Management of inguinal lymph nodes of vulvar cancer

Management after inguinal node dissection

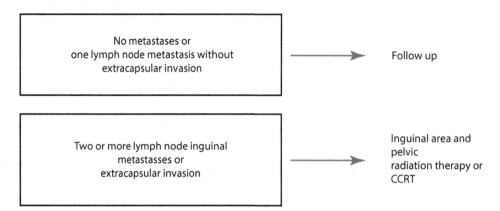

In the GOG 101 study, 73 patients underwent chemoradiation before surgery and a residual disease was just detected in 3% of patients treated [12].

An analysis of NCDB data (2004–2012) compared the outcomes of 2046 women with locally advanced vulvar carcinoma who underwent chemotherapy or chemoradiation treatment before surgery. Patients who underwent surgery after the combination treatment had a higher OS compared to patients that received chemotherapy alone [13].

Many other studies assessed the efficacy and safety of a preoperative surgery in a locally advanced disease, and the preferred chemotherapy regimens used were cisplatin and 5-fluorouracil and mitomycin and 5-fluorouracil.

■ **Recurrent and Metastatic Disease**
According to NCCN guidelines, the preferred chemotherapy regimens used in the recurrent/metastatic setting are represented by cisplatin and carboplatin as single agents, as well as the combination of cisplatin or carboplatin with paclitaxel, with or without bevacizumab.

Cisplatin is used as a radiosensitizing agent and it has been demonstrated that short- and long-term complication rates were acceptable, with a promising OS and DFS. Additionally, due to the lack of tissue toxicity, this strategy allowed physicians to surgically treat regional lymph node recurrence safely [14].

Carboplatin can be a valid alternative to cisplatin. The JCOG0505 randomized phase III trial assessed that carboplatin-based regimen was non-inferior to cisplatin-based regimen [15].

Prospective trials confirmed that the prognosis for inguinofemoral recurrence is poor. If this event occurs, radiotherapy or concomitant chemotherapy and radiation therapy can be considered. Re-excision for inguinal node recurrence is not a standard of care but can be performed in selected patients [16].

Paclitaxel can also be used as single agent in patients not eligible for locoregional treatment. A phase II study (EORTC-GCG, European Organisation for Research and Treatment of Cancer – Gynaecological Cancer Group) demonstrated that taxol administered once every 3 weeks in patients with metastatic/recurrent vulvar cancer, not amenable for locoregional treatment, had moderate activity for local control. The study registered an ORR of 13.8% and a median PFS of 2.6 months (median follow-up was 24 months).

Immunotherapy has been recently introduced in trial enrolling patients with vulvar cancer. In fact, pembrolizumab has been studied and approved for a second-line therapy for PDL-1-positive or MSI (microsatellite instability) cervical cancers [17]. KEYNOTE-158 is an ongoing trial that is enrolling patients with advanced vulvar cancer to receive pembrolizumab as second-line treatment (NCT02628067).

54.1.5 Follow-Up

Most recurrences of vulvar cancer occur within the first 1 or 2 years. A retrospective analysis of 330 patients with vulvar cancer at Mayo Clinic was conducted and showed that the higher rates of treatment failure were registered in patients with inguinofemoral node involvement, within a 2-year follow up, suggesting that the node involvement is one of the most important prognostic factors. In 35% of patients, disease occurred 5 years or more after diagnosis; this last information suggests the importance of a long-term follow-up [18].

The recommended surveillance is based on the disease stage. History and physical examination should be performed for all patients every 2–3 months for the first 2 years and every 6 months for another 3–5 years. Patients with high risk of recurrence (stage III) can be assessed more frequently. Annual cervical/vaginal cytology can be indicated in order to detect lower tract dysplasia. Imaging techniques such as CT, PET-CT, and MRI are indicated for suspicious examination findings or symptoms.

54.2 Vaginal Cancer

54.2.1 Overview

Vaginal cancer is a rare disease (1% of the gynecological cancers). The commonest histology is the squamous cell carcinoma, while only 5–10% is adenocarcinoma. The risk factors are similar to the cervical cancer ones; in particular HPV infection and age are involved (PMID: 26411952).

The most common sites for vaginal cancer are the upper third of the vagina (56%) followed by the lower third (31%) and the middle third (13%) [19].

The upper two-thirds of the vagina are drained into pelvic nodes while the lower third drains into the inguinal nodes so that the metastatic routes depend on the site of the primary tumor.

The surgical approach is chosen based on the site of the primary tumor and the surgeon should consider the removal of both the primary tumor and the regional lymph nodes.

Recurrences are usually treated with chemotherapy; however, due to the rarity of this disease, there are few studies in this setting [19].

54.2.2 Histopathological Approaches

The most common histology of vaginal cancer is the squamous cell carcinoma (SCC).

SCC can be histologically divided into five different types: keratinizing, non-keratinizing, basaloid, verrucous, and warty. HPV infection is detected in 80% of cases of vaginal cancer, mostly in the non-keratinizing variant [20].

As for cervical intraepithelial neoplasia (CIN), there is a vaginal intraepithelial neoplasia that is defined as the presence of atypical squamous cells within the vagina epithelium that is not accompanied by interstitial infiltrate. Vaginal intraepithelial neoplasia (VAIN) is classified into three grades: VAIN 1, VAIN 2, and VAIN 3. The largest part of VAIN is caused by HPV infection. VAIN 1 is also called LSIL while VAIN 2 and 3 correspond to HSIL [21].

A less frequent histology is the adenocarcinoma of the vulva that is frequently diagnosed in women who had been exposed in utero to synthetic non-steroid estrogens such as diethylstilbestrol (DES). It was typically used in pregnant women in the 1950s and many cases of vaginal cancers were diagnosed in their young children in the 1970s [22, 23].

The staging of vaginal cancer is performed according to the FIGO classification. In stage I and II the carcinoma is limited at vaginal and subvaginal tissue, in stage III it is extended to the pelvic wall, and in stage IV it is extended beyond the true pelvis and invades bladder and/or rectal mucosa (IVa) or is spread to distant organs (IVb) [23].

54.2.3 Management

■ **Principles of Surgical and Radiation Therapy**

Surgery remains the gold standard for resectable vaginal cancer. The type of surgery depends on the site of the disease and on its extension. If the tumor occurs in the upper third of the vagina, surgery consists of hysterectomy extended to the vagina. If vaginal cancer also presents VAIN, a total vaginectomy is recommended. Moreover, pelvic exenteration could represent an option in selected cases [24]. In particular, surgery is recommended for stage I disease and tumor localized in the upper third of the vagina [23]. If the tumor has a large extension and it is mainly localized in the lower part of the vagina, radiation therapy is preferred. If the tumor is small and is localized in the lower third of the vagina, surgery remains highly recommended [24].

Extended surgery such as pelvic exenteration may be considered if the patient has the invasive tumor to the rectum or urinary bladder, a rectovaginal or vesicovaginal fistula, or local recurrent tumors after radiation therapy.

A retrospective study performed by the Magee Hospital of Pittsburgh reported a better prognosis for patients that underwent surgery than irradiation therapy alone in stage I and II disease with an upper third vagina localization [25].

Additionally, the histological features of the disease can determine the treatment strategy; the majority of vaginal cancer has a squamous histopathology while a minority is adenocarcinoma. It has been reported that the adenocarcinoma is poorly sensitive to radiation therapy; thus, surgical therapy is recommended.

Due to the rarity of the disease, there is a lack of randomized trials and only retrospective studies are reported. According to these reports, relevant prognostic factors are tumor size and lymph node involvement.

Radiation therapy is recommended to preserve the function of adjacent organs, when the disease is locally advanced. Methods of irradiation therapy include brachytherapy and more recently image-guided brachytherapy (IMBT). External beam irradiation based on 3D treatment planning using CT and MRI has become a standard [23, 26].

More specifically, stage I disease may benefit from brachytherapy alone or in combination with external beam irradiation (with tumor thickness <5 mm, while for tumor thickness greater than 5 mm or at stages II to IVA, external beam irradiation is recommended). Also, concurrent chemotherapy with carboplatin or cisplatin may be considered [27].

Concurrent chemo- and radiation therapy is performed using sensitizing agents such as cisplatin and 5-fluorouracil. Because of the rarity of this disease, it is hard to find out the real efficacy of combining treatments. Given that, it is reasonable to apply results of clinical trials regarding cervical cancer, based on similarities of organ sites, risk factors, and histopathology. Physicians must consider concurrent use of chemotherapy in combination with radiation therapy if the tumor is stage III or IVA, >4 cm in diameter, or positive for lymph node metastasis [23, 27, 28] (see ◘ Tables 54.2 and 54.3).

54.2.4 Follow-Up

History and physical examination, cytology, chest X-ray examination, tumor markers, and CT should be performed every 2–3 months for the first 2 years, every 6 months through the fifth year, and once a year for the sixth and subsequent years.

The higher risk of recurrence has been registered in the first 2 years after the diagnosis. The recurrence rates decrease after 5 years [29].

Recurrence can be confirmed using cytology and biopsy and CT, MRI, and PET are indicated for suspicious findings.

The first choice for locoregional relapse is radiation therapy; when distant metastases occur, chemotherapy is the treatment selected [23].

54.3 Summary: Conclusion

Vulvar and Vaginal cancer are considered rare diseases with a low incidence but a relative increase in the most industrialized countries. surgery is the recommended primary treatment for localized vulvar and vaginal cancer (stage I), while locally advanced diseases may benefit of concurrent chemo and radiation therapy. The preferred chemotherapy regimens are cisplatin or carboplatin and 5FU. Immunotherapy (Pembrolizumab) is still under investigation in the second line treatment of metastatic vulvar cancer.

◘ **Table 54.2** Primary treatment for early-stage vaginal cancer

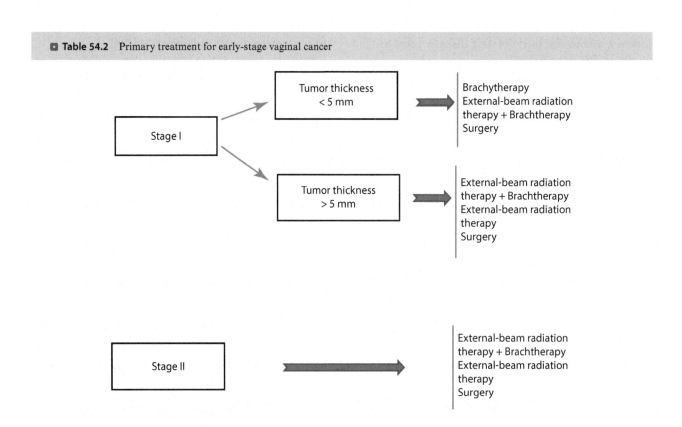

Table 54.3 Primary treatment for locally advanced and metastatic vaginal cancer

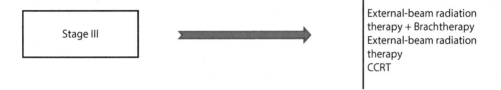

Stage III → External-beam radiation therapy + Brachtherapy
External-beam radiation therapy
CCRT

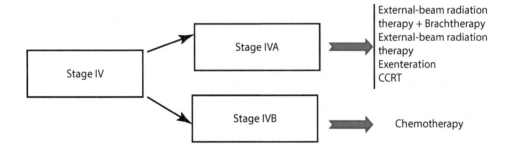

Stage IV → Stage IVA → External-beam radiation therapy + Brachtherapy
External-beam radiation therapy
Exenteration
CCRT

Stage IVB → Chemotherapy

Key Points

- Vulvar and vaginal cancer are considered rare diseases with a low incidence but a relative increase in the most industrialized countries. The main risk factors are HPV infection, age, disadvantaged socio-economic conditions, and cigarette smoking.
- The instrumental diagnostic approach in case of suspected disease is represented by clinical examination, cytology, and biopsy. A more specific evaluation must be carried out using the TC and the MRI; in some circumstances, PET integration can be helpful.
- Currently surgery is the recommended primary treatment for localized vulvar and vaginal cancer (stage I), while locally advanced diseases may benefit from concurrent chemo- and radiation therapy. The preferred chemotherapy regimens are cisplatin or carboplatin and 5-FU. The addition of bevacizumab can be considered in the treatment of metastatic vulvar cancer.
- Local recurrence/persistence: Radiation therapy should be considered for local recurrence. Re-excision of inguinofemoral lymph nodes is discouraged because of postoperative complications.
- Immunotherapy: Pembrolizumab is still under investigation in the second-line treatment of metastatic vulvar cancer.

Case Study: Vulvar Cancer In Situ

Woman, 55 years old
- *Family history:* Negative for malignancy
- *APR:* Nothing to report
- *APP:* Bleeding and itchiness on her vulva
- *Objective examination:* Papules, plaques, and ulcerated lesions on the vulva

Question

What action should be taken?
    (1) Surgery. (2) Biopsy and/or cytology. (3) Others

Answer

Biopsy and path: Usual-type VIN, warty subtype, with HPV changes

Question

What action should be taken?
    (1) Surgery. (2) Medical therapy. (3) Clinical staging

Answer

Surgery: Wide local excision of the lesions
    Path: VIN 2 (HSIL)

Question

What would you do next?

(1) Surgery. (2) Medical therapy. (3) Follow-up

Answer

Follow-up: Clinical examination every 6 months for the first 2 years

Key Points

- The importance of a correct diagnosis: Attention to rectal masses
- Symptoms often nonspecific
- The importance of the management of a locally advanced disease

Case Study: Metastatic Vaginal Cancer

Woman, 70 years old

- *Family history:* Negative for malignancy
- *APR*: Negative
- *APP*: Asthenia, bleeding on the vagina
- *Blood tests*: Hb 9,2 g/dl
- *Objective examination*: Wide ulcerative and bleeding lesion on her vagina
- *Chest and abdominal CT scan*: Multiple lung lesions
- *Biopsy*: Squamous cell carcinoma of the vagina

Question

What action should be taken?

(1) Surgery. (2) Metastasectomy. 3) Chemotherapy

Answer

Chemotherapy with 5-FU and cisplatin

Question

Is metastasectomy on lung lesions recommended?

(1) Yes, after four cycles of chemotherapy. (2) Surgery is not indicated for the metastatic setting. (3) Others

Answer:

No evidence supports resection of metastatic disease.

Key Points

- The importance of a correct diagnosis: Attention to rectal masses
- Importance of the right management for metastatic disease

Expert Opinion
Domenica Lorusso

Key Points

It is estimated that approximately 27.000 and 15000 women worldwide are diagnosed with vulvar cancer and vaginal cancer, respectively, each year thus meaning that both diseases represent rare conditions for which solid literature evidences about treatment are hard to be produced.

Both conditions are, at some extent, related to HPV infections and, in this case, are associated to a better prognosis than non-HPV-related tumors. As such, HPV vaccines represent the best form of primary prevention for both tumors, and last-generation 9-valent HPV vaccine has been calculated to be able to eradicate 90% of HPV-driven cases. Both tumors are preceded by pre-invasive conditions (VIN and VAIN) whose treatment represents a tool to reduce the risk of developing invasive cancer (secondary prevention).

Stage of disease represents the most important prognostic factor with 5-year survival ranging from 80% to 15% for stage I and IV, respectively, for vulvar cancer and from 60 to less than 10% for vaginal cancer.

For vulvar cancers, the mainstay of treatment is represented by the surgical excision of the primary tumor providing free radical 1 cm margins and the surgical assessment of the inguinofemoral nodes through the excision of sentinel lymph node (SLN) in less than 4 cm lateral tumors and by bilateral linguino-femoral lymphadenectomy in all other cases. The role of SLN in tumors larger than 4 cm need to be addressed in future clinical trials.

Radiotherapy and chemoradiation represent the standard of care for more advanced disease when free radical margins are impossible to obtain without extremely demolitive surgical procedures and the adjuvant treatment for node positive patients after radical surgery.

In vaginal cancers, surgery (radical local excision and pelvic lymphadenectomy) has a role limited to stage I disease involving the upper posterior vagina, while radiation or chemoradiotherapy represents the standard of care for most patients.

Chemotherapy has a palliative role in recurrent disease. Most used drugs are platinum, paclitaxel, gemcitabine, and 5-fluorouacil with response rate of about 10–15% and median PFS of less than 3 months. No biological agent has been approved for the treatment of both diseases, but a strong scientific rationale and preliminary clinical data suggest that antiangiogenic agents, tyrosine kinase inhibitors, and EGFR receptor inhibitors may play a role in the treatment of the disease. New agents and new treatment strategies are needed to improve outcome in such setting, and immunotherapy may represent a potent tool particularly for HPV–related tumors as recently reported during the last ASCO meeting.

In most cases, vulvar and vaginal tumors are squamous: to further complicate the scenario, the presence of several rarest histotypes in both the anatomical locations (adenocarcinomas, melanomas, sarcomas) make treatment evidences even more scanty.

The major difficulties in producing strong scientific evidences in these diseases leading to new drug approval is represented by the infrequency of the tumors. I strongly believe this is an area in which international cooperation of groups involved in clinical research may play a fundamental role in ameliorating treatment outcome. Moreover, as for all rare cancers, different study designs and simplified drug approval procedures are mandatory.

In conclusion, vulvar and vaginal cancers are rare malignancies that need to be treated in tertiary referral centers where these diseases can be managed through a multidisciplinary approach.

Key Message

- Vaginal and vulvar cancer are rare diseases that need to be managed in tertiary referral centers in a multidisciplinary approach.
- Most part of these tumors are HPV related and can be prevented by HPV vaccines (primary prevention).

- Both the tumors are anticipated by premalignant lesions that can be cured in order to reduce the incidence of malignant disease (secondary prevention).
- Radical surgery with clear margins and inguinofemoral lymph node evaluation is the mainstay of treatment in early stage vulvar cancers
- Radiotherapy/chemoradiation is the treatment of choice in most part of vaginal cancer and in advanced stage vulvar cancer.
- Chemotherapy has a palliative role in recurrent disease; no biological agents have been approved for the treatment of these rare tumors.
- International collaboration is mandatory in producing evidences for the management of rare tumors.

Discussion Points

- The role of sentinel lymph node in larger than 4 cm tumors need to be addressed.
- The role of isolated tumor cells and micrometastasis on prognosis need to be better clarified.
- New biological agents (antiangiogenic agents, tyrosine kinase inhibitors, and EGFR receptor inhibitors) need to be studied and possibly approved for the management of advanced disease where prognosis remains dismal.
- Different study designs and simplified drug approval procedures are mandatory in rare disease.

Summary of Clinical Recommendations

- *NCCN*
  - ▶ https://www.nccn.org/professionals/physician_gls/pdf/vulvar_blocks.pdf
- *ESGO*
  - ▶ https://guidelines.esgo.org/media/2016/08/ESGO-Vulvar-cancer-Complete-report-fxd2.pdf
- *AIOM*

References

1. Carter JS, Downs LS. Vulvar and vaginal cancer. Obstet Gynecol Clin N Am. 2012;39:213–31.
2. Burger MP, Hollema H, Emanuels AG, Krans M, Pras E, Bouma J. The importance of the groin node status for the survival of T1 and T2 vulval carcinoma patients. Gynecol Oncol. 1995;57:327–34.
3. Landrum LM, Lanneau GS, Skaggs VJ, Gould N, Walker JL, McMeekin DS, Gold MA. Gynecologic Oncology Group risk groups for vulvar carcinoma: improvement in survival in the modern era. Gynecol Oncol. 2007;106:521–5.
4. Slomovitz BM, Coleman RL, Oonk MH, van der Zee A, Levenback C. Update on sentinel lymph node biopsy for early-stage vulvar cancer. Gynecol Oncol. 2015;138:472–7.
5. Arvas M, Kahramanoglu I, Bese T, Turan H, Sozen I, Ilvan S, Demirkiran F. The role of pathological margin distance and prognostic factors after primary surgery in squamous cell carcinoma of the vulva. Int J Gynecol Cancer. 2018;28:623–31.
6. Woelber L, Eulenburg C, Grimm D, Trillsch F, Bohlmann I, Burandt E, Dieckmann J, Klutmann S, Schmalfeldt B, Mahner S, Prieske K. The risk of contralateral non-sentinel metastasis in patients with primary vulvar cancer and unilaterally positive sentinel node. Ann Surg Oncol. 2016;23:2508–14.
7. Van der Zee AG, Oonk MH, De Hullu JA, Ansink AC, Vergote I, Verheijen RH, Maggioni A, Gaarenstroom KN, Baldwin PJ, Van Dorst EB, Van der Velden J, Hermans RH, van der Putten H, Drouin P, Schneider A, Sluiter WJ. Sentinel node dissection is safe in the treatment of early-stage vulvar cancer. J Clin Oncol. 2008;26:884–9.

8. Stehman FB, Bundy BN, Thomas G, Varia M, Okagaki T, Roberts J, Bell J, Heller PB. Groin dissection versus groin radiation in carcinoma of the vulva: a Gynecologic Oncology Group study. Int J Radiat Oncol Biol Phys. 1992;24:389–96.

9. Swanick CW, Eifel PJ, Huo J, Meyer LA, Smith GL. Challenges to delivery and effectiveness of adjuvant radiation therapy in elderly patients with node-positive vulvar cancer. Gynecol Oncol. 2017;146:87–93.

10. Boronow RC. Combined therapy as an alternative to exenteration for locally advanced vulvo-vaginal cancer: rationale and results. Cancer. 1982;49:1085–91.

11. Han SC, Kim DH, Higgins SA, Carcangiu ML, Kacinski BM. Chemoradiation as primary or adjuvant treatment for locally advanced carcinoma of the vulva. Int J Radiat Oncol Biol Phys. 2000;47:1235–44.

12. Lupi G, Raspagliesi F, Zucali R, Fontanelli R, Paladini D, Kenda R, di Re F. Combined preoperative chemoradiotherapy followed by radical surgery in locally advanced vulvar carcinoma. A pilot study. Cancer. 1996;77:1472–8.

13. Berek JS, Heaps JM, Fu YS, Juillard GJ, Hacker NF. Concurrent cisplatin and 5-fluorouracil chemotherapy and radiation therapy for advanced-stage squamous carcinoma of the vulva. Gynecol Oncol. 1991;42:197–201.

14. Bellati F, Angioli R, Manci N, Angelo Zullo M, Muzii L, Plotti F, Basile S, Panici PB. Single agent cisplatin chemotherapy in surgically resected vulvar cancer patients with multiple inguinal lymph node metastases. Gynecol Oncol. 2005;96:227–31.

15. Kitagawa R, Katsumata N, Shibata T, Kamura T, Kasamatsu T, Nakanishi T, Nishimura S, Ushijima K, Takano M, Satoh T, Yoshikawa H. Paclitaxel plus carboplatin versus paclitaxel plus cisplatin in metastatic or recurrent cervical cancer: the open-label randomized phase III trial JCOG0505. J Clin Oncol. 2015;33:2129–35.

16. Salom EM, Penalver M. Recurrent vulvar cancer. Curr Treat Options in Oncol. 2002;3:143–53.

17. Frenel JS, Le Tourneau C, O'Neil B, Ott PA, Piha-Paul SA, Gomez-Roca C, van Brummelen EMJ, Rugo HS, Thomas S, Saraf S, Rangwala R, Varga A. Safety and efficacy of Pembrolizumab in advanced, programmed death ligand 1-positive cervical cancer: results from the phase Ib KEYNOTE-028 trial. J Clin Oncol. 2017;35:4035–41.

18. Gonzalez Bosquet J, Magrina JF, Gaffey TA, Hernandez JL, Webb MJ, Cliby WA, Podratz KC. Long-term survival and disease recurrence in patients with primary squamous cell carcinoma of the vulva. Gynecol Oncol. 2005;97:828–33.

19. Foroudi F, Bull CA, Gebski V. Primary invasive cancer of the vagina: outcome and complications of therapy. Australas Radiol. 1999;43:472–5.

20. Creasman WT, Phillips JL, Menck HR. The National Cancer Data Base report on cancer of the vagina. Cancer. 1998;83:1033–40.

21. Bogani G, Ditto A, Ferla S, Paolini B, Lombardo C, Lorusso D, Raspagliesi F. Treatment modalities for recurrent high-grade vaginal intraepithelial neoplasia. J Gynecol Oncol. 2019;30:e20.

22. Herbst AL, Ulfelder H, Poskanzer DC, Longo LD. Adenocarcinoma of the vagina. Association of maternal stilbestrol therapy with tumor appearance in young women. 1971. Am J Obstet Gynecol. 1999;181:1574–5.

23. Saito T, Tabata T, Ikushima H, Yanai H, Tashiro H, Niikura H, Minaguchi T, Muramatsu T, Baba T, Yamagami W, Ariyoshi K, Ushijima K, Mikami M, Nagase S, Kaneuchi M, Yaegashi N, Udagawa Y, Katabuchi H. Japan Society of Gynecologic Oncology guidelines 2015 for the treatment of vulvar cancer and vaginal cancer. Int J Clin Oncol. 2018;23:201–34.

24. Creasman WT. Vaginal cancers. Curr Opin Obstet Gynecol. 2005;17:71–6.

25. Stock RG, Chen AS, Seski J. A 30-year experience in the management of primary carcinoma of the vagina: analysis of prognostic factors and treatment modalities. Gynecol Oncol. 1995;56:45–52.

26. Beriwal S, Demanes DJ, Erickson B, Jones E, De Los Santos JF, Cormack RA, Yashar C, Rownd JJ, Viswanathan AN, Society AB. American Brachytherapy Society consensus guidelines for interstitial brachytherapy for vaginal cancer. Brachytherapy. 2012;11:68–75.

27. Murakami N, Kasamatsu T, Sumi M, Yoshimura R, Takahashi K, Inaba K, Morota M, Mayahara H, Ito Y, Itami J. Radiation therapy for primary vaginal carcinoma. J Radiat Res. 2013;54:931–7.

28. Frank SJ, Jhingran A, Levenback C, Eifel PJ. Definitive radiation therapy for squamous cell carcinoma of the vagina. Int J Radiat Oncol Biol Phys. 2005;62:138–47.

29. Chyle V, Zagars GK, Wheeler JA, Wharton JT, Delclos L. Definitive radiotherapy for carcinoma of the vagina: outcome and prognostic factors. Int J Radiat Oncol Biol Phys. 1996;35:891–905.

Cancer of the Adrenal Gland

Mélanie Claps, Deborah Cosentini, Elisa Roca, and Alfredo Berruti

Endocrine Cancers

Contents

© Springer Nature Switzerland AG 2021
A. Russo et al. (eds.), *Practical Medical Oncology Textbook*, UNIPA Springer Series,
https://doi.org/10.1007/978-3-030-56051-5_55

Learning Objectives

By the end of the chapter the reader will
- have reached in-depth knowledge of biology and clinical presentation of paraganglioma/pheochromocytoma and adrenocortical carcinoma
- have learned the basic concepts of diagnosis and natural history of these rare diseases be able to put acquired knowledge to select the best treatment strategies for every patient bearing these rare diseases.

55.1   Introduction

The adrenal gland is composed of two embryological and functional distinct organs (◘ Fig. 55.1). The inner adrenal medulla is derived from neural ectoderm, and in the adult, it is a mediator of the acute stress response through secretion of catecholamines. The adrenal cortex is derived from intermediate mesoderm, and it is organized into three distinct concentric zones with three distinct functions [1]. The outer zona glomerulosa synthesizes and secretes mineralocorticoids that function to maintain sodium balance and intravascular volume, the zona fasciculate synthesizes glucocorticoids that function to regulate energy storage, and the zona reticularis synthesizes sex-steroid precursors.

Tumors may arise both from medulla and cortex. The majority of them are benign. Pheochromocytomas are tumors derived from the chromaffin cells of the embryonic neural crest [2]. Chromaffin cells are postganglionic parasympathetic and sympathetic neurons which are located in the adrenal medulla or along the paravertebral and para-aortic axes (◘ Fig. 55.2). Sympathetic paraganglia have a neck-to-pelvis distribution and produce catecholamines, while parasympathetic paraganglia, which do not produce catecholamines, are found almost exclusively in the neck and skull base, along the branches of glossopharyngeal and vagus nerve. Tumors arising from extra-adrenal chromaffin cells are termed paragangliomas.

Tumors deriving from malignant transformation of adrenal cortex are either adenoma or adrenocortical carcinoma.

55.2   Epidemiology

Pheochromocytomas (PCCs) and paragangliomas (PGLs) are rare diseases with an estimated incidence in Western countries between 2 and 8 new cases per million population per year [3]. Many cases are discovered incidentally by computed tomography or magnetic resonance imaging. The peak age of occurrence is in the third to fifth decade of life with almost equal distribution among male and female patients. About 10–20 % occur in pediatric patients. Between 5 % and 20 % of PCCs and 15 % and 35 % of sympathetic PGLs is malignant with the occurrence of metastatic disease either at diagnosis or during the natural history of the disease.

Adrenocortical neoplasms are relatively frequent, with an estimated incidence in the general population ranging from 3 % to 10 % [4]. A large Italian study showed that of 380 operated adrenal incidetalomas, the 52 % were adenomas [5].

The incidence of adrenocortical carcinoma (ACC) in Western countries is between 0.5 and 2 new cases per

The same gland, two different tumors

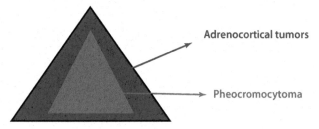

◘ **Fig. 55.1** Adrenal gland is composed of two different organs. Pheochromocytomas derived from the inner medulla, instead adrenocortical tumors from the outer zones

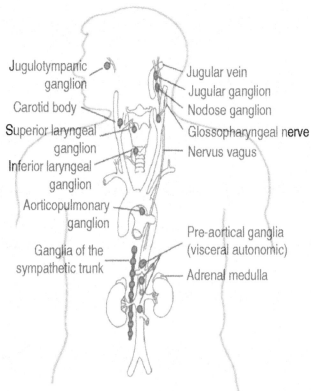

◘ **Fig. 55.2** Potential sites of paragangliomas and pheochromocytomas

million population per year. The male/female ratio is 1/1.5, and according to age, there is a bimodal distribution with 2 peaks in childhood and young adults between 4th and 5th decade [6].

55.3 Heritability

PCCs and PGLs are mainly sporadic, but they may also be associated with specific familiar disorders. More than 30% of PCCs/PGLs present with germline mutations being associated with hereditary syndromes [7], that is, multiple endocrine neoplasia type 2 (MEN2), neurofibromatosis type 1 (NF), von Hippel–Lindau syndrome (VHL), and pheochromocytoma-paraganglioma syndrome (PGL 1, 3, and 4) (◘ Table 55.1).

Since this group of tumors is the most strongly inherited among all human tumors, genetic screening is recommended, particularly in case of young age of tumor appearance, positive family history, bilaterally multifocal tumors, and recurrence or malignancy.

Genetic disorders associated with ACC are Li-Fraumeni and Beckwith-Wiedemann syndromes. Less clear is the association of ACC with familial adenomatous polyposis, multiple endocrine neoplasia 1, and neurofibromatosis [8] (◘ Table 55.1). Genetic tests for ACC are not routinely recommended but may be performed in selected young patients.

55.4 Adrenal Incidentaloma

Adrenal incidentaloma (AI) is an asymptomatic adrenal mass detected on imaging not performed for suspected adrenal disease. With modern imaging techniques, AIs are increasingly detected, and based on published literature, the frequencies of the different underlying tumor types are adrenocortical adenomas in 80 % (75 % of them are nonfunctioning, and the majority of functioning are cortisol secreting), adrenocortical carcinoma in 8 %, pheochromocytomas in 7 %, and metastatic tumors in 5 %. In surgical series, the distribution is as follows: adenoma 55 % (nonfunctioning 69 %, cortisol-secreting 10 %, aldosterone-secreting 6 %), pheochromocytoma 10 %, adrenocortical carcinoma 11 %, myelolipoma 8%, cyst 5%, ganglioneuroma 4 %, and metastasis 7 % [11].

The prevalence of adrenal adenomas decreases with the tumor size in favor of ACC that represents a minor part of AI if they are less than 4 cm (2 % of cases) or 4–6 cm (6 % of cases) in size. However, their prevalence increases substantially, and among adrenal tumors >6 cm, it can be up to 25 %.

According to the guidelines of the European Society of Endocrinology, surgical treatment of AI should be considered in an individualized approach; the appropriateness of surgical intervention should be guided by the likelihood of malignancy, the presence and degree of hormone excess, age, general health, and patient preference.

55.5 Clinical Features

The vast majority of symptoms and signs of PCCs are due to the associate excess of catecholamines released by tumors either continuously or paroxysmally [12]. The most frequent symptoms and sign is hypertension typically sustained, paroxysmal, or sustained with paroxysms. The paroxysmal release of catecholamines constitutes the characteristic classic triad of episodic headache, sweating, and palpitations. This may be triggered by anesthesia and tumor manipulation; positional change, exercise, and various medications (e.g., tricyclic antidepressants, opiates, metoclopramide, and radiographic contrast agents) are other possible precipitating factors. Frequently, the episodes occur in a random pattern with no clearly defined precipitating event. Other symptoms associated to PCCs are anxiety, dyspnea, chest, abdominal or flank pain, nausea and vomiting, tremor, flushing, dizziness, visual symptoms such as blurred vision, and paresthesia. Persistent vasoconstriction in patients with pheochromocytoma declines the blood volume leading to orthostatic hypotension. Chronic exposure to catecholamine may lead to irreversible myocardial fibrosis [13].

The majority of ACC are functioning at presentation; according to the Orbassano and Brescia database, 52 % of ACC at diagnosis are hormone secreting (◘ Fig. 55.3). Cortisol either alone or in association with androgens is the hormone most frequently secreted, so Cushing syndrome is the most frequent clinical manifestation. Less frequently, the tumors may produce androgens or other hormones such as estrogens or mineral corticoid hormones, and consequently, the symptoms and signs can be amenorrhea and virilization or hypertension with hypokalemia, respectively (◘ Table 55.2).

Both malignant PCCs and ACC patients may suffer from symptoms and signs related to malignancy such as weight loss and fatigue and symptoms related to primary tumor mass and/or relevant metastases.

55.6 Pathological Features

The pathological differential diagnosis of adrenal neoplasias is still largely based on morphological features requiring an experienced pathologist.

There is no histological system that is currently endorsed for the biological aggressiveness of PCCs/

Table 55.1 Hereditary syndromes in PCC, PGL, and ACC

Adrenal Tumor	Syndrome	Mutation	Prevalence in general population	Clinical features
PCC	Von Hippel-Lindau	VHL	1:36.000	Hemangioblastomas of the brain, spinal cord, and retina, renal cysts and clear cell renal cell carcinoma, pheochromocytoma, pancreatic cysts, and neuroendocrine tumors, endolymphatic sac tumors, and epididymal and broad ligament cysts
PCC	MEN2A MEN2B	RET	1–9:100.000	MEN2A: Medullary thyroid carcinoma, pheochromocytoma, parathyroid adenoma or hyperplasia. MEN2B: Medullary thyroid carcinoma, pheochromocytoma, mucosal neuromas of the lips and tongue, distinctive facies with enlarged lips, ganglioneuromatosis of the gastrointestinal tract, and a "marfanoid" habitus
PCC	Pheochromocytoma-paraganglioma syndrome	SDHA SDHB SDHC SDHD SDHAF2	1:30.000–100.000	Leigh syndrome, late-onset optic atrophy, ataxia and myopathy, PGLs High malignant potential extra-adrenal PGLs, adrenal PCCs and HNPGLs HNPGLs, rare cases of adrenal PCCs and extra-adrenal PGLs Multifocal HNPGLs, adrenal PCCs and extra-adrenal PGLs (usually benign) Young age onset multifocal HNPGLs
PCC and ACC	Von Recklinghausen	NF1	1:3.000	Malignant peripheral nerve sheet tumor, pheochromocytoma, café au lait spots, neurofibroma, optic glioma, Lisch nodule, skeletal abnormalities
ACC	Li-Fraumeni syndrome	TP53	1:20.000–1.000.000	Sarcoma, choroid plexus tumor, brain cancer, early breast cancer, leukemia, lymphoma
ACC	Lynch syndrome	MSH2, MSH6, MLH1, PMS2	1:440	Colorectal cancer, endometrial cancer, sebaceous neoplasms, ovarian cancer, pancreatic cancer, brain cancer
ACC	MEN1	MENIN	1:30.000	Foregut neuroendocrine tumors, pituitary tumors, parathyroid hyperplasia, collagenoma, angiofibroma, adrenal adenoma/hyperplasia
ACC	Beckwith-Wiedemann syndrome	IGF2, CDKN1C, H19 locus changes on 11p15	1:13.000	Wilms' tumor, hepatoblastoma, macrosomia, adrenocortical cytomegaly, adrenal adenoma, adrenal cyst, hemihypertrophy, macroglossia, omphalocele, ear pits
ACC	FAP	APC	1:30.000	Intestinal polyps, colon cancer, duodenal carcinoma, thyroid cancer, desmoid tumor, adrenal adenoma, supernumerary teeth, congenital hypertrophy of the retina, osteoma, epidermoid cysts
ACC	Carney complex	PRKAR1A	700 cases worldwide	Primary pigmented nodular adrenal disease, large-cell calcifying Sertoli cell tumors, thyroid adenoma, myxoma, somatotroph pituitary adenoma, lentigines

VHL von Hippel-Lindau, *MEN1* Multiple endocrine neoplasia type 1, *MEN2* Multiple endocrine neoplasia type 2, *RET* rearranged during transfection proto-oncogene, *SDH* succinate dehydrogenase, *HNPGLs* head and neck region paragangliomas, *FAP* familial adenomatous polyposis, *NF1* neurofibromatosis type 1
Modified from [9, 10]

55

PGLs. The certainty of malignant behavior is done by the presence of metastases. According to the last WHO classification [14], all pheochromocytomas could have metastatic potential. Several histologic features such as invasion (vascular, capsular, and/or periadrenal adipose tissue), large nests or diffuse growth, focal or confluent necrosis, high cellularity, tumor cell spindling, cellular monotony, increased and/or atypical mitotic figures, profound nuclear pleomorphism, and hyperchromasia included in the Pheochromocytoma Adrenal gland Scaled Score (PASS) have been associated with malignancy. However, the validity of this scoring system is a matter of controversy.

Several markers have been introduced to establish the adrenocortical origin of adrenal masses, with steroidogenesis factor-1 immunohistochemistry and

Melan-A being particularly useful. The differential diagnosis between adrenocortical adenoma versus carcinoma may be challenging.

The most widely used diagnostic score has been introduced by Weiss et al. [15] and includes the following parameters: mitosis, atypical mitosis, necrosis, venous invasion, sinusal invasion, capsular invasion, nuclear atypia, diffuse architecture, and clear cell. A score of ≥3 suggests malignancy. Ki67 as a marker of proliferative activity is useful particularly as independent prognostic factor.

55.7 Molecular Biology

The inherited basis of PCCs/PGLs has been well characterized since many years. About 12 % to 16 % of them have SDHx or FH mutations. The gene encoding subunit B of the SDH complex is by far the most important contributor to a hereditary malignant disease. Between 1 % and 13 % of PCCs/PGLs have germline VHL mutations, whereas the frequency of RET, NF1, TMEM, and MAX considered together is between 1 % and 11 %. Sporadic PCCs/PGLs may retain the same driver genes as seen in inherited tumors; however, the number of driver genes has grown to more than 20 over the past decade suggesting great complexity of these diseases. A comprehensive molecular analysis, recently published, revealed that PCCs/PGLs have a low genome alteration rate with a remarkable diversity of driver alterations including germline and somatic mutations and somatic fusion genes. New driver genes were discovered including a Wnt-altered subtype driven by a MAML3 fusion gene and CSDE1 somatic mutation [16]. Put these new data in the context of the established literature five molecular subtypes of both inherited and sporadic PCCs/PGLs have been identified: (1) pseudohypoxic

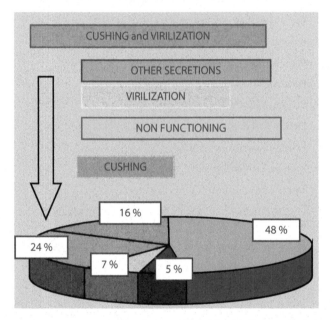

CUSHING and VIRILIZATION

OTHER SECRETIONS

VIRILIZATION

NON FUNCTIONING

CUSHING

16 %

48 %

24 %

7 %

5 %

Fig. 55.3 Adrenocortical cancer. Clinical presentation

Table 55.2 Hormone syndromes related to secreting ACC and PCC

Syndrome	Incidence	Hormone profile	Signs and symptoms
Cushing's syndrome	50–80 % of cases	Hypercortisolism, suppressed ACTH levels	Plethora, dorsal fat hump, diabetes mellitus, muscle weakness/atrophy, osteoporosis, hypokalemia, hypertension, mood alterations, insomnia, skin atrophy, higher susceptibility to infectious diseases
Hyperandrogenism	40–60 % of cases	Excess of dehydroepiandrosenedione sulfate, 17-hydroxyprogesterone, testosterone, androstenedione	In women: hirsutism, virilization, menstrual irregularities, temporal balding, acne.
Pheochromocytoma	All cases	Paroxysmal and chronic release of catecholamines	Classic triad: episodic headache, sweating, and palpitations; anxiety, dyspnea, chest, abdominal or flank pain, nausea and vomiting, tremor, flushing, dizziness, blurred vision, and paresthesia, orthostatic hypotension, irreversible myocardial fibrosis.

☐ Table 55.3 Clusters and driven alterations

Cluster	Driven alteration	Degree hereditary	Altered pathways
Pseudohypoxia	TCA cycle-related	100 %	Mitochondrial dysfunction (*SDHA, SDHB, SDHC, SDHD, SDHAF2, FH*) and pseudohypoxia
Pseudohypoxia	VHL/EPAS1-related	25 %	Pseudohypoxia (*VHL, EPAS1*)
Wnt signaling	CSDE1, MAML3-fusion	0 %	Wnt-signaling (*CSDE1, MAML3*)
Kinase signaling	NF1> HRAS> RET> TMEM127 > MAX	20 %	MYC (*MAX*), MAPK (*RET, NF1, HRAS*), mTOR (*TMEM127*)

PCCs/PGLs, (2) pseudohypoxic PCCs/PGLs, TCA cycle-related, (3) pseudohypoxic PCCs/PGLs, VHL, and EPAS1-related, (4) Wnt signaling PCCs/PGLs, and (5) Kinase signaling PCCs/PGLs (☐ Table 55.3). This molecular classification provides opportunities for prognostic stratifications and future targeted therapies [17].

Numerous genetic and molecular studies have recently been performed on adrenocortical tumors, including carcinoma. These studies have detected nine driver genes CTNNB1, ZNRF3, TP53, RB1, CDKN2A, MEN1, DAXX, TERT, and MED12 and the involvement of three major pathways, including the p53, Wnt/b-catenin, and IGFII pathways. Alteration in microRNA (miRNA) profiling or hypermethylation of the CpG island methylator phenotype in up to 50 % of cases of ACC was also described [8].

55.8 Diagnosis

55.8.1 Hormone and Biochemical Assessment

Since both PCCs/PGLs and ACC are hormone secreting, a comprehensive hormonal analysis is recommended when an adrenal mass is diagnosed. The ACC working group of the European Network for the Study of Adrenal Tumors [18] suggests a preoperative hormonal work-up including basal cortisol, ACTH, dehydroepiandrostenedione sulfate, 17-hydroxyprogesterone, testosterone, androstenedione, estradiol, urinary free cortisol, and dexamethasone suppression test [19, 20]. The endocrine assessment is essential in order to confirm a suspected hormonal excess and to establish the origin (cortex or medulla) and nature (malignant or benign) of the adrenal lesion, i.e., the coexistence of cortisol and androgen hypersecretion is a sign of malignancy [11, 14, 19] (☐ Table 55.4). The best screening test for initial assessment of PCCs/PGLs is measurement of free plasma and urinary fractionated metanephrines

☐ Table 55.4 Homonal work-up for adrenal cancers

Glucocorticoid excess (minimum of 3 of 4 tests)

Dexamethasone suppression test (1 mg, 23:00 h)

Excretion of free urinary cortisol (24 h urine)

Basal cortisol (serum)

Basal ACTH (plasma)

Sexual steroids and steroid precursor

DHEA-S (serum)

17-OH-progesterone (serum)

Androstenedione (serum)

Testosterone (serum)

17-beta-estradiol (serum, only in men and postmenopausal women)

24-h urine steroid metabolite examination

Mineralocorticoid excess

Potassium (serum)

Aldosterone/renin ratio (only in patients with arterial hypertension and /or hypokalemia)

Catecholamine excess

Normetanephrine, metanephrine, and methoxytyramine (plasma)

Alternatively: fractionated metanephrine excretion (24 h urine)

[21]. Although elevation of plasma or urinary normetanephrines slightly above the upper reference range only marginally increases the probability of PCs/PGLs, a more than fourfold elevation is associated with a 100 % probability [22].

In metastatic PCs/PGLs, any increment of normetanephrines indicates disease relapse and activity often before the onset of symptoms [23]. Plasma methoxytyramine is another useful marker. Elevated levels (more than fourfold higher the normal range) are associated with SDHB mutations and extra-adrenal disease and can be predictive of malignancy [22]. Plasma chromogranin (CgA) levels may be elevated in both benign and metastatic PCCs/PGLs although it is significantly higher in metastatic tumors and associated with poor prognosis. CgA is a valuable complementary in malignant PCCs/PGLs since supranormal levels are frequently found in patients with metastatic disease and normal normetanephrine levels [24].

55.8.2 Imaging

The role of imaging procedures is of paramount importance to differentiate benign and malignant adrenal lesions and to correctly stage the disease. Computed tomography (CT) scan is the first choice imaging technique [19]. Tumor size, lipid content of the mass, and the velocity of the washout of contrast medium are the best criteria for diagnosing ACC [25].

As previously mentioned, the risk for malignancy increases for lesions >4 cm (sensitivity, 97 %; specificity, 52 %) and >6 cm (sensitivity, 91 %; specificity, 80 %) [26], while a density mass ≤10 Hounsfield Unit (HU) in unenhanced CT scan is significant for a lipid-rich content and, thus, for the benign nature of the lesion [11, 20]. In case of basal density >10 HU, a rapid contrast-medium washout (>50 %) is diagnostic for the benignity of the tumor [19, 20]. ACCs are usually irregular large masses, with heterogeneous enhancement for the presence of necrotic, calcific, and hemorrhagic areas in the solid component [20, 25]. Local invasion and tumor extension into the inferior vena cava are indicative of malignant behavior [19]. A chest CT scan must be performed to exclude the presence of lung metastases before surgery [19, 20].

Magnetic resonance imaging (MRI) of the abdomen is considered as effective as CT scan in detecting ACCs [19]. Adrenal carcinomas appear isointense to hypointense on T1-weighted images and hyperintense on T2-weighted images and show a heterogeneous signal drop on chemical shift [27, 28]. In radiologically indeterminate adrenal lesions, functional imaging can be a helpful integrative diagnostic tool, as a high uptake at the ^{18}F-fluorodeoxyglucose-positron emission tomography (FDG-PET) is suggestive for ACC [29, 30]. To prove the adrenocortical origin of a lesion, a new tracer can be used: metomidate ([11C]MTO). It specifically binds to adrenocortical CYP11B, key step enzymes in steroid synthesis. ACCs show a higher uptake at [11C]MTO-PET compared to normal gland [31].

CT scanning of the abdomen and pelvis is the recommended initial imaging modality also for pheochromocytoma [5]. CT provides high tomographic resolution with a localization sensitivity between 88 % and 100 %.

On CT imaging, PCCs can be homogeneous or heterogeneous, solid or cystic, and with or without calcification. MRI is another useful tool in localizing PCCs. The most common MR imaging appearance of a PCC is of low signal intensity on T1 imaging and high signal intensity on T2-weighted imaging. Although MRI lacks the superior spatial resolution of CT, it is useful to detect skull base and neck paragangliomas. Contrast-enhanced ultrasound has attracted interest, but there are insufficient data to recommend it for PPGL screening [32].

Functional imaging is another widely used imaging modality for pheochromocytomas. Meta-iodobenzylguanidine (MIBG) is a radiopharmaceutical agent that accumulates preferentially in catecholamine-producing cells. ^{123}I-labelled MIBG has a sensitivity between 85 % and 88 % for PCCs and between 56 % and 75 % for PGLs. Its specificity ranges from 70–100 % to 84–100 %, respectively [33, 34, 35, 36]. ^{123}I-MIBG is the recommended agent for functional imaging in patients with PCC. Its major diagnostic uses are confirmation that an adrenal lesion is a PCC, the identification of metastases, and assessing suitability for ^{131}I-MIBG therapy. Prior to ^{123}I-MIBG imaging, thyroid uptake of radioactive iodine must be blocked with potassium iodide.

In addition to MIBG, several other functional imaging modalities have been identified including PET scanning using 18Ffluorodopamine, 18F-fluorodihydroxy-phenylalanine (^{18}F-DOPA), or ^{18}F-fluoro-deoxy-glucose (FDG). FDG-PET is especially used in paragangliomas or metastatic; it is a highly sensitive disease in tumors showing SDH mutations [37]. ^{68}Ga-DOTATATE PET/CT was recently found to be superior to ^{123}I-MIBG and SRS and is considered as the first-line investigation in high-risk patients of metastatic PCCs/PGLs and familial PGLs harboring SHDB mutations [38].

55.9 Differential Diagnosis

Tumors which should be considered in the differential diagnosis of adrenal pheochromocytomas and adrenal adenoma/carcinoma include myelolipoma, cyst, ganglioneuroma, and metastasis.

55.10 Prognostic Factors

The progression of PCCs/PGLs is strongly influenced by genetics. Currently, the only reliable predictor of malignancy is the SDHB gene germline mutation as it is found in more than 40 % of metastatic PCCs/PGLs (especially extra-adrenal PGLs) [39]. There is no staging system for malignant PCCs/PGLs. The survival rate depends mainly on the tumor size and primary tumor location (extra-adrenal location is associated with poor prognosis) [19]. Short-term survivors (<5 years) are patients with metastases to the liver and lungs, whereas long-term survivors have bone metastases [40].

The most important prognostic factors in early ACC are the disease stage, margin-free resection, age, the proliferation marker Ki67, and the glucocorticoid excess [19]. In patients with metastatic disease, the prognosis is generally poor, but it is more heterogeneous than previously believed, and long-term survivors are rarely seen. The number of tumor organs (☐ Table 55.5) has a major prognostic role together with four other parameters grouped together under the label GRAS, defined by grade (Weiss score <6 or >6 or Ki67 <20 % or >20 %), resection status of the primary, age younger than or older than 50 years, and the absence or presence of tumor-related or hormone-related symptoms at diagnosis. The GRAS parameters are defined favorable if Ki67 < 20 %, primary R0 resection is performed, age <50 years, and there is the absence of symptoms at diagnosis (either related to cortisol hypersecretion or tumor mass). The GRAS parameters are classified as pejorative in case of grading as defined by Ki67 >20 % and/or primary R1-2 resection status [41].

☐ **Table 55.5** mENSAT + GRAS classification of ACC

Stage	mENSAT + GRAS
I	T1–2, favorable GRAS[a]
II	II-A: T1–2, unfavorable GRAS
	II-B: T1–2, pejorative GRAS
III	III-A: T3, or T4, N0, M0, and favorable GRAS
	III-B: T3, or T4, N0, M0, and unfavorable GRAS
	III-C: T3, or T4, N0, M0, and pejorative GRAS
IV	IV-A: 2 or 3 tumor organs[b] and favorable GRAS
	IV-B: 2 or 3 tumor organs and unfavorable GRAS
	IV-C: 2 or ≥3 tumor organs and pejorative GRAS

[a]GRAS parameters are considered favorable if grading defined by Ki67 is <20 %, primary R0 resection status performed, age <50 y, and there is the absence of symptoms at diagnosis. GRAS parameters are classified unfavorable in case of age >50 y, or the presence of symptoms at diagnosis. GRAS parameters are classified as pejorative in case of grading as defined by Ki67 >20 % and/or primary R1-2 resection status.
[b]Tumor organ counts include the primary and lymph nodes if not resected (Baudin E. et al., 2015)

55.11 Treatment

Surgery is the mainstay of therapy in the management of both ACC and pheochromocytoma with local regional disease. It is advisable that adrenal surgery should be performed in referenced centers with a documented number for adrenal cancer per year (>10 adrenalectomies) [19]. Open surgery is the standard treatment of ACC patients when complete resection can be achieved. Laparoscopic adrenalectomy is the standard procedure for pheochromocytoma and for a selected group of patients with small ACCs without preoperative evidence for invasiveness and adrenal masses (e.g., incidentalomas) that are judged as only potentially malignant.

The major principles of the management of metastatic PCCs/PGLs include control of symptoms related to catecholamine overproduction and of tumor growth, but no curative treatment is achievable. Treatment choices include a wait-and-see policy, locoregional therapies, systemic chemotherapy, and radiopharmaceutical agents. The decision on the best treatment for each individual patient is often complex and requires a multidisciplinary approach.

Phenoxybenzamine, a long-acting nonselective (alpha1 and alpha-2), noncompetitive alpha-adrenergic blocker, and doxazosin, a selective alpha-1-adrenergic blocker, are the most frequently used drugs to obtain symptom control and prepare patients for surgery. In patients with PCC and secreting PGL, in fact, exposure to high levels of circulating catecholamines during surgery could cause hypertensive crises and arrhythmias. Therefore, a preoperative preparation with an alpha-adrenergic blocker at least 10–14 days before surgery is required [42].

As regards the antineoplastic therapy, the wait-and-see strategy could be an option for selected patients with slowly progressive tumors, while active therapeutic intervention is generally required in the presence of uncontrolled hormone- or tumor-related symptoms, high tumor burden, or significant radiographic progression [43].

Cytoreductive (R2) resection in malignant PCC may sometimes improve the quality of life and survival by reducing the tumor burden and controlling hormonal hypersecretion [40].

^{131}I-MIBG therapy should be considered as a first-line approach in patients with significant tumor burden, slowly progressive disease, and adequate ^{131}I-MIBG uptake on diagnostic imaging. With ^{131}I-MIBG therapy, a disease stabilization and partial hormonal responses can be achieved in 50 % and 40 % of patients. Although objective responses are common, complete response

rates are low [44]. The use of ^{131}I-MIBG therapy may be limited by hematologic toxicity [45] and by the need of a prolonged inpatient admission for radiation safety purposes.

Because a significant number of metastatic sites express SSRTs, peptide receptor radionuclide therapy (PRRT) using ^{90}Y-DOTATOC and ^{177}Lu-DOTATOC can be potentially used.

The results of a retrospective study on 20 consecutive advanced PCCs/PGLs patients, in which PRRT was administered, showed disease regression in 36 % of patients (29 % partial and 7 % minor response), while 50 % had stable disease. Eight of 14 patients treated for uncontrolled secondary hypertension obtained the reduction of medication doses [46].

Combination chemotherapy with cyclophosphamide, vincristine, and dacarbazine (CVD) administered to malignant PCCs/PGLs can obtain 37 % tumor response and 40 % hormonal response; complete remissions are rare [47]. Temozolomide is a 3-methyl analogue of mitozolomide developed as an oral alternative to intravenous dacarbazine. A retrospective study on 15 consecutive patients with metastatic PCs/PGLs showed five partial responses (33 %), seven stable (47 %), and three progressive diseases (20 %). Interestingly, disease responses were confined to the 10 patients carrying a mutation in SDHB [48].

In cases of unresectable liver metastases, transarterial-(chemo)-embolization (TACE) has been shown to reduce metastatic deposits and catecholamine and CgA levels [49]. Other options include radiofrequency ablation and alcohol injection to unresectable lesions.

Approximately 70 % of patients with metastatic PCCs/PGLs develop bone metastases that are mainly lytic. These patients require a combination of therapeutic modalities including antiresorptive medications such as bisphosphonates or RANKL inhibitors, externalbeam irradiation and radiofrequency ablation of bone metastases or surgical stabilization, and cementation [49]. ◘ Table 55.6 summarizes the treatment options for PCCs/PGLs.

Surgical series have shown that up to 80 % of ACC patients are destined to develop locoregional recurrence or distant metastases after an apparent complete surgical excision [50, 51]. On these bases, there is a strong rationale for the use of adjuvant therapy in ACC patients. The evidence in favor of this therapeutic option, however, is still limited since the results of prospective randomized clinical trials are lacking.

Mitotane is the only drug approved by international pharmaceutical agencies for treatment of advanced ACC. A large retrospective case-control study reported that patients treated with adjuvant mitotane had a significantly longer recurrence-free survival (RFS) and overall

◘ **Table 55.6** Therapeutic algorithm for the primary treatment of metastatic PCCs and PGLs

Disease status	Medical Treatment	Therapeutic Options
If resectable tumor	Alpha blockade ± alpha-methyltyrosine ± beta blockade (pre-operatively)	Resection (laparoscopic preferred when safe and feasible)
If unresectable locally	Alpha blockade ± alpha-methyltyrosine ± beta blockade (pre-operatively)	If possible cytoreductive (R2) resection and/or
		Local radiotherapy
If distant metastasis	Alpha blockade ± alpha-methyltyrosine ± beta blockade (pre-operatively)	If possible cytoreductive (R2) resection and/or
		^{131}I-MIBG (if positive MIBG scan with dosimetry) or SSR analogs if positive receptors or
		Systemic chemotherapy (CVD) or TMZ or
		Clinical Trial
If asymptomatic tumor without significant radiographic progression (RECIST)		Wait and see strategy Active radiological surveillance (at 3, 6 months, 1 year)

survival (OS), compared with two independent groups of patients untreated after surgery [52]. Recently, the same group has updated the follow-up of these cohorts of patients with almost 10 years of additional observation, confirming that adjuvant mitotane treatment is associated with a significant benefit in terms of RFS regardless of the hormone secretory status [53]. Advantage on OS is less evident, but this may be explained by different treatment of ACC recurrence between groups and the introduction of a landmark analysis. Despite its retrospective nature, this study remains the most informative piece of evidence on the topic, and it represents a reference for decision making in ACC patients. On the basis of the results of this study, adjuvant mitotane therapy is currently recommended by international guidelines [19].

The management of patients under long-term mitotane therapy is not easy and requires experienced endocrinologists or medical oncologists. The most common side effects are gastrointestinal (nausea, vomiting, diarrhea, anorexia, and mucositis) and neurological (lethargy, somnolence, vertigo, ataxia, confusion, depression, dizziness, decreased memory, and polyneuropathy) (◘ Table 55.7). The management of them is complicated by the long half-life of drug plasma levels (40 days). The maintenance of mitotane serum levels within the so-called therapeutic range (14–20 mg/L) allows the attainment of the best benefit from the drug and the prevention of side effects (neurological, in particular) in most cases [54].

About 50 % of newly diagnosed ACC patients present with metastatic or unresectable disease [19].

Moreover, despite initial complete resection of ACC, up to 70–80 % of patients are destined to develop recurrent or metastatic disease [6]. The management of these patients is mainly centered on systemic therapy that since many years include mitotane alone or mitotane in combination with chemotherapy. The standard chemotherapy regimen for advanced ACC is EDP (etoposide, doxorubicin, and cisplatin) plus mitotane (EDP-M) [55]. The efficacy of the EDP-M regimen was demonstrated by the results of a prospective randomized clinical trial in which 304 patients were prospectively enrolled in about 6 years and randomized to receive either EDP-M or streptozotocyn plus mitotane (Sz-M). Patients with disease progression to the first-line treatment received the alternate regimen. EDP-M was supe-

◘ **Table 55.7** Side effects of mitotane therapy

System organ class	Very common	Common	Rare	Very rare
Nervous system disorders	Dizziness, somnolence, vertigo, depression, decreased memory	Lethargy, ataxia, confusion, polyneuropathy		
Gastrointestinal disorders	Nausea, vomiting, diarrhea, mucositis			
Blood and lymphatic system disorders		Leucopenia	Thrombocytopenia, anemia	
Endocrine disorders	Adrenal insufficiency	Primary hypogonadism in men		
Skin and subcutaneous tissue disorders		Rash, gynecomastia		
Metabolism and nutrition disorders	Anorexia; hypercholesterolemia, hypertriglyceridemia			
Cardiac disorders				Hypertension
Hepatobiliary disorders	Increase in hepatic enzymes (mostly GGT); hepatic microsomal enzyme induction			
Immune-related adverse reaction			Autoimmune hepatitis	
Eye disorders				Blurred vision, double vision, toxic retinopathy, macular edema, cataract
Renal and urinary disorders				Hemorrhagic cystitis, hematuria, albuminuria
Investigations	Increase in hormone binding globulins (CBG, SHBG, TBG, vitamin D binding protein); reduction of fT4;			

55

rior to Sz-M both in terms of disease response rate and progression-free survival (PFS). Analysis of OS also favored patients initially randomized to receive EDP-M, but due to the attenuating effect of the crossover to EDP-M of patients randomized to the Sz-M at disease progression, the difference just failed to attain statistical significance [56].

In addition to systemic therapy, also local regional therapies, i.e., radiofrequency ablation (RFA) [57] and chemoembolization [58, 59], can be taken into consideration in a selected patient population.

Finally, the morbidity caused by ACC and the prognosis derives not only from the spread of malignant cells into other organs, but also from the consequences of hormone excess. Consequently, the goals of treatment in ACC include both control of tumor growth and mitigation of the effects derived from hormone excess in patients with clinical and biochemical finding of hormone hyperscretion. Patients with metastatic ACC that exhibits autonomous steroid secretion should be treated with steroidogenic inhibitors to ameliorate the effects of excessive mineralocorticoids (hypertension and hypokalemia) and glucocorticoids (hypertension, hyperglycemia, hypokalemia, and muscle atrophy). The management of hormone excess in patients with metastatic ACC is often challenging. The presence of Cushing syndrome may consistently increase the toxicity of chemotherapy since it is associated by immune depression that favors infections particularly in the neutropenia phase. Therefore, a rapid control of hormone hypersecretion is mandatory. Mitotane has both antisecretive and antiproliferative activities; however, the slow onset of its activity is a main limitation for the management of Cushing's syndrome [6]. Faster drug in lowering the serum cortisol levels is needed. Ketoconazole is more rapid than mitotane in controlling Cushing syndrome [60], but it requires several weeks, and its clinical employment is hampered by the hepatic toxicity. Metyrapone (Cormeto) is an adrenolytic molecule targeting the 11-beta-hydroxylase. In a recently published experience by our group, metyrapone was associated upfront to the EDP-M regimen, and this combination was very well tolerated and led to a rapid control of Cushing's syndrome induced by cortisol secreting ACC [61]. In patients with advanced ACC with severe Cushing syndrome, the EDP-M plus metyrapone regimen (EDP-MM) is the best treatment strategy.

55.12 Follow-up

Patients who underwent successful surgery for nonmetastatic PCC/PGL are at risk of malignant recurrence and require long-term clinical (adrenergic symptoms and blood pressure levels) and biochemical follow-up [19]. The follow-up is especially important for patients with extra-adrenal primary disease, tumor size >5 cm, or SDHB mutations. Biochemical testing (plasma or urinary metanephrine, normetanephrine, chromogranin A, and methoxythyramine) should be repeated ~14 days following surgery to check for remaining disease and thereafter every 3–4 months for 2–3 years. This should subsequently be repeated every 6 months. Patients with new events (high blood pressure, adrenergic symptoms, or pain) and/or elevated circulating or urinary biochemical tests should undergo imaging that includes thorax and abdomen CT and best functioning imaging (PET FDG in most cases).

For patients with ACC after complete resection, a regular follow-up every 3 months including abdominal CT (or MRI), thoracic CT, and monitoring of initially elevated steroids is recommended. After 2 years, intervals may be gradually increased. In case of long-term persistence of the disease-free status, follow-up should be continued for at least 10 years [19].

1. *Man, 57 years old*
2. *Family history:* Negative for malignancies
3. *APR:* Negative
4. *APP:* Insomnia, palpitation

5. *Objective examination*: Moon face, central obesity, buffalo hump, hypertension
6. *Blood tests*: Hyperglycemia, hypokalemia;
7. *TC abdomen mdc*: Adrenal lesion of $10 \times 9 \times 9$ cm. few lung lesions (maximum diameter of 3 cm)

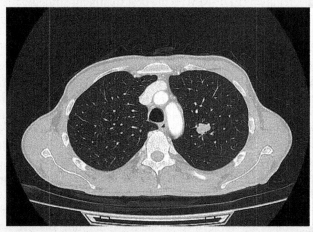 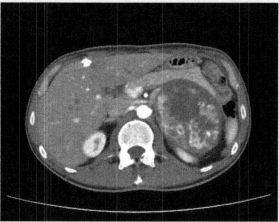

Question

What action should be taken?

(1) Surgery. (2) Hormonal assessment and biopsy. (3) Biopsy alone

Answer

Hormonal assessment and biopsy

8. *Baseline hormonal assessment*: hypercortisoluria, hypercortisolemia, ACTH suppression, negative metanephrine and normetanephrine.
9. *Lung biopsy*
Histological examination: Adrenocortical carcinoma. MART-1 +, MELAN-A +inhibin +, Ki67 30 %.

Question

What action should be taken?

(1) Surgery. (2) Chemotherapy plus Mitotane. (3) Chemotherapy plus Mitotane plus Metyrapone

Answer

Chemotherapy plus Mitotane plus Metyrapone

10. *Chemotherapy* with Etoposide, Doxorubicin and Cisplatin (EDP scheme) plus Mitotane and Metyrapone.
11. *Hormonal assessment after one month*: normalization of cortisoluria, cortisolemia, and ACTH
12. *Response evaluation after 5 cycles of chemotherapy (EDP scheme) plus Mitotane:* Partial response

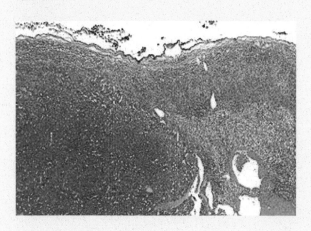

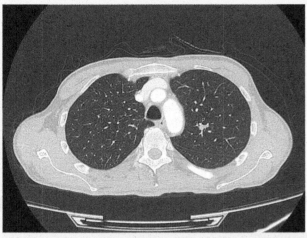
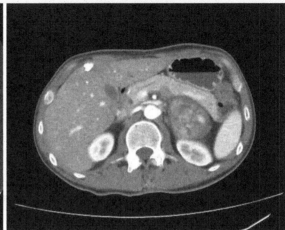

13. *Response evaluation after 7 cycles of chemotherapy (EDP scheme) plus mitotane:*

Partial response

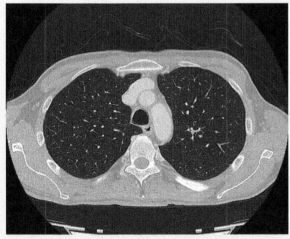
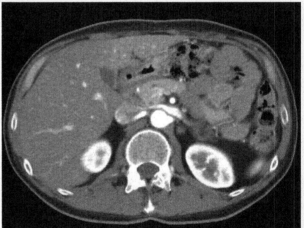

Question

What action should be taken?

  (1) Continue chemotherapy. (2) Continue only Mitotane. (3) Surgery

Answer

Surgery

14. Surgery: Left surrenectomy and lymphadenectomy of the renal hilum.
    Histological examination: Adrenocortical carcinoma. Negative lymph nodes. R0.

Question

What action should be taken?

  (1) Continue chemotherapy plus mitotane. (2) Continue only mitotane. (3) Follow-up

Answer

Continue only mitotane and perform an instrumental follow-up

15. The patient is actually treated with mitotane. A periodic follow-up with a CT scan is performed every 3–4 months.

Key Points

- The importance of a correct approach of metastatic ACC with Cushing syndrome:
  - Complete hormonal assessment to evaluate the concomitant secretion of other hormones in addition to cortisol
  - Biopsy of one lesion to confirm the diagnosis
- The importance to obtain the rapid control of Cushing syndrome by adding metyrapone to the EDP-M scheme
- The importance of a correct monitoring to evaluate the response
- The potential positive impact of resection of primary adrenal disease in a patient with oligo metastatic ACC
- The importance to individualize the treatment length in order to obtain the maximum cytoreductive effect

Advanced Pheochromocytoma: A Clinical Case

Man, 56 years old

1. *Family history:* father and mother deceased for a not specified abdominal malignancy
2. *Comorbidities:* arterial hypertension since 15 years
3. *Recent history:* recurrent hypertensive crisis and episodes of hypotension requiring access to the emergency response service
4. *CT scan:* right adrenal mass, diameter max 8.5 cm, inhomogeneous. No evidence of metastases.

Question

What should be done first?
- Biopsy
- Surgery
- Antihypertensive therapy

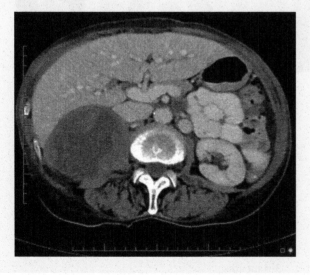

Answer

Anti-hypertensive therapy

2 weeks before surgery, the patient was treated with noncompetitive alpha-adrenoreceptor antagonist. In suspected pheochromocytomas, fine needle biopsy is contraindicated.

- *Surgery:* right adrenalectomy
- *Pathology:* IHC positive for CgA, NSE, synaptophyisin, and CD56 and negative for CEA, S100, Melan A, cytokeratins, alpha-inhibin, and vimentin
- *Follow-up:* periodic clinical, abdominal US sonography and tumor markers (CgA and NSE) evaluations, with no evidence of disease recurrence for 6 years
- *Disease recurrence after 6 years. Laboratory analysis:* NSE 34.8 ng/ml (nv < 16); CgA 1066 ng/mL (nv), metanephrine 0.660 mg/24 h (nv), normetanephrine 39,390 mg/24 h (nv), 3-metossithyramine 1.865 mg/24 h (nv)
- *Abdominal US sonography:* in the retroperitoneum; in para-aortic; in the presence of multiple, voluminous, and confluent formations; in hypoechoic; and in compatible with adenopathy
- *Total body CT scan:* multiple confluent retroperitoneal adenopathy, 10 cm in diameter, and bulky thoracic mass, with necrotic areas

55

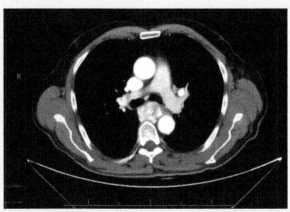
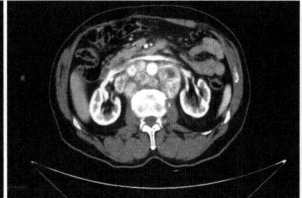

Question

What should be done now?

- Surgery
- Medical therapy
- Metabolic imaging

Answer

Metabolic Imaging:

- *68Ga-DOTA-NOC PET/TC:* Multiple high intensity uptakes of radionuclide in mediastinum, bilateral lung ilus, Barety lymph nodes, carenal and paraesophageal adenopathy, precardiac area, and common iliac lymph nodes. The presence of intense uptake also in inferior left and right lung lobes

- *MIBG-Scintigraphy:* Evidence of bulky abdominal and thoracic disease with high intensity uptake of MIBG

55

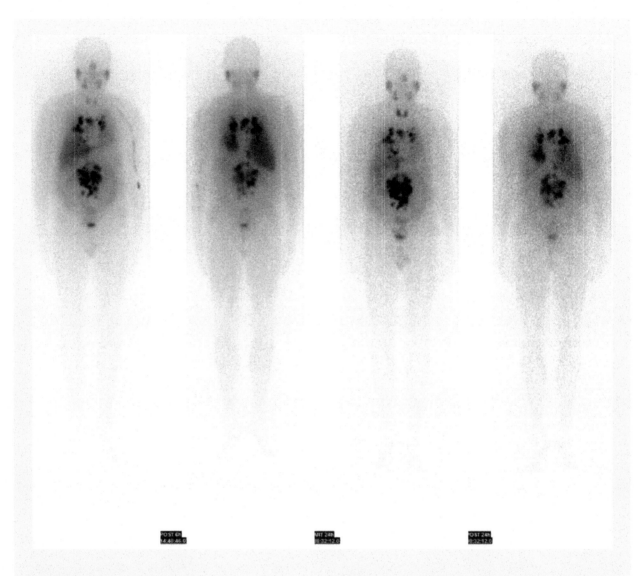

POST 6H
14:40:46.0

ANT 24h
8:32:12.0

POST 24h
8:02:12.0

Question

Which therapy for this patient?
- Radionuclide therapy
- Chemotherapy
- Clinical Trial

Answer

Radionuclide therapy with MIBG: The patient was treated with 1850 MBq MIBG I-131. The MIBG-scintigraphy evaluation 4 months after the PRRT showed the reduction of the metabolic activity of all the metastatic sites.

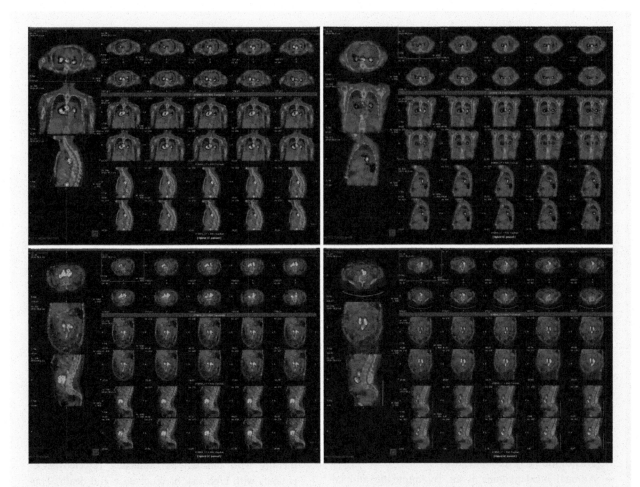

Key Points

1. The importance of a correct study of an incidental adrenal mass.
2. The importance of long-term follow-up and the diagnosis of malignancy of pheochromocytoma are extremely difficult at diagnosis and are done in case of metastatic disease.
3. Multidisciplinary management of patients affected with pheochromocytoma.
4. The role of radionuclides for diagnosis and treatment.

Expert Opinion
Alfredo Berruti

Key Points

- The adrenal gland is composed of two embryological and functional distinct organs: medulla and cortex. The majority of adrenal tumors are benign. Malignant transformation is rare. Tumors arising from adrenal chromaffin cells of the medulla are called pheochromocytomas (PCCs), whereas those arising from extraadrenal chromaffin cells are termed paragangliomas (PGLs). Tumors deriving from the transformation of adrenal cortex are either adenoma or adrenocortical carcinoma (ACC).

- PCCs and PGLs are rare diseases with an estimated incidence in Western countries between 2 and 8 new cases per million population per year. Benign adrenocortical neoplasms (adenomas) are frequent, whereas ACC is extremely disease with an estimated incidence between 0.5 and 2 new cases per million population per year.

- PCCs and PGLs are mainly sporadic. Thirty percent of them, however, are associated with specific familiar disorders. Therefore, genetic counseling is recommended in all PCCs and PGLs patients. This is not the case of ACC patients that are rarely associated to genetic disorders. In these latter patients, genetic tests are not routinely recommended.

- Adrenal incidentaloma is an asymptomatic adrenal mass detected on imaging not performed for suspected adrenal disease. A surgical treatment should be considered individually, on the basis of the likelihood of malignancy (i.e., tumor size >4 cm), the presence and degree of hormone excess, age, general health, and patient preference.

- The most frequent symptoms and sign of PCCs is hypertension that is associated to an excess of catecholamines released by tumors either continuously or paroxysmally. Forty to sixty percent of ACC are functioning at presentation, being cortisol hypersecretion (Cushing syndrome) the most frequent clinical manifestation.

- Since both PCCs/PGLs and ACC are hormone secreting, a comprehensive hormonal analysis is recommended when an adrenal mass is diagnosed in order to establish the origin (cortex or medulla) and nature (malignant or benign) of the lesion. Hormone monitoring is essential also during follow-up as hormone increase may indicate early disease relapse. Moreover, plasma chromogranin levels could be additionally evaluated in PCCs/PGLs.

- No histological system currently available can predict the biological aggressiveness of PCCs/PGLs. The certainty of malignant behavior is done by the evidence of metastases. The Weiss score is widely used to discriminate benign versus malignant ACC.

- Imaging procedures are fundamental to both differentiate benign and malignant adrenal lesions and to correctly stage the disease. Computed tomography scan is the first choice imaging technique for PCCs/PGLs and ACC. FDG PET scan could be of help in the staging of both PCCs and PGLs. Functional imaging techniques, such as ^{123}I MIBG and ^{68}Ga-DOTATATE PET/CT, offer both diagnostic and theranostic information and are widely used for PCCs/PGLs.

- In PCCs/PGLs, the only reliable predictor of malignancy is the SDHB gene germline mutation. There is no staging system for malignant PCCs/PGLs. The most important prognostic factors in early ACC are the disease stage, margin-free resection, age, the proliferation marker Ki67, and the glucocorticoid excess. Additional prognostic factors in metastatic patients may be mENSAT stage and GRAS parameters, but they are not validated yet.

- Surgery is the mainstay of therapy in the management of both ACC and PCCs/PGLs with local regional disease. It is advisable that adrenal surgery should be performed in referenced centers.

- Currently available guidelines recommend adjuvant therapy with mitotane in radically resected ACC patients with high risk of recurrence and death. This recommendation, however, is based on a weak evidence, since it is not supported by the results of prospective randomized clinical trials.

- The major principles in the management of metastatic PCCs/PGLs include control of symptoms related to catecholamine overproduction and tumor growth, but no curative treatment is achievable. Treatment choices include locoregional therapies, systemic chemotherapy, and radiopharmaceutical agents, and a wait-and-see policy in case of indolent disease with low tumor burden. The decision on the best treatment for each individual patient is often complex and requires a multidisciplinary approach.

- In metastatic ACC patients, the goals of treatment include both tumor growth control and mitigation of the effects derived from hormone excess when there is a biochemical and clinical evidence of hormone hyperscretion. Mitotane and metirapone play a major role in the control of Cushing syndrome. The standard first-line approach in ACC patients is mitotane alone or mitotane in combination with EDP chemotherapy scheme (etoposide, doxorubicin, and cisplatin). In addition to systemic therapy also local regional therapies, that is, radiofrequency ablation and chemoembolization can be taken into consideration in a selected patient population.

- A hormonal, clinical, and imaging follow-up is suggested after surgery in both PCCs/PGLs and ACC patients.

Summary of Clinical Recommendation
ESMO

- ACC is defined by a Weiss score of 3 or more. Malignant pheochromocytomas/paragangliomas are defined by the presence of metastasis.
- Patients suspected to harbor primary adrenal tumors should undergo a standardized diagnostic work-up consisting of endocrine assessment for excess hormone production and modern imaging (CT/MRI of abdomen, chest CT, and in selected cases supplemented by isotope functional imaging mainly FDG-PET). The diagnostic work-up differs between ACC and pheochromocytoma.
- Guided biopsies of potentially resectable primary adrenal tumors are not informative in most cases, but these are potentially harmful and should be avoided.
- The ENSAT TNM staging system should be used for ACC staging.
- Histological diagnosis should be done by an experienced pathologist and should rely on morphological, mitotic, and immunohistochemical parameters.
- Complete surgical extirpation of localized and locally advanced ACC or pheochromocytoma (R0 resection) is the mainstay of potentially curative approaches. Additionally, a locoregional lymphadenectomy is suggested for ACC.
- In pheochromocytoma, cytoreductive surgery might be considered. In advanced ACC, this approach is only reasonable for patients with severe hormone excess.
- Meticulous perioperative management of hormonal, glucose, electrolytes, cardiac, and fluid/blood pressure abnormalities is a critical component of patient care.
- Despite the limited literature evidence, adjuvant systemic mitotane is recommended for patients with ACC and incomplete resection (R1, Rx stage III) or in the presence of high-risk features (Ki67>10 %). R1 and Rx ACC resections may be followed by additional adjuvant radiotherapy to the tumor bed.
- Fit patients with inoperable ACC, high tumor volume, and rapid disease progression should be treated with combination cytotoxic chemotherapy plus mitotane (EDP-M). Less fit patients and/or patients with low tumor burden and slow progression can (first) be managed with mitotane monotherapy combined or not with locoregional options.

- Disease and symptom control is the main treatment goal for patients with inoperable pheochromocytoma and can be attempted by radiopharmaceuticals (^{131}I-MIBG), locoregional ablative procedures, and/or combination chemotherapy (CVD) in selected cases.
- Wait-and-see policy is recommended in low tumor burden and asymptomatic malignant pheochromocytoma and paraganglioma.
- Patients with resected ACC or pheochromocytoma should be followed at regular intervals with clinical, imaging, and biochemical screens for at least 10 years. Lifelong surveillance with an increased interval of time is favored in malignant pheochromocytoma/paraganglioma.
- The follow-up of patients with inoperable disease should be performed every 2–4 months for ACC and every 3–6 months for pheochromocytoma/paraganglioma during the first year of follow-up and then adjusted.

NCCN
1. PCC
    1. For the correct diagnosis and tumor staging, it is recommended to measure plasma-free or 24-hour urine fractionated metanephrines and to perform a chest CT with or without contrast and abdominal/pelvic multiphasic CT or MRI. The genetic counseling recommended too.
    2. For metastatic disease, tumor staging should include MIBG scan, somatostatin receptor-based imaging (i. e., see Primary Treatment (PHEO-2) somatostatin receptor scintigraphy or gallium-68 dotatate PET/Ctg), FDG-PET/CT (skull base to mid-thigh), and bone scan (if bone symptoms).
    3. Medical therapy should include alpha blockade with volume repletion and high salt diet for 7–14 days or until stable.
    4. Resectable disease should undergo surgery, preferring the laparoscopic approach when feasible
    5. Locally unresectable disease should continue medical therapy and should be referred to multidisciplinary center and then evaluated for radiotherapy with or without cytoreductive resection (R2) when possible; if positivity to MIBG scan, 131I-MIBG should be considered
    6. Metastatic disease should continue medical therapy and should receive one of the following therapies:
        - Cytoreductive resection (R2) when possible.
        - 131I-MIBG (if positivity to MIBG scan).
        - Clinical trial.
        - Systemic chemotherapy.
        - Palliative RT for bone metastases.

- Surveillance program should be offered both to resected and metastatic patients and comprises every 3–12 months H&P, blood pressure, markers, chest CT ± contrast, and abdominal/pelvic CT or MRI with contrast or FDG-PET/CT.

2. ACC
   - The basal evaluation of an adrenal mass should include the following:
     - Adrenal protocol for morphologic evaluation: CT with contrast or MRI with/without contrast to determine size, heterogeneity, lipid content (MRI), contrast washout (CT), and margin characteristics.
     - A functional evaluation, in order to identify functioning or nonfunctioning tumors. The hormonal work-up is specific for hyperaldosterism, Cushing's syndrome, and pheochromocytoma.
   - When a carcinoma is suspected (greater dimension >4 cm or inhomogeneous, irregular margins, local invasion or other malignant imaging characteristics), it is necessary to complete the staging with chest CT with or without contrast and abdominal/pelvic CT or MRI with/without contrast to evaluate for metastases and local invasion.
   - Localized disease should undergo surgery. Open adrenalectomy is recommended.
   - If high risk of recurrence, consider adjuvant mitotane therapy and external-beam RT to tumor bed.
   - In metastatic disease, consider observation with chest CT with or without contrast and abdominal/pelvic CT or MRI with contrast for clinically indolent disease every 3 months and biomarkers (if tumor initially functional).
   - If primary tumor and >90 % of metastases are removable, the surgical resection should be considered, particularly if functional
   - In metastatic disease, systemic therapy should be considered, preferably in clinical trial:
     - Cisplatin/carboplatin + etoposide ± doxorubicin ± mitotane.
     - Streptozocin ± mitotane.
     - Mitotane monotherapy.
   - After disease, resection consider chest CT with or without contrast and abdominal/pelvic CT or MRI with contrast and biomarkers (if tumor initially functional) every 3–12 months up to 5 years.

Hints for Deeper Insight
Pheochromocytomas and Paragangliomas
- *International guidelines*
  Berruti A, Baudin E, Gelderblom H, Haak HR, Porpiglia F, Fassnacht M, Pentheroudakis G; ESMO Guidelines Working Group. Adrenal cancer: ESMO Clinical Practice Guidelines for diagnosis, treatment and follow-up. Ann Oncol. 2012 Oct;23 Suppl 7:vii131–8. PMID: 22997446.
  Lenders JW, Duh QY, Eisenhofer G. Pheochromocytoma and paraganglioma: an endocrine society clinical practice guideline. J Clin Endocrinol Metab. 2014 Jun;99(6):1915–42. PMID: 24893135.
- *Prognostic stratifications and future targeted therapies.*
  Crona J, Taïeb D, Pacak K. New Perspectives on Pheochromocytoma and Paraganglioma: Toward a Molecular Classification. Endocr Rev. 2017 Dec 1;38(6):489–515. PMID: 28938417.
- *Perioperative Management of PCCs and PGLs.*
  Naranjo J, Dodd S, Martin YN. Perioperative Management of Pheochromocytoma. J Cardiothorac Vasc Anesth. 2017 Aug;31(4):1427–1439. Epub 2017 Feb 4. PMID: 28392094.
- *Novel targeted therapy in PCCs and PGLs*
  Pandit-Taskar N, Modak S. Norepinephrine Transporter as a Target for Imaging and Therapy. J Nucl Med. 2017 Sep;58(Suppl 2):39S-53S. PMID: 28864611.

Adrenocortical carcinoma:
- *International guidelines*
  Fassnacht M, Dekkers OM, Else T, Baudin E, Berruti A, de Krijger R, Haak HR, Mihai R, Assie G, Terzolo M. European Society of Endocrinology Clinical Practice Guidelines on the management of adrenocortical carcinoma in adults, in collaboration with the European Network for the Study of Adrenal Tumors. Eur J Endocrinol. 2018 Oct 1;179(4):G1-G46. PMID: 30299884.
  Berruti A, Baudin E, Gelderblom H, Haak HR, Porpiglia F, Fassnacht M, Pentheroudakis G; ESMO Guidelines Working Group. Adrenal cancer: ESMO Clinical Practice Guidelines for diagnosis, treatment and follow-up. Ann Oncol. 2012 Oct;23 Suppl 7:vii131–8. PMID: 22997446.
- *Prognostic factors in ACC.*
  Baudin E. Adrenocortical carcinoma. Endocrinol Metab Clin North Am. 2015 Jun;44(2):411–34. Review. PMID: 26038209.
- *Therapeutic range in mitotane treatment.*
  Hermsen IG, Fassnacht M, Terzolo M, et al. Plasma concentrations of o,p'DDD, o,p'DDA, and o,p'DDE as predictors of tumor response to mitotane in adrenocortical carcinoma: results of a retrospective ENS@T multicenter study. J. Clin. Endocrinol. Metab. 2011;96:1844–1851. PMID: 21470991.
- *Targeted therapies and immunotherapy in ACC.*
  Konda B, Kirschner LS. Novel targeted therapies in adrenocortical carcinoma. Curr Opin Endocrinol Diabetes Obes. 2016; 23(3):233–41. PMID: 27119750.

Cosentini D, Grisanti S, Dalla Volta A, et al Immunotherapy failure in adrenocortical cancer: where next? Endocr Connect. 2018 Nov 1. pii: EC-18–0398. R1. PMID: 30400026.

Suggested reading

Pheochromocytomas and Paragangliomas

1. Angelousi A, Kassi E, Zografos G et al. Metastatic pheochromocytoma and paraganglioma.Eur J Clin Invest 2015;45(9):986–997. PMID: 26183460.
2. Lenders JW, Pacak K, Walther MM et al. Biochemical diagnosis of pheochromocytoma: which test is best? JAMA 2002;287:1427–34. PMID: 11903030.
3. Janssen I, Blanchet EM, Adams K, et al. Superiority of [68 Ga]-DOTATATE PET/CT to other functional imaging modalities in the localization of SDHB-associated metastatic pheochromocytoma and paraganglioma. Clin Cancer Res 2015;14:2751. PMID: 25873086.
4. Baudin E, Habra MA, Deschamps F, et al. Therapy of endocrine disease: treatment of malignant pheochromocytoma and paraganglioma. Eur J Endocrinol 2014;171:111–22. PMID: 24891137.

5. Kong G, Grozinsky-Glasberg S, Hofman MS, et al. Efficacy of Peptide Receptor Radionuclide Therapy for Functional Metastatic Paraganglioma and Pheochromocytoma. J Clin Endocrinol Metab. 2017; 102(9):3278–328. PMID: 28605448.

Adrenocortical carcinoma:

1. Terzolo M, Baudin AE, Ardito A, et al Mitotane levels predict the outcome of patients with adrenocortical carcinoma treated adjuvantly following radical resection. Eur J Endocrinol. 2013 Jul 29;169(3):263–70. PMID: 23704714.
2. Berruti A, Terzolo M, Sperone P, et al Etoposide, doxorubicin and cisplatin plus mitotane in the treatment of advanced adrenocortical carcinoma: a large prospective phase II trial. Endocr Relat Cancer. 2005; 12(3):657–66. P MID: 16172198.
3. Fassnacht M, Terzolo M, Allolio B, et al Combination chemotherapy in advanced adrenocortical carcinoma. N Engl J Med. 2012 Jun 7;366(23):2189–97. PMID: 22551107.
4. Terzolo M, Daffara F, Ardito A, et al. Management of adrenal cancer: a 2013 update. J Endocrinol Invest. 2014;37(3):207–217. PMID: 24458831.

References

1. Yates R, Katugampola H, Cavlan D, et al. Adrenocortical development, maintenance, and disease. Curr Top Dev Biol. 2013;106:239–312.
2. Lam KY, Lo CY. Composite pheochromocytoma-ganglioneuroma of the adrenal gland: an uncommon entity with distinctive clinicopathologic features. Endocr Pathol. 1999; 10:343–52.
3. Gunawardane Kavinga PT, Grossman A. Phaeochromocytoma and paraganglioma. Adv Exp Med Biol. 2016; https://doi.org/10.1007/5584_2016_76.
4. Mansmann G, Lau J, Balk E, Rothberg M, Miyachi Y, Bornstein SR. The clinically inapparent adrenal mass: up- date in diagnosis and management. Endocr Rev. 2004;25:309–40.
5. Mantero F, Terzolo M, Arnaldi G, et al. A survey on adrenal incidentaloma in Italy. Study Group on Adrenal Tumors of the Italian Society of Endocrinology. J Clin Endocrinol Metab. 2000;85:637–44.
6. Terzolo M, Daffara F, Ardito A, et al. Management of adrenal cancer: a 2013 update. J Endocrinol Investig. 2014;37(3):207–17.
7. Dahia PL. Pheochromocytoma and paraganglioma pathogenesis: learning from genetic heterogeneity. Nat Rev Cancer. 2014;14(2):108–19.
8. Assié G, Letouzé E, Fassnacht M, et al. Integrated genomic characterization of adrenocortical carcinoma. Nat Genet. 2014;46(6):607–12.
9. Else T, Kim AC, Sabolch A, et al. Adrenocortical Carcinoma. Endocr Rev. 2014;35:282–326.
10. Angelousi A, Kassi E, Zografos G, et al. Metastatic pheochromocytoma and paraganglioma. Eur J Clin Investig. 2015;45(9):986–97.

11. Fassnacht M, Arlt W, Bancos I, et al. Management of adrenal incidentalomas: european society of endocrinology clinical practice guideline in collaboration with the European Network for the Study of Adrenal Tumors. Eur J Endocrinol. 2016;175(2): G1–G34.
12. Lam AK. Update on Paragangliomas and Pheochromocytomas. Turk Patoloji Derg. 2015;31(Suppl 1):105–12.
13. Ferreira VM, Marcelino M, Piechnik SK, et al. Pheochromocytoma is characterized by catecholamine-mediated myocarditis, focal and diffuse myocardial fibrosis, and myocardial dysfunction. J Am Coll Cardiol. 2016;67(20):2364–74.
14. Lam AK. Update on adrenal tumours in 2017 World Health Organization (WHO) of endocrine tumours. Endocr Pathol. 2017;28(3):213–27.
15. Weiss LM, Medeiros LJ, Vickery AL Jr. Pathologic features of prognostic significance in adrenocortical carcinoma. Am J Surg Pathol. 1989;13:202–6.
16. Fishbein L, Leshchiner I, Walter V, et al. Cancer Genome Atlas Research Network. Comprehensive molecular characterization of pheochromocytoma and paraganglioma. Cancer Cell. 2017;31(2):181–93.
17. Crona J, Taïeb D, Pacak K. New perspectives on Pheochromocytoma and Paraganglioma: toward a molecular classification. Endocr Rev. 2017;38(6):489–515.
18. European Network for Adrenal Tumors (ENS@T): www.ensat.org.
19. Berruti A, Baudin E, Gelderblom H, et al. on behalf of the ESMO guidelines working group. Adrenal cancer: ESMO clinical practice guidelines for diagnosis, treatment and follow-up. Ann Oncol. 2012;23(Suppl 7):vii131–vii138.
20. Libè R. Adrenocortical carcinoma (ACC): diagnosis, prognosis, and treatment. Front Cell Dev Biol. 2015;3:45.

21. Lenders JW, Pacak K, Walther MM, et al. Biochemical diagnosis of pheochromocytoma: which test is best? JAMA. 2002;287:1427–34.

22. Eisenhofer G, Lenders JW, Siegert G, et al. Plasma methoxytyramine: a novel biomarker of metastatic pheochromocytoma and paraganglioma in relation to established risk factors of tumour size, location and SDHB mutation status. Eur J Cancer. 2012;48:1739–49.

23. Amar L, Peyrard S, Rossignol P, et al. Changes in urinary total metanephrine excretion in recurrent and malignant pheochromocytomas and secreting paragangliomas. Ann N Y Acad Sci. 2006;1073:383–91.

24. Zuber S, Wesley R, Prodanov T, et al. Clinical utility of chromogranin A in SDHx-related paragangliomas. Eur J Clin Investig. 2014;44:365–71.

25. Hahner S, Caoili E, Else T. 5th international ACC symposium: imaging for diagnosis and surveillance of adrenal tumors - new advances and reviews of old concepts. Horm Canc. 2016;7:40–3.

26. Sturgeon C, Shen WT, et al. Risk assessment in 457 adrenal cortical carcinomas: how much does tumor size predict the likelihood of malignancy? J Am Coll Surg. 2006;202:423–30.

27. Elsayes KM, Mukundan G, Narra VR, et al. Adrenal masses: mr imaging features with pathologic correlation. Radiographics. 2004;24(Suppl.1):S73–86.

28. Bharwani N, Rockall AG, et al. Adrenocortical carcinoma: the range of appearances on CT and MRI. Am J Roentgenol. 2011;196:W706–14.

29. Boland GW, et al. Characterization of adrenal masses by using FDG PET: a systematic review and meta-analysis of diagnostic test performance. Radiology. 2011;259:117–26.

30. Deandreis D, Leboulleux S, Caramella C, et al. FDG PET in the management of patients with adrenal masses and adrenocortical carcinoma. Horm Cancer. 2014;2:354–62.

31. Hahner S, Stuermer A, Kreiss, et al. [123 I]Iodometomidate for molecular imaging of adrenocortical cytochrome P450 family 11B enzymes. J Clin Endocrinol Metab. 2008;93:2358–65.

32. Rednam SP, Erez A, Druker H, et al. Von Hippel–Lindau and hereditary pheochromocytoma/paraganglioma syndromes: clinical features, genetics, and surveillance recommendations in childhood. Clin Cancer Res. 2017;23(12):e68–75.

33. Berglund AS. Hulthe'n UL, Manhem P, et al. Metaiodobenzylguanidine (MIBG) scintigraphy and computed tomography (CT) in clinical practice. Primary and secondary evaluation for localization of phaeochromocytomas. J Intern Med. 2001;249:247–51.

34. Bhatia KS, Ismail MM, Sahdev A, et al. 123I- metaiodobenzylguanidine (MIBG) scintigraphy for the detection of adrenal and extra-adrenal phaeochro- mocytomas: CT and MRI correlation. Clin Endocrinol. 2008;69:181–8.

35. Jacobson AF, Deng H, Lombard J, et al. 123I -metaiodobenzylguanidine scintigraphy for the detection of neuroblastoma and pheochromo- cytoma: results of a meta-analysis. J Clin Endocrinol Metab. 2010;95:2596–606.

36. Mozley PD, Kim CK, Mohsin J, et al. The efficacy of iodine-123-MIBG as a screening test for pheochromocytoma. J Nucl Med. 1994;35:1138–44.

37. Timmers HJ, Chen CC, Carrasquillo JA, et al. Comparison of 18F-fluoro-L-DOPA, 18F-fluoro- deoxyglucose, and 18F-fluorodopamine PET and 123I-MIBG scintigraphy in the localization of pheo- chromocytoma and paraganglioma. J Clin Endocrinol Metab. 2009;94:4757–67.

38. Janssen I, Blanchet EM, Adams K, et al. Superiority of [68 Ga]-DOTATATE PET/CT to other functional imaging modalities in the localization of SDHB-associated metastatic pheochromocytoma and paraganglioma. Clin Cancer Res. 2015;14:2751.

39. Comino-Mendez I, Gracia-Aznarez FJ, Schiavi F, et al. Exome sequencing identifies MAX mutations as a cause of hereditary pheochromocytoma. Nat Genet. 2011;43:663–7. 48.

40. Pacak K, Eisenhofer G, Ahlman H, et al. International symposium on Pheochromocytoma. Pheochromocytoma: recommendations for clinical practice from the first international symposium. Nat Clin Pract Endocrinol Metab. 2007;3:92–102.

41. Baudin E. Adrenocortical carcinoma. Endocrinol Metab Clin N Am. 2015;44(2):411–34.

42. Cosentini D, Badalamenti G, Grisanti S, et al. Activity and safety of temozolomide in advanced adrenocortical carcinoma patients. Eur J Endocrinol. 2019;181(6):681–9. https://doi.org/10.1530/EJE-19-0570.

43. Baudin E, Habra MA, Deschamps F, et al. Therapy of endocrine disease: treatment of malignant pheochromocytoma and paraganglioma. Eur J Endocrinol. 2014;171:111–22.

44. van Hulsteijn LT, Niemeijer ND, Dekkers OM, et al. (131) IMIBG therapy for malignant paraganglioma and phaeochromocytoma: systematic review and meta-analysis. Clin Endocrinol. 2014;80:487–501.

45. Gonias S, Goldsby R, Matthay KK, et al. Phase II study of high-dose [131I]metaiodobenzylguanidine therapy for patients with metastatic pheochromocytoma and paraganglioma. J Clin Oncol. 2009;27(25):4162–8.

46. Kong G, Grozinsky-Glasberg S, Hofman MS, et al. Efficacy of peptide receptor radionuclide therapy for functional metastatic paraganglioma and pheochromocytoma. J Clin Endocrinol Metab. 2017;102(9):3278–328.

47. Niemeijer ND, Alblas G, van Hulsteijn LT, et al. Chemotherapy with cyclophosphamide, vincristine and dacarbazine for malignant paraganglioma and pheochromocytoma: systematic review and meta-analysis. Clin Endocrinol. 2014;8:642–51.

48. Hadoux J, Favier J, Scoazec JY, et al. SDHB mutations are associated with response to temozolomide in patients with metastatic pheochromocytoma or paraganglioma. Int J Cancer. 2014;135(11):2711–20.

49. Hidaka S, Hiraoka A, Ochi H, et al. Malignant pheochromocytoma with liver metastasis treated by transcatheter arterial chemo-embolization (TACE). Intern Med. 2010;49:645–51.

50. Bellantone R, Ferrante A, Boscherini, et al. Role of reoperation in recurrence of adrenal cortical carcinoma: results from 188 cases collected in the Italian National Registry for Adrenal Cortical Carcinoma. Surgery. 1997;122:1212–8.

51. Schulick RD, Brennan MF. Long-term survival after complete resection and repeat resection in patients with adrenocortical carcinoma. Ann Surg Oncol. 1999;6:719–26.

52. Terzolo M, Angeli A, Fassnacht M, et al. Adjuvant mitotane treatment for adrenocortical carcinoma. N Engl Med. 2007;356:2372–80.

53. Berruti A, Grisanti S, Pulzer A, et al. Long-term outcomes of adjuvant Mitotane therapy in patients with radically resected adrenocortical carcinoma. J Clin Endocrinol Metab. 2017;102(4):1358–65.

54. Hermsen IG, Fassnacht M, Terzolo M, et al. Plasma concentrations of o,p'DDD, o,p'DDA, and o,p'DDE as predictors of tumor response to mitotane in adrenocortical carcinoma: results of a retrospective ENS@T multicenter study. J Clin Endocrinol Metab. 2011;96:1844–51.

55. Berruti A, Terzolo M, Sperone P, et al. Etoposide, doxorubicin and cisplatin plus mitotane in the treatment of advanced adreno-cortical carcinoma: a large prospective phase II trial. Endocr Relat Cancer. 2005;12:657–66.

56. Fassnacht M, Terzolo M, Allolio B, et al. Combination chemo-therapy in advanced adrenocortical carcinoma. N Engl J Med. 2012;366:2189–97.

57. Deschamps F, Farouil G, Ternes N, et al. Thermal ablation tech-niques: a curative treatment of bone metastases in selected patients? Eur Radiol. 2014;24(8):1971–80.

58. Wood BJ, Abraham J, Hvizda JL, et al. Radiofrequency ablation of adrenal tumors and adrenocortical carcinoma metastases. Cancer. 2003;97(3):554–60.

59. Wong E, Jacques S, Bennett M, et al. Complete response in a patient with stage IV adrenocortical carcinoma treated with adjuvant trans-catheter arterial chemo-embolization (TACE). Asia Pac J Clin Oncol. 2017; in press

60. Kamenický P, Droumaguet C, Salenave S, et al. Mitotane, metyrapone, and ketoconazole combination therapy as an alter-native to rescue adrenalectomy for severe ACTH-dependent Cushing's syndrome. J Clin Endocrinol Metab. 2011;96(9): 2796–804.

61. Claps M, Cerri S, Grisanti S, et al. Adding metyrapone to che-motherapy plus mitotane for Cushing's syndrome due to advanced adrenocortical carcinoma. Endocrine. 2018; in press

Cancer of the Thyroid

Valerio Gristina, Nadia Barraco, Silvio Buscemi, Lorena Incorvaia, and Alfredo Berruti

Endocrine Cancers

Contents

Authors Valerio Gristina, Nadia Barraco, and Silvio Buscemi should be considered equally co-first authors.

© Springer Nature Switzerland AG 2021
A. Russo et al. (eds.), *Practical Medical Oncology Textbook*, UNIPA Springer Series,
https://doi.org/10.1007/978-3-030-56051-5_56

Learning Objectives

By the end of the chapter, the reader will:
- Be able to apply diagnostic and therapeutic procedures in thyroid cancer
- Have learned the basic concepts of thyroid cancer
- Have reached in depth knowledge of thyroid cancer management
- Be able to put acquired knowledge into clinical practice

56.1 Introduction

Thyroid cancers are the most common endocrine neoplasms, accounting for more than 90% of the total newly diagnosed endocrine cancers [1] while representing <1% of all human tumors and about 3% of visceral malignancies.

Thyroid cancers are basically derived from either follicular cells (papillary, follicular, anaplastic and poorly differentiated carcinoma) or parafollicular cells (medullary carcinoma) and share a common classification based on differentiation (well, intermediate, and poor differentiated). Nevertheless, thyroid carcinoma can be additionally categorized by increasing clinical aggressiveness reflecting the wide range of clinical behavior from low mortality and long-term survival in most cases of well and intermediately differentiated tumors to frequently incurable poorly differentiated cancers.

Both papillary and follicular cancers, grouped together under the header of "well-differentiated thyroid cancer" (WDTC), account for 95% of cases and are effectively treated with surgery, radioactive iodine (RAI), and thyroid-stimulating hormone suppressive therapy unless patients present with advanced disease [2]. Medullary thyroid cancer (MTC) is less common constituting between 2 and 5% of all thyroid malignancies but much more clinically aggressive whenever surgery is not feasible. Anaplastic carcinoma (ATC) is one of the most aggressive cancers in humans and fortunately appears to be declining over time. Poorly differentiated thyroid carcinoma (PDTC) was introduced as a separate entity in 2004 in the WHO Classification of Tumors [3] showing an intermediate prognosis between differentiated and undifferentiated neoplasms (◻ Table 56.1).

In recent years, the development of targeted therapy has led to the approval of different multikinase inhibitors for iodine refractory-DTC (sorafenib and lenvatinib) and for progressive or metastatic MTC (cabozantinib and vandetanib).

◻ **Table 56.1** Frequency and mortality rates in thyroid cancers

Thyroid cancer	Frequency	Mortality
Papillary (PTC)	85–90%	1–2% at 20 years
Follicular (FTC)	10–15%	10–20% at 10 years
Midollary (MTC)	2–5%	25–50% at 10 years
Poorly differentiated (PDTC)	1–3%	60% at 5 years
Anaplastic (ATC)	1%	90% at 5 years

56.2 Epidemiology and Etiology

The incidence of thyroid cancers has tripled over the past 30 years varying considerably by geographic area, age, and sex.
- The incidence of thyroid cancers is increasing worldwide probably due to two coexisting processes: increased detection of (apparent increase) and increased number of cases (true increase) due to unrecognized thyroid-specific carcinogens [4, 5].
- Nearly 60–80% of thyroid carcinomas detected nowadays are micropapillary thyroid carcinomas (<1 cm in size).
- WDTCs have a greater incidence in whites than in blacks of both genders.
- Both papillary and follicular thyroid carcinomas are approximately 2.5 times more common in females with an earlier median age at diagnosis that tends to be even earlier for papillary cancer as compared to follicular cancer in either gender.
- Older patients are more likely to have higher risk PTC variants, PDTC or ATC.
- The incidence rates of MTC and ATC do not show any substantial differences by race/ethnicity. Up to 75% of MTC cases occur sporadically with other distinct familial syndromes accounting for the remainder. Occasionally, ATC may arise via dedifferentiation of prior WDTC.
- Radiation exposure, age, gender, family history, and low iodine intake are known risk factors for WDTC and probably for ATC while autoimmune thyroiditis and obesity remain controversial. MTC is not associated with radiation exposure but significantly related to hereditary conditions.

56.3 Histopathology Overview

The cellular consistency of the normal thyroid gland is made up of two main parenchymal cell types: follicular (◘ Fig. 56.1) and parafollicular cells. While the former line colloid follicles, concentrate on iodine and produce thyroid hormones giving rise to both DTC and ATC, the latter produce the hormone calcitonin and are the cells of origin for MTC. Immune cells and stromal cells are responsible for extremely rare lymphoma [5] and sarcoma [6] of the thyroid, respectively.

56.4 Clinical Features

While thyroid nodules are common in the general population, the risk of malignancy is rare (approximately 5–10%) and easily assessed by obtaining information from the history and physical exam.

The vast majority of thyroid cancers presents as a palpable neck mass which may represent a primary tumor or metastatic lymphadenopathy, detected either by the patient or by clinician's physical examination. Conversely, patients first present with a non-palpable mass diagnosed incidentally with neck imaging.

On physical exam, particular attention to the firmness, mobility, irregularities, and size of the nodules, their adherence to the surrounding structures, and the presence of lymphadenopathy are significant clues to the presence of carcinoma.

The presence of a solitary nodule and evolution of symptoms such as rapid growth of the mass, worsening of dysphagia and breathing, hoarseness, fatigue, and weight loss should be queried albeit these features do lack specificity for malignancy. Vocal cord paralysis is generally associated with advanced disease (◘ Fig. 56.2).

Most differentiated thyroid cancers are clinically indolent and have a favorable outcome with two-thirds of patients exhibiting gross disease localized to the thyroid at presentation. Conversely, approximately 10% of patients have recurrent or persistent disease with follicular carcinoma (FTC) showing more of a propensity to spread to distant sites (such as bone and lung) than papillary carcinoma (PTC), which tends to metastasize to lymph nodes [7]. However, prognosis seems to be similar in age-matched and disease stage-matched patients [8].

Alternatively, MTC may present either as an asymptomatic mass or as a bulky disease with high levels of serum calcitonin and severe secretory diarrhea. If not metastatic or relapsed, the natural history of localized and regional MTC is generally indolent with many patients having excellent long-term outcomes. Moreover, an increasing number of patients have been identified in one of the familial settings (◘ Table 56.2).

◘ **Fig. 56.1** Normal thyroid follicular cells and parafollicular cells. (Photos by courtesy of Prof. A. Martorana, Department of Health Promotion, Mother and Child Care, Internal Medicine and Medical Specialties, Pathologic Anatomy Unit-University of Palermo, University of Palermo)

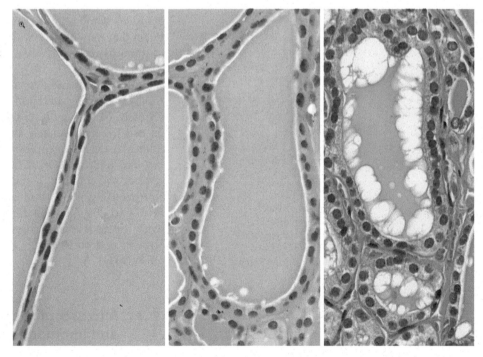

Fig. 56.2 Main clinical features suggestive for thyroid malignancies

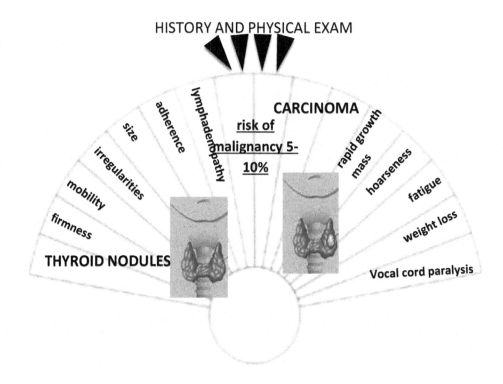

56

Table 56.2 Clinical and genetic characteristics of familial medullary thyroid cancer syndromes

Syndrome	Characteristics Features
FMTC	MTC
MEN-2A	MTC Adrenal medulla (pheochromocytoma) Parathyroid hyperplasia
MEN-2A with cutaneous lichen amyloidosis	MEN-2A and a priuritic cutaneous lesion located over the upper back
MEN-2A or FMTC with Hirschsprung disease	MEN-2A or FMTC with Hirschsprung disease
MEN-2B	MTC Adrenal medulla (pheochromocytoma) Intestinal and mucosal ganglioneuromatosis Characteristic Marfanoid habitus

FMTC familial medullary thyroid cancer, *MEN* multiple endocrine neoplasia, *MTC* medullary thyroid carcinoma

On the contrary, ATC and PDTC uniformly present with a large and hard palpable mass invading the neck and often causing rapid compressive symptoms. To date, the majority of patients affected by ATC primarily die from upper airway respiratory failure. Regardless of treatment strategy, survival after diagnosis is unfortunately very poor.

56.5 Pathological Features

56.5.1 Macroscopic Aspect

PTCs show a variable appearance from minute subcapsular white scars to large tumors greater than 5 to 6 cm that may present with cystic change, calcification, or even ossification grossly invading surrounding structures.

FTC usually presents as unifocal and thickly encapsulated showing invasion of the capsule or vessels. Grossly, MTC may be circumscribed or infiltrative and is usually encapsulated and white-yellow. PDTC is a follicular-derived neoplasm that usually presents with a large infiltrative mass and a solid growth pattern, grossly showing intraglandular lymphatic and vascular spread. However, certain examples are encapsulated, at least partially. ATCs are large, extrathyroidal, and fleshy with obvious hemorrhage, necrosis, and aggressive growth pattern that may replace all previous evidence of WDTC.

56.5.2 Microscopic Aspects and Immunohistochemical

Microscopically, PTCs are characterized by the presence of papillae with ground glass nuclei and necrotic changes ("psammoma bodies"), but some variants are totally follicular in pattern and are identified as a follicular variant. Further subtypes are tall cell variant (TCV), columnar cell variant (CCV), diffuse scleroting variant (DSV), solid variant (SV), and hobnail variant [9].

FTCs show trabecular or solid pattern of follicles with nuclear atypia, focal splinded areas, mitotic figures, and no necrosis. Oncocytic carcinoma (OTC or Hurtle cell carcinoma) is considered a variant of follicular neoplasms (■ Fig. 56.3).

MTC cells are monomorphic with round, oval, or spindle shape and a low nuclear/cytoplasmatic ratio often containing a characteristic amyloid substance (deposit from calcitonin). PDTCs usually present with a solid, trabecular, or insular pattern with at least one of the following: convoluted nuclei, >3 mitotic figures/10 HPF, and tumor necrosis [10]. ATC displays three patterns often mixed with better differentiated cells: large pleomorphic, spindle, or squamoid cells rarely showing rhabdoid inclusions (■ Fig. 56.4).

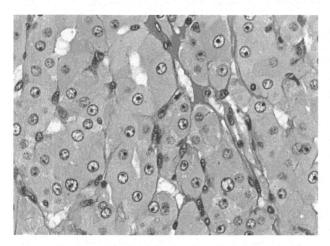

■ Fig. 56.3 Hurtle cell carcinoma microscopic aspect. (Photos by courtesy of Prof. A. Martorana, Department of Health Promotion, Mother and Child Care, Internal Medicine and Medical Specialties, Pathologic Anatomy Unit-University of Palermo, University of Palermo)

56.6 Diagnosis, Classification, and Staging Systems

Based on cancer statistics, incidence of thyroid tumors has been largely and globally increasing during the last decades. The diagnostic evaluation of thyroid cancer is mainly based on neck ultrasonography (US) encompassing the thyroid as well as the central and lateral neck compartments (■ Fig. 56.5a, b).

Specifically, some US parameters are traditionally associated with high risk of malignancy but poorly predictive when evaluated singly (■ Table 56.3). Moreover, US determination of tissue stiffness (elastography) has been recently suggested to detect malignancy in thyroid nodules with high sensitivity and specificity [11]. Nevertheless, larger prospective studies are needed for routine clinical use. Other imaging modalities (such as CT, MRI and PET) are less sensitive in diagnosing thyroid malignancies but important for eventually staging the extrathyroidal spread of the disease.

Fine needle aspiration (FNA) along with US is proved to be the most sensitive, reliable, and cost-effective technique in the evaluation of the thyroid nodules. FNA cytology (FNAC) plays an important role in the diagnostic work-up by estimating the risk of malignancy of the nodule in order to prevent unnecessary surgeries for benign conditions and avoid missing malignant nodules (■ Fig. 56.6). In particular, any patients affected by thyroid nodule >1 cm or <1 cm if there is any clinical or ultrasonographic suspicion of malignancy should undergo FNAC [12].

However, several factors can affect the diagnostic value of FNA including sampling error, heterogeneity of the nodule, physician's experience, and follicular neoplasia [13]. Furthermore, considering also the confusion related to diagnostic terminology between cytopa-

■ Fig. 56.4 Histologic subtypes of thyroid cancers. (Photos by courtesy of Prof. A. Martorana, University of Palermo)

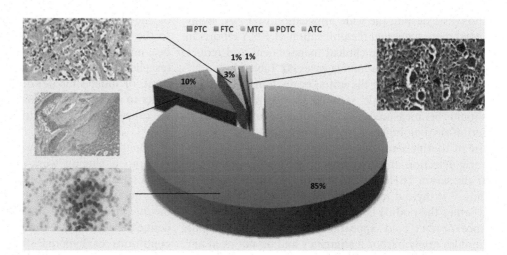

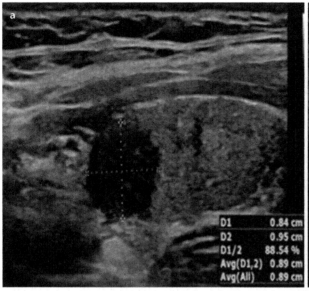
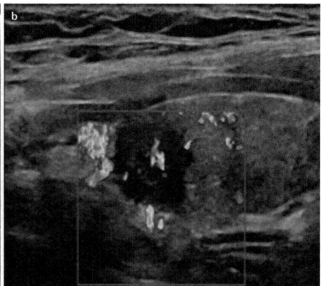

D1	0.84 cm
D2	0.95 cm
D1/2	88.54 %
Avg(D1,2)	0.89 cm
Avg(All)	0.89 cm

Fig. 56.5 *Thyroid US*: **a** Ultrasound scan shows a well-defined, homogeneous, solid hypoechoic oval-shaped nodule with irregular margins in upper left thyroid lobe suggestive for PTC; **b** Color-Doppler mode scan shows peripheral and intranodular vascularity. (Photos by courtesy of Department of Radiology, University of Palermo)

56

Table 56.3 US features suggestive of malignancy in thyroid cancers

Thyroid nodule features	Lymphnode features
Microcalcifications	Microcalcifications
Hypoechogenicity, absence of halo	Hyperechogenicity
Irregular margins (infiltrative, microlobulated or spiculated)	Peripheral vascularity
Shape "taller than wide" on transverse view	Rounded shape
Solid aspect	Cystic aspect

thologists despite the wide application of FNA, many researchers suggested the unification of FNA reports in order to improve the clinical management and reduce the number of indeterminate cases (■ Table 56.4).

Moreover, during the initial evaluation of a patient with a thyroid nodule, serum thyrotropin (TSH) level should be measured while routine measurement of serum thyroglobulin (Tg) is not recommended and the use of routine serum calcitonin (CT), even if crucial for early detection and screening in MTC, is still debated. If the serum TSH is subnormal, a radionuclide (preferably ^{123}I) thyroid scan should be obtained to document whether the nodule is hyperfunctioning ("hot" appearance) or not ("cold" appearance) since hyperfunctioning nodules rarely harbor malignancy and do not need any further cytologic evaluation. Conversely, a higher serum TSH level is associated with increased risk of malignancy as well as more advanced stage thyroid cancer [14].

Although several systems have been proposed and validated for staging differentiated thyroid cancers without any clear superiority (■ Table 56.5), TNM (tumor-node-metastasis) staging system is internationally adopted providing a good risk stratification while failing to predict the risk of recurrence and the individual response to treatment in DTC [15].

In order to adequately predict the risk of disease recurrence/permanence in DTC, first initial risk evaluation should be carried out postoperatively according to American Thyroid Association (ATA) guidelines (■ Fig. 56.7). Since the risk of recurrence and disease-specific mortality can change over time as a function of the clinical course of the disease and the response to therapy, a dynamic risk stratification (DRS) should be continually assessed according to treatment response (excellent, incomplete biochemical, incomplete structural, or indeterminate) during the whole follow-up in order to avoid overtreatment in low-risk patients and on the other hand undertreatment in high-risk subjects [12, 16].

Finally, all patients with suspicious MTC should undergo a staging work-up before surgery including basal serum CT, CEA, calcium, and plasma metanephrines and normetanephrines, or 24-h urine collection for metanephrines and normetanephrines. The goal is to define the extent of disease and to identify the comorbid conditions of hyperparathyroidism and/or pheochromocytoma in the case of hereditary forms.

Fig. 56.6 Algorithm for evaluation and management of patients with thyroid nodules based on FNAC

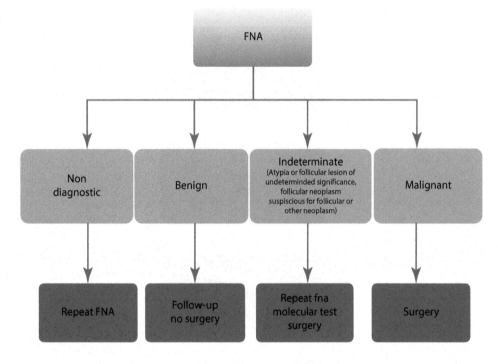

Table 56.4 Recommended diagnostic categories according to Italian (SIAPEC-IAP, AIT, AME, SIE), American (The Bethesda System for Reporting Thyroid Cytopathology), and UK (UKRCP) cytopathology classification

Diagnostic Category	Risk of malignancy	Clinical management
Not diagnostic, cystic	–	Repeat FNA
Not malignant, Benign	0–3	Clinical follow-up
Low risk undetermined lesion, atypia or follicular lesion of undetermined significance	5–15	Repeat FNA
High risk undetermined lesion, follicular neoplasia or suspicious	15–30	Surgical lobectomy
Suspicious for malignancy	60–75	Near-total thyroidectomy or lobectomy
Malignant	97–99	Near-total thyroidectomy

Table 56.5 Prognostic classification systems in DTC

System	Criteria
AGES	Age, Grade of tumor, Extent, Size
AMES	Age, Metastasis, Extent, Size
MACIS	Mestasis, Age, Completeness of resection. Invasion, Size
Ohio State	Size, Cervical metastasis. Multiplicity, Invasion, Size
Sloan-Kettering	Age, Histology, Size, Extension, Metastasis
NCTTS	Size, Multifocality, invasion. Differentiation, Metastasis
TNM	Size, Extension, Nodal metastasis. Distant metastasis

56.7 Molecular Biology

Several studies demonstrated that traditional histopathological features of WDTCs, ATCs, and PDTCs are associated with genetic changes indicating how molecular alterations in thyroid cancer could closely correlate with specific stages in a multistep tumorigenic process. MTC, whether sporadic or inherited, has a detectable association with mutations of the rearranged during transfection (RET) proto-oncogene; mutations in RET are associated with autosomal dominant syndromes including MEN2A, MEN2B, and familial MTC and are found in approximately 50% of sporadic cases (Fig. 56.8).

Although ultrasound and ultrasound-guided FNA remain the first-line diagnostic tools for detecting and characterizing thyroid tumors, cytology alone fails to define thyroid nodules in 15–30% of cases [17] probably due to the high heterogeneous nature of the lesions and

Fig. 56.7 Initial risk evaluation in DTC according to 2015 American Thyroid Association guidelines

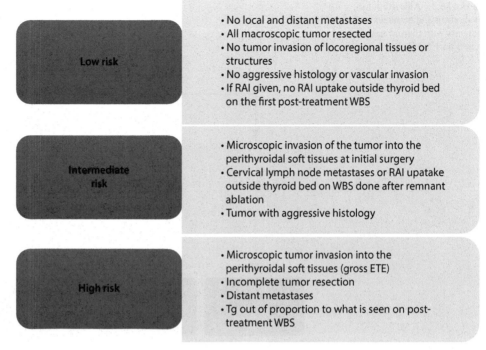

- No local and distant metastases
- All macroscopic tumor resected
- No tumor invasion of locoregional tissues or structures
- No aggressive histology or vascular invasion
- If RAI given, no RAI uptake outside thyroid bed on the first post-treatment WBS

Low risk

- Microscopic invasion of the tumor into the perithyroidal soft tissues at initial surgery
- Cervical lymph node metastases or RAI upatake outside thyroid bed on WBS done after remnant ablation
- Tumor with aggressive histology

Intermediate risk

- Microscopic tumor invasion into the perithyroidal soft tissues (gross ETE)
- Incomplete tumor resection
- Distant metastases
- Tg out of proportion to what is seen on post-treatment WBS

High risk

56

Fig. 56.8 Multistep tumorigenesis in thyroid cancer

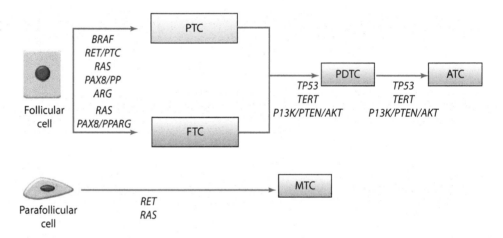

the lack of specific markers. Taking into account the need to reduce unnecessary diagnostic thyroid surgery for indeterminate thyroid nodules, molecular testing has been also studied to help define prognosis and improve precise personalized treatments.

Specifically, two main pathways (RAS/RAF/MEK/ERK and PI3K/AKT/mTOR) seem to be involved in the propagation of signals from the cell membrane tyrosine kinase receptors (RET, EGF, VEGF, PDGF) into the nucleus. Gene alteration in the RAF/ RAS/ MEK pathway leads to promotion of cell proliferation, cell growth, and angiogenesis and loss of differentiation, while mutation in the PI3K/AKT/mTOR pathway results in tumor progression [17].

Recently, the application of the next-generation sequencing (NGS) technique has detected common molecular alterations, such as BRAF p.V600E, RAS point mutations, fusion oncogenes (RET/PTC, PAX8/PPARγ), and other aberrations of the MAPK and PI3K–PTEN–AKT signaling (■ Table 56.6), as strong indicators of malignancy because ~97% of mutation-positive nodules had confirmed malignant diagnosis at histology [18, 19].

Moreover, two update gene panels using NGS have been developed to rule-in PTC and FTC with high specificity and positive predictive value (PPV) in the case of cytologically indeterminate nodules and rule-out malignancies with high negative predictive value (NPV) in benign nodules [20]. Nevertheless, considering the relative high percentage of false negatives, the lack of long-term outcomes, and the standardization of these molecular tests, further research into the implications on

Table 56.6 Principal genes detected by NGS in thyroid tumors

Gene	Expression	Main Alteration	Tumor
AKT1	Ubiquitous	Activating mutation	PDTC
BRAF	Ubiquitous	Activating mutation in exon 15 (95% p.V600E)	PTC (40–80%) PDTC (5–35%) ATC (10–50%)
NTRK1	Nervous system, not in normal follicular cell	Rearrangement with TMP53 and TGF	PTC (0–10%)
PIK3CA	Ubiquitous	Activating mutations, copy number gain	FTC (0–10%) PDT (0–15%) ATC (5–25%)
PPARG	High levels in adipose tissue, low levels in follicular cells	Rearrangement with PAX8	FTC (20–50%)
RAS	Ubiquitous	Activating mutation	FTC (30–50%) PTC (0–10%) PDTC (20–50%) ATC (10–50%)
RET	*Normally expressed in C-cells, not in follicular cells*	Activating mutation, rearrangement with PTC	PTC (5–25%) MTC

treatment decisions, disease prognosis, and risk stratification is warranted.

Additionally, more clinical studies are needed in order to validate miRNAs as effective molecular markers in the diagnosis and prognosis of thyroid cancer in serum samples [21].

56.8 Prognostic Factors

As previously described, different staging and scoring systems exist and appear to be essential for accurate prognostic evaluation and treatment algorithms. Despite the variability between these systems, both patient and tumor characteristics were found to be independently associated with survival and therefore considered "widely accepted" prognostic factors.

While tumor size, distant metastasis, lymph node involvement, and clinical stage were all found to have definite prognostic value, both the result of histologic grade and the number of clinically positive lymph nodes seemed to show a controversial effect on survival. Moreover, gender and age should be reconsidered as prognostic factors since several studies have shown contradictory results regarding male gender as a negative prognostic factor and a different cutoff point than 45 years may be more accurate for prognosis [15].

Concerning DTC, a number of new factors with potential prognostic implications have recently emerged, including clinical factors (postoperative radiation, LN ratio, postoperative Tg levels, and positive PET-CT findings) and molecular markers (BRAF, Ki67, P53, PAX8-PPARγ), but yet to be included in new predicting systems.

56.9 Treatment

Whereas in WDTC combination of surgery, adjuvant radioactive iodine (RAI) ablation and TSH-suppressive therapy enable high rates of cure even in cases of extrathyroidal tumor manifestation [15], in PDTC and in MTC surgical resection may represent the only definitive therapy. Unfortunately, in ATC there is not yet a standardized and efficient treatment that could improve survival [22].

In WDTCs, the treatment for thyroid cancer is predominantly surgical considering also that the completeness of resection has been associated with less recurrence and improved survival [23]. Total thyroidectomy, removing both lobes and the isthmus (plus the pyramidal lobe, if present), is considered the mainstay of curative-intent therapy. The key decisions in the surgical management of differentiated tumors basically are whom to operate and how extensive a resection to perform.

Surgery is usually followed by the administration of ^{131}I, a selective and targeted approach for delivering tumoricidal doses of radiation to thyroid tumors, which showed reductions in both recurrence and cause-specific mortality in several large retrospective studies [24, 25]. The aim of RAI is to destroy any residual thyroid tissue preventing locoregional recurrence especially in high-

56

risk patients and to facilitate long-term surveillance with whole-body iodine scans or stimulated thyroglobulin measurements.

Postoperative thyroid hormone therapy should be immediately initiated with the aim to replace the thyroid hormone deficiency (replacement therapy) or suppress the potential growth stimulus of TSH on tumor cells (suppressive therapy).

Although about one-third of advanced DTC have metastatic lesions with low avidity for iodine at the time of diagnosis, relapsed or metastatic DTC is frequently ^{131}I-enriched and responds well to RAI. External beam radiation therapy (EBRT) should be only considered for critical metastasis and when complete surgical excision is not possible or when there is no significant radioiodine uptake in the tumor. In iodine-refractory WDTC, the role of chemotherapy has been limited, while two new drugs, sorafenib and lenvatinib, recently demonstrated prolongation of PFS compared with placebo in the phase III trials, DECISION and SELECT [26, 27].

Likewise WDTC, surgery is the primary treatment of MTC and can result in cure in locoregional recurrences whenever feasible. Postoperative thyroid hormone replacing therapy should be given to maintain serum TSH concentration within the normal range while no indications exist for RAI therapy. The results of EBRT and chemotherapy in patients affected by metastatic MTC are disappointing. Two drugs, vandetanib and cabozantinib, have been approved for use in progressive or metastatic MTC.

PDTC and ATC generally do not take up RAI and may not secrete Tg, and their proliferative activity may not be influenced by TSH. In this setting, surgery is indicated to improve the local control. A comprehensive and aggressive multimodal approach including high-dose EBRT and chemotherapy is the current treatment of choice in highly selected patients.

The role of neoadjuvant chemotherapy or targeted therapy in thyroid cancer is not well established [28], although this approach can be of benefit in selected cases.

56.9.1 Localized Disease

In the management of localized thyroid cancer, a long-standing controversy exists among international guidelines regarding the extent of surgical resection, the use of RAI therapy, the intensity and length of follow-up, and the degree of TSH suppression, particularly in DTCs.

There is a clear trend in the evolution of guidelines addressing surgical management of WDTC de-escalation, with recommendations recognizing the role of active surveillance of low-risk disease, higher thresholds for surgery, and acceptance of less than total thy-

roidectomy when surgery is recommended [29]. Indeed, active surveillance can be a safe and effective option for small subcentimetric PTCs [30], while three single observational cohort studies suggested that for WDTC between >1 cm and <4 cm, without extrathyroidal extension, and without clinical evidence of lymph node metastases (cN0), thyroid lobectomy alone may be sufficient as initial treatment [31–33]. As a matter of fact, these studies comparing lobectomy with total thyroidectomy did not show any substantial differences in overall survival and disease-specific survival rates contradicting a previous study by Bilimoria et al. in whom total thyroidectomy for PTC >1 cm was found to provide an overall survival advantage. Despite offering several advantages over thyroidectomy such as lower rate of both permanent hypoparathyroidism and hypothyroidism with subsequent lifelong levothyroxine (LT4) replacement therapy and bilateral recurrent laryngeal nerve palsy, it is worth noting that lobectomy was associated with higher risk of disease recurrence [23, 34]. Furthermore, there is international consensus that lobectomy (instead of total thyroidectomy) could be offered to low-risk small tumors, while a therapeutic lymph node dissection is necessary with clinically positive nodal (N1) disease in the central or lateral neck compartment. However, prophylactic lymph node dissection is still controversial. No guidelines actively recommend routine prophylactic lateral neck dissection, though some previous retrospective studies have considered it [35, 36].

Following surgical resection, radioiodine (RAI) ablation is recommended for selected patients with primary tumors measuring 1–4 cm and clinical-histologic features predicting intermediate to high risk of tumor recurrence (◘ Fig. 56.9). RAI treatment is performed 1–6 months following thyroidectomy, while patients are significantly hypothyroid (low iodine diet of approximately 1–2 weeks suggested) or iatrogenically stimulated (with recombinant human TSH, rhTSH), in order to deliver a targeted ablative dose to any remnant thyroid tissue within the thyroid bed and/or elsewhere (e.g., thyroglossal duct tract and/or metastatic foci). Additionally, the dosing of ^{131}I is somewhat controversial even if in the recent years it has become increasingly apparent that successful thyroid ablation may be achieved using low radioiodine activities [37, 38]. Acute adverse effects of RAI are represented by nausea, neck pain, lacrimal gland dysfunction, salivary gland dysfunction, and altered taste, while the long-term toxicities include secondary primary malignancy, sialadenitis, nasolacrimal duct obstruction, and infertility [39].

Adjuvant thyroid hormone suppression therapy is indicated in high-risk patients (initial TSH suppression to below 0.1 mU/L is recommended) in whom it may decrease progression of metastatic disease, thus reducing cancer-related mortality (◘ Fig. 56.10).

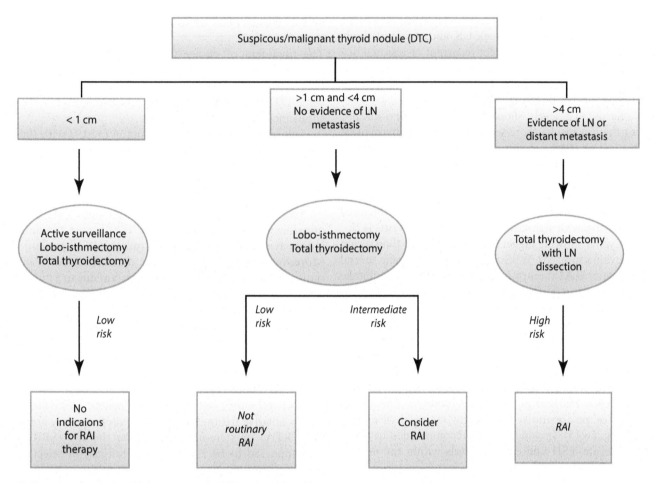

Fig. 56.9 Surgical and RAI treatment in differentiated thyroid cancers

Low risk	TSH 0.5-2 MU/L, if not evidence of disease
Intermediate risk	TSH 0.1-0.5 MU/L
High risk	TSH < 0,1 MU/L

Fig. 56.10 Risk-stratified management of thyroid hormone therapy

The drug of choice is levothyroxine (LT4). While for intermediate-risk thyroid cancer patients initial TSH suppression to 0.1–0.5 mU/L is recommended, no substantial benefits are demonstrated in low-risk patients [40]. Adverse effects of TSH suppression may include the known consequences of subclinical thyrotoxicosis, including exacerbation of angina in patients with ischemic heart disease, increased risk for atrial fibrillation in older patients, and increased risk of osteoporosis in postmenopausal women.

Likewise WDTC, the cornerstone of local treatment of MTC is surgical resection consisting of total thyroidectomy with dissection of central lymph node compartment and resection of the involved lateral compartment. Total thyroidectomy is also indicated in the sporadic setting because a small portion of lesions may be bilateral and because at the time of diagnosis it may not be clear whether the patient is affected by a familial disease or a true sporadic case. Unlike differentiated tumors, where the iodine avidity of follicular cells makes even metastatic DTC amenable to treatment, parafollicular cells do not concentrate iodine. Little randomized control data support the use of adjuvant radiotherapy for microscopic or macroscopic residual disease, extrathyroidal extension or extensive lymph node metastases, and in cases where there is a concern for airway obstruction [41]. Preoperative serum calcitonin levels and neck imaging findings should guide the initial surgical approach, since some retrospective cohort studies demonstrated the clinical benefit of elective neck dissection with serum calcitonin levels.

Unfortunately, in ATC complete resection does not significantly correlate with longer overall survival and cannot be even performed in most cases because of extensive disease.

Assessment and Management After Initial Treatment

Serum Tg determination, neck US, and ^{131}I whole-body scan (WBS) specifically detect recurrent or residual disease in most patients affected by DTCs who have undergone total thyroid ablation with thyroidectomy and remnant ablation (■ Fig. 56.11)

Serum Tg levels should be assessed periodically, but the test results more sensitive when the thyroxine is stopped or when recombinant human TSH (rhTSH) is given to increase the serum TSH [41]. However, patients dislike periodic hormone therapy withdrawal because of symptomatic hypothyroidism; intramuscular administration of rhTSH represents a safe and well-tolerated alternative with significantly fewer adverse events [42].

Even if showing higher false-negative rate than serum Tg evaluation, ^{131}I WBS should be performed several days after RAI therapy is given to assess iodine uptake by the tumor. Posttreatment imaging appeared to be much more sensitive in patients younger than 45 years old who previously had received RAI-therapy [42].

Concerning MTC, calcitonin (CT) is the only hormone produced by parafollicular cell, thus resulting crucial for postoperative surveillance. Measurements of both serum CEA and calcitonin are established prognostic markers in MTC and represent the cornerstone of postoperative assessment for residual disease (■ Fig. 56.15). In addition, it is recommended to maintain serum TSH and calcium levels within the normal range 4–6 weeks after surgery.

56.9.2 Recurrent or Metastatic Disease

The treatment of choice for localized thyroid cancer recurrences remains surgery, performed according to the type of thyroid cancer, the stage, and the patient's age. In some DTCs at high risk of recurrence, surgery may be supplemented by RAI treatment.

Tumor relapses are not uncommon (~20%) with the most frequent sites of distant metastases for WDTC occurring in the lung (50%), bone (25%), brain, liver, and skin. Liver is a major site of distant metastasis for MTC.

Treatment for metastatic WDTC includes TSH suppression and RAI therapy since the disease remains iodine avid and sensitive in the two-thirds of patients. Moreover, one-third of these tumors considered to be radiosensitive eventually become resistant due to a mutation of the sodium-iodide symporter (NIS) gene [43]. Specifically, tumors considered to be iodine refractory are those having some of the following characteristics: persistent neoplastic tissue that does not take up RAI, disease characterized by heterogeneous RAI uptake, or disease that progresses after RAI treatment despite RAI uptake (■ Fig. 56.12).

RAI-refractory patients should benefit from other locally ablative treatments such as radiofrequency ablation (RFA) or stereotactic radiation therapy (SBRT) that appeared to be as effective as surgery in selected patients, improving local tumor control and delaying the initiation of systemic treatment. To a lesser extent,

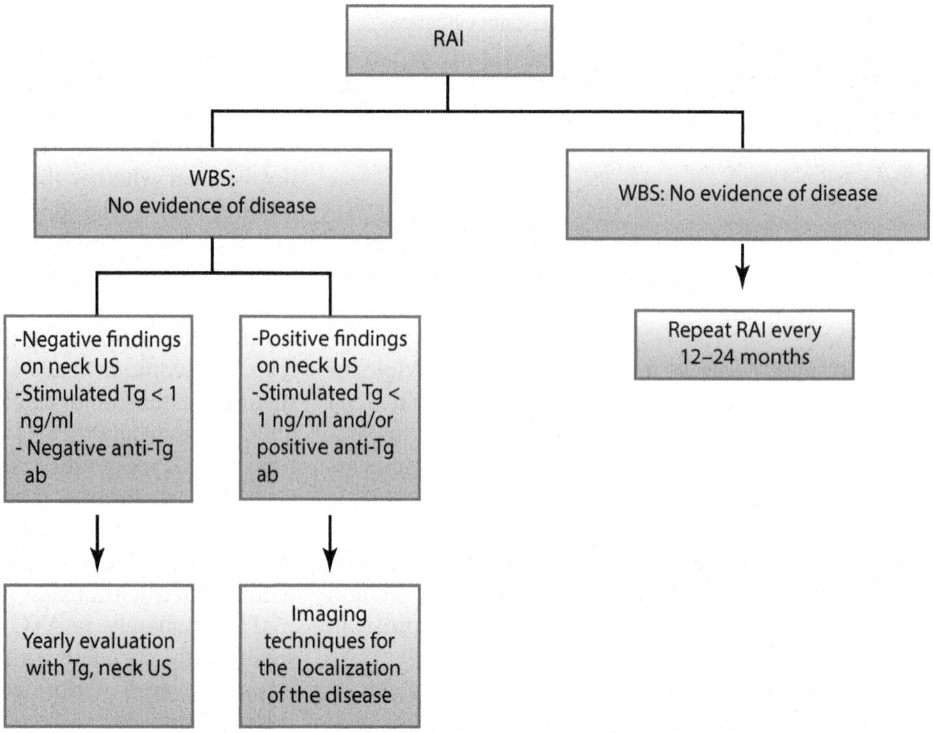

■ **Fig. 56.11** Assessment algorithm at the time of the first control post-initial treatment in RAI-treated patients with differentiated thyroid carcinoma (DTC)

☐ Fig. 56.12 Treatment algorithm for locally advanced or metastatic DTC

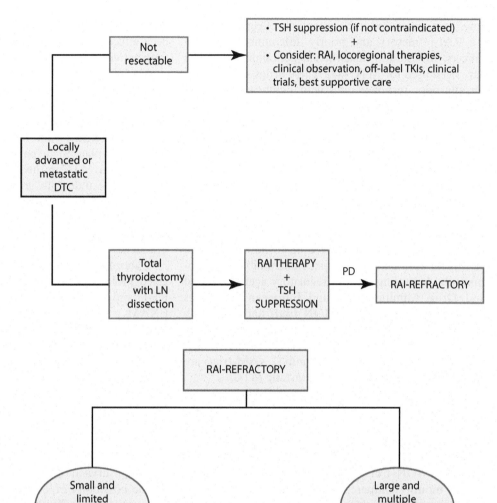

☐ Fig. 56.13 Treatment options for progressive RAI-refractory DTC

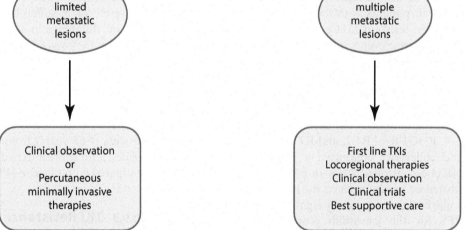

these local treatments are indicated for symptomatic or imminently symptomatic disease, even in the presence of RAI uptake. EBRT may be indicated when complete surgical excision is not feasible or when there is no significant radioiodine uptake in the tumor, as also in the case of ATC.

When disease progression occurs at multiple sites where other better tolerated and more accessible local treatments have been exhausted and when target lesions appear to be radiologically measurable and in progression over the previous 12–14 months (as defined by RECIST criteria), treatment with tyrosine kinase inhibitors (TKIs) should be considered (☐ Fig. 56.13).

For several decades, chemotherapy was the only option for treating patients with metastatic thyroid cancer. Several chemotherapeutic agents, including platinum compounds, bleomycin, doxorubicin, and paclitaxel, either administered alone or in combination, have been considered to be potentially effective in treating RAI-refractory and poorly differentiated thyroid cancers. In addition, dacarbazine-containing regimens have been used for MTC [44]. These drugs showed universally poor response rates with significant toxicities and had short, if any, duration of effect [45].

Serine (BRAF) and tyrosine kinases (RAS, RET) act in tumors as intermediaries in cell signaling stimulating tumor proliferation and angiogenesis and favoring the capacity for invasion and metastasis. Therefore, the discovery of the antiangiogenic and antiproliferative effect of multitarget TKIs has led to the approval of four molecules that block these inappropriately activated pathways within the cancer cells. Four phase III studies have been conducted up to now showing a benefit for sorafenib, lenvatinib, vandetanib, and cabozantinib. According to drug regulatory agencies (Food and Drug Administration and European Medicines Agency), sorafenib (DECISION trial) and lenvatinib (SELECT trial) are approved for the use in progressive radioiodine-refractory PTC and FTC, while vandetanib (ZETA trial) and cabozantinib (EXAM trial) are approved for the treatment of metastatic MTC.

Sorafenib is a multitargeted kinase inhibitor targeting vascular endothelial growth factor receptor (VEGFR)-2 and (VEGFR)-3, platelet-derived growth factor receptor (PDGFR)-β, fibroblast growth factor receptors (FGFRs) 1–4, c-KIT, BRAF, and RET. In the DECISION trial, sorafenib showed a mean PFS of 10.8 months compared to 5.8 months in the placebo group in patients with locally advanced or metastatic radiation-resistant DTCs. 98.6% of the patients experienced adverse events (fatigue, hand–foot syndrome, and diarrhea) with 37.2% of these being grade 3 or higher [26].

Lenvatinib is an oral molecule capable of inhibiting receptors involved in the modulation of angiogenesis and lymphangiogenesis such as VEGFRs 1–3, FGFRs 1–4, PDGFR-α, RET, and KIT. In 2015, Schlumberger and colleagues conducted a phase III, double-blind, placebo-controlled study in patients affected by a pretreated or non-pretreated RAI-resistant DTC, showing a marked and statistically significant increase in median PFS for the lenvatinib group (18.3 months versus 3.6 months) while achieving a high clinical benefit. In the SELECT trial, lenvatinib showed a higher PFS (18.3 vs 10.8 months) and higher percentage of partial response (63.2% vs 12.2%) than sorafenib with some cases of complete response. However, 97.3% of patients mostly presented grade 3 or higher adverse events (hypertension, proteinuria, thromboembolism or renal failure), and a higher number of deaths were described for lenvatinib. Notwithstanding this, the shorter PFS observed in the placebo arm with respect to the PFS in the placebo arm of DECISION study (3.6 vs 5.8 months) suggested

that patients enrolled in the SELECT study could have been affected by a more severe disease. Recently, lenvatinib activity has been also evaluated in ATC preclinical studies [46].

Vandetanib is also an oral multikinase inhibitor molecule mainly targeting the VEGFR, the epidermal growth factor receptor (EGFR), and RET-tyrosine kinase. The efficacy and safety of this drug was compared with placebo in patients with locally advanced or metastatic MTC in the ZETA trial [47]. The median PFS in the vandetanib group was not reached, but it was estimated at 30.5 months; it was 19.3 months in the placebo group. Frequent adverse events were diarrhea, rash, nausea, hypertension, dry skin, dry mouth, and headache.

Cabozantinib is an oral, small-molecule, multitargeted TKI with potent activity against VEGFRs, MET, RET, and the c-KIT, TIE2, and FLT3 genes. In the EXAM trial [48], a statistically significant prolongation in median progression-free survival was observed in patients with documented radiographic progression of MTC treated with cabozantinib (11.2 months vs 4.0 months in the placebo group). Most frequent adverse events include stomatitis, hypertension and diarrhea, fatigue, weight loss, and palmar-plantar erythrodysesthesia syndrome.

All TKI phase III studies have demonstrated significant improvement in progression-free survival, but not in overall survival (◘ Table 56.7). This can be explained by the possibility of crossover in most of the studies. However, in a subgroup analysis, a statistically significant difference in overall survival (44.3 months vs. 18.9 months) was observed in patients with MTC and somatic RET M918T mutations who received cabozantinib compared with placebo [27]; similarly, patients with sporadic MTCs harboring a somatic *M918T* mutation had a higher response rate to vandetanib in the ZETA trial. In another subgroup, analysis of older patients (>65 years) from the SELECT trial who were treated with lenvatinib had an improved overall survival compared with placebo [49].

56.9.3 TKI Resistance: The "Escape Phenomenon"

The main limitation of targeted therapy is the development of an escape mechanism, called "escape phenomenon," that allows cancer cells to grow after a variable period of time from the beginning of the treatment. Resistance to TKI-based treatment is almost always present, regardless of TKI efficacy or tumor type [50–52].

This is likely due to the method of action of TKIs, which are cytostatic and not cytotoxic molecules, implying that tumoral cells are not killed but made quiescent

◻ Table 56.7 Phase III studies in locally advanced or metastatic thyroid cancers resistant to radioiodine

Trial	Treatment	Phase study	Cell type	Prior treatments	Crossover	Number of patients	Response rate	PFS
DECISION	Sorafenib	III	DTC	No	Yes	207		10.8
	Placebo					210		5.8
SELECT	Lenvatinib	III	DTC	Yes	Yes	261	64%	18.3
	Placebo					131	1.5%	3.6
ZETA	Vandetanib	III	MTC	Yes	Yes	231	45%	30.5
	Placebo					100	13%	19.3
EXAM	Cabozantinib	III	MTC	Yes	No	219	283%	11.2
	Placebo					111	0%	4.0

DTC differentiated thyroid carcinoma, *HR* hazard ratio, *MTC* medullary thyroid carcinoma, *OS* overall survival, *PFS* progression-free survival

and not proliferative. Therefore, surviving cells can develop a mechanism of drug resistance determined by both the activation or upregulation of alternative pro-angiogenic pathways and the selective pressures of the microenvironment during malignant progression.

Since TKIs are cytostatic drugs, they should be indefinitely continued until there is clear evidence of disease progression or severe side effects occur; however, if the progression appears to be somehow limited, it is clinically reasonable to continue the administration of the drug until the possibility of substitution with another drug. There is also some evidence that once the TKI is stopped, the disease progresses even rapidly.

There are two main types of resistance: a "primary" or intrinsic resistance that is already present before targeted treatment is begun and a "secondary" resistance that develops after a variable period of definite response. An example of primary resistance is represented by *RET V804M* and *V804L* gatekeeper mutations that appeared to confer resistance to vandetanib in MTC by preventing the binding of the drug to the receptor in vitro studies [53]. Examples of secondary resistance in thyroid cancer treated with TKIs are still unknown but possibly due to secondary site mutations that are usually located downstream from the TKI target or in parallel pathways, as observed in some in vitro models [54].

■ **Strategies to Overcome Resistance**

A genotype-directed therapy using a TKI that acts via more than one pathway is one way of countering resistance. This can be explained by the sustained therapeutic effect of cabozantinib that effectively blocks the onset of MET-driven evasive resistance by inhibiting both MET and VEGFR2, unlike agents targeting the VEGF pathway alone. Similarly, the administration of another TKI with other mechanisms of action seemed to be able to revert the trend of growth after the escape

mainly considering that in the SELECT trial lenvatinib showed efficacy in prolonging PFS also in patients previously treated with other TKIs (no data available on the use of Sorafenib as second line in patients who develop resistance to other TKIs).

Furthermore, addition of a synergistic agent is another way of evading resistance since dual inhibition of the MAPK and mTOR pathways or the MEK and mTOR pathways showed an interesting and effective inhibitory synergism in thyroid cancer cell lines, including ATC [55, 56]. Since early mutation of BRAF and RAS has been reported in almost one-third of ATC cases, a phase II open-label basket trial was conducted in patients with BRAF V600E-positive malignancies (including 16 with ATC), showing an acceptable safety profile and an objective response rate of 69% (11/16; 95% CI 41–89%) when administering the BRAF inhibitor dabrafenib plus the MEK inhibitor trametinib.

Another way of overcoming drug resistance mechanism and/or enhancing drug efficacy is the combination of targeted therapy with chemotherapy or radiotherapy that resulted to be safe and tolerable in ATC and PTC patients in phase I trials [57, 58].

■ **Alternative TKIs**

Pazopanib, a multikinase inhibitor mainly acting against VEGF 1–3, PGDF, FGFR, and RET, found to have activity against MTCs in preclinical studies. Likewise, sunitinib showed efficacy in phase II trials though not without adverse effects (asthenia, mucosal and cutaneous toxicities, hand–foot syndrome, and cardiac events).

No phase III clinical trials of axitinib (a second-generation VEGFR1–3 inhibitor) are available, but in a phase II trial, a progression-free survival of 15 months was observed with a 93% rate of adverse events, the most common being diarrhea, nausea, and hypertension [59]. In 2008, this molecule was first evaluated in a phase II trial showing partial responses and stable diseases in 60 subjects affected by advanced thyroid cancer including 11 MTC patients [60].

Furthermore, current experimental strategies aim to target oncogenic signaling pathways that diminish iodide avidity in thyroid cancer. As previously described, oncogenic activation of the mitogen-activated protein kinase (MAPK) signaling pathway (RET/RAS/RAF/MEK/ERK), suppressing the expression of follicular cell-specific genes that are responsible for iodide uptake (e.g., the sodium-iodine symporter, or NIS) and metabolism, is a central event for the development of the majority of thyroid malignancies. Hence, MAPK pathway inhibition can enhance RAI incorporation and efficacy in a subset of RAI-refractory patients: selumetinib, a MEK 1/2 inhibitor, was found to reverse refractoriness to RAI in patients with metastatic DTC in combination with therapeutic radioiodine [61].

Moreover, the understanding of this biology provides the molecular basis of the well-established clinical observation that BRAF mutant tumors present with more aggressive clinical behavior and are more often RAI-refractory. For BRAF mutant patients, treatment with dabrafenib, a BRAF inhibitor, increased iodide incorporation in 6 of 10 BRAF mutant patients, resulting in tumor shrinkage after subsequent treatment with I-131 in 5 of the 6 patients [62]. In patients with ATC and BRAF V600F mutation, a study with the selective BRAF inhibitor vemurafenib was also done [63].

■ **Immunotherapy and Other Agents**

In the presence of nondruggable mutations, immunotherapy could represent an alternative approach, even if inclusion of targeted therapy, immunotherapy, chemotherapy, and/or radiotherapy, administered in combination or sequentially, should be tested within the context of a clinical trial. Few data are available with antibodies targeting programmed cell death 1 (PD-1) receptor or programmed cell death ligand-1 (PD-L1). The anti-PD-1 monoclonal antibody spartalizumab was tested in 41 heavily pretreated patients with advanced ATC, and responses were observed in 19.5%.

Patients who undergo PET/CT scan with tumor lesions having strong avidity for Ga-DOTATATE may benefit from a new type of radionuclide-based therapy, a technique called peptide receptor radionuclide therapy (PRRT). This is a molecule of lutetium-177 or yttrium-90 linked to a somatostatin analog that has high affinity for the overexpressed somatostatin type 2 receptors (SSTR) in MTC. Several series reported a good response rate and a beneficial effect on QOL for both DTCs and MTCs [64].

Histone deacetylase inhibitors (HDACIs), such as valproic acid or romidepsin, cause selective cell death of tumor cells since HDAC exert a pro-oncogenic effect by keeping genes involved in apoptosis in a transcriptionally quiescent state [65]. Though several HDACIs have not yet shown clinical benefit, these small molecule inhibitors are good potential therapeutic agents and under trial for all advanced thyroid cancers, including MTC.

The rise of immunotherapy may further alter the fate of patients with thyroid carcinoma, whether differentiated, medullary, or anaplastic. Chowdhury and colleagues showed that overexpression of PD-L1, involved in controlling the immune response of T cells, is associated with an increased risk of relapse and, thus, is a marker of poor prognosis in PTCs. In addition, Zwaenepoel and colleagues described this overexpression in about one-third of ATCs. The first two checkpoint inhibitors developed targeting PD-1 are pembrolizumab and nivolumab whose responses observed are encouraging in terms of continuing research on the subject.

56.10 Follow-up

The aim of follow-up is to define the absence of persistent tumor 6–12 months after the primary treatment, ascertaining whether or not the patient is free of disease and eventually leading to the early discovery and treatment of persistent or recurrent locoregional or distant disease.

No evidence of disease (NED) is defined by the absence of both clinical and imaging evidence of tumor, undetectable Tg levels (during either THS suppression or TSH stimulation) and the absence of anti-Tg antibodies.

Regarding DTC, patients treated with RAI therapy may be followed with unstimulated Tg annually and periodic neck US if they have negative clinical and ultrasound findings, stimulated Tg less that 1 ng/ml with negative anti-Tg antibodies, and negative whole body scan (◘ Fig. 56.11). The trend in Tg levels over time, which should be assessed with the same laboratory and same assay, can help indicate those patients with a clinically significant residual disease that should be studied using further imaging techniques. However, when basal serum Tg is ≤ 0.1 ng/ml and neck US is unremarkable, patients may be clinically considered free of disease and are able to avoid an rhTSH stimulation; conversely, rhTSH stimulation testing may still be informative on the absence or presence of disease when basal serum Tg is >0.1 ng/ml but <1.0 ng/ml. If thyroid function tests (FT3, FT4, TSH) additionally confirm the adequacy of hormone suppressive or substitutive therapy after 3–6 months from the initial treatment, patients may be considered in complete remission with a very low subsequent recurrence rate ($<1.0\%$ at 10 years). RAI scans may be used to characterize the functional status of structural disease and are recommended every 12–24 months until no clinically significant response to RAI is seen. Non-RAI imaging (such as CT and or FDG-PET/TC) might be considered if negative RAI imaging and rising stimulated Tg levels.

On the contrary, diagnostic total body ^{131}I imaging is less often used for low-risk patients and absolutely not specific for thyroid cancer in patients who have not undergone remnant ablation. These patients may be followed with periodic neck US and Tg level measurements (▣ Fig. 56.14).

Regarding MTC, if serum CT after a provocative (pentagastrin or calcium) test results undetectable from 1 to 3 month after surgery, no other diagnostic test is warranted, and serum CT should be repeated every 6 months for the first 2–3 years and annually thereafter. In patients with serum CT concentration <150 pg/ml, localization of disease should be limited to a careful examination by neck US. Patients with basal CT >150 pg/ml should be screened for distant metastases (▣ Fig. 56.15)

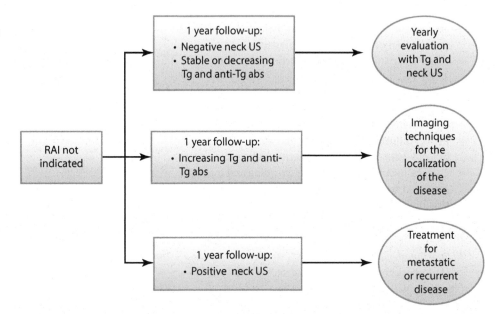

▣ **Fig. 56.14** Follow-up algorithm in DTC patients not previously treated with RAI therapy

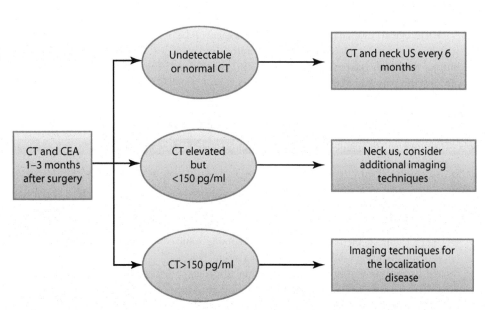

▣ **Fig. 56.15** Diagnostic algorithm based on calcitonin levels obtained 1–3 months after initial surgery in patients with medullary thyroid carcinoma

Case Study: Management of a Patient with a Progressive Metastatic Papillary Thyroid Cancer

Female, 45 years old
- *Family history* negative for malignancies
- *APR:* prior exposure to ionizing radiation for Hodgkin's lymphoma
- *APP:* Incidental US finding of an asymptomatic and painless mass located on the thyroid left lobe, unintentional weight loss, no skin changes on the overlying skin, no obstructive symptoms, no swellings
- *Objective examination*: solitary and palpable nodule with firm consistency, fixed in respect to surrounding tissues and mobile with the trachea at swallowing; absence of hoarseness, cervical lymphadenopathies and tracheal or esophageal compression
- *Blood tests*: normal thyroid function tests (fT4, fT3, TSH)
- *Ultrasonography*: well-defined, homogeneous, solid hypoechoic oval-shaped nodule measuring up to 4 cm in diameter with irregular margins in upper left thyroid lobe
- *FNAC*: cellular smears with papillary fronds composed of cells with enlarged oval nuclei with intranuclear grooves, inclusions with nuclear crowding and overlapping, and background "chewing-gum" colloid suggestive for classical PTC

Question

What action should be taken?
   (1) Lobectomy. (2) Total thyroidectomy. (3) Total thyroidectomy with LN dissection

Answer

Total thyroidectomy (in light of the radiation history, the size of the tumor and the absence of involved lymph nodes)
   Histological examination confirmed classical PTC with lymphovascular invasion, with a high mitotic index (5 mitosis × 10 high power fields) and high Ki67 expression (15%) (Foto papillare Martorana)

WBS ⇨ residual disease in the thyroid bed

Question

What action should be taken postoperatively?
   (1) Substitutive hormone therapy. (2) RAI therapy + suppressive hormone therapy. (3) Active surveillance

Answer

RAI therapy + suppressive hormone therapy
   ⇩
RAI therapy until radioiodine uptake is completely absent + initial TSH suppression to 0.1– 0.5 mU/L (intermediate risk patient)
   Follow-up at 1 year: positive findings on neck US and rising TG serum levels. Total body CT and PET scans revealed the new appearance of pulmonary and vertebral osteolytic lesions

Question

What action should be taken?
   (1) Axitinib. (2) RAI therapy. (3) Lenvatinib

Answer

Begins Lenvatinib 24 mg cp daily with significant reduction of bone lesion volume

Key Points

- Start with medical history, physical examination and diagnostic work-up
- Surgery remains the cornerstone of thyroid cancer initial treatment
- The importance of the postoperative risk-stratified management in DTC
- Consider TKIs in the progressive life-threatening metastatic disease

Case Study Management of MTC in a Patient Affected by MEN2A

Female, 30 years old
- *Family history* positive for malignancy (mother's history of pheochromocytoma)
- *APR*: negative
- *APP*: Lump at the base of the neck becoming more prominent during swallowing, episodic sweating, hypertensive crisis in the last weeks, no intestinal disorders
- *Objective examination*: dominant thyroid nodule at the base of the neck; nontender palpable left lateral cervical lymph node; elevated blood pressure and heart rate; no mucosal neuromas in the tongue, lips or eyelids; no musculoskeletal abnormalities.
- *Laboratory tests*: serum calcium, parathyroid hormone, TSH and cathecolamines within reference range; rising levels of both serum calcitonin (420 pg/ml) and CEA; 24 h urinary cathecolamine was 1100 nmol/24 h (normal range < 230 nmol/24 h); 24 h urinary vanillylmandelic acid weakly positive.
- *US*: hypoechogenic mass with diameter of 2.3 cm x 1.5 cm on the left lobe of the thyroid

Question

What action should be taken?

(1) Surgery. (2) CT scan. (3) FNAB

Answer

Total body *CT scan* did not detect metastatic disease and confirmed the presence of a right adrenal pheochromocytoma. Avoid FNAC since the diagnosis could be consistent with MEN2A and biopsy could increase the possibility of tumor spread.

Question

What action should be taken?

(1) Surgery. (2) RAI therapy. (3) Other

Answer

Surgery: right total adrenalectomy followed by total thyroidectomy with lymph nodes dissection to both central and latero-cervical compartments

Question

What action should be taken?

(1) Hormone substitutive therapy + Genetic screening for RET. (2) Other. (3) Follow-up

Answer

Administer *hormone replacement therapy* and perform *genetic screening for RET* mutation to the patient and the family members (parents, siblings, and children)

Key Points

— The importance of both family history assessment and proper clinical management in MTC
— Consider lab tests and imaging techniques for differential diagnosis
— Understand the use of RET testing in families with MEN2 as a part of strategy to prevent MTC

Expert Opinion
Alfredo Berruti

Key Points

— The cellular origin of the thyroid tumor has important implications for prognosis and planning the therapeutic and follow-up strategies.
— Differentiated tumor cells, both papillary and follicular, are able to take up iodine and to secrete thyroglobulin (Tg) under stimulus from thyrotropin-stimulating hormone (TSH).
— Medullary thyroid cancer (MTC) derived from parafollicular C cells, which are not involved in iodine metabolism and are not TSH dependent. MTC is not able to concentrate 131I and does not produce Tg. It instead produces Calcitonin
— Both differentiated thyroid cancer and MTC can be cured by surgery, that is the mainstay of therapy.
— Postoperative radioactive iodine (131I) therapy can improve the cure rate of differentiated thyroid cancers.
— Tg is an important and useful marker in the follow-up to early detect recurrent or residual disease. Calcitonin and carcinoembryonic antigen (CEA) are the reference tumor markers for MTC.
— The prognosis of patients affected by thyroid cancer is highly variable and depend on the histotype and the degree of differentiation. The survival perspective of non metastatic patients with differentiated thyroid cancer is very good, while it is poor in patients with poorly differentiated and anaplastic tumors. The survival perspective of MTC is generally poorer than that of differentiated tumors.
— Recurrences of differentiated thyroid cancer can be identified early and tcured by measuring the basal and/or TSH-stimulated serum Tg levels and via neck ultrasound.
— Serum calcitonin is a sensitive marker in the follow-up of MTC patients. Diagnostic imaging could be negative in patients with calcitonin levels <150 pg/ml, whereas the probability of detecting metastases increases with growing of calcitonin and CEA levels.
— In about one-third of advanced differentiated thyroid cancers, the metastatic lesions have a very low avidity for iodine, and 131I therapy has no effects. Anaplastic and poorly differentiated thyroid cancers are no longer able to take up iodine, secrete Tg, or respond to TSH stimulus.
— The increasing knowledge about the molecular alterations underlying thyroid cancer has provided the rationale for the use of targeted cancer therapies that represent newer options for patients with advanced thyroid cancer.
— Randomized prospective clinical trials have shown that sorafenib and lenvatinib are efficacious in the management of metastatic differentiated thyroid cancer that are radioiodine refractory, while vandetanib and cabo-

zantinib are efficacious in metastatic MTC. All these molecular target agents improved progression-free survival but not overall survival, and their administration is associated with relevant (although manageable) toxicity. The prescription of these drugs on individual patients should be done taking carefully into account the cost/benefit balance.

- Since both differentiated thyroid cancers and MTC may follow and indolent disease course, it is not always clear which patient needs a systemic therapy. Discussion within a multidisciplinary team is of paramount importance to guarantee the best therapeutic approach to these patients.

- The therapeutic strategies actually available have had only a limited impact on survival of metastatic patients with both differentiated thyroid cancer and MTC, and the management of anaplastic and poorly differentiated malignancies still remains challenging. Moreover, risk stratification is currently based mainly on clinic pathologic risk factors. New drugs and new prognostic parameters are therefore needed.

Summary of Clinical Recommendations

- Lobectomy (instead of total thyroidectomy) could be offered to low-risk small DTCs, while a therapeutic lymph node dissection is necessary with clinically positive nodal (N1) disease in the central or lateral neck compartment. Preoperative serum calcitonin levels and neck imaging findings should guide the initial surgical approach of MTC. In ATC, complete resection cannot be even performed in most cases because of extensive disease.

- RAI administration is not recommended for small (≤1 cm) intrathyroidal DTC with no evidence of locoregional metastases (classified as low-risk cases), may be considered in intermediate-risk patients, and is recommended for patients at high risks of recurrence.

- In DTCs, high-sensitivity assays of basal Tg can be used in testing to verify the absence of disease (excellent response), whereas serial measurements of basal Tg should be obtained in patients with residual thyroid tissue and following lobectomy; neck US is the most effective tool for detecting structural disease in the neck, and other Imaging studies are indicated if locoregional and/or distant metastases are clinically suspected or in patients with known metastases; TSH should be suppressed when structural disease persists or when high-risk patients have a less-than-excellent response to therapy. As regards MTC, CT and CEA monitoring along with multimodality imaging should be included in the early and long-term postoperative staging work-ups

- DTC patients with distant metastases should receive radioactive iodine after TSH stimulation; non-RAI-avid lesions and those that lose their ability to concentrate RAI or progress despite RAI avidity should be considered RAI-refractory; lenvatinib and sorafenib should be considered the first-line systemic therapy for RAI-refractory DTC. Cabozantinib and vandetanib should be considered the first-line systemic therapy for MTC patients; in patients with RETM918T or RAS-mutant MTCs, cabozantinib offers significant PFS and OS advantages over wild-type cancers. Patients with BRAF V600E-positive ATCs should be treated with the BRAF inhibitor dabrafenib plus the MEK inhibitor trametinib; clinical trial enrolment should be encouraged for patients with good clinical PS.

Hints for Deeper Insight and Suggested Reading

1. S Filetti, C Durante, D Hartl, S Leboulleux, LD Locati, K Newbold, MG Papotti, A Berruti, ESMO Guidelines Committee, Thyroid cancer: ESMO Clinical Practice Guidelines for diagnosis, treatment and follow-up, Annals of Oncology, mdz400, ▶ https://doi.org/10.1093/annonc/mdz400
2. AIOM Guidelines (Associazione Italiana Oncologia Medica)- Tumori della Tiroide 2017/2018. ▶ https://www.aiom.it/tumori-della-tiroide-2017/
3. NCCN Clinical Practice Guidelines in Oncology-Thyroid Carcinoma

Bibliography

1. Chen AY, Jemal A, Ward EM. Increasing incidence of differentiated thyroid cancer in the United States, 1988-2005. Cancer. 2009;115(16):3801–7.
2. Newbold KL, Flux G, Wadsley J. Radioiodine for high risk and radioiodine refractory thyroid cancer: current concepts in management. Clin Oncol (R Coll Radiol). 2017;29(5):307–9.
3. Perren A, Schmid S, Locher T, et al. BRAF and endocrine tumors: mutations are frequent in papillary thyroid carcinomas, rare in endocrine tumors of the gastrointestinal tract and not detected in other endocrine tumors. Endocr Relat Cancer. 2004;11(4):855–60.
4. Davies L, Morris LG, Haymart M, et al. American Association of Clinical Endocrinologists and American College of Endocrinology Disease State clinical review: the increasing incidence of thyroid cancer. Endocr Pract. 2015;21(6):686–96.
5. Vigneri R, Malandrino P, Vigneri P. The changing epidemiology of thyroid cancer: why is incidence increasing? Curr Opin Oncol. 2015;27(1):1–7.

6. Kabata P, Kaniuka-Jakubowska S, Kabata W, et al. Primary Ewing sarcoma of the thyroid-eight cases in a decade: a case report and literature review. Front Endocrinol (Lausanne). 2017;8:257.

7. Acquaviva G, Visani M, Repaci A, et al. Molecular pathology of thyroid tumours of follicular cells: a review of genetic alterations and their clinicopathological relevance. Histopathology. 2018;72(1):6–31.

8. Brennan MD, Bergstralh EJ, van Heerden JA, McConahey WM. Follicular thyroid cancer treated at the Mayo Clinic, 1946 through 1970: initial manifestations, pathologic findings, therapy, and outcome. Mayo Clin Proc. 1991;66(1):11–22.

9. Baloch ZW, LiVolsi VA. Special types of thyroid carcinoma. Histopathology. 2018;72(1):40–52.

10. Volante M, Collini P, Nikiforov YE, et al. Poorly differentiated thyroid carcinoma: the Turin proposal for the use of uniform diagnostic criteria and an algorithmic diagnostic approach. Am J Surg Pathol. 2007;31(8):1256–64.

11. Cosgrove D, Piscaglia F, Bamber J, et al. EFSUMB guidelines and recommendations on the clinical use of ultrasound elastography. Part 2: clinical applications. Ultraschall Med. 2013;34(3):238–53.

12. Pacini F, Castagna MG, Brilli L, Pentheroudakis G, Group EGW. Thyroid cancer: ESMO clinical practice guidelines for diagnosis, treatment and follow-up. Ann Oncol. 2012;23(Suppl 7):vii110–9.

13. Siadati S, Rabiee SM, Alijanpour E, Bayani MA, Nikbakhsh N. The diagnostic value of fine needle aspiration in comparison with frozen section in thyroid nodules: a 20-year study. Caspian J Intern Med. 2017;8(4):301–4.

14. Haugen BR, Alexander EK, Bible KC, et al. 2015 American Thyroid Association management guidelines for adult patients with thyroid nodules and differentiated thyroid cancer: the American Thyroid Association guidelines task force on thyroid nodules and differentiated thyroid cancer. Thyroid. 2016;26:1):1–133.

15. Glikson E, Alon E, Bedrin L, Talmi YP. Prognostic factors in differentiated thyroid cancer revisited. Isr Med Assoc J. 2017;19(2):114–8.

16. Krajewska J, Chmielik E, Jarząb B. Dynamic risk stratification in the follow-up of thyroid cancer: what is still to be discovered in 2017? Endocr Relat Cancer. 2017;24(11):R387–402.

17. Cibas ES, Ali SZ. The Bethesda system for reporting thyroid cytopathology. Thyroid. 2009;19(11):1159–65.

18. Nikiforov YE, Steward DL, Robinson-Smith TM, et al. Molecular testing for mutations in improving the fine-needle aspiration diagnosis of thyroid nodules. J Clin Endocrinol Metab. 2009;94(6):2092–8.

19. Cantara S, Capezzone M, Marchisotta S, et al. Impact of proto-oncogene mutation detection in cytological specimens from thyroid nodules improves the diagnostic accuracy of cytology. J Clin Endocrinol Metab. 2010;95(3):1365–9.

20. Roth MY, Witt RL, Steward DL. Molecular testing for thyroid nodules: review and current state. Cancer. 2018;124(5):888–98.

21. Mahmoudian-Sani MR, Mehri-Ghahfarrokhi A, Asadi-Samani M, Mobini GR. Serum miRNAs as biomarkers for the diagnosis and prognosis of thyroid cancer: a comprehensive review of the literature. Eur Thyroid J. 2017;6(4):171–7.

22. Wendler J, Kroiss M, Gast K, et al. Clinical presentation, treatment and outcome of anaplastic thyroid carcinoma: results of a multicenter study in Germany. Eur J Endocrinol. 2016;175(6):521–9.

23. Bilimoria KY, Bentrem DJ, Ko CY, et al. Extent of surgery affects survival for papillary thyroid cancer. Ann Surg. 2007;246(3):375–381; discussion 381-374.

24. Sawka AM, Thephamongkhol K, Brouwers M, Thabane L, Browman G, Gerstein HC. Clinical review 170: a systematic review and metaanalysis of the effectiveness of radioactive iodine remnant ablation for well-differentiated thyroid cancer. J Clin Endocrinol Metab. 2004;89(8):3668–76.

25. Cooper DS, Doherty GM, Haugen BR, et al. Revised American Thyroid Association management guidelines for patients with thyroid nodules and differentiated thyroid cancer. Thyroid. 2009;19(11):1167–214.

26. Brose MS, Nutting CM, Jarzab B, et al. Sorafenib in radioactive iodine-refractory, locally advanced or metastatic differentiated thyroid cancer: a randomised, double-blind, phase 3 trial. Lancet. 2014;384(9940):319–28.

27. Schlumberger M, Tahara M, Wirth LJ, et al. Lenvatinib versus placebo in radioiodine-refractory thyroid cancer. N Engl J Med. 2015;372(7):621–30.

28. Dang RP, McFarland D, Le VH, et al. Neoadjuvant therapy in differentiated thyroid cancer. Int J Surg Oncol. 2016;2016:3743420.

29. Kovatch KJ, Hoban CW, Shuman AG. Thyroid cancer surgery guidelines in an era of de-escalation. Eur J Surg Oncol. 2017;44:297.

30. Miyauchi A. Clinical trials of active surveillance of papillary microcarcinoma of the thyroid. World J Surg. 2016;40(3):516–22.

31. Mendelsohn AH, Elashoff DA, Abemayor E, St John MA. Surgery for papillary thyroid carcinoma: is lobectomy enough? Arch Otolaryngol Head Neck Surg. 2010;136(11):1055–61.

32. Barney BM, Hitchcock YJ, Sharma P, Shrieve DC, Tward JD. Overall and cause-specific survival for patients undergoing lobectomy, near-total, or total thyroidectomy for differentiated thyroid cancer. Head Neck. 2011;33(5):645–9.

33. Adam G, Cınar C, Akbal E. Rare thyroid cartilage involvement of multiple myeloma visualized on F-18 FDG-PET/CT imaging: 3 case reports. Indian J Surg Oncol. 2014;5(3):194–5.

34. Macedo FI, Mittal VK. Total thyroidectomy versus lobectomy as initial operation for small unilateral papillary thyroid carcinoma: a meta-analysis. Surg Oncol. 2015;24(2):117–22.

35. Sugitani I, Fujimoto Y, Yamada K, Yamamoto N. Prospective outcomes of selective lymph node dissection for papillary thyroid carcinoma based on preoperative ultrasonography. World J Surg. 2008;32(11):2494–502.

36. Ito Y, Miyauchi A. Is surgery necessary for papillary thyroid microcarcinomas? Nat Rev Endocrinol. 2011;8(1):9; author reply 9.

37. Pilli T, Brianzoni E, Capoccetti F, et al. A comparison of 1850 (50 mCi) and 3700 MBq (100 mCi) 131-iodine administered doses for recombinant thyrotropin-stimulated postoperative thyroid remnant ablation in differentiated thyroid cancer. J Clin Endocrinol Metab. 2007;92(9):3542–6.

38. Chianelli M, Todino V, Graziano FM, et al. Low-activity (2.0 GBq; 54 mCi) radioiodine post-surgical remnant ablation in thyroid cancer: comparison between hormone withdrawal and use of rhTSH in low-risk patients. Eur J Endocrinol. 2009;160(3):431–6.

39. Andresen NS, Buatti JM, Tewfik HH, Pagedar NA, Anderson CM, Watkins JM. Radioiodine ablation following thyroidectomy for differentiated thyroid cancer: literature review of utility, dose, and toxicity. Eur Thyroid J. 2017;6(4):187–96.

40. Hovens GC, Stokkel MP, Kievit J, et al. Associations of serum thyrotropin concentrations with recurrence and death in differentiated thyroid cancer. J Clin Endocrinol Metab. 2007;92(7):2610–5.

41. Wells SA, Asa SL, Dralle H, et al. Revised American Thyroid Association guidelines for the management of medullary thyroid carcinoma. Thyroid. 2015;25(6):567–610.

42. Ladenson PW, Braverman LE, Mazzaferri EL, et al. Comparison of administration of recombinant human thyrotropin with withdrawal of thyroid hormone for radioactive iodine scanning in patients with thyroid carcinoma. N Engl J Med. 1997;337(13):888–96.

43. Salavati A, Puranik A, Kulkarni HR, Budiawan H, Baum RP. Peptide receptor radionuclide therapy (PRRT) of medullary and nonmedullary thyroid cancer using radiolabeled somatostatin analogues. Semin Nucl Med. 2016;46(3):215–24.

44. Orlandi F, Caraci P, Berruti A, et al. Chemotherapy with dacarbazine and 5-fluorouracil in advanced medullary thyroid cancer. Ann Oncol. 1994;5(8):763–5.

45. Sherman SI. Cytotoxic chemotherapy for differentiated thyroid carcinoma. Clin Oncol (R Coll Radiol). 2010;22(6):464–8.

46. Tohyama O, Matsui J, Kodama K, et al. Antitumor activity of lenvatinib (e7080): an angiogenesis inhibitor that targets multiple receptor tyrosine kinases in preclinical human thyroid cancer models. J Thyroid Res. 2014;2014:638747.

47. Wells SA, Robinson BG, Gagel RF, et al. Vandetanib in patients with locally advanced or metastatic medullary thyroid cancer: a randomized, double-blind phase III trial. J Clin Oncol. 2012;30(2):134–41.

48. Elisei R, Schlumberger MJ, Müller SP, et al. Cabozantinib in progressive medullary thyroid cancer. J Clin Oncol. 2013;31(29):3639–46.

49. Martinez FJ, Calverley PM, Goehring UM, Brose M, Fabbri LM, Rabe KF. Effect of roflumilast on exacerbations in patients with severe chronic obstructive pulmonary disease uncontrolled by combination therapy (REACT): a multicentre randomised controlled trial. Lancet. 2015;385(9971):857–66.

50. Ding T, Zhou F, Chen X, et al. Continuation of gefitinib plus chemotherapy prolongs progression-free survival in advanced non-small cell lung cancer patients who get acquired resistance to gefitinib without T790M mutations. J Thorac Dis. 2017;9(9):2923–34.

51. Arao T, Matsumoto K, Furuta K, et al. Acquired drug resistance to vascular endothelial growth factor receptor 2 tyrosine kinase inhibitor in human vascular endothelial cells. Anticancer Res. 2011;31(9):2787–96.

52. Finke J, Ko J, Rini B, Rayman P, Ireland J, Cohen P. MDSC as a mechanism of tumor escape from sunitinib mediated antiangiogenic therapy. Int Immunopharmacol. 2011;11(7):856–61.

53. Carlomagno F, Santoro M. Identification of RET kinase inhibitors as potential new treatment for sporadic and inherited thyroid cancer. J Chemother. 2004;16(Suppl 4):49–51.

54. Isham CR, Netzel BC, Bossou AR, et al. Development and characterization of a differentiated thyroid cancer cell line resistant to VEGFR-targeted kinase inhibitors. J Clin Endocrinol Metab. 2014;99(6):E936–43.

55. Jin N, Jiang T, Rosen DM, Nelkin BD, Ball DW. Dual inhibition of mitogen-activated protein kinase kinase and mammalian target of rapamycin in differentiated and anaplastic thyroid cancer. J Clin Endocrinol Metab. 2009;94(10):4107–12.

56. Liu D, Xing J, Trink B, Xing M. BRAF mutation-selective inhibition of thyroid cancer cells by the novel MEK inhibitor RDEA119 and genetic-potentiated synergism with the mTOR inhibitor temsirolimus. Int J Cancer. 2010;127(12):2965–73.

57. Smallridge RC, Copland JA, Brose MS, et al. Efatutazone, an oral PPAR-γ agonist, in combination with paclitaxel in anaplastic thyroid cancer: results of a multicenter phase 1 trial. J Clin Endocrinol Metab. 2013;98(6):2392–400.

58. Lin Z, Wu VW, Lin J, Feng H, Chen L. A longitudinal study on the radiation-induced thyroid gland changes after external beam radiotherapy of nasopharyngeal carcinoma. Thyroid. 2011;21(1):19–23.

59. Cohen EE, Tortorici M, Kim S, Ingrosso A, Pithavala YK, Bycott P. A phase II trial of axitinib in patients with various histologic subtypes of advanced thyroid cancer: long-term outcomes and pharmacokinetic/pharmacodynamic analyses. Cancer Chemother Pharmacol. 2014;74(6):1261–70.

60. Cohen EE, Rosen LS, Vokes EE, et al. Axitinib is an active treatment for all histologic subtypes of advanced thyroid cancer: results from a phase II study. J Clin Oncol. 2008;26(29):4708–13.

61. Ho AL, Grewal RK, Leboeuf R, et al. Selumetinib-enhanced radioiodine uptake in advanced thyroid cancer. N Engl J Med. 2013;368(7):623–32.

62. Rothenberg SM, Daniels GH, Wirth LJ. Redifferentiation of iodine-refractory BRAF V600E-mutant metastatic papillary thyroid cancer with Dabrafenib-response. Clin Cancer Res. 2015;21(24):5640–1.

63. Rosove MH, Peddi PF, Glaspy JA. BRAF V600E inhibition in anaplastic thyroid cancer. N Engl J Med. 2013;368(7):684–5.

64. Vaisman F, Rosado de Castro PH, Lopes FP, et al. Is there a role for peptide receptor radionuclide therapy in medullary thyroid cancer? Clin Nucl Med. 2015;40(2):123–7.

65. Brest P, Lassalle S, Hofman V, et al. MiR-129-5p is required for histone deacetylase inhibitor-induced cell death in thyroid cancer cells. Endocr Relat Cancer. 2011;18(6):711–9.

56

Cutaneous Melanoma and Other Skin Cancers

Paola Queirolo, Andrea Boutros, and Enrica Teresa Tanda

Skin Cancers

Contents

© Springer Nature Switzerland AG 2021
A. Russo et al. (eds.), *Practical Medical Oncology Textbook*, UNIPA Springer Series,
https://doi.org/10.1007/978-3-030-56051-5_57

🎓 **Learning Objectives**

By the end of the chapter, the reader will:

− Have notions of incidence, mortality, and the main risk factors for cutaneous melanoma
− Have learned the basic concepts of pathogenesis of melanoma
− Be able to identify a suspected skin lesion for melanoma
− Know the staging of melanoma
− Have learned basic concepts on melanoma therapy
− Be able to put acquired knowledge into clinical practice.

57.1 Cutaneous Melanoma

Paola Queirolo and Andrea Boutros

57.1.1 Introduction

The majority of melanomas arise from the skin, but other types, with substantially different pathogenesis and biological behavior, include mucosal or uveal melanoma too. This chapter will focus essentially on cutaneous melanoma.

Cutaneous melanoma is the deadliest form of skin cancer, despite being relatively rare, representing less than 5% of all skin cancers.

According to the American Cancer Society, cutaneous melanoma is the fifth leading type of cancer in the United States, with about 96 000 new estimated cases and about 7 000 expected deaths in 2019 [1].

Before the introduction of immunotherapy and targeted therapy, the median survival of patients with stage IV disease was less than 1 year [2–5]. For more than 30 years, the standard of care for advanced melanoma was chemotherapy, but in the last decade, significant therapeutic achievements were obtained in patients with advanced melanoma thanks to targeted therapy and immunotherapy.

In this chapter, data from the most relevant clinical trials in early-stage and advanced melanoma will be discussed with some insight on the treatment of real-world patients.

57.1.2 Epidemiology and Risk Factors

According to the Centers for Disease Control and Prevention (CDC), in 2015 in the United States, a total of 80 442 new cases of cutaneous melanoma were observed. The CDC reported a total of 22 new cases and 2 deaths for every 100 000 people [6].

Melanoma tends to be more frequent in fair-skinned people who tends to develop sunburns more easily [7].

Indeed, sunburns, especially early in life, are considered a crucial risk factor in the tumor genesis of melanoma [8]. In particular, ultraviolet lights in the UVB spectrum (290–320 nm) are the principal ones to be associated to sunburns, leading to DNA damage, inflammation, and local immunosuppression.

Other risk factors include the total number of melanocytic nevi, family history of melanoma or any other skin cancer, immunosuppression, male sex, and age. Even if the average age at diagnosis is around 60 years old, cutaneous melanoma is not uncommon among young adults [9].

57.1.3 Pathogenesis

The two most important predisposing factors to the development of cutaneous melanoma are sun exposure and genetic susceptibility. Indeed, cutaneous melanoma occurs more commonly on sun-exposed areas of the back in men, and of the extremities in women, with an overall increased risk for fair-skinned subjects versus dark-skinned subjects. However, the relationship between melanoma and sun exposure is not as evident as it is in other non-melanoma skin tumors, since melanoma can also occur on dark-skinned people and in non-photo-exposed areas (acral melanoma).

57.1.3.1 Familial Melanoma

Familiarity is another very important risk factor, since it is estimated that about 10–15% of all melanomas occur on a genetic basis.

The main mutations observed are involved in the decreased activity of the retinoblastoma (RB) tumor suppressor proteins and may also be involved in the pathogenesis of sporadic melanoma, such as CDKN2A and cyclin-dependent kinase 4 (CDK4).

In particular, the CDKN2A gene encodes three different oncosuppressors (p15/INK4b, p16/INK4a, and p14/ARF), and it is involved in an autosomal dominant inherited mutation. In particular, p16/INK4a increases the activity of the tumor suppressor proteins of the RB family by inhibiting CDK4, while p14/ARF increases the activity of the p53 oncosuppressor by inhibiting the activity of the MDM2 oncoprotein. These mutations lead to an increase in uncontrolled melanocyte proliferation [9].

The CDKN2A germline mutation has been associated with the multiple mole/melanoma/pancreatic cancer syndrome [10].

Other rare familial melanomas have been associated with mutations of the MITF susceptibility gene, involved in the development of melanoma and renal cell carcinoma [11].

Other predisposing conditions are xeroderma pigmentosum, dysplastic nevus syndrome, and family history of melanoma (even without the evidence of pathogenetic mutations).

57.1.3.2 Sporadic Melanoma

Melanoma may occur sporadically on somatic mutations that inhibit the activity of tumor suppressor proteins (e.g., CDK4 and CDKN2A), or on mutations that increase the activity of signal-transduction oncoproteins (RAS and PI-3K/AKT), leading to increased cell growth and survival.

About half of melanoma patients bear the BRAF mutation, a gene encoding a serine/threonine kinase downstream of RAS, and about 10% carry the NRAS mutation. Melanomas that arise in non-sun-exposed areas, on the other hand, can lead to activating mutations of the C-KIT receptor tyrosine kinase. These somatic mutations have today become a fundamental therapeutic target.

Note that these mutations are probably necessary, but not sufficient for the development of melanoma, since even the melanocytic nevi carry the same activating mutations as NRAS and BRAF, without having an evolution in malignancy [9].

57.1.4 Clinical Presentation

Melanoma occurs classically according to the acronym ABCDE:
- Asymmetry.
- Border irregularity.
- Color: variegated and uneven with streaks of black, red-brown, gray, blue.
- Dimensions more than 6 mm in diameter.
- Evolution. The early recognition of suspicious skin lesions is important, as melanoma can assume a rapidly progressive behavior and give distant metastasis [12].

However, not all melanomas occur according to the ABCDE rule. In many cases, it may present as a nodular symmetrical lesion; in other cases, it may not be pigmented; and in others, it may have small dimensions. On the other hand, in subjects with dysplastic nevus syndrome, most nevi fall within the characteristics of ABCDE, without being melanoma. For this reason, it is important to integrate the ABCDE rule with the sign of the "ugly duckling," where lesions presenting uneven characteristics that deviate from all the other patient's nevi pattern must be considered as suspect [12].

Usually, melanoma is an asymptomatic lesion, but sometimes it can cause itching, local pain, or bleeding [9].

57.1.5 Diagnosis

Biopsy is the only valid way to diagnose melanoma. Furthermore, biopsy is essential for proper staging.

The excisional biopsy must include all the lesion in all its thickness (without necessarily including the subcutis) and a narrow margin of about 1 mm.

When an excisional biopsy is not possible (large lesions, lesions of the face or genital mucosa), an incisional biopsy is taken from a representative site.

In ungual lesions, a punch biopsy can be the first diagnostic step [12].

57.1.5.1 Histopathology

In its early stage, melanoma may present a horizontal diffusion within the epidermis and superficial dermis (radial growth phase). After a variable period of time, melanoma can begin to grow vertically (vertical growth phase). Having acquired the ability to metastasize, melanoma can invade the deeper dermal layers in this phase.

The Breslow thickness has a strong prognostic value, and it represents the distance from the granular layer of the epidermis to the deeper intradermal tumor cells. Other factors are the presence of ulceration and the number of mitoses.

Melanoma cells are larger than normal melanocytes and contain large nuclei, condensed chromatin, and prominent nucleoli [9].

The different histological variants of melanoma are described in Table 57.1 [12].

Table 57.1 Melanoma histologic subtypes

Superficial spreading melanoma	The most frequent type of melanoma. It occurs mainly on trunk and extremities (except on acral sites). This variant is the mainly associated with sun exposure.
Nodular melanoma	The second histotype in frequency, associated with a worse prognosis due to its thickness at time of diagnosis.
Acral melanoma	Relatively rare variant, despite being the most common in dark-skinned subjects. It arises in the acral sites (palms, plants, subungual).
Lentigo maligna melanoma	Lesion that typically occurs on the face of elderly subjects, characterized by a very long phase of radial growth.
Desmoplastic melanoma	Uncommon variant. Histologically it presents melanocytes in the dermis with intense stromal infiltrate. Often clinically unpigmented.

[12]

57.1.6 **Staging**

A correct staging is a fundamental step in the planning of the appropriate diagnostic-therapeutic strategy. The approved classification is the TNM by the American Joint Committee on Cancer (AJCC), 8th edition, reported in ◘ Table 57.2 [13].

◘ Table 57.2   Melanoma staging system, AJCC 8th edition

T	Breslow thickness	Ulceration	
Tx	Not applicable because the primary tumor thickness cannot be assessed	Not applicable	Not applicable
T0	Not applicable	Not applicable	Unknown primary or complete regression
Tis	Not applicable Melanoma in situ	Not applicable	Stage 0
T1	T1a: <0.8 mm	Absent	Stage I
	T1b: <0.8	Present	
	T1b: 0.8–1.0 mm	Absent	
T2	T2a: >1.0–2.0 mm	Absent	
	T2b: >1.0–2.0 mm	Present	Stage II
T3	T3a: >2.0–4.0 mm	Absent	
	T3b: >2.0–4.0 mm	Present	
T4	T4a: >4.0 mm	Absent	
	T4b: >4.0 mm	Present	
N	No. of involved regional lymph nodes	In transit metastasis, satellite, and/or microsatellitosis	
Nx	Not assessed	No	
N0	Not detected	No	
N1	N1a: one clinically occult	No	Stage III
	N1b: one clinically detected	No	
	N1c: not detected	Yes	
N2	N2a: 2–3 clinically occult	No	
	N2b: 2–3, at least one clinically detected	No	
	N2c: one clinically occult or clinically detected	Yes	
N3	N3a: ≥4 clinically occult	No	
	N3b: ≥4, at least one clinically detected or any number of matted nodes	No	
	N3c: ≥2 clinically occult or clinically detected and/or any number of matted nodes	Yes	
M	Anatomic site of distant metastasis	LDH level	
M0	Nonevident distant metastasis	Not applicable	
M1	M1a: skin, soft tissue, and/or nonregional lymph nodes	(0) Not elevated (1) Elevated	Stage IV
	M1b: lung	(0) Not elevated (1) Elevated	
	M1c: non-central nervous system (CNS) visceral sites	(0) Not elevated (1) Elevated	
	M1d: CNS	(0) Not elevated (1) Elevated	

57

The most significant prognostic factors are the Breslow thickness and the presence of ulceration.

In fact, the 5-year survival goes from 99% for melanomas <1 mm to 90% for those >4 mm [13]. Ulceration has a similar impact, especially in thicker melanomas, ranging from a 5-year survival of 94% and 90% in pT3a and pT4a melanomas to 86% and 82%, respectively, in pT3b and pT4b [13].

The number of mitoses per mm^2 has a real impact on survival for values greater than 4 [13].

Stage III 5-year survival ranges from 82% in N1 melanoma, to 76% in N2, and 57% in N3 [13].

In stage IV disease, serum LDH level is a clinically significant factor with a predictive and prognostic value [13].

57.1.7 Treatment of Early-Stage Disease

57.1.7.1 Surgery

Early-stage melanoma has an excellent long-term prognosis [13]: surgical excision is the standard treatment, with a 5-year survival rates at 98% for stage I and ranging from 96% to 82% for stage II disease [13]. Wide local excision is the definitive approach. Several meta-analyses [14] summarized the evidence regarding width of excision margins for primary cutaneous melanoma. In particular, recommended excision margins are as follows:

- 5 mm in melanoma in situ
- 10 mm if Breslow's thickness <2 mm
- 20 mm if Breslow's thickness ≥2 mm

When Breslow's thickness is ≥0.8 mm, a sentinel lymph node biopsy (SLNB) is indicated. In fact, the risk of lymph node metastatic involvement is proportional to depth. The SLNB is a minimally invasive procedure that confers prognostic information regarding risk stratification.

Risk stratification, as shown in a recent meta-analysis, should be based on ulceration (present/absent) of the primary tumor and SN tumor burden (high > 1 mm/low < 1 mm) as shown by Rotterdam criteria for Sentinel Node Tumor Load [15].

This risk stratification is in line with the recent evidence that the complete lymph node dissection (CLND) does not have a significant impact on survival [16], with an important and unnecessary exposure to morbidity over time.

57.1.7.2 Adjuvant Setting

Patients with thick and/or ulcerated-primary melanoma and/or regional lymph node involvement at diagnosis (stage III) have higher risk of recurrence after surgical resection. So, in this category of patients, there is strong indication to start an adjuvant treatment, in order to improve the risk of relapse. The main adjuvant clinical studies are summarized in ▣ Table 57.3.

▣ Figure 57.1 shows a therapeutic algorithm for melanoma at high risk of relapse.

57.1.7.3 Interferon Alpha

During the last two decades [17], the only approved treatment in the adjuvant setting was interferon alpha. Different doses and schedules were studied in different nations.

In terms of event-free survival (EFS) an improvement has been observed, leading to absolute increases in 5- and 10-year EFS of 3.5% and 2.7%, respectively,

▣ **Table 57.3** A summary of the main clinical studies in the adjuvant setting in melanoma

Study	Treatment	Stage	HR$_{RFS}$	HR$_{OS}$
Interferon alpha meta-analyses [17]	Interferon – different regimens	IIB-IIIC	**0.82** *vs.* placebo	**0.89**
EORTC 18071/ CA184-029 [18]	Ipilimumab (10 mg/kg; q3w × 4 → q3m) vs. placebo	IIIA(>1mm)/IIIB/IIIC	**0.76** *vs.* placebo	**0.72**
CheckMate-238 [19]	Nivolumab (3 mg/kg; q2w) vs. ipilimumab (10 mg/kg; q3w × 4 → q12w)	IIIB/IIIC/resected IV	**0.65** *vs.* ipilimumab	Not available
KEYNOTE 054 [20]	Pembrolizumab (200 mg/kg; q3w) vs. placebo	IIIA(>1mm)/IIIB/IIIC	**0.57** *vs.* placebo	Not available
BRIM-8 [22]	Vemurafenib (960 mg bid) vs. placebo	IIC/IIIA(>1mm)/IIIB/IIIC	**0.65** *vs.* placebo **0.80** IIIC **0.54** IIC-IIIB	Not available
Combi-AD [21]	Dabrafenib + trametinib (150 mg bid + 2 mg qd) vs. placebo	IIIA(>1mm)/IIIB/IIIC	**0.47** *vs.* placebo	**0.57**

Fig. 57.1 A therapeutic algorithm for melanoma at high risk of relapse

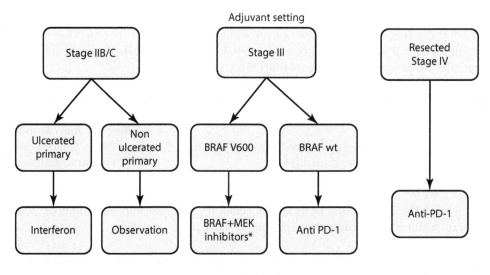

with a significantly greater benefit in ulcerated primary tumor patients. Note that disease stages I and II were also included in those clinical trials.

In the recent years, great progress has been made in the immunologic treatment of metastatic melanoma. Now we see the same progress in the adjuvant setting.

Available drugs are anti-CTLA4 ipilimumab, and anti-PD-1 nivolumab and pembrolizumab.

57.1.7.4 Ipilimumab

EORTC 18071/CA184-029 [18] is a phase 3, randomized trial where ipilimumab – administered at 10 mg/kg dose every 21 days, for 4 cycles, followed by maintenance doses every 3 months up to 3 years – was compared to placebo. Ipilimumab showed greater efficacy than placebo in terms of relapse-free survival with a 5-year RFS of 41% for the ipilimumab arm and 30% for the placebo and in terms of distant metastases-free survival (DMFS), where, at 5 years, ipilimumab showed superior data compared to placebo: 48% were alive metastases-free in the ipilimumab arm versus 39% in the placebo arm.

In particular, the superiority of ipilimumab was more evident in the ulcerated-primary and >3 positive lymph nodes subgroups.

However, the treatment arm showed a higher toxicity profile (high incidence of grade >3 adverse events), which occurred in more than a half of the ipilimumab arm patients. In order to overcome this issue, another study was designed to compare ipilimumab 10 mg/kg and ipilimumab 3 mg/kg, with no significant difference in terms of efficacy and with an improvement of the severe adverse event (SAE) rate.

57.1.7.5 Nivolumab

CheckMate 238 [19] is a phase 3, double-blind study, which enrolled completely resected stage IIIB, IIIC, and IV patients to receive nivolumab 3 mg/kg every 2 weeks for 1 year or ipilimumab 10 mg/kg every 3 weeks for four cycles. This trial compared an anti-PD-1 to an anti-CTLA4 (which efficacy was already demonstrated versus placebo).

RFS at 24 months was 63% and 50%, respectively, in the nivolumab and the ipilimumab arm, with a more favorable toxicity profile in the nivolumab group.

57.1.7.6 Pembrolizumab

Pembrolizumab is another anti-PD-1 agent, approved in the advanced disease, that was also experimented in the adjuvant setting KEYNOTE-054 [20] clinical study.

Patients were randomized to receive pembrolizumab 200 every 3 weeks or placebo up to 1 year or placebo. RFS and toxicity profile were as manageable and tolerable as shown in the metastatic setting and substantially the same of nivolumab.

57.1.7.7 Dabrafenib Plus Trametinib

As for the immune checkpoint inhibitors, BRAF and MEK inhibitors have been tested as well in the adjuvant setting, both in monotherapy and in combination.

In particular, the COMBI-AD [21] study, presented in 2017, investigated the efficacy of BRAF and MEK inhibitors in combination. Patients with completely resected, high risk stage III (lymph node metastasis > 1 mm), BRAF V600-mutated cutaneous melanoma were enrolled and randomized in two arms: placebo or dabrafenib 150 mg bid plus trametinib 2 mg qd, for maximum 1 year. RFS showed a highly significant superiority of the experimental arm. After 36 months of follow-up, DMFS was 71% in the treatment group versus 57% in the placebo arm.

57.1.8 Treatment of Advanced Stage Disease

1. *Targeted Therapy*

- **Molecular Basis of Targeted Therapy**

The MAPK (RAS-RAF-MEK-ERK) signaling pathway is a critical regulator of cellular growth, tissue invasion, and survival.

Nearly half of patients with metastatic melanoma harbor a BRAF V600-mutation [23] (most commonly V600E or V600K). The analysis of anatomic subtypes showed that BRAF mutations are common in cutaneous melanoma (43%) and less commonly observed in patients whose tumors arise from sun-damaged skin (e.g., lentigo maligna melanoma), from mucosal (6%) and uveal (<2%) sites. Among cutaneous melanomas, BRAF mutations are more frequently found in superficial spreading melanomas (53%) and less frequently present in acral melanoma (18%) and lentigo maligna melanoma (9%).

This somatic mutation activates the MAPK signaling pathway. In particular, mutated BRAF signals as a monomer, becoming independent of upstream growth stimuli and constitutively activated as well as insensitive to negative feedback signals.

BRAF V600-mutation has been implicated in different mechanisms of melanoma progression [23]:

- Activation of the downstream MEK/ERK signaling pathway and unchecked tumor replication
- Evasion from apoptosis and cellular senescence mechanisms
- Increased MEK-dependent angiogenesis
- Evasion from the immunologic surveillance
- Metastatic potential through upregulation of proteins involved in cellular migration.

The BRAF inhibitors vemurafenib and dabrafenib were both approved as single agents by the US Food and Drug Administration (FDA) and the European Medicines Agency (EMA) in 2011 and 2013, for the treatment of unresectable or metastatic BRAF V600-mutated melanoma. These BRAF inhibitors are able to reduce MAPK pathway activation and prevent melanoma cell growth.

However, chronic BRAF inhibition can lead to acquired resistance through various mechanisms, such as the following:

1. Reactivation of MAPK pathway signaling
2. Activation of PI3K-Akt-mTOR pathway signaling
3. NRAS mutation

In addition, rapid responses are often short-lived, and recurrent tumors are often more aggressive.

These issues led to preclinical studies and clinical investigations of combination therapy with MEK inhibitors. In ◘ Table 57.4, those clinical studies are summarized.

In 2014, the randomized, phase 3 coBRIM [4] study evaluated the combination of the BRAF inhibitor vemurafenib and the MEK inhibitor cobimetinib versus vemurafenib single-agent first-line treatment, in patients with unresectable, BRAF V600-mutated, melanoma. The combination treatment showed a significant advantage (2016 update [24]) in terms of median progression-free survival (PFS), the primary endpoint of the study 12.3 months for cobimetinib and vemurafenib versus 7.2 months for placebo and vemurafenib (HR = 0.58, CI 0.46–0.72, $p < 0.0001$), and in terms of overall survival (HR = 0.70, CI 0.55–0.90), with a median OS of 22.3 and 17.4 months, respectively, in the combination and single-agent arms.

◘ **Table 57.4** A summary of the main clinical studies of targeted therapy in melanoma

Study	Treatment	ORR (%)	mPFS (months)	3-year OS (%)	Grade 3/4 AEs (%)
coBRIM [24]	Vemurafenib (960 mg; bid) + cobimetinib (60 mg; qd) vs. vemurafenib + placebo	68 45	12.3 7.3	38.5 31	62 52
COMBI-v [5]	Dabrafenib (150 mg; bid) + trametinib (2 mg; qd) vs. vemurafenib (960 mg; bid)	64 51	11.4 7.3	45 32	52 63
COMBI-d [25]	Dabrafenib (150 mg; bid) + trametinib (2 mg; qd) vs. dabrafenib (150 mg; bid) + placebo	67 51	9.3 8.8	44 32	48 50
COLUMBUS [26, 27]	Encorafenib + binimetinib (450 mg + 45 mg; qd) vs. vemurafenib (960 mg; qd) or encorafenib (300 mg; qd)	64 41 52	14.9 7.3 9.6	47 – –	58 63 66

In the same year, the randomized, open-label, phase 3, COMBI-v [5] trial showed the efficacy of the combination of dabrafenib and trametinib, compared with vemurafenib alone, in patients with previously untreated unresectable melanoma with BRAF V600E or V600K mutations. The combination significantly improved the OS (HR = 0.69, CI 0.53–0.89, p = 0.005) and the PFS (HR = 0.56, CI 0.46–0.69, p<0.001).

COMBI-d [25] is another phase 3, randomized, double-blind, clinical trial showing the superiority of dabrafenib and trametinib versus dabrafenib single agent. The 2017 update showed significant advantage for the combination arm in terms of 3-year PFS (22% vs. 12%), HR = 0.71 (CI 0.57–0.88).

COLUMBUS [26, 27] is a two-part, randomized, open-label, phase 3, clinical trial investigating efficacy and safety of the combination of encorafenib, a BRAF inhibitor and binimetinib, a MEK inhibitor, in unresectable stage III or IV, BRAF V600 mutated melanoma.

In Part 1, encorafenib (450 mg) plus binimetinib combination was compared to encorafenib (300 mg) alone and vemurafenib alone. The primary endpoint was PFS of encorafenib plus binimetinib versus vemurafenib. The combination arm showed median PFS of 14.9 months versus 7.3 of the vemurafenib single-agent arm (HR = 0.54. CI 0.41–0.71, p < 0.0001). In addition, the combination arm showed an advantage in terms of median OS: 33.6 months versus 16.9 months (HR = 0.61, 0.47–0.79). The 3-year OS was 47% in the encorafenib + binimetinib arm.

In Part 2, encorafenib (300 mg) plus binimetinib was compared to encorafenib (300 mg) alone. The combination treatment showed superiority in terms of PFS (HR = 0.77. CI 0.61–0.97, p = 0.029).

Note that in the COLUMBUS trial, a lesser number of patients had baseline LDH > ULN.

Targeted therapy is well tolerated as confirmed by all clinical trials. Some toxicities, such as skin toxicity, arthralgia, fatigue, and gastrointestinal adverse events, are common to all BRAF and MEK inhibitors.

In particular, photosensitivity and diarrhea are more common with vemurafenib plus cobimetinib, while fever and chills are more common with dabrafenib plus trametinib.

Type and severity of these toxicities vary considerably and may influence the choice of drug.

■ **C-KIT**

Mutations in the KIT proto-oncogene – arising on mucosal, acral, and chronically sun-damaged (CSD) skin melanomas – could be responsive to the tyrosine kinase inhibitor imatinib mesylate [28]. In fact, three phase 2 studies demonstrated a clinical efficacy of imatinib targeting KIT, with a median time to progression (TTP) of 4 months in the KIT-mutated (exons 9, 11, and 13) group of patients.

2. *Immunotherapy*

Melanoma has always been described as an immunogenic tumor. In fact, before the immune checkpoint inhibitors (ICIs), many immunomodulatory drugs have been tested, such as high-dose interleukin-2 (IL-2) [29].

ICIs showed survival benefits with several randomized clinical trials, leading to the approval by the FDA (Food and Drug Administration) and the EMA (European Medicines Agency) of the anti-CTLA-4 (cytotoxic T-lymphocyte antigen 4) antibody ipilimumab and the anti-PD-1 (programmed cell death protein 1) antibodies nivolumab and pembrolizumab. ■ Table 57.5 shows the main clinical studies on immunotherapy in melanoma.

■ **Table 57.5** A summary of the main clinical studies of immunotherapy in melanoma

Study	Treatment	ORR (%)	mPFS (months)	3-year OS (%)	Grade 3/4 AEs (%)
CA184-024 [3]	Ipilimumab (10 mg/kg; q3w) + dacarbazine (DTIC) vs. DTIC (850 mg/m²; q3w)	15.2 10.3	3 3	20.8 12.2	56.3 27.5
KEYNOTE-002 [35]	Pembrolizumab (2 mg/kg or 10 mg/kg; q3w) vs. ChT	21–25 4	2.9 2.7	– 	11–14 26
KEYNOTE-006 [32]	Pembrolizumab (10 mg/kg; q2w or q3w) vs. ipilimumab (3 mg/kg; q3w)	36–37 13	5.6–4.1 2.8	48.1 37.8	17 20
CheckMate 037 [30]	Nivolumab (3 mg/kg; q2w) vs. ChT	31.7 10	3.1 3.7	– 	14 34
CheckMate 066 [31]	Nivolumab (3 mg/kg; q2w) vs. DTIC (1000 mg/m²; q3w)	40 14	5.1 2.2	51.2 21.6	11.7 17.6
CheckMate 067 [33]	Nivolumab + ipilimumab (1 mg/kg + 3 mg/kg; q3w × 4 → nivolumab 3 mg/kg; q2w) vs. nivolumab (3 mg/kg; q2w) or ipilimumab (3 mg/kg; q3w)	58 44 19	11.5 6.9 2.9	58 52 34	59 21 28

57

Ipilimumab showed in two main phase 3 clinical trials (CA 184-002 [2], comparing ipilimumab 3 mg/kg vs. gp100 vaccine therapy in pre-treated patients and CA 184-024 [3], ipilimumab 10 mg/kg plus dacarbazine vs. dacarbazine alone, in treatment-naïve patients) an improvement in terms of long-term benefit, with a 3-year OS of 21% and with a plateau on the OS curve, representing a long-term responders subgroup.

However, the CTLA-4 blockage is associated with an increased risk of developing autoimmune disorders, known as immune-related adverse events (irAEs). In fact, 10–26% presented grade ≥3 irAEs, principally enterocolitis, hepatitis, dermatitis, and endocrinopathies.

Currently, ipilimumab as single agent has an uncertain role in the treatment of melanoma due to the superiority, in terms of both clinical activity and safety, showed in clinical trials by the anti-PD-1 agents.

In particular, the phase 3 CheckMate 037 [30] trial compared the ORR of nivolumab 3 mg/kg every 2 weeks with investigator's choice chemotherapy in pre-treated patients who progressed on BRAF inhibitors or ipilimumab. The ORR was higher in the nivolumab arm: 31.7% versus 10.6%. The CheckMate 066 [31] showed its superiority in the first-line setting as well. Compared with dacarbazine in BRAF wild-type melanoma patients, nivolumab obtained a 3-year OS of 51% versus 22%, with an ORR of 40% versus 14%.

KEYNOTE-006 [32] is a phase 3 study designed to compare pembrolizumab 10 mg/kg (every 2 weeks or every 3 weeks) with ipilimumab 3 mg/kg every 3 weeks. Results showed a median PFS of 5.6 and 4.1 months for each schedule of pembrolizumab versus 2.8 months in the ipilimumab arm, with an ORR of 36% and 37% versus 13%, also showing an advantage in the pembrolizumab arms; 4-year OS was 42% in the pooled pembrolizumab arms and 34% in the ipilimumab arm.

As in the case of ipilimumab, the anti-PD-1 treated patients show a prolonged clinical response, as seen mainly in the KEYNOTE-006 study. This potential is leading to take in consideration the question of how long to continue treatment in these patients.

In addition, pembrolizumab and nivolumab showed a more favorable safety profile as well when compared with ipilimumab. In fact, the observed incidence of grade ≥3 irAEs with an anti-PD-1 agent was about 10–16% versus 19–27% with ipilimumab. The most common anti-PD-1 adverse events are fatigue, rash and pruritus, diarrhea, and endocrinopathies.

■ **Combination of Immune Checkpoint Inhibitors**

In order to improve the ORR, several clinical trials were designed to investigate the combination of different ICI. In particular, the CheckMate 067 [33] is a phase 3 clinical trial that randomly assigned, in a 1:1:1 ratio, treatment-naïve patients to receive nivolumab 1 mg/kg plus ipilimumab 3 mg/kg every 3 weeks for four cycles, followed by nivolumab 3 mg/kg every 2 weeks; nivolumab 3 mg/kg every 2 weeks plus placebo; or ipilimumab 3 mg/kg every 3 weeks for four cycles plus placebo.

ORR and PFS were significantly higher for the combination arm: the observed ORR were 58% versus 44% and 19% in the nivolumab and ipilimumab arms, respectively; with a median PFS of 11.5 months in the combination arm versus 7 and 3 months for nivolumab and ipilimumab alone, respectively. In addition, a recent 3-year OS update showed that 58% of patients who received nivolumab plus ipilimumab were alive at 3 years, versus 52% of the nivolumab single-agent group and 34% of the ipilimumab group.

However, these encouraging results were obtained with a high toxicity profile: grade 3/4 adverse events have been observed in 58% of patients in the combination arm.

Despite the poor safety profile, the combination regimen of ipilimumab plus nivolumab was approved by the regulatory authorities.

In order to decrease the incidence of grade ≥3 irAEs, a combination of pembrolizumab and reduced-dose ipilimumab (1 mg/kg) was studied in the phase 1 study KEYNOTE-029 [34], with an incidence of grade 3–4 AEs of 42%, with no difference in term of ORR (57%).

3. *Radiation Therapy*

Melanoma has a variable spectrum of radiosensitivity; therefore, it should be considered as a radioresistant neoplasm and requires high doses of radiation to show efficacy [37].

Its application is mainly in the treatment of encephalic lesions through stereotaxis or whole brain radiation [38, 39], and of bone lesions through an 8 Gy single fraction radiation therapy [40, 41]. However, potentially any metastatic localization can be irradiated in a palliative setting or to increase local disease control (◘ Fig. 57.2).

Fig. 57.2 A therapeutic algorithm for advanced stage disease setting melanoma

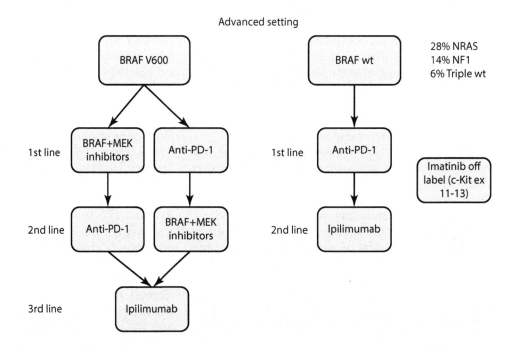

Case Study

A 43-year-old man comes to your attention after having surgically removed a suspect pigmented skin lesion of the back with the following histological report:

Histological report 1

Sample of skin of 23 mm × 9 mm
Superficial spreading melanoma
Breslow thickness: 1.2 mm
Ulceration: present
Mitoses/mm²: 2

Question 1

What action should be taken?
(a) Start an adjuvant treatment with nivolumab + ipilimumab
(b) Wide excision with 10-mm margins
(c) Wide excision with 5-mm margins
(d) Wide excision with 10-mm margins + sentinel lymph node biopsy

Answer

Wide excision with 10-mm margins + sentinel lymph node biopsy.

The patient also performs a CT that shows no evidence of distant metastases. He shows you the report of the wide excision and sentinel lymph node biopsy:

Histological report 2

Margins: free
Left axillary sentinel lymph node: presence of 1 micrometastasis.
Molecular biology
Primitive melanoma BRAF V600E positive

Question 2

What is the TNM stage?
(a) pT1b pN0 M0
(b) pT2b pN1a M0
(c) pT2a pN1a M0
(d) pT1a pN1a M0

Answer 2

pT2b pN1a M0

Question 3

What action should be taken?
(a) Start a 1-year adjuvant treatment with vemurafenib.
(b) Start a 2-year adjuvant treatment with pembrolizumab.
(c) Start a 1-year adjuvant treatment with dabrafenib + tramentinib.
(d) Perform a left axillary complete lymph node dissection and start an 18-months adjuvant treatment with interferon.

Answer 3

Start a 1-year adjuvant treatment with dabrafenib + tramentinib.

After 1 year, the patient has completed the adjuvant therapy without any particular adverse event, with the exception of some febrile peaks. At the follow-up CT, there is no evidence of distant metastasis.

Expert Opinion
Paola Queirolo

Key Points

1. Cutaneous melanoma represents less than 5% of all skin cancers but it is regarded as the deadliest. The main risk factors are fair skin, male sex, age, sunburns in early life, total number of melanocytic nevi, family history of melanoma, and immunosuppression. Mutations in CDKN2A and MITF genes are associated to the predisposition of melanoma's onset, together with other conditions such as xeroderma pigmentosum and dysplastic nevus syndrome. Other important mutations regard BRAF and c-KIT genes.

2. Melanoma usually appears as an asymmetric nodule with border irregularity, variegated and uneven with streaks of black, red-brown, gray or blue coloration, more than 6 mm in diameter and with a rapidly progressive behavior (ABCDE). Local pain or bleeding can be present.

3. Excisional biopsy (with a narrow margin of about 1 mm), is the golden standard; in case of big nodules or particular sites, an incisional biopsy can be done. In order to understand the main features and risk of melanoma evolution, the Breslow's thickness (BT) must be evaluated. There are different histologic subtypes: superficial spreading, nodular (linked to the worst prognosis), acral, lentigo maligna, and desmoplastic melanoma.

4. In case of early-stage melanoma, wide local excision is the definitive approach, according to the BT: 5 mm in melanoma in situ, 10 mm (when BT is <2 mm), and 20 mm (when >2 mm). A sentinel lymph node is indicated when BT is >0.8 mm.

5. Adjuvant therapy consists in interferon (stage IIB/C for ulcerated primary lesions), BRAF and MEK inhibitors (stage III and mutation in BRAF V600), nivolumab, pembrolizumab (stage III and BRAF wild type and stage IV). Nivolumab and pemrbolizumab are anti-PD-1 antibodies (immune checkpoint inhibitors) which have shown good responses in this setting of patients, alone or in combination. Vemurafenib and dafrafenib are a group of tyrosine kinase inhibitors, which can be used in case of BRAF mutations for unresectable or metastatic melanoma. MEK inhibitors such as trametinib and cobimetinib are also used in this setting of patients. Some trials have shown better responses in case of combination treatments, that is dabrafenib + trametinib or encorafenib + binimetinib. C-KIT inhibitors can be otherwise used in case of KIT mutations.

Suggested Reading

Haanen JBaG. et al. Management of toxicities from immunotherapy: ESMO Clinical Practice Guidelines for diagnosis, treatment and follow-up. Ann Oncol Off J Eur Soc Med Oncol. 2017;28, iv119–iv142.

Immunotoxicity is a new field of Medicine, born with the increasingly use of immune checkpoint inhibitors in clinical practice in oncology. It is therefore important to know the main manifestations, the diagnostic and therapeutic approach, and the natural course of these conditions [36].

Recommendations

- AIOM
- ▶ www.aiom.it/wp-content/uploads/2020/10/2020_LG_AIOM_Melanoma.pdf
- ESMO
- ▶ www.esmo.org/Guidelines/Melanoma/Cutaneous-Melanoma

The Word to the Expert

The awareness about cutaneous melanoma and its risks has increased in the last years thanks to prevention campaigns among the population. Although more and more must be done above all among young people that tend to ignore the major risk factors linked to this neoplasm such as unprotected sun exposure. In case of suspected lesions, a dermatology expert should be consulted, in order to exclude the presence of cutaneous melanoma. The most interesting results concerning the therapeutic successes, regard the use of tyrosine kinase inhibitors (TKIs) and immunotherapy, which have modified the natural history of this cancer. Nowadays more attention is given to the possible relapses after the end of immunotherapy and in those patients who do not response to this category of drugs. In conclusion, it is essential that in case of advanced disease the patient is addressed to a reference center, which has a good experience in managing TKIs, immunotherapy, and its possible side effects.

Hints for a Deeper Insight

- Cutaneous melanoma: From pathogenesis to therapy (Review): ▶ https://www.ncbi.nlm.nih.gov/pubmed/29532857
- Advances in Immunotherapy for Melanoma: A Comprehensive Review: ▶ https://www.ncbi.nlm.nih.gov/pubmed/28848246
- Acral lentiginous melanoma: differences in survival compared to other subtypes: ▶ https://www.ncbi.nlm.nih.gov/pubmed/31628856
- Pericardial effusion under nivolumab: case-reports and review of the literature: ▶ https://www.ncbi.nlm.nih.gov/pubmed/31627742

57.2 Nonmelanoma Skin Cancer

Paola Queirolo Andrea Boutros, and Enrica Teresa Tanda

57.2.1 Introduction

Nonmelanoma skin cancer (NMSC) is a huge group of skin tumors that constitutes the most common form of human cancer, with an estimated incidence >3 million new cases each year in the US, with about 2000 estimated deaths each year [42, 43].

The main risk factor for NMSC is ultraviolet (UV A, UV B) rays exposure, and its incidence increases with age [44].

Many NMSC present as an erythematous lesion or a nodule. Definitive diagnosis can be obtained by shave, punch, or excisional biopsy.

57.2.2 Actinic Keratosis

AKs are common precancerous lesions that mainly occur in fair-skinned individuals as a result of cumulative sun exposure. AKs may potentially undergo spontaneous regression or progress into in situ or invasive SCC [45, 46].

Pathogenesis of AK includes UVB light exposure, DNA instability (e.g., xeroderma pigmentosum), albinism, age, and history of immunosuppression.

AKs present as a reddish-pink hyperkeratotic surface on a sun-exposed area (mainly head and neck, forearms).

There are many histologic subtypes: hyperplastic, atrophic, Bowenoid, acantholytic, and pigmented, with common features, such as atypical keratinocytes and nuclear atypia [47].

57.2.2.1 Treatment

Firstly, preventive measures consist of avoidance of excessive sun exposure and sun protection. AKs have low but actual SCC transformation potential; this is the reason why therapy is recommended. The approach can be lesion-directed or field-directed.

Lesion-directed therapy is suitable in case of few clinically visible AKs and consists mainly in cryotherapy. A multicenter study evaluated the efficacy of cryotherapy for AKs of the face and scalp, with an average response rate of 67% per patient [48].

Field-directed therapy offers an advantage [45] when a huge amount of clinically evident and subclinical lesions are present. In this case, treatment may also have a role in terms of prevention.

- *PDT*. AK is currently the only FDA-approved indication for PDT. When topically applied, 5-aminolevulinic acid (ALA) and methylaminolevulinic acid (MAL) accumulate in malignant and premalignant cells and are metabolized to protoporphyrin IX, a photoactive agent that promotes the generation of free radicals when irradiated with an appropriate light source, leading to irreversible cell damage, and precancerous cell death [49, 50].
- *Cryotherapy*. This technique exposes a precancerous lesion to temperatures reaching −60 °C, provoking tissue damage, and a thermal shock leading to premalignant cell death. Cryotherapy does not allow a precise margin control [48].
- *5-FU*. A systematic review of randomized clinical trials showed that 5-FU 0.5% resulted in an average reduction of lesions of 86%, with a higher compliance profile from lower side effect rate [51].
- *Imiquimod*. The FDA-approved protocol is twice weekly for 16 weeks. When compared to cryotherapy and 5-FU [52], imiquimod showed similar efficacy but higher sustained response at 1 year [45].

Another possible option is diclofenac 3% gel, with similar outcomes [53].

57.2.3 Basal Cell Carcinoma

BCC is the most common human cancer, accounting for 25% of all cancers in the US. It typically develops from sun-exposed areas, but it has been reported in non-exposed regions too [54]. BCC is a slow-growing tumor originating from the basal layer of epidermis, with a poor metastasizing potential, but a locally invasive behavior. Extensive sun exposure, age, and immunosuppression are the most important risk factors [44].

57.2.3.1 Clinical Presentation

Many hereditary syndromes can manifest through multiple BCCs. Among these, the nevoid BCC syndrome (NBCC, also known as Gorlin syndrome, autosomal dominant mutation of PTCH1 gene, with broad nasal root, odontogenic keratocysts, palmo-plantar pits, calcification of the falx cerebri, medulloblastomas, multiple skeletal abnormalities, and multiple BCCs) [55–57], Bazex syndrome (X-linked, follicular atrophoderma, hypotrichosis, hypohidrosis, milia, epidermoid cysts, facial BCCs), Rombo syndrome (similar to Bazex), xeroderma pigmentosum (autosomal recessive, DNA repair defect, multiple NMSC, and melanomas), Rasmussen, Darier, and albinism.

BCC is clinically variable and includes many subtypes: superficial, infiltrative, nodular (the most common subtype, accounting approximately 50% of all variants), morpheaform, pigmented, and fibroepithelioma of Pinkus [58, 59].

Superficial BCC is a well-defined erythematous-pink macule. It is difficult to differentiate from AK. Nodular BCC is a pearly papule with telangiectasias. History of central ulceration or easy bleeding is not rare. *Morpheaform* (also known as sclerosing) BCC presents as an indurated, firm, not well-demarcable, scar-like lesion. The actual extension of the tumor is often greater than its clinical appearance. Fibroepithelioma of Pinkus is a rare variant of BCC, presenting as a pink dome-shaped or pedunculated papule or nodule [60]. It may be difficult to distinguish from amelanotic melanoma.

57.2.3.2 Treatment

Radical surgical excision – when applicable – is the treatment of choice for BCC [61]. In fact, surgery gives advantage in terms of histologic evaluation of the excised specimen. In case of anatomic sites requiring maximal tissue conservation (i.e., face), Mohs micrographic surgery (MMS) allows an optimal margin control.

Imiquimod, 5-FU, and PDT are FDA-approved local treatments for superficial BCC. A clinical study randomized 601 patients with superficial BCC to receive MAL PDT, imiquimod, or 5-FU. Complete clinical response at 1 year was 73% in the PDT arm, 83% in the imiquimod arm, and 80% for 5-FU. However, imiquimod and 5-FU showed higher rates of local side effects [62].

Radiation therapy has a role when surgery is contraindicated (such as relapse or extensive, unresectable BCC).

Systemic therapy is indicated in case of unresectable or metastatic BCC, when both radiation therapy and surgery are not anymore suitable. The only available systemic therapy in the past for metastatic disease was chemotherapy, but no randomized clinical trial has been conducted.

A clinical study showed the efficacy of systemic retinoids, but with unacceptable toxicity rates.

Currently, new treatment options targeting the "Hedgehog" pathway are available: vismodegib is a smoothened (SMO) inhibitor (approved in 2012 by the FDA) showing, in a clinical trial, an objective response rate of 67% in locally advanced disease patients and of 38% in metastatic disease patients [63]. Most common adverse events are muscle spasms, alopecia, and dysgeusia (leading to weight loss and malnutrition) [64–67].

Case Study

A 53-year-old woman comes to your attention presenting the lesion shown in ▪ Fig. 57.3. She tells you that the lesion evolved very slowly over a decade.

Question 1

What action should be taken?
(a) Try to perform a radical surgery
(b) Start a radiation therapy
(c) Obtain an incisional biopsy
(d) Put on antibiotics for 14 days

Answer 1

Obtain an incisional biopsy.
The patient returns with the following histological report:

Histological report

Infiltrative basal cell carcinoma
Infiltrating the fascia
Perineural invasion: present
Lymphovascular invasion: present

Question 2

What action should be taken?
(a) Try to perform a radical surgery
(b) Start a radiation therapy
(c) Start a systemic treatment with vismodegib
(d) Mohs micrographic surgery

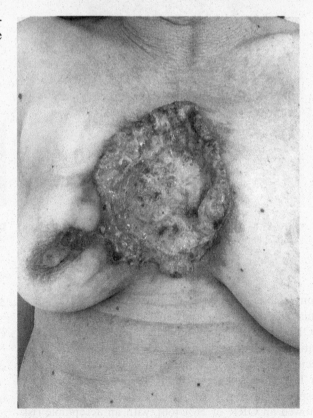

▪ **Fig. 57.3** Huge carcinomatous lesion of the chest in a 53-year-old woman

Answer 2

Start a systemic treatment with vismodegib.

The patient returns for an 8-week check. She has always taken her medications without adverse events. The lesion is shown in ◘ Fig. 57.4.

Question 3

What action should be taken?
(a) Try to perform a radical surgery
(b) Start an adjuvant radiation therapy
(c) Continue with the current treatment with vismodegib
(d) Switch to chemotherapy

Answer 3

Continue with the current treatment with vismodegib

The patient returns again after other 8 weeks of treatment. She continued her treatment with no adverse events. The lesion is shown in ◘ Fig. 57.5.

Patient's locally advanced basal cell carcinoma is responding successfully to treatment. You decide to continue until disease progression or unacceptable toxicity.

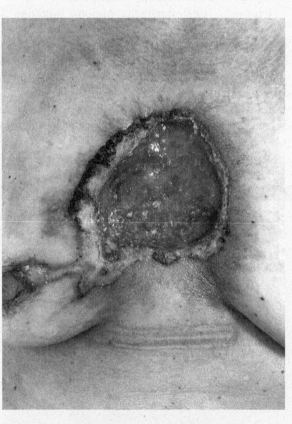

◘ Fig. 57.4 Partial response after 8 weeks of treatment with vismodegib

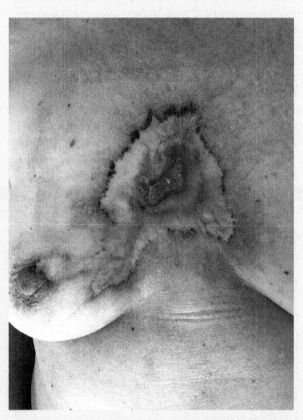

◘ Fig. 57.5 Further response after 16 weeks of treatment with vismodegib

Sonidegib is another FDA-approved oral SMO antagonist that showed efficacy in the multicenter phase 2 BOLT trial for locally advanced or metastatic BCC patients who are not suitable for surgery or RT, or for recurrent locally advanced BCC following surgery or RT. The primary endpoint was an objective tumor response rate (ORR) point estimate of ≥30%. Sonidegib showed an ORR of 56% [68], with an acceptable risk profile and comparable adverse events to that observed in vismodegib [69].

57.2.4 Squamous Cell Carcinoma

Cutaneous SCC (cSCC) is one of the most common NMSCs [70], originating from epidermal keratinizing cells [43].

In the USA, 2.1 million new cases have been registered in 2017, making it the second most common human cancer after BCC. Anyway, it is difficult to estimate the exact incidence and mortality due to the absence of cSCC in the US tumor registers. European data show that incidence of this tumor ranges from 9 to 96 per 100.000 ab. in male, and 5 to 68 per 100.000 in female. In Australia [71], the incidence in 2002 was 499 per 100.000 in male and 291 per 100.000 in female. In 2011, the cSCC mortality incidence in Australia was 2 per 100.000. Higher data coming from a Danish [72] study showed that disease-specific mortality was 2–4% in 1984.

Principal risk factors are cumulative sun exposure over life (especially in fair-skinned subjects), age, immunosuppression, HPV chronic infection, and male sex (3:1 ratio). However, among black subjects, cSCC arises more often on sites of preexisting inflammatory conditions, with a high mortality rate, because of delayed diagnosis [73]. Other risk factors are chemical (petroleum, coal, arsenic) and physical (ionizing radiations) agents and smoking.

57.2.4.1 Histology

CSCC originates from epidermis (or follicles) as atypical single cells or cellular nests [74]. In situ cSCC is an intraepidermal carcinoma (isolated to the epidermis) that seldom progresses to an invasive disease. Dermal invasion differentiates invasive SCC from in situ SCC. Invasive SCC is characterized by large cellular size, nuclear hyperchromatism, and the presence of mitotic figures. In well-differentiated SCC, the presence of keratin pearls is a sign of cytoplasmic keratinization.

Generally, the prognosis of cSCC is excellent, but it has been estimated that almost 3% of patients develop a metastatic disease. In 2012, a study suggested that from 5.604 to 12.572 people with cSCC developed nodal metastasis in the USA [70]. In particular, tumors arising from chronically inflamed skin, at mucocutaneous junction, presenting perineural invasion, diameter >40 mm, depth >4 mm, or a locally recurrent lesion, have a high risk (10–30%) of progression to metastatic disease.

Many distinct histologic subtypes of cSCC already exist; most of them are well-known, but their malignant potential is still not adequately well-recognized.

Previous classifications were not based on malignant potential. Ackerman defined cSCCs as "one entity with many faces" in 1978, when he described cSCC arising from actinic keratoses and carcinoma in situ, as well as keratotic, pseudoglandular (adenoid), pale-cell (clear cell), necrotizing, verrucous, spindle cell, and keratoacanthoma (KA)-like variants of SCC [75]. This histopathologic classification was not based on the malignant potential.

Cassarino divided in 2006 invasive cSCC into low (<3%), intermediate (3–10%), and high risk (>10%), based on risk rated of recurrence and metastasis [76, 77].

57.2.4.2 Low-Risk Invasive cSCC

Most of cSCC have an indolent behavior. The majority arise from AKs, sun-damaged skin of elderly people. Low-grade variants include the following:

— *Arising on AK*. About 95% of invasive cSCC arise from AKs, but the estimated rate of AKs leading to invasive cSCC is 0.2–10% per year. This variety of cSCC is often superficially invasive and well differentiated, with a low risk of metastasis, and it could be considered cured by surgical excision.

— *Verrucous carcinoma and other HPV-related cSCC.* A group of cSCC variants including verrucous carcinoma, oral (florid papillomatosis), anogenital (giant condyloma of Buschke-Lowenstein), plantar (epithelioma cuniculatum), epidermodysplasia verruciformis (genetic autosomal recessive disorder), sporadic, and HIV-related forms. It is a low-grade group of tumors, with an eso-/endophytic growth, associated to chronic HPV-6 and HPV-11 (epithelioma cuniculatum) and HPV-16 and HPV-18 (oral florid papillomatosis and giant condyloma of Buschke-Lowenstein) infection. Radiation therapy is not recommended, as it has been reported to lead the tumor to dedifferentiation and higher-grade SCC.

— *Spindle cell/sarcomatoid SCC (nonradiation associated)*. Uncommon variant, usually arising on sun-damaged skin, head, and neck. Cases related to radiation or arising on scars have a more aggressive behavior, and these will be discussed under the section on radiation-induced SCC. This tumor is usually composed of poorly differentiated dermal spindle cells.

— *Trichilemmal carcinoma (TLC)*. Rare subtype of cSCC arising upon sun-damaged skin of elderly people. Excellent prognosis.

— *Keratoacanthoma (KA)*. KA is a low malignant potential variant of cSCC characterized by its rapid growth and – often – a clinical spontaneous regression. KA presents clinically as a dome-shaped papule with a crateriform architecture. It should be treated as a variant of cSCC because it is impossible to predict which lesions regress and which progress.

57.2.4.3 Intermediate Risk Invasive cSCC

The following are less common group of tumors with a controversial prognosis:

— *Acantholytic/adenoid*. Arising on sun-exposed skin, mainly of elderly males. Its malignant potential ranges between 3% and 19% of distant metastasis rate.

— *Lymphoepithelioma-like carcinoma of the skin (LELCS)*. Rare tumor arising on sun-exposed skin in elderly people, not EBV-related as the nasopharyngeal LELC. Its malignant potential is still not totally known.

- *Intraepidermal epithelioma (IEE)/Borst-Jadassohn tumor with invasion.* This tumor has been described as "the most controversial entity in dermatopathology." However, its malignant potential, ranging 6–10% of distant metastasis, should not be underestimated.

57.2.4.4 High-Risk Invasive cSCC

Many of these skin cancers are rare tumors with few large studies able to determine their real malignant potential.

- *Invasive Bowen's disease.* Rapidly growing ulcerated tumor occurring in a scaly or erythematous patch. About 5% of Bowen's disease may become invasive and 13–20% of those develop distant metastasis.
- *Desmoplastic.* Aggressive variant arising principally on sun-damaged skin of elderly males, characterized by high rates of recurrence and distant metastasis (22–77%). Histologically composed by cords of spindled cells in a desmoplastic stroma, with frequent perineural invasion.
- *Malignant proliferating pilar tumor (PPT)/cyst.* Rare tumor arising on the scalp of elderly men, presenting as a cystic mass that may be ulcerate. PTTs are benign tumors but with a high recurrence potential, while malignant PTT/SCC arising in PTT is highly aggressive and metastatic in about 30%.
- *De novo SCC.* Uncommon variant arising on both sun-exposed and non-exposed skin, presenting as an erythematous nodule or induration with crusting or ulceration. 8–15% rate of local or distant metastasis.
- *Adenosquamous cell carcinoma.* Highly aggressive, rare tumor arising in the head and neck or genitalia of elderly patients, characterized by frequent recurrences and distant metastasis (up to 50%) associated with high tumor-related death. Histologically characterized by mucin-producing cuboid-columnar cells.
- *Arising in association with radiation, burn scars, chronic conditions, and immunosuppression.* Generally, cSCC arises more often in chronically injured skin affected by chronic inflammatory disorders, or immunosuppressed skin, including ulcers, burns, organ-transplanted patients, discoid lupus, lichen sclerosus, lichen planus, dystrophic epidermolysis bullosa, and lupus vulgaris. These tumors bear an aggressive behavior with high rates of invasion, recurrence, and metastatic potential.
  1. Burn scar SCC (Marjolin's ulcer). Arising on a scar with a latency period ranging from 4 months to 35 years. Characterized by a high metastatic rate (35–50%)
  2. SCC arising in discoid lupus. Common among African-Americans. High metastatic rate (30%)

  3. Radiation-induced. Radiations lead to a 3 times increased risk. Any histologic subtype is possible, but spindle cell is the most common. Tumors are aggressive and frequently metastatic
  4. Immunosuppression-related. Related to degree and duration of immunosuppression

Based on these data, the National Comprehensive Cancer Network (NCCN) [78] identified key risk factors for recurrence (summarized in ◘ Table 57.6 [79]).

Some sites are considered high-risk factors independently of size, such as area H, where optimal tumor clearance is not always possible.

These risk criteria have been revised by Schmults in a multivariate analysis of 256 high-risk cSCC, in another four risk factors:

1. Tumor diameter 2 cm or greater
2. Depth of invasion beyond subcutaneous fat
3. Poor differentiation
4. Perineural invasion [80]

In conclusion, cSCC includes distinct subtypes of varying malignant potential. This is the reason why it is recommended that the pathology report includes the following:

1. Histologic subtype
2. Degree of differentiation [81]. Poorly differentiated cSCC (Broder's grades III–IV) has a higher risk of developing distant metastasis than well and moderately differentiated (33% vs 9%).
3. Approximate depth of invasion [82]. The metastatic potential is related to depth of invasion: <2 mm (about 0% of metastasis rate), 2–6 mm (4.5% of metastasis rate), >6 mm (15% of metastasis rate).
4. Perineural invasion [81]. It is associated with about 50% of recurrence and metastasis rate.
5. Hematolymphatic invasion.

57.2.4.5 Treatment

There are four general approaches to treat cSCC:

- *Surgical excision.* Surgical excision using margins of 4 mm and 6 mm for low-risk and high-risk tumors, respectively, is the treatment of choice for cSCC. Traditional surgery showed lower recurrence rates than Mohs micrographic surgery [83].
- *Cautery or electrodesiccation.* This technique is suitable only in case of low-risk cSCC due to the impossibility to have a complete histopathology review of the tumor and the risk of residual foci of invasive tumor [84].
- *Radiation therapy.* RT is the treatment of choice in case of special sites (such as lip) or advanced SCC. In addition, advanced cutaneous carcinomas may be treated with surgery and adjuvant RT when

Table 57.6 A summary of the key risk factors of cSCC recurrence identified by the NCCN [79]

		Low risk	High risk
History and physical examination	Location/size	Area L (trunk and extremities) <20 mm Area M (cheeks, forehead, scalp, neck, pretibial) <10 mm	Area L ≥ 20 mm Area M ≥ 10 mm Area H (face, genitalia, hands, feet)
	Borders	Well-defined	Poorly-defined
	Primary vs. recurrent	Primary	Recurrent
	Immunosuppression	No	Yes
	Site of prior RT or chronic inflammatory process	No	Yes
	Rapidly growing tumor	No	Yes
	Neurologic symptoms	No	Yes
Pathology	Degree of differentiation	G1 – G2	G3
	Acantholytic (adenoid), adenosquamous (mucin production), desmoplastic, or metaplastic (carcinosarcomatous)	No	Yes
	Depth/level of invasion	≤6 mm	>6 mm
	Perineural, lymphatic, vascular invasion	No	Yes

the possibility of residual disease is high. Indications for postsurgical RT are as follows:

- Positive margins
- Perineural invasion
- Multiple recurrences
- Underlying tissue invasion

In case of regional lymph node involvement, treatment may include local RT, lymphadenectomy, or both.

Unresectable cSCC is treated with RT alone [85].

Electrochemotherapy (ECT)   This recent therapeutic technique is used in primary and metastatic skin tumors. The procedure exploits high intensity electric pulses, applicated on the tumoral mass, in order to increase the permeability of cell membrane to a systemically infused chemotherapeutic agent. In particular, bleomycin and cisplatin local cytotoxicity is significantly augmented by the electroporation [86].

Medical treatment   Treatment of metastatic disease may include chemotherapy, treatment with targeted therapy, or – from few months – immunotherapy.

In particular, *platinum*-based chemotherapy showed to have a radio-sensitizing effect in this setting, as showed in two retrospective studies [87, 88].

Cetuximab is a chimeric monoclonal antibody that inhibits the EGFR signaling pathway and used off-label for treatment of unresectable or metastatic cSCC. A phase 2 clinical study showed that cetuximab monotherapy obtained an overall response rate of 22% [89]. Other

reports showed that, when combined with adjuvant RT, cetuximab reached 50% of complete responses [90].

Cemiplimab is an FDA-approved anti-PD-1 immunotherapeutic agent that has shown interesting results in two clinical trials in a group of patients with locally advanced disease without surgical indications or with metastatic disease. The overall responses were 50% and 48% in both cases, respectively. The toxicity profile was not different from that of immune-checkpoint inhibitors when used in monotherapy, in both trials.

Among 108 patients with advanced cSCC, including metastatic ($N = 75$) or locally advanced ($N = 33$) disease, the overall response rate (ORR) was 47% (95% CI: 38, 57). 61% of responses were 6 months durable or longer.

Observed severe adverse events were principally immune-related in both trials (pneumonitis, hepatitis, colitis, adrenal insufficiency, hypo- and hyperthyroidism, diabetes mellitus, and nephritis).

Among patients with advanced cSCC, cemiplimab induced a response in approximately half the patients and was associated with adverse events that usually occur with immune checkpoint inhibitors [91].

57.2.5 Merkel Cell Carcinoma

Merkel cell carcinoma (MCC) is a rare, primary, and highly aggressive neuroendocrine skin tumor, described for the first time by Toker in 1972 as a "trabecular carcinoma of the skin" [92]. Some cytological characteristics like the presence of neurosecretory granules led to identify the Merkel cells, cutaneous mechanoreceptors, as the cells of origin of this tumor. For this reason, the name of this malignancy was redefined as MCC in the early 1980s.

57.2.5.1 Epidemiology and Risk Factors

The incidence of MCC is increasing more rapidly than other skin tumors, such as malignant melanoma, probably due to longevity, improved detection, and increased reporting. Indeed, the incidence rate passed from 0.22 to 0.79 cases per 100.000/year in the USA [93], from 0.13 to 0.35 in Europe, and reaching the highest rate in Australia [94]. In a recent study by Paulson and colleagues, the total number of cases reported annually showed a 95.2% increase (from 334 cases in 2000 to 652 cases in 2013) [95].

Several demographic factors are associated to this phenomenon. First of all, the incidence of MCC increases dramatically with age, by approximately 10-fold between 40–44 and 60–64 years and 10-fold again between 60–64 and 85 years. Indeed, data about the incidence rate (from 2011 to 2013) are consistent: 0.1 cases/100,000 person-years among subjects of 40–44 years and 9.8/100,000 person-years for people older than 85.

Incidence is higher among men, with a men/women ratio of 2–3:1, and this effect is most pronounced among the oldest age groups.

Most frequently, MCC presents with local disease, but regional lymph node and distant metastases may be present in up to 30% of new cases. In a minority of cases, MCC is diagnosed as a lymph node metastasis without an identifiable primary lesion, which may have spontaneously regressed or be occult [96]. MCC is highly aggressive, with a disease-related mortality rate of 46%, higher than the one seen among melanoma patients, but the stage at diagnosis strongly influences this parameter [97].

The main risk factor for the development of MCC includes infection with the Merkel cell polyomavirus (MCPyV), ultraviolet radiation exposure (UVB irradiation), and immunosuppression [98, 99].

Approximately 80% of MCCs are caused by a ubiquitous virus called Merkel cell polyomavirus (MCPyV) [100]. In these cases, carcinogenesis is caused by the clonal integration of the MCPyV into the host genome: we will talk more extensively about the role of MCPyV in the pathogenesis of MCC in the dedicated section.

UV exposure is a significant risk factor for MCC and may contribute by causing immunosuppression and mutagenesis [101]. Several observations support this data. First of all, there is a great difference in incidence between non-Hispanic white individuals and other ethnical groups, with a white–black ratio of 20:1. Secondly, MCC commonly arise on chronically sun-exposed skin and/or in individuals treated with UVA photochemo-

therapy. Moreover, usually MCC patients have a history of other skin cancers associated with sun exposure like melanoma or cutaneous SCC. Finally, a molecular UV signature (DNA mutations that are typically caused by UV damage) has been demonstrated in MCPyV-negative MCCs [102].

A separate category is represented by immunocompromised people, such as organ transplant recipients, HIV-infected subjects, people using immunosuppressant medications, and those with lymphoproliferative disorders or other malignancies. In this group, a younger age and higher mortality are observed. This emphasizes the crucial role of the efficient immune surveillance [103]. On the other hand, chronic inflammatory disorders such as rheumatoid arthritis are also associated with higher incidence of MCC [104].

57.2.5.2 Histopathology

Even though MCCs share some morphologic and histologic features with normal Merkel cells (MCs), emerging data suggest that MCs are not the cells of origin.

One of the most accredited hypotheses affirm that MCC could originate from an immature totipotential stem cell with neuroendocrine features acquired during malignant transformation [105]. Other fascinating hypothesis sees the pre-pro B cell or fibroblasts as the origin cell.

The pre-pro B-cell origin is based on the expression of some elements that are normally restricted to early B cells, like Paired Box 5 (PAX-5), Terminal deoxynucleotidyl Transferase (TdT), and immunoglobulins rearrangement, and are expressed in MCCs [106]. Finally, the discovery that human dermal fibroblasts support productive MCPyV infection has generated the hypothesis that fibroblast could be the origin cell [107].

Even if no clinically significant differences have been described, we recognize three histologic form of MCC:

- Trabecular, rare, and less aggressive
- Intermediate, more common, and with a high number of mitotic figures
- Small cell MCC, indistinguishable from small cell carcinoma of other origin (e.g., lung)

The histopathologic differential includes basal cell carcinoma, melanoma, Ewing sarcoma, neuroblastoma, leukemia cutis, and poorly differentiated carcinoma (e.g., metastatic small cell lung cancer).

The definitive diagnosis of MCC is based on immunohistochemistry: MCC is positive for EMA, CK20 with a distinctive pattern, neurofilament, and neuroendocrine markers including synaptophysin and chromogranin.

Several histological parameters can be used as independent prognostic factors: first of all, the tumor thickness that reflects the deep invasion of MCCs is measured from the granular layer to the deepest extent of the tumor. This data is associated with decreased survival, like higher mast cell counts, and vascular density in the tumor and surrounding stroma. Infiltrative tumor growth pattern ($p = 0.001$) and lymphovascular invasion ($p = 0.007$) are also features associated with more aggressive tumor behavior. Moreover, nodular growth pattern, shallow invasion, and the absence of lymphovascular invasion are associated with longer survival [108].

Also, immunohistochemical features such as p53 and p63 immunopositivity have been shown to negatively predict survival, with p63 expression showing the greatest prognostic value [109].

Finally, several small studies since 2010 have shown that MCV-positive MCC confers a better prognosis than its MCV-negative counterpart [110].

57.2.5.3 Clinical Presentation

Clinically, MCC usually presents as an asymptomatic erythematous or violaceous nodule.

The surface can be ulcerated or crusted (especially among "old" lesions, ◘ Fig. 57.3), lucid or opaque, and dome-shaped with multiple peripheral telangiectasia.

To better summarize the clinical presentation of MCC, in 2007 Heath et al. [101] analyzed 106 patients and identified some clinical characteristics which appeared more frequent. On the basis of this observation, it has been created an acronym (AEIOU) that resumes the most significative characters. As we said, MCC often presents as follows:

(A) Asymptomatic nodule with a rapid
(E) Evolution; more frequently affects
(I) Immunosuppressed patients
(O) Older people over 70 years old and strongly exposed to
(U) UV radiation

At presentation, 65% of patients have skin-limited disease, 26% have nodal involvement, and 8% have distant metastases [111]. The most common sites of metastases are regional nodal basins (inguinal, axillary, or head and neck nodes), distant skin, lung, bone, and brain.

Spontaneous regression of the primary has occasionally been seen on re-excision specimens with a dense lymphocytic infiltrate of T cells around the site of the prior biopsy [112]. Metastatic MCC with no known primary has also been reported and represents 4% of all MCC cases.

57.2.5.4 Staging

Once the diagnosis of MCC has been established on clinical and histopathologic grounds, appropriate staging should be performed.

First of all, sentinel lymph node biopsy (SLNB) is recommended for all MCC patients because approximately one-third of patients without clinical nodal involvement have microscopic involvement detected by SLNB [97].

The impact of SLNB on survival has been mixed in the literature: patients with a negative SLNB had about 85% 5-year MCC-specific survival rate compared with about 55% of patients with positive nodes [113].

57.2.5.5 Treatment

The rarity of MCC has made clinical studies of treatment difficult to perform. The absence of univocal information generated a lack of consensus around the most effective treatment algorithm.

The treatment depends on the stage of the disease, the tumor site, and any comorbid conditions.

57.2.5.6 Local Disease

Complete surgical excision of the primary site with 1–2 cm negative margins with sentinel lymph node biopsy is the first step in treating localized MCC [114]. The rate of local recurrence ranges from 25% to 40% [115–118]. Retrospective studies showed that also Mohs micrographic surgery could be an effective surgical option, even if prospective clinical trials comparing MMS to wide local excision have not been performed [117, 119–121].

Radiation monotherapy could be an alternative to surgery for patients who are poor surgical candidates or for those in whom surgery would result in significant functional compromise [122, 123]. However, the outcomes of radiation monotherapy may be inferior compared to complete surgical resection. Higher doses of radiation are typically recommended for radiation monotherapy as compared to doses used for adjuvant therapy. The NCCN guidelines recommend doses of 60 to 66 Gy for curative-intent radiation, with a wide treatment margin (5 cm) around the primary site [114].

In patients with *negative SLNBs* (stage II), if the primary tumor is less than 1 cm, widely excised with negative resection margins, and contains no high-risk features (lymphovascular invasion, location on the head and neck, immunosuppression), data suggest that no adjuvant therapy is needed [114]. On the other hand, patients with high-risk tumors should undergo 50 Gy to 66 Gy of adjuvant radiation to the primary site [122, 124]. Data from a retrospective analysis of 6908 cases from the National Cancer Database demonstrate that a combination between adjuvant radiation and surgery could reduce local recurrence and improve survival compared to surgery alone [125, 126].

Patients with *positive SLNBs* (stage III) should be discussed in a multidisciplinary tumor board because optimal management has not been established. Standard treatment options include CLND, definitive nodal radiation, or a combination of the two. Actually, most studies have not sufficient power to draw meaningful conclusions. In this landscape, two independent studies found no difference in regional recurrence or overall survival between groups treated with CLND, definitive radiation, or combination therapy [127]. However, NCCN recommends adjuvant radiation to the draining nodal basin after CLND in the presence of multiple involved nodes or extracapsular extension of tumor [114].

57.2.5.7 Advanced Disease

Patients with distant metastatic disease should be referred expediently to a multidisciplinary tumor board. They may benefit from a combination of surgical excision for local debulking, radiation for palliation of symptoms or nodal disease, and/or systemic therapy, often through clinical trials.

Chemotherapy regimens were based on small cell lung cancer protocols, due to the similar neuroendocrine properties to MCC. The most common regimens are carboplatin (or cisplatin) and etoposide or a combination of cyclophosphamide, doxorubicin (or epirubicin), and vincristine. All these chemotherapic regimens are associated with considerable toxicity, especially in patients older than 65, and can worse immunosuppression.

MCC is chemosensitive, with initial response rates that range from 53% to 76%, but these responses tend not to be durable, with a usually short median progression-free survival (3–8 months) and progressive disease developing in 90% of patients at 10 months [128–130]. The few real-world, retrospective studies which assessed second-line or later chemotherapy showed low objective response rates (ORRs; from 8.8 to 23.0% with no complete responses) and very limited durability (1.3–3.3 months) [131].

57.2.5.8 Immune Checkpoint Inhibitors

Nowadays, considerable evidence suggests that immunosuppression contributes significantly to develop of MCC, and this consideration implies that therapeutic agents might be beneficial in this neoplasm.

Advancements in immunotherapy have greatly extended survival for patients with metastatic disease, particularly with the use of checkpoint immunotherapy involving the PD-1 (programmed death) and PD-L1 (programmed death-ligand) pathways. Both avelumab (MSB0010718C; anti-PD-L1) and pembrolizumab (anti-PD-1) have shown great results in clinical trials performed on patients with metastatic MCC. Results of these trials led to the addition of ICIs in the most recent update of the National Comprehensive Cancer Network (NCCN) Clinical Practice guidelines as a treatment option for stages III–IV MCC, and these agents are now the standard, first-line agents for metastatic MCC [114].

Avelumab, a monoclonal antibody that specifically inhibits PD-L1, is the first systemic immunotherapy for use in metastatic MCC. In the international multicenter phase II JAVELIN Merkel 200 trial, 88 patients with stage IV chemotherapy refractory MCC were treated in a single arm with avelumab 10 mg/kg every 2 weeks until confirmed disease progression or unacceptable toxicity [132]. After 1 year of follow-up, avelumab demonstrated an overall response rate (primary endpoint) of 33% with 11.4% of complete response rate and a disease control rate of 43.2%. 1-year progression-free survival (PFS) rate was 29%, and an overall survival (OS) was 52% [133]. Updated analysis, published during ASCO 2018, showed 2-year PFS rate of 26% and 2-year OS of 36%. This trial gave a lot of information regarding also the great safety profile of avelumab, with just 9.1% grade 3 adverse events and 4.5% grade 3 immunorelated adverse events, no grade 4 adverse events, or treatment-related deaths. The most common adverse events were fatigue (24%), infusion-related reactions (IRRs) (17%), diarrhea, and nausea (9% each). However, five patients developed serious adverse events leading to permanent discontinuation: elevated aminotransferases, enterocolitis, IRRs, chondrocalcinosis, synovitis, and interstitial nephritis. Based on these results and on the safety profile, the FDA accelerated approval to avelumab for the treatment of patients with metastatic MCC, in the first- and second-line settings.

Data from an interim analysis of avelumab as first-line treatment in patients with metastatic MCC have been recently published [134]. First-line avelumab treatment was associated with early and durable responses and a manageable safety profile.

Pembrolizumab, an anti-PD-1 monoclonal antibody, has been tested in a multicenter, phase II non-controlled study of 25 systemic therapy-naive patients. Preliminary results of this study, after 33 weeks of median follow-up, showed 6-month PFS of 67% and median PFS of 9 months [135].

Updated results after a median follow-up of 6.8 months, published during ASCO 2018, demonstrated a median PFS of 16.8 months and an 18-month OS of 68%. The disease control rate was 66% with an ORR of 56% and 24% of complete response. Among 21 confirmed responders, median response duration was not reached (range 3.9–25.6 months). The safety analysis confirmed the good safety profile of pembrolizumab with a rate of grade 3–4 adverse events of 30%.

The largest study of *nivolumab* to date consisted of a single-arm, open-label trial with nivolumab 240 mg every 2 weeks, for 25 systemic therapy-naive and previously treated patients [136]. After a median follow-up of 26 weeks, 22 patients responded, with a higher percentage occurring in treatment-naive patients and a PFS of 82%. ORR was 73% among treatment-naive population and 50% in pretreated population. Survival analysis showed a 3-month OS of 92%. Regarding safety, the rate of grade 3–4 adverse events was 24%.

In all these studies, response was seen in both virus-positive and virus-negative tumors, although studies have suggested that PD-L1 expression is higher on virus positive tumors [137].

Other immune checkpoint inhibitors investigated by clinical trials are ipilimumab, atezolizumab, durvalumab, tremelimumab, and daratumumab.

Finally, combinations of immunotherapeutic options are being evaluated: a lot of attention has been generated around *talimogene laherparepvec* (TVEC), a genetically altered herpes simplex type I virus that selectively replicates in tumor cells and express human granulocyte-macrophage colony-stimulating factor, which activates dendritic cells to present tumor antigens and encourage an innate cell-mediated host response. There have been a few reported cases regarding the success of TVEC in treating advanced locoregional MCC in elderly patients who were not good surgical or chemotherapy candidates [138]. Primary nodules regressed and did not recur for 7 months to 11 months after the last dose. A multicenter phase II trial is under way to further investigate its success in treating MCC and other cutaneous tumors.

57.2.5.9 Target Therapies

Finally, targeted therapies remain an area of research for MCCs dominated by specific mutations. Several different pathways have been identified as potential targets of therapy. One case of complete response to idelalisib in a PI3K/AKT-mutated MCC and one in a stage IV MCC patient has been reported since now [139]. MLN0128 is a target of the mTOR pathway currently in phase II trial for advanced MCC. Pazopanib was reported to induce partial remission in a case report [140].

57.2.6 Dermatofibrosarcoma Protuberans

DFSP is a rare (incidence: 3 per million) soft tissue sarcoma of histiocytic origins [141] and arising from the dermis, with a locally aggressive potential to deeper soft tissues. DFSP represents 1% of all sarcomas, and it principally affects young subjects in their mid-30s. Blacks have slightly higher incidence than whites; men and women are equally affected [142].

57.2.6.1 Histopathology

Histologically, DFSP is composed of monomorphous, dense, spindle cells, arranged in a storiform pattern that takes over the dermis. This tumor is characterized by tentacle-like projections, and often, no defined border can be recognized between the tumor and normal tissue. This may be the reason why the incidence of local recurrence is so high.

A pigmented variant of DFSP – also known as Bednar tumor – presents melanin-containing dendritic cells. The juvenile form – called giant cell fibroblastoma – is characterized by loose hypocellular areas that resemble mature DFSP.

Immunohistochemistry helps to differentiate DFSP from dermatofibroma (DF) through the exclusive expression of the human progenitor cell antigen CD34 in DFSP.

More than 90% of DFSP bear a particular translocation between chromosomes 17 and 22, provoking the fusion of the collagen type I-alfa1 gene (COL1A1) to the platelet-derived growth factor (PDGF) beta-chain gene (PDGFB). This fusion results in the deletion of exon 1 of PDGFB, leading to the constitutive activation of PDGF receptor (PDGFR) protein tyrosine kinase, providing signals for the cells to proliferate.

57.2.6.2 Clinical Presentation

DFSP is a slow-growing tumor (most commonly occurring on the trunk and proximal extremities), starting as a small asymptomatic firm, indurated papule, or patch, and it may gradually evolve into a nodule or a sclerotic plaque; ulceration may be present in case of accelerated growth.

Possible differential diagnoses may include cutaneous melanoma, dermatofibroma, keloid, and morphea.

57.2.6.3 Treatment

Surgery Wide excision without elective lymph node dissection is the standard of care for DFSP. A study suggested a 5 cm margin of excision in order to prevent local recurrences, as the likelihood of local recurrence is directly proportional to the adequacy of surgical margins [143].

Radiation therapy is an alternative treatment option to surgery, as this can lead the neoplasm to have a more aggressive behavior. RT is used, in particular, if surgical resection was not possible, or would result in major cosmetic or functional loss, with good local response. In addition, RT may be recommended in case of positivity of the margins of resection or in an adjuvant setting.

The complete RT dose ranges from 50 to 70 Gy [144].

A medical treatment option in case of advanced or metastatic disease may include *imatinib mesylate*, a BCR/ABL (the fusion product responsible of chronic myelogenous leukemia), and a specific tyrosine kinase (including c-kit and PDGF receptors) inhibitor. Imatinib has been used in DFSP based on the central role of the constitutively activated PDGFB-PDGFBR signaling pathway in the proliferation of DFSP cells, showing a clinical success.

In 2006, the US Food and Drug Administration approved imatinib mesylate for treatment of unresectable, recurrent, and/or metastatic DFSP. Note that a small group of DFSP patients lacking the t (17;22) translocation have no response to imatinib.

Recent studies showed a decreased tumor load using imatinib in a neoadjuvant setting.

Conventional chemotherapy is rarely used to treat DFSP [145, 146].

57.2.7 Kaposi Sarcoma

Kaposi sarcoma (KS) was described first in 1872 by the Hungarian dermatologist Moritz Kaposi. KS is a spindle-cell tumor deriving from endothelial cell lineage. KS can be categorized into four types:

1. *Epidemic.* The epidemic type is the most commonly observed in the USA. This form tends to have an aggressive behavior, and it is considered to be typically AIDS related. Positivity to human herpesvirus 8 (HHV-8) has been associated to this form, and the infection can predate the epidemic KS by about 10 years [147].
2. *Iatrogenic.* Principally related to immunosuppressive treatments, especially in transplant patients [148]. The observed time to development of KS following transplantation ranges 15–30 months. In these cases, the disease shows an aggressive behavior with visceral involvement, but withdrawal of immunosuppression may cause regression of the disease [149].
3. *Classic, sporadic.* This form, typical of the Mediterranean and Eastern European elderly men, has a more indolent course, with rare lymph nodes or visceral involvement. Its development may be due to aging immune dysregulation (subsequent immune suppression and reactivation), history of other neoplasm, and possible concomitant infections, as malaria. Cigarette smoking has been noted to have a protective effect [150].
4. *Endemic, African.* This entity occurs in African HIV-seronegative people. It represents the first form of cancer observed in men in the African countries of Malawi, Swaziland, Uganda, Zambia, and Zimbabwe (9% of all cancers in Ugandan males) and the second cancer in women. The high prevalence of shoeless people in these areas has been associated with an increase of endemic KS, possibly related to chronic lymphatic obstruction in the lower limbs from fine soil particles. The endemic form has a more common lymph node involvement than the classic variant [151].

The involvement of HHV-8 (identified by polymerase chain reaction in more than 90% of all subtypes of KS

lesion), HIV infection, immunologic dysregulation, and environmental factors requires further investigation to understand the complex pathogenesis of KS.

KS cutaneous lesions are typically brown-violaceous nodules and typically concentrated on the lower extremities and the head and neck. KS nodules may be single or symmetrically distributed, following Langer lines.

Mucous membrane involvement is not uncommon (oral cavity, conjunctiva). The bulky tumor mass may interfere with speech or mastication.

57.2.7.1 Treatment

Epidemic KS In the AIDS-associated form, the treatment of choice is always centered on the highly active antiretroviral therapy (HAART). In some high-risk patients, a combination of HAART and chemotherapy is still needed. However, no data are still available to show that treatment improves overall survival [152].

Classic KS In this indolent form, surgical excision may be enough especially for patients with small lesions. However, local recurrence is very common.

Local treatment by RT may be effective in a palliative setting, against bleeding and pain.

Other topical treatment options include intralesional therapy with vinca alkaloids, cryotherapy, laser therapy, and topical retinoids [153].

In case of visceral involvement, symptomatic disease, or rapidly progressive mucocutaneous disease, chemotherapy can be used with a palliative intent. The chemotherapy protocol of choice is doxorubicin, bleomycin, and vincristine (ABV). Single drug (in liposomal preparation) regimens have also been approved in AIDS-related KS [152].

A recent study with imatinib mesylate has shown response in 4 of 5 patients [154]. In another small trial of nine patients with AIDS-related KS, immune-checkpoint inhibition with nivolumab or pembrolizumab leads to partial responses in six patients and complete response in one patient, with a low toxicity profile [155].

Finally, study of the complex multiple pathways of pathogenesis may lead to develop inhibitors of the principal tumor growth-stimulating factors. Recent ongoing studies are now involving the VEGF, the basic fibroblast growth factor (bFGF) pathways, as the matrix metalloproteinases and oligonucleotides, showing good preliminary results [156].

Topical Treatment Insights

The general approach to management of skin cancer depends on the biologic aggressiveness of the tumor. Surgical options are generally considered the gold standard treatment, including excision and Mohs surgery. In case of superficial tumors or precancerous lesions, many other options can include curettage, cautery/electrodessication, cryosurgery, photodynamic therapy (PDT), and laser surgery, with limited efficacy. Other options are topical therapy (such as imiquimod, diclofenac, or 5-fluorouracil) and radiation therapy (RT).

Imiquimod

Imiquimod is an imidazoquinoline-binding toll-like receptors (TLR) 7 and 8 acting as an immunomodulator. This effect promotes tumor regression by the cell-mediated immune response (CD4 T-helper 1 and CD8-T cytotoxic lymphocytes) through the upregulation of interferon (IFN)-α, IFN-γ, and proinflammatory interleukins (IL)-8, 6, 12, by the innate immunity cells.

Imiquimod has been approved by the US Food and Drug Administration (FDA) for treatment of low-risk skin cancers, such as actinic keratosis (AK) and superficial basocellular carcinoma (BCC). Variable results were obtained in case of nodular BCC, in situ squamous cell carcinoma (SCC), or melanoma in situ.

Imiquimod 5% cream should be administered for 6–12 weeks, and it may show several adverse events including application site reactions, but also systemic flu-like syndromes [157, 158].

5-Fluorouracil

5-FU is a chemotherapeutic agent that inhibits the DNA synthesis, blocking the thymidylate synthetase. It is approved by the FDA for AKs and superficial BCC [159]. The main adverse event is application site reaction.

Diclofenac

Diclofenac is a nonsteroidal anti-inflammatory agent, characterized by a high affinity for cyclo-oxygenase-2 (COX-2), a prostaglandin-producing enzyme, frequently elevated in AK, NMSC, and melanoma, involved in the UV-induced skin damage [160]. Diclofenac inhibits the prostaglandin-mediated UV-induced mutagenic effect also by the reduction of proinflammatory cytokines such as IL-1 and TNF-α [161].

Photodynamic Therapy

PDT is effective in the treatment of certain NMSCs. 5-aminolevulinic acid (ALA) and methyl-aminolevulinic acid (MAL), when topically applicated, accumulate in malignant and premalignant cells and metabolized to protoporphyrin IX, a photoactive agent, generating reactive oxygen species when exposed to a specific wavelength of light (from 400 nm to infrared). This leads to irreversible damage and cancerous cell death [162].

PDT is currently approved by the FDA for AKs, but many off-label uses in other dermatologic conditions are currently under investigation [49].

Postprocedural scarring are depigmentation are rare adverse events [162].

Radiation Therapy

RT is a treatment option in many NMSCs, such as Merkel cell carcinoma, cutaneous lymphomas, BCC, and cutaneous SCC, especially when surgery is precluded due to poor patients' performance status, or in case of unresectable tumors.

Another important indication of RT is in the adjuvant setting, in case of the following:

- Positive surgical margins
- Perineural invasion
- Locoregional nodal metastasis

RT can be delivered as electrons or superficially penetrating photons (X-rays) [163, 164].

Postprocedural adverse events may be acute and chronic radiation dermatitis or necrosis, epidermal atrophy, telangiectasias, altered pigmentation, alopecia, and secondary NMSCs [165].

Expert Opinion

Paola Queirolo

Key Points

1. Nonmelanoma skin cancer are heterogeneous group of neoplasms which affect primarily the skin. They can have a different biological behavior and risk factors. Most frequently, they are associated to sun exposure, prior skin neoplasm, previous treatments, and genetic conditions.

2. Actinic keratosis (AK) are cutaneous precancerous lesions as a result of sun exposure, and they can evolve into in situ or invasive SCC. Usually they appear as reddish-pink hyperkeratotic surface on a sun-exposed area. Treatment can consist in photodynamic therapy, cryotherapy, and the use of 5-FU or imiquimod. Obviously, it is recommended to avoid further sun exposure.

3. Basal cell carcinoma is the most common human cancer, and it is characterized by a locally invasive

behavior. It is associated to some genetic syndromes such as the nevoid BCC (Gorlin syndrome) or to the Bazex syndrome. It usually appears as a well-defined erythematous-pink macule, quite difficult to differentiate from AK. There are different subtypes such as superficial, infiltrative, nodular (the most frequent), morpheaform, fibroepithelioma of Pinkus, and the pigmented one. Treatment is based on radical surgery excision, imiquimod, 5-FU, and PDT. In case of inoperable or metastatic cancers, a new drug is represented by vismodegib, approved in 2012 by FDA *and sonidegib.*

4. Cutaneous squamous cell carcinoma (cSCC) arises from epidermal keratinizing cells. The most important risk factors are sun exposure, age, immunosuppression, HPV chronic infection, and male sex. Prognosis of cSCC is excellent, but sometimes a metastatic diffusion of this neoplasm is possible. Thanks to dermal invasion, it is possible to differentiate an in situ cSCC from an invasive one, which can be divided according to the risk of recurrence and metastases in three categories: low (<3%), intermediate (3–10%), and high risk (>10%). As the cSCC includes different subtypes of varying malignant potential, the pathology should report the following: histologic subtype, degree of differentiation, depth of invasion, perineural invasion, and hematolymphatic invasion. Treatment is based on surgical excision, cautery or electrodesiccation, radiation therapy, electrochemotherapy, and chemotherapy in case of metastatic disease (platinum-based regimens, cetuximab, cemiplimab).

5. Merkel cell carcinoma is a rare neuroendocrine cancer of the skin. Its incidence has increased in the last years, probably for a better knowledge of this neoplasm. It is associated to advanced age, previous UV exposure, immunodeficiency, and Merkel cell polyomavirus (MCPyV). Clinical presentation consists in cutaneous erythematous or violaceous nodules with possible ulcerations. Metastases can occur, most frequently in locoregional lymph nodes; distant sites are bone, distant skin, lung, and brain. After the excisional surgery, when possible, adjuvant radiotherapy (RT), complete local nodal dissection or both are recommended in case of positive sentinel lymph-node biopsy or in high-risk patients (in this setting just RT can be sufficient). In advanced stages, platinum agents and etoposide chemotherapy were the main treatment options before the use of avelumab, a PD-L1 inhibitor, which has shown successful results in controlling neoplastic proliferation. New drugs under investigation are other immunotherapy drugs and some targeted therapies (idelasib and pazopanib).

6. Dermatofibrosarcoma protuberans is a soft tissue sarcoma arising from histiocytic cells. It tends to recur locally, and the treatment is a surgical excision with almost 5 cm of margin. In case of positivity of the margins or when surgery is not practicable, RT is recommended. For unresectable, recurrent or metastatic disease, imatinib is a possible treatment.

7. Kaposi sarcoma is characterized by brown-violaceous nodules typically localized in lower extremities. There are four types with a different population distribution: epidemic (HIV-correlated), iatrogenic (caused by iatrogenic immunodeficiency as in case of organ transplants), sporadic (in elderly men of Mediterranean and Eastern European areas), and endemic (in African regions). Classic form can be surgically treated; radiotherapy can have an effective palliative intent and other possible topic approaches are cryotherapy, intralesional therapy with vinca alkaloids, or laser therapy. In case of visceral involvement, symptomatic disease or rapidly progressive mucocutaneous disease, chemotherapy with doxorubicin, bleomycin, and vincristine is recommended. Targeted therapies and immunotherapy are under study, and some trials are on-going.

Recommendations

— American Academy of Dermatology
— ► https://www.aad.org/news/guidelines-to-treat-nonmelanoma-skin-cancer

Hints for a Deeper Insight

— Understanding the Molecular Genetics of Basal Cell Carcinoma: ► https://www.ncbi.nlm.nih.gov/pubmed/29165358
— Patient-centered management of actinic keratosis. Results of a multi-center clinical consensus analyzing non-melanoma skin cancer patient profiles and field-treatment strategies: ► https://www.ncbi.nlm.nih.gov/pubmed/31625770
— Kaposi sarcoma herpesvirus pathogenesis: ► https://www.ncbi.nlm.nih.gov/pubmed/28893942
— Efficacy and Safety of First-line Avelumab Treatment in Patients With Stage IV Metastatic Merkel Cell Carcinoma: A Preplanned Interim Analysis of a Clinical Trial: ► https://www.ncbi.nlm.nih.gov/pubmed/29566106

References

Cutaneous Melanoma

1. https://www.cancer.org/cancer/melanoma-skin-cancer/about/key-statistics.html#references. On March 30, 2019.
2. Hodi FS, et al. Improved survival with ipilimumab in patients with metastatic melanoma. N Engl J Med. 2010;363:711–23.
3. Robert C, et al. Ipilimumab plus dacarbazine for previously untreated metastatic melanoma. N Engl J Med. 2011;364:2517–26.
4. Larkin J, et al. Combined vemurafenib and cobimetinib in BRAF-mutated melanoma. N Engl J Med. 2014;371:1867–76.
5. Robert C, et al. Improved overall survival in melanoma with combined dabrafenib and trametinib. N Engl J Med. 2015a;372:30–9.
6. https://gis.cdc.gov/Cancer/USCS/DataViz.html. On March 30, 2019. Off. Fed. Stat. Cancer Incid. Deaths Prod. Cent. Dis. Control Prev. CDC Natl. Cancer Inst. NCI, 2019.
7. Gandini S, et al. Meta-analysis of risk factors for cutaneous melanoma: III. Family history, actinic damage and phenotypic factors. Eur J Cancer Oxf Engl 1990. 2005a;41:2040–59.
8. Gandini S, et al. Meta-analysis of risk factors for cutaneous melanoma: II. Sun exposure. Eur J Cancer Oxf Engl 1990. 2005b;41:45–60.
9. Kumar V, Abbas AK, Fausto N, Aster JC. Robbins & Cotran pathologic basis of disease. 8th ed: Elsevier: Amsterdam, Netherlands; 2010.
10. Bartsch D, et al. Clinical and genetic analysis of 18 pancreatic carcinoma/melanoma-prone families. Clin Genet. 2010;77:333–41.
11. Yokoyama S, et al. A novel recurrent mutation in MITF predisposes to familial and sporadic melanoma. Nature. 2011;480:99–103.
12. DeVita VT, Lawrence TS, Rosenberg SA. Cancer principles & practice of oncology: Lippincott Williams & Wilkins: Philadelphia, Pennsylvania, United States of America; 2016.
13. Gershenwald JE, et al. Melanoma staging: Evidence-based changes in the American Joint Committee on Cancer eighth edition cancer staging manual: Melanoma Staging: AJCC 8 th$ Edition. CA Cancer J Clin. 2017;67:472–92.
14. Sladden MJ, et al. Surgical excision margins for primary cutaneous melanoma. Cochrane Database Syst Rev. 2009:CD004835. https://doi.org/10.1002/14651858.CD004835.pub2.
15. van Akkooi ACJ, et al. Sentinel Node Tumor Burden According to the Rotterdam Criteria Is the Most Important Prognostic Factor for Survival in Melanoma Patients: A Multicenter Study in 388 Patients With Positive Sentinel Nodes. Ann Surg. 2008;248:949–55.
16. Faries MB, et al. Completion Dissection or Observation for Sentinel-Node Metastasis in Melanoma. N Engl J Med. 2017;376:2211–22.
17. Ives NJ, et al. Adjuvant interferon-α for the treatment of high-risk melanoma: An individual patient data meta-analysis. Eur J Cancer. 2017;82:171–83.
18. Eggermont AMM, et al. Adjuvant ipilimumab versus placebo after complete resection of high-risk stage III melanoma (EORTC 18071): a randomised, double-blind, phase 3 trial. Lancet Oncol. 2015;16:522–30.
19. Weber J, et al. Adjuvant Nivolumab versus Ipilimumab in Resected Stage III or IV Melanoma. N Engl J Med. 2017;377:1824–35.
20. al E e. Adjuvant Pembrolizumab in Resected Stage III Melanoma. N Engl J Med. 2018;379:593–5.
21. Long GV, et al. Adjuvant Dabrafenib plus Trametinib in Stage III BRAF -Mutated Melanoma. N Engl J Med. 2017a;377:1813–23.
22. Maio M, et al. Adjuvant vemurafenib in resected, BRAF V600 mutation-positive melanoma (BRIM8): a randomised, double-blind, placebo-controlled, multicentre, phase 3 trial. Lancet Oncol. 2018;19:510–20.
23. Ascierto PA, et al. The role of BRAF V600 mutation in melanoma. J Transl Med. 2012;10:85.
24. Ascierto PA, et al. Cobimetinib combined with vemurafenib in advanced BRAF(V600)-mutant melanoma (coBRIM): updated efficacy results from a randomised, double-blind, phase 3 trial. Lancet Oncol. 2016;17:1248–60.
25. Long GV, et al. Dabrafenib and trametinib versus dabrafenib and placebo for Val600 BRAF-mutant melanoma: a multicentre, double-blind, phase 3 randomised controlled trial. Lancet Lond Engl. 2015;386:444–51.
26. Dummer R, et al. Encorafenib plus binimetinib versus vemurafenib or encorafenib in patients with BRAF-mutant melanoma (COLUMBUS): a multicentre, open-label, randomised phase 3 trial. Lancet Oncol. 2018a;19:603–15.
27. Dummer R, et al. Overall survival in patients with BRAF-mutant melanoma receiving encorafenib plus binimetinib versus vemurafenib or encorafenib (COLUMBUS): a multicentre, open-label, randomised, phase 3 trial. Lancet Oncol. 2018b;19:1315–27.
28. Hodi FS, et al. Imatinib for melanomas harboring mutationally activated or amplified KIT arising on mucosal, acral, and chronically sun-damaged skin. J Clin Oncol Off J Am Soc Clin Oncol. 2013;31:3182–90.
29. Atkins MB, et al. High-dose recombinant interleukin 2 therapy for patients with metastatic melanoma: analysis of 270 patients treated between 1985 and 1993. J Clin Oncol Off J Am Soc Clin Oncol. 1999;17:2105–16.
30. Weber JS, et al. Nivolumab versus chemotherapy in patients with advanced melanoma who progressed after anti-CTLA-4 treatment (CheckMate 037): a randomised, controlled, open-label, phase 3 trial. Lancet Oncol. 2015;16:375–84.
31. Robert C, et al. Nivolumab in previously untreated melanoma without BRAF mutation. N Engl J Med. 2015b;372:320–30.
32. Robert C, et al. Pembrolizumab versus Ipilimumab in Advanced Melanoma. N Engl J Med. 2015c;372:2521–32.
33. Larkin J, et al. Combined Nivolumab and Ipilimumab or Monotherapy in Untreated Melanoma. N Engl J Med. 2015;373:23–34.
34. Long GV, et al. Standard-dose pembrolizumab in combination with reduced-dose ipilimumab for patients with advanced melanoma (KEYNOTE-029): an open-label, phase 1b trial. Lancet Oncol. 2017b;18:1202–10.
35. Ribas A, et al. Pembrolizumab versus investigator-choice chemotherapy for ipilimumab-refractory melanoma (KEYNOTE-002): a randomised, controlled, phase 2 trial. Lancet Oncol. 2015;16:908–18.
36. Haanen JB a G, et al. Management of toxicities from immunotherapy: ESMO Clinical Practice Guidelines for diagnosis, treatment and follow-up. Ann Oncol. 2017;28:iv119–42.
37. Stevens G, McKay MJ. Dispelling the myths surrounding radiotherapy for treatment of cutaneous melanoma. Lancet Oncol. 2006;7:575–83.
38. Ajithkumar T, Parkinson C, Fife K, Corrie P, Jefferies S. Evolving treatment options for melanoma brain metastases. Lancet Oncol. 2015;16:e486–97.
39. Peacock KH, Lesser GJ. Current therapeutic approaches in patients with brain metastases. Curr Treat Options Oncol. 2006;7:479–89.

40. Lutz S, et al. Palliative Radiotherapy for Bone Metastases: An ASTRO Evidence-Based Guideline. Int J Radiat Oncol. 2011;79:965–76.

41. Nielsen OS, Bentzen SM, Sandberg E, Gadeberg CC, Timothy AR. Randomized trial of single dose versus fractionated palliative radiotherapy of bone metastases. Radiother Oncol J Eur Soc Ther Radiol Oncol. 1998;47:233–40.

Nonmelanoma Skin Cancer

42. Stern RS. Prevalence of a history of skin cancer in 2007: results of an incidence-based model. Arch Dermatol. 2010;146:279–82.

43. Rogers HW, Weinstock MA, Harris AR, et al. Incidence estimate of nonmelanoma skin cancer in the United States, 2006. Arch Dermatol. 2010;146:283–7.

44. Madan V, Lear JT, Szeimies R-M. Non-melanoma skin cancer. Lancet Lond Engl. 2010;375:673–85.

45. Berman B, Amini S, Valins W, Block S. Pharmacotherapy of actinic keratosis. Expert Opin Pharmacother. 2009;10:3015–31.

46. Schwartz RA. The actinic keratosis. A perspective and update. Dermatol Surg. 1997;23:1009–19; quiz 1020–1.

47. Roewert-Huber J, Stockfleth E, Kerl H. Pathology and pathobiology of actinic (solar) keratosis - an update. Br J Dermatol. 2007;157(Suppl 2):18–20.

48. Thai K-E, Fergin P, Freeman M, et al. A prospective study of the use of cryosurgery for the treatment of actinic keratoses. Int J Dermatol. 2004;43:687–92.

49. Lehmann P. Methyl aminolaevulinate-photodynamic therapy: a review of clinical trials in the treatment of actinic keratoses and nonmelanoma skin cancer. Br J Dermatol. 2007;156:793–801.

50. Szeimies RM, Karrer S, Radakovic-Fijan S, et al. Photodynamic therapy using topical methyl 5-aminolevulinate compared with cryotherapy for actinic keratosis: a prospective, randomized study. J Am Acad Dermatol. 2002;47:258–62.

51. Pearlman DL. Weekly pulse dosing: effective and comfortable topical 5-fluorouracil treatment of multiple facial actinic keratoses. J Am Acad Dermatol. 1991;25:665–7.

52. Krawtchenko N, Roewert-Huber J, Ulrich M, Mann I, Sterry W, Stockfleth E. A randomised study of topical 5% imiquimod vs. topical 5-fluorouracil vs. cryosurgery in immunocompetent patients with actinic keratoses: a comparison of clinical and histological outcomes including 1-year follow-up. Br J Dermatol. 2007;157(Suppl 2):34–40.

53. Rivers JK, Arlette J, Shear N, Guenther L, Carey W, Poulin Y. Topical treatment of actinic keratoses with 3.0% diclofenac in 2.5% hyaluronan gel. Br J Dermatol. 2002;146:94–100.

54. Kyrgidis A, Vahtsevanos K, Tzellos TG, et al. Clinical, histological and demographic predictors for recurrence and second primary tumours of head and neck basal cell carcinoma. A 1062 patient-cohort study from a tertiary cancer referral hospital. Eur J Dermatol EJD. 2010;20:276–82.

55. Epstein EH. Basal cell carcinomas: attack of the hedgehog. Nat Rev Cancer. 2008;8:743–54.

56. Grossman D, Leffell DJ. The molecular basis of nonmelanoma skin cancer: new understanding. Arch Dermatol. 1997;133:1263–70.

57. Situm M, Buljan M, Bulat V, Lugović Mihić L, Bolanca Z, Simić D. The role of UV radiation in the development of basal cell carcinoma. Coll Antropol. 2008;32(Suppl 2):167–70.

58. Raasch BA, Buettner PG, Garbe C. Basal cell carcinoma: histological classification and body-site distribution. Br J Dermatol. 2006;155:401–7.

59. Saldanha G, Fletcher A, Slater DN. Basal cell carcinoma: a dermatopathological and molecular biological update. Br J Dermatol. 2003;148:195–202.

60. Ackerman AB, Gottlieb GJ. Fibroepithelial tumor of pinkus is trichoblastic (basal-cell) carcinoma. Am J Dermatopathol. 2005;27:155–9.

61. Wolf DJ, Zitelli JA. Surgical margins for basal cell carcinoma. Arch Dermatol. 1987;123:340–4.

62. Arits AHMM, Mosterd K, Essers BA, et al. Photodynamic therapy versus topical imiquimod versus topical fluorouracil for treatment of superficial basal-cell carcinoma: a single blind, non-inferiority, randomised controlled trial. Lancet Oncol. 2013;14:647–54.

63. Lupi O. Correlations between the Sonic Hedgehog pathway and basal cell carcinoma. Int J Dermatol. 2007;46:1113–7.

64. Ionescu DN, Arida M, Jukic DM. Metastatic basal cell carcinoma: four case reports, review of literature, and immunohistochemical evaluation. Arch Pathol Lab Med. 2006;130:45–51.

65. Jefford M, Kiffer JD, Somers G, Daniel FJ, Davis ID. Metastatic basal cell carcinoma: rapid symptomatic response to cisplatin and paclitaxel. ANZ J Surg. 2004;74:704–5.

66. Sekulic A, Migden MR, Basset-Seguin N, et al. Long-term safety and efficacy of vismodegib in patients with advanced basal cell carcinoma: final update of the pivotal ERIVANCE BCC study. BMC Cancer. 2017;17:332.

67. Von Hoff DD, LoRusso PM, Rudin CM, et al. Inhibition of the hedgehog pathway in advanced basal-cell carcinoma. N Engl J Med. 2009;361:1164–72.

68. Chen L, Aria AB, Silapunt S, Lee H-H, Migden MR. Treatment of advanced basal cell carcinoma with sonidegib: perspective from the 30-month update of the BOLT trial. Future Oncol. 2018;14:515–25.

69. Burness CB, Scott LJ. Sonidegib: a review in locally advanced basal cell carcinoma. Target Oncol. 2016;11:239–46.

70. Karia PS, Han J, Schmults CD. Cutaneous squamous cell carcinoma: estimated incidence of disease, nodal metastasis, and deaths from disease in the United States, 2012. J Am Acad Dermatol. 2013;68:957–66.

71. Staples MP, Elwood M, Burton RC, Williams JL, Marks R, Giles GG. Non-melanoma skin cancer in Australia: the 2002 national survey and trends since 1985. Med J Aust. 2006;184:6–10.

72. Osterlind A, Hjalgrim H, Kulinsky B, Frentz G. Skin cancer as a cause of death in Denmark. Br J Dermatol. 1991;125:580–2.

73. Mora RG, Perniciaro C. Cancer of the skin in blacks. I. A review of 163 black patients with cutaneous squamous cell carcinoma. J Am Acad Dermatol. 1981;5:535–43.

74. McGuire JF, Ge NN, Dyson S. Nonmelanoma skin cancer of the head and neck I: histopathology and clinical behavior. Am J Otolaryngol. 2009;30:121–33.

75. Wade TR, Ackerman AB. The many faces of squamous-cell carcinomas. J Dermatol Surg Oncol. 1978;4:291–4.

76. Cassarino DS, Derienzo DP, Barr RJ. Cutaneous squamous cell carcinoma: a comprehensive clinicopathologic classification. Part one. J Cutan Pathol. 2006a;33:191–206.

77. Cassarino DS, Derienzo DP, Barr RJ. Cutaneous squamous cell carcinoma: a comprehensive clinicopathologic classification-part two. J Cutan Pathol. 2006b;33:261–79.

78. Miller SJ. The National Comprehensive Cancer Network (NCCN) guidelines of care for nonmelanoma skin cancers. Dermatol Surg. 2000;26:289–92.

79. NCCN Clinical Practice Guidelines in Oncology - Squamous Cell Skin Cancer https://www.nccn.org/professionals/physician_gls/pdf/squamous.pdf. On April 1, 2019. NCCN.org.

80. Schmults CD, Karia PS, Carter JB, Han J, Qureshi AA. Factors predictive of recurrence and death from cutaneous squamous cell carcinoma: a 10-year, single-institution cohort study. JAMA Dermatol. 2013;149:541–7.

81. Rowe DE, Carroll RJ, Day CL. Prognostic factors for local recurrence, metastasis, and survival rates in squamous cell carcinoma of the skin, ear, and lip. Implications for treatment modality selection. J Am Acad Dermatol. 1992;26:976–90.

82. Breuninger H, Black B, Rassner G. Microstaging of squamous cell carcinomas. Am J Clin Pathol. 1990;94:624–7.

83. Brodland DG, Zitelli JA. Surgical margins for excision of primary cutaneous squamous cell carcinoma. J Am Acad Dermatol. 1992;27:241–8.

84. Honeycutt WM, Jansen GT. Treatment of squamous cell carcinoma of the skin. Arch Dermatol. 1973;108:670–2.

85. Jambusaria-Pahlajani A, Miller CJ, Quon H, Smith N, Klein RQ, Schmults CD. Surgical monotherapy versus surgery plus adjuvant radiotherapy in high-risk cutaneous squamous cell carcinoma: a systematic review of outcomes. Dermatol Surg. 2009;35:574–85.

86. Di Monta G, Caracò C, Simeone E, et al. Electrochemotherapy efficacy evaluation for treatment of locally advanced stage III cutaneous squamous cell carcinoma: a 22-cases retrospective analysis. J Transl Med. 2017;15:82.

87. Guthrie TH, Porubsky ES, Luxenberg MN, Shah KJ, Wurtz KL, Watson PR. Cisplatin-based chemotherapy in advanced basal and squamous cell carcinomas of the skin: results in 28 patients including 13 patients receiving multimodality therapy. J Clin Oncol. 1990;8:342–6.

88. Jarkowski A, Hare R, Loud P, et al. Systemic therapy in advanced Cutaneous Squamous Cell Carcinoma (CSCC): the Roswell Park experience and a review of the literature. Am J Clin Oncol. 2016;39:545–8.

89. Maubec E, Petrow P, Scheer-Senyarich I, et al. Phase II study of cetuximab as first-line single-drug therapy in patients with unresectable squamous cell carcinoma of the skin. J Clin Oncol. 2011;29:3419–26.

90. Wollina U. Cetuximab in non-melanoma skin cancer. Expert Opin Biol Ther. 2012;12:949–56.

91. Migden MR, Rischin D, Schmults CD, et al. PD-1 blockade with Cemiplimab in advanced cutaneous squamous-cell carcinoma. N Engl J Med. 2018;379:341–51.

92. Toker C. Trabecular carcinoma of the skin. Arch Dermatol. 1972;105:107–10.

93. Fitzgerald TL, Dennis S, Kachare SD, Vohra NA, Wong JH, Zervos EE. Dramatic increase in the incidence and mortality from Merkel cell carcinoma in the United States. Am Surg. 2015;81:802–6.

94. Youlden DR, Soyer HP, Youl PH, Fritschi L, Baade PD. Incidence and survival for Merkel cell carcinoma in Queensland, Australia, 1993-2010. JAMA Dermatol. 2014;150:864–72.

95. Paulson KG, Park SY, Vandeven NA, et al. Merkel cell carcinoma: current US incidence and projected increases based on changing demographics. J Am Acad Dermatol. 2018;78:457–463.e2.

96. Deneve JL, Messina JL, Marzban SS, et al. Merkel cell carcinoma of unknown primary origin. Ann Surg Oncol. 2012;19:2360–6.

97. Lemos BD, Storer BE, Iyer JG, et al. Pathologic nodal evaluation improves prognostic accuracy in Merkel cell carcinoma: analysis of 5823 cases as the basis of the first consensus staging system. J Am Acad Dermatol. 2010;63:751–61.

98. Hodgson NC. Merkel cell carcinoma: changing incidence trends. J Surg Oncol. 2005;89:1–4.

99. Prewett SL, Ajithkumar T. Merkel cell carcinoma: current management and controversies. Clin Oncol R Coll Radiol G B. 2015;27:436–44.

100. Feng H, Shuda M, Chang Y, Moore PS. Clonal integration of a polyomavirus in human Merkel cell carcinoma. Science. 2008;319:1096–100.

101. Heath M, Jaimes N, Lemos B, et al. Clinical characteristics of Merkel cell carcinoma at diagnosis in 195 patients: the AEIOU features. J Am Acad Dermatol. 2008;58:375–81.

102. Goh G, Walradt T, Markarov V, et al. Mutational landscape of MCPyV-positive and MCPyV-negative Merkel cell carcinomas with implications for immunotherapy. Oncotarget. 2016;7:3403–15.

103. Clarke CA, Robbins HA, Tatalovich Z, et al. Risk of merkel cell carcinoma after solid organ transplantation. J Natl Cancer Inst. 2015;107 https://doi.org/10.1093/jnci/dju382.

104. Sahi H, Sihto H, Artama M, Koljonen V, Böhling T, Pukkala E. History of chronic inflammatory disorders increases the risk of Merkel cell carcinoma, but does not correlate with Merkel cell polyomavirus infection. Br J Cancer. 2017;116:260–4.

105. Tilling T, Wladykowski E, Failla AV, Houdek P, Brandner JM, Moll I. Immunohistochemical analyses point to epidermal origin of human Merkel cells. Histochem Cell Biol. 2014;141:407–21.

106. Sauer CM, Chteinberg E, Rennspiess D, Kurz AK, Zur Hausen A. Merkel cell carcinoma: cutaneous manifestation of a highly malignant pre–/pro-B cell neoplasia? : Novel concept about the cellular origin of Merkel cell carcinoma. Hautarzt Z Dermatol Venerol Verwandte Geb. 2017;68:204–10.

107. Liu W, Yang R, Payne AS, et al. Identifying the target cells and mechanisms of Merkel cell polyomavirus infection. Cell Host Microbe. 2016;19:775–87.

108. Andea AA, Coit DG, Amin B, Busam KJ. Merkel cell carcinoma: histologic features and prognosis. Cancer. 2008;113:2549–58.

109. Husein-ElAhmed H, Ramos-Pleguezuelos F, Ruiz-Molina I, et al. Histological features, p53, c-kit, and Poliomavirus status and impact on survival in Merkel cell carcinoma patients. Am J Dermatopathol. 2016;38:571–9.

110. Sihto H, Kukko H, Koljonen V, Sankila R, Böhling T, Joensuu H. Clinical factors associated with Merkel cell polyomavirus infection in Merkel cell carcinoma. J Natl Cancer Inst. 2009;101:938–45.

111. Harms KL, Healy MA, Nghiem P, et al. Analysis of prognostic factors from 9387 Merkel cell carcinoma cases forms the basis for the new 8th edition AJCC staging system. Ann Surg Oncol. 2016;23:3564–71.

112. Vesely MJJ, Murray DJ, Neligan PC, Novak CB, Gullane PJ, Ghazarian D. Complete spontaneous regression in Merkel cell carcinoma. J Plast Reconstr Aesthetic Surg JPRAS. 2008;61:165–71.

113. Allen PJ, Bowne WB, Jaques DP, Brennan MF, Busam K, Coit DG. Merkel cell carcinoma: prognosis and treatment of patients from a single institution. J Clin Oncol. 2005;23:2300–9.

114. Bichakjian CK, Olencki T, Aasi SZ, et al. Merkel cell carcinoma, version 1.2018, NCCN clinical practice guidelines in oncology. J Natl Compr Cancer Netw JNCCN. 2018;16:742–74.

115. Ratner D, Nelson BR, Brown MD, Johnson TM. Merkel cell carcinoma. J Am Acad Dermatol. 1993;29:143–56.

116. Gollard R, Weber R, Kosty MP, Greenway HT, Massullo V, Humberson C. Merkel cell carcinoma: review of 22 cases with surgical, pathologic, and therapeutic considerations. Cancer. 2000;88:1842–51.

117. O'Connor WJ, Roenigk RK, Brodland DG. Merkel cell carcinoma. Comparison of Mohs micrographic surgery and wide excision in eighty-six patients. Dermatol Surg. 1997;23:929–33.

118. Haag ML, Glass LF, Fenske NA. Merkel cell carcinoma. Diagnosis and treatment. Dermatol Surg. 1995;21:669–83.

119. Snow SN, Larson PO, Hardy S, et al. Merkel cell carcinoma of the skin and mucosa: report of 12 cutaneous cases with 2 cases arising from the nasal mucosa. Dermatol Surg. 2001;27:165–70.

120. Boyer JD, Zitelli JA, Brodland DG, D'Angelo G. Local control of primary Merkel cell carcinoma: review of 45 cases treated

with Mohs micrographic surgery with and without adjuvant radiation. J Am Acad Dermatol. 2002;47:885–92.

121. Kline L, Coldiron B. Mohs micrographic surgery for the treatment of Merkel cell carcinoma. Dermatol Surg. 2016;42:945–51.

122. Harrington C, Kwan W. Radiotherapy and conservative surgery in the Locoregional Management of Merkel cell carcinoma: the British Columbia Cancer Agency experience. Ann Surg Oncol. 2016;23:573–8.

123. Veness M, Foote M, Gebski V, Poulsen M. The role of radiotherapy alone in patients with merkel cell carcinoma: reporting the Australian experience of 43 patients. Int J Radiat Oncol Biol Phys. 2010;78:703–9.

124. Miller NJ, Bhatia S, Parvathaneni U, Iyer JG, Nghiem P. Emerging and mechanism-based therapies for recurrent or metastatic Merkel cell carcinoma. Curr Treat Options in Oncol. 2013;14:249–63.

125. Bhatia S, Storer BE, Iyer JG, et al. Adjuvant radiation therapy and chemotherapy in Merkel cell carcinoma: survival analyses of 6908 cases from the National Cancer Data Base. J Natl Cancer Inst. 2016;108 https://doi.org/10.1093/jnci/djw042.

126. Hasan S, Liu L, Triplet J, Li Z, Mansur D. The role of postoperative radiation and chemoradiation in merkel cell carcinoma: a systematic review of the literature. Front Oncol. 2013;3:276.

127. Fields RC, Busam KJ, Chou JF, et al. Recurrence after complete resection and selective use of adjuvant therapy for stage I through III Merkel cell carcinoma. Cancer. 2012;118:3311–20.

128. Tai PT, Yu E, Winquist E, et al. Chemotherapy in neuroendocrine/Merkel cell carcinoma of the skin: case series and review of 204 cases. J Clin Oncol. 2000;18:2493–9.

129. Voog E, Biron P, Martin JP, Blay JY. Chemotherapy for patients with locally advanced or metastatic Merkel cell carcinoma. Cancer. 1999;85:2589–95.

130. Crown J, Lipzstein R, Cohen S, et al. Chemotherapy of metastatic Merkel cell cancer. Cancer Investig. 1991;9:129–32.

131. Iyer JG, Blom A, Doumani R, et al. Response rates and durability of chemotherapy among 62 patients with metastatic Merkel cell carcinoma. Cancer Med. 2016;5:2294–301.

132. Kaufman HL, Russell J, Hamid O, et al. Avelumab in patients with chemotherapy-refractory metastatic Merkel cell carcinoma: a multicentre, single-group, open-label, phase 2 trial. Lancet Oncol. 2016;17:1374–85.

133. Kaufman HL, Russell JS, Hamid O, et al. Updated efficacy of avelumab in patients with previously treated metastatic Merkel cell carcinoma after ≥1 year of follow-up: JAVELIN Merkel 200, a phase 2 clinical trial. J Immunother Cancer. 2018;6:7.

134. D'Angelo SP, Russell J, Lebbé C, et al. Efficacy and safety of first-line Avelumab treatment in patients with stage IV metastatic Merkel cell carcinoma: a preplanned interim analysis of a clinical trial. JAMA Oncol. 2018;4:e180077.

135. Nghiem PT, Bhatia S, Lipson EJ, et al. PD-1 blockade with Pembrolizumab in advanced Merkel-cell carcinoma. N Engl J Med. 2016;374:2542–52.

136. Topalian SL, Bhatia S, Hollebecque A, et al. Abstract CT074: non-comparative, open-label, multiple cohort, phase 1/2 study to evaluate nivolumab (NIVO) in patients with virus-associated tumors (CheckMate 358): efficacy and safety in Merkel cell carcinoma (MCC). Cancer Res. 2017;77:CT074.

137. Lipson EJ, Vincent JG, Loyo M, et al. PD-L1 expression in the Merkel cell carcinoma microenvironment: association with inflammation, Merkel cell polyomavirus and overall survival. Cancer Immunol Res. 2013;1:54–63.

138. Blackmon JT, Dhawan R, Viator TM, Terry NL, Conry RM. Talimogene laherparepvec for regionally advanced Merkel cell carcinoma: a report of 2 cases. JAAD Case Rep. 2017;3:185–9.

139. Nardi V, Song Y, Santamaria-Barria JA, et al. Activation of PI3K signaling in Merkel cell carcinoma. Clin Cancer Res. 2012;18:1227–36.

140. Davids MS, Davids M, Charlton A, et al. Response to a novel multitargeted tyrosine kinase inhibitor pazopanib in metastatic Merkel cell carcinoma. J Clin Oncol. 2009;27:e97–100.

141. Shindo Y, Akiyama J, Takase Y. Tissue culture study of dermatofibrosarcoma protuberans. J Dermatol. 1988;15:220–3.

142. Kampshoff JL, Cogbill TH. Unusual skin tumors: Merkel cell carcinoma, eccrine carcinoma, glomus tumors, and dermatofibrosarcoma protuberans. Surg Clin North Am. 2009;89:727–38.

143. D'Andrea F, Vozza A, Brongo S, Di Girolamo F, Vozza G. Dermatofibrosarcoma protuberans: experience with 14 cases. J Eur Acad Dermatol Venereol JEADV. 2001;15:427–9.

144. Sun LM, Wang CJ, Huang CC, et al. Dermatofibrosarcoma protuberans: treatment results of 35 cases. Radiother Oncol J Eur Soc Ther Radiol Oncol. 2000;57:175–81.

145. Scheinfeld N, Schienfeld N. A comprehensive review of imatinib mesylate (Gleevec) for dermatological diseases. J Drugs Dermatol JDD. 2006;5:117–22.

146. Sjöblom T, Shimizu A, O'Brien KP, et al. Growth inhibition of dermatofibrosarcoma protuberans tumors by the platelet-derived growth factor receptor antagonist STI571 through induction of apoptosis. Cancer Res. 2001;61:5778–83.

147. Jacobson LP, Jenkins FJ, Springer G, et al. Interaction of human immunodeficiency virus type 1 and human herpesvirus type 8 infections on the incidence of Kaposi's sarcoma. J Infect Dis. 2000;181:1940–9.

148. Penn I. Cancer in the immunosuppressed organ recipient. Transplant Proc. 1991;23:1771–2.

149. Sarid R, Olsen SJ, Moore PS. Kaposi's sarcoma-associated herpesvirus: epidemiology, virology, and molecular biology. Adv Virus Res. 1999;52:139–232.

150. Goedert JJ, Vitale F, Lauria C, et al. Risk factors for classical Kaposi's sarcoma. J Natl Cancer Inst. 2002;94:1712–8.

151. Ruocco E, Ruocco V, Tornesello ML, Gambardella A, Wolf R, Buonaguro FM. Kaposi's sarcoma: etiology and pathogenesis, inducing factors, causal associations, and treatments: facts and controversies. Clin Dermatol. 2013;31:413–22.

152. PDQ Adult Treatment Editorial Board. Kaposi sarcoma treatment (PDQ®): health professional version. In: PDQ cancer information summaries. Bethesda: National Cancer Institute (US); 2002. http://www.ncbi.nlm.nih.gov/books/NBK65897/. Accessed 3 Feb 2019.

153. Tsao MN, Sinclair E, Assaad D, Fialkov J, Antonyshyn O, Barnes E. Radiation therapy for the treatment of skin Kaposi sarcoma. Ann Palliat Med. 2016;5:298–302.

154. Koon HB, Bubley GJ, Pantanowitz L, et al. Imatinib-induced regression of AIDS-related Kaposi's sarcoma. J Clin Oncol. 2005;23:982–9.

155. Galanina N, Goodman AM, Cohen PR, Frampton GM, Kurzrock R. Successful treatment of HIV-associated Kaposi sarcoma with immune checkpoint blockade. Cancer Immunol Res. 2018;6:1129–35.

156. Cianfrocca M, Cooley TP, Lee JY, et al. Matrix metalloproteinase inhibitor COL-3 in the treatment of AIDS-related Kaposi's sarcoma: a phase I AIDS malignancy consortium study. J Clin Oncol. 2002;20:153–9.

157. Nouri K, O'Connell C, Rivas MP. Imiquimod for the treatment of Bowen's disease and invasive squamous cell carcinoma. J Drugs Dermatol JDD. 2003;2:669–73.

158. Junkins-Hopkins JM. Imiquimod use in the treatment of lentigo maligna. J Am Acad Dermatol. 2009;61:865–7.

159. Love WE, Bernhard JD, Bordeaux JS. Topical imiquimod or fluorouracil therapy for basal and squamous cell carcinoma: a systematic review. Arch Dermatol. 2009;145:1431–8.

160. Zhan H, Zheng H. The role of topical cyclo-oxygenase-2 inhibitors in skin cancer: treatment and prevention. Am J Clin Dermatol. 2007;8:195–200.

161. Iraji F, Siadat AH, Asilian A, Enshaieh S, Shahmoradi Z. The safety of diclofenac for the management and treatment of actinic keratoses. Expert Opin Drug Saf. 2008;7:167–72.

162. Tierney E, Barker A, Ahdout J, Hanke CW, Moy RL, Kouba DJ. Photodynamic therapy for the treatment of cutaneous neoplasia, inflammatory disorders, and photoaging. Dermatol Surg. 2009;35:725–46.

163. Wang Y, Wells W, Waldron J. Indications and outcomes of radiation therapy for skin cancer of the head and neck. Clin Plast Surg. 2009;36:335–44.

164. Halpern JN. Radiation therapy in skin cancer. A historical perspective and current applications. Dermatol Surg. 1997;23:1089–93.

165. Fitzgerald TJ, Jodoin MB, Tillman G, et al. Radiation therapy toxicity to the skin. Dermatol Clin. 2008;26:161–72, ix.

Soft Tissue Sarcomas (STS)

Giuseppe Badalamenti, Bruno Vincenzi, Massimiliano Cani, and Lorena Incorvaia

Soft Tissue Sarcoma, GIST and Neuroendocrine Neoplasms

Contents

© Springer Nature Switzerland AG 2021
A. Russo et al. (eds.), *Practical Medical Oncology Textbook*, UNIPA Springer Series,
https://doi.org/10.1007/978-3-030-56051-5_58

Learning Objectives

By the end of the chapter, the reader will:

- Have learned the basic concepts of epidemiology, histological subtype, and molecular profile of STS.
- Have reached in-depth knowledge of diagnosis, staging, and clinical management of STS.
- Be able to put acquired knowledge on STS into clinical practice

58.1   Introduction

Soft tissue sarcomas (STSs) represent a rare and heterogeneous group of solid tumors derived from mesenchymal progenitors and account for 1% of all adult malignancies [1]. Approximately 80% of sarcomas arise from soft tissue and viscera, whereas the remaining 20% originate from bone. STSs potentially may occur at all body anatomic sites, even though the majority arise from the extremities.

As classified by the World Health Organization (WHO), the group of STSs comprise more than 100 different histologies according to the presumptive tissue in origin [2]. Histological diagnosis is crucial in order to define staging and prognosis and to deliver appropriate therapy. Unfortunately, sometimes it causes a diagnostic challenge for pathologist, particularly when the diagnostic material is a small biopsy and when clinical information is incomplete. After the development of distant metastasis, the median overall survival (OS) is 12–19 months, and almost 20% of patients are still alive at 3 years [3].

58.1.1   Diagnosis and Pathology

There is agreement on the recommendation that the pathological diagnosis of STM should contain the following information:

- Macroscopic description
- Status of margins, so as to allow the attribution of surgical intervention to the categories "radical," "broad," "marginal," and "intralesional"
- Histotype according to WHO 2013

The malignancy grade is described by the classification of the French Federation of Cancer Centers:

- Grade 1: Low grade
- Grade 2: Intermediate grade
- Grade 3: High grade

The WHO 2013 classification of mesenchymal tumors distinguishes (1) benign lesion, (2) lesion with intermediate biological behavior, and (3) lesion with malignant biological behavior.

Intermediate lesions are defined as follows:

- Locally aggressive but not metastasizing tumors (e.g., aggressive fibromatosis)
- Tumors with a metastasis rate of less than 2% (e.g., plexiform fibrohistiocytic tumor)

58.1.2   Staging and Risk Assessment

Available staging classifications have limited relevance and should be improved. The Union for International Cancer Control (UICC) stage classification system, eighth edition, stresses the importance of the malignancy grade in sarcoma [4]. In general, in addition to grading, other prognostic factors are tumor size and tumor depth for limb sarcomas. Of course, site, tumor resectability, and the presence of metastases are also important. Nomograms are available, which can help personalize risk assessment and thus clinical decision-making, especially on adjuvant/neoadjuvant treatments [5, 6].

58.2   STS Management

58.2.1   Essential Elements Prior to the Initiation of Therapy

According to major national and international guidelines, the optimal therapeutic strategy of all soft tissue sarcomas (STS) patients should be discussed within multidisciplinary teams. Disease histology, stage, anatomical localization, and patient preferences are the most important elements for a correct decisional process [7, 9]. Notably, compliance to guidelines and relapse-free survival of sarcoma patients are significantly better when the initial treatment is guided by a pretherapeutic specialized multidisciplinary tumor board [10].

Adequate imaging of primary tumor, i.e., MRI with and without contrast +/− CT with contrast, is necessary to provide details about the size of the tumor and its contiguity to nearby visceral and neurovascular structures. A chest spiral CT scan without contrast is recommended in the US guidelines [1] and mandatory in the European ones [2]. In selected circumstances, other imaging studies might be required.

Histological diagnosis prior to therapy should be acquired whenever possible. Core needle biopsy or incisional biopsy usually provides sufficient tissue to perform a correct pathological and molecular diagnosis e must always be carried out in the case of lesions over 5 cm in diameter (□ Fig. 58.1).

The STS clinical presentation can be very different in relation to the place of origin. In the case of a limbs or trunk localization, the sarcoma is presented as a clini-

Fig. 58.1 The role of biopsy for all lesions greater than 5 cm. (Diagnosis: flow chart)

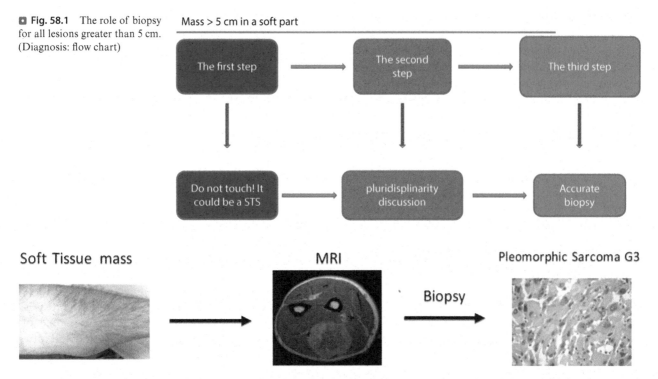

Fig. 58.2 Soft tissue mass of the forearm compatible with sarcoma; magnetic resonance imaging confirms the suspicion and the biopsy confirm pleomorphic sarcoma G3

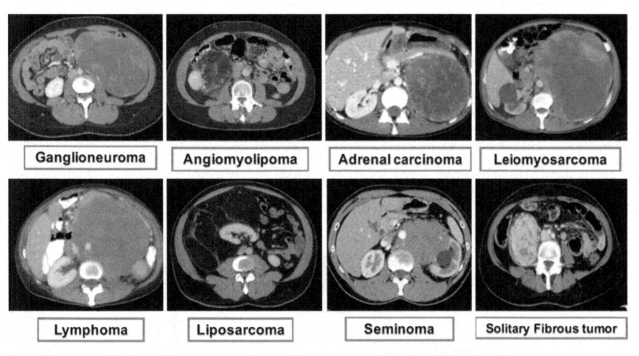

Fig. 58.3 The retroperitoneum may be the site of different type of cancers and imaging does not allow a differential diagnosis

cally evident swelling, with stretched-elastic consistency and rapid growth. In this case, only biopsy can confirm the diagnosis and define the histotype (■ Fig. 58.2).

Retroperitoneal sarcomas, on the other hand, can reach considerable size because they are very often asymptomatic. In this case, as in the case of the sarcomas of the limbs and of the trunk, the biopsy is mandatory. The retroperitoneum may also be the site of different type of cancers, and imaging does not allow a differential diagnosis (■ Fig. 58.3).

Finally, visceral sarcomas, which are much rarer and are clinically similar to the most frequent carcinomas.

Pathological review by national and international STS experts should be obtained in all cases where the histological, immunohistochemical, and molecular data do not allow a straightforward diagnosis. In fact, selected histologic subtypes characteristically display unusual biological behaviors. For example, epithelioid hemangioendothelioma is often indolent, whereas visceral Ewing(–like) sarcomas tend to be particularly aggressive. These histologic subtypes do not usually follow the principles of therapy hereby discussed.

58.2.2 Principles of Multidisciplinary Therapeutic Approach

58.2.2.1 Surgery

Surgical resection with appropriately negative margins is the standard treatment for most patients with STS. Dissection should be through grossly normal tissue planes uncontaminated by tumor and should be performed by a surgeon specifically trained in the treatment of STS. In fact, the volume and expertise of the center where the surgery is conducted does significantly impact overall and progression-free survival [4]. The biopsy site should be excised en bloc with the definitive surgical specimen, to minimize the risk of seeding. Currently, there is no universal agreement on the dimensions of the margins, ideally >2 cm. Closer margins might be necessary to preserve bones, joints, major vessels, or nerves, especially in extremity STS. Surgical clips might be placed to mark the periphery of the surgical field to help guide potential future radiotherapy, particularly for retroperitoneal and abdominal sarcomas.

58

In extremity STS, limb-sparing surgery should be performed, whenever possible. Stage I disease of the extremities should be treated with radical surgery and oncologically appropriate margins. In case of appropriate margins, patients should be evaluated for rehabilitation and start clinical and radiological follow-up. In case of positive surgical margins, surgical re-resection is strongly advised; if the reintervention does not significantly affect organ function [5], adjuvant RT should be considered. Patients with stage II, III resectable disease might follow several therapeutic strategies according to size, histologic subtype, and localization.

Appropriate multimodal strategies include the following:

1. Surgery followed by adjuvant RT +/– chemotherapy
2. Preoperative (chemo)RT followed by surgery +/– adjuvant chemotherapy
3. Preoperative chemotherapy followed by surgery + adjuvant RT +/– chemotherapy.

Preoperative RT and/or chemotherapy should be considered to reduce the likelihood of a local relapse and to improve the outcomes of surgery [6]. In selected cases, either resectable with adverse functional outcome or unresectable, regional limb therapy (perfusion and infusion) with chemotherapy +/– TNF-alpha can be considered in institutions with experience [7]. Amputation should be performed for patient preference or if the gross total resection of the tumor is expected to render the limb nonfunctional [8].

For STS of the retroperitoneum, the standard surgical treatment is multi-visceral en bloc resection, often including nephrectomy, partial colectomy, and resection of vascular and muscular structures. This type of surgery is considered safe when carried out at a specialist sarcoma center. High-risk resections should be carefully considered on an individual basis and weighed against anticipated disease biology [9].

Notably, patients with limited metastasis confined to a single organ and limited tumor bulk that are amenable to local therapy should receive primary tumor management as described for stage II or III tumors and consider metastasectomy +/– chemotherapy +/– RT [10] (◘ Fig. 58.4).

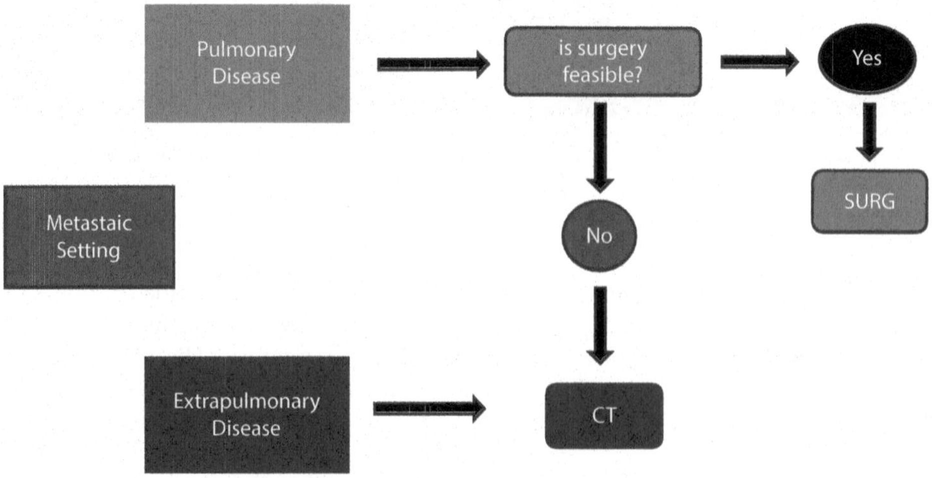

◘ **Fig. 58.4** Therapeutic approach in advanced disease

58.2.2.2 Radiotherapy

Radiotherapy is widely used in the treatment of STS patients. Adjuvant (i.e., postoperative) external beam RT (50 Gy + a variable boost dose based on margin status) should be considered for a close soft tissue margin (10–16 Gy boost) or a microscopically positive margin on bone, major blood vessels, or a major nerve (16–18 Gy boost). Randomized clinical trial data support the use of adjuvant RT to reduce local relapse, although there is no clear improvement in overall survival rates [11]. Preoperative RT is believed to reduce the risk of seeding due to surgical manipulation of the tumor. It is usually administered at a dosage of 50 Gy in 1.8–2 Gy fractions. Preoperative and adjuvant RT does not differ in terms of local or global disease control. Compared to adjuvant RT, preoperative RT is associated to greater risk of wound complications [12], but usually targets smaller radiation fields, reducing side effects, such as fibrosis, joint stiffness, and oedema [13]. A recent meta-analysis combining 16 studies also supports the use of external beam RT (both pre- and postoperative) for local tumor control in patients with resectable STS, both in the extremities and in the retroperitoneum [14]. Brachytherapy can also be considered in selected patients as an alternative to external beam RT [15].

58.3 Medical Therapy

58.3.1 Neoadjuvant Chemotherapy

The cornerstone of the medical therapy for most STS patients in all settings is represented by anthracyclines (doxorubicin and epirubicin), alone or in association to other drugs.

In the last few years, the efficacy of neoadjuvant treatment has been evaluated in different trials. The advantages of a neoadjuvant treatment are different: tumor shrinkage with the possibility of a conservative surgery, early control of micrometastases, and in vivo evaluation of treatment activity (◘ Fig. 58.5).

In this setting, the data are conflicting and the benefit of chemotherapy seems to be limited to patients with high-grade large tumours [16]. Importantly, in patients with high-risk localized STS, three cycles of full-dose pre-

---

Neoadjuvant treatment:
Theoretical advantages

- Tumor cytoreduction
- Immediate treatment of micrometastases
- Early indication as to the effectiveness of chemotherapy/radiotherapy

◘ **Fig. 58.5** Theoretical advantages of neoadjuvant treatment

---

operative CT are not inferior to five cycles [17]. Recently, it was reported that neoadjuvant full-dose epirubicin + ifosfamide was superior to histotype-tailored chemotherapy for most histological STS subtypes [18]. Among the histology-driven regimens, the use of trabectedin in high-grade myxoid liposarcoma has shown particularly interesting results, with response rates comparable to the standard epirubicin regimen [18]. Neoadjuvant therapy is proposed in experienced centers high risk to patients where primary surgical treatment would not be feasible or would be only feasible with adverse functional outcome.

In specific histologies, neoadjuvant chemoradiotherapy treatment may be particularly active and must be considered before surgery (◘ Fig. 58.6).

58.3.2 Adjuvant Chemotherapy

The finality of adjuvant treatment in STS is to improve overall survival (OS) and relapse-free survival (RFS) (◘ Fig. 58.7).

The role of adjuvant chemotherapy in STS therapy is debatable [19]. Large meta-analysis including several trials conducted up to the year 2000 showed a statistically significant 6–10% increase in recurrence-free survival at 10 years, associated to a non significant 4% increase in overall survival [20]. In a 2001 Italian trial, restricted selection criteria for high-risk cases and high-dose intensities of doxorubicin and ifosfamide resulted in a positive impact on the disease-free survival and overall survival [21]. A second, updated meta-analysis published in 2008 confirmed a significant, although marginal, efficacy of chemotherapy in localized resectable soft-tissue sarcoma with respect to local recurrence, distant recurrence, overall recurrence and overall survival. These benefits are further improved with the addition of ifosfamide to doxorubicin-based regimens, but must be weighed against associated toxicities [22]. Notably, in 2012, the randomized clinical trial EORTC 62931 showed no significant benefit deriving from an adjuvant chemotherapy with doxorubicin, ifosfamide, and granulocyte colony-stimulating factor [23]. This study, however, was limited by a long period of accrual, a large number of ineligible patients, inadequate dosing of ifosfamide, and inclusion of patients with leiomyosarcoma, an histology known to be poorly responsive to ifosfamide. Currently, adjuvant chemotherapy is generally considered for young fit patients with high-grade disease after discussion of risk-benefit ratio [24].

The Italian AIOM guidelines and European ESMO guidelines suggest an adjuvant treatment in the case of lesions greater than 5 centimeters in diameter, G3, and with deep localization.

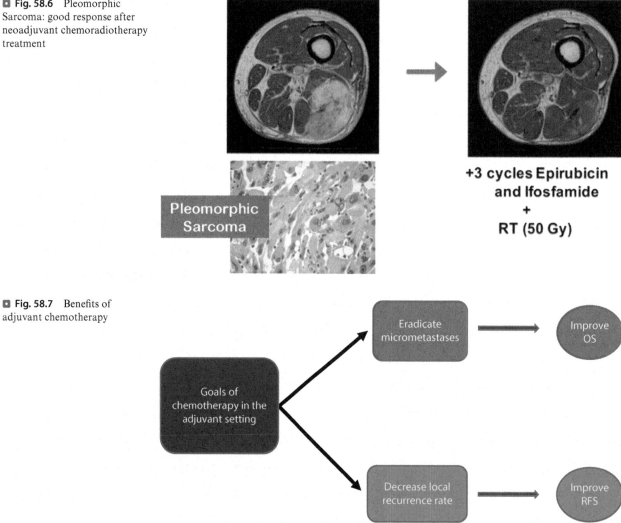

Fig. 58.6 Pleomorphic Sarcoma: good response after neoadjuvant chemoradiotherapy treatment

Fig. 58.7 Benefits of adjuvant chemotherapy

Age, performance status, and sensitivity to chemotherapy are further parameters to be evaluated (☐ Fig. 58.8).

58.3.3 Palliative Chemotherapy

The benefit of doxorubicin in metastatic STS patients was first reported by Benjamin et al. in 1975 [25]. Median survival for patients with metastatic STS treated with doxorubicin-containing regimens is however only 12–16 months, and the 2-year survival rate is ~30% [26, 27]. It must be noted that the addition of ifosfamide to doxorubicin does not significantly increase overall survival, but is associated to higher response rates and longer progression-free survival, with usually manageable increases in toxicity [26].

Two other chemotherapeutic regimens, i.e., doxorubicin + evofosfamide, a hypoxia-activated prodrug similar to ifosfamide [28], and gemcitabine + docetaxel [29],

have been recently studied as potential first-line therapies in randomized controlled phase III trials, both with no benefit in survival compared to doxorubicin alone. Alternative regimens should be proposed if anthracyclines are contraindicated (e.g., in case of reached cumulative dose due to previous chemotherapy for other cancers, in presence of known cardiologic morbidity) or based on patient preference [30].

In second line, based on the specific histologic subtypes, other drugs and regimens can be chosen (see), for example, gemcitabine+/−docetaxel or dacarbazine in leiomyosarcomas [31, 32], trabectedin in liposarcoma and leiomyosarcoma [33], and the multi-tyrosine kinase inhibitor pazopanib for non-adipocytic sarcomas [35]. Among these agents, eribuline showed impressive results with improved overall survival, particularly in liposarcomas [34].

Moreover, in selected histologies, targeted therapies should be considered based on their molecular specificity [36], e.g., in dermatofibrosarcoma protuberans (a subtype driven by PDGF-β/PDGFR signaling), the multi-tyrosine kinase inhibitor imatinib has strong activity [37, 38]; and in myofibroblastic inflammatory tumor, a subtype often driven by ALK translocation, ALK inhibitors can be used [39, 40] (■ Table 58.1).

Immunotherapy in STS is not approved yet, although recently promising results have been observed with pembrolizumab in a limited number of histologies. [41]

■ Figure 58.9 shows the treatment flow chart in the case of metastatic disease (■ Fig. 58.10).

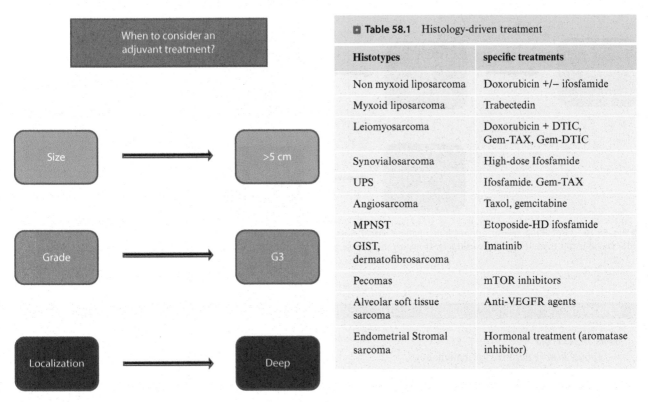

■ **Table 58.1** Histology-driven treatment

Histotypes	specific treatments
Non myxoid liposarcoma	Doxorubicin +/− ifosfamide
Myxoid liposarcoma	Trabectedin
Leiomyosarcoma	Doxorubicin + DTIC, Gem-TAX, Gem-DTIC
Synovialosarcoma	High-dose Ifosfamide
UPS	Ifosfamide. Gem-TAX
Angiosarcoma	Taxol, gemcitabine
MPNST	Etoposide-HD ifosfamide
GIST, dermatofibrosarcoma	Imatinib
Pecomas	mTOR inhibitors
Alveolar soft tissue sarcoma	Anti-VEGFR agents
Endometrial Stromal sarcoma	Hormonal treatment (aromatase inhibitor)

■ **Fig. 58.8** Indications for adjuvant treatment

■ **Fig. 58.9** Flow chart treatment in metastatic setting

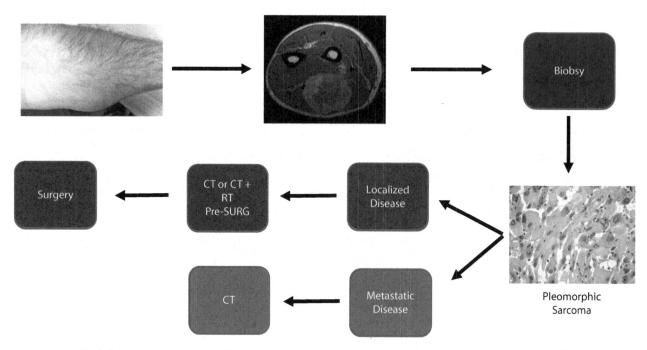

Fig. 58.10 Global therapeutic approach in a patient with a mass of soft tissues. First, biopsy. Second, staging. If localized disease, consider neoadjuvant treatment and then surgery. If metastatic disease, palliative chemotherapy

58

Case Study

Man, 50 years old
— *Family history* negative for malignancy
— *APR:* hypertension
— *APP:* contusive trauma on the left forearm with the appearance of a rapidly growing lesion

— *Objective examination:* stretch-elastic swelling of soft parts
— *Blood tests:* normal blood tests

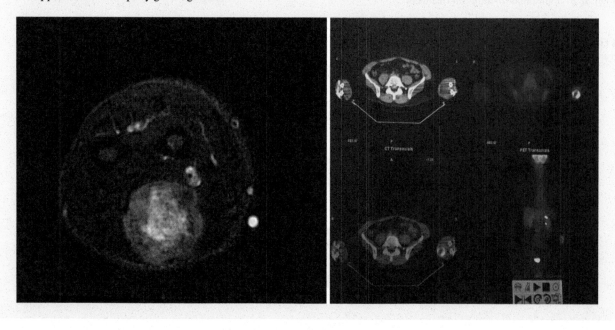

- *RMI mdc*: In correspondence of the proximal third of the fly side of the forearm, round formation with sharp margins. DT max 3.8 cm × 5.6 cm
- *FDG-PET:* metabolic radiocomposed localized in correspondence of the left forearm, with a diameter of 38 mm and with an SUV = 12.1
- *CT-scan: negative for distant metastases*

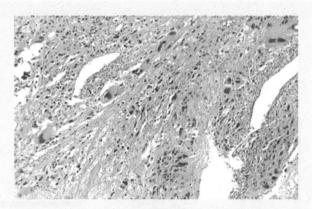

Question

What action should be taken?

1. Surgery
2. Biopsy
3. Other

Answer

Biopsy
Pleomorphic saroma G3

Question

What action should be taken?
1. Surgery
2. Neoadjuvant treatment

Answer

Neoadjuvant treatment
- *Response evaluation after three cycles with epirubicin and ifosfamide:* partial response (Choi criteria)

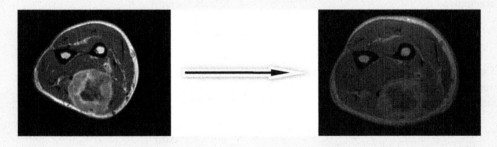

Question

What action should be taken?
1. Surgery
2. Radiotherapy
3. Continue chemotherapy

Answer

Surgery: Undifferentiated pleomorphic sarcoma with a high degree of malignancy, largely necrotic, with residual groups of vital cellular elements. Necrosis 95%. HWOS grade 3.

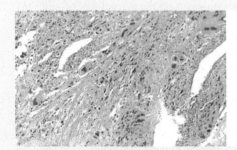
Pre-chemotherapy

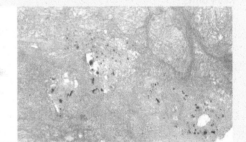
Post-chemotherapy

Key Points

- The importance of a correct diagnosis: biopsy is essential
- Considers a neoadjuvant treatment in the case of high grade sarcomas over 5 cm in diameter

Man, 45 years old
- *Family history* negative for malignancy
- *APR:* 2 years ago, surgery for a leiomyosarcoma of the right arm followed by adjuvant chemotherapy

- *APP:* in the course of the follow up finding of a single growing pulmonary nodule

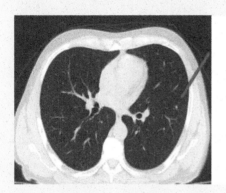 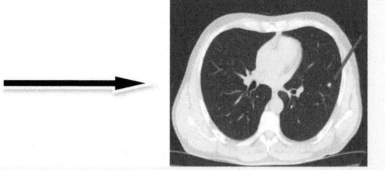

Question

What action should be taken?
1. Surgery
2. Radiotherapy
3. Chemotherapy
4. Biopsy

Answer

Surgery: Thoracotomy and transsegmental resection of the left lower lobe with diagnosis of metastases from leiomyosarcoma G2

Question

What action should be taken?
1. Follow up
2. Radiotherapy
3. Chemotherapy

Answer

Follow up

Key Points

- In case of single pulmonary metastases, consider surgery
- After pulmonary metastasectomy, chemotherapy is not a standard

58

Expert Opinion
Giuseppe Badalamenti

Key Points
- Soft tissue sarcomas (STSs) include over 80 histological rare entities, with even more molecular subsets, characterized by a low to very low incidence in all populations.
- A multidisciplinary approach is mandatory in all cases, involving pathologists, radiologists, surgeons, radiation therapists, medical oncologists, and pediatric oncologists, as well as nuclear medicine specialists and organ-based specialists.
- Surgery is the standard treatment of all patients with an adult type, localized STS. The standard surgical procedure is a wide excision with negative margins (no tumor at the margin, R0).

- Surgery (wide excision) can be completed with adjuvant RT in case of STS >5 cm diameter, G3, and deep localization.
- There is no consensus on the current role of adjuvant chemotherapy. Study results are conflicting, though some data available from smaller studies suggesting that adjuvant ChT might improve, or at least delay, distant, and local recurrence in high-risk patients. The choice of an adjuvant treatment must therefore be individualized especially in the case of chemosensitive histology.
- In the advanced/metastatic disease, the goal is palliative, and the decision-making is complex, depending on diverse presentations and histologies and should always be multidisciplinary. Monotherapy with anthracyclin remains the gold standard. The histology-driven treatment is an option in particular cases.

— (Ref. ESMO Clinical Practice Guidelines – Soft Tissue and Visceral Sarcomas)

Hints for Deeper Insight and Suggested Reading
— Soft Tissue and Visceral Sarcomas: ESMO-EURACAN Clinical Practice Guidelines for Diagnosis, Treatment and Follow-up. P.G. Casali, N. Abecassis et al., on behalf of the ESMO Guidelines Committee and EURACAN. Annals of Oncology 29 (Supplement 4): iv51–iv67, 2018. ► https://doi.org/10.1093/annonc/mdy096. Published online 28 May 2018; updated 04 October 2018.
— AIOM (Associazione Italiana di Oncologia Medica) Guidelines. Sarcomi dei Tessuti Molli e GIST. ► https://www.aiom.it/linee-guida-aiom-2018-sarcomi-dei-tessuti-molli-e-gist/
— NCCN Clinical Practice Guidelines in Oncology – Soft Tissue Sarcoma.

Bibliography

1. Siegel RL, Miller KD, Jemal A. Cancer statistics, 2017. CA Cancer J Clin. 2017;67(1):7–30.
2. Jo VY, Fletcher CD. WHO classification of soft tissue tumours: an update based on the 2013 (4th) edition. Pathology. 2014;46(2):95–104.
3. Judson I, Verweij J, Gelderblom H, Hartmann JT, Schöffski P, Blay JY, Kerst JM, Sufliarsky J, Whelan J, Hohenberger P, Krarup-Hansen A, Alcindor T, Marreaud S, Litière S, Hermans C, Fisher C, Hogendoorn PC, des Tos AP, van der Graaf WT, European Organisation and Treatment of Cancer Soft Tissue and Bone Sarcoma Group. Doxorubicin alone versus intensified doxorubicin plus ifosfamide for first-line treatment of advanced or metastatic soft-tissue sarcoma: a randomised controlled phase 3 trial. Lancet Oncol. 2014;15(4):415–23.
4. Brierley JD, Gospodarowicz MK, Wittekind C (eds). TNM classification of malignant tumours, 8th edn. Oxford: Wiley 2016.
5. Callegaro D, Miceli R, Bonvalot S, et al. Development and external validation of two nomograms to predict overall survival and occurrence of distant metastases in adults after surgical resection of localised soft-tissue sarcomas of the extremities: a retrospective analysis. Lancet Oncol. 2016;17:671–80.
6. Haas RL, Gronchi A, van de Sande MAJ, et al. Perioperative management of extremity soft tissue sarcomas. J Clin Oncol. 2018;36:118–24.
7. Neuwirth MG, Song Y, Sinnamon AJ, et al. Isolated limb perfusion and infusion for extremity soft tissue sarcoma: a contemporary systematic review and meta-analysis. Ann Surg Oncol. 2017;24:3803–10.
8. Rizzo A, Nannini M, Astolfi A, et al. Impact of chemotherapy in the adjuvant setting of early stage uterine leiomyosarcoma: a systematic review and updated meta-analysis. Cancers (Basel). 2020;12(7):1899. Published 2020 Jul 14. https://doi.org/10.3390/cancers12071899.
9. MacNeill AJ, Gronchi A, Miceli R, et al. Postoperative morbidity after radical resection of primary retroperitoneal sarcoma: a report from the transatlantic RPS working group. Ann Surg. 2018;267(5):959–64.
10. Marulli G, Mammana M, Comacchio G, et al. Survival and prognostic factors following pulmonary metastasectomy for sarcoma. J Thorac Dis. 2017;9:S1305–15.
11. Yang JC, Chang AE, Baker AR, et al. Randomized prospective study of the benefit of adjuvant radiation therapy in the treatment of soft tissue sarcomas of the extremity. J Clin Oncol. 1998;16:197–203.
12. O'Sullivan B, Davis AM, Turcotte R, et al. Preoperative versus postoperative radiotherapy in soft-tissue sarcoma of the limbs: a randomised trial. Lancet. 2002;359:2235–41.
13. Davis AM, O'Sullivan B, Turcotte R, et al. Late radiation morbidity following randomization to preoperative versus postoperative radiotherapy in extremity soft tissue sarcoma. Radiother Oncol. 2005;75:48–53.
14. Albertsmeier M, Rauch A, Roeder F, et al. External beam radiation therapy for resectable soft tissue sarcoma: a systematic review and meta-analysis. Ann Surg Oncol. 2018;25(3):754–67.
15. Naghavi AO, Fernandez DC, Mesko N, et al. American Brachytherapy Society consensus statement for soft tissue sarcoma brachytherapy. Brachytherapy. 2017;16:466–89.
16. Grobmyer SR, Maki RG, Demetri GD, et al. Neo-adjuvant chemotherapy for primary high-grade extremity soft tissue sarcoma. Ann Oncol. 2004;15:1667–72.
17. Gronchi A, Frustaci S, Mercuri M, et al. Short, full-dose adjuvant chemotherapy in high-risk adult soft tissue sarcomas: a randomized clinical trial from the Italian Sarcoma Group and the Spanish Sarcoma Group. J Clin Oncol. 2012;30:850–6.
18. Gronchi A, Ferrari S, Quagliuolo V, et al. Histotype-tailored neoadjuvant chemotherapy versus standard chemotherapy in patients with high-risk soft-tissue sarcomas (ISG-STS 1001): an international, open-label, randomised, controlled, phase 3, multicentre trial. Lancet Oncol. 2017;18:812–22.
19. Rizzo A, Nannini M, Astolfi A, Impact of Chemotherapy in the Adjuvant Setting of Early Stage Uterine Leiomyosarcoma: A Systematic Review and Updated Meta-Analysis. Cancers (Basel). 2020;12(7):1899. https://doi.org/10.3390/cancers12071899. PMID: 32674439.
20. Sarcoma Meta-analysis C. Adjuvant chemotherapy for localised resectable soft tissue sarcoma in adults. Cochrane Database Syst Rev. 2000:CD001419.
21. Frustaci S, Gherlinzoni F, De Paoli A, et al. Adjuvant chemotherapy for adult soft tissue sarcomas of the extremities and girdles: results of the Italian randomized cooperative trial. J Clin Oncol. 2001;19:1238–47.
22. Pervaiz N, Colterjohn N, Farrokhyar F, et al. A systematic meta-analysis of randomized controlled trials of adjuvant chemotherapy for localized resectable soft-tissue sarcoma. Cancer. 2008;113:573–81.
23. Woll PJ, Reichardt P, Le Cesne A, et al. Adjuvant chemotherapy with doxorubicin, ifosfamide, and lenograstim for resected soft-tissue sarcoma (EORTC 62931): a multicentre randomised controlled trial. Lancet Onol. 2012;13:1045–54.
24. Napolitano A, Mazzocca A, Spalato Ceruso M, et al. Recent advances in desmoid tumor therapy. Cancers (Basel).

2020;12(8):2135. Published 2020 Aug 1. https://doi.org/10.3390/cancers12082135.

25. Benjamin RS, Wiernik PH, Bachur NR. Adriamycin: a new effective agent in the therapy of disseminated sarcomas. Med Pediatr Oncol. 1975;1:63–76.

26. Judson I, Verweij J, Gelderblom H, et al. Doxorubicin alone versus intensified doxorubicin plus ifosfamide for first-line treatment of advanced or metastatic soft-tissue sarcoma: a randomised controlled phase 3 trial. Lancet Oncol. 2014;15:415–23.

27. Judson I, Verweij J, Gelderblom H, et al. Doxorubicin alone versus intensified doxorubicin plus ifosfamide for first-line treatment of advanced or metastatic soft-tissue sarcoma: a randomised controlled phase 3 trial. Lancet Oncol. 2015;15:415–23.

28. Tap WD, Papai Z, Van Tine BA, et al. Doxorubicin plus evofosfamide versus doxorubicin alone in locally advanced, unresectable or metastatic soft-tissue sarcoma (TH CR-406/SARC021): an international, multicentre, open-label, randomised phase 3 trial. Lancet Oncol. 2017;18:1089–103.

29. Seddon B, Strauss SJ, Whelan J, et al. Gemcitabine and docetaxel versus doxorubicin as first-line treatment in previously untreated advanced unresectable or metastatic soft-tissue sarcomas (GeDDiS): a randomised controlled phase 3 trial. Lancet Oncol. 2017;18:1397–410.

30. Cannella R, Tabone E, Porrello G, et al. Assessment of morphological CT imaging features for the prediction of risk stratification, mutations, and prognosis of gastrointestinal stromal tumors [published online ahead of print, 2021 Apr 21]. Eur Radiol. 2021;10.1007/s00330-021-07961-3. https://doi.org/10.1007/s00330-021-07961-3.

31. Pautier P, Floquet A, Penel N, et al. Randomized multicenter and stratified phase II study of gemcitabine alone versus gemcitabine and docetaxel in patients with metastatic or relapsed leiomyosarcomas: a Federation Nationale des Centres de Lutte Contre le Cancer (FNCLCC) French Sarcoma Group Study (TAXOGEM study). Oncologist. 2012;17:1213–20.

32. Maki RG, Wathen JK, Patel SR, et al. Randomized phase II study of gemcitabine and docetaxel compared with gemcitabine alone in patients with metastatic soft tissue sarcomas: results of

sarcoma alliance for research through collaboration study 002 [corrected]. J Clin Oncol. 2007;25:2755–63.

33. Demetri GD, von Mehren M, Jones RL, et al. Efficacy and safety of trabectedin or dacarbazine for metastatic liposarcoma or leiomyosarcoma after failure of conventional chemotherapy: results of a phase III randomized multicenter clinical trial. J Clin Oncol. 2016;34:786–93.

34. Schoffski P, Chawla S, Maki RG, et al. Eribulin versus dacarbazine in previously treated patients with advanced liposarcoma or leiomyosarcoma: a randomised, open-label, multicentre, phase 3 trial. Lancet. 2016;387:1629–37.

35. van der Graaf WT, Blay JY, Chawla SP, et al. Pazopanib for metastatic soft-tissue sarcoma (PALETTE): a randomised, double-blind, placebo-controlled phase 3 trial. Lancet. 2012;379:1879–86.

36. Napolitano A, Mazzocca A, Spalato Ceruso M, Recent Advances in Desmoid Tumor Therapy. Cancers (Basel). 2020;12(8):2135. https://doi.org/10.3390/cancers12082135. PMID: 32752153.

37. Rubin BP, Schuetze SM, Eary JF, et al. Molecular targeting of platelet-derived growth factor B by imatinib mesylate in a patient with metastatic dermatofibrosarcoma protuberans. J Clin Oncol. 2002;20:3586–91.

38. Badalamenti G, Messina C, De Luca I, Musso E, Casarin A, Incorvaia L. Soft tissue sarcomas in the precision medicine era: new advances in clinical practice and future perspectives. Radiol Med. 2019;124(4):259–65. https://doi.org/10.1007/s11547-018-0883-6.

39. Butrynski JE, D'Adamo DR, Hornick JL, et al. Crizotinib in ALK-rearranged inflammatory myofibroblastic tumor. N Engl J Med. 2010;363:1727–33.

40. Badalamenti G, Incorvaia L, Messina C, et al. One shot NEPA plus dexamethasone to prevent multiple-day chemotherapy in sarcoma patients [published correction appears in Support Care Cancer. 2019 May 14]. Support Care Cancer. 2019;27(9):3593–7. https://doi.org/10.1007/s00520-019-4645-3.

41. Tawbi HA, Burgess M, Bolejack V, et al. Pembrolizumab in advanced soft-tissue sarcoma and bone sarcoma (SARC028): a multicentre, two-cohort, single-arm, open-label, phase 2 trial. Lancet Oncol. 2017;18:1493–501.

Gastrointestinal Stromal Tumors (GISTs)

Lorena Incorvaia, Giuseppe Badalamenti, Sergio Rizzo, Viviana Bazan, Antonio Russo, Alessandro Gronchi, and Sinziana Dumitra

Soft Tissue Sarcoma, GIST and Neuroendocrine Neoplasms

Contents

Lorena Incorvaia and Giuseppe Badalamenti should be considered equally co-first authors.

© Springer Nature Switzerland AG 2021
A. Russo et al. (eds.), *Practical Medical Oncology Textbook*, UNIPA Springer Series,
https://doi.org/10.1007/978-3-030-56051-5_59

59.1 The Role of Medical Treatment in the Management of GIST

Lorena Incorvaia, Giuseppe Badalamenti,
Sergio Rizzo Viviana Bazan and Antonio Russo

59.1.1 Introduction

GISTs, while *relatively rare*, are the most common primary mesenchymal neoplasms of the gastrointestinal tract.

GISTs are typically *highly resistant to conventional chemotherapy*; the discovery of activating mutations in the *proto-oncogene KIT* and the development of *tyrosine kinase inhibitors (TKI)*, such as imatinib, first introduced in 2002, revolutionized the treatment strategy for GISTs, by making possible to target the specific molecular events that are key events for pathogenesis of the disease.

- GISTs can arise at *any age*, with a median of diagnosis *around 60–65 years.*
- More than 80% of the patients are older than 50 years.
- Occurrence in children is rare, and pediatric GIST represents a distinct subset, with the absence of KIT/platelet-derived growth factor alpha (PDGFRA) mutations, female predominance, and multifocal pattern of gastric GISTs [1, 2].
- GISTs can be found *anywhere in the gastrointestinal tract*, but the most frequent location is stomach (55%), followed by small intestine (30%). Less frequent are colon/ rectum (5%) and esophagus (<1%).
- Exceptionally rarely, GISTs can occur outside the gastrointestinal tract, such as in the omentum, mesentery, or retroperitoneal (<5%) (▣ Fig. 59.1).

59.1.2 Origin

For many years, GISTs were initially classified as smooth muscle sarcomas, such as leiomyoma, leiomyoblastoma, or leiomyosarcomas.

59

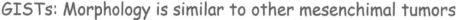

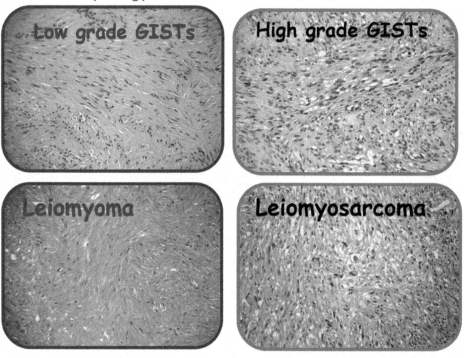

GISTs: Morphology is similar to other mesenchimal tumors

Low grade GISTs

High grade GISTs

Leiomyoma

Leiomyosarcoma

Further studies identified similarity to a cell population in the gastrointestinal tract called *interstitial cells of Cajal (ICCs)*, present in the wall of the gut. These cells facilitate the communication between the nervous system and the smooth muscle and work as pacemaker cells that cause peristaltic contractions in the GI tract. Data proving this relationship are based on similar histological findings and above all on the common expression of certain antigens such as CD117, the product of the oncogene c-KIT, and myoid antigens [3].

GISTs: Cellular origin
Interstitial Cells of Cajal (ICCs)

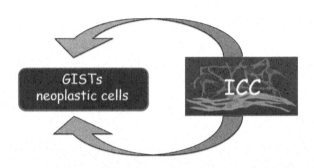

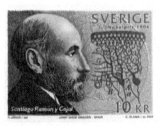

GISTs neoplastic cells

ICC

IC of Cajal of the wall of the gut
-Facilitate the communication between the nervous system and the smooth muscle
-Work as pacemaker cells that cause peristaltic contractions in the GI tract
KIT positive like GISTs

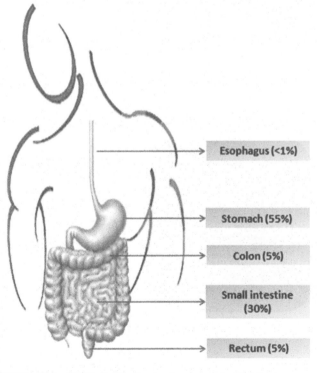

Esophagus (<1%)

Stomach (55%)

Colon (5%)

Small intestine (30%)

Rectum (5%)

☐ **Fig. 59.1** GISTs distribution on the gastrointestinal tract

59.1.3 Pathological Features

Pathologically, the diagnosis of GIST relies on morphology and immunohistochemistry.

59.1.3.1 Macroscopic Aspects (☐ Fig. 59.2)

59.1.3.2 Microscopic Aspects and Immunohistochemistry (IHC)

A. Microscopic evaluation reveals *three principal subtypes of GIST* depending on the cytomorphology: spindle cell, epithelioid cell, and the less frequent GISTs with mixed morphology, both spindle and epithelioid cells (☐ Fig. 59.3).

B. Approximately, the *95% GISTs are immunohistochemically positive for the tyrosine kinase receptor KIT (CD117)*. About 5% of GISTs are, instead, negative for detectable KIT expression [4].

C. In the diagnosis of c-kit-negative cases, DOG1 expression is a new immunohistochemical marker with unknown functions selectively expressed in GISTs.

Fig. 59.2 Macroscopic appearance of a small bowel GIST. (Courtesy of Dr. A. Gronchi)

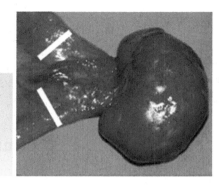

Macroscopic aspect

- Well-circumscribed
- Highly vascular
- May show hemorrhagic foci, central cystic degenerative changes or necrosis

Fig. 59.3 Histological subtype of GISTs

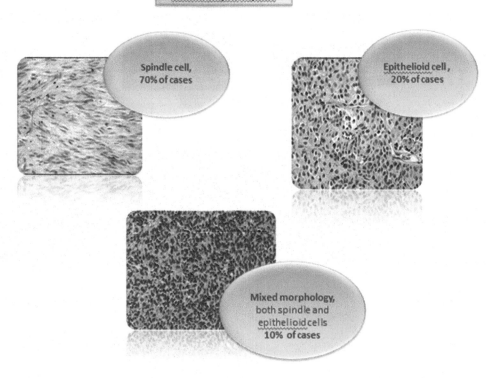

Microscopic aspect

Spindle cell, 70% of cases

Epithelioid cell, 20% of cases

Mixed morphology, both spindle and epithelioid cells 10% of cases

Because the receptor KIT (CD117) is commonly expressed on GIST cells, it represents an important feature for a correct histological diagnosis [5]. Other antigens to be studied are CD34, an antigen common in hematopoietic stem cells, endotheliocytes, and fibroblasts, positive in 70–80% of GISTs, smooth muscle actin (SMA) positive in around 30% of GISTs, and usually reciprocal to CD34 and vimentin, while S100 and desmin expression is usually rare [2, 3].

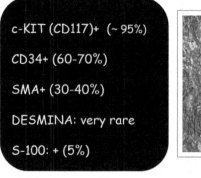

GISTs: Immunohistochemistry

c-KIT (CD117)+ (~95%)

CD34+ (60-70%)

SMA+ (30-40%)

DESMINA: very rare

S-100: + (5%)

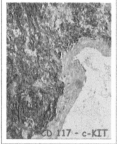

CD 117 - c-KIT

59.1.4 Molecular Biology

The identification of *activating mutations in the proto-oncogene KIT* in 1998 triggered a sea change in our understanding of the GIST pathogenesis and has resulted in a new paradigm for the use of molecular genetic diagnostics to guide targeted therapies.

KIT gain-of-function mutations, together with those in *platelet-derived growth factor receptor A (PDGFRA)*, are now well established as the *driver mutations* in the majority of GISTs [3, 6].

While pediatric and Mendelian inheritance-based GISTs are often wild type for PDGFRα and C-KIT and may be mutated in other genes such as *SDH*, sporadic GISTs often need a mutation of these genes as a fundamental step in their pathogenesis [7].

However, KIT and PDGFRα mutations are not sufficient for the development of a high-risk GIST since it seems other mutations or chromosomal aberrations are required. In fact, similar to the carcinogenetic model hypothesized for colon cancer by Vogelstein, a model of tumor evolution has also been proposed for GIST, that is, the high-risk GIST commonly seen in clinical practice would be the result of the evolution of a micro-GIST, usually characterized by the mutation of C-KIT or PDGFRα, to a low-risk GIST by acquiring new mutations such as secondary point mutations or epigenetic alterations and then to a clinically evident disease by new KIT or PDGFRα activating mutations, telomerase activation, or chromosomal aberrations [8].

Furthermore, the so-called micro-GISTs are probably extremely common in the population – about 30% in different studies – though only a very small number of these will progress to low- and then high-risk GISTs [9, 10].

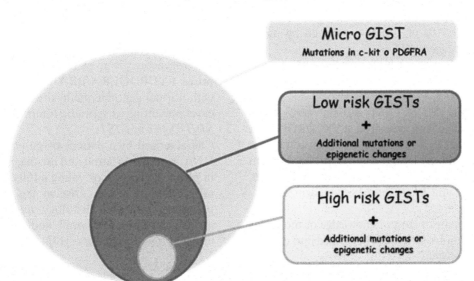

GISTs Epidemiology

Micro GIST
Mutations in c-kit o PDGFRA

Low risk GISTs
+
Additional mutations or epigenetic changes

High risk GISTs
+
Additional mutations or epigenetic changes

Only a few % of microGISTs become low grade GIST and eventually high grade GISTs

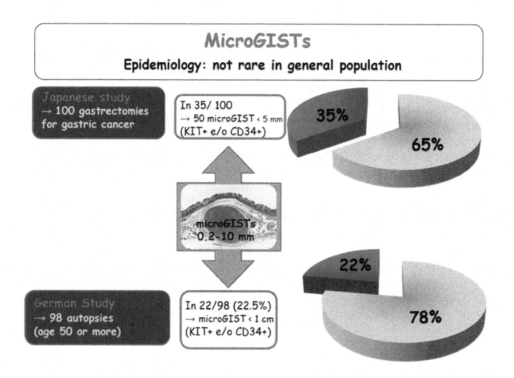

59

The *frequency* of mutations in KIT and PDGFRA is different, and the mutations are mutually exclusive [11]:
- *Approximately 70%* of GISTs are driven by mutations in the *oncogene KIT.*
- Of those GISTs without KIT mutations, the majority harbor mutations in the gene encoding (*PDGFRA*) (15%).
- The remaining 15% of GISTs initially were genetically unclassified and described as KIT/PDGFRA "wild-type" GISTs. Today, with the expansion of our knowledge about molecular profile, further different and less frequent genetic mutations in other genes, such as *BRAF* and *KRAS,* have been recognized.

Therefore, at the state of current knowledge of molecular spectrum of mutations, GISTs can be divided into two dis-tinct clusters: *succinate dehydrogenase (SDH)-competent* and *SDH-deficient subgroups,* each with distinct clinical and genetic characteristics (Fig. 59.4) [3, 12].

1. *SDH-Competent GISTs*
   Heterogeneous group of tumors that primarily comprises KIT/PDGFRA/BRAF/NF1-mutated GISTs with normal genomic methylation patterns, in most cases presenting as sporadic tumors.
2. *SDH-Deficient GISTs*
   Characterized by a pattern of global, genome-wide DNA hypermethylation and are diagnosed primarily in pediatric patients or young adults. SDH-deficient GISTs almost always arise in the stomach, show prevalent epithelioid histology, and undergo early metastasis to liver and lymph nodes, with a relatively indolent long-term course [13].

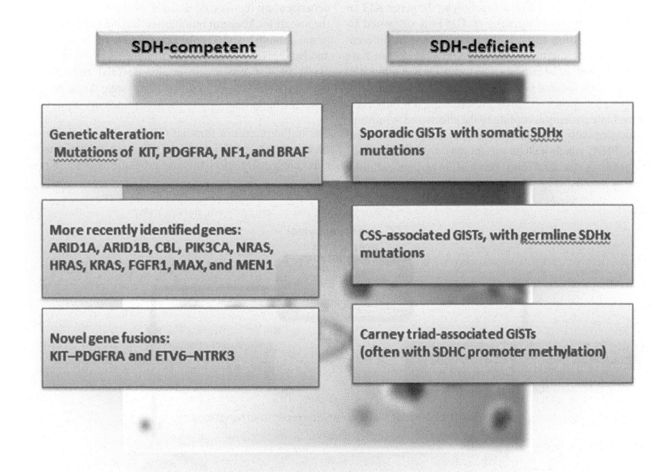

SDH-competent

SDH-deficient

Genetic alteration:
 Mutations of KIT, PDGFRA, NF1, and BRAF

Sporadic GISTs with somatic SDHx mutations

More recently identified genes:
ARID1A, ARID1B, CBL, PIK3CA, NRAS,
HRAS, KRAS, FGFR1, MAX, and MEN1

CSS-associated GISTs, with germline SDHx mutations

Novel gene fusions:
KIT–PDGFRA and ETV6–NTRK3

Carney triad-associated GISTs
(often with SDHC promoter methylation)

Fig. 59.4 Succinate dehydrogenase (SDH)-competent and SDH-deficient subgroups of GISTs

Features	Carney's triad	Carney's-Stratakis diad
GISTs	yes	yes
Paraganglioma	yes	yes
Pulmonary chondroma	yes	No
Hereditary	No	yes
Gender	> F	F = M
c-Kit or PDGFRA mutations	yes	No
Mutations on the SDH subunits SDHD, SDHC and SDHB	yes	In 9/11 families
SDH gene loss	In some cases	In some cases

Biology of Familial GISTs   The initial role of mutations leading to the acquisition of function by the genes KIT or PDGFRA in the oncogenesis of GISTs is suggested by their transmission through the germinal line in different familial cases. Germinal mutations in these genes have been observed in 14 families. The mean age at diagnosis in patients with familial GISTs is 46 years. This familial form is not so common in children. Nevertheless, it is important to evaluate patients according to the effects and symptoms associated with germinal mutations in the genes KIT and PDGFRA, which include melanomas, freckles, urticaria pigmentosa, perioral and perianal hyperpigmentation, and achalasia. The various clinical manifestations in patients with germinal mutations in KIT are closely dependent on the specific domain of the KIT involved in the mutation. Aberrant mutations affecting the juxtamembrane domain (exon 11) are associated with mastocytosis and hyperpigmentation, apart from the generalized hyperplasia of the progenitor intestinal Cajal cells (ICC). Nevertheless, such symptoms do not seem to be present when the mutation involves the kinasic activity domain.

The initial phases of familial GISTs appear biologically similar to those of sporadic GISTs, with similar cytogenetic progression mechanisms and genic expression profiles.

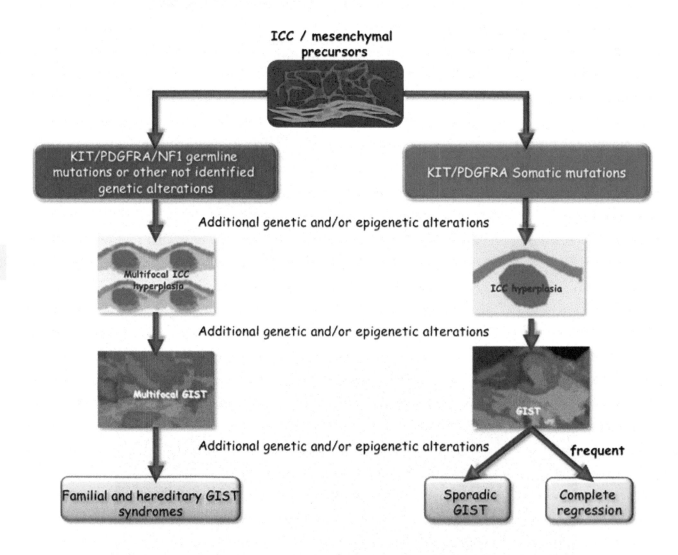

In familial GISTs, germinal mutations in KIT and PDGFRA are mostly similar to those found in sporadic forms. Two mutations which have never been found in sporadic GISTs, Asp419del in KIT and Tyr555Cys in PDGFRA, have, however, been identified in two families presenting hereditary GISTs. Furthermore, a recent study reports the case of a patient who developed lipomas and GISTs and who showed the germinal mutation Asp561Val in PDGFRA.

Two very similar models of transgenic mice have been developed in an attempt to identify the germinal mutations of KIT found in familial GIST syndromes

63. Such mutations are exactly the same as those found in patients with sporadic GISTs. Transgenic mice with these mutations maintain both their vitality and fertility and develop GISTs with a penetrance of about 100% 64.

The first case of familial GIST observed involved a Japanese family where the deletion of one of the two consecutive residues of valine (codon 559 or 560, GTTGTT) in exon 11 of KIT was identified throughout three generations. The subjects affected presented perianal hyperpigmentation and developed both malignant and benign multiple GISTs 65. A germinal mutation in the kinasic domain I of KIT has been identified in France in a 67-year-old woman and her 40-year-old son. Both these patients presented a dozen duodenal and jejunal GISTs and presented a constitutive substitution (K642E) in exon 13 of KIT 66 [10].

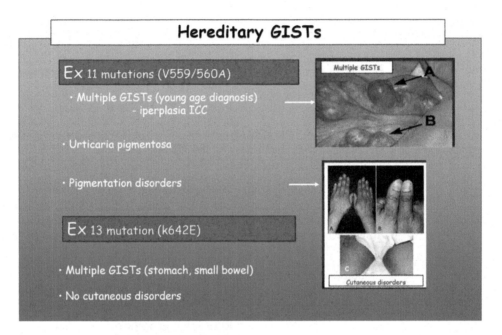

GISTs are not often diagnosed in children. Up till now, pediatric forms make up only 1% of all the identified cases. The current know-how regarding adult GISTs and correlated tumors, for example, paragangliomas, together with the development of new methods, such as microarray techniques, have led to remarkable progress in the comprehension of the rare pediatric forms. These may, however, show a different pathogenesis from that of adult GISTs, since apparently no mutations of KIT and PDGFRA are present (*wild-type* GIST). This might indicate that there exist other activation mechanisms of KIT or oncogenic *pathways* which are not linked to the gene and which are active within the cells. In the majority of pediatric GISTs examined, no other cytogenetic anomaly or alterations of exons 9, 11, or 13 of KIT have been identified. Of the 64 pediatric GISTs undergoing mutational analysis reported in literature, only 7 (11%) show a mutation in the genes *KIT* and *PDGFRA*. These mutations were equally distributed between exons 11 and 9 of *KIT* and were relatively common in *PDGFRA*. A homozygous punctiform mutation in exon 9 of *KIT* (C>T): Pro456Ser and a nonsense mutation in exon 18

of *PDGFRA* were found in two different cases of pediatric GISTs. This is a different model from that observed in adult sporadic GISTs, where *KIT* mutations are ten times as common as *PDGFRA* mutations.

59.1.4.1 KIT and PDGFRA

As mentioned before, the main initial event in GIST tumorigenesis are often gain-of-function mutations in *KIT* or *PDGFRA* genes, located on the long arm of chromosome 4 (4q12) (◘ Figs. 59.5 and 59.6).

— In GIST, the most common mutations are found in *KIT exon 11* (60–70%) that affects the juxtamembrane domain (Corless et al., 2011). The most frequent types of mutation are in-frame deletions, followed by single nucleotide substitution, resulting in constitutive activity of the kit receptor. Approximately 80% of exon 11-mutated tumors are located in the stomach and typically show more spindled than epithelioid histology.

— Mutations in *KIT exon 9* are the second most common following the exon 11 mutations. Account for 8–10% of GISTs, affecting the extracellular domain

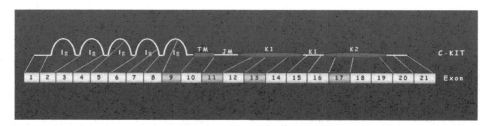

Fig. 59.5 C-KIT oncogene gene structure. The members of type III tyrosine kinase receptor family consist of a ligand-binding extracellular domain of 5 immunoglobulin (Ig) regions, an autoinhibitory intracellular juxtamembrane domain, and a kinase domain of an amino terminal ATP-binding region (activation loop)

Fig. 59.6 KIT and PFGFRA signaling pathways

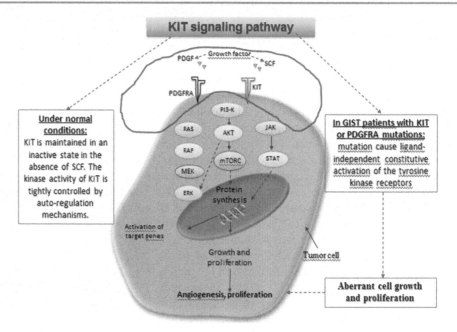

KIT and PDGFRA genes encode transmembrane glycoprotein receptor tyrosine kinase **(RTK).**

The **ligands** of KIT and PDGFRA are stem cell factor **(SCF)** and platelet-derived growth factor **(PDGF),** respectively.

Binding to the receptors results in **kinase activation**, initiating downstream signaling pathways, mainly through phosphoinositide 3-kinase (PI3K)/AKT, RAS/RAF/mitogen-activated protein kinase (MAPK) and signal transducer and activator of transcription 3 (STAT3) pathways, that promote cell **proliferation** and **survival**. PMID: 24267995

Mutations in the **KIT or PDGFRA genes** may result in expression of a protein with constitutive RTK activity and **aberrant cell growth and proliferation.** (Fig 1.6)

and 95% are duplications of codons 502 and 503 (Lux et al., 2000). These tumors have a higher prevalence in the small or large bowel.

Generally uncommon are the mutations is in *exons 13 and 17* of KIT (Corless et al., 2011).

- About 10% of GISTs harbor *PDGFRA mutations* (Heinrich et al., 2003b; Hirota et al., 2003). PDGFRA and KIT mutations are mutually exclusive. The majority of PDGFRA-mutated GISTs occur in the stomach, usually with epithelioid or mixed epithelioid and spindle cell histology. Although the activated pathways downstream are identical to KIT mutations, PDGFRA-mutated GISTs tend to have a lower risk of recurrence, and among metastatic GISTs, only 2.1% showed PDGFRA mutation compared with 82.8% in those with KIT mutations.

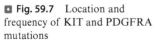

Fig. 59.7 Location and frequency of KIT and PDGFRA mutations

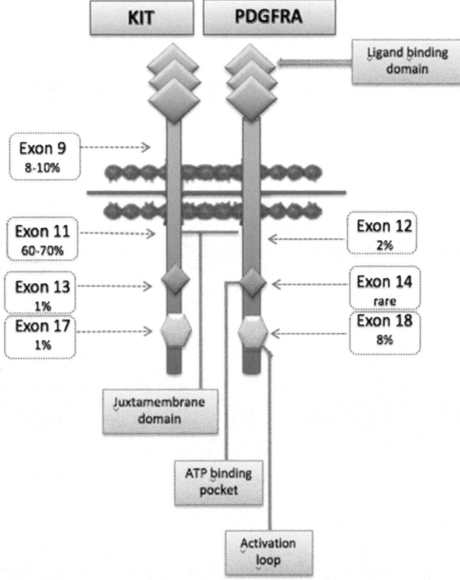

PDGFRA-mutated GISTs showed a variability of response to medical treatment. Most PDGFRA mutations in GISTs have been identified in *exon 18*: the most frequent mutation, *D842V*, represents 70% of PDGFRA mutations and 5% of metastatic GISTs and is the most common cause of primary resistance to therapy. The second most frequent mutation of exon 18, instead, the *deletion of codons 842 to 845*, confers imatinib sensitivity [14, 15] (■ Fig. 59.7).

59.1.5 Clinical Features

Unlike gastrointestinal carcinoma that has epithelial origin, GISTs are tumors of ▶ connective tissue, and therefore, most commonly grow extrinsically from the wall of GI tract. For this submucosal location, the GISTs achieve usually a large size without causing gastrointestinal obstruction or other symptoms typical of epithelial cancers (■ Fig. 59.8).

The *clinical presentation* of GIST is not characteristic and depends on the localization and the size of the tumor.

In contrast with epithelial carcinoma of the GI tract, which has an irregular mucosal or polypoidal growth with or without intestinal obstruction, GIST has a predominant *exophytic component* and displaces rather than invades the surrounding structures.

The GISTs *tumor size* at the time of diagnosis varies widely, from small nodules <2 cm to large masses, up to 30 cm in size (Corless et al., 2002).

The small tumors are, frequently, *asymptomatic* or associated with *nonspecific symptoms* and often diag-

◻ Fig. 59.8 Pattern of growth

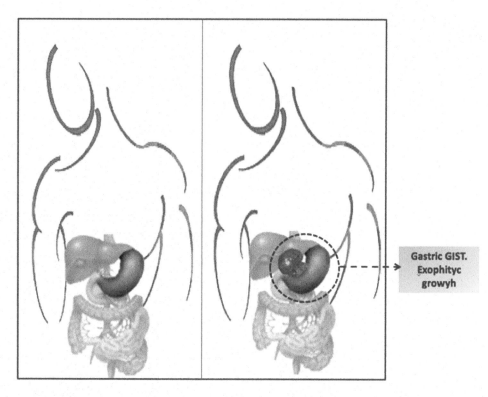

Gastric GIST. Exophityc growyh

nosed incidentally during endoscopic/surgical procedures or during radiologic studies performed to investigate manifestations of gastrointestinal tract disease.

Also for the voluminous tumors, the *symptoms* associated with GISTs are nonspecific and can include the following:

− Abdominal pain
− Nausea and early satiety
− Vomiting
− Anorexia and Weight loss
− Epigastric fullness

Localization of the tumor	Several clinical symptoms depending on localization of the tumor: for example, the esophageal tumors are present with dysphagia, odynophagia, retrosternal pain, and hematemesis; gastric tumors may cause epigastric pain, anorexia, nausea, vomiting, and weight loss
Obstruction	GISTs may also produce site-specific symptoms secondary to obstruction, for intraluminal growth of the tumors or for exophytic luminal compression (e.g., constipation in colorectal GIST or obstructive jaundice in duodenal GISTs)
GI bleeding	It can be produced by pressure and ulceration of the overlying mucosa with resultant blood loss and fatigue

In loss frequent cases, especially for large GISTs, the *GIST rupture* can occur into the abdominal cavity with life-threatening intraperitoneal hemorrhage [17].

59.1.6 Diagnosis

The diagnostic evaluation of gastrointestinal stromal tumors is based on imaging techniques, but the most important diagnostic tools remain the histology with the immunohistochemical examinations.

Small, asymptomatic lesions are usually discovered accidentally during endoscopy, ultrasonography, or computer tomography performed for other indications.

Endoscopy	Usually describes GIST as submucosal changes, in the majority of cases as oval protrusion, observed through the gastrointestinal lumen, with a covering mucosa often intact
Computed tomography	Shows these lesions as a solid mass with exophytic growth from the muscularis propria that displays contrast enhancement and may contain areas of necrosis (◻ Fig. 59.9)
Endoscopic ultrasonography (EUS)	Besides endoscopy and computer tomography, it plays an important role in the diagnostic work-up of GISTs. Frequently, EUS shows GIST as hypoechogenic mass originating from different layers of the gastrointestinal tract wall, usually from the muscularis propria and muscularis mucosa, with an irregular outer margin and nonhomogeneous echo pattern

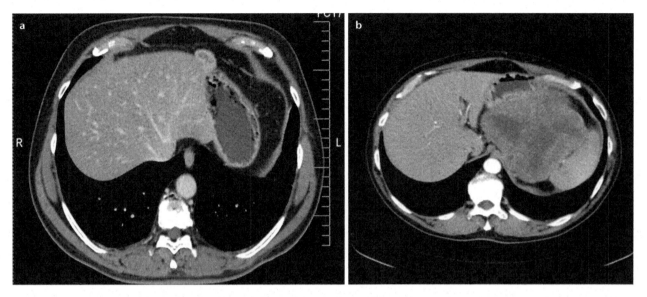

▣ Fig. 59.9   a Small Gastric GIST. **b** Heterogeneously enhancing mass in the stomach, with necrosis

Magnetic resonance imaging (MRI)	May be an alternative to abdominal and pelvic CT scan. For rectal GISTs, MRI provides better preoperative staging information.

The final diagnosis is established on the basis of *histological examination of biopsy* with *immunohistochemical investigations.*

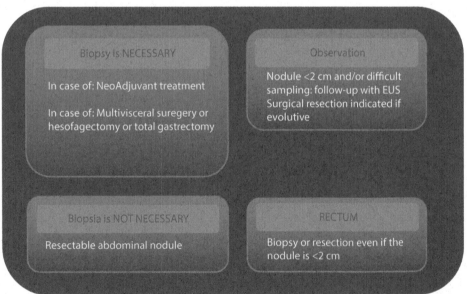

The evaluation of fluorodeoxyglucose (FDG) uptake using an FDG-positron emission tomography *(PET) scan*, or FDG-PET–CT, is useful mainly for early detection of the tumor response to molecular-targeted therapy [3, 17] (▣ Fig. 59.10).

59.1.7 Prognostic Factors

Current ESMO guidelines do not recommend the use of TNM system for the classification and staging of GIST, due to the limitations of this system.

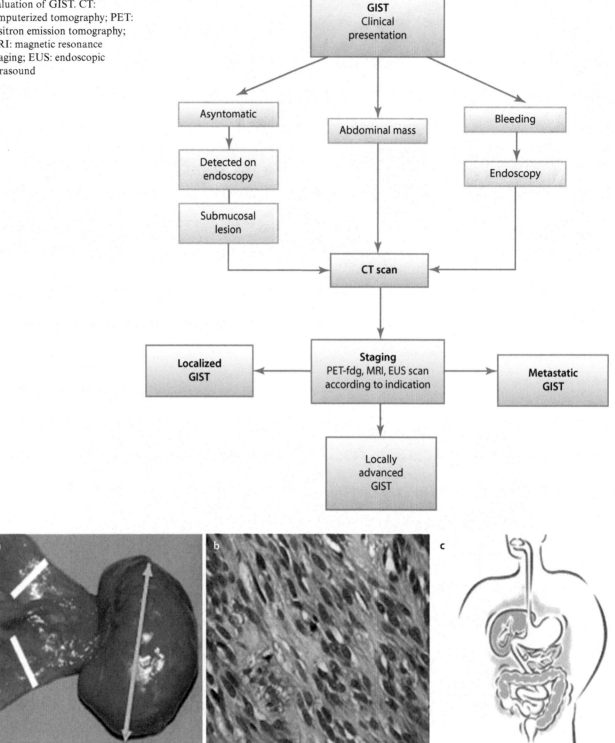

◘ Fig. 59.10 Diagnostic evaluation of GIST. CT: computerized tomography; PET: positron emission tomography; MRI: magnetic resonance imaging; EUS: endoscopic ultrasound

59

◘ Fig. 59.11 Prognostic factors **a** tumor size; **b** mitotic activity; **c** anatomic site

Prognostic factors used for risk assessment affect the primary tumor site (◘ Fig. 59.11):
- *Mitotic index*
- *Tumor size*

- *Tumor site: gastric* GISTs have a better prognosis than *small bowel or rectal* GISTs.
- *Tumor rupture* is an additional adverse prognostic factor.

This version of the risk assessment scheme is based on several large series published by Mietinnen and colleagues (2006) (■ Fig. 59.12), after integrated by Joensuu (■ Fig. 59.13).

More recently, prognostic heat and contour maps have been developed which should address issues associated with the nonlinear continuous variables of tumor size, mitotic index, and tumor rupture (■ Fig. 59.12).

■ **Fig. 59.12** Joensuu's risk stratification for gastrointestinal stromal tumors

Risk category	Tumor size (cm)	Mitotic index (5 HPF)	Primary tumor site
Very low-risk	>2	<5	Any
Low-risk	2.1-5	<5	Any
Intermediate-risk	<5 5-10	6-10 <5	Gastric Gastric
High-risk	Any >10 Any >5 5.1-10	Any Any >10 >5 >5	Tumor rupure Any Any Non-gastric Non-gastric

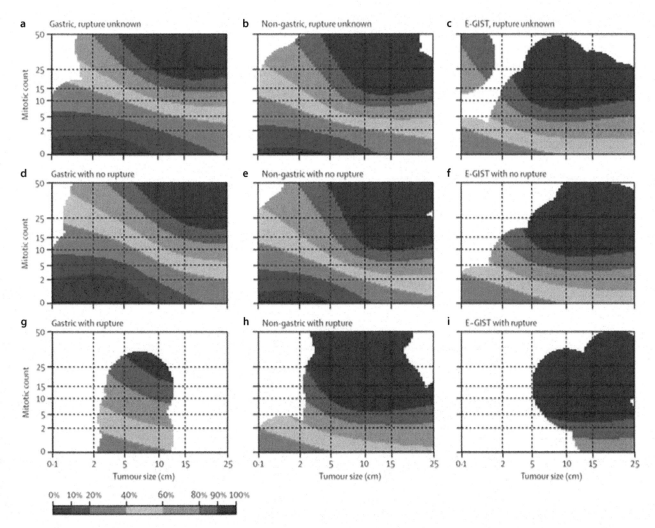

■ **Fig. 59.13** Prognostic heat map for the risk assessment

In the future, also the *molecular profiling* of GISTs should be considered in risk classification systems. For example, GIST with exon 11 mutation has a higher risk of relapse than GIST WT.

Tumor mutational status is particularly important in GIST because it is predictive of response to TKI treatment, but has also a prognostic value: the type of mutation affects prognosis in metastatic disease. Patients with advanced GISTs and *KIT exon 11 mutation* have the superior prognosis and the longest progression-free survival (PFS) compared with *exon 9 mutations* or patients lacking both KIT and PDGFRA, who have less favorable PFS [15].

59.1.8 GIST Management

Prior to the advent of the tyrosine kinase inhibitors (TKIs), there were few treatment options available to patients with advanced GIST; the response rate to conventional chemotherapy agents was extremely low and the survival generally measured in few months [16].

Advances in understanding the molecular background of GIST allow the identification of abnormal receptor tyrosine kinase (RTK) signaling and the development of specific TKI, such as the first approved imatinib, that has become a paradigm for molecularly targeted therapies in solid tumors [17].

59.1.8.1 Focus on Imatinib (◘ Fig. 59.14)

59.1.9 The Medical Treatment

59.1.9.1 Advanced and Metastatic GIST

In locally advanced inoperable and metastatic GIST patients, imatinib is the standard first-line treatment. The standard dose of imatinib is 400 mg daily. A higher dosage (800 mg/day) demonstrated a PFS advantage for KIT exon 9-mutated GISTs, despite no difference in overall survival (OS) and is endorsed by the NCCN, ESMO, and AIOM guidelines.

> Treatment should be continued indefinitely, since treatment interruption is generally followed by relatively rapid tumor progression.
>
> Imatinib achieved disease control in 70–85% of patients, but, despite the high response rate, the median time to progression (TTP) is approximately 24 to 30 months.
>
> Median OS is approximately 57–60 months
>
> 5–23% of patients show a durable response lasting for more than 10 years.
>
> 10–15% of patients show progressive disease to imatinib within 3/6 months of starting therapy (primary resistance) and show stronger correlation with certain genotypes. These tumors most commonly are those with mutations in PDGFRA, particularly the D842V mutation in exon 18, or those lacking mutations in either KIT or PDGFRA.

— Despite the high efficacy of imatinib, virtually all metastatic GISTs will become resistant due to additional acquired mutation in KIT.
Secondary or acquired resistance to imatinib, it develops in the large proportion of patients who demonstrate disease control and ultimately develop progressive disease, usually within 2–3 years [18].

59.1.9.2 Molecular Profile of Primary and Secondary Resistance

> The **primary resistance** arises in GSTs with no identifiable KIT or PDGFRA mutations is likely due to different mechanisms causing the disease development and activation of alternative signaling pathways. Therefore, treatment of these GISTs with the targeted agents other than imatinib, such as VEGFR, BRAF or MEK inhibitors, might be a better clinical alternative
> (Janeway et al, 2009)

In 1996, Druker and colleagues published their identification of a small molecule TKI, now known as imatinib, that can *selectively block the ABL kinase activity and induce cell death of BCR-ABL positive chronic myeloid lymphoma (CML) cells* (Druker et al, 1996).

Concurrently imatinib was shown **not only specific to BCR-ABL,** but *also blocks the enzymatic activity of the trasnmembrane receptor tyrosine kinases KIT and PDGFRA.* (Buchdunger, 2000; Heinrich, 2000a)

Imatinib binds to the ATP-binding site located in the amino-terminal lobe of the kinase domain that **competitively blocks ATP binding and consequent phosphorylation of KIT** (fig. 1.11).

Inhibition of mutant receptor KIT by imatnib led to GIST cell growth arrest and apoptosis (Tuveson, 2001).

Therafter, clinical development of imatinib for GIST therapy repidly progressed and has been considered the **standard first-line therapy** *for inoperable or metastatic GISTs since its approval in 2002.*

*IN 2008, FDA approved **adjuvant use of imatinib** for patients with high risk of recurrence.*

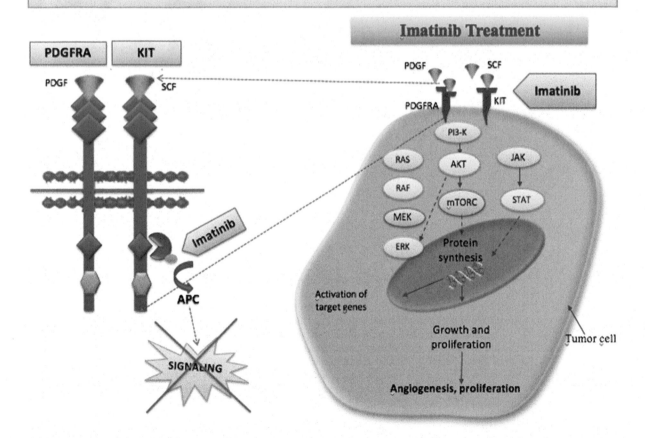

Fig. 59.14 Mechanism of action of imatinib

- Mutations in *exon 9* affect the extracellular KIT domain, mimicking the conformation change when SCF binds to the receptor, which induces higher degree of dimerization (Yuzawa et al., 2007). Since this mutation does not interfere with the kinase domain, exon 9 mutated KIT has the kinase domain same as the wild-type KIT, in which decreased sensitivity to imatinib was observed in vitro compared to exon 11 mutant KIT (Corless et al., 2011). Dose escalation is suggested for treatment of GISTs harboring these mutations (MetaGIST, 2010).

- Both clinical and in vitro studies have reported that *PDGFRA D842V mutation* is strongly resistant to imatinib (Corless et al., 2005; Heinrich et al., 2008a; Weisberg et al., 2006). This mutation results in a change in the kinase activation loop that strongly favors the active conformation of the kinase domain, which consequently disfavors imatinib binding (Gajiwala et al., 2009; Heinrich et al., 2003a). Patients with D842V-mutant GISTs show low response rates and short progression-free and overall survival during imatinib treatment (Biron et al., 2010).

- In addition to mutations, *gene amplification of KIT or PDGFRA* was shown as a potential mechanism leading to either primary or secondary resistance (Debiec-Rychter et al., 2005; Liegl et al., 2008; Miselli et al., 2007).

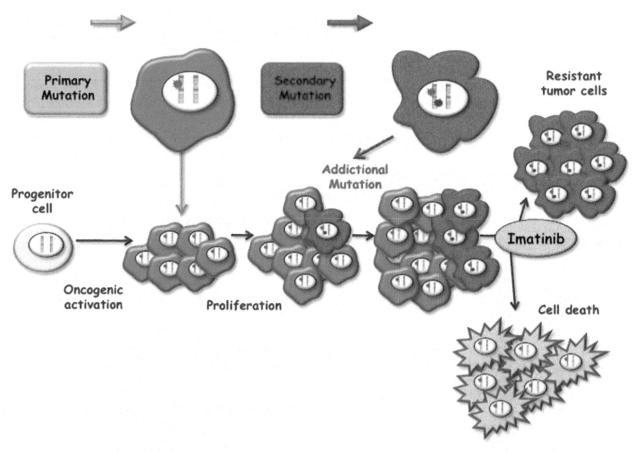

Secondary mutations is the main known mechanism for deveoping imatinib acquired resistance (Antonescu et al, 2005; Grimpen et al, 2005; Heinrich et al. 2006).
The most common mechanism is the occurrence of secondary mutations in the same gane that was originally activated and that render these clones resistant to imatinib (clonal evolution).
The most common secondary mutations occur in the ATP-binding pocket (encoded by exon 13 and 14) and in the kinase activation loop (encoded by exons 17 and 18).

59.1.9.3 Type of Progression

Most of the imatinib-resistant tumors exhibit inter- and intratumor heterogeneity (Liegl et al., 2008; Loughrey et al., 2006; Wardelmann et al., 2006): different types of secondary mutations across the multiple nodules of the same patient, and in different areas of the same tumor, cause the onset of resistant subclones.

This heterogeneity has important implications onto the efficacy of second-line TKI therapy after the first-line imatinib treatment.

The type of progression disease (PD) evaluated with CT scan can be distinguished into different groups:

- *Dimensional PD*: characterized exclusively by dimensional growth of pre-existing lesions
- *Numerical PD*: characterized by the occurrence of new lesions
- *Mixed PD*: characterized by both dimensional and numerical PD
- Exists also a "focal progression" into a lesion in previous response to the treatment, the so-called nodule in the nodule (Fig. 59.15)

59.1.9.4 Strategies to Overcome the Resistance

- *Second-line treatment*
  For GIST patients who progress on the standard dose of imatinib (400 mg daily), both imatinib dose escalation (800 mg daly) and sunitinib are feasible options.

- *Imatinib 800* mg daily should be considered for patients who was started on first-line imatinib 400 mg daily and experienced disease progression, on the basis of two large dose finding randomized phase III trials 14–15.
- *Sunitinib*, an oral multitarget tyrosine kinase inhibitor with high selectivity for KIT and PDGFRα, is an alternative strategy to overcome resistance for imatinib-refractory patients. In a randomized phase III trial, sunitinib 50 mg 4 weeks on and 2 off improved significantly PFS over placebo in second-line setting for those patients who had progression to first-line imatinib 17. However, sunitinib 37.5 mg continuously seems to be similarly effective and safe to sunitinib standard dose.
  The degree of disease control, including length of PFS and median OS, is significantly higher in patients whose GIST is with primary exon 9 mutation in KIT or those with no mutations in either KIT or PDGFRA.
- *Third-line treatment*
  Regorafenib is a recent third-line standard of care for metastatic GISTs resistant to both imatinib and sunitinib [19].
  Besides KIT and PDGFRA, this TKI also inhibits VEGFR1–3, TEK, RET, RAF1, BRAF, and BRAFV600E and FGFR (Wilhelm et al., 2011). Similar to sunitinib, regorafenib delayed the progression of patients for only 3.9 months compared to the placebo treatment (Demetri et al., 2013).

 Fig. 59.15 Type of progression to imatinib in metastatic disease

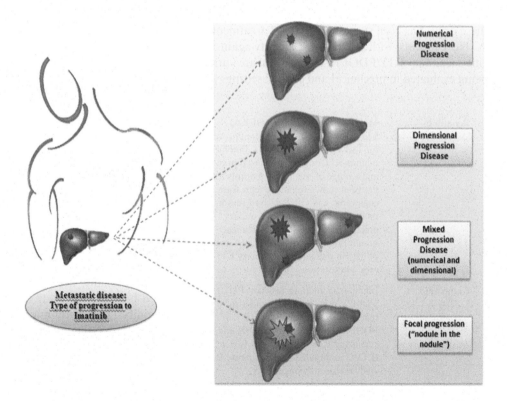

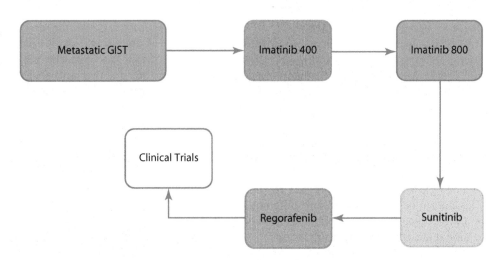

◘ Fig. 59.16 Therapeutic algorithm for Metastatic GIST

For patients progressing to regorafenib, inclusion in clinical trials is indicated. In the absence of clinical trials, an option may be the treatment rechallenge with imatinib [20, 21] (◘ Fig. 59.16).

59.1.9.5 New Therapeutic Targets and Treatments to Overcome Resistance to TKI

Several alternative TKI targeting KIT/PDGFRA (nilotinib, masatinib, sorafenib, dovitinib, pazopanib), multiple RTK (crizotinib, cabozantinib), or downstream signaling pathways (buparlisib, alpelisib, binimetinib) were studied in GIST patients with resistance to approved TKI.

Many clinical trials testing the compounds alone and in combination are ongoing, but unfortunately, none of these drugs has been registered for GIST treatment.

Novel agents, with an enhanced activity against specific secondary KIT/PDGFRA mutations, are currently being evaluated in preclinical and clinical settings [22].

Ponatinib	Multitarget inhibitor (PDGFRA, VEGFR2, FGFR1, and Src) approved for TKI-refractory leukemia. Potently inhibits KIT exon 11 primary mutants and a range of secondary mutants and has been shown to induce regression in engineered and GIST-derived tumor models containing these secondary mutations. Demonstrated a clinical benefit rate (CR, PR, or SD ≥16 weeks) of 55% in patients with primary KIT exon 11 mutation
Crenolanib	Inhibits the imatinib-resistant PDGFRA p.D842V-mutated kinase and also reduced the expression of KIT/PDGFRA by inhibiting MAPK and stabilizing ETS translocation variant 1 (ETV1) in mutated GIST. A phase III study is currently ongoing

BLU-285 (a vapritinib)	Highly selective inhibitor of KIT exon 17 mutations was also found to inhibit PDGFRA p.D842V mutant activity. Preliminary data from clinical trial showed a tumor reduction in all PDGFRA p.D842V-mutated patients
PLX9486 (Plexxikon)	Had an inhibitory effect on proliferation in a TKI-resistant PDX model (KIT exon 11 + 17), where its activity was more pronounced than imatinib. Currently, is evaluated alone and also in combination with pexidartinib
DCC-2618 (ripretibib)	Switch-control tyrosine kinase inhibitor active against a broad spectrum of KIT and PDGFRA mutations, under evaluation in clinical trials

59.1.9.6 Role of Medical Treatment in Localized Disease

Given the efficacy of imatinib in the metastatic setting, the use of imatinib has been extended to the *adjuvant setting* for the treatment of adult patients following GIST resection.

Risk stratification is essential to identify and better define the patients with GIST who are most likely to benefit from adjuvant imatinib therapy.

Three randomized phase III clinical trials have examined the use of imatinib 400 mg daily as an adjuvant for 1, 2, and 3 years; all three showed that it extends recurrence-free survival (RFS) in comparison with placebo or surveillance.

Additionally, the initial and long-term results provided by the AIO study demonstrated that 3 years of imatinib significantly improves RFS and OS compared with 1 year of therapy.

According to survival findings in the AIO trial, 3 years of adjuvant imatinib therapy are recommended for patients with GIST with high-risk features.

59

Fig. 59.17 Treatment strategy for GIST; LR: Low risk; IR: intermediate risk; HR: high risk; Njd:

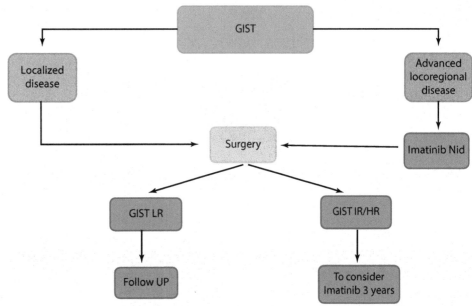

Moreover, two randomized trials are ongoing in high-risk GIST patients: a Scandinavian study comparing 5 years with 3 years and a French study comparing 6 years to 3 years of imatinib.

The use of adjuvant imatinib is not recommended for low risk and very low risk, but there is no consensus for intermediate risk. In this situation, the risks and benefits of treatment should be shared with the patient.

In the *neoadjuvant setting,* its preoperative use is proposed in tumor bulk reduction in order to ease complete surgical resection or make organ preservation more likely in initially unresectable or borderline resectable disease. Imatinib should be continued for 6–9 months but not extended beyond 12 months because of the risk of imatinib resistance and of usually minor additional tumor shrinkage

If an adjuvant or neoadjuvant treatment is indicated, the mutational analysis is required to predict the response to treatment with imatinib [23, 24] (Fig. 59.17).

neoadjuvant

59.1.10 **Response Evaluation**

Response evaluation is complex, and early progression should be confirmed by an experienced team. Antitumor activity translates into tumor shrinkage in the majority of patients, but some patients may show changes only in tumor density on CT scan, or these changes may precede delayed tumor shrinkage. These changes in tumor radiological appearance should be considered as the tumor response. Even increase in the tumor size, in particular, may be indicative of the tumor response if the tumor density on CT scan is decreased. Even the "appearance" of new lesions may be due to their being more evident when becoming less dense [25].

Therefore, both tumor size and tumor density on CT scan, or consistent changes in MRI or contrast-enhanced ultrasound, should be considered as criteria for tumor response. An FDG-PET scan has proved to be highly sensitive in early assessment of tumor response and may be useful in cases where there is doubt, or when early prediction of the response is particularly useful (e.g., preoperative cytoreductive treatments) (Fig. 59.18).

A small proportion of GISTs have no FDG uptake, however. The absence of tumor progression at 6 months after months of treatment also amounts to a tumor response. On the other hand, tumor progression may not be accompanied by changes in the tumor size. In fact, some increase in the tumor density within tumor lesions may be indicative of tumor progression. A typical progression pattern is the "nodule within the mass," by which a portion of a responding lesion becomes hyperdense [24, 26].

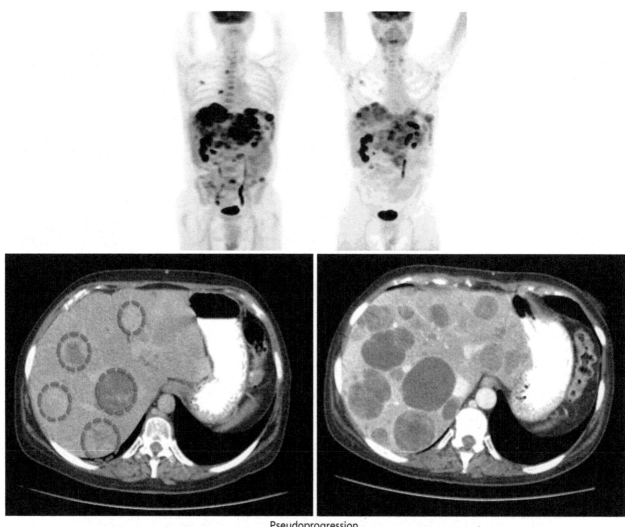

Pseudoprogression

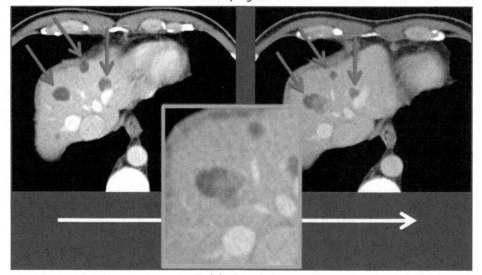

Nodular Progression

Fig. 59.18 Effect of imatinib therapy using positron emission tomography on fluorodeoxyglucose (FDG) levels: tumors that had a robust response to imatinib present a significant decrease in FDG signal, even within 24 hours of the first dose (Van den Abbeele & Badawi, 2002)

59

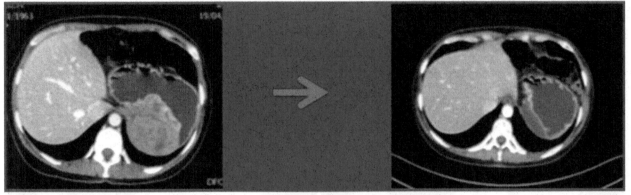

RECIST Response

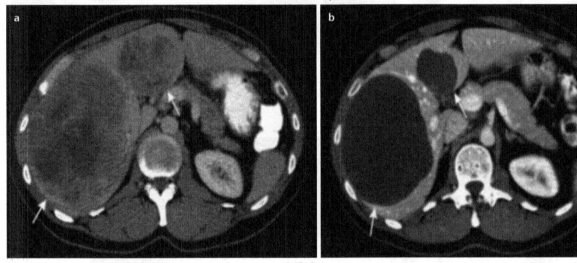

CHOI Response

◻ **Fig. 59.18** (continued)

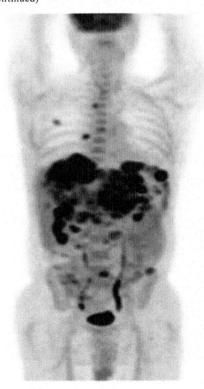
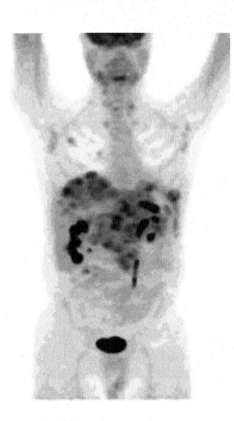

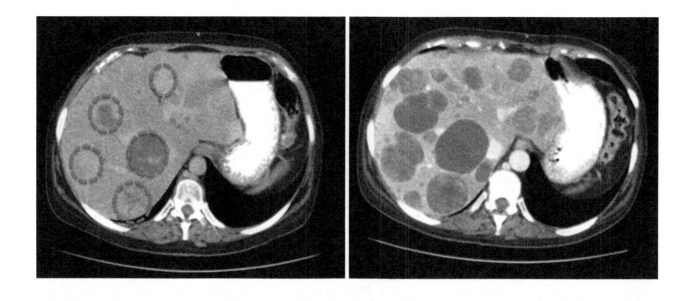

Pseudoprogression

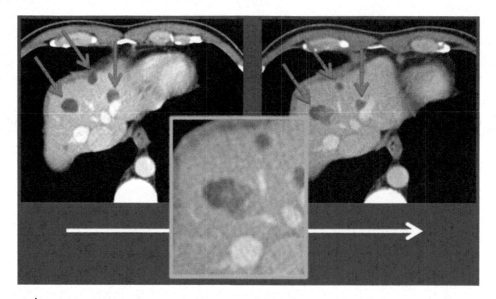

59

Nodular Progression

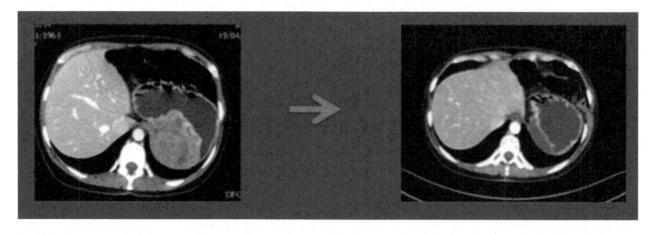

RECIST Response

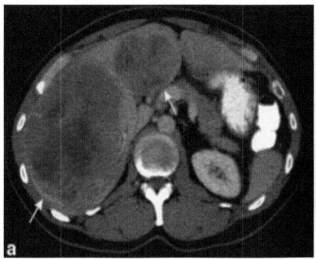 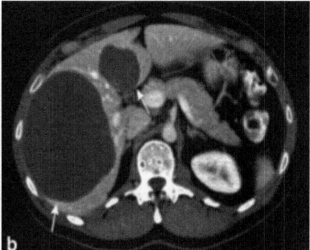

CHOI Response

59.2 The Role of Surgery in the Management of GIST

Sinziana Dumitra and Alessandro Gronchi

59.2.1 Introduction

While the management and ultimately survival of GIST was revolutionized at the dawn of the twenty-first century with the discovery of the *c-kit* tyrosine kinase mutations [27, 28] and that of targeted therapy [29], allowing disease control in a historically difficult to manage disease [30–36], surgical management remains the cornerstone of GISTs management and is based on the phase of disease at presentation. While a well-established and valid staging system is not currently in use for GIST, however a practical way to conceptualize this disease and its surgical management is to think of it as localized, locally advanced, or metastatic disease.

59.2.2 Localized GIST

Much of the surgical management of GIST truly depends on the primary site of disease occurrence; the most common site being stomach (50%), followed by small bowel (25%), and colon and rectum (10%) [37–41]. There are some reports of less common locations of GIST, namely, omentum, mesentery, and retroperitoneum [42]. The overall disease prognosis depends on size, location, mitotic count, and tumor rupture [43]. While the surgical options might differ based on location, the principles of an oncologic surgical resection

remain the same. First of all, it is important to thoroughly inspect the abdomen to ensure absence of peritoneal metastases. Secondly, achieving negative resection margins over the organ of origin is recommended, even if a clear association between quality of surgical margins and disease free and overall survival has not been demonstrated [37], save for rectal GIST. This is mainly due to the variety of presentations, with the majority of GIST having an intra-abdominal growth. When the tumor is confined to the GI wall, quality of surgical margins is likely to be more critical. A main advantage in GIST is that compared to other sarcomas and adenocarcinomas margins need be less wide, allowing for less extensive and morbid surgery. Thirdly, surgeons should manipulate GISTS with great care as not to rupture these friable tumors. Lastly, given that these stromal tumors rarely metastasize to lymph nodes, a lymphadenectomy is not performed routinely unless the presence of suspicious nodes is detected preoperatively.

59.2.3 Gastric GIST

Adequate preoperative assessment includes imaging as well as upper endoscopy. In the stomach, GIST often presents as an exophytic mass that can be easily resected or wedged out with the aid of a stapler (◘ Fig. 59.19, panel a). While the authors believe that all GISTs should be resected given the fact, some have argued for potential observation at smaller sizes (<2 cm) after discussion with the patient [44]. It is important to highlight that symptomatic GIST (e.g., bleeding, perforation, obstruction) should undergo resection. Emerging endoscopic techniques have also been successful in adequately

Panel A   Panel B   Panel C

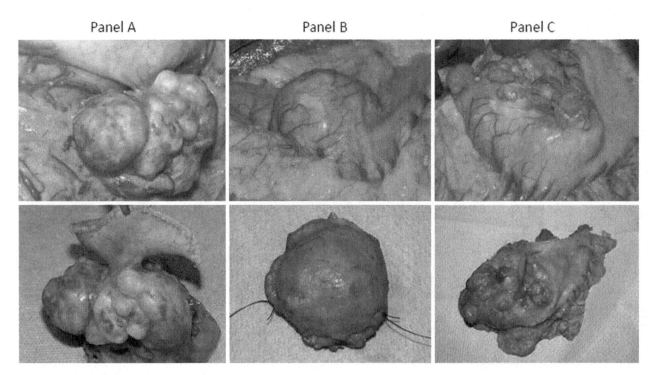

◘ Fig. 59.19 Macroscopic appearance of gastric GIST and its implication for surgical management: extraluminal growth, which can be resected with a wedge mechanical suture in panel **a**; intralumi-nal growth, which can be resected conservatively with a wedge manual suture in panel **b**; multinodular growth, which can only be resected with a conventional subtotal/total gastrectomy in panel **c**

removing gastric small (i.e., <2 cm) GIST [45, 46]. These are particularly useful in patients with multiple comorbidities who could not undergo a surgical procedure or as an alternative to active surveillance.

If larger non-exophytic GISTs are encountered often times, a large resection can be avoided by simply incising the gastric wall and resecting the tumor with an adequate margin, under direct vision, and subsequently closing the gastric wall by approximating the edges (◘ Fig. 59.19, panel b). This allows for a controlled gastric wedge, while avoiding resecting a large portion of the stomach. A particular case where great care needs to be taken when resecting a gastric GIST is one at or close to the gastroesophageal (GE) junction; a 32 French bougie should be utilized to ensure that the GE junction remains patent and sufficiently wide after wedge resection. These patients need to be carefully assessed in the preoperative setting and if a gastoesophageal resection would be necessary in order to obtain negative margins; then neoadjuvant targeted therapy should be considered in order to spare such an extensive resection and anastomosis. Very rarely is a subtotal or total gastrectomy required for GIST. Likewise multivisceral resections, including pancreas, spleen, and liver, are rarely required, as the tumor can often be separated from surrounding organs. However, when this is anticipated not to be the case, a preoperative therapy with imatinib should be considered, unless the tumor harbors an insensitive

mutation, such as PDGFRA D842V, or belongs to the SDH-deficient subgroup, both insensitive to imatinib and all other approved TKIs. Finally, SDH-deficient GIST is predominantly located to the stomach and is multifocal (◘ Fig. 59.19, panel c). As a result of this specific subgroup, subtotal/total gastrectomy is more often required, along with regional lymphadenectomy, as lymph node metastases are more common.

An important surgical modality to discuss is the utilization of laparoscopic surgery in GIST that allows for a faster recovery, shorter hospital stay, and decreased overall costs of care. Recent studies and meta-analyses did not identify oncologic outcome differences when using laparoscopic surgery when compared to open [47–49]. Even in studies assessing larger GIST >5 cm, oncologic results were similar [50]. The authors do caution in case of large tumors to ensure the extraction site is large enough and suggest the tumor be extracted in a specimen bag as to avoid rupture and spillage. Of note, imatinib therapy can be used to downsize the tumor and allow a laparoscopic procedure.

59.2.4 Duodenal GIST

The surgical management of duodenal GISTs can be more challenging and greatly depends on size as well as the portion of the duodenum affected. The most com-

☐ Fig. 59.20 Macroscopic appearance of a duodenal GIST occurring on the 2nd portion of the duodenum and its implication for surgical management: antimesenteric growth, which can be resected conservatively with a wedge manual primary suture (or at times with a jejunal loop interposition) in panel **a**; mesenteric growth, which can be resected only with a pancreaticoduodenectomy and a Whipple reconstruction (pancreatic [A], biliary [B] and gastrointestinal [C] anastomoses) in panel **b**

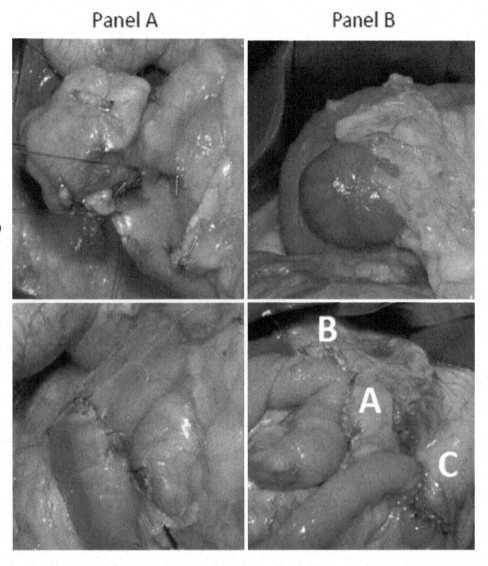

mon site of duodenal GIST occurrence is the second portion followed by the third, fourth, and finally the first portion of the duodenum [51, 52].

Another important limitation that might not allow for a local excision is whether the tumor occurs on the mesenteric or non-mesenteric side [52]. Given the risk of duodenal stricture, after an extensive Kocher maneuver, we suggest a wedge excision under direct vision and primary closure (☐ Fig. 59.20, panel a). If necessary, the common bile duct can be identified by using a pediatric feeding tube. More specific reconstructions are mandated by the size of the defect and the location (☐ Fig. 59.20, panel b).

As with GE junction tumors if they occur at the insertion of the bile duct in the D2 or D2-D3 area, for which a pancreaticoduodenectomy might be required to obtain an adequate negative margin excision, then neo-adjuvant therapy is suggested in order to downsize the tumor and allow for a less morbid resection. In our experience, the extent of surgery does not confer a disease-free or survival advantage [53].

59.2.5 Small Bowel GIST

Small bowel GISTs can have widely varying presentations such as palpable masses, obstruction, bleeding, and rupture, and more increasingly often they present incidentally based on imaging or endoscopy. Their prognosis varies widely based on size and mitotic count [54]. Surgery upfront should be offered upfront when disease is limited. Often time small bowel GIST is easily amenable to resection and can even be considered for laparoscopic resection [55]. Often times it is much easier to proceed to a segmental resection and primary anastomosis rather than perform a wedge resection (☐ Fig. 59.21, panel a). GIST associated to neurofibromatosis type 1 is predominantly located to the small bowel and is virtually always multifocal (☐ Fig. 59.21, panel b). Their risk does not depend in the number of lesions, while it depends on the features of the most aggressive one. Surgical resection may be directed only to remove the one or the ones at high risk, as removing

Fig. 59.21 Macroscopic appearance of a small bowel GIST and its implication for surgical management: single nodule, which can be resected with a simple small bowel segmental resection in panel **a**; multiple nodules (typical scenario in Neurofibromatosis type 1 patients), which can be resected with a more extended small bowel resection

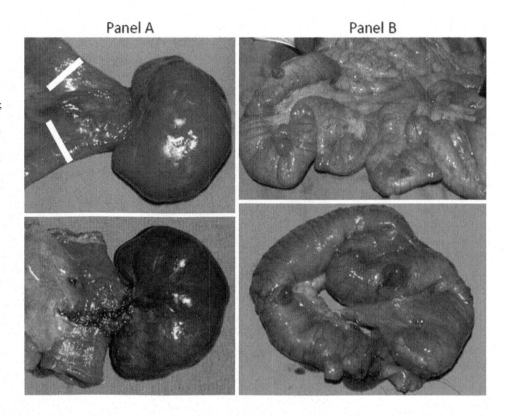

Panel A   Panel B

all lesions may at times require an extended procedure followed by short bowel syndrome.

59.2.6 Rectal GIST

The most common site of presentation of colonic GIST is the lower rectum. Rectal GIST, while rare, often displays a more aggressive behavior than GISTs occurring in other locations [56]; indeed even small GISTs <2 cm with mitotic activity can recur and even metastasize [57]. Indeed, local recurrence rates are much higher than at other locations even after correcting for number of mitoses. Studies have shown that obtaining R0 margins of resection is paramount in rectal cancer for disease-free survival and overall survival. Neoadjuvant treatment with imatinib is associated with improved survival [58]. Depending on the size of the tumor, local approach to resection can be performed via transanal, transarcral, or perineal approaches (Fig. 59.22, panel a). It is important when performing a resection to achieve a complete removal of the tumor-bearing rectal wall and the tumor-covering tissue layer as GISTs originate from the muscularis propria and not the mucosa [58]. Often times if rectal GISTs are large and not amenable to local resection, abdominal resection or abdominoperineal resections should be undertaken (Fig. 59.22, panel b). There have been some case reports of laparoscopic techniques being used in rectal tumor resection, but the

authors believe it should be undertaken only in small tumors when rupture-free and negative resection can be achieved.

59.2.7 Locally Advanced GIST

Perhaps, one of the important indications for neoadjuvant treatment is in the case of locally advanced borderline resectable GIST. Indeed, the conceptual advantage of therapy in these patients is twofold: first, the potential to avoid a multiorgan resection and organ preservation, thanks to tumor downstaging and the increased ability to obtain R0-negative resection margins (Fig. 59.23, panel a, b). Another advantage is the fact that treatment can render the tumor less vascular and friable allowing for easier manipulation and decreased risk of rupture which is key especially in larger or difficult to access tumors (Fig. 59.23, panel c, d) [59]. The use of imatinib prior to surgical intervention was based initially on institutional series demonstrating good radiologic responses of 60–70% with disease-free survival rates of 70% at 3 years [59]. In the radiation therapy oncology group, RTOG 0132 trial assesses the use of neoadjuvant imatinib in patients with locally advanced disease among others. Despite the short duration of neoadjuvant treatment in this cohort, the rate of R0 resection was 77%, quiet high in this fairly high-risk group [60]. A much larger 10 center retrospective study

Fig. 59.22 Macroscopic appearance of a rectal GIST and its implication for surgical management: small nodule, which can be resected with a local approach in panel **a**; big tumor, occupying the whole pelvis, which can only be removed with an abdominoperineal resection in panel **b**

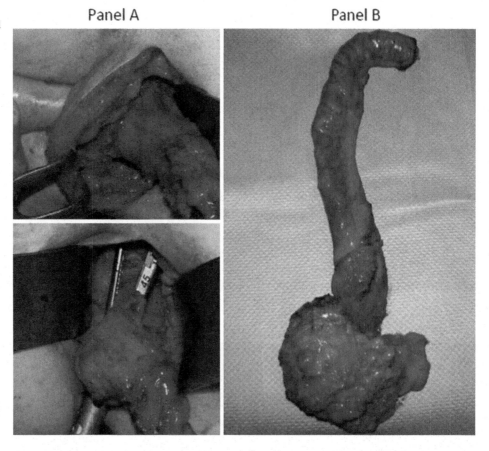

Panel A   Panel B

of neoadjuvant treatment with imatinib until maximal response was achieved or the lesion was no longer borderline. While the rate of R0 resection was of 80%, the rate of recurrence was 23% at 46 months [61].

There are particular clinical scenarios where neoadjuvant treatment is particularly important as tumor location might require an extensive, morbid resection with more complex long-term effects. In GISTs of the gastroesophageal junction, a two-cavity approach may be avoided by downstaging the tumor as it would be the case for duodenal GISTs where three patient might be spared a pancreaticoduodenectomy with all the possible morbidity it entails. Another important scenario is that of rectal GISTs where sphincter might be preserved and continence maintained, improving the patient's quality of life.

As impressive as the results obtained with neoadjuvant therapy, it is paramount for the surgeons to regularly assess the response to treatment. Indeed while the duration of preoperative treatment varies widely in the literature between 12 and 40 weeks and it does seem that optimal time for intervention is situated somewhere between 6 and 12 months. It is critical to assess response to treatment at the initiation of therapy and to continue this assessment regularly as not to miss the window of

resectabilty. Moreover, the resection should occur ideally before the development of clonal resistance to the drug given.

59.2.8 Metastatic GIST

The main goal in the treatment of metastatic GIST at presentation is disease control, and the only way to do so is via systemic treatment as can be demonstrated by historical series where debulkings were attempted with dismal results with 25% median survival at 5 years [62]. While there remains a fervent debate on the utility of surgery in the setting of metastatic disease, there are some clinical scenarios in which patients might benefit from metastasectomy. The main rationale behind cytoreductive surgery in the era of third and even fourth line systemic therapy for GISTs is the concept of clonal resistance and the delay of subsequent lines of therapy [59]. It is important to recall that imatinib and other targeted therapies are not cytotoxic; rather, they produce cell senescence; they thus do not provide a cure for GIST.

Multiple institutional series have described promising results in disease control [63, 64]; however, patient

Panel A

Panel C

Panel B

Panel D

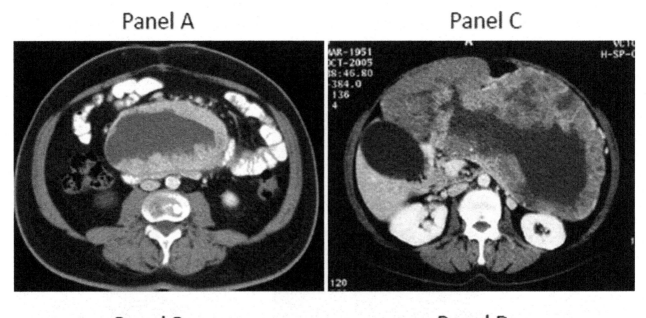

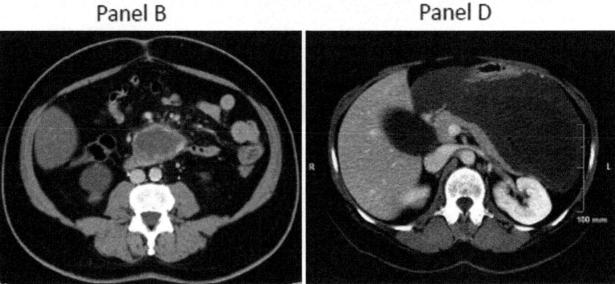

☐ Fig. 59.23 Contrast enhanced CT scan, venous phase, of a primary large duodenal GIST abutting superior mesenteric vessels before (panel **a**) and after (panel **b**) 12 months of medical therapy with Imatinib: a major shrinkage has occurred, improving quality of surgical margins. Contrast enhanced CT scan, venous phase, of a primary large necrotic and highly vascularized gastric GIST before (panel **c**) and after (panel **d**) 12 months of medical therapy with Imatinib: no shrinkage has occurred, but an important change in tumor density has taken place with a significant reduction of vascularization, which makes tumor resection much less at risk of tumor rupture and safer

selection and optimal intervention timing are key when performing metastasectomies [65]. Indeed, patients with localized, persistent, and slow-growing metastases seem to benefit from surgical intervention much more than those with multifocal progression [59]. This might be secondary to the limited ability to obtain a complete debulkings in patients with multifocal disease. In a the large multicenter study by Bauer et al., an important prognosis factor in the patients selected for resection is site of disease with disease limited to the liver surviving significantly longer than those with peritoneal disease

[63]. As with localized disease, the widow of opportunity after initiation of treatment with imatinib seems to be 6–12 months (☐ Fig. 59.24, panel a, b) [63].

Some groups have suggested that cytoreductive surgery should be offered at the outset in order to clear all macroscopic disease. However, retrospective series did not find a survival advantage of initiating the treatment sequence with surgery. Moreover, surgery at the outset did not delay the initiation of second-line treatment [66]. Indeed starting the treatment sequence with imatinib allows for disease biology to declare itself and enables

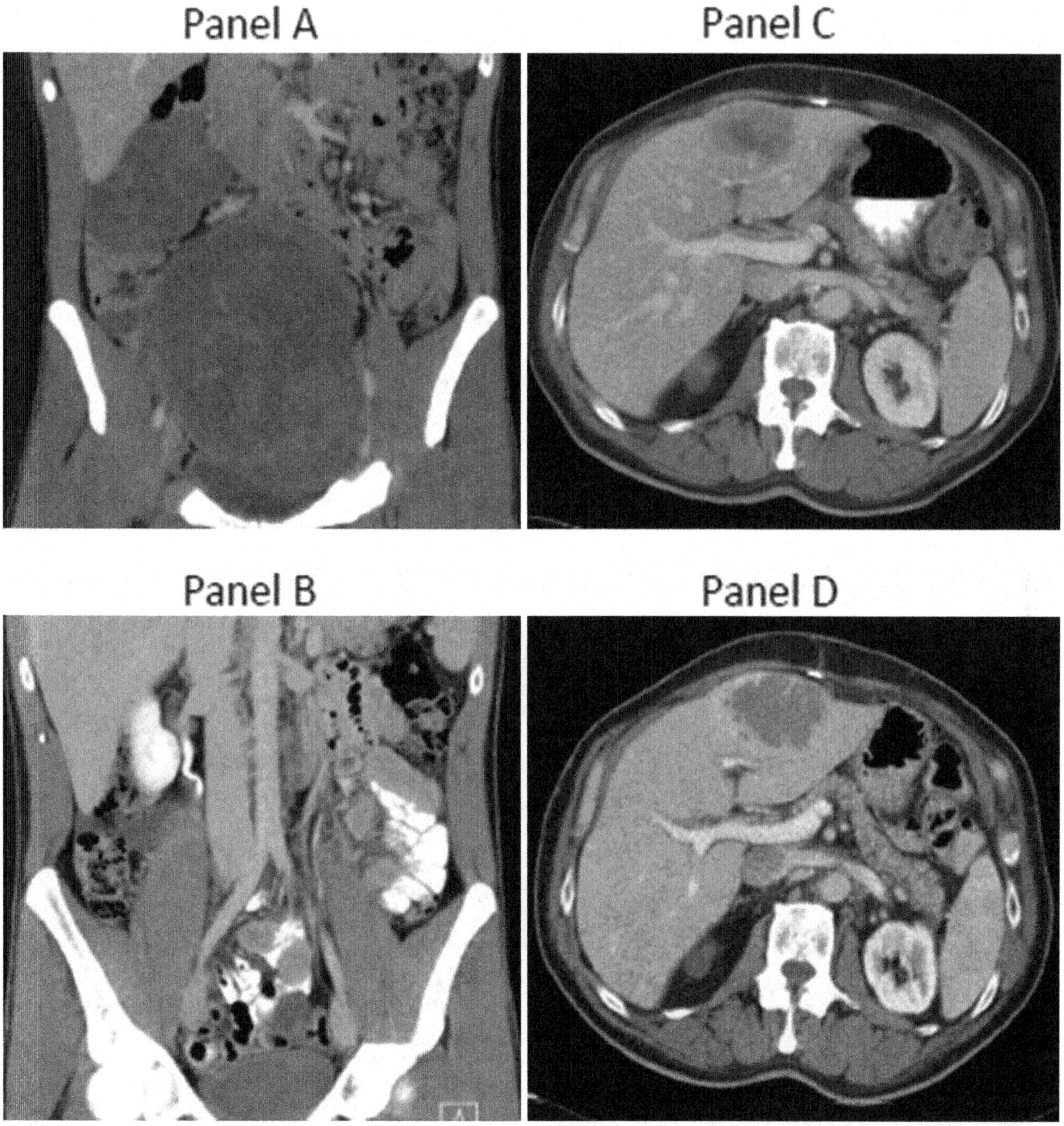

Panel A

Panel C

Panel B

Panel D

Fig. 59.24 Contrast enhanced CT scan, venous phase, of a large small bowel GIST metastatic to the peritoneum before (panel **a**) and after (panel **b**) 12 months of medical therapy with Imatinib: a major shrinkage has occurred of both primary and metastatic sites. Con-trast enhanced CT scan, venous phase, of a single GIST liver metas-tasis before (panel **c**) and after (panel **d**) progressing on Imatinib: surgical resection of the single liver nodule is an option to consider

selecting patients that will have a favorable response to intervention. Another important factor in the choice of timing of intervention is disease progression. Indeed, patients undergoing interventions at the time of pro-gression have shorter disease-free intervals postopera-tively than those in remission at the time of intervention [64]. However, the use of surgery in limited progression may be of help to postpone the switch to a further line

therapy, as this may maximize the time a patient stay on the given drug and therefore the control of the disease (■ Fig. 59.24, panel c, d) [63–65].

Another juncture when surgery could be considered for metastatic GIST is at the time of second-line therapy. In a study assessing survival in patients undergoing sur-gery for metastatic disease while on sunitinib, surgery was much less successful when compared to results described in patients on first-line therapy, with lower macroscopically negative excision rates, higher complication rates, and lower survival [67].

Finally, surgery may play a role in the subgroup of TKI-insensitive GIST (PDGFRA D842V-mutated GIST or SDH-deficient GIST), as the natural history is usually more indolent and patients may survive several years with metastatic disease. The same does not apply to metastatic NF1-associated GIST, the prognosis of which is generally very poor.

59.2.9 Conclusion

Surgery remains the cornerstone treatment modality in GIST and the only one to provide a cure. Surgical techniques and their roles in the continuum of care are dictated by disease location and stage. With the advent of targeted therapies has been an increased utilization of neo-adjuvant imatinib in the treatment of localized disease leading to increased rates of complete resection and an associated disease free survival benefit. While surgery for metastatic GIST does remain controversial, there are certain patients that may benefit from resection especially when the disease is stable on systemic treatment and limited or an isolated progression has occurred.

> **Summary of Clinical Recommendations**
> — *Linee Guida dell'Associazione Italiana di Oncologia Medica (AIOM)*
> — *Sarcomi dei Tessuti molli e GIST. Edizione 2019.*
> — *ESMO Clinical Practice Guidelines. Sarcoma and GIST.*
> — *Annals of Oncology 2018*
> — *NCCN (National Comprehensive Cancer Network) GUIDELINES FOR TREATMENT OF CANCER BY SITE-2018: Soft Tissue Sarcoma and GIST.*

Case Study Author: Please Indicate the Clinical Case TITLE Here

Man, 56 years old
- *Family history* negative for malignancy
- *APR:* Diabetes Mellitus type II
- *APP:* For nearly 2 months nausea and asthenia; diffuse abdominal pain
- *Objective examination*: Globose abdomen; mild tenderness on deep palpation (quadrant sup.sx); Palpable mass in the left hip
- *Blood tests*: Hb 9,1 g/dl; mildly impaired liver function tests (GOT; GPT)
- *Esofagogastroduodenoscopy*: Normal mucosa; compression of the gastric wall

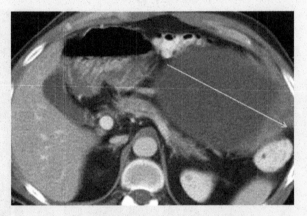

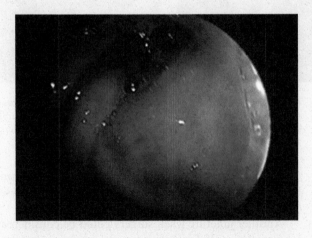

- *TC abdomen mdc*: Lesion of 34 × 23 × 10 cm in continuity with small curvature, no cleavage plane from the gastric wall
- No lymphadenopathies
- Peritoneal implants and multiple liver metastases

Question

What action should be taken?
  (1) Surgery (2) Biopsy (3) Other

Answer

Ecoendoscopy with biopsy
  Histological examination:
  GIST spindle cell; gastric origin
  CD 117+; 2 mitosis/50 hpf

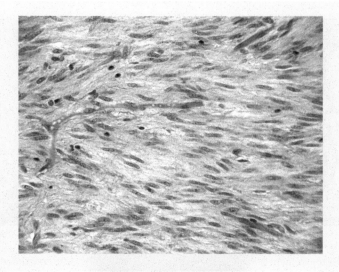

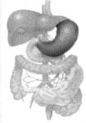

Gastric GIST   ⇨   Metastasis to liver and peritoneum   ⇨ Symptomatic patient

Question

What action should be taken?
(1) Surgery (2) Medical therapy (3) Mutational analysis

Answer

Mutational analysis: Exon 9 KIT mutation

⇩

Medical therapy: Imatinib 800 mg/die
Response evaluation after 3 months of therapy with Imatinib 800 mg/die: Complete metabolic response to PET-FDG

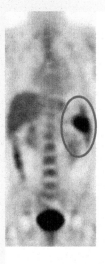 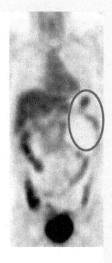

⇨

Before Imatinib   After 3 months of Imatinib

Response evaluation after 12 months of therapy with Imatinib 800 mg/die: Appears "nodule in nodule" that increases in size after a further 2 months (14 months of therapy with Imatinib 800 mg/die)

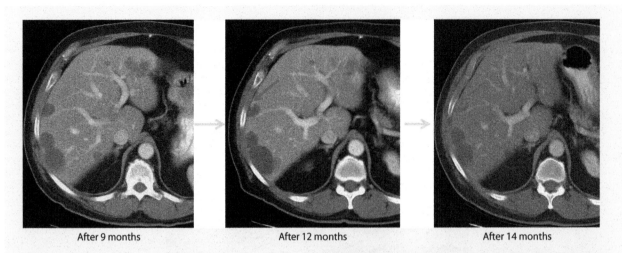

After 9 months   After 12 months   After 14 months

Question

What action should be taken?

(1) Sunitinib (2) Regorafenib (3) Continues Imatinib 800

Answer

Begins Sunitinib 37.5 mg/die

Response evaluation after 3 months of therapy with Sunitinib 37.5 mg/die:

Tissue response to TC

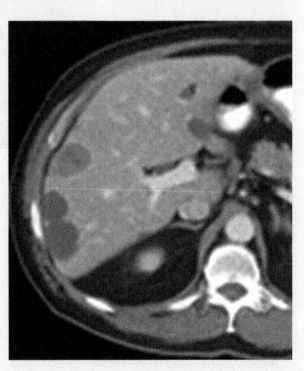

Key Points

— The importance of a correct diagnosis: attention to the large bowel masses
— Symptoms often nonspecific; mucosa normally not involved
— The importance of a correct evaluation of the response
— Importance of mutational analysis in the therapeutic choice

Man, 56 years old

- *Family history* negative for malignancy
- *APR*: negative
- *APP*: asthenia, dyspepsia, change in bowel habit
- *Blood tests*: Hb 9,2 g/dl
- *TC Abdomen mdc*: Voluminous abdominal lesion of 10 × 9.5 × 8 cm. located between stomach, spleen, pancreas, transverse colon and the first ileal loops. (localized disease)

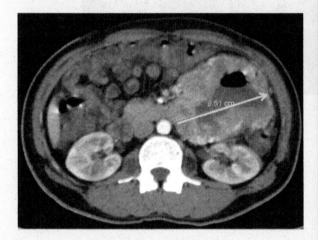

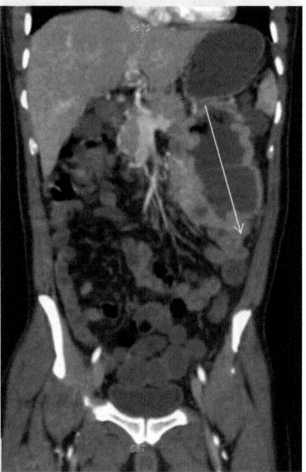

Question

What action should be taken?
   (1) Surgery (2) Biopsy (3) Other

Answer

Biopsy: GIST spindle cell, CD 117 + Mutational analysis: Exon 11 Kit mutation

Question

What action should be taken?
   (1) Surgery (2) Medical therapy (3) Other

Answer

Preoperative treatment: Imatinib 400 mg/die

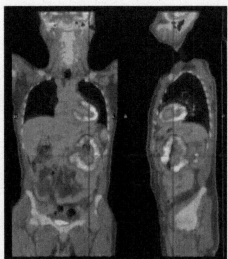 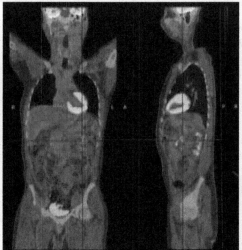

Before treatment   After 1 month of Imatinib

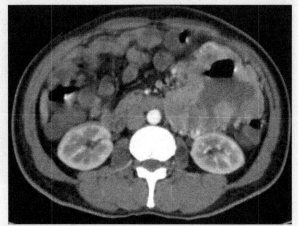

After 6 months of Imatinib: SD

Question

What action should be taken?
    (1) Surgery (2) Continues Imatinib (3) Other

Answer

Surgery: R0

Key Points

- Importance of preoperative biopsy:
- Differential diagnosis with other neoplasia: Other sarcomas, germ cell tumors and lymphomas not need the same surgery!
- Possibility of medical treatment preoperative: it would be desirable to know the mutated exon before deciding whether or not to initiate a preoperative treatment
- Is appropriate to assess early response by PET
- The maximum response is obtained after 6–12 month

59

Expert Opinion
Giuseppe Badalamenti

Key Points

GISTs are rare cancer that originate from the gastrointestinal tract; the most frequent location is stomach (55%), followed by small intestine (30%). Less frequent are colon/rectum (5%) and esophagus (<1%).

- Approximately 70% of GISTs are driven by mutations in the oncogene KIT; of those GISTs without KIT mutations, the majority harbor mutations in the gene encoding (PDGFRA) (15%). The remaining 15% of GISTs were described as KIT/PDGFRA "wild-type" GISTs.
- The mutational analysis is essential to predict the response to treatment with imatinib
- Surgery is the standard treatment in operable localized disease; locally advanced borderline resectable GIST or avoid multi-organ resection are the important indications for neoadjuvant treatment with imatinib. Surgery should be proposed between 6 and 12 months after starting a neoadjuvant treatment.
- In the case of high-risk GIST, an adjuvant treatment with imatinib for 3 years is the standard; in this case, the mutational analysis is mandatory to identify GISTs sensitive to imatinib.

- In metastatic setting, imatinib 400 mg is the standard treatment; in the case of GIST, exon 9 mutated, the treatment with imatinib high doses might be preferred. In the case of mutations resistant to imatinib, a clinical trial should be proposed.
- For GIST resistant to imatinib, sunitinib is indicated in the second line and regorafenib in the third line.
- Given the rarity of the pathology and the opportunity to participate in clinical trials, the patient's reference to highly experienced centers is always recommended.

Hints for Deeper Insight and Suggested Reading

- Recommendations for the implementation of mutational analysis and management of gastrointestinal stromal tumor (GIST) patients. Raccomandazioni 2019 per l'implementazione dell'analisi mutazionale e la gestione del paziente con Tumore Stromale Gastrointestinale (GIST). October 2019.
- Position paper of Italian Scientific Societies (AIOM – Fondazione AIOM – ISG – SIAPEC-IAP – SIBIOC – SICO – SIF). ▶ www.aiom.it
- Tailored management of primary gastrointestinal stromal tumors. Etherington MS, DeMatteo RP. Cancer. 2019. doi: 10.1002/cncr.32067.

References

The Role of Medical Treatment in the Management of GIST

1. De Matteo RP, Lewis JJ, Leung D, et al. Two hundred gastrointestinal stromal tumors: recurrence patterns and prognostic factors for survival. Ann Surg. 2000;231:51–8.
2. ESMO Guidelines Committee and EUROCAN. Soft tissue and visceral sarcomas: ESMO–EURACAN Clinical Practice Guidelines for diagnosis, treatment and follow-up. Ann Oncol. 2018;29(Suppl 4):iv1–iv17.
3. Fletcher CD, Berman JJ, Corless C, et al. Diagnosis of gastrointestinal stromal tumors: a consensus approach. Hum Pathol. 2002;33(5):33459–65.
4. Nannini M, Nigro MC, Vincenzi B, et al. Personalization of regorafenib treatment in metastatic gastrointestinal stromal tumours in real-life clinical practice. Ther Adv Med Oncol. 2017;9(12):731–9. https://doi.org/10.1177/1758834017742627.
5. Badalamenti G, Barraco N, Incorvaia L, et al. Are long noncoding rnas new potential biomarkers in gastrointestinal stromal tumors (GISTs). The role of H19 and MALAT1. J Oncol. 2019;2019:5458717. Published 2019 Nov 15. https://doi.org/10.1155/2019/5458717.

6. Vincenzi B, Nannini M, Badalamenti G, et al. Imatinib rechallenge in patients with advanced gastrointestinal stromal tumors following progression with imatinib, sunitinib and regorafenib. Ther Adv Med Oncol. 2018;10:1758835918794623. Published 2018 Aug 29. https://doi.org/10.1177/1758835918794623.
7. Fanale D, Incorvaia L, Badalamenti G, et al. Prognostic role of plasma PD-1, PD-L1, pan-BTN3As and BTN3A1 in patients affected by metastatic gastrointestinal stromal tumors: can immune checkpoints act as a sentinel for short-term survival?. Cancers (Basel). 2021;13(9):2118. Published 2021 Apr 27. https://doi.org/10.3390/cancers13092118.
8. Incorvaia L, Fanale D, Vincenzi B, et al. Type and Gene Location of KIT Mutations Predict Progression-Free Survival to First-Line Imatinib in Gastrointestinal Stromal Tumors: A Look into the Exon. Cancers (Basel). 2021;13(5):993. Published 2021 Feb 27. https://doi.org/10.3390/cancers13050993.
9. Corless C, Fletcher JA, Heinrich MC. Biology of gastrointestinal stromal tumors. J Clin Oncol. 2004;22:3813–25.
10. Miettinen M, Lasota J. Gastrointestinal stromal tumors. Review on morphology, molecular pathology, prognosis, and differential diagnosis. Arch Pathol Lab Med. 2006;130:1466–78.
11. del Cerro M, Ison JR, Bowen GP, Lazar E, del Cerro C. Intra-retinal grafting restores visual function in light-blinded rats. Neuroreport. 1991;2(9):529–32. https://doi.org/10.1097/00001756-199109000-00008.

12. Miettinen M, Lasota J. Gastrointestinal stromal tumors: pathology and prognosis at different sites. Semin Diagn Pathol. 2006;23:70–83.

13. Miettinen M, Killian JK, Wang ZF, Lasota J, et al. Immunohistochemical loss of succinate dehydrogenase subunit A (SDHA) in gastrointestinal stromal tumors (GISTs) signals SDHA germline mutation. Am J Surg Pathol. 2013;37:234–40.

14. Indio V, Astolfi A, Tarantino G, Urbini M, Patterson J, Nannini M, Saponara M, Gatto L, Santini D, Do Valle IF, Castellani G, Remondini D, Fiorentino M, Von Mehren M, Brandi G, Biasco G, Heinrich MC, Pantaleo MA. Integrated molecular characterization of gastrointestinal stromal tumors (GIST) harboring the rare D842V mutation in PDGFRA gene. Int J Mol Sci. 2018;19:732.

15. Dematteo RP, Heinrich MC, El-Rifai WM, Demetri G. Clinical management of gastrointestinal stromal tumors: before and after STI-571. Hum Pathol. 2002;33:466–77.

16. Pantuso G, Macaione I, Taverna A, et al. Surgical treatment of primary gastrointestinal stromal tumors (GISTs): Management and prognostic role of R1 resections. Am J Surg. 2020;220(2):359–64. https://doi.org/10.1016/j.amjsurg.2019.12.006.

17. Gold JS, Gönen M, Gutiérrez A, et al. Development and validation of a prognostic nomogram for recurrence-free survival after complete surgical resection of localised primary gastrointestinal stromal tumour: a retrospective analysis. Lancet Oncol. 2009;10:1045–52.

18. Dematteo RP, Heinrich MC, El-Rifai WM, Demetri G. Clinical management of gastrointestinal stromal tumors: before and after STI-571. Hum Pathol. 2002;33:466–77.

19. Nannini M, Rizzo A, Nigro MC, et al. Standard versus personalized schedule of regorafenib in metastatic gastrointestinal stromal tumors: a retrospective, multicenter, real-world study [published online ahead of print, 2021 Aug 2]. ESMO Open. 2021;6(4):100222. https://doi.org/10.1016/j.esmoop.2021.100222.

20. Vincenzi B, Nannini M, Badalamenti G, et al. Imatinib rechallenge in patients with advanced gastrointestinal stromal tumors following progression with imatinib, sunitinib and regorafenib. Ther Adv Med Oncol. 2018;10 https://doi.org/10.1177/1758835918794623.

21. Nannini M, Nigro MC, Vincenzi B, et al. Personalization of regorafenib treatment in metastatic gastrointestinal stromal tumours in real-life clinical practice. Ther Adv Med Oncol. 2017;9(12):731–9. https://doi.org/10.1177/1758834017742627. PMID: 29449894.

22. Rubin BP, Blanke CD, Demetri GD, et al. Protocol for the examination of specimens from patients with gastrointestinal stromal tumor. Arch Pathol Lab Med. 2010;134:165–70.

23. Rossi S, Miceli R, Messerini L, et al. Natural history of imatinib-naive GISTs: a retrospective analysis of 929 cases with long-term follow-up and development of a survival nomogram based on mitotic index and size as continuous variables. Am J Surg Pathol. 2011;35:1646–56.

24. Linee Guida AIOM 2018-Sarcomi dei Tessuti Molli e GIST.

25. Cannella R, Tabone E, Porrello G, et al. Assessment of morphological CT imaging features for the prediction of risk stratification, mutations, and prognosis of gastrointestinal stromal tumors. Eur Radiol. 2021. https://doi.org/10.1007/s00330-021-07961-3. PMID: 33881567.

26. Joensuu H, Vehtari A, Riihimäki J, et al. Risk of recurrence of gastrointestinal stromal tumor after surgery: an analysis of pooled population-based cohorts. Lancet Oncol. 2012;13:265–74.

The Role of Surgery in the Management of GIST

27. Hirota S, Isozaki K, Moriyama Y, et al. Gain-of-function mutations of c-kit in human gastrointestinal stromal tumors. Science. 1998;279:577–80.

28. Nakahara M, Isozaki K, Hirota S, et al. A novel gain-of-function mutation of c-kit gene in gastrointestinal stromal tumors. Gastroenterology. 1998;115:1090–5.

29. Joensuu H, Roberts PJ, Sarlomo-Rikala M, et al. Effect of the tyrosine kinase inhibitor STI571 in a patient with a metastatic gastrointestinal stromal tumor. N Engl J Med. 2001;344:1052–6.

30. Verweij J, Casali PG, Zalcberg J, et al. Progression-free survival in gastrointestinal stromal tumours with high-dose imatinib: randomised trial. Lancet. 2004;364:1127–34.

31. Dematteo RP, Ballman KV, Antonescu CR, et al. Adjuvant imatinib mesylate after resection of localised, primary gastrointestinal stromal tumour: a randomised, double-blind, placebo-controlled trial. Lancet. 2009;373:1097–104.

32. Joensuu H, Eriksson M, Sundby Hall K, et al. One vs three years of adjuvant imatinib for operable gastrointestinal stromal tumor: a randomized trial. JAMA. 2012;307:1265–72.

33. Blanke CD, Demetri GD, von Mehren M, et al. Long-term results from a randomized phase II trial of standard- versus higher-dose imatinib mesylate for patients with unresectable or metastatic gastrointestinal stromal tumors expressing KIT. J Clin Oncol. 2008;26:620–5.

34. Cassier PA, Fumagalli E, Rutkowski P, et al. Outcome of patients with platelet-derived growth factor receptor alpha-mutated gastrointestinal stromal tumors in the tyrosine kinase inhibitor era. Clin Cancer Res. 2012;18:4458–64.

35. Miettinen M, Wang ZF, Sarlomo-Rikala M, et al. Succinate dehydrogenase-deficient GISTs: a clinicopathologic, immunohistochemical, and molecular genetic study of 66 gastric GISTs with predilection to young age. Am J Surg Pathol. 2011;35:1712–21.

36. Bauer S, Joensuu H. Emerging agents for the treatment of advanced, imatinib-resistant gastrointestinal stromal tumors: current status and future directions. Drugs. 2015;75:1323–34.

37. DeMatteo RP, Lewis JJ, Leung D, et al. Two hundred gastrointestinal stromal tumors: recurrence patterns and prognostic factors for survival. Ann Surg. 2000;231:51–8.

38. Miettinen M, Sarlomo-Rikala M, Sobin LH, Lasota J. Gastrointestinal stromal tumors and leiomyosarcomas in the colon: a clinicopathologic, immunohistochemical, and molecular genetic study of 44 cases. Am J Surg Pathol. 2000;24:1339–52.

39. Schneider-Stock R, Boltze C, Lasota J, et al. High prognostic value of p16INK4 alterations in gastrointestinal stromal tumors. J Clin Oncol. 2003;21:1688–97.

40. Miettinen M, Sobin LH, Lasota J. Gastrointestinal stromal tumors of the stomach: a clinicopathologic, immunohistochemical, and molecular genetic study of 1765 cases with long-term follow-up. Am J Surg Pathol. 2005;29:52–68.

41. Miettinen M, Makhlouf H, Sobin LH, Lasota J. Gastrointestinal stromal tumors of the jejunum and ileum: a clinicopathologic, immunohistochemical, and molecular genetic study of 906 cases before imatinib with long-term follow-up. Am J Surg Pathol. 2006;30:477–89.

42. Reith JD, Goldblum JR, Lyles RH, Weiss SW. Extragastrointestinal (soft tissue) stromal tumors: an analysis of 48 cases with emphasis on histologic predictors of outcome. Mod Pathol. 2000;13:577–85.

43. Joensuu H, Vehtari A, Riihimäki J, et al. Risk of recurrence of gastrointestinal stromal tumour after surgery: an analysis of pooled population-based cohorts. Lancet Oncol. 2012;13(3):265–74.

44. Gronchi A, Colombo C, Raut CP. Surgical management of localized soft tissue tumors. Cancer. 2014;120:2638–48.

45. Wang H, Feng X, Ye S, et al. A comparison of the efficacy and safety of endoscopic full-thickness resection and laparoscopic-assisted surgery for small gastrointestinal stromal tumors. Surg Endosc. 2016;30:3357–61.

46. An W, Sun PB, Gao J, et al. Endoscopic submucosal dissection for gastric gastrointestinal stromal tumors: a retrospective cohort study. Surg Endosc. 2017;31:4522–31.

47. Pelletier JS, Gill RS, Gazala S, Karmali S. A systematic review and meta-analysis of open vs. laparoscopic resection of gastric gastrointestinal stromal tumors. J Clin Med Res. 2015;7:289–96.

48. Ye L, Wu X, Wu T, et al. Meta-analysis of laparoscopic vs. open resection of gastric gastrointestinal stromal tumors. PLoS One. 2017;12:e0177193.

49. Xiong H, Wang J, Jia Y, et al. Laparoscopic surgery versus open resection in patients with gastrointestinal stromal tumors: An updated systematic review and meta-analysis. Am J Surg. 2017;214:538–46.

50. Lian X, Feng F, Guo M, et al. Meta-analysis comparing laparoscopic versus open resection for gastric gastrointestinal stromal tumors larger than 5 cm. BMC Cancer. 2017;17:760.

51. Miettinen M, Kopczynski J, Makhlouf HR, et al. Gastrointestinal stromal tumors, intramural leiomyomas, and leiomyosarcomas in the duodenum: a clinicopathologic, immunohistochemical, and molecular genetic study of 167 cases. Am J Surg Pathol. 2003;27:625–41.

52. Lee SY, Goh BK, Sadot E, et al. Surgical strategy and outcomes in duodenal gastrointestinal stromal tumor. Ann Surg Oncol. 2017;24:202–10.

53. Colombo C, Ronellenfitsch U, Yuxin Z, et al. Clinical, pathological and surgical characteristics of duodenal gastrointestinal stromal tumor and their influence on survival: a multi-center study. Ann Surg Oncol. 2012;19:3361–7.

54. Grover S, Ashley SW, Raut CP. Small intestine gastrointestinal stromal tumors. Curr Opin Gastroenterol. 2012;28:113–23.

55. Tabrizian P, Sweeney RE, Uhr JH, et al. Laparoscopic resection of gastric and small bowel gastrointestinal stromal tumors: 10-year experience at a single center. J Am Coll Surg. 2014;218:367–73.

56. Dematteo RP, Gold JS, Saran L, et al. Tumor mitotic rate, size, and location independently predict recurrence after resection of primary gastrointestinal stromal tumor (GIST). Cancer. 2008;112:608–15.

57. Miettinen M, Lasota J. Gastrointestinal stromal tumors: review on morphology, molecular pathology, prognosis, and differential diagnosis. Arch Pathol Lab Med. 2006;130:1466–78.

58. Jakob J, Mussi C, Ronellenfitsch U, et al. Gastrointestinal stromal tumor of the rectum: results of surgical and multimodality therapy in the era of imatinib. Ann Surg Oncol. 2013;20:586–92.

59. Ford SJ, Gronchi A. Indications for surgery in advanced/metastatic GIST. Eur J Cancer. 2016;63:154–67.

60. Eisenberg BL, Harris J, Blanke CD, et al. Phase II trial of neoadjuvant/adjuvant imatinib mesylate (IM) for advanced primary and metastatic/recurrent operable gastrointestinal stromal tumor (GIST): early results of RTOG 0132/ACRIN 6665. J Surg Oncol. 2009;99:42–7.

61. Rutkowski P, Gronchi A, Hohenberger P, et al. Neoadjuvant imatinib in locally advanced gastrointestinal stromal tumors (GIST): the EORTC STBSG experience. Ann Surg Oncol. 2013;20:2937–43.

62. Gold JS, van der Zwan SM, Gonen M, et al. Outcome of metastatic GIST in the era before tyrosine kinase inhibitors. Ann Surg Oncol. 2007;14:134–42.

63. Bauer S, Rutkowski P, Hohenberger P, et al. Long-term follow-up of patients with GIST undergoing metastasectomy in the era of imatinib -- analysis of prognostic factors (EORTC-STBSG collaborative study). Eur J Surg Oncol. 2014;40:412–9.

64. Raut CP, Posner M, Desai J, et al. Surgical management of advanced gastrointestinal stromal tumors after treatment with targeted systemic therapy using kinase inhibitors. J Clin Oncol. 2006;24:2325–31.

65. Fairweather M, Balachandran VP, Li GZ, et al. Cytoreductive surgery for metastatic gastrointestinal stromal tumors treated with tyrosine kinase inhibitors: a 2-institutional analysis. Ann Surg. 2017;268(2):296–302. https://doi.org/10.1097/SLA.0000000000002281.

66. An HJ, Ryu MH, Ryoo BY, et al. The effects of surgical cytoreduction prior to imatinib therapy on the prognosis of patients with advanced GIST. Ann Surg Oncol. 2013;20:4212–8.

67. Raut CP, Wang Q, Manola J, et al. Cytoreductive surgery in patients with metastatic gastrointestinal stromal tumor treated with sunitinib malate. Ann Surg Oncol. 2010;17:407–15.

Neuroendocrine Neoplasms (NENs)

Nicola Fazio, Francesca Spada, Roberta Elisa Rossi, Valentina Ambrosini,
Lorena Incorvaia, Francesco Passiglia, Massimiliano Cani,
and Giuseppe Badalamenti

Soft Tissue Sarcoma, GIST and Neuroendocrine Neoplasms

Contents

© Springer Nature Switzerland AG 2021
A. Russo et al. (eds.), *Practical Medical Oncology Textbook*, UNIPA Springer Series,
https://doi.org/10.1007/978-3-030-56051-5_60

■ **Learning Objectives**
  − Have learned the basic concepts of neuroendocrine neoplasms (NENs).
  − Have reached in-depth knowledge about terminology, classification, diagnostic, and therapeutic features of gastroenteropancreatic and lung NENs.

60.1 Terminology/Classification

Neuroendocrine neoplasms (NENs) represent a rare and heterogeneous group of malignancies which can develop in many different sites of our body. They originate from the cells of the diffuse neuroendocrine system.

The main classification of NENs is based on their pathology features.

60.1.1 GEP NENs

Gastroenteropancreatic (GEP) NENs are classified according to the grade of differentiation and proliferation index.

Particularly, they are named neuroendocrine tumors (NETs) when they are well differentiated (WD) whereas neuroendocrine carcinomas (NECs) when they are poorly differentiated (PD).

Gastroenteropancreatic NENs were classified in four categories, including NETs G1 (WD with <3% Ki-67), NETs G2 (WD with 3–20% Ki-67), NETs G3 (WD with >20% Ki-67), and NECs (PD with >20% Ki-67) in accordance with the 2019 WHO classification [1].

Gastroenteropancreatic NENs can be differently named on the basis of their biological and clinical features as low/intermediate grade of malignancy (comprising NET G1,G2) and high grade of malignancy (NET G3 and NEC) (■ Table 60.1).

60.1.2 Lung NENs

Lung NENs were classified on the basis of some pathological parameters, such as mitosis and necrosis. In accordance with the latest WHO classification, 2015 edition, they are distinguished in small cell lung cancer (SCLC), large cell neuroendocrine carcinoma (LCNEC), atypical carcinoid (AC), and typical carcinoid (TC) (■ Table 60.2) [2].

The two forms of carcinoids, such as TC and AC, are also called lung NETs, and they have low/intermediate grade of malignancy. Large cell NEC and SCLC are

■ **Table 60.1** GEP NENs WHO/IARC classification

Type	Ki-67 (%)	Mitosis	Grade of malignancy
NET G1	<3	<2	Low
NET G2	3–20	2–20	Intermediate
NET G3	>20	>20	High
NEC	>20	>20	High

■ **Table 60.2** Lung NENs WHO classification

Type	Mitosis	Necrosis	Grade of malignancy
SCLC	>10	Present	High
LCNEC	>10	Present	High
AC	2–10	Focal, if any	Intermediate
TC	<2	None	Low

both called lung NECs, and they have a high grade of malignancy.

60.1.3 Clinical Classification of NENs

From a clinical perspective, it is critical to distinguish GEP NENs in functioning and nonfunctioning [3]. The former regards the presence of a clinical syndrome related to the production of one or more substances or hormones by the tumor, whereas the latter indicates the absence of a clinical syndrome related to the tumor although the patient can be symptomatic due to mass-effect symptoms related to the tumor and/or the tumor can secrete some substances without any clinical implication. The majority of GEP NETs are nonfunctioning.

The most common NEN-related clinical syndrome is the carcinoid syndrome. This is associated mainly with WD, small bowel origin, and metastatic stage NETs. A carcinoid syndrome has been reported in around 20% of all NETs, ranging from 8% of lung to 32% of small intestine NETs [4].

A further manner to classify GEP NENs is the distinction into sporadic and inherited. The most common inherited syndromes which can be associated with GEP NENs are multiple endocrine neoplasia type 1 (MEN-1) and von Hippel-Lindau (VHL) syndrome. Much rarely, GEP NENs can be associated with neurofibromatosis

◘ Table 60.3 Genetic syndromes associated with GEP NENs

Syndrome	NET
MEN-1 (Wermer's syndrome)	Pituitary adenoma PanNET Thymic NET Lung NET Gastric, type 2, NET (ZES related)
Von Hippel-Lindau (VHL)	PanNET Pheocromocytoma
Neurofibromatosis (NF-1)	Periampullary NET Pheocromocytoma
Tuberous sclerosis complex (TSC)	PanNET

type 1 (NF-1) and tuberous sclerosis complex (TSC) syndromes (◘ Table 60.3).

60.2 Epidemiology

60.2.1 GEP NENs

Epidemiologic data about NENs are fragmented and derive from different sources all over the world. One of the richest registry database is the surveillance, epidemiology, and end results (SEER). This is a comprehensive source of population-based information initiated in 1973 and updated annually. The current (SEER 18) registry grouping now includes approximately 30% of the US population. Based on the latest updated publication [5], incidence of GEP NENs was 3.56 per 100,000 persons per year, with small intestine and rectum representing the most common sites (1.05 and 1.04 per 100,000 persons, respectively) and pancreas much rarer (0.48 per 100,000 persons).

Interestingly, prevalence of all NENs is clearly increasing due to the good prognosis of most of them. This is particularly important if it is considered that GEP NENs were reported as the second type of malignancy of the digestive system in terms of prevalence just after colorectal cancer.

Low-grade (G1) and early-stage (localized) GEP NENs showed the most increasing incidence. This can be referred to the <2 cm pancreatic incidentalomas and small GI polyps, especially in the rectum, probably related to increasing use of imaging procedure in clinical practice.

Gastroenteropancreatic NECs are extremely rare. They represent around 3% of extrapulmonary NEC that are about 9% of all NECs. The vast majority of NEC are represented by small cell lung cancer (SCLC) [6].

With regard to survival rectum and appendix, NETs showed a median survival (24.6 and >30 years, respectively) much better than panNETs (3.6 years). Of course survival resulted related to the stage and grade. Metastatic small intestine NETs had the best survival (5.8 years) and metastatic colon NET the worst (4 months).

Globally, the updated SEER database data showed that incidence of NENs increased 6.4 folds from 1973 to 2012, with stomach and rectum representing the highest rate (fifteenfold and ninefold, respectively). Also survival improved over time, especially for metastatic panNET, probably due to improvements of therapy.

60.2.2 Lung NENs

Lung NENs represent around 25% of all lung cancers. Unlike GEP NENs that are for the vast majority WD, lung NENs are dominated by the PD forms. Small cell lung cancer (SCLC) represents roughly 20% of all lung cancers, LCNEC 3%, AC 0.3%, and TC 2%.

Epidemiology of lung NETs can be different if considered from two different points of view. Indeed while in clinical practice of a lung cancer medical oncologist lung NET represents a very rare entity (<3% of all lung cancers), they are quite frequent in the clinical practice of a NET-dedicated medical oncologist, representing around one third of all low-/intermediate-grade NEN (◘ Fig. 60.1).

Lung NET, particularly TC, can be associated to a clinical syndrome. Carcinoid syndrome is the most frequently associated syndrome, and it regards around 10% of lung NET; ectopic ACTH and acromegaly are the two other possible syndromes [7].

Lung NET can be associated in very rare cases to an inherited syndrome, mainly MEN-1.

60.3 Diagnostic Features of the Functioning and Nonfunctioning GEP NETs

The diagnosis of GEP NENs is based on multiple features including clinical presentation, biochemical markers, imaging, and endoscopy. However, in any case of suspected GEP NEN, a histological confirmation is required to define the diagnosis and to plan a proper multidisciplinary management.

60.3.1 Clinical Presentation

The clinical manifestations of GEP NENs are heterogeneous as these malignancies may be asymptomatic or

☐ Fig. 60.1 Lung NET represent <3% of all lung cancers and 25% of all NET. (References Rekhtman N et al. Arch Pathol Lab Med 2010; 134:1628-38; Modlin IM et al. Cancer 2003; 97:934-959; Halperin, D.M.; Shen, C.; Dasari, A.; et al. Lancet Oncol. 2017, 18, 525–534; and Ejaz, S.; Vassilopoulou-Sellin, R.; Busaidy, N.L. et al. Cancer 2011, 117, 4381–4389)

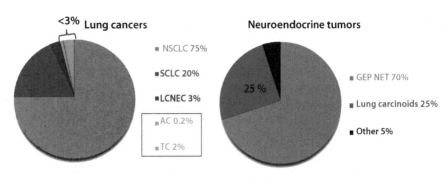

may cause nonspecific or obstructive symptoms, particularly in those cases where metastases are already present at the first diagnosis. However, functioning tumors show typical syndromes which are the consequence of hormonal hypersecretion.

60.3.2 Gastrointestinal Neuroendocrine Neoplasms (GI NENs)

Patients with GI NENs are often asymptomatic, although these neoplasms might be responsible for nonspecific symptoms, which are often confused with irritable bowel syndrome (abdominal pain/discomfort, change in bowel movements). Moreover, intestinal NENs can cause obstructive symptoms due to a local fibrotic reaction; thus their prompt diagnosis with consequent surgical resection of the primary tumor is needed. Intestinal tumors with liver metastases can be responsible for the typical carcinoid syndrome, present in 18% of patients with jejunal-ileal carcinoids [3], and characterized by flushing, diarrhea, abdominal pain, and more rarely from tearing, profuse sweating, telangiectasia, cardiac fibrosis, and cutaneous manifestations. It depends on the release of serotonin, which is not any more metabolized in the liver, together with other molecules (tachykinins, prostaglandins, bradykinin) [4].

Appendicular NETs are usually small, well differentiated, and often incidentally found during appendectomy, with a frequency of 3–9/1000 appendectomy [8].

Gastric NETs, which are rare malignancies of the stomach that develop from enterochromaffin-like (ECL) cells in the gastric wall, represent 0.5–1.7% of all gastric cancers and 7.1% of all GI NETs [9]. Three distinct tumor types have been proposed: type 1, which develops as a consequence of hypergastrinemia secondary to achlorhydria in type A chronic atrophic gastritis (CAG), usually not metastatizing; type 2, which is associated with Zollinger–Ellison syndrome in multiple endocrine neoplasia (MEN) type 1, potentially metastatizing; and type 3, which is not associated with hypergastrinemia (sporadic gastric NETs) and is often malignant with frequent metastases to regional nodes (55%) and liver (24%) [6–8]. These tumors are generally asymptomatic, and they are often incidentally discovered during gastroscopy; however, they can rarely give an atypical carcinoid syndrome with prolonged flushing, sialorrhea, sweating, tearing, hypotension, and widespread itching.

Neuroendocrine tumors of the colon (8.6% of all carcinoids) are often voluminous [10]. Finally, rectal NENs (1: 1000–2500 endoscopies) are usually small, nonfunctional, and rarely metastatic.

60.3.3 Pancreatic Neuroendocrine Neoplasms (PanNENs)

Neuroendocrine neoplasms of the pancreas (PanNENs) are a heterogenous, malignant disease with varying tumor biology and clinical presentation. The annual incidence of all PanNENs is 0.8/100,000, which includes both functioning and nonfunctioning PanNENs [11].

Nonfunctioning tumors contribute 60% of all PanNENs. Functioning PanNENs with specific clinical syndromes include [12] the following:

1. Insulinoma, which is characterized by hypoglycemia-related symptoms.
2. Zollinger–Ellison syndrome which includes diarrhea, recurrent peptic ulcers, gastroesophageal reflux symptoms and pain.
3. Verner–Morrison syndrome (VIPoma syndrome), characterized by diarrhea, hypokalemia, and hypochloridia.
4. Glucagonoma which is characterized by the so-called 4D syndrome consisting of diabetes, dermatitis, deep vein thrombosis, and depression.
5. Somatostatinoma which includes diarrhea, diabetes mellitus, and cholelithiasis.
6. ACTH-producing PanNENs which is characterized by the Cushing syndrome.

60.3.4 Biochemical Markers

There are generic and specific biochemical markers for GEP NENs.

Chromogranin A (CgA), which is an acidic glycoprotein of 439 amino acids and a molecular mass of 48 kDa, is found throughout the diffuse neuroendocrine system and shows a sensitivity of 96% and 75% in functioning and nonfunctioning NENs, respectively, and a specificity of 68–100% [13–17]. However, CgA is not highly specific to GEP NENs since it can be found in other malignancies and other non-tumor-related conditions [18–20] and during proton pump inhibitor (PPI) therapy. In addition, blood CgA is also elevated in other neoplasms of non-endocrine origin [18–20] and is not increased in all patients with NENs. Even if CgA does not seem to be particularly accurate as a biomarker in the diagnosis of NENs, it may be useful in the follow-up of patients with NENs [17, 21–27].

Nevertheless, over the last decades new biomarkers have been developed, and they may overcome CgA, NETest being the most studied one, that is, an RNA transcript panel of peripheral blood [28, 29].

In the cases of carcinoid syndrome, the specific marker is the urinary 5-hydroxyindolacetic acid (5-HIAA), serotonin metabolite, which is characterized by a sensitivity of 65–75%, with a specificity of 90–100% [30]. The 5-HIAA dosage can be influenced by some foods or drugs that should be avoided in 3–5 days prior to urine collection.

Regarding functioning NENs, the diagnosis should be based on the following serological tests, summarized in ◘ Table 60.4.

60.3.5 Radiological Techniques and Nuclear Medicine Tests

Conventional radiological techniques including abdomen ultrasound (US), computed tomography (CT) scan, and magnetic resonance imaging (MRI) are useful to localize both the primary tumor and possible metastases. However, the identification of a small bowel primary NEN on CT and MRI either via the standard technique or in combination with enteroclysis is challenging [31]; thus in this specific subgroup of patients, endoscopy plays a pivotal role [32]. Computed tomography or MRI scans should be also repeated during the follow-up to assess tumor recurrence/progression after therapy.

In recent years, PET/CT with ^{68}Ga-labeled somatostatin analogues *(SSAs)* has shown the highest sensitivity for localizing NENs and also a high specificity. According to several studies, the sensitivity varied from 86 to 100% and the specificity from 79% to 100% [11], except insulinomas, in which case the sensitivity was only 25% [33].

◘ Table 60.4 Diagnostic and clinical features of functioning PanNENs

Functioning PanNENs	Diagnosis	Main manifestations
Insulinoma	Plasma glucose <55 mg/dl, insulin ≥3.0 μU/ml, C-peptide ≥0.6 ng/ml and proinsulin ≥5.0 pmol/l	Hypoglycemia-related symptoms
Gastrinoma	Gastrin levels >1000 ng/l with a gastric pH <2. Positive secretin test	Zollinger–Ellison syndrome: diarrhea, recurrent peptic ulcers, gastroesophageal reflux symptoms, pain
VIPoma	Increased VIP	Verner-Morrison syndrome: diarrhea, hypokalemia, hypochloridia
Glucagonoma	Increased glucagon	4D syndrome: diabetes, dermatitis, deep vein thrombosis, depression
Somatostatinoma	Increased somatostatin	Diarrhea, diabetes mellitus, cholelithiasis
ACTH-producing PanNENs	Increased ACTH	Cushing syndrome

PET/CT with ^{68}Ga-labeled SSAs is therefore the method of choice to fully stage and localize the extent of disease in patients with NENs, except for insulinoma [34, 35].

60.3.6 Endoscopy

Digestive tract endoscopy allows to identify and to diagnose, by targeted biopsy, mucosal and submucosal NENs located in all the sites of the digestive tract reachable from the endoscope. The diagnosis of small bowel NENs may be challenging with upper and lower GI endoscopy, and their diagnosis has improved with the advent of capsule endoscopy (CE) and double balloon enteroscopy (DBE), which allow for direct visualization of the entire small bowel. CE and DBE may be complementary and show a similar diagnostic yield even if their role in routine staging needs further clarification, also considering the lack of data on potential procedural risks of these methods in NENs [35]. Endoscopic ultrasound (EUS) is the modality of choice for diagnosing PanNENs and for the locoregional staging of gastric, duodenal, pancreatic, and rectal NETs. In the setting of PanNENs, it has demonstrated higher accuracy in tumor detection than other imaging modalities with sensitivity ranging up to 94%. The sampling adequacy rate of EUS-fine needle aspiration has been reported to be of 83–93%, with an overall complication rate of about 1–2% [36–38].

The diagnostic yield of combined EUS imaging and cytology is significantly better than EUS imaging alone. Moreover, the preoperative availability of the Ki-67 index of a pancreatic lesion may help to decide between typical and atypical resection, and EUS may also have a potential role in the surveillance of multiple endocrine neoplasia type 1 (MEN-1) patients [39, 40].

As regards gastric NENs, the ENETS guidelines suggest to perform EUS in case of lesions >1 cm [7]. A staging EUS is frequently performed to confirm the appropriateness of endoscopic resection, usually endoscopic mucosal resection (EMR). EUS is important also for the staging of duodenal NENs as the exclusion of any locoregional lymph node metastases by EUS is required prior to EMR [41]. Finally, EUS plays a key role in the staging of rectal tumors, especially if >20 mm, with muscularis propria invasion or aggressive histological features, as EUS allows to accurately assess the depth of invasion and the possible presence of locoregional lymph node metastases.

The role of endoscopic technique in the diagnosis of GEP NENs is summarized in ◘ Table 60.5.

60.3.7 Histology

The definitive diagnosis of GEP NENs is based on histopathological examination, which is also essential for NEN classification and allocation to therapy [1].

However, obtaining adequate tissues by endoscopic forceps biopsy is often difficult due to the location of gastrointestinal NENs in the deep mucosa and submucosa. Moreover, even if biopsy is successful, the diagnosis may be difficult due to small specimen size or "crush" artifacts, which can lead to misdiagnosis [42].

A complete histopathological examination, which should be performed by histopathologists with a proper expertise in this specific field, must consider the size of the tumor, the number of mitosis, the presence of cellular atypia, the proliferative index, angioinvasiveness, and local invasiveness.

The histological diagnosis of NENs is generally confirmed by immunohistochemical demonstration of neuroendocrine markers [43]. Several general neuroendocrine markers are known: chromogranin-A (CgA), synaptophysin, protein cell product 9.5, neural cell adhesion molecule (NCAM/CD56), neuron-specific enolase (NSE), and Leu 7. However, CgA and synaptophysin are the most common markers to confirm the endocrine nature of the neoplastic cells.

60.4 Diagnostic Features of Lung NETs

In accordance with the 2015 World Health Classification (WHO), lung NENs include four morphological entities: typical carcinoid (TC), atypical carcinoid (AC), large cell neuroendocrine carcinoma (LCNEC), and small cell lung carcinoma (SCLC) [2]. They have specific pathological and clinical features as shown in ◘ Table 60.6.

The distinction between TC and AC requires a surgical sample and cannot be reliably assigned to a cytological or biopsy sample [2]. From a clinical point of view, it is essential to not confuse a lung carcinoid, either typical or atypical, with a poorly differentiated neuroendocrine carcinoma (NECs), be it small or large cells

◘ **Table 60.5** The role of endoscopic technique in the diagnosis of GEP NENs

Neoplasm	Gastroscopy	Colonoscopy	DBE/CE	EUS
Gastric neoplasms	*Yes*	/	/	For the staging of lesions >1 cm
Duodenal neoplasms	*Yes*	/	/	For the locoregional staging of all duodenal neoplasms
Small bowel neoplasms	Yes	Yes	*Yes*	/
Colorectal neoplasms	/	*Yes*	/	For the staging of rectal tumors, if >20 mm, with muscularis propria invasion or aggressive histological features
PanNENs	/	/	/	*Yes*

Table 60.6 Clinical and pathological features of lung NENs

		TC	AT	LCNEC	SCLC
Age	Mean	45 ys	55 ys	65	65
	Decade	IV–V	V–VI	VI–VII	VI–VII
Sex		F > M	M > F	M > F	M > F
Prevalence		1–2%	0.2%	3%	15%
Smoke		No	Yes (or past)	Yes	Yes
MEN-1		5%	Rare	No	No
Metastases		10–15%	45–50%	50–70%	>80%
Grade		Low	Intermediate	High	High
Morphology		Well–diff.	Well–diff.	Poorly–diff.	Poorly–diff
Mitosis (x 2 mm^2)		<2	2–10	>10 (median 70)	>10 (median 80)
Necrosis		No	Yes (focal)	Yes (extended)	Yes (extended)

60.4.1 Minimum Requirements of an Anatomopathological Report of Lung Neuroendocrine Neoplasms (NENs)

Mitotic counts, the presence of necrosis, and Ki-67 labeling index (LI) should be indicated in the pathological diagnosis of a surgical or biopsy (noncytological) sample for at least two reasons: (a) mitosis and necrosis are integral parts of the current diagnostic-classification criteria, they allow comparative crossed studies and, for mitotic counts, identify CA with different prognosis; (b) although Ki-67 LI has no recognized diagnostic role in lung NEN, many studies have suggested a prognostic role in the carcinoid category (TC and AC), even in the individual subcategories, in addition to orienting the clinician to one or the other extreme of the clinical-pathological spectrum of pulmonary NETs.

60.4.2 Role of Ki67 in Pulmonary NEN

The role of Ki-67 LI is not yet well codified in the lung NEN [44]. However, its scopes of use can be exemplified as follows:

(a) Utility in distinguishing CT and CA from poorly differentiated NE carcinomas, in particular, SCLC, in limited diagnostic material (cytology and biopsies) [45].

(b) Unreliability as the sole diagnostic criterion in individual cases, although there are significant differences in mean or median distribution values between the different subtypes of pulmonary NET.

(c) Possibility of using Ki-67 LI as a prognostic criterion (various "cut-offs" have been proposed in the literature) within carcinoids, even with independent value in multivariate analysis, while there are no data in poorly differentiated NECs.

(d) Nonuniformity of literature data on the methodologies to be followed to calculate Ki-67 [44].

60.4.3 Immunohistochemistry (IHC) in Lung NENs

Immunohistochemical characterization of neuroendocrine differentiation markers (chromogranin A, synaptophysin, and CD56/NCAM and, in some cases, hormones) may be useful to confirm the neuroendocrine nature of neoplastic proliferation or the origin of the tumour, especially in poorly differentiated NENs or when the diagnostic material (biopsy or cytology) is limited where the neuroendocrine nature may not be immediately evident [2]. In case of metastatic sample, the positivity for TTF1 may suggest the lung origin of a TC or AC, while there is often an unfaithful expression of nuclear transcription factors (TTF1, CDX-2, Isl-1, PAX-8, WT1) in NECs independently by the original anatomical site.

60.4.4 Endoscopic Diagnosis

Endoscopic procedures (flexible bronchoscopy) represent the first choice to get a cytohistological diagnosis of patients with suspected airway tumor [46]. Neuroendocrine neoplasms may present as typical carcinoids with endobronchial lesions, endoscopically visible, and well-delimited, regular surface, sometimes polypoid and easily bleeding upon contact with the instrument. *Large cell neuroendocrine carcinomas* often present as invasive lesions of the airways, necrotic, with evident infiltration of the bronchial wall and, sometimes, of adjacent mediastinal structures. *Atypical carcinoids* have intermediate endoscopic characteristics between TC and LCNECs with variable degree of invasiveness of the bronchial wall and adjacent structures. Currently, EBUS-TBNA is the most used method for the diagnosis and staging of pulmonary neoplasms; it presents high diagnostic performance and guarantees a quality of sampling sufficient for different immunohistochemical analyses and differentiation between different types of neuroendocrine tumors [47, 48]. Invasive staging methods of pulmonary neoplasms (mediastinoscopy, video thoracoscopy, mediastinotomy) are only indicated in cases of highly suspicious lymph nodes if EBUS-TBNA is negative for malignancy [49].

60.4.5 Radiological Imaging

The radiological diagnosis is based on two main procedures: multislices computed tomography (MSCT) and magnetic resonance (MR).

Pulmonary carcinoids in MSCT occur as well-circumscribed nodular alterations, usually <5 cm in size, often associated with the presence of a perihilar mass.

In most cases, the carcinoid has a central location, while less commonly it is located in the peripheral pulmonary site [50]. With MSCT, it is possible to identify the location of the disease to undergo biopsy. Percutaneous CT-guided biopsy is the best technique for histological diagnosis of both medial and pulmonary solid lesions. Indeed, in addition to providing adequate material for a reliable histological diagnosis [51], the needle gauge used (18 Gauge) to perform the sampling does not significantly affect the percentage of expected complications as for other body districts [52]. The LCNEC shows radiological characteristics very similar to those of the NSCLC, so it is difficult to distinguish them on the only morphological basis. The LCNEC [53] develops peripherally in the vast majority of cases, while, in a minority of cases, it is found in the central lung, with concomitant atelectasis. The margins are usually well defined often with lobulations, but there are also presentations with nodules with spiculated margins, with cavitations, aerial bronchogram in their context, and central necrosis [52, 53]. A characteristic contrast enhancement for this type of injury is not appreciated. The SCLC develops centrally, and the diagnosis is almost always made when the disease is in an advanced stage.

Patients who cannot undergo CT (i.e., allergy to iodine m.d.c.) can be studied with MR for the abdominopelvic evaluation. In this case, it is recommended to use standard weighted T1 and T2 sequences for the study of the abdomen and multiphase dynamic sequences during and after the injection of hepato-specific m.d.c. (Gd -EOB -DTPA) [54–56]. Moreover, MR is more sensitive than MSCT in recognizing very small lesions in the liver [57, 58].

60.5 Molecular Biology Features

60.5.1 Gastroenteropancreatic Neuroendocrine Neoplasms (GEP NENs)

In the last years, the development of new technologies has allowed the study of innovative aspects about tumors and their mechanisms, e.g., their genesis, growth, and strategies of resistance to chemotherapy. This new awareness has taken importance on the landscape of the biological features of tumours and allowed the research and the use of new key strategies. The classical therapies are now joined by new drugs known as "targeted therapies" which actually are more effective and characterized by a different and lower toxicity. This is the reason why it is important not just studying but also understanding which are the genetic and epigenetic features of a tumor; the knowledge about the molecular aspects of GEP NENs is not so deep unlike other neoplasms, above all for their low frequency and their heterogeneous behavior; what we know is that the majority of mutations which lead the tumorigenesis are expressed in those genes which usually regulate in a negative sense the growth and the proliferation of cells; they are known as "suppressor genes." This is an atypical aspect as in other tumors, the uncontrolled cell proliferation starts from activating mutations which involve other types of genes (proto-oncogene).

Classically, it is possible to divide the mutations in two main categories: the germline and the somatic ones.

60.5.2 Germline Mutations

They account for about 5% of NENs and above all pancreatic ones, even if they can be involved also in the midgut. There are different genes implicated, in particular, MEN1, VHL, NF1, TSC1, and TSC2 [59]. Mutations in these genes are present not only in GEP NENs' tumorigenesis but also in more complex and multiple organ diseases in which GEP NENs are just a part of the syndrome.

60.5.2.1 MEN1 and Menin

MEN-1 (11q) by the expression of its protein interacts with several transcription factors such as JUN-D (resulting in a negative control of cell-proliferation), c-Myb and c-Myc, and NF-kB; furthermore menin controls TGF-beta, Wnt and Hedgehog, and PI3K/AKT signals; its role implies also the regulation of RNA and, in particular, of miRNA [60]. Considering these pathways is possible to understand the role of menin as negative controller of cell cycle. The synthetic view of ◘ Fig. 60.2 shows how complicated is the role of menin and how many pathways can be modified by its mutation.

Clinically, MEN-1 mutations lead to a condition characterized by at least two of these three tumors: pancreatic NENs, parathyroid adenomas, and anterior pituitary adenomas, even if there are lots of other manifestations like adrenal cortical tumor or skin alterations (facial angiofibroma) [62].

60.5.2.2 VHL (Von Hippel Lindau)

VHL gene codifies for a protein, VHL, which contributes to regulate the cell proliferation: in particular, it interacts with elongin C, forming a complex which allows the degradation (via ubiquitinylation) of HIF-alpha (hypoxia-induced factor), a transcript factor of genes like VEGF, EPO, TGF-alpha, and PDGF-beta [63]. Von Hippel Lindau disease can be distinguished into two types, and both of them are associated to the development of NENs of pancreas (type 1 and subtype 2B) [64].

60.5.2.3 NF1 (Neurofibromatosis-1)

Neurofibromin 1 (17q11) has an important role in inhibiting RAS protein, thanks to its GTPase activity. Germline mutation of NF1 causes a particular disease characterized by skin alteration like "café au lait" spots, neurofibromas, malignant peripheral nerve sheath tumor, and rarely neuroendocrine tumors [65].

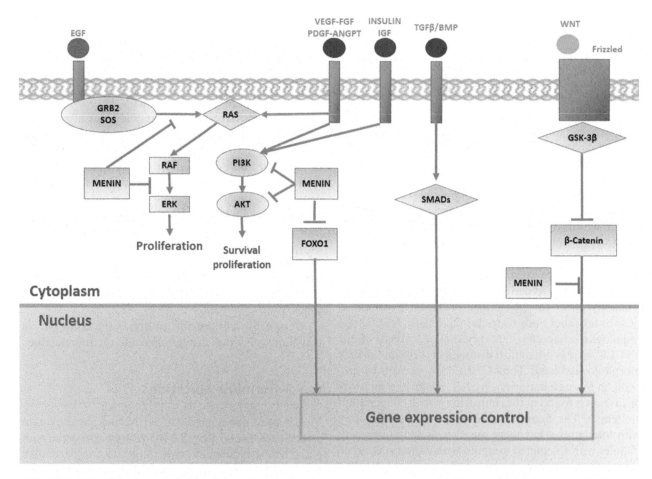

◘ **Fig. 60.2** Role of Menin: modified from "Towards a new classification of gastroenteropancreatic neuroendocrine neoplasms" [61]

60.5.2.4 TSC (Tuberous Sclerosis)1 and 2

Tuberous sclerosis complex 1 and 2 codes for hamartin and tuberin; their role involves the regulation of cell adhesion, thanks to the interaction with PI3K/AKT/mTOR pathways [66]. Some clinical manifestations consist in skin lesions (hypomelanotic macules), ungueal fibromas, renal angiolipomas, and hamartomas [59].

For a synthetic view, see ◘ Table 60.7.

60.5.3 Somatic Mutations

Between PanNENs and small-intestinal NENs, there are some differences regarding the types and the frequency of somatic mutations.

The most frequent genetic alteration in PanNENs consists in the loss of heterozygosis (LOH) of MEN1; other alterations include YY1 (ying-yang 1) which is a transcriptional repressor involved in the control of some factors of the mTOR pathway; it is correlated to a more advanced age at the diagnosis, and it accounts for about 30% of patients with sporadic insulinomas [67].

Death domain-associated protein (DAXX) and ATRX are other two factors implied in the tumorigenesis of NETs. ATRX (involved also in an inherited X-linked disease characterized by alpha-thalassemia and mental retardation), with DAXX, forming a histone H3.3 chaperone, contributes to regulate most aspects of cell regulation-like apoptosis and transcription.

In particular, it seems that they are linked to the chromosome instability (CIN) when their levels are lower than normal, and it is also correlated with tumor stage and the presence of metastasis [68].

Some tumors are characterized by the presence of specific alteration, like MEN1 for gastrinomas or YY1 for insulinomas [67, 69].

Usually, NENs of small intestine are genetically stable, and it was not possible to find somatic alterations in MEN1, ATRX, or DAXX. Although the biological landscape presents some modifications like the mutation of CDKN1B, it encodes for cyclin-dependent kinase inhibitor 1B (p27KIP1), and its inactivation leads to a worse prognosis.

Other mutations which have been discovered in small intestine NENs regard SDHD gene (involved in a hypoxic response when mutated and already studied for the onset of paraganglioma); it has been proved a loss of heterozygosis of this gene, and this correlates with a possible role of hypoxia in small intestine tumor [70].

60.5.4 Role of Chromosomes

Understanding the chromosomal alterations is another strategy to study the biological aspect of tumors to find and at the same time new criteria useful to classify GEP NENs.

It is possible to identify two kinds of events: a chromosome or a microsatellite instability. The latter is actually not well-known, and it seems to be correlated to a better prognosis; differently, CIN is a well-known mechanism in both types of NENs (pancreatic and small intestinal): loss of chromosomes is more frequent, and probably during the development of the tumor, there is an accumulation of chromosomal alteration [35]. Some alterations in PanNENs regard [61] the following:

— Deletion of chromosome 9p: It leads to the loss of CDKN2A, which expresses p16 and p14, two tumor-suppressor proteins.

— Deletion of chromosome 16p: In this case, there is the loss of expression of TSC2, involved in the regulation of PI3K/AKT/mTOR pathway.

— Deletion of chromosome 10p: Found more in malignant lesions, it leads to a deregulation of AKT/mTOR pathway.

◘ **Table 60.7** Genetic syndromes

Syndrome	Gene	Localization	Main manifestations
Multi-endocrine neoplasia 1	MEN	11q13	Pancreatic NENs, parathyroid adenomas and anterior pituitary adenomas, adrenal cortical tumor or skin alterations (facial angiofibroma), lipomas, collagenomas, meningiomas
Von Hippel Lindau disease	VHL	3p25–26	Angiomiomatosis, pheochromocytoma, renal cell carcinoma, NENs, hemangioblastomas
Neurofibromatosis (Von Recklinghausen's disease)	NF1	17q11	Café au lait spots, neurofibromas, malignant peripheral nerve sheath tumor, neuroendocrine tumors
Tuberous sclerosis complex	TSC1 TSC2	9q34 16p13.3	Skin lesions (hypomelanotic macules), ungueal fibromas, renal angiolipomas, hamartomas

60.5.5 Mechanism of Methylation

Methylation of CpG islands is a known mechanism, not just for colorectal carcinoma but also for GEP NENs; in particular, this process involves different loci like MGMT, RASSF1A, MLH, and CDKN2A [22]. The most remarkable aspect regards the methylation status of MGMT: it correlates with a better response to alkylating agents like dacarbazine or temozolomide [38]. Methylation mechanism is more common among midgut NENs than pancreatic ones [61].

60.5.6 Gene Expression Patterns

As a result of what is reported until now, it could be useful to remind the necessity of classifying NENs considering the biological aspects of the tumors. Some studies have already done this: Duerr et al. have identified, using DNA microarray analyses, two categories of PanNENs: a benign and a malignant form; the latter is characterized by the overexpression of the genes ADCY2, FEV, GADD45beta, and NR4A2 and is compared to the well-differentiated NENs. Other genes like PDGFR are expressed in the two subtypes [71].

60.6 Molecular Pathways and Biological Drugs

See related paragraph.

60.6.1 Bases of Treatment

60.6.1.1 Gastroenteropancreatic Neuroendocrine Neoplasms (GEP NENs)

Each patient with a GEP NEN or suspicious for that should be referred as soon as possible to a referral center for NENs.

First of all, it is extremely important that pathological diagnosis of GEP NEN is reliable, that means that the neoplasm should be a *pure* NEN. Indeed, a *non-pure* GEP NEN might be an adenocarcinoma with *neuroendocrine differentiation* or a mixed neuroendocrine/non-neuroendocrine neoplasm (MiNEN) that are two entities distinct from NENs and therefore requiring a different clinical management [1].

Tumor staging and characterization Fig. 52.5 - See below "Lung neuroendocrine neoplasm staging" are two critical steps. Clinical staging should be performed by means of morphological (radiological) tools, such as contrast-medium computed tomography (CT) scan of

the chest and abdomen or abdominal magnetic resonance imaging (MRI) + chest CT scan. Pathological staging is related to the TNM eighth edition (*AJCC Cancer Staging Manual, eighth ed, Amin MB (Ed), Springer, Chicago 2017*). Somatostatin receptor subtype 2 (SSTR-2)-related imaging should be performed in patients with low-/intermediate-grade GEP NET. Metabolic imaging with 18-fluorodeoxyglucose (FDG)-positron emission tomography (PET) should be considered for high- and intermediate-grade GEP NEN.

60.6.1.2 Local/Locally Advanced Stage

For patients presenting a pure G1–G2 GEP NET at a local or locally advanced radically resectable stage, an upfront surgical approach should be discussed within the MDT.

For patients presenting a pure G3 GEP NEC at a local or locally advanced radically resectable stage, a chemotherapy +/- radiotherapy should be discussed integrated with a possible surgical approach and its timing.

For patients presenting a pure G3 GEP NET at a local or locally advanced radically resectable stage, an upfront surgical approach versus an upfront medical treatment should be discussed within the MDT.

60.6.1.3 Advanced Stage

In patients with advanced GEP NETs, no specific sequence or integration of therapies has been validated so far. Therapeutic decision about the single-line therapy depends on a number of factors, including level of evidence, regulatory aspects, guidelines, local expertise/experience, logistics, and clinical trials availability. Furthermore, it should be linked to a number of tumor-related factors, such as the presence of a clinical syndrome, inherited condition, tumor grade, and SSTR-2 functional expression. The metastatic tumor burden, tumor primary site, resectability, patient symptomaticity (tumor's mass effect), and rate and pattern of tumor progression are also important factors to be considered for the therapeutic choice (Tables 60.8 and 60.9).

It is therefore clear that ideally each clinical case should be discussed within a NEN-dedicated multispecialist team and that early and late therapeutic goals should be shared. Different goals and strategies can induce distinct therapeutic choices for therapies with different level of evidence in the same clinical settings (Fig. 60.3).

Locoregional treatments, mainly in the liver, can be discussed in selected cases, such as monofocal or oligofocal liver progression, minimal residual disease after tumor response on systemic therapies, or within a global debulking strategy. However, the level of evidence is quite low, coming mostly from retrospective analyses [72].

Table 60.8 Main criteria for therapeutic choice

Clinical syndrome	Functioning vs. nonfunctioning
Tumor grade	Histology (morphology + Ki-67)
Tumor stage	Clinical (morphological and functional imaging) or pathologic (TNM)
Tumor primary site	Midgut, pancreas, other GI, unknown primary
SSTR-2 imaging	^{68}Ga-SSA-PET/CT
Genetic syndrome	Sporadic vs. inherited

Table 60.9 Further criteria for therapeutic choice

Tumor related symptoms (mass-effect)	Symptomatic vs. asymptomatic
Performance status	0 vs >0 (ECOG)
Comorbidity	
Tumor status	Stable vs. slowly progressing vs. rapidly progressing
Tumor burden	Radiological imaging
Goal of the single therapy	Syndrome control vs. symptoms control vs. tumor growth control Cytoreduction vs. stabilization
Goal of the therapeutic strategy	Debulking (partial or absolute) vs. tumor growth control over time (QoL)

Bases of therapeutic approach to GEP NET patients

◆ Involvement of a NET referral center

◆ Multidisciplinary discussion (1° step of diagnostic-therapeutic management)

◆ The MDTshould be composed by NEN-dedicated specialists

◆ The MDT should share a therapeutic strategy rather than the single therapy

Fig. 60.3 Key-points of clinical management of patients with GEP NET

In advanced *nonfunctioning* pNET, an SSA can be considered as first-line therapy.

For the so-called GEP *NET G3*, there is no absolute evidence about a specific first-line therapy and sequencing. As

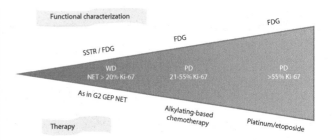

Fig. 60.4 Functional characterization of high-grade GEP NENs

they are *high-grade* neoplasms, a chemotherapy is usually considered, with alkylating-based regimens or fluoropyrimidines/oxaliplatin combinations preferred to platinum/etoposide [73]. However, EVE and SUN can be evaluated in advanced pancreatic NETs G3 considering that tumor morphology rather than proliferation index was the inclusion criterion for the regulatory trials. Furthermore, some recent reports indicated specific activity of EVE and SUN in panNET G3 [74, 75], and recommendations [76] suggest that clinicians should manage NET G3 in a different manner than the NEC G3 even considering therapeutic options usually discussed in the G2.

In a patient with an advanced GEP NEC, the SSTR-2 imaging does not have a role, whereas ^{18}FDG-PET/CT should be considered to stage and characterize the disease.

In this latter context chemotherapy represents the universally shared option. Historically, a combination of cisplatin or, less commonly, carboplatin plus etoposide was proposed (◘ Fig. 60.4).

60.6.1.4 Lung Neuroendocrine Neoplasms (GEP NENs)

Staging and Characterization (◘ Fig. 60.5)
Local or Locally Advanced Stage

A patient with a resectable locally advanced lung NET should be considered for resective surgery.

A patient with a locally advanced high-grade lung LCNEC should be considered for upfront or delayed resection, including neo-/adjuvant chemotherapy +/− radiotherapy.

A patient with locally advanced SCLC should be considered for chemotherapy +/− radiotherapy.

Advanced Stage

Patientis with a metastatic lung NET can receive two general types of therapies, comprising locoregional and systemic therapies. Among the former, there are palliative surgical resection of the primary site or metastatic disease, palliative external beam radiotherapy, palliative interventional radiology procedures including liver transarterial embolization (TAE), thermoablation radiofrequency (TARF), and liver transarterial radioem-

Fig. 60.5 Staging and characterization of lung neuroendocrine neoplasms

Lung neuroendocrine neoplasm staging

Type of lung NEN	Morphological imaging	Functional imaging	Circulating markers
Well differentiated Very low Ki-67 Low grade TC	Total-body CT scan	68GaPET-CT-DOTA-peptide	CgA
Well/moderately differentiated Intermediate Ki-67 (e.g. 3–20) AC	Total-body CT scan	68GaPET-CT-DOTA-peptide + 18FDGPET-CT	CgA + NSE
Poorly differentiated, High Ki-67 (e.g. > 20%) LCNEC/SCLC	Total-body CT scan	18FDGPET-CT	N SE

Caplin ME, et al. Ann Oncol. 2015; 26:1604-20. Gasparri R, et al. Q J Nucl Med Mol Imaging. 2015;59:446-54. Wolin ME. Oncologist. 2015;20:1123-31.

bolization (TARE) with ^{90}Yttrium. The latter category comprises somatostatin receptor 2 (SSTR-2)-directed therapies, including somatostatin analogs (SSAs) and peptide receptor radionuclide therapy (PRRT), molecular targeted agents (MTAs) like Everolimus, chemotherapy (several regimens), and interferon (IFN).

Criteria for choosing therapy and therapeutic strategy in lung NET are similar to those of GEP NET.

60.7 Theragnostic Role of Nuclear Medicine

Nuclear medicine has acquired a central role for the management of NEN, mainly as a consequence of several factors including a high diagnostic accuracy and clinical availability of different radiopharmaceuticals (which may prove more valuable in specific clinical settings) and for the possibility to employ the same compounds for target therapy. In fact, being very heterogeneous both at presentation and during the disease natural course, NEN still represents a challenge for the clinicians.

PET/CT presents several advantages including a higher spatial resolution [77, 78], the possibility to semi-quantify the tracer uptake in the region of interest (SUVmax) [77, 78], lower costs [79], and shorter image acquisition protocol (2 hours vs acquisitions at 4-24 hours). Moreover, several β+ emitting radiopharmaceuticals are currently available for PET/CT imaging to study either somatostatin receptor (SSTR) expression (68Ga-DOTA-peptides, the most frequently employed tracers in well differentiated NEN) or metabolism (18F-DOPA, 18F-FDG).

60.7.1 β+ Emitting Radiopharmaceuticals Employed for PET/CT Imaging

68Ga-DOTA-peptides (DOTA-TATE, DOTA-NOC, DOTA-TOC): are somatostatin receptor analogues, internalized after binding. The currently available compounds differ for the affinity to SSTR subtypes (DOTA-TATE shows higher affinity for SSTR-2; DOTA-NOC shows the wider SSTR subtype affinity, binding to SSTR-2,3,5) [80]. Sensitivity and specificity for the detection of well-differentiated NEN lesions is very high (90–98% and 92–98, respectively) [80–82], and a very high interobserver agreement has been reported [83].

Indications include evaluation of disease extension (staging/restaging) (■ Fig. 60.6), detection of relapse, selection for targeted therapy (with either cold or hot SSAs), and identification of the unknown primary tumour site in pts. with proven NEN metastatic lesions [80].

Potential utility of SSA therapy withdrawal has been suggested (1 day is suggested for short-lived molecules and at least 3–4 weeks for long-acting SSAs I.V.); however, there is no consensus;

18F-DOPA [80]: at present, the clinical setting in which 18F-DOPA is most frequently employed is the detection of NEN presenting with low/variable SR-expression (neuroblastoma, pheochromocytoma, paraganglioma-abdominal, medullary thyroid cancer).

18F-FDG [84]: is the most frequently employed radiopharmaceutical in oncology; its uptake reflects cell glucose metabolism and is therefore an indirect measure of dedifferentiation and aggressiveness of tumour cells. Most solid tumors are FDG-avid.

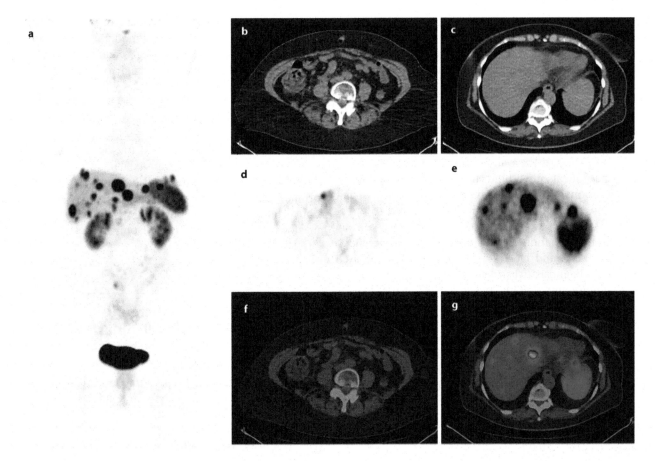

Fig. 60.6 PET/CT MIP **a**, low dose CT **b**, **c**, PET **d**, **e** and fused PET/CT **f**, **g** transaxial images of a patient with multiple metastatic liver NEN lesions **e**, **g** and ileal primary **d**, **f**. All lesions show high SR expression. Of note: ileal NEN may present with very small lesions that may be better appreciated in PET only images

60.7.2 Choice of the Radiopharmaceutical

The choice of the radiopharmaceutical to employ first is guided by evaluation of several factors: tracer availability in the nuclear medicine center, SSTR expression (some histotypes are known to show low/variable SSTR expression), and differentiation grade (SSTR expression is higher in well-differentiated forms).

The 2017 EANM (European Association of Nuclear Medicine) guidelines [80] indicated in the primary tumor site a fundamental criterion choice (▶ https://www.eanm.org/publications/guidelines/): in particular, 68Ga-DOTA-peptides should be considered as first choice for the assessment of NEN of the foregut and midgut and for paragangliomas of the head and neck. On the contrary, 18F-DOPA is to be considered first choice for abdominal paragangliomas, while 18F-FDG should be employed before 68Ga-DOTA-peptides to study NEN of the hindgut.

Additional factors to be considered when assessing the potential additional role of FDG are tumor grade and whether the detection of the presence of a more aggressive (dedifferentiated and therefore FDG-avid)

clone is mandatory. In particular, much attention has been devoted to the potentially complimentary role of 68Ga-DOTA-peptides and 18F-FDG [80, 85]. On one side, obtaining images with both tracers could provide a complete biological characterization of the whole tumor burden: confirming both a significant SR expression (which would drive somatostatin target therapy) and detecting if aggressive clones are also present (providing prognostic patients stratification). On the other side, there is no international consensus on whether FDG should be performed regardless of tumor grading (therefore in all NEN grades) [80, 85] and how often it should be repeated during the disease natural history (taking into account that the generally better prognosis of NEN as compared with other solid tumors corresponds to a longer life expectancy). International experts agree however that, if positive, FDG is prognostic, allowing the idnetification of patients with more aggressive disease tumors. Although the current approach to FDG/DOTA-peptides combined imaging is different across centers and countries, based on current knowledge [80, 85], experts agree that FDG should be the first choice for NEC and it may provide additional clinically useful information in G3 (ki67 values 21–55%) and G2 (ki67 values 3–20%) NEN. The most accurate approach seems to plan combined imaging based on accurate evaluation on the clinical case and on multidisciplinary discussion.

60.7.3 Radionuclide Target Therapy (PRRT)

PRRT consists of the systemic administration of radiopharmaceuticals that bind to SR (overexpressed on NEN lesions) and that are labeled with isotopes that can deliver a cytotoxic radiation (β-emission) to target cells, resulting in target radiotherapy. The short pathway of emitted radiation ensures a target cytotoxic effect. DOTA-TATE and DOTA-TOC can therefore be used for both diagnosis (when labeled with the β+ emitting 68Gallium) and therapy (when labeled with 90Y or 177Lu), acquiring a theranostic role in NEN management.

Critical organs are represented by the kidneys (infusion of positively charged amino acids can reduce radiation to kidneys of approximately 60%) and the bone marrow (including late hematologic toxicity).

However, mainly due to regulatory issues, PRRT has been employed up to now only as an experimental treatment. In 2013, the EANM published the first procedural guidelines for PRRT in NEN (detailed schemes and doses can be found at ► https://www.eanm.org/publications/guidelines/). In 2017, the first international phase 3 multicenter trail was published [86]. This latter study evaluated the efficacy and safety of 177Lu-DOTA-TATE as compared with high-dose octreotide long acting in patients with advanced, progressive, SR–positive mid-gut NEN. The study reported how PRRT with 177Lu-DOTA-TATE resulted in markedly longer progression-free survival and a significantly higher response rate as compared to the arm treated with high-dose octreotide. Severe adverse effects were minor.

Current ENETS guidelines [85] consider PRRT for treatment of patients with positive expression of SR-2, or metastatic or inoperable, after failure of other treatment or at progression. There is an open debate on when to position PRRT in the NEN management flow chart and to what extent is the impact of potential late complications (e.g., hematologic toxicity) on subsequent treatment options.

60.7.3.1 Contraindications to PRRT

Absolute: pregnancy, severe acute concomitant illnesses/unmanageable psychiatric disorders.

Relative: breast feeding (if not discontinued), severely compromised renal function (especially when 90Y-labeled

compounds are employed, while for 177Lu-labeled radiopharmaceuticals, a mild-/moderate-grade renal impairment can be tolerated, e.g., creatinine ≤1.7 mg/dl); severely compromised bone marrow (EANM suggested reference values are WBC <3000/µl, with absolute neutrophil count <1000/µl, PLT <75,000/µl for 177Lu-DOTATATE, <90,000/µl for 90Y-DOTATOC, RBC <3,000,000/µl).

Figure legend: PET/CT MIP **a**, low-dose CT **b**, **c**, PET **d**, **e**, and fused PET/CT **f**, **g** transaxial images of a patient with multiple metastatic liver NEN lesions **e**, **g** and ileal primary **d**, **f**. All lesions show high SR expression. Of note: ileal NEN may present with very small lesions that may be better appreciated in PET only images

60.8 Chemotherapy

60.8.1 Gastroenteropancreatic Neuroendocrine Neoplasms (GEP NENs)

Chemotherapy has been used for several decades in NEN patients, although no clear evidence about its survival impact was demonstrated. Since no validated and universally shared predictors of response and efficacy has been found so far, clinical and tumor features are the only drivers for chemotherapeutic regimens and schedules choice.

60.8.1.1 Chemotherapy in Neuroendocrine Carcinomas (NECs)

Chemotherapy is the most common option proposed in advanced NECs. Although these neoplasms appear relatively chemosensitive, their prognosis remains dismal. Cisplatin (CDDP)/etoposide (VP-16) is the regimen of choice based on the assumption that the clinical behavior of NECs is similar to that of SCLC. The literature, however, is quite scant and limited to studies rather dated and not specifically designed to clarify this topic [87–90].

Carboplatin (CBDCA) has been reported as a valid alternative to CDDP and irinotecan to VP16 for lung NECs [91, 92].

According to the latter point, it has been reported that patients with <55% Ki67 GEP NECs had a low response rate but lived longer than those with >55% Ki67 [93].

Oral etoposide has been reported safe and efficient in treating G3 GEP NEN patients scheduled for cisplatin/carboplatin + etoposide therapy [1, 94].

Over the latest years, the heterogeneity of high-grade category has been deeply explored [93, 95, 96].

O^6-methylguanine

Active MGMT

Consumed MGMT

Guanine

Among GEP NENs G3 (WHO 2010), a particular subgroup is represented by morphologically well-differentiated and Ki67 > 20% and/or mitosis >20 HPF NENs. Recent reports suggest that these neoplasms have a better prognosis than the other GEP NECs and respond less to conventional chemotherapies [93, 95, 97].

On these bases in patients with Ki67 < 55% NEC, it is possible to consider chemotherapeutic regimens alternative to those containing platinum.

60.8.1.2 Chemotherapy in Neuroendocrine Tumors (NETs)

In NETs, chemotherapy has been widely used as single-agent or combination regimens.

Evidence came from retrospective and phase II studies, mostly using alkylating agents [streptozotocin (STZ), dacarbazine (DTIC), temozolomide (TMZ)], antimetabolites [5-fluorouracil (5-FU), capecitabine)], and, more recently, oxaliplatin.

Dacarbazine has been reported active as single agent and combination [98, 99].

Temozolomide is the latest compound from this category; it is an oral agent, usually well tolerated. A number of retrospective and prospective studies with TMZ were published as single agent and combination; although a specific combination regimen was not defined, TMZ + capecitabine is one of the most proposed. The methylguanine-methyltransferase (MGMT) enzyme can methylate the oxygen in 8-guanine position allowing the repair of the DNA damage induced by alkylating agents as TMZ. Therefore, it is supposed that the expression of MGMT is inversely proportional to the response to the TMZ itself (■ Fig. 60.7). However, so far no absolute validation of this concept in clinical practice was done.

Among the other type of chemotherapy, oxaliplatin has been largely used all around the world [100–106].

Lung Neuroendocrine Neoplasms (NENs)

There is no standard chemotherapy regimen for lung NETs [107].

Five-FU, CDDP, carboplatin, irinotecan, TMZ, gemcitabine, VP-16, doxorubicin, STZ, dacarbazine, paclitaxel, docetaxel, and pemetrexed were the mostly drugs used as single agent. Polychemotherapy was able to produce a radiological PR in only 5–10% of patients, but with symptomatic responses in 40–60% of cases.

A retrospective study on just lung NETs [108] reported activity of TMZ as monotherapy in 31 patients (66% ORR) and good tolerability. Oxaliplatin has been reported active and potentially effective in retrospective analyses of patients with metastatic lung NETs alone or lung NETs mixed with other primary sites, treated with GEMOX, CAPOX, or FOLFOX regimens [101, 105, 109].

60.9 Systemic Biological Therapies

60.9.1 Gastroenteropancreatic Neuroendocrine Neoplasms (GEP NENs)

Biological systemic therapies investigation was limited to GEP NETs. Some molecular pathways represented the targets, including somatostatin receptor (*SSR*), phosphoinositide 3-kinase (*PI3K*)/protein kinase B also known as *AKT*/mammalian target of rapamycin (*mTOR),* insulin-like growth factor receptor (*IGFR)*/epidermal growth factor receptor (*EGFR),* and vascular endothelial growth factor and vascular endothelial growth factor receptor (*VEGF*/*VEGFR)*. Understanding these pathways is a key strategy to a correct use of new therapeutic approaches.

60.9.2 Somatostatin Receptors (SSTRs)

The PROMID trial was a placebo-controlled phase III study, demonstrating the efficacy of using octreotide 30 mg every 4 weeks in metastatic functionally active or inactive neuroendocrine midgut NETs. In particular, median time to tumor progression (TTP) in octreotide LAR and placebo groups was 14.3 and 6 months, respectively; after 6 months of treatment, stable disease was observed in 66.7% of patients treated with octreotide LAR and 32.7% of placebo groups [110].

The randomized double-blind CLARINET study compared lanreotide 120 mg every 4 weeks with placebo in patients with nonfunctioning enteropancreatic advanced NENs with a Ki-67 < 10%. After 24 months, estimated rates of progression-free survival (PFS) were 65.1% in the Lanreotide group and 33.0% in the placebo group: concluding that treatment with somatostatin analogue (SSA) was associated with prolonged PFS [111].

60.9.3 mTOR Pathway

The serine/threonine kinase mTOR and its complexes (mTORC 1 and 2) contribute to the regulation of cell growth, protein synthesis, and autophagy, thanks to the interaction with lots of stimuli such as nutrition availability which involves AMPK or insulin and IGF1/IGF2 [61] that can activate PI3K and AKT signals; both pathways lead to the activation of mTORC 1–2 [61]. Some studies have shown that the expression and the activation of this pathway is higher in PanNENs than in small intestine NETs. According to this, in PanNENs there is also a lower expression of tuberin (TSC2), an inhibitor of mTOR signaling, and this leads to a more aggressive behavior of the tumor with a worse prognosis. The PI3K/AKT/mTOR pathway is regulated also by the phosphate PTEN which acts as inhibitor; its levels are lower in NECs and in the most aggressive forms, and the loss of its expression might correlate with sensibility to mTOR inhibitors [112–114].

For a general view of mTOR pathway, see the image below.

The RADIANT-4 trial has studied the activity of a rapalog inhibitor of mTORC1, Everolimus, in progressive nonfunctioning NENs of lung and GI tract. The results of the trial have demonstrated the significant improvement in PFS in the group of patients treated with Everolimus compared to the placebo group [115].

Sunitinib, which is a multitargeted tyrosin-kinase inhibitor (VEGFR-PDGFR), is a possible strategy since a randomized phase III trial in patients with progressive pancreatic NENs has proven its efficacy (PFS 11.4 months against 5.5 in the placebo group) [116]. Thanks to that, sunitinib is recommended in progressive PanNENs with a high grade of recommendation. Predictors of efficacy to sunitinib can be IL-8 and VEGFR3 levels [117].

For a short view on the biological mechanisms of NENs, see ▣ Table 60.10 and ▣ Fig. 60.8.

▣ **Table 60.10** An easy view on the biological pathway of NENs

Molecular target	Role	Drugs	Trials	Notes
SSR	Inhibitory effects on cell-growth and proliferation and on protein synthesis.	SSA: lanreotide or octreotide	PROMID/ CLARINET	–
mTOR	Regulation of cell growth, protein synthesis, and autophagy	Everolimus	RADIANT	–
VEGFR/ EGFR	Proliferation of new vessels, PI3K/AKT/mTOR signal, TGF-beta and the connective tissue growth factor	Sunitinib	NCT00428597	–

Fig. 60.8 mTOR pathway 1

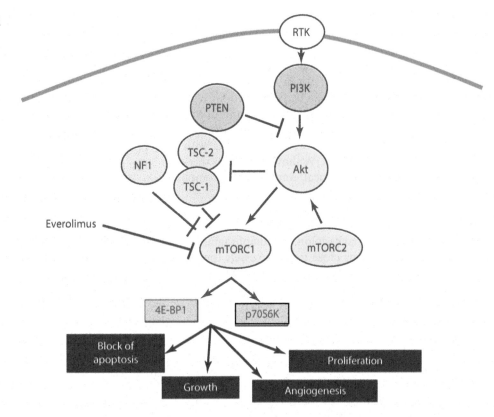

60.9.4 Lung NETs

Somatostatin analogues (SSAs) such as octreotide or lanreotide were compared to placebo and showed antiproliferative effects in midgut carcinoids, including patients with lung tumors, with a progression-free survival (PFS) increase from 6 months to 14 months [110]. These agents are also recommended to control symptoms caused by secretion of biologically active peptides or amine, occurring in 60% of patients with lung carcinoids. Recently, the subgroup analysis of the phase III randomized RADIANT-4 trial demonstrated that everolimus led to a median PFS improvement of 5.6 months preserving overall health-related quality of life as compared to placebo in patients with advanced, nonfunctional, lung carcinoids, emerging as new standard of care in this subgroup of patients [115, 118, 119]. The phase II randomized LUNA trial compared the long-acting SRA pasireotide versus everolimus versus pasireotide plus everolimus in patients with advanced lung carcinoids, showing that the proportion of patients progression-free at month 9 were 39%, 33.3%, 58.5%, respectively, with tolerability consistent with the known safety profiles of these agents [120]. The results of this study indicate that combination therapy of an SSA with everolimus would need further clinical investigation in this rare subset of patients.

60.10 Liver-Directed Treatments

Liver-directed treatments (LDTs) are mostly represented by interventional radiology procedures. They include ablative and vascular treatments.

60.10.1 Ablative Treatments

Local ablative techniques play an important role in the treatment of liver metastases when there is no surgical indication as for location and/or number and/or size of lesions.

Although more ablative treatments are available such as cryotherapy, microwave ablation, laser, or electroporation, the most common technique is the *radiofrequency thermal ablation (RFA)*. In well-selected patients, this method allows to reach results quite overlapping to surgery [121].

This type of treatment should be proposed to patients with localized and limited or residual disease after other therapies. Radiofrequency thermal ablation acts by converting the energy of radiofrequency waves into heat: a high-frequency alternating current, approximately 460 kHz, passes through the tip of a needle-electrode, spreading into the surrounding tissue and causing an ionic vibration. The vibration in turn determines the progressive heating of the cell walls of the tumor tissue surrounding the electrode and resulting in cell death at temperatures of 60–90 °.

In patients with liver metastases from GEP-NETs or lung NETs, RFA is effective both in symptom control and tumor growth control; it can be performed through both a percutaneous and surgical approach and in this latter case by both an open and laparoscopic technique [122]. A published large series of NEN patients with liver metastases treated with RFA showed that this therapy could provide effective local control with prompt symptomatic improvement [123].

One of the RFA limits is the treatment of liver lesions close to vital organs, or superficial metastases in contiguity with the stomach, colon, and diaphragm.

In case of liver lesions close to large vessels (portal venous branches or hepatic veins), there is a high risk of disease recurrence after thermal ablation due to a "cooling" effect induced by the blood flow which dissipates the heat induced by electrode.

Although surgical resection represents the treatment of choice in patients with low liver tumor burden, RFA could replace the surgery itself, particularly in patients in whom the metastases are unresectable or when the surgical access is particularly difficult. The combination of the surgical resection with the RFA may give the opportunity to completely treat the metastatic liver metastases in case of lesions less than 3 cm diameter and when the number of them is limited.

Microwave ablation (MWA) over the last years has been spreading a lot due to a better efficiency of the equipment available. Microwave generators use electromagnetic energy at a minimum of 900 MHz to cause thermal ablation of tumor cells, reaching a temperature of 160 °C. Compared to RFA, MWA acts with energy release in the active tissue, determining the dehydration and carbonization of the tissue and generally completing the treatment in a much shorter time than RFA. Moreover, due to the differences in energy release, MWA is involved in the "cooling" effect of the tissue caused by the surrounding vasculature less than RFA.

The most important limit for both RFA and MWA is liver lesion size, even though it has been described the possibility of performing the thermoablation also of large lesions by the multi-positioning of the needle in the context of the same metastasis and during the same session. However, it is difficult to radically treat a liver lesion greater than 3 cm, obtaining an adequate thermo-induced necrosis margin in the surrounding healthy hepatic parenchyma (comparable to the surgical resection margin).

60.10.2 Vascular Treatments

The hepatic transarterial embolization (TAE) is performed under radiological control, and it is based on the Seldinger percutaneous technique and on the principle that liver metastases and primary tumors in NENs are vascularized by the hepatic arterial circulation, whereas the nonpathological hepatocytes are mainly supplied by the portal vein [124–127].

The procedure requires the hepatic artery or its anatomical variants catheterization for an angiographic study of the hepatic arterial circle and to evaluate which arterial branches are involved in the pathological circle of the lesion. Then with a superselective technique, a slow infusion of embolizing microspheres (tens to hundreds microns in size) carries on through the arterial branches belonging to the lesion.

The main purpose of this procedure is to embolize the pathological arterial path as distally as possible with the embolizing material to induce ischemia and tissue necrosis (Fig. 60.9).

The treatment can be repeated after 1–3 months for several sessions.

From a clinical point of view, TAE could reduce tumor-related symptoms and induce a tumor debulking in order to improve the efficacy of systemic treatments or surgery inside a multidisciplinary strategy.

The chemoembolization (TACE) differs from TAE only for the type of material infused which is a chemotherapy (adriamycin, streptozotocin) mixed to an embolizing agent like an oil (Lipiodol) or microparticles with different composition based on the chosen material. The utility of this procedure is increasing tissue damage induced by ischemia through a chemotherapy [128].

These treatments are often associated with a postembolization syndrome, characterized by transient liver failure which may be caused by treatment-induced necrosis. The clinical symptoms are fever, nausea, vomiting, and, in particular, after TACE, abdominal pain. It is generally lasting for 24–48 hours, and the therapy is based on hydration, antibiotics, and antipyretics; in case of patients with functioning tumor, an infusion treatment with somatostatin analogs (SSAs) should be considered.

The selective internal radiation therapy (SIRT) is another treatment with a vascular approach [25, 26], and it can be performed by intra-arterial infusion of microspheres preloaded with Ittrio90 (90Y), in patients with unresectable liver metastases, who already underwent TAE and/or TACE.

Its efficacy seems independent by the neoplastic tissue already treated, while it is dependent by the doses administered which, in turn, depends on the relationship between liver disease and liver healthy. Higher this ratio is, higher should be the dose delivered to the lesion compared to the healthy liver parenchyma. Contraindications to SIRT are the same for TAE and TACE.

Based on the observed results (PR or CR in 63% of patients and median OS of 36–70 months), long-term clinical results should be performed and encouraged.

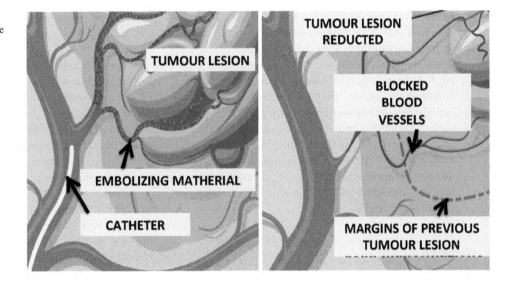

◘ **Fig. 60.9** TAE: The embolizing materials block the blood flow and the lesion reduction

---

Expert Opinion
Nicola Fazio

Key Points

1. Neuroendocrine neoplasms (NENs) are a group of heterogeneous malignancies raising from cells of the diffuse neuroendocrine system. Neuroendocrine neoplasms are rare cancers as their incidence is <6 new cases/100.000 × year.

2. Gastroenteropancreatic (GEP), which are the most common among NENs, are classified according to tumor morphology + ki-67 and/or number of mitosis into four categories: neuroendocrine tumors (NET) G1, NET G2, NET G3, and neuroendocrine carcinomas (NEC). Neuroendocrine tumors are the well differentiated, whereas NEC represent the poorly differentiated. In case of mixed forms, they will be indicated as mixed neuroendocrine non ndocrine neoplasm (MiNEN).

Lung NENs are the second most frequent subgroup of NENs; they are classified into typical and atypical carcinoids, which are the well differentiated, and small cell and large cell neuroendocrine carcinomas, which are the poorly differentiated.

3. Clinical presentation of NENs is heterogeneous. Particularly, NENs comprise functioning and nonfunctioning types, depending on the presence or absence of a clinical syndrome due to hormones or other substances produced by the tumor. The most frequent syndrome is the carcinoid syndrome, more often characterized by diarrhea and facial flushing.

4. Morphological (cross-sectional) and functional (somatostatin receptor, metabolic) imaging are indicated for diagnosis, staging, and characterization of a NEN. Upper and lower digestive endoscopy +/− endoscopic ultrasound (EUS) are tools to diagnose, to stage, and to treat NENs from the stomach, duodenum, and rectum. Pancreatic EUS is useful for

diagnosis of pancreatic NEN. However, a pathologic diagnosis, preferably histologic, should always be obtained.

5. Therapeutic approach to NENs is various. Localized low-grade NETs can be removed endoscopically or surgically. Radical surgery should be performed in locally advanced radically resectable NETs. In the advanced setting, systemic medical therapies, surgical or interventional radiology debulking, and primary tumor removal should all be discussed within an NEN-dedicated multidisciplinary team (MDT). Somatostatin analogs (SSA), sunitinib, everolimus, peptide receptor radionuclide therapy (PRRT), and various chemotherapeutic regimens can be proposed in clinical practice to patients with advanced NENs.

6. Liver-directed treatments, including surgical and nonsurgical approaches, are usually discussed within the NEN-dedicated MDT for patients with metastatic GEP or lung NETs.

Recommendations

- ESMO
- ▶ https://www.esmo.org/Guidelines/Endocrine-and-Neuroendocrine-Cancers/Neuroendocrine-Bronchial-and-Thymic-Tumours
- ▶ https://www.esmo.org/Guidelines/Endocrine-and-Neuroendocrine-Cancers/Neuroendocrine-Gastroenteropancreatic-Tumours

The knowledge about NENs has been hugely increasing over the last three decades. Although this led to a wider awareness about this disease, improved diagnostic work-up and characterization, and a higher number of therapeutic options, unfortunately currently there is no validated predictive factor of efficacy to some therapy or specific sequence/integration of the different treatments. This may be due on the one hand to the limitations of our research approach and on the other hand to the biological and clinical heterogeneity of NENs. On this basis, it looks clear that the key of a successful therapy for a patient with a NEN should be his/her management within a NEN-dedicated MDT. Luckily, several centers all over the world constituted the own internal NEN MDT, many of them certified by the European Society of Neuroendocrine Tumors (ENETS) as Centers of Excellence for GEP NEN. The NEN-dedicated MDT involvement is critical to individualize the therapeutic strategy in line with the tumor/patient characteristics and goals of treatment.

Guidelines from the main scientific societies may give some help in terms of algorithm of clinical thinking, but it should be always kept in mind that the level of evidence is often very low and therefore exposed to bias. The NEN-dedicated MDT makes less difficult to contextualize the evidence, experience, approvals, and investigations into the specific clinical context of the patient who should be treated.

Although the aforementioned limitations basic and clinical research on NEN have been clearly improved over the last decades by leading to important new insights and laying solid foundations for practice-changing future investigations.

Hints for a Deeper Insight

- Anti-tumour effects of lanreotide for pancreatic and intestinal neuroendocrine tumours: the CLARINET open-label extension study: ▶ https://www.ncbi.nlm.nih.gov/pubmed/26743120
- Everolimus for the treatment of advanced, nonfunctional neuroendocrine tumours of the lung or gastrointestinal tract (RADIANT-4): a randomised, placebo-controlled, phase 3 study: ▶ https://www.ncbi.nlm.nih.gov/pubmed/26703889
- Non-conventional doses of somatostatin analogs in patients with progressing well differentiated neuroendocrine tumor: ▶ https://www.ncbi.nlm.nih.gov/pubmed/31545377
- Therapeutic schemes in 177Lu and 90Y-PRRT: radiobiological considerations: ▶ https://www.ncbi.nlm.nih.gov/pubmed/26576734

Case Study: A Huge Abdominal Mass

Woman, 35 years old
- *Family history* negative for malignancy
- *APR:* Rheumatic heart disease (mitral valve)
- *APP:* Frequent episodes of nausea and vomiting with abdominal pain
- *Objective examination*: Mild tenderness on deep palpation of the abdomen and a palpable mass in the mesogastric area
- *Blood tests*: Normal blood test
- *CT abdomen mdc*: Evidence of a retroperitoneal mass (DT max: 14 × 13.7 × 6.7 cm) originating from pancreatic tissue with a consistent compressive effect on the surrounding structures. Negative for distant metastases

Question

What action should be taken?
  (1) Surgery. (2) Biopsy. (3) Other

Answer

Biopsy
  Neuroendocrine tumor (NET) G2, chromogranin A+, ki67: 10%, 7/10 mitosis HPF.

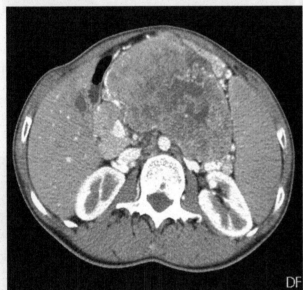
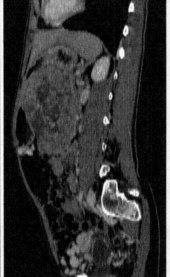

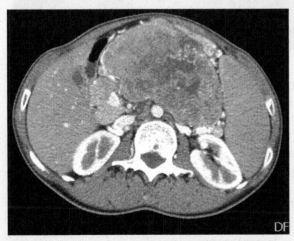
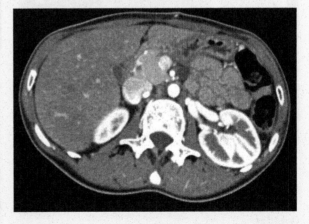

Before surgery

After surgery

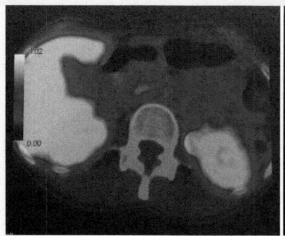

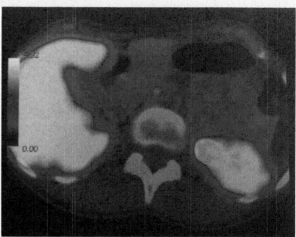

Question

What action should be taken?

   (1) Surgery. (2) Medical therapy. (3) Other

Answer

Surgery.

   Distal splenopancreatectomy. Histopathological examination: neuroendocrine tumor, G2, ki67: 12% Nine months later, at the CT scan, evidence of a new nodule on the left suprarenal region. (DT max 6 mm).

Answer

The patient begins somatostatin analogues (SSA) at standard dose.

   At the next CT scan evaluation, evidence of progression disease of the previous nodule (DT max 13 mm), and arising of a new hepatic lesion (DT max 8 mm).

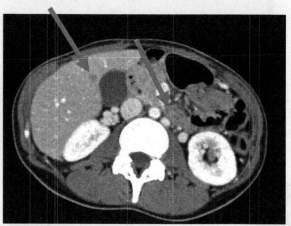

Question

What action should be taken?

   (1) Everolimus. (2) Sunitinib. (3) Other

Answer

Everolimus 10 mg.

Key Points

- The importance of a correct surgical approach
- Symptoms often nonspecific
- The main role of the targeted therapies (i.e., everolimus).

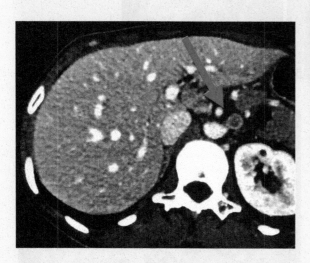

68Ga-PET: Positive uptake in the celiac region.

Question

What action should be taken?

   (1) Somatostain analogues. (2) Sunitinib. (3) Other

60

Case Study: The Importance of PRRT

Woman, 72 years old
- *Family history* negative for malignancy
- *APR:* Hysterectomy, for leiomyoma, appendectomy, major depressive disorder
- *APP:* Intense acute abdominal pain
- *Objective examination*: Tenderness on palpation of the abdomen
- *Blood tests*: Normal blood test
- *CT abdomen MDC*: Evidence of enlarged mesenteric lymph nodes
- *Colonoscopy:* Negative
- *Esophagogastroduodenoscopy:* Negative

An exploratory laparotomy is performed in the critical surgery unit: resection of a small tract of the bowel. Histopathological examination: neuroendocrine tumor, ki67: 7%, 3/10 mitosis HPF, G2.
- *Octreoscan*: Negative
- One year later, after a suspicious CT scan and because of the presence of abdominal pain, a ^{68}Ga-PET is performed with the positive uptake of the tracer at some mesenteric lymph nodes and small tracts of bowel.

Question

What action should be taken?
  (1) Surgery. (2) Biopsy. (3) Other

Answer

Surgery.
  Resection of lymph nodes and the involved tracts of bowel.
  Histopathological examination: Neuroendocrine tumor (NET) G1, ki67: <2%
- As the presence of symptoms like nausea, vomiting, abdominal pain, the patient is treated with somatostatin analogs at standard dose with a relief of the symptoms.
- After six years, at a follow-up CT scan, multiple mesenteric lymph nodes appear bigger and suspicious.

Question

What action should be taken?
  (1) Watchful waiting. (2) ^{68}Ga-PET. (3) Other

Answer

^{68}Ga-PET.
  Uptake of the tracer in multiple mesenteric and supradiaphragmatic lymph nodes. Evidence of doubtful uptake in the liver.

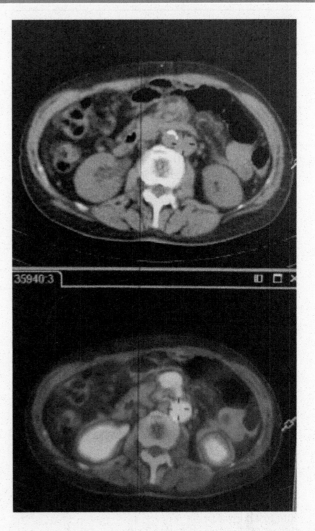

35940:3

Question

What action should be taken?
  (1) Surgery. (2) Medical therapy. (3) Other

Answer

Other: Peptide receptor radionuclide therapy (PRRT)

Key Points

- The possibility of acute presentation of neuroendocrine neoplasms (bowel obstruction)
- The importance of a correct follow-up
- The role of peptide receptor radionuclide therapy in a multidisciplinary approach

Bibliography

1. Nagtegaal ID, Odze RD, Klimstra D, Paradis V, Rugge M, Schirmacher P, et al. The 2019 WHO classification of tumours of the digestive system. Histopathology. 2020;76(2):182–8.

2. Travis WD, Brambilla E, Burke AP, Marx A, Nicholson AG. Introduction to the 2015 World Health Organization classification of tumors of the lung, pleura, thymus, and heart. J Thorac Oncol. 2015;10(9):1240–2.

3. Modlin IM, Oberg K, Chung DC, Jensen RT, de Herder WW, Thakker RV, et al. Gastroenteropancreatic neuroendocrine tumours. Lancet Oncol. 2008;9(1):61–72.

4. Halperin DM, Shen C, Dasari A, Xu Y, Chu Y, Zhou S, et al. Frequency of carcinoid syndrome at neuroendocrine tumour diagnosis: a population-based study. Lancet Oncol. 2017;18(4):525–34.

5. Dasari A, Shen C, Halperin D, Zhao B, Zhou S, Xu Y, et al. Trends in the incidence, prevalence, and survival outcomes in patients with neuroendocrine tumors in the United States. JAMA Oncol. 2017;3(10):1335–42.

6. Dasari A, Mehta K, Byers LA, Sorbye H, Yao JC. Comparative study of lung and extrapulmonary poorly differentiated neuroendocrine carcinomas: a SEER database analysis of 162,983 cases. Cancer. 2018;124(4):807–15.

7. Caplin ME, Baudin E, Ferolla P, Filosso P, Garcia-Yuste M, Lim E, et al. Pulmonary neuroendocrine (carcinoid) tumors: European Neuroendocrine Tumor Society expert consensus and recommendations for best practice for typical and atypical pulmonary carcinoids. Ann Oncol. 2015;26(8):1604–20.

8. Pape UF, Niederle B, Costa F, Gross D, Kelestimur F, Kianmanesh R, et al. ENETS consensus guidelines for neuroendocrine neoplasms of the appendix (excluding goblet cell carcinomas). Neuroendocrinology. 2016;103(2):144–52.

9. Modlin IM, Kidd M, Latich I, Zikusoka MN, Shapiro MD. Current status of gastrointestinal carcinoids. Gastroenterology. 2005;128(6):1717–51.

10. Ramage JK, De Herder WW, Delle Fave G, Ferolla P, Ferone D, Ito T, et al. ENETS consensus guidelines update for colorectal neuroendocrine neoplasms. Neuroendocrinology. 2016;103(2):139–43.

11. Falconi M, Eriksson B, Kaltsas G, Bartsch DK, Capdevila J, Caplin M, et al. ENETS consensus guidelines update for the management of patients with functional pancreatic neuroendocrine tumors and non-functional pancreatic neuroendocrine tumors. Neuroendocrinology. 2016;103(2):153–71.

12. Oberg K. Management of functional neuroendocrine tumors of the pancreas. Gland Surg. 2018;7(1):20–7.

13. Kidd M, Bodei L, Modlin IM. Chromogranin A: any relevance in neuroendocrine tumors? Curr Opin Endocrinol Diabetes Obes. 2016;23(1):28–37.

14. Baudin E, Bidart JM, Bachelot A, Ducreux M, Elias D, Ruffie P, et al. Impact of chromogranin a measurement in the work-up of neuroendocrine tumors. Ann Oncol. 2001;12(Suppl 2):S79–82.

15. Zatelli MC, Torta M, Leon A, Ambrosio MR, Gion M, Tomassetti P, et al. Chromogranin a as a marker of neuroendocrine neoplasia: an Italian Multicenter Study. Endocr Relat Cancer. 2007;14(2):473–82.

16. Arnold R, Wilke A, Rinke A, Mayer C, Kann PH, Klose KJ, et al. Plasma chromogranin A as marker for survival in patients with metastatic endocrine gastroenteropancreatic tumors. Clin Gastroenterol Hepatol. 2008;6(7):820–7.

17. Nehar D, Lombard-Bohas C, Olivieri S, Claustrat B, Chayvialle JA, Penes MC, et al. Interest of Chromogranin A for diagnosis and follow-up of endocrine tumours. Clin Endocrinol. 2004;60(5):644–52.

18. Marotta V, Nuzzo V, Ferrara T, Zuccoli A, Masone M, Nocerino L, et al. Limitations of Chromogranin A in clinical practice. Biomarkers. 2012;17(2):186–91.

19. Khan MO, Ather MH. Chromogranin A–serum marker for prostate cancer. J Pak Med Assoc. 2011;61(1):108–11.

20. Nobili E, Pezzilli R, Santini D, Campidelli C, Calculli L, Casadei R, et al. Autoimmune pancreatitis associated with high levels of chromogranin a, serotonin and 5-hydroxyindoleacetic Acid. Case Rep Gastroenterol. 2008;2(1):11–7.

21. Bajetta E, Ferrari L, Martinetti A, Celio L, Procopio G, Artale S, et al. Chromogranin A, neuron specific enolase, carcinoembryonic antigen, and hydroxyindole acetic acid evaluation in patients with neuroendocrine tumors. Cancer. 1999;86(5):858–65.

22. Jensen KH, Hilsted L, Jensen C, Mynster T, Rehfeld JF, Knigge U. Chromogranin A is a sensitive marker of progression or regression in ileo-cecal neuroendocrine tumors. Scand J Gastroenterol. 2013;48(1):70–7.

23. Wang YH, Yang QC, Lin Y, Xue L, Chen MH, Chen J. Chromogranin a as a marker for diagnosis, treatment, and survival in patients with gastroenteropancreatic neuroendocrine neoplasm. Medicine (Baltimore). 2014;93(27):e247.

24. Nikou GC, Marinou K, Thomakos P, Papageorgiou D, Sanzanidis V, Nikolaou P, et al. Chromogranin A levels in diagnosis, treatment and follow-up of 42 patients with non-functioning pancreatic endocrine tumours. Pancreatology. 2008;8(4–5):510–9.

25. Modlin IM, Gustafsson BI, Moss SF, Pavel M, Tsolakis AV, Kidd M. Chromogranin A–biological function and clinical utility in neuro endocrine tumor disease. Ann Surg Oncol. 2010;17(9):2427–43.

26. Belli SH, Oneto A, Aranda C, O'Connor JM, Domenichini E, Roca E, et al. Chromogranin A as a biochemical marker for the management of neuroendocrine tumors: a multicenter study developed in Argentina. Acta Gastroenterol Latinoam. 2009;39(3):184–9.

27. Massironi S, Rossi RE, Casazza G, Conte D, Ciafardini C, Galeazzi M, et al. Chromogranin A in diagnosing and monitoring patients with gastroenteropancreatic neuroendocrine neoplasms: a large series from a single institution. Neuroendocrinology. 2014;100(2–3):240–9.

28. Cwikla JB, Bodei L, Kolasinska-Cwikla A, Sankowski A, Modlin IM, Kidd M. Circulating transcript analysis (NETest) in GEP-NETs treated with somatostatin analogs defines therapy. J Clin Endocrinol Metab. 2015;100(11):E1437–45.

29. Modlin IM, Frilling A, Salem RR, Alaimo D, Drymousis P, Wasan HS, et al. Blood measurement of neuroendocrine gene transcripts defines the effectiveness of operative resection and ablation strategies. Surgery. 2016;159(1):336–47.

30. Ramage JK, Ahmed A, Ardill J, Bax N, Breen DJ, Caplin ME, et al. Guidelines for the management of gastroenteropancreatic neuroendocrine (including carcinoid) tumours (NETs). Gut. 2012;61(1):6–32.

31. Bader TR, Semelka RC, Chiu VC, Armao DM, Woosley JT. MRI of carcinoid tumors: spectrum of appearances in the gastrointestinal tract and liver. J Magn Reson Imaging. 2001;14(3):261–9.

32. Rossi RE, Conte D, Elli L, Branchi F, Massironi S. Endoscopic techniques to detect small-bowel neuroendocrine tumors: a literature review. United European Gastroenterol J. 2017;5(1):5–12.

33. Sharma P, Arora S, Karunanithi S, Khadgawat R, Durgapal P, Sharma R, et al. Somatostatin receptor based PET/CT imaging with 68Ga-DOTA-Nal3-octreotide for localization of clinically and biochemically suspected insulinoma. Q J Nucl Med Mol Imaging. 2016;60(1):69–76.

34. Treglia G, Castaldi P, Rindi G, Giordano A, Rufini V. Diagnostic performance of Gallium-68 somatostatin receptor PET and PET/CT in patients with thoracic and gastroenteropancreatic neuroendocrine tumours: a meta-analysis. Endocrine. 2012;42(1):80–7.

35. Sundin A. Radiological and nuclear medicine imaging of gastroenteropancreatic neuroendocrine tumours. Best Pract Res Clin Gastroenterol. 2012;26(6):803–18.

36. Niederle B, Pape UF, Costa F, Gross D, Kelestimur F, Knigge U, et al. ENETS consensus guidelines update for neuroendocrine neoplasms of the jejunum and ileum. Neuroendocrinology. 2016;103(2):125–38.

37. Gornals J, Varas M, Catala I, Maisterra S, Pons C, Bargallo D, et al. Definitive diagnosis of neuroendocrine tumors using fine-needle aspiration-puncture guided by endoscopic ultrasonography. Rev Esp Enferm Dig. 2011;103(3):123–8.

38. Pais SA, Al-Haddad M, Mohamadnejad M, Leblanc JK, Sherman S, McHenry L, et al. EUS for pancreatic neuroendocrine tumors: a single-center, 11-year experience. Gastrointest Endosc. 2010;71(7):1185–93.

39. van Asselt SJ, Brouwers AH, van Dullemen HM, van der Jagt EJ, Bongaerts AH, Kema IP, et al. EUS is superior for detection of pancreatic lesions compared with standard imaging in patients with multiple endocrine neoplasia type 1. Gastrointest Endosc. 2015;81(1):159–67 e2.

40. Thomas-Marques L, Murat A, Delemer B, Penfornis A, Cardot-Bauters C, Baudin E, et al. Prospective endoscopic ultrasonographic evaluation of the frequency of nonfunctioning pancreaticoduodenal endocrine tumors in patients with multiple endocrine neoplasia type 1. Am J Gastroenterol. 2006;101(2):266–73.

41. Yamamoto C, Aoyagi K, Suekane H, Iida M, Hizawa K, Kuwano Y, et al. Carcinoid tumors of the duodenum: report of three cases treated by endoscopic resection. Endoscopy. 1997;29(3):218–21.

42. Brenner B, Tang LH, Klimstra DS, Kelsen DP. Small-cell carcinomas of the gastrointestinal tract: a review. J Clin Oncol. 2004;22(13):2730–9.

43. Yazawa N, Imaizumi T, Okada K, Matsuyama M, Dowaki S, Tobita K, et al. Nonfunctioning pancreatic endocrine tumor with extension into the main pancreatic duct: report of a case. Surg Today. 2011;41(5):737–40.

44. Pelosi G, Rindi G, Travis WD, Papotti M. Ki-67 antigen in lung neuroendocrine tumors: unraveling a role in clinical practice. J Thorac Oncol. 2014;9(3):273–84.

45. Pelosi G, Rodriguez J, Viale G, Rosai J. Typical and atypical pulmonary carcinoid tumor overdiagnosed as small-cell carcinoma on biopsy specimens: a major pitfall in the management of lung cancer patients. Am J Surg Pathol. 2005;29(2):179–87.

46. Varela-Lema L, Fernandez-Villar A, Ruano-Ravina A. Effectiveness and safety of endobronchial ultrasound-transbronchial needle aspiration: a systematic review. Eur Respir J. 2009;33(5):1156–64.

47. Nakajima T, Yasufuku K. How I do it--optimal methodology for multidirectional analysis of endobronchial ultrasound-guided transbronchial needle aspiration samples. J Thorac Oncol. 2011;6(1):203–6.

48. Detterbeck FC, Lewis SZ, Diekemper R, Addrizzo-Harris D, Alberts WM. Executive Summary: Diagnosis and management of lung cancer, 3rd ed: American College of Chest Physicians evidence-based clinical practice guidelines. Chest. 2013;143(5 Suppl):7S–37S.

49. Rosado de Christenson ML, Abbott GF, Kirejczyk WM, Galvin JR, Travis WD. Thoracic carcinoids: radiologic-pathologic correlation. Radiographics. 1999;19(3):707–36.

50. Guimaraes MD, de Andrade MQ, da Fonte AC, Chojniak R, Gross JL. CT-guided cutting needle biopsy of lung lesions–an effective procedure for adequate material and specific diagnose. Eur J Radiol. 2011;80(3):e488–90.

51. Rizzo S, Preda L, Raimondi S, Meroni S, Belmonte M, Monfardini L, et al. Risk factors for complications of CT-guided lung biopsies. Radiol Med. 2011;116(4):548–63.

52. Oshiro Y, Kusumoto M, Matsuno Y, Asamura H, Tsuchiya R, Terasaki H, et al. CT findings of surgically resected large cell neuroendocrine carcinoma of the lung in 38 patients. AJR Am J Roentgenol. 2004;182(1):87–91.

53. Jung KJ, Lee KS, Han J, Kwon OJ, Kim J, Shim YM, et al. Large cell neuroendocrine carcinoma of the lung: clinical, CT, and pathologic findings in 11 patients. J Thorac Imaging. 2001;16(3):156–62.

54. Semelka RC, Custodio CM, Cem Balci N, Woosley JT. Neuroendocrine tumors of the pancreas: spectrum of appearances on MRI. J Magn Reson Imaging. 2000;11(2):141–8.

55. Kelekis NL, Semelka RC. MRI of pancreatic tumors. Eur Radiol. 1997;7(6):875–86.

56. Macera A, Lario C, Petracchini M, Gallo T, Regge D, Floriani I, et al. Staging of colorectal liver metastases after preoperative chemotherapy. Diffusion-weighted imaging in combination with Gd-EOB-DTPA MRI sequences increases sensitivity and diagnostic accuracy. Eur Radiol. 2013;23(3):739–47.

57. Dromain C, de Baere T, Baudin E, Galline J, Ducreux M, Boige V, et al. MR imaging of hepatic metastases caused by neuroendocrine tumors: comparing four techniques. AJR Am J Roentgenol. 2003;180(1):121–8.

58. Sundin A, Vullierme MP, Kaltsas G, Plockinger U, Mallorca Consensus Conference P, European Neuroendocrine Tumor S. ENETS Consensus Guidelines for the Standards of Care in Neuroendocrine Tumors: radiological examinations. Neuroendocrinology. 2009;90(2):167–83.

59. Camilli M, Papadimitriou K, Nogueira A, Incorvaia L, Galvano A, D'Antonio F, et al. Molecular profiling of pancreatic neuroendocrine tumors (pNETS) and the clinical potential. Expert Rev Gastroenterol Hepatol. 2018;12(5):471–8.

60. Feng Z, Ma J, Hua X. Epigenetic regulation by the menin pathway. Endocr Relat Cancer. 2017;24(10):T147–T59.

61. Kidd M, Modlin I, Oberg K. Towards a new classification of gastroenteropancreatic neuroendocrine neoplasms. Nat Rev Clin Oncol. 2016;13(11):691–705.

62. Agarwal SK. The future: genetics advances in MEN1 therapeutic approaches and management strategies. Endocr Relat Cancer. 2017;24(10):T119–T34.

63. Nielsen SM, Rhodes L, Blanco I, Chung WK, Eng C, Maher ER, et al. Von Hippel-Lindau disease: genetics and role of genetic counseling in a multiple neoplasia syndrome. J Clin Oncol. 2016;34(18):2172–81.

64. Varshney N, Kebede AA, Owusu-Dapaah H, Lather J, Kaushik M, Bhullar JS. A review of Von Hippel-Lindau syndrome. J Kidney Cancer VHL. 2017;4(3):20–9.

65. Kiuru M, Busam KJ. The NF1 gene in tumor syndromes and melanoma. Lab Investig. 2017;97(2):146–57.

66. Au KS, Williams AT, Gambello MJ, Northrup H. Molecular genetic basis of tuberous sclerosis complex: from bench to bedside. J Child Neurol. 2004;19(9):699–709.

67. Cao Y, Gao Z, Li L, Jiang X, Shan A, Cai J, et al. Whole exome sequencing of insulinoma reveals recurrent T372R mutations in YY1. Nat Commun. 2013;4:2810.

68. Marinoni I, Kurrer AS, Vassella E, Dettmer M, Rudolph T, Banz V, et al. Loss of DAXX and ATRX are associated with chromosome instability and reduced survival of patients with pancreatic neuroendocrine tumors. Gastroenterology. 2014;146(2):453–60. e5

69. Zhuang Z, Vortmeyer AO, Pack S, Huang S, Pham TA, Wang C, et al. Somatic mutations of the MEN1 tumor suppressor

gene in sporadic gastrinomas and insulinomas. Cancer Res. 1997;57(21):4682–6.

70. Kidd M, Modlin IM, Drozdov I. Gene network-based analysis identifies two potential subtypes of small intestinal neuroendocrine tumors. BMC Genomics. 2014;15:595.

71. Duerr EM, Mizukami Y, Ng A, Xavier RJ, Kikuchi H, Deshpande V, et al. Defining molecular classifications and targets in gastroenteropancreatic neuroendocrine tumors through DNA microarray analysis. Endocr Relat Cancer. 2008;15(1):243–56.

72. de Mestier L, Zappa M, Hentic O, Vilgrain V, Ruszniewski P. Liver transarterial embolizations in metastatic neuroendocrine tumors. Rev Endocr Metab Disord. 2017;18(4):459–71.

73. Coriat R, Walter T, Terris B, Couvelard A, Ruszniewski P. Gastroenteropancreatic well-differentiated grade 3 neuroendocrine tumors: review and position statement. Oncologist. 2016;21(10):1191–9.

74. Panzuto F, Rinzivillo M, Spada F, Antonuzzo L, Ibrahim T, Campana D, et al. Everolimus in pancreatic neuroendocrine carcinomas G3. Pancreas. 2017;46(3):302–5.

75. Pavel M, O'Toole D, Costa F, Capdevila J, Gross D, Kianmanesh R, et al. ENETS consensus guidelines update for the management of distant metastatic disease of intestinal, pancreatic, bronchial neuroendocrine neoplasms (NEN) and NEN of unknown primary site. Neuroendocrinology. 2016;103(2):172–85.

76. Fazio N, Milione M. Heterogeneity of grade 3 gastroenteropancreatic neuroendocrine carcinomas: new insights and treatment implications. Cancer Treat Rev. 2016;50:61–7.

77. Srirajaskanthan R, Kayani I, Quigley AM, Soh J, Caplin ME, Bomanji J. The role of 68Ga-DOTATATE PET in patients with neuroendocrine tumors and negative or equivocal findings on 111In-DTPA-octreotide scintigraphy. J Nucl Med. 2010;51(6):875–82.

78. Etchebehere EC, de Oliveira SA, Gumz B, Vicente A, Hoff PG, Corradi G, et al. 68Ga-DOTATATE PET/CT, 99mTc-HYNIC-octreotide SPECT/CT, and whole-body MR imaging in detection of neuroendocrine tumors: a prospective trial. J Nucl Med. 2014;55(10):1598–604.

79. Schreiter NF, Brenner W, Nogami M, Buchert R, Huppertz A, Pape UF, et al. Cost comparison of 111In-DTPA-octreotide scintigraphy and 68Ga-DOTATOC PET/CT for staging enteropancreatic neuroendocrine tumours. Eur J Nucl Med Mol Imaging. 2012;39(1):72–82.

80. Bozkurt MF, Virgolini I, Balogova S, Beheshti M, Rubello D, Decristoforo C, et al. Guideline for PET/CT imaging of neuroendocrine neoplasms with (68)Ga-DOTA-conjugated somatostatin receptor targeting peptides and (18)F-DOPA. Eur J Nucl Med Mol Imaging. 2017;44(9):1588–601.

81. Geijer H, Breimer LH. Somatostatin receptor PET/CT in neuroendocrine tumours: update on systematic review and meta-analysis. Eur J Nucl Med Mol Imaging. 2013;40(11):1770–80.

82. Skoura E, Michopoulou S, Mohmaduvesh M, Panagiotidis E, Al Harbi M, Toumpanakis C, et al. The impact of 68Ga-DOTATATE PET/CT imaging on management of patients with neuroendocrine tumors: experience from a National Referral Center in the United Kingdom. J Nucl Med. 2016;57(1):34–40.

83. Fendler WP, Barrio M, Spick C, Allen-Auerbach M, Ambrosini V, Benz M, et al. 68Ga-DOTATATE PET/CT interobserver agreement for neuroendocrine tumor assessment: results of a prospective study on 50 patients. J Nucl Med. 2017;58(2):307–11.

84. Boellaard R, Delgado-Bolton R, Oyen WJ, Giammarile F, Tatsch K, Eschner W, et al. FDG PET/CT: EANM procedure guidelines for tumour imaging: version 2.0. Eur J Nucl Med Mol Imaging. 2015;42(2):328–54.

85. Sundin A, Arnold R, Baudin E, Cwikla JB, Eriksson B, Fanti S, et al. ENETS consensus guidelines for the standards of care in neuroendocrine tumors: radiological. Nucl Med Hybrid Imag Neuroendocrinol. 2017;105(3):212–44.

86. Strosberg J, El-Haddad G, Wolin E, Hendifar A, Yao J, Chasen B, et al. Phase 3 trial of (177)Lu-dotatate for midgut neuroendocrine tumors. N Engl J Med. 2017;376(2):125–35.

87. Moertel CG, Kvols LK, O'Connell MJ, Rubin J. Treatment of neuroendocrine carcinomas with combined etoposide and cisplatin. Evidence of major therapeutic activity in the anaplastic variants of these neoplasms. Cancer. 1991;68(2):227–32.

88. Mitry E, Baudin E, Ducreux M, Sabourin JC, Rufie P, Aparicio T, et al. Treatment of poorly differentiated neuroendocrine tumours with etoposide and cisplatin. Br J Cancer. 1999;81(8):1351–5.

89. Fjallskog ML, Granberg DP, Welin SL, Eriksson C, Oberg KE, Janson ET, et al. Treatment with cisplatin and etoposide in patients with neuroendocrine tumors. Cancer. 2001;92(5):1101–7.

90. Iwasa S, Morizane C, Okusaka T, Ueno H, Ikeda M, Kondo S, et al. Cisplatin and etoposide as first-line chemotherapy for poorly differentiated neuroendocrine carcinoma of the hepatobiliary tract and pancreas. Jpn J Clin Oncol. 2010;40(4):313–8.

91. Rossi A, Di Maio M, Chiodini P, Rudd RM, Okamoto H, Skarlos DV, et al. Carboplatin- or cisplatin-based chemotherapy in first-line treatment of small-cell lung cancer: the COCIS meta-analysis of individual patient data. J Clin Oncol. 2012;30(14):1692–8.

92. Lu ZH, Li J, Lu M, Zhang XT, Li J, Zhou J, et al. Feasibility and efficacy of combined cisplatin plus irinotecan chemotherapy for gastroenteropancreatic neuroendocrine carcinomas. Med Oncol. 2013;30(3):664.

93. Sorbye H, Welin S, Langer SW, Vestermark LW, Holt N, Osterlund P, et al. Predictive and prognostic factors for treatment and survival in 305 patients with advanced gastrointestinal neuroendocrine carcinoma (WHO G3): the NORDIC NEC study. Ann Oncol. 2013;24(1):152–60.

94. Ali AS, Gronberg M, Langer SW, Ladekarl M, Hjortland GO, Vestermark LW, et al. Intravenous versus oral etoposide: efficacy and correlation to clinical outcome in patients with high-grade metastatic gastroenteropancreatic neuroendocrine neoplasms (WHO G3). Med Oncol. 2018;35(4):47.

95. Velayoudom-Cephise FL, Duvillard P, Foucan L, Hadoux J, Chougnet CN, Leboulleux S, et al. Are G3 ENETS neuroendocrine neoplasms heterogeneous? Endocr Relat Cancer. 2013;20(5):649–57.

96. Milione M, Maisonneuve P, Spada F, Pellegrinelli A, Spaggiari P, Albarello L, et al. The clinicopathologic heterogeneity of grade 3 gastroenteropancreatic neuroendocrine neoplasms: morphological differentiation and proliferation identify different prognostic categories. Neuroendocrinology. 2017;104(1):85–93.

97. Heetfeld M, Chougnet CN, Olsen IH, Rinke A, Borbath I, Crespo G, et al. Characteristics and treatment of patients with G3 gastroenteropancreatic neuroendocrine neoplasms. Endocr Relat Cancer. 2015;22(4):657–64.

98. Bajetta E, Rimassa L, Carnaghi C, Seregni E, Ferrari L, Di Bartolomeo M, et al. 5-Fluorouracil, dacarbazine, and epirubicin in the treatment of patients with neuroendocrine tumors. Cancer. 1998;83(2):372–8.

99. Walter T, Bruneton D, Cassier PA, Hervieu V, Pilleul F, Scoazec JY, et al. Evaluation of the combination 5-fluorouracil, dacarbazine, and epirubicin in patients with advanced well-differentiated neuroendocrine tumors. Clin Colorectal Cancer. 2010;9(4):248–54.

100. Kulke MH, Hornick JL, Frauenhoffer C, Hooshmand S, Ryan DP, Enzinger PC, et al. O6-methylguanine DNA methyltransferase deficiency and response to temozolomide-based therapy in patients with neuroendocrine tumors. Clin Cancer Res. 2009;15(1):338–45.

101. Bajetta E, Catena L, Procopio G, De Dosso S, Bichisao E, Ferrari L, et al. Are capecitabine and oxaliplatin (XELOX) suitable treatments for progressing low-grade and high-grade neuroendocrine tumours? Cancer Chemother Pharmacol. 2007;59(5):637–42.

102. Cassier PA, Walter T, Eymard B, Ardisson P, Perol M, Paillet C, et al. Gemcitabine and oxaliplatin combination chemotherapy for metastatic well-differentiated neuroendocrine carcinomas: a single-center experience. Cancer. 2009;115(15):3392–9.

103. Ferrarotto R, Testa L, Riechelmann RP, Sahade M, Siqueira LT, Costa FP, et al. Combination of capecitabine and oxaliplatin is an effective treatment option for advanced neuroendocrine tumors. Rare Tumors. 2013;5(3):e35.

104. Dussol AS, Joly MO, Vercherat C, Forestier J, Hervieu V, Scoazec JY, et al. Gemcitabine and oxaliplatin or alkylating agents for neuroendocrine tumors: comparison of efficacy and search for predictive factors guiding treatment choice. Cancer. 2015;121(19):3428–34.

105. Spada F, Antonuzzo L, Marconcini R, Radice D, Antonuzzo A, Ricci S, et al. Oxaliplatin-based chemotherapy in advanced neuroendocrine tumors: clinical outcomes and preliminary correlation with biological factors. Neuroendocrinology. 2016;103(6):806–14.

106. Faure M, Niccoli P, Autret A, Cavaglione G, Mineur L, Raoul JL. Systemic chemotherapy with FOLFOX in metastatic grade 1/2 neuroendocrine cancer. Mol Clin Oncol. 2017;6(1):44–8.

107. Lim E, Goldstraw P, Nicholson AG, Travis WD, Jett JR, Ferolla P, et al. Proceedings of the IASLC international workshop on advances in pulmonary neuroendocrine tumors 2007. J Thorac Oncol. 2008;3(10):1194–201.

108. Crona J, Bjorklund P, Welin S, Kozlovacki G, Oberg K, Granberg D. Treatment, prognostic markers and survival in thymic neuroendocrine tumours. A study from a single tertiary referral centre. Lung Cancer. 2013;79(3):289–93.

109. Walter T, Planchard D, Bouledrak K, Scoazec JY, Souquet PJ, Dussol AS, et al. Evaluation of the combination of oxaliplatin and 5-fluorouracil or gemcitabine in patients with sporadic metastatic pulmonary carcinoid tumors. Lung Cancer. 2016;96: 68–73.

110. Rinke A, Muller HH, Schade-Brittinger C, Klose KJ, Barth P, Wied M, et al. Placebo-controlled, double-blind, prospective, randomized study on the effect of octreotide LAR in the control of tumor growth in patients with metastatic neuroendocrine midgut tumors: a report from the PROMID Study Group. J Clin Oncol. 2009;27(28):4656–63.

111. Caplin ME, Pavel M, Cwikla JB, Phan AT, Raderer M, Sedlackova E, et al. Lanreotide in metastatic enteropancreatic neuroendocrine tumors. N Engl J Med. 2014;371(3):224–33.

112. Kasajima A, Pavel M, Darb-Esfahani S, Noske A, Stenzinger A, Sasano H, et al. mTOR expression and activity patterns in gastroenteropancreatic neuroendocrine tumours. Endocr Relat Cancer. 2011;18(1):181–92.

113. Han X, Ji Y, Zhao J, Xu X, Lou W. Expression of PTEN and mTOR in pancreatic neuroendocrine tumors. Tumour Biol. 2013;34(5):2871–9.

114. Wang L, Ignat A, Axiotis CA. Differential expression of the PTEN tumor suppressor protein in fetal and adult neuroendocrine tissues and tumors: progressive loss of PTEN expression in poorly differentiated neuroendocrine neoplasms. Appl Immunohistochem Mol Morphol. 2002;10(2):139–46.

115. Yao JC, Fazio N, Singh S, Buzzoni R, Carnaghi C, Wolin E, et al. Everolimus for the treatment of advanced, non-functional neuroendocrine tumours of the lung or gastrointestinal tract (RADIANT-4): a randomised, placebo-controlled, phase 3 study. Lancet. 2016;387(10022):968–77.

116. Raymond E, Dahan L, Raoul JL, Bang YJ, Borbath I, Lombard-Bohas C, et al. Sunitinib malate for the treatment of pancreatic neuroendocrine tumors. N Engl J Med. 2011;364(6):501–13.

117. Zurita AJ, Khajavi M, Wu HK, Tye L, Huang X, Kulke MH, et al. Circulating cytokines and monocyte subpopulations as biomarkers of outcome and biological activity in sunitinib-treated patients with advanced neuroendocrine tumours. Br J Cancer. 2015;112(7):1199–205.

118. Fazio N, Buzzoni R, Delle Fave G, Tesselaar ME, Wolin E, Van Cutsem E, et al. Everolimus in advanced, progressive, well-differentiated, non-functional neuroendocrine tumors: RADIANT-4 lung subgroup analysis. Cancer Sci. 2018;109(1):174–81.

119. Pavel ME, Singh S, Strosberg JR, Bubuteishvili-Pacaud L, Degtyarev E, Neary MP, et al. Health-related quality of life for everolimus versus placebo in patients with advanced, non-functional, well-differentiated gastrointestinal or lung neuroendocrine tumours (RADIANT-4): a multicentre, randomised, double-blind, placebo-controlled, phase 3 trial. Lancet Oncol. 2017;18(10):1411–22.

120. Ferolla P, Brizzi MP, Meyer T, Mansoor W, Mazieres J, Do Cao C, et al. Efficacy and safety of long-acting pasireotide or everolimus alone or in combination in patients with advanced carcinoids of the lung and thymus (LUNA): an open-label, multicentre, randomised, phase 2 trial. Lancet Oncol. 2017;18(12):1652–64.

121. Mazzaglia PJ, Berber E, Milas M, Siperstein AE. Laparoscopic radiofrequency ablation of neuroendocrine liver metastases: a 10-year experience evaluating predictors of survival. Surgery. 2007;142(1):10–9.

122. Basuroy R, Srirajaskanthan R, Ramage JK. A multimodal approach to the management of neuroendocrine tumour liver metastases. Int J Hepatol. 2012;2012:819193.

123. Maire F, Lombard-Bohas C, O'Toole D, Vullierme MP, Rebours V, Couvelard A, et al. Hepatic arterial embolization versus chemoembolization in the treatment of liver metastases from well-differentiated midgut endocrine tumors: a prospective randomized study. Neuroendocrinology. 2012;96(4):294–300.

124. Carrasco CH, Charnsangavej C, Ajani J, Samaan NA, Richli W, Wallace S. The carcinoid syndrome: palliation by hepatic artery embolization. AJR Am J Roentgenol. 1986;147(1):149–54.

125. Ajani JA, Carrasco CH, Charnsangavej C, Samaan NA, Levin B, Wallace S. Islet cell tumors metastatic to the liver: effective palliation by sequential hepatic artery embolization. Ann Intern Med. 1988;108(3):340–4.

126. Eriksson BK, Larsson EG, Skogseid BM, Lofberg AM, Lorelius LE, Oberg KE. Liver embolizations of patients with malignant neuroendocrine gastrointestinal tumors. Cancer. 1998;83(11):2293–301.

127. Brown KT, Koh BY, Brody LA, Getrajdman GI, Susman J, Fong Y, et al. Particle embolization of hepatic neuroendocrine metastases for control of pain and hormonal symptoms. J Vasc Interv Radiol. 1999;10(4):397–403.

128. O'Toole D, Ruszniewski P. Chemoembolization and other ablative therapies for liver metastases of gastrointestinal endocrine tumours. Best Pract Res Clin Gastroenterol. 2005;19(4):585–94.

Supplementary Information

© Springer Nature Switzerland AG 2021
A. Russo et al. (eds.), *Practical Medical Oncology Textbook*, UNIPA Springer Series,
https://doi.org/10.1007/978-3-030-56051-5

Index

Printed by Printforce, United Kingdom